Ophthalmic Signs in Practice of Medicine

Amod Gupta • Reema Bansal
Aman Sharma • Arun Kapil

Ophthalmic Signs in Practice of Medicine

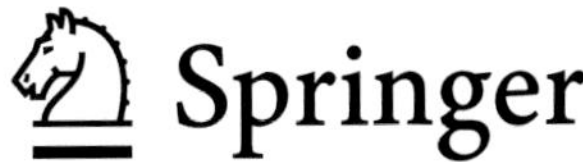

Amod Gupta
Advanced Eye Centre, Chandigarh
Post Graduate Institute of Medical
Education and Research
Chandigarh, India

Reema Bansal
Advanced Eye Centre, Chandigarh
Post Graduate Institute of Medical
Education and Research
Chandigarh, Chandigarh, India

Aman Sharma
Department of Internal Medicine
Post Graduate Institute of Medical
Education and Research
Chandigarh, India

Arun Kapil
Advanced Eye Centre, Chandigarh
Post Graduate Institute of Medical
Education and Research
Chandigarh, India

ISBN 978-981-99-7925-7 ISBN 978-981-99-7923-3 (eBook)
https://doi.org/10.1007/978-981-99-7923-3

This Springer imprint is published by the registered company Springer Nature Singapore Pte Ltd.
The registered company address is: 152 Beach Road, #21-01/04 Gateway East, Singapore 189721, Singapore

Paper in this product is recyclable.

Dedicated to my wife Gunita, daughter Sumedha, and son-in-law Sachin for always standing by me; my students for keeping me au courant for more than 45 years of my academic career and above all, my patients, who reposed their complete trust in my ability to serve them and learn from them.
—Amod Gupta

Dedicated to my mentor, Prof Amod Gupta, who taught and inspired me at every step of my training in uveitis and vitreo-retina, for his constant support and motivation; my family for being proud of me and for being my pillar of strength; my friends for their love and trust; and my patients for believing me and my abilities to treat them, and for also being a constant source of my learning.
—Reema Bansal

Dedicated to my father, Balbir Parkash Sharma, my guiding light; my mother, Sudesh Sharma, my pillar of strength; my sister, Kusum Sharma, who thinks her brother can do anything; my wife, Sushmita Sharma, who always stood by me and dealt with my absence without any complaints and my loving daughters, Ananya and Sharanya, who are my lifelines.
—Aman Sharma

To my Mentor, Prof. Amod Gupta for raising me to believe that anything is possible. I feel blessed and proud of working under his guidance for over 30 years. To Prof. Vishali Gupta, Retina Head, for her continuous motivation.

To my wife, Suman Kapil, for continuous support and encouragement in every step of my life. To my daughter, son-in-law, son, daughter-in-law, family and friends, and grandsons.
—Arun Kapil

Foreword

The quest to become an ophthalmologist has become increasingly popular and competitive. This may be because vision is our most precious sense. An ophthalmologist has the skill to preserve vision and, in some instances, to restore vision with just a few delicate motions in an operating theatre. The attraction lies in the fact that ophthalmology has a major role in some of the greatest recent medical advances, such as gene therapy and the application of technology to image anatomy and pathology. For many, ophthalmology affords the rewards of internal medicine and surgery. The cornea's clarity allows the retina and brain to process light and the curious physician to look inward. And if that physician is knowledgeable and prepared, properly examining a tiny space, 2.5 cm from cornea to optic nerve, might reveal many secrets hidden elsewhere in the body.

In *Ophthalmic Signs in the Practice of Medicine*, four experts from the Postgraduate Institute of Medical Education and Research in Chandigarh, India, share their considerable wisdom and experience so that others may also skilfully interrogate the eye for clues to diagnosis and therapy. It is vital to understand that this is an interdisciplinary group led by Amod Gupta, a distinguished emeritus Professor of Ophthalmology. He is assisted by another talented ophthalmologist, Reema Bansal, a prolific rheumatologist, Aman Sharma, and an expert in capturing images of the eye, Arun Kapil. Their insights provide a comprehensive resource which will be of value to the experienced practitioner who has examined the eye for decades, the internist who wishes to understand more fully the secrets of the eye, or the novice who is still in training and unsure if ophthalmology is the discipline most attractive to pursue.

We should be grateful to these authors for the considerable effort to assemble this volume. I am confident that patients will be among the many beneficiaries of their insights.

Legacy Devers Eye Institute
Portland, OR, USA, Corvus Pharmaceuticals
Burlingame, CA, USA
February 28, 2023

James T. Rosenbaum

Foreword

Ophthalmology is one of the areas more internists find most difficult to assess and interpret. This book *Ophthalmic Signs in the Practice of Medicine* is a much-needed book for all general physicians and internists.

The eye is an organ that offers a window into many disease processes. The absence of ophthalmic signs in many books on Medicine is serious lacunae that the authors are addressing with this book.

The book authored by Amod Gupta, Reema Bansal, Aman Sharma, and Arun Kapil is nicely structured with chapters on all signs. The extensive emphasis on retinal vasculature is excellent and offers the reader clear guidance on interpreting these signs.

The extensive use of high-quality illustrations makes this book stand out for me.

Ophthalmic signs are spotters; like skin, clinical examination skills are paramount. Ophthalmology is the last bastion where clinical examination skills still reign supreme as the rest of Medicine is taken over by emphasis on laboratory tests and imaging over clinical examination skills.

This book is of value to medical students, postgraduate trainees in general medicine, trainees in ophthalmology and general practitioners.

The authors are to be congratulated for bringing this book to help diagnose and assess ocular signs. In the new era of "precision medicine", it is more important that clinicians (internists and ophthalmologists) understand each other's language and work closely to improve the outcome of multisystem disease with ocular manifestations.

Paediatric Rheumatology, Bristol Royal Hospital for Children
Athimalaipet V. Ramanan,
Bristol, UK
February 27, 2023

Foreword

It gives me great pleasure to write the foreword to *Ophthalmic Signs in the Practice of Medicine* not only because one of the authors, Professor Amod Gupta, is a friend of many years but also because this book enables us to share the vast knowledge and expertise of an internationally renowned authority in the fields of uveitis and retinal diseases. He is joined by prolific contributors to the medical sciences, Prof. Reema Bansal, a professor of Ophthalmology; Prof. Aman Sharma, a Professor of Rheumatology and internal medicine and Arun Kapil, one of the most experienced clinical photographers.

Whereas most ophthalmic textbooks are organised according to anatomic or pathogenetic classifications, this takes a different approach. Each chapter focuses on a specific sign (e.g. cotton wool spots) and describes its significance, clinical features and pathogenesis. A differential diagnosis of the sign itself (e.g. cotton wool spots versus medullated nerve fibres) is followed by the list of ocular or systemic conditions associated with the presence of the sign in question. Most of these conditions are listed and the subject of a comprehensive overview of their pathogenesis, clinical features and, when relevant, therapeutic possibilities. Therefore, more than being a guide to the differential diagnosis of retinal conditions based on clinical signs, this book also doubles as an excellent and up-to-date treatise of retinal diseases. For instance, reading and absorbing the chapters on cotton wool spots, hard exudates, microaneurysms and new vessels will provide the reader with solid knowledge of the pathogenesis, clinical features and treatment of diabetic retinopathy.

Each chapter is extensively referenced and profusely illustrated. The many recent papers from 2020, 2021 and 2022 testify to the authors' successful effort to include the most recent knowledge. The high quality of the illustrations (colour photographs, wide field fundus imaging, fluorescein angiography, OCT and OCT-A) substantially adds to the book's quality.

Without hesitation, I would recommend this textbook to train residents: starting from observing a clinical sign in their patient, this textbook will take them on a fascinating journey to explore the rich world of retinal pathology.

The established practitioner who wants to update his or her knowledge on retinal pathology will not find a better source. As an additional bonus, he or she will benefit from the many clinical pearls the authors share with the reader, wisdom collected during distinguished careers as clinician-scientists.

University of Ghent
Ghent, Belgium
March 26, 2023

Philippe Kestelyn,

Preface

The human eyes are often called the windows to the body in health and disease. Eyes provide an extraordinary insight into our overall health. The eyes are the only part of the body where a physician, using non-invasive tools, can directly visualize pathology as it is evolving, often decades before manifesting as a grave systemic disorder.

Within these small, though intricate organs lies a world of valuable information that can provide vital insights into a person's well-being. Ophthalmic signs, the tell-tale indicators in the eyes, are remarkable signatures of underlying systemic diseases. From the subtlest of changes to the most pronounced abnormalities, these signs can offer a glimpse into the intricate workings of the human body.

Artificial compartmentalization and increasing sub-specialization in every field of medicine, beginning in the latter half of the twentieth century, rapidly created silos of excellence that can deal successfully with the most complicated diseases, often at the cost of missing clues to the earliest onset of the disease. Unlike when the ophthalmic examination was an integral part of the patient workup, heavy demand on the trainees' time in different subspecialties has dramatically reduced the captive time for exposure to ophthalmology and the ophthalmic signs.

Ophthalmology is a highly visual science wherein such signs can be easily learnt, objectively documented, and used in clinical practice to improve quality of care, early diagnosis, and appropriate referrals. In medicine, recognizing and interpreting ophthalmic signs has proven to be an invaluable tool.

The eyes are integral to the body's systems and share structural, physiological, immunological, biochemical, neurological, and biological homology and pathways. The eyes often reveal the consequences of systemic disorders, chronic diseases, and genetic disorders. Not only do these signs aid in diagnosing ocular disorders, but they can also serve as early warning signals for a myriad of systemic diseases.

This book, profusely illustrated, delves into the fascinating realm of ophthalmic signs, exploring their diverse manifestations and significance in medicine. Through an in-depth exploration of various eye conditions, their associated signs and pathogenetic mechanisms, we aim to empower clinicians, family physicians, medical students, residents, and fellows in training with the knowledge and skills necessary to detect, evaluate, and interpret these invaluable clues.

Drawing upon the latest research and clinical experiences, this book seeks to enhance the understanding of ophthalmic signs as a crucial component of the diagnostic process. By highlighting the interplay between ocular health and systemic well-being, we hope to foster a holistic approach to patient care and encourage collaboration between ophthalmologists, general practitioners, internists, endocrinologists, neurologists, and specialists from various other medical disciplines.

Embark on this enlightening journey through the captivating realm of ophthalmic signs and witness how the eyes are extraordinary indicators of our overall health.

Chandigarh, India Amod Gupta
Chandigarh, India Reema Bansal
Chandigarh, India Aman Sharma
Chandigarh, India Arun Kapil

Acknowledgements

We want to acknowledge several eminent ophthalmologists' and researchers' generosity in sharing their precious images with us, without which this book would have remained incomplete.

Dr Manphool Singhal, Department of Radiodiagnosis and Imaging, Postgraduate Institute of Medical Education and Research, Chandigarh, India, for figures 1.13 and 18.7

Dr Alok Sen Sadguru Netra Chikitsalya, Chitrakoot, MP, India, for figures 3.12, 3.18, 10.9B

Dr Simar Rajan Singh, Advanced Eye Centre, Postgraduate Institute of Medical Education and Research, Chandigarh, India, for figures 6.18 to 6.21

Prof Anjali Agarwal, Head, Department of Anatomy, Postgraduate Institute of Medical Education and Research, Chandigarh, for figures 8.1, 15.1, 16.2, 20.1

Dr Anuradha V K, Head of Uveitis Services, Aravind Eye Hospital, Coimbatore, India, for Fig. 10.8A

Prof Ramandeep Singh, Advanced Eye Centre, Postgraduate Institute of Medical Education and Research, Chandigarh, India, for Fig. 10.8B

Dr Padmamalini Mahendradas, Uveitis and Ocular Oncology, Narayana Nethralaya, Bangalore, India, for figures 10.22 to 10.24

Dr Anita Agarwal, West Coast Retina Medical Group, San Francisco, CA 94109, for figures 13.1, 13.7, 13.8, 13.10 to 13.15.

Dr Chirag Ahuja, Department of Radiodiagnosis and Imaging, Postgraduate Institute of Medical Education and Research, Chandigarh, India, for the interpretation of Fig. 1d.

Prof Daisy Sahni (Ex-Professor) Department of Anatomy, Postgraduate Institute of Medical Education and Research, Chandigarh, India, for Fig. 15.1

Dr SS Pandav, Professor and Head, Advanced Eye Centre, Postgraduate Institute of Medical Education and Research, Chandigarh, India, for figures 15.3, 15.16

Dr Rithambra Nada, Prof of Pathology, Postgraduate Institute of Medical Education and Research, Chandigarh, India, for figures 15.20 and 18.8B

Dr Chintan Malhotra, Professor, Cornea, Lens and Refractive Surgery Services, Advanced Eye Centre, Postgraduate Institute of Medical Education and Research, Chandigarh, India, for figures 17.3 to 17.13

Dr Anandita Sinha, Department of Radiodiagnosis and Imaging, Postgraduate Institute of Medical Education and Research, Chandigarh, India, for figures. 17.14B and 17.17 (d, e)

Prof Pradeep Bambery, Ex-Professor of Medicine, Postgraduate Institute of Medical Education and Research, Chandigarh, India, for Fig. 18.16

Dr Amit Gupta, Professor, Cornea, Lens and Refractive Surgery Services, Advanced Eye Centre, Postgraduate Institute of Medical Education and Research, Chandigarh, India, for figures 17.14 b–d, 18.6

Dr Kanwar Mohan, Dr Kanwar Mohan's Squint Centre, Chandigarh, India, for figures 19.5, 19.7, 19.15, 19.16, 19.18, 19.19, 19.20, 20.1b

Dr Manpreet Singh, Advanced Eye Centre, Postgraduate Institute of Medical Education and Research, Chandigarh, India, for figures 19.8c, 19.11e, 20.2, 20.6, 20.7

Dr Ali G. Hamedani, Department of Neurology, Hospital of the University of Pennsylvania, Philadelphia, PA, United States, for figures 19.10 and 19.12

Dr Anja K E Horn, Professor, Ludwig-Maximilian University Munich, Germany, for Fig. 19.21

Prof. Usha Singh, Advanced Eye Centre, Postgraduate Institute of Medical Education and Research, Chandigarh, India, for figures 20.4, 20.5, 20.8, 20.13, 20.17, 20.18, 20.19

Dr Pankaj Gupta, Advanced Eye Centre, Postgraduate Institute of Medical Education and Research, Chandigarh, India, for Fig. 20.9

Dr Shweta Chaurasia, Advanced Eye Centre, Postgraduate Institute of Medical Education and Research, Chandigarh, India, for figures 20.10 to 20.12, 20.14, 20.15

Dr Kasturi Bhattacharjee, Sri Sankaradeva Nethralaya, Guwahati, India, for figures 20.16, 20.20

Kritika Thakur for graphics—figures 15.2; 16.3 to 16.6; 16.8 to 16.10; 19.1 to 19.4; 19.6; 19.8 a, b; 19.9; 19.11a–d; 19.13; 19.14; 19.22 to 19.26

We want to thank several publishers who allowed us to reuse our images published over several years in the past.

Publishers of Frontiers of Medicine for reusing Fig. 3.11 from our publication Bansal et al. (2021) Frontiers of Medicine 8:681942. doi: 10.3389/fmed.2021.681942.

Publishers of Neurology for allowing us to reuse Fig. 5.15 from our publication Takkar et al. Neurology 2013,81:e40

Springer Singapore for allowing us to reuse Fig. 6.5 and Fig. 16.1 from our publication Gupta A (2022). Bench-to-Bedside Research in Ophthalmology. In: Sobti, R., Ganju, A.K. (eds) Biomedical Translational Research. Springer, Singapore. https://doi.org/10.1007/978-981-16-8845-4_5

Elsevier for allowing us to reuse Fig. 6.17 published by Chiang et al. (2021) in Ophthalmology. 2021 Oct;128(10):e51–e68. doi: 10.1016/j.ophtha.2021.05.031

Publisher for allowing us to reuse figures 10.10C and 10.11B from our publication, Bansal et al. (2012) Expert Review of Ophthalmology, 7(4), 341–349. doi:10.1586/eop.12.42

Springer Berlin for Fig. 10.11C from our publication Gupta A (2016) in Zierhut et al. (eds) Intraocular Inflammation. Springer, Berlin, Heidelberg. https://doi.org/10.1007/978-3-540-75387-2_105

Figure 12.7C from Singh et al. (2012) Medicine (Baltimore). 2012 Jul;91(4):179–194. doi: 10.1097/MD.0b013e3182574a0b. PMID: 22732948

Figure 14.12, Gupta A and Gupta V (2009) Paediatric uveitis in Gupta A et al. (eds) Uveitis: Text and Imaging 1st Edn. Jaypee Brothers Medical Publishers (P) Ltd., New Delhi. P 518

Fig. 15.15 from Gupta et al. (2012) BMJ Case Rep. 2012 Aug 21;2012:bcr2012006718. doi: 10.1136/bcr-2012-006718. PMID: 22914240

Figure 16.7 with permission from NeurOptics, inc. (Irvine, CA92612, USA)

Figure 17. 14a, 17.16a, 17.19, 17.20, 18.8, 18.15b, c, d from Bambery et al. (2009) Systemic examination and imaging in Gupta et al. (eds) Uveitis: Text and Imaging 1st Edn. Jaypee Brothers Medical Publishers (P) Ltd., New Delhi

Figure 17.18 from Gupta et al. (2009) Gupta et al. (eds). Uveitis: Text and Imaging 1st Edn. Jaypee Brothers Medical Publishers (P) Ltd., New Delhi

Figure 17.24 EyeNet Magazine, Agarwal AK et al., Pigmented Keratic Precipitates in Herpes Simplex Virus Anterior Uveitis November 2018

Figure 17.27 EyeNet Magazine, Gupta AK, et al. September 2014

Figure 18.1, 18.13 from Sharma et al. In: Sharma A (ed).Textbook of Systemic Vasculitis, 1st Edn. Jaypee Brothers Medical Publishers (P) Ltd., New Delhi

We also thank publishers for allowing us to adapt/reuse material from their publications to create boxes for various chapters in our book.

Publishers to allow us to reuse/adapt from various publications for

Boxes 10.1 from Holland, 1994

Box 10.2. from Standardization of Uveitis Nomenclature (SUN) Working Group. Classification Criteria for Acute Retinal Necrosis Syndrome 2021

Box 10.3 from Standardization of Uveitis Nomenclature (SUN) Working Group. Classification Criteria for Cytomegalovirus Retinitis, 2021

Box 10.4 and 10.5 from Gupta et al. (2015) Classification of intraocular tuberculosis. Ocul Immunol Inflamm. 2015 Feb;23(1):7–13. doi: 10.3109/09273948.2014.967358

Box 10.6 from Fig. 2 by Aringer et al. (2019)

Box 10.7 from Korsten et al. (2018)

Box 10.8 from Standardization of Uveitis Nomenclature (SUN) Working Group

Box 10.9 Classification Criteria for Sarcoidosis-Associated Uveitis, 2021 from Standardization of Uveitis Nomenclature (SUN) Working Group. Classification Criteria for Behçet Disease Uveitis, 2021

Box 10.9 from Criteria for diagnosis of Behçet's disease. International Study Group for Behçet's Disease, 1990.

Box 10.10 from O'Keefe and Rao from Surv Ophthalmol. 2017 Jan-Feb;62(1):1–25. doi: 10.1016/j.survophthal.2016.05.002. Epub 2016 May 27. PMID: 27241814

Box 14.1 from Lonser et al. (2003)

Box 14.2 from VHL Alliance, Boston, MA, 02284-4682 and 14.3 from Ophthalmology. 2006 Dec;113(12):2276–80. doi: 10.1016/j.ophtha.2006.06.018

Box 15.1 from Petzold et al. Lancet Neurol. 2022 Dec;21(12):1120–1134. doi: 10.1016/S1474-4422(22)00200-9

Box 15.2 Reproduced under the Creative Commons Attribution license (CC BY) from Szekeres and Othman Front Med (Lausanne). 2022 Dec 13;9:1066503. doi: 10.3389/fmed.2022.1066503. PMID: 36582285

Box 19.1 from Jaretzki et al. 2000. Myasthenia gravis: recommendations for clinical research standards. Task Force of the Medical Scientific Advisory Board of the Myasthenia Gravis Foundation of America. Ann Thorac Surg. 2000 Jul;70(1):327–34. doi: 10.1016/s0003-4975(00)01595-2. PMID: 10921745

Reviewers: We want to thank Dr Anita Agarwal, West Coast Retina Medical Group, San Francisco, CA, for the review of Chapters 7, 12, and 13 and Dr Aastha Takkar for the review of Chapters 15 and 16. We highly appreciate their valuable comments to improve the quality of our book.

Finally, we like to express our gratitude to Prof Jim Rosenbaum MD, Chair, Emeritus Legacy Devers Eye Institute, Portland, OR, USA, Prof Athimalaipet V Ramanan, FRCP, Professor of Paediatric Rheumatology, Bristol Royal Hospital for Children, Bristol, UK, and Prof Philippe Kestelyn, Emeritus Professor University of Ghent, Belgium, for finding time from their extremely busy schedule to review our manuscript and write forewords for this book.

We like to thank Ms Sinchu Mohan, Ms Jagjit Kaur Saini, and Mr Naren Agarwal of Springer Team India for giving a final shape to our book

Amod Gupta MBBS; MS, Emeritus Professor, Advanced Eye Centre, Postgraduate Institute of Medical Education and Research, Chandigarh, India

Reema Bansal MBBS, MS, PhD. Professor of Ophthalmology, Advanced Eye Centre, Postgraduate Institute of Medical Education and Research, Chandigarh, India

Aman Sharma MD, FRCP (London). Professor of Medicine, Clinical Immunology and Rheumatology, Program Director, Centre of Excellence in HIV/AIDS,

Postgraduate Institute of Medical Education and Research, Chandigarh, India

Arun Kapil Senior ophthalmic technician, Chief, Digital Retina Imaging Laboratory, Advanced Eye Centre, Postgraduate Institute of Medical Education and Research, Chandigarh, India

Chandigarh

Contents

Part I

Intraocular Signs

1 Retinal Capillary Microaneurysms

1.1 Introduction

Microaneurysms (MAs) are one of the most significant intraocular signs of an underlying systemic disease. Retinal MAs are the earliest lesion seen in patients with diabetic retinopathy and the sine qua non of diabetic retinopathy. The early stages of diabetic retinopathy and the associated comorbidities are completely asymptomatic and require regular screening and prompt control. The patients become aware only when the vision is affected due to macular oedema, or they are at the threshold of severe visual loss or have already lost vision from complications of diabetic retinopathy. As the disease carries significant morbidity and mortality, it must be detected by purposeful screening to detect the early stages of retinopathy (Box 1.1). See Box 1.2 for clinical clues for diabetes and other diseases that may cause MAs.

Box 1.1 Common Causes of Retinal Capillary Microaneurysms

1. Diabetes mellitus is the most common
2. Hypertension
3. Carotid atherosclerosis
4. Takayasu's arteritis
5. Ocular ischaemic syndrome (OIS)
6. Branch retinal vein occlusion
7. Central retinal vein occlusion
8. Coats' disease
9. Type 1 macular telangiectasia
10. Radiation retinopathy

Box 1.2 Key Points in History and Clinical Examination in Diabetes and MAs Related Disorders

1. Duration and control of diabetes
2. Check blood pressure in both upper arms
3. History of smoking
4. Nocturnal obstructive sleep apnea
5. Check for body mass index
6. Check for asymmetry/absence of peripheral pulses and for the presence of arterial bruits or tenderness over the carotids (Takayasu's arteritis)

A. Gupta et al., *Ophthalmic Signs in Practice of Medicine*,
https://doi.org/10.1007/978-981-99-7923-3_1

7. Detailed neurological examination, including vibration sense and joint position sense in patients with diabetes having MAs
8. Palpate for vessel wall thickness as a clue to atherosclerosis

Abbreviation: *MAs* microaneurysms

Often the detection of MAs in the retina may be the first clue toward diagnosing type 2 diabetes mellitus (DM). Patients with type 2 diabetes mellitus have an insidious onset and remain asymptomatic till they get detected by a routine laboratory test carried out in the context of other illnesses. Thus, the duration of type 2 DM is not known. MAs in the retina indirectly show that type 2 DM has been present for at least 5 years. Detection of retinal microaneurysms should prompt a thorough clinical history, examination, and laboratory workup to detect DM and other causes of MAs. Depending upon the cause of the MAs, minimum laboratory investigations that should be done are listed in Box 1.3.

Box 1.3 Lab Investigations to Be Considered Based upon the Underlying Condition

1. Check for fasting blood sugar, HbA1C, lipidogram, Hb
2. APLA workup and procoagulant workup for BRVO and CRVO
3. Urinalysis to look for microalbuminuria/proteinuria in patients with diabetes to look for nephropathy
4. Arterial Doppler examination of carotid arteries

Abbreviations: *HbA1C* glycosylated haemoglobin, *Hb* haemoglobin, *APLA* anti-phospholipid antibodies, *BRVO* branch retinal vein occlusion, *CRVO* central retinal vein occlusion

DM affects practically all organs of the body. DM co-morbidities compound each other, and it is essential that all DM patients undergo regular screening for early detection of these for prompt management (see Box 1.4). For detailed information on the current screening, diagnostic, and therapeutic guidelines of diabetes and comorbidities, the readers are advised to consult the American Diabetic Association guidelines [1].

Box 1.4 Key Points in Screening for Diabetes and Comorbidities

1	DM is diagnosed if FBSL is >126 mg/dL or HbA1c is >6.5%, or random BSL or OGTT at 2 h is >200 mg/dL
2	Screening for diabetic retinopathy should be done at diagnosis of DM type 2 and 5 years after the onset of DM type 1. An ophthalmologist should do screening in a dilated eye or tele-screening using a non-mydriatic camera
3	If no DR is detected, screening is done every 2 years. More frequently if MAs are detected. If sight-threatening DR is detected, refer immediately to an ophthalmologist for treatment
4	Screen for co-morbidities at least annually—anaemia, nephropathy, peripheral neuropathy, and foot sensations. Anaemia is often overlooked in patients with DM/DR
5	Control of BSL, lipid, and blood pressure. Blood pressure should be checked every visit with a target BP <130/80 if ASCVD[a] risk is >15%. DM patients most often require statins. Control of these factors delays the onset of diabetic retinopathy and if present, reduces the severity of DR and the need for interventions
6	Encourage physical activity, weight control, a Mediterranean diet, and no smoking

Abbreviations: *Dm* diabetes mellitus, *FBSL* fasting blood sugar level, *HbA1c* glycosylated haemoglobin, *OGTT* oral glucose tolerance test, *DR* diabetic retinopathy, *ASCVD* atherosclerotic cardiovascular disease

[a]https://www.acc.org/Tools-and-Practice-Support/Mobile-Resources/Features/2013-Prevention-Guidelines-ASCVD-Risk-Estimator

If the patients are detected to be suffering from DM, the guidelines for follow-up and referral for diabetic retinopathy should be meticulously adhered to.

1.2 Anatomical Considerations of the Retina

The retina is a highly organized, multi-layered innermost lining of the eyeball. It converts photons into electrical signals to transmit to the visual cortex located in the occipital lobes of the brain for ultimately transforming reflected light from the objects around into their 3-D visual perception. Maintaining the light path transparency is critical to achieving sharp and high-resolution images. Several anatomical and physiological factors must work in perfect harmony to project a sharp image of the object on the photoreceptors. The retina consists of two layers, the transparent neurosensory retina anteriorly and a dark retinal pigment epithelial (RPE) layer posteriorly, separated by a potential space. The neurosensory retina is a multi-layered structure consisting of several highly organized cells of neural and glial origin and their processes. The light has to pass through from front to back, the internal limiting membrane (footplates of the macroglia, the Muller cells), the retinal nerve fibre layer (RNFL, the axons of the retinal ganglion cells), retinal ganglion cells (RGC), the inner plexiform layer (the synaptic junction of the dendrites of the RGC, amacrine cells, and the axons of the bipolar cells), the bipolar cell layer (it also has the cell bodies of the Muller cells, amacrine, and horizontal cells), the outer plexiform layer (the synaptic junctions of the dendrites of the bipolar cells and the axons of the photoreceptor rods and cones; with horizontal cell processes controlling transmission), the external limiting membrane (Muller cell apical processes joining each other and the inner segments of the photoreceptors), the outer nuclear layer (ONL), and the cell bodies of the rods and cones. The neurosensory retina is further divided into an inner retina up to the outer border of the inner nuclear layer and the outer retina, from the outer plexiform layer (OPL) to the photoreceptor layer. The neural cells and fibres are tightly packed in all the layers and are oriented vertically in the outer retina but become near parallel in the anterior retina. The blood supply of the retina is also layered. The anterior neurosensory retina gets its blood supply from the central retinal vessels that run their course in the RNFL and supply the inner retina through four capillary plexuses. The superficial plexus (SCP) in the ganglion cells layer, the intermediate plexus (ICP) at the inner border of the inner nuclear layer (INL), and the deep plexus (DCP) at the outer border of the INL (Fig. 1.1). The radial capillaries from the optic disc supply the RNFL peripapillary retina. If the cilioretinal artery is present, it supplies nutrients and oxygen to all the layers of the macula.

The retinal capillaries do not cross beyond the inner one-third of the OPL, also known as the middle limiting membrane. The OPL in the fovea is known as the Henle fibre layer. The cones and the Muller cell fibres have a radial orientation in this zone. The retinal vessels have tight endothelial junctions (inner blood-retinal barrier) and do not allow macromolecules, cellular elements, and fluid movement into the extravascular space. The central 400–500 μm of the anterior neurosensory retina is called the foveal avascular zone and is a vessel-free zone. The outer retina is avascular and receives nutrition and oxygen requirements from the choroid. The OPL is avascular and falls in the watershed zone of the two vascular supply systems. The dark RPE at the back of the neurosensory retina has tight junctions and maintains the outer blood–retina barrier. The vertebrate outer limiting membrane (OLM) also has adherent and tight junction proteins. It provides a partial semipermeable barrier function that allows diffusion of only small protein molecules (<35 radius Angstrom units) that are present in the extracellular space around the photoreceptors [2].

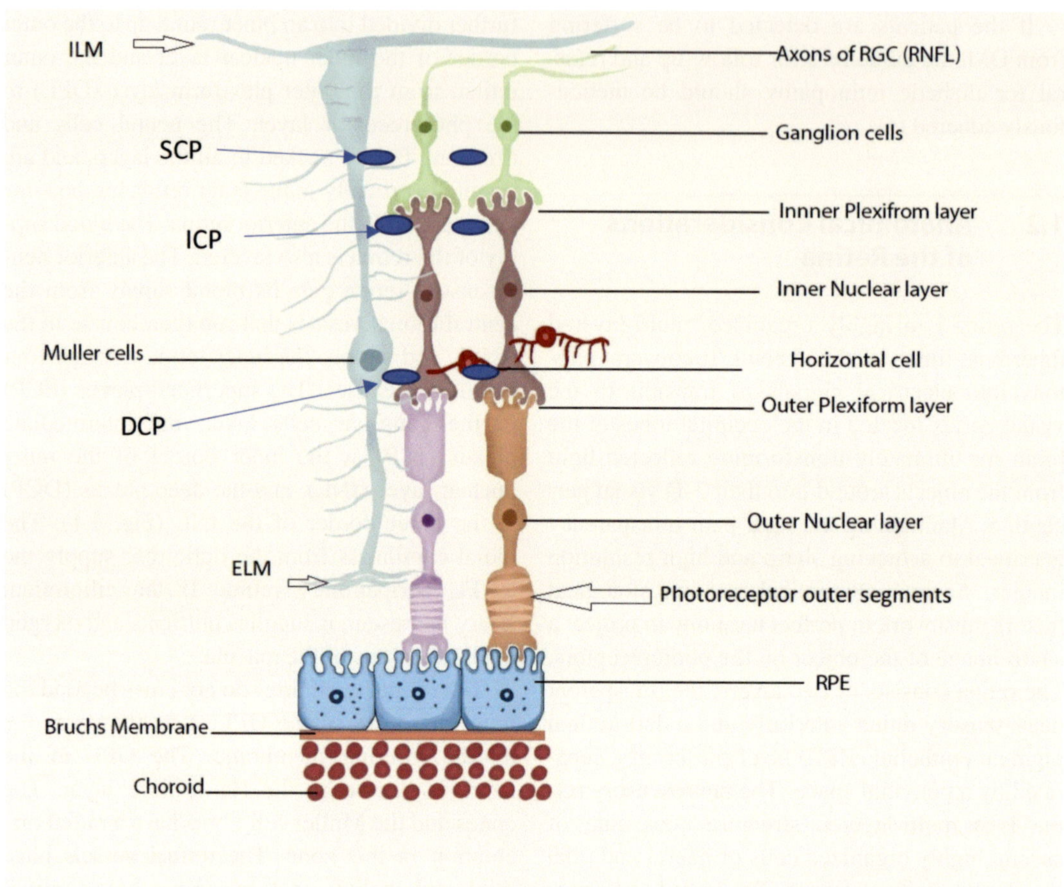

Fig. 1.1 A highly schematic representation of the retina's microstructure shows the retinal capillary plexuses limited to the anterior retina. (Modified from Fig. 5.4 Gupta A. Bench-to-Bedside research in Ophthalmology. in Biomedical translational research-From disease diagnosis to treatment. Sobti RC and Ganju AK (Eds). With permission of the publisher. Springer Nature, Singapore Pte Ltd. 2022)

1.3 Pathogenesis of Retinal Capillary Microaneurysm Formation in Diabetic Retinopathy

The earliest change in diabetic retinopathy is the thickening of the capillary basement membrane (BM) across all body organs, most pronounced in the retina. The thickening of the BM is due to the deposition of the extracellular matrix proteins by the non-enzymatic glycation of proteins in long-term hyperglycaemia. The thickened BM leads to the loss of cell-to-cell talk between the pericytes and the endothelial cells and the resultant loss of the pericyte–endothelial cell ratio. This leads to loss of contact and control by the pericyte over the endothelial cell. In normal retinal capillaries, the ratio of pericyte to endothelial cells is maintained at 1:1. Along with the Muller cells, these form a neurovascular unit that plays a major role in maintaining metabolic homeostasis in the retina [3]. Once there is a loss of contact between the Muller cells, pericytes, and endothelial cells, normal homeostasis is lost, activating the retinal microglia, which release proinflammatory cytokines. There is an overexpression of hypoxia-inducible factor 1-α (HIF-1α) in the endothelial and Muller cells. HIF-1α is a regulator of vascular endothelial growth factor (VEGF). Hypoxic Muller cells also produce VEGF, which promotes endothelial cell proliferation and break down of the tight endothelial junctions [4]. Unlike endothelial cells, pericytes do not have the potential to regenerate. Microaneurysms (MAs) are usually formed around the area of acellular capillaries by a fusiform or saccular dilation of the capillaries, which may be cellular or acellular. The endothelial cells lining the MAs lack junctional proteins and leak fluid and macromolecules like lipoproteins.

1.4 Historical Perspective on the Detection of Retinal Capillary Microaneurysms

Photographic documentation of the retinal vasculature by injecting a bolus of fluorescein dye into the antecubital vein called the fundus fluorescein angiography (FFA) was a disruptive technological breakthrough since the discovery of a direct ophthalmoscope more than 100 years ago. The technique gave a major fillip to the study of retinal involvement in several systemic and ophthalmological disorders. [5, 6]. Although initially the dye was injected into the antecubital vein, attempts were made for a short while to perform FFA by intraarterial cannulation of the innominate artery [7]. It was believed that injecting fluorescein dye directly into the innominate artery allowed the dye bolus to reach the retinal arterioles, followed by the retinal capillaries, and finally move on to the retinal veins. The brachial artery was punctured in the antecubital fossa of the right arm and cannulated with a 60-cm polyethylene tube. A small bolus of heparinized sucrose was injected to determine that the cannula had reached the innominate artery. When the patient felt the sweet taste on the right side of the tongue, they knew that it had reached the innominate artery and then the fluorescein sodium dye was injected. Using this technique, Eva Kohner erroneously believed that MAs in diabetes were located on the venous end of the capillaries [8]. It was undoubtedly a highly cumbersome technique and soon reverted to the original technique of Novotny and Alvis of dye injection through the antecubital vein, a technique so simplified that it is followed till now. The availability of FFA made it possible to visualize, in vivo, MAs and the areas of retinal perfusion, which till then had been seen and documented only on trypsin digestion studies of the retina obtained from the harvested eyes of patients with DM.

1.5 Retina Examination to Detect Retinal Capillary Microaneurysms

MAs are seen as red dot-like focal dilatations of the retinal capillaries. These are 10–100 μm in size. Normal retinal capillaries and microaneurysms less than 30 μm in diameter cannot be visualized on clinical examination. However, MAs larger than 30 μm can be easily seen by physicians with a monocular direct ophthalmoscope (15× magnification). Using a +60D, +78, or +90D lens remains the most prevalent clinical technique for the stereoscopic fundus examination on a slit lamp. It is convenient but provides a lower resolution than a contact lens. The high plus objective lens provides a real, inverted, and laterally reversed image of the macula in front of this lens and needs experience to master the technique. A +90 D lens provides a field of view of ~90°, a working distance of 7 mm from the cornea, and a magnification factor of 0.76×. Choosing a 10× magnification on the slit lamp, a final retinal image magnification of 7.6× (cf. 15× from direct ophthalmoscope) can be obtained. Because of the lens's small diameter and metallic ring, it is convenient to hold it for a long time and can be used even in an undilated pupil. A wider area of the retina can be screened by asking the patient to move his eye in different directions. The +78D lens is bigger and can have a field of view of 81/97° and a magnification factor of 0.93× at 8 mm from the cornea. However, it requires a dilated pupil and may be tiring if required to hold for a long time.

However, MAs and retinal capillaries can be easily visualized on fundus fluorescein angiography (FFA). This invasive technique involves injecting a 3 mL bolus of a water-soluble fluorescent dye (fluorescein sodium 20%) intravenously and taking fundus photographs through a special camera equipped with matched narrow-band excitation and barrier filters. As the dye flows in the retinal vessels, it is excited by the blue light and emits light in the green spectrum, which has a higher wavelength. This phenomenon was earlier captured on a photographic B&W film that required processing in a dark room. Digital cameras have completely replaced film-based systems. The fluorescein angiogram is instantly available for review by the ophthalmologist as soon as the images are saved.

1.6 Differentiating Retinal Capillary Microaneurysms and Dot Haemorrhages

Clinically, it is difficult to differentiate MAs from dot haemorrhages, a common accompaniment in diabetic retinopathy. MAs are globular with a regular contour and show a shiny reflex from their surface. On the other hand, dot haemorrhages result from the extravasation of red blood cells (RBCs) from the MAs in the various capillary plexuses. A careful examination would reveal dot haemorrhages to be dull red in colour that neither have a globular shape nor show a light reflex from their surface (Fig. 1.2). These leaked RBCs assume a dot-like shape because they are in a tightly packed inner nuclear layer or

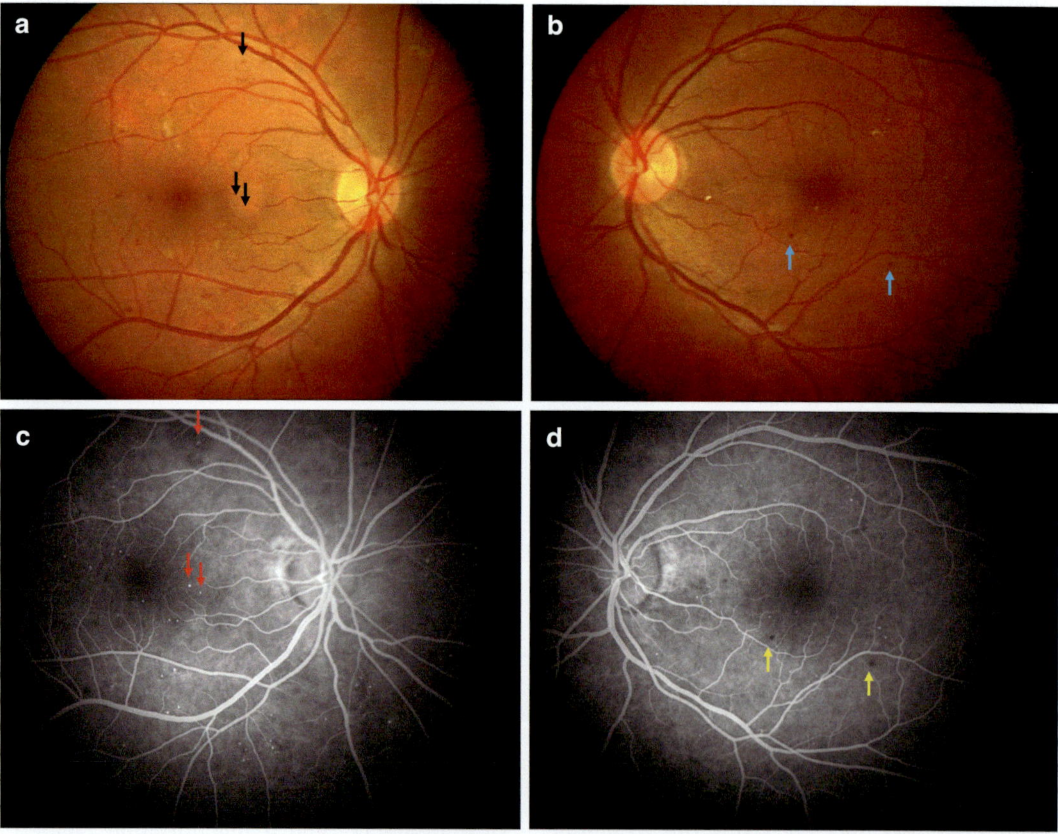

Fig. 1.2 Colour fundus photograph of the right eye (**a**) showing microaneurysms (black arrows) and of the left eye (**b**) showing dot haemorrhages (blue arrows). Fundus fluorescein angiography of the right eye (**c**) shows hyperfluorescent lesions (red arrows) corresponding to microaneurysms, while in the left eye (**d**), the dot haemorrhages appear hypofluorescent (yellow arrows) due to blocked fluorescence

the ganglion cell layer (GCL). The normal retina is tightly packed with cellular elements with only a potential extracellular space in the inner and outer plexiform layers.

1.7 Location of Retinal Microaneurysms

It is now believed that the MAs in DM are located on the arterial end of the capillaries. In the diabetic retina, the MAs are not distributed uniformly. These are located preferentially in the posterior pole, with a majority seen in the upper and temporal sectors of the macula (Fig. 1.3). The left eye shows more MAs than the right [9]. There are areas of the retina with an entirely normal capillary bed and areas with a loss of the retinal capillary bed. MAs are clustered around capillary non-perfusion, as seen on fundus fluorescein angiography (FFA). In flat-mount trypsin digestion studies, these are seen as hollow acellular tubes. Many more MAs are seen on FFA than are visible on clinical examination (Fig. 1.4).

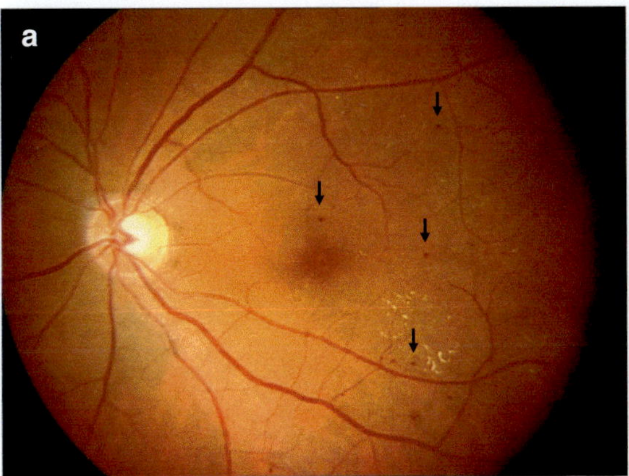

Fig. 1.3 Left eye colour fundus photograph (**a**) showing microaneurysms in the posterior pole, more along temporal and superior macula (black arrows), which are more prominently seen as hyperfluorescent lesions (blue arrows) on fundus fluorescein angiography (**b**)

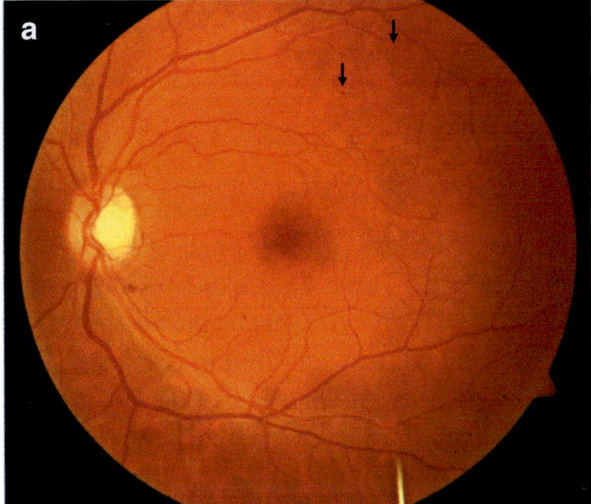

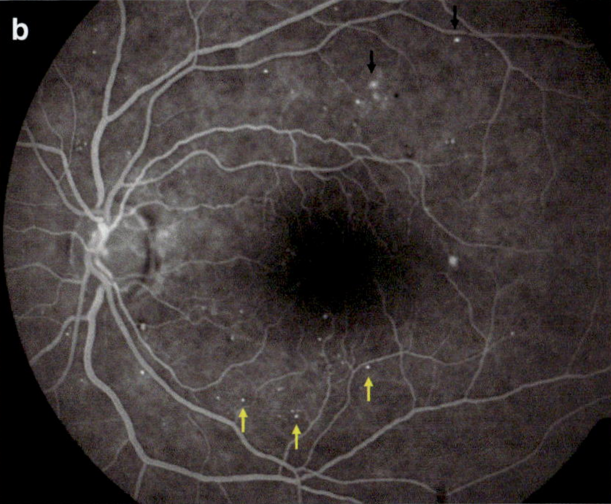

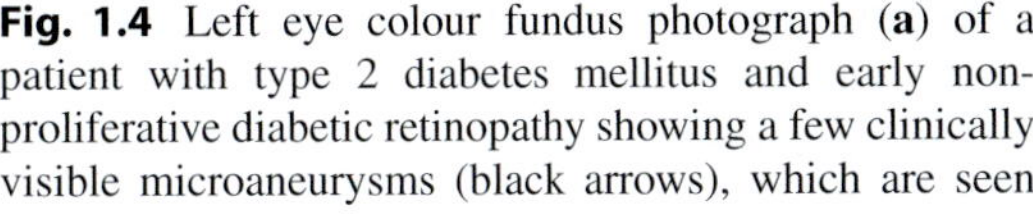

Fig. 1.4 Left eye colour fundus photograph (**a**) of a patient with type 2 diabetes mellitus and early non-proliferative diabetic retinopathy showing a few clinically visible microaneurysms (black arrows), which are seen much more in number on fundus fluorescein angiography (**b**), the black arrows corresponding to clinically visible microaneurysms, and yellow arrows corresponding to those seen only on FFA

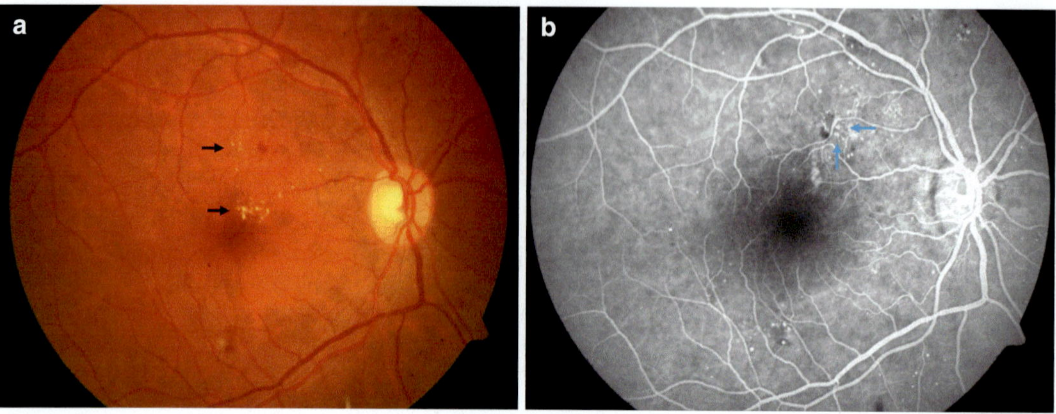

Fig. 1.5 Hard exudates appear as shiny deposits (black arrows) on fundus examination (**a**) and the causative microaneurysms (blue arrows) can be seen more clearly on FFA (**b**)

Some clinically seen MAs but not seen on FFA are either dot haemorrhages or thrombosed MAs [5].

MAs are present in the superficial and the inner (located in the ganglion cell layer) and the deep capillary plexus of the retina (located on either side of the inner nuclear layer). It is impossible to discern whether a specific microaneurysm is in the superficial or deep capillary plexus on fundoscopy or even on FFA. However, their location can be determined using advanced imaging techniques such as optical coherence tomography angiography (Fig. 1.9).

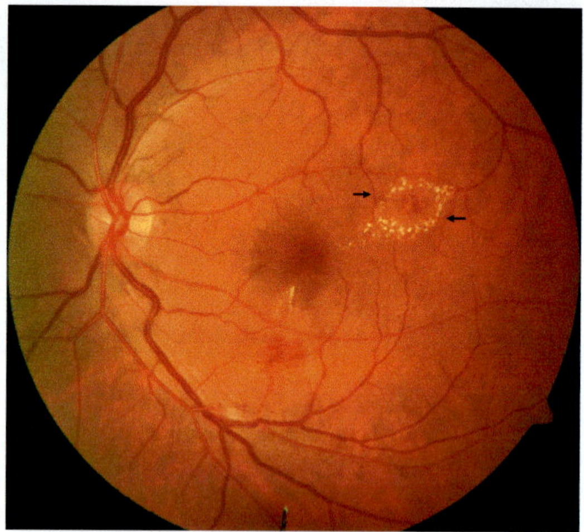

Fig. 1.6 A complete ring of hard exudates, the circinate ring (arrows), marks the outer boundary of the leaking microaneurysms

1.8 Leakage from the Retinal Capillary Microaneurysms

Leakage from the MAs leads to the formation of hard exudates. In the normal retina, endothelial cells lining the retinal vessels have tight junctions that do not allow the movement of fluid and macromolecules into the extravascular space. Once the MAs are formed in the retinal capillary bed, the endothelial tight junctions are lost, with consequent leakage of fluid and lipoproteins into the extravascular space that results in the thickening of the retina and accumulation of lipoproteins seen as bright shiny hard exudates (Fig. 1.5). The leaked fluid gets absorbed by the adjacent normal capillary bed. However, the large lipoprotein exudates cannot move back into the intravascular space. These stay in the extravascular space and mark the boundary of the normal and abnormal capillary beds. These hard exudates are carted away by the phagocytes, but as the new exudates keep forming and an equilibrium is reached, any change in the number and size of these hard exudates may not be readily appreciated. Complete or incomplete rings of hard exudates (circinate rings) mark the outer boundary of the leaking microaneurysms (Fig. 1.6). It was the basis of focal laser photocoagulation to destroy the leaking microaneurysms.

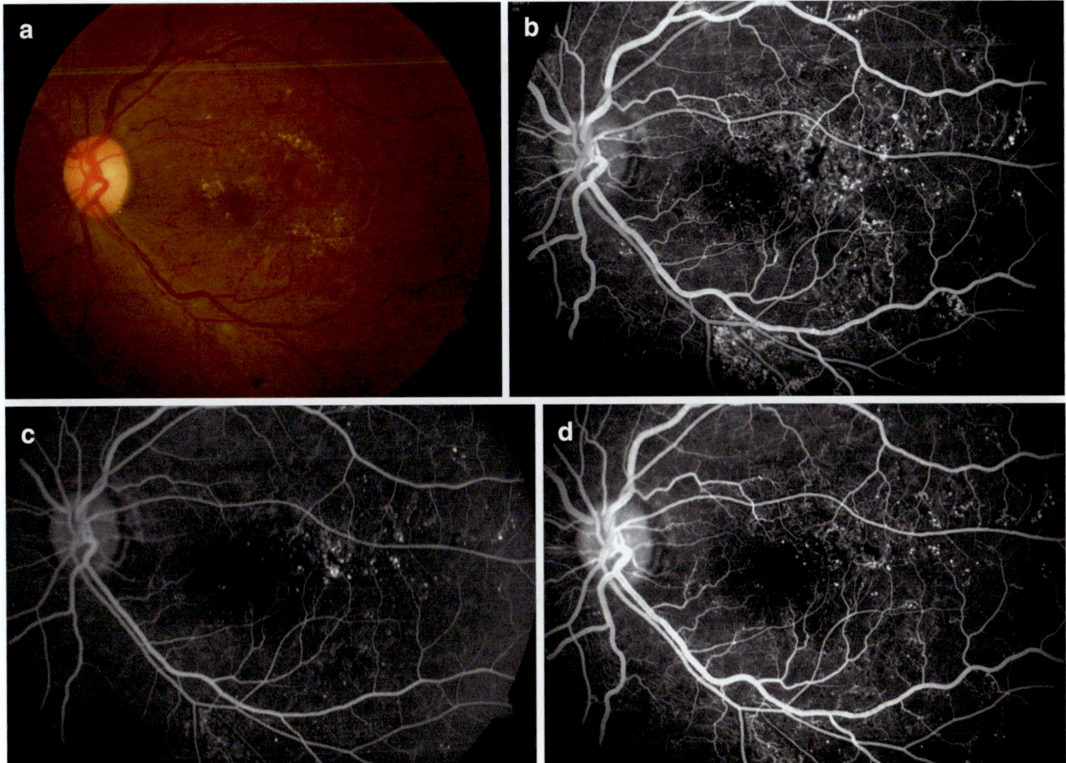

Fig. 1.7 A 20-year-old type 1 woman with non-proliferative diabetic retinopathy (**a**) with many microaneurysms on FFA in the macula (**b**), 3 months following intravitreal injection of Ozurdex, most microaneurysms have regressed (**c**). However, as the effect of Ozurdex injection wanes off by 4 months, many microaneurysms have reappeared (**d**)

1.9 Life Cycle of Retinal Capillary Microaneurysms

Once formed, the MAs in diabetes show a gradual increase in their numbers and over the years, some of them become involute while the new ones continue to form. The course of the MAs is stable; once formed, they disappear at ~3% per month when seen over a long follow-up. The formation of new MAs is a sign of the progression of diabetic disease and the number of MAs indicates the severity of diabetic retinopathy [10]. An increase in MAs by a factor of 16× from baseline to the 4-year follow-up increased the 10-year risk of proliferative diabetic retinopathy by 4.6 times and clinically significant macular oedema by 9.1 times [11]. Compared to the standard 7-field 30° stereoscopic colour fundus images (early treatment diabetic retinopathy study), a single field 200° ultrawide fundus image detects ~50% more MAs/dot haemorrhages [12]. In experimental models, an intravitreal injection of VEGF led to the formation of MAs mimicking diabetic retinopathy [13]. The use of anti-VEGF injections, including ranibizumab and aflibercept for treating diabetic macular oedema, reduces retinal thickening and causes the regression of pre-existing MAs and fewer new MAs to form [14–16]. We have seen a similar regression of MAs with intravitreal corticosteroids (Fig. 1.7). This effect is responsible for the apparent reversal of diabetic retinopathy. However, it is important to realize that the non-perfused areas persist despite the disappearance of the MAs following intravitreal injections of anti-VEGF agents [14]. Anaemia was recently recognized as a risk factor

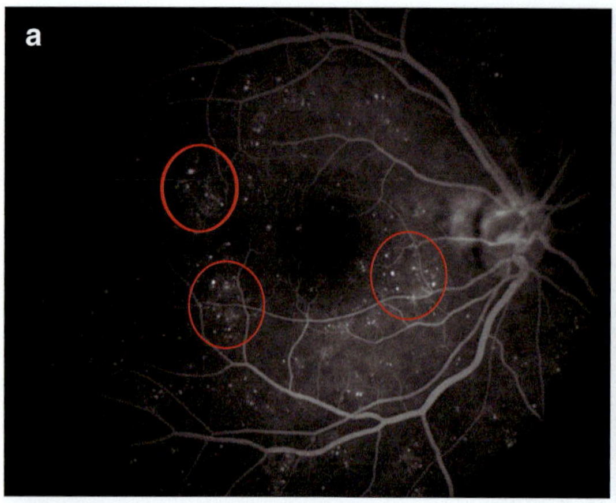

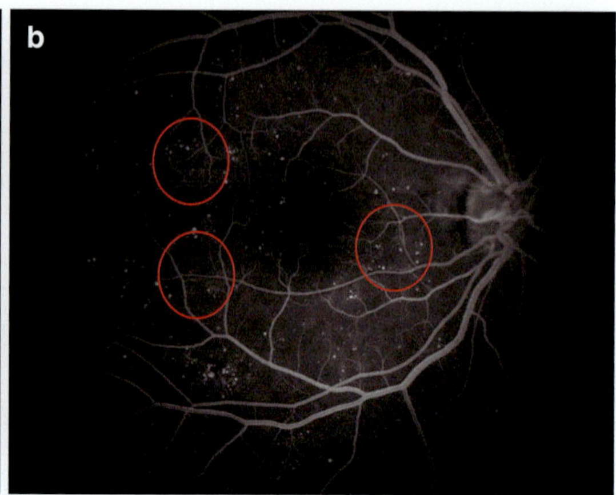

Fig. 1.8 A 35-year-old woman with type 2 DM for 10 years from a pre-anti-VEGF era. Had uncontrolled BSL and Hb 9.1 gm%. Fundus fluorescein angiography revealed multiple microaneurysms; some are encircled (**a**). She was advised of multifactorial control of her metabolic parameters. She was treated with iron supplementation. Over the next 9 months, her BSL were controlled, and the Hb increased to 11.1 gm%. Note the disappearing microaneurysms (**b**)

for the progression of diabetic retinopathy independent of chronic kidney disease [17, 18] Reversal of hypoxia by the correction of coexisting anaemia may cause complete disappearance of MAs [19] (Fig. 1.8).

1.10 Imaging of Retinal Capillary Microaneurysms

Fundus imaging is fundamental in tele-screening strategies for the early detection of diabetic retinopathy. The fundus images also serve as a document for future changes in the retina, determine the need for therapeutic interventions, and assess the outcome of those interventions. In the past, 30° standard 7-field, colour film-based fundus photography through a dilated pupil was done to document retinal diseases and objectively document the effect of the therapeutic interventions on retinal pathology, including MAs. The seven fields included the one centered on the optic disc, macula, and temporal to the macula. Four images were taken tangentially to lines forming a cross passing at the upper and lower poles of the optic disc. Non-simultaneous stereoscopic pictures were taken of all the fields. In recent years, there have been revolutionary changes in the multiple ways by which the retina is imaged, termed multimedia imaging. Exploiting the various reflectance properties of various retinal structures, the scanning laser ophthalmoscope in digital cameras can obtain blue reflectance (for superficial structures like epiretinal membranes), green reflectance (for blood vessels, MAs, RNFL and exudates), and near-infrared reflectance (for deeper retina and choroidal structures) images to highlight retinal structures located in the different layers of the retina. Besides, these systems now obtain a wide angle (retinal field of view including vortex vein ampulla) or ultra-wide (includes retina field of view anterior to the entry of vortex veins) image of the entire retina (~200°) in a single exposure. The need for stereoscopic retina imaging is obviated by using optical coherence tomography (OCT) for microstructural retina (1–3 μm axial resolution) imaging and visualizing the cross-sectional or enface details.

1.10.1 Imaging of Retinal Capillary Microaneurysms: Morphology

Using adaptive optics scanning laser ophthalmoscope (AOSLO) at least six morphological types of MAs are recognized. These are focal bulging, saccular, fusiform, mixed saccular/fusiform, pedunculated, and irregularly shaped [20]. The morphological shape rather than the size of the MAs is responsible for leakage. The irregular, mixed type, and fusiform are more likely to leak than the saccular and pedunculated MAs [21]. Moreover, saccular MAs are more likely to be thrombosed than fusiform MAs [22]. Simulation studies have shown that reduced inlet velocity of the feeding vessel of the saccular MAs leads to increased adherence of the platelets to the aneurysmal wall where the blood is more stagnant and initiates thrombus formation. Reduced bold flow velocity may also lead to thrombus formation in some fusiform MAs [17, 18]. It may be noted that before the development of retinopathy, the blood flow velocity in type 1 DM is reduced and is dependent on the blood glucose levels, but with the development of non-proliferative diabetic retinopathy there is an increase in the flow velocity [23]. It is likely that this increase in flow velocity may be mediated through vascular endothelial growth factor (VEGF) [17, 18, 24].

1.10.2 Imaging of Retinal Capillary Microaneurysms: OCT

On optical coherence tomography (OCT), MAs show either a complete, incomplete, or no ring. Compared to those with no or incomplete rings, MAs with complete rings are less likely to be associated with cystic spaces in the retina. The complete ring likely indicates a thickened and hyalinized basement membrane. Hyperreflectivity in the MAs indicates the presence of cellular elements and is often seen in those without rings [25].

1.10.3 Imaging of Retinal Capillary Microaneurysms: OCTA

Optical coherence tomography angiography (OCTA) allows 3-D enface visualization of the various segmented layers of the retina with a caveat that all microaneurysms may not be visible on OCTA [26]. On a 3-D rotational OCTA, most MAs are fusiform in shape and seem to arise from the DCP in the inner nuclear layer (Fig. 1.9). Some of these are also present in the SCP and on the capillaries connecting the SCP and the DCP. MAs are also seen in the outer plexiform layer [27, 28]. Most MAs are associated with two vessels originating in the DCP and, less commonly, from the SCP. Those arising from the DCP are in the inner nuclear layer, those from the SCP occupy the ganglion cell layer, and others may be seen in the outer plexiform layer and rarely in the outer nuclear layer [27].

In OCTA, two reflectivity patterns are discernible in the MAs, hyporeflective and hyperreflective. Hyporeflective MAs are unlikely to be visible on OCTA because of a very slow blood flow or thrombosis, while the hyperreflective MAs are visible due to increased blood flow in these MAs which may damage the wall of the MAs, causing extravasation and retinal thickening [28] (Fig. 1.10).

The last few years have seen a very aggressive application of artificial intelligence using deep learning algorithms for the automated detection of the earliest diabetic retinopathy changes, namely, the MAs and dot haemorrhages [29].

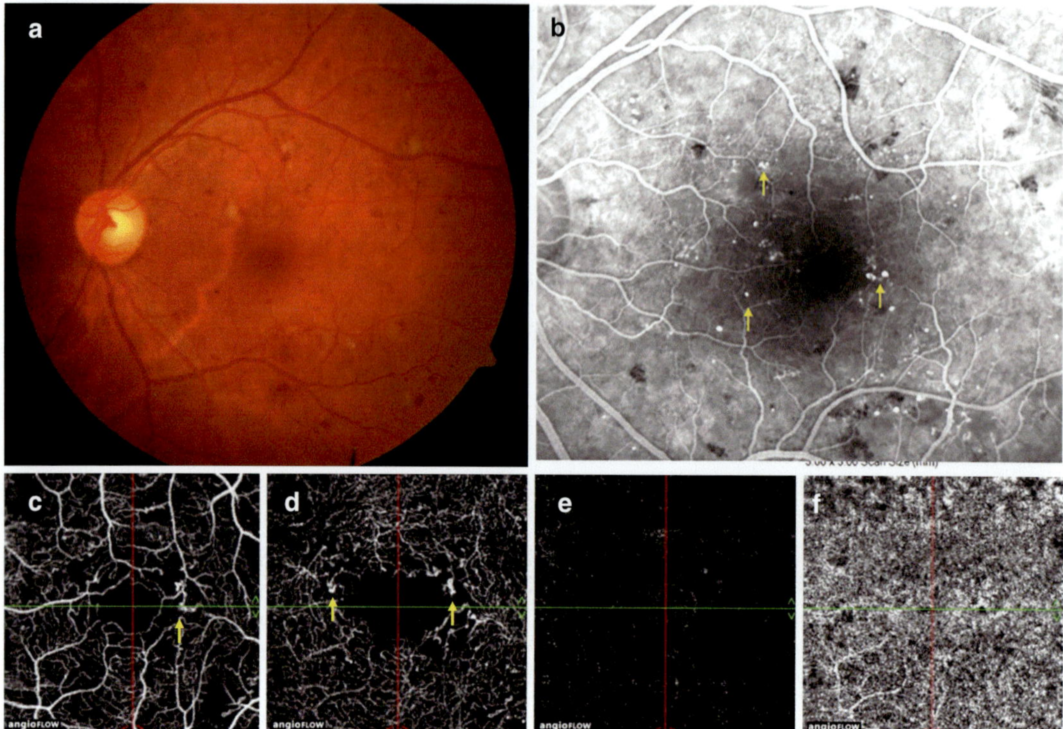

Fig. 1.9 Colour Fundus photograph of the left eye (**a**) showing moderate non-proliferative diabetic retinopathy (microaneurysms, retinal haemorrhages and cotton wool spots). Fluorescein angiogram (**b**) showing leaking microaneurysms (yellow arrows) and retinal haemorrhages. The bottom panel shows the OCT angiography (macular scan 3.00 × 3.00 mm scan) with microaneurysms seen in the superficial capillary plexus (SCP) (yellow arrows) (**c**), as well as deep capillary plexus (DCP) as fusiform dilatations (yellow arrows) (**d**). The microaneurysms are absent in the outer retina (**e**) and choriocapillaris (**f**) layers

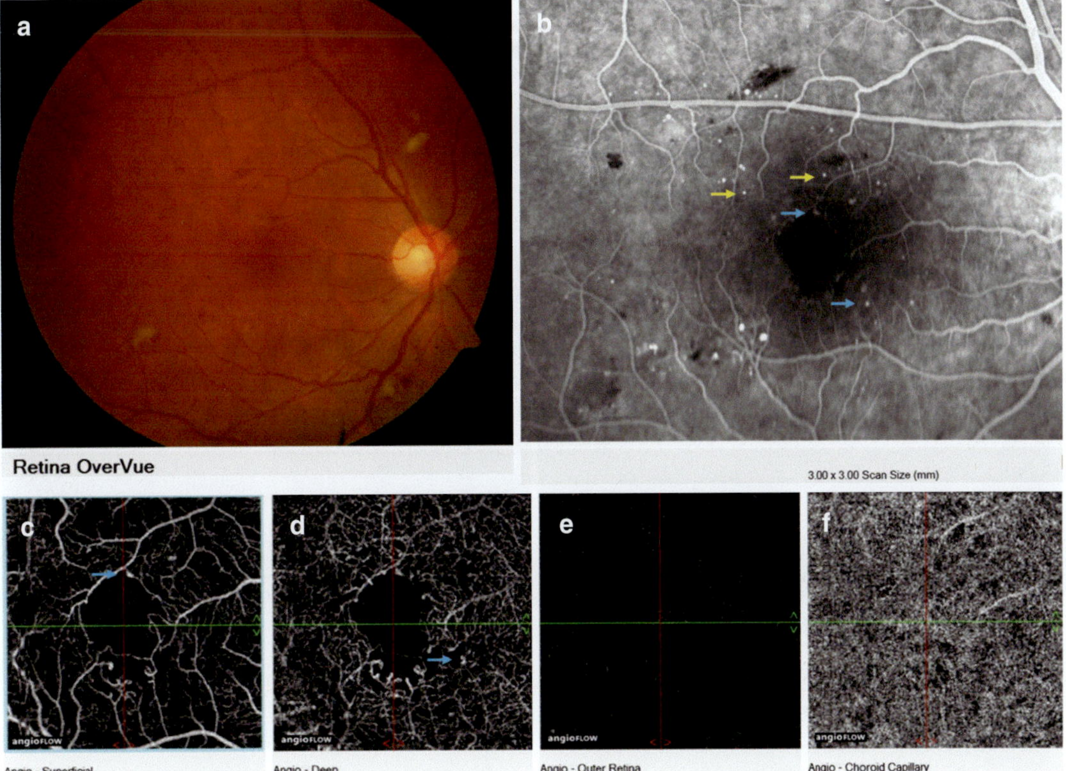

Fig. 1.10 Colour Fundus photograph of the right eye (**a**) showing moderate NPDR (microaneurysms, retinal haemorrhages and cotton wool spots). Fluorescein angiogram (**b**) showing leaking microaneurysms, some of which are visible (blue arrows) on OCT angiography (bottom panel) in superficial capillary plexus (SCP) (**c**) or deep capillary plexus (DCP) (**d**). In contrast, some on FFA (yellow arrows) are not visible on OCT angiography. The microaneurysms are not seen in the outer retina (**e**) and choriocapillaris (**f**) layers

1.11 Other Causes of Retinal Capillary Microaneurysms

Retinal microaneurysms are formed in response to hypoxia of the retina. In patients with hypertensive retinopathy, microaneurysms are seen surrounding cotton-wool spots formed by the occlusion of precapillary arterioles. These microaneurysms last only a few weeks and disappear with the disappearance of the cotton wool spots. Besides diabetes and hypertension, microaneurysms may be seen in carotid atherosclerosis (carotid insufficiency). In contrast to diabetes, where MAs are predominantly seen in the posterior pole, in carotid insufficiency, MAs are seen in the retinal periphery. Likewise, these may be seen in Takayasu's arteritis (TA) if the arteries involve the common or the internal carotid artery (Figs. 1.11 and 1.12). In the latter, MAs are seen all over the retina and are accompanied by a cattle-trucking of the blood cells in both retinal arterioles and the veins. Low intraocular pressure can be an additional clue to diagnosing TA in these two situations. Patients may also complain of dizziness on suddenly getting up (Fig. 1.13).

Microaneurysms may also be seen in longstanding branch retinal vein occlusion (BRVO) (Fig. 1.14) and central retinal vein occlusion (CRVO). These are also seen in congenital retinal vasculature abnormalities such as Coats' disease which mostly affects young boys' left eye. Large microaneurysm dilatations on telangiectatic retinal vessels characterize the latter. These profusely leak fluid and lipoproteins, forming massive deposits of hard exudates. Limited MAs are also seen in type 1 macular telangiectasia (Mac Tel type 1). The formation of MAs also characterizes radiation retinopathy.

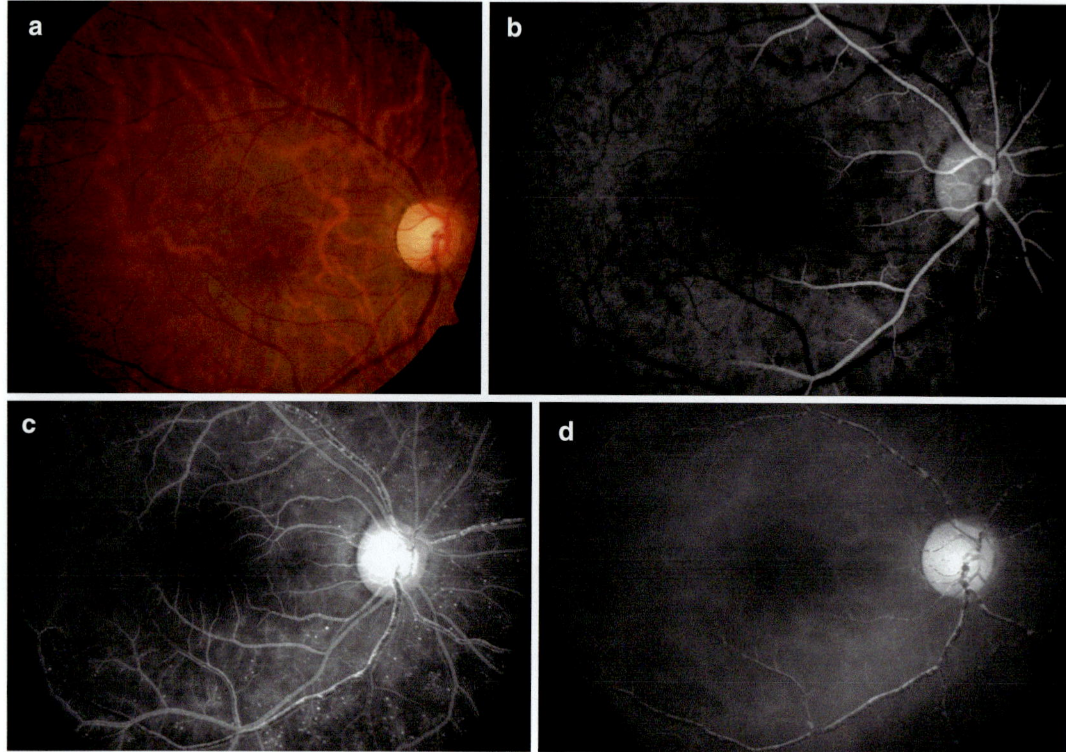

Fig. 1.11 A 28-year-old woman complained of giddiness on standing. Brachial pulse was absent. She had bilateral symmetrical changes. The right showed venous fullness with few visible microaneurysms (**a**). On FFA, there was a remarkable delay in the perfusion of the dye in the retinal arterioles with several microaneurysms (**b**), which are absent in the macula but prominent along the vessels. Cattle trucking can be seen in the major veins (**c** and **d**). She also complained of giddiness which recovered on lowering of head. Her physical exam was significant for absent radial and brachial pulses. On ocular examination she had visual acuity of 6/36 OU. Her intraocular pressures were 6 and 7 mm in the right and left eye, respectively. There were no iris neovessels. Pupil reactions were sluggish. She underwent CT angio of arch of aorta and its branches was suggestive of Type 4 Takayasu arteritis involving the ascending aorta, arch of aorta, descending aorta, left pulmonary artery, bilateral common carotid artery, brachiocephalic trunk, bilateral subclavian and axillary arteries

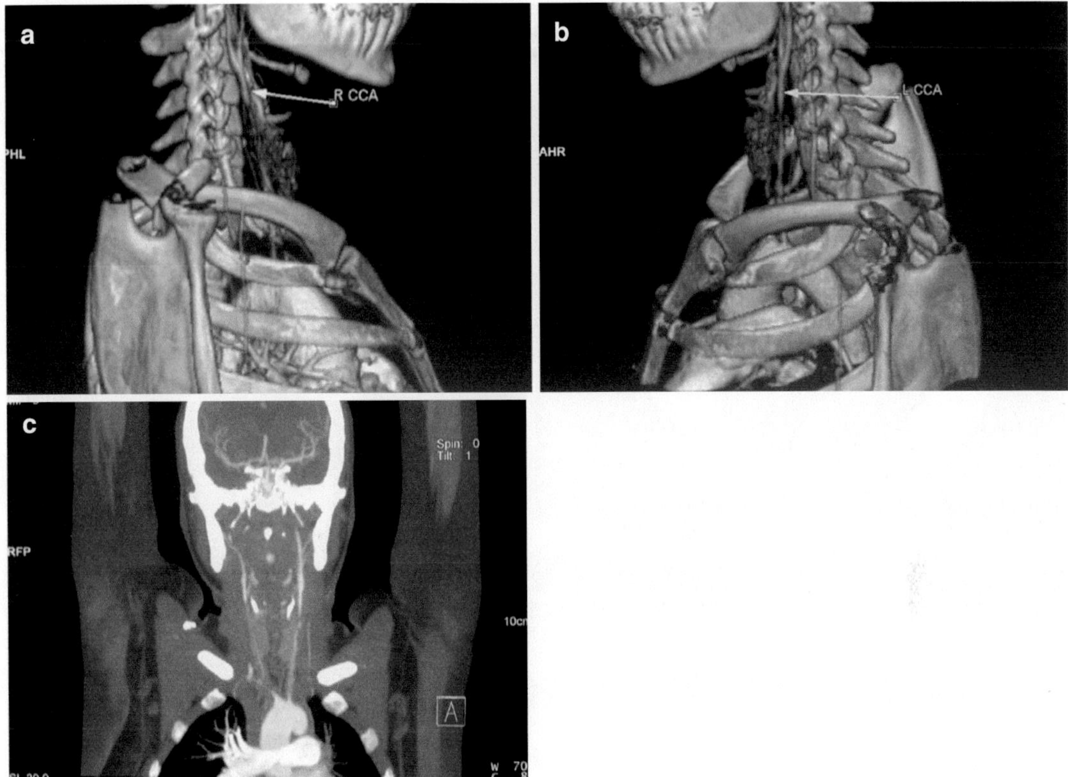

Fig. 1.12 CT angio of the same patient shown in Fig. 1.11, shows involvement of ascending aorta, arch of aorta, left pulmonary artery, bilateral common carotid arteries, brachiocephalic trunk, bilateral subclavian and axillary arteries

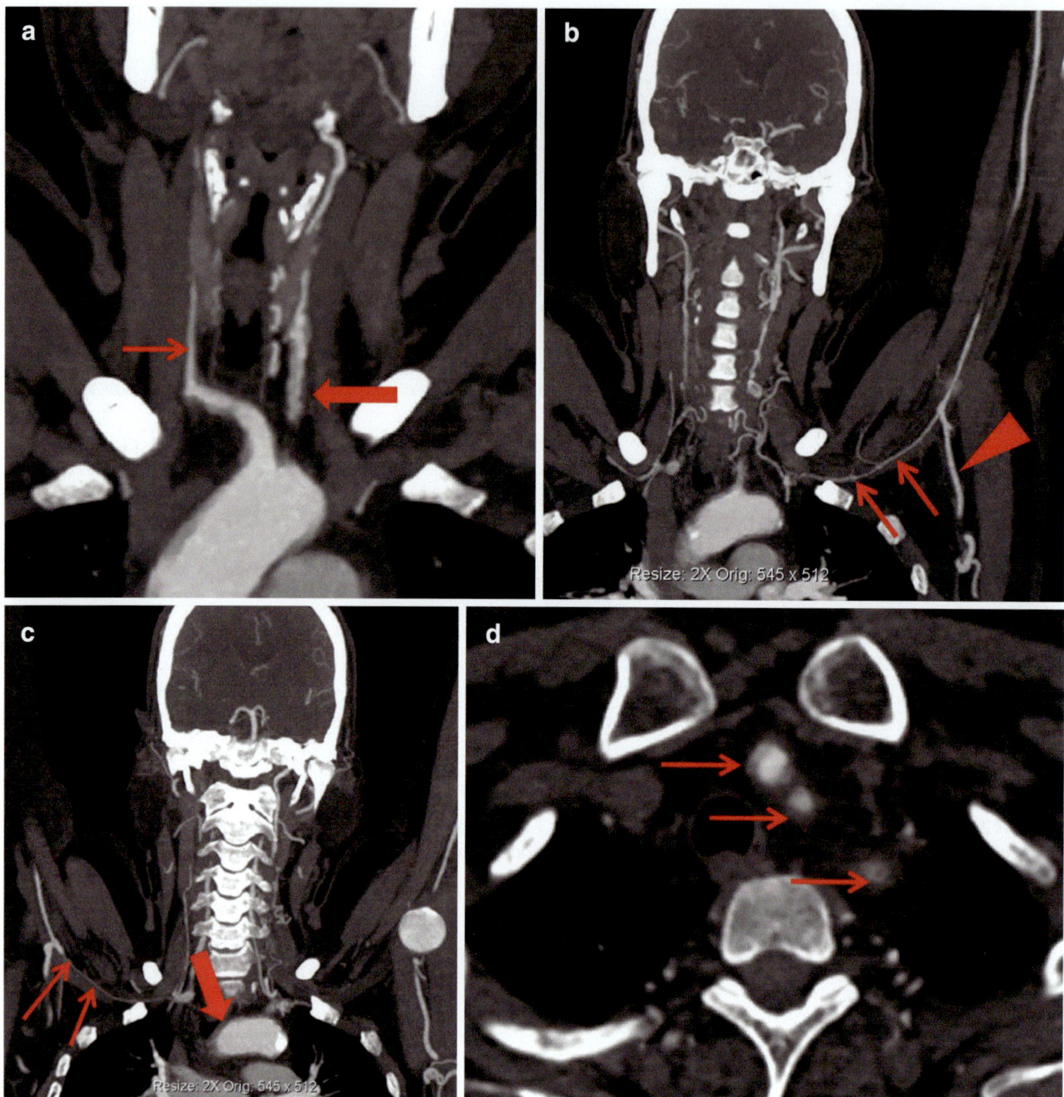

Fig. 1.13 A 43-year-old female with a history of upper limbs claudication and syncope show (**a**) attenuation of both common carotid arteries-CCA (right > left) [thin arrow—right CCA, thick arrow—left CCA], (**b**) attenuated osteo-proximal left subclavian (thin arrows) and (**c**) attenuated osteo-proximal right subclavian (thin arrows) arteries on reconstructed coronal CT angiography images. Note prominent collateral in (**b**) and circumferential mural thickening of the arch of the aorta (thick arrow in **c**). Axial image (**d**) shows circumferential symmetric mural thickening with attenuation of the calibre of the brachiocephalic trunk, left CAA and left subclavian arteries. *Images courtesy of DR Manphool Singhal. Department of Radiodiagnosis, Post Graduate Institute of Medical Education and Research, Chandigarh. India*

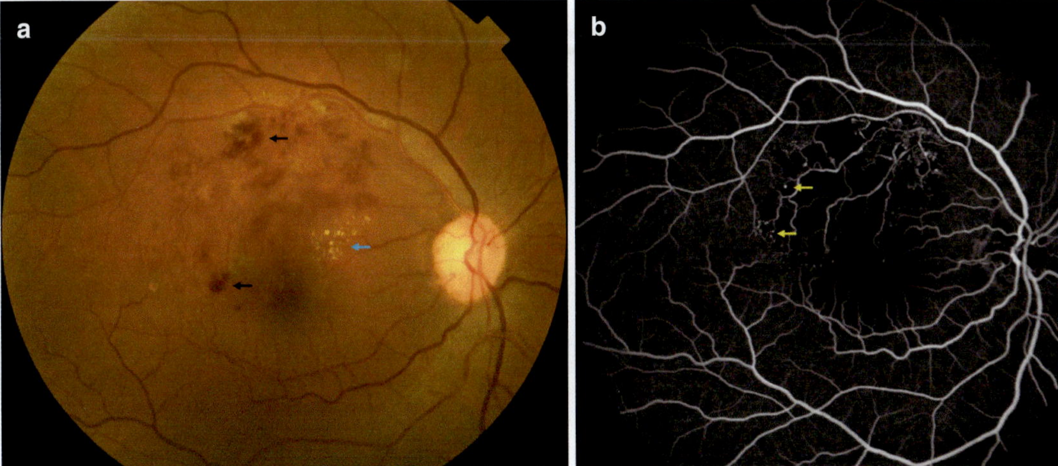

Fig. 1.14 Colour fundus photograph (**a**) of the right eye of a patient with macular branch retinal vein occlusion (BRVO), showing retinal haemorrhages (black arrows) and hard exudates (blue arrow) in the macula. Fundus fluorescein angiography (**b**) showed microaneurysms (yellow arrows) that were not visible clinically

1.12 Significance of Retinal Capillary Microaneurysms

1. Sighting of retinal MAs in patients with diabetes indicates that the patients have had out-of-range glycemic control for at least 5 years. It should be noted that in patients who have the onset of type 1 diabetes before puberty, MAs are not seen till the onset of puberty.
2. Besides being now the leading cause of blindness, the presence of MAs in patients with diabetes (diabetic retinopathy) should prompt a search for associated diabetic nephropathy. Both are microangiopathy manifestations of long-standing diabetes. Diabetic nephropathy is now the leading cause of end-stage renal disease requiring renal replacement therapy. Diabetic retinopathy is an independent risk factor for the outcome of diabetic nephropathy [30].
3. In the elderly population, retinal MAs are an independent risk factor for the progressive worsening of renal functions [31].
4. Patients with impaired glucose tolerance or impaired fasting glucose who have peripheral neuropathy are four times more likely to have retinopathy and twice more often albuminuria than those with no peripheral neuropathy [32].
5. All three microvascular complications of diabetes, namely, retinopathy, nephropathy, and peripheral neuropathy, are intimately related. Detecting retinopathy should lead to a search for peripheral neuropathy and peripheral arterial disease (PAD). Diabetes is a major risk factor for the acceleration of atherosclerotic PAD. Coupled with diabetic peripheral polyneuropathy, it is the leading cause of amputation of limbs/toes/feet [33].
6. Irrespective of the associated diabetes or hypertension, MAs and dot haemorrhages are more likely to be seen in patients with acute coronary syndrome than stable angina. Thus, a useful adjunct in risk assessment requiring a closer watch [34].
7. There is mounting evidence that retinal microvascular lesions, including MAs/Ha, irrespective of known risk factors, diabetes, hypertension, smoking etc., are markers of subclinical microangiopathy in the brain and can be used to predict future events like stroke [35].
8. Increasing the number of diabetic microvascular complications (retinopathy, nephropathy, and peripheral neuropathy) is related to an increased risk of cardiovascular events and all-cause mortality in type 1 diabetes [36].

9. Diffusely scattered MAs indicate the presence of an underlying systemic atherosclerotic disease if it involves the internal carotid artery in the elderly or Takayasu's arteritis in younger patients.

References

1. American Diabetes Association. Standards of Medical Care in Diabetes—2022 abridged for primary care providers. Clin Diabetes. 2022;40(1):10–38. https://doi.org/10.2337/cd22-as01. PMID: 35221470; PMCID: PMC8865785.
2. Omri S, Omri B, Savoldelli M, Jonet L, Thillaye-Goldenberg B, Thuret G, Gain P, Jeanny JC, Crisanti P, Behar-Cohen F. The outer limiting membrane (OLM) revisited: clinical implications. Clin Ophthalmol. 2010;4:183–95. https://doi.org/10.2147/opth.s5901. PMID: 20463783; PMCID: PMC2861922.
3. Lechner J, O'Leary OE, Stitt AW. The pathology associated with diabetic retinopathy. Vis Res. 2017;139:7–14. https://doi.org/10.1016/j.visres.2017.04.003. Epub 2017 Apr 29. PMID: 28412095.
4. Rodrigues M, Xin X, Jee K, Babapoor-Farrokhran S, Kashiwabuchi F, Ma T, Bhutto I, Hassan SJ, Daoud Y, Baranano D, Solomon S, Lutty G, Semenza GL, Montaner S, Sodhi A. VEGF secreted by hypoxic Müller cells induces MMP-2 expression and activity in endothelial cells to promote retinal neovascularization in proliferative diabetic retinopathy. Diabetes. 2013;62(11):3863–73. https://doi.org/10.2337/db13-0014. Epub 2013 Jul 24. PMID: 23884892; PMCID: PMC3806594.
5. Dollery CT, Hodge JV, Engel M. Studies of the retinal circulation with flourescein. Br Med J. 1962;2(5314):1210–5. https://doi.org/10.1136/bmj.2.5314.1210. PMID: 14028474; PMCID: PMC1926224.
6. Novotny HR, Alvis DL. A method of photographing fluorescence in circulating blood in the human retina. Circulation. 1961;24:82–6. https://doi.org/10.1161/01.cir.24.1.82. PMID: 13729802.
7. Hill DW, Dollery CT, Mailer CM, Oakley NW, Ramalho PS. Arterial fluorescein studies in diabetic retinopathy. Proc R Soc Med. 1965;58(7):535–7. PMID: 19994430; PMCID: PMC1898598.
8. Kohner EM, Dollery CT, Paterson JW, Oakley NW. Arterial fluorescein studies in diabetic retinopathy. Diabetes 1967;16(1):1–10. https://doi.org/10.2337/diab.16.1.1. PMID: 6015679.
9. Munuera-Gifre E, Saez M, Juvinyà-Canals D, Rodríguez-Poncelas A, Barrot-de-la-Puente JF, Franch-Nadal J, Romero-Aroca P, Barceló MA, Coll-de-Tuero G. Analysis of the location of retinal lesions in central retinographies of patients with type 2 diabetes. Acta Ophthalmol. 2020;98(1):e13–21. https://doi.org/10.1111/aos.14223. Epub 2019 Aug 30. PMID: 31469507.
10. Kohner EM, Sleightholm M. Does microaneurysm count reflect severity of early diabetic retinopathy? Ophthalmology. 1986;93(5):586–9. https://doi.org/10.1016/s0161-6420(86)33692-3. PMID: 3725317.
11. Klein R, Meuer SM, Moss SE, Klein BE. Retinal microaneurysm counts and 10-year progression of diabetic retinopathy. Arch Ophthalmol. 1995;113(11):1386–91. https://doi.org/10.1001/archopht.1995.01100110046024. PMID: 7487599.
12. Silva PS, El-Rami H, Barham R, Gupta A, Fleming A, van Hemert J, Cavallerano JD, Sun JK, Aiello LP. Hemorrhage and/or microaneurysm severity and count in ultrawide field images and early treatment diabetic retinopathy study photography. Ophthalmology. 2017;124(7):970–6. https://doi.org/10.1016/j.ophtha.2017.02.012. Epub 2017 Mar 20. PMID: 28336057.
13. Tolentino MJ, Miller JW, Gragoudas ES, Jakobiec FA, Flynn E, Chatzistefanou K, Ferrara N, Adamis AP. Intravitreous injections of vascular endothelial growth factor produce retinal ischemia and microangiopathy in an adult primate. Ophthalmology. 1996;103(11):1820–8. https://doi.org/10.1016/s0161-6420(96)30420-x. PMID: 8942877.
14. Couturier A, Rey PA, Erginay A, Lavia C, Bonnin S, Dupas B, Gaudric A, Tadayoni R. Widefield OCT-angiography and fluorescein angiography assessments of nonperfusion in diabetic retinopathy and edema treated with anti-vascular endothelial growth factor. Ophthalmology. 2019;126(12):1685–94. https://doi.org/10.1016/j.ophtha.2019.06.022. Epub 2019 Jun 26. PMID: 31383483.
15. Leicht SF, Kernt M, Neubauer A, Wolf A, Oliveira CM, Ulbig M, Haritoglou C. Microaneurysm turnover in diabetic retinopathy assessed by automated RetmarkerDR image analysis—potential role as biomarker of response to ranibizumab treatment. Ophthalmologica. 2014;231(4):198–203. https://doi.org/10.1159/000357505. Epub 2014 Mar 19. PMID: 24662930.
16. Sugimoto M, Ichio A, Mochida D, Tenma Y, Miyata R, Matsubara H, Kondo M. Multiple effects of intravitreal Aflibercept on microvascular regression in eyes with diabetic macular edema. Ophthalmol Retina. 2019;3(12):1067–75. https://doi.org/10.1016/j.oret.2019.06.005. Epub 2019 Jun 15. PMID: 31446029.
17. Li H, Sampani K, Zheng X, Papageorgiou DP, Yazdani A, Bernabeu MO, Karniadakis GE, Sun JK. Predictive modelling of thrombus formation in diabetic retinal microaneurysms. R Soc Open Sci. 2020a;7(8):201102. https://doi.org/10.1098/rsos.201102. PMID: 32968536; PMCID: PMC7481715.
18. Li Y, Yu Y, VanderBeek BL. Anaemia and the risk of progression from non-proliferative diabetic retinopathy to vision threatening diabetic retinopathy. Eye

(Lond). 2020b;34(5):934–41. https://doi.org/10.1038/s41433-019-0617-6. Epub 2019 Oct 4. PMID: 31586167; PMCID: PMC7182576.
19. Singh R, Gupta V, Gupta A, Bhansali A. Spontaneous closure of microaneurysms in diabetic retinopathy with treatment of co-existing anaemia. Br J Ophthalmol. 2005;89(2):248–9. https://doi.org/10.1136/bjo.2004.050252. PMID: 15665369; PMCID: PMC1772514.
20. Dubow M, Pinhas A, Shah N, Cooper RF, Gan A, Gentile RC, Hendrix V, Sulai YN, Carroll J, Chui TY, Walsh JB, Weitz R, Dubra A, Rosen RB. Classification of human retinal microaneurysms using adaptive optics scanning light ophthalmoscope fluorescein angiography. Invest Ophthalmol Vis Sci. 2014;55(3):1299–309. https://doi.org/10.1167/iovs.13-13122. PMID: 24425852; PMCID: PMC3943418.
21. Schreur V, Domanian A, Liefers B, Venhuizen FG, Klevering BJ, Hoyng CB, de Jong EK, Theelen T. Morphological and topographical appearance of microaneurysms on optical coherence tomography angiography. Br J Ophthalmol. 2018:bjophthalmol-2018-312258. https://doi.org/10.1136/bjophthalmol-2018-312258. Epub ahead of print. PMID: 29925511.
22. Bernabeu MO, Lu Y, Abu-Qamar O, Aiello LP, Sun JK. Estimation of diabetic retinal microaneurysm perfusion parameters based on computational fluid dynamics modeling of adaptive optics scanning laser ophthalmoscopy. Front Physiol. 2018;9:989. https://doi.org/10.3389/fphys.2018.00989. PMID: 30245632; PMCID: PMC6137139.
23. Bursell SE, Clermont AC, Kinsley BT, Simonson DC, Aiello LM, Wolpert HA. Retinal blood flow changes in patients with insulin-dependent diabetes mellitus and no diabetic retinopathy. Invest Ophthalmol Vis Sci. 1996;37(5):886–97. PMID: 8603873.
24. Clermont AC, Aiello LP, Mori F, Aiello LM, Bursell SE. Vascular endothelial growth factor and severity of nonproliferative diabetic retinopathy mediate retinal hemodynamics in vivo: a potential role for vascular endothelial growth factor in the progression of nonproliferative diabetic retinopathy. Am J Ophthalmol. 1997;124(4):433–46. https://doi.org/10.1016/s0002-9394(14)70860-8. PMID: 9323935.
25. Horii T, Murakami T, Nishijima K, Sakamoto A, Ota M, Yoshimura N. Optical coherence tomographic characteristics of microaneurysms in diabetic retinopathy. Am J Ophthalmol. 2010;150(6):840–8. https://doi.org/10.1016/j.ajo.2010.06.015. Epub 2010 Sep 19. PMID: 20855054.
26. Spaide RF, Klancnik JM Jr, Cooney MJ. Retinal vascular layers imaged by fluorescein angiography and optical coherence tomography angiography. JAMA Ophthalmol. 2015;133(1):45–50. https://doi.org/10.1001/jamaophthalmol.2014.3616. PMID: 25317632.
27. Borrelli E, Sacconi R, Brambati M, Bandello F, Querques G. In vivo rotational three-dimensional OCTA analysis of microaneurysms in the human diabetic retina. Sci Rep. 2019;9(1):16789. https://doi.org/10.1038/s41598-019-53357-1. PMID: 31728070; PMCID: PMC6856183.
28. Querques G, Borrelli E, Battista M, Sacconi R, Bandello F. Optical coherence tomography angiography in diabetes: focus on microaneurysms. Eye (Lond). 2021;35(1):142–8. https://doi.org/10.1038/s41433-020-01173-7. Epub 2020 Sep 4. PMID: 32887935; PMCID: PMC78526765.
29. Rageh A, Ashraf M, Fleming A, Silva PS. Automated microaneurysm counts on ultrawide field color and fluorescein angiography images. Semin Ophthalmol. 2021;36(4):315–21. https://doi.org/10.1080/08820538.2021.1897852. Epub 2021 Mar 28. PMID: 33779483.
30. Zhang J, Wang Y, Li L, Zhang R, Guo R, Li H, Han Q, Teng G, Liu F. Diabetic retinopathy may predict the renal outcomes of patients with diabetic nephropathy. Ren Fail. 2018;40(1):243–51. https://doi.org/10.1080/0886022X.2018.1456453. PMID: 29633887; PMCID: PMC6014304.
31. Edwards MS, Wilson DB, Craven TE, Stafford J, Fried LF, Wong TY, Klein R, Burke GL, Hansen KJ. Associations between retinal microvascular abnormalities and declining renal function in the elderly population: the cardiovascular health study. Am J Kidney Dis. 2005;46(2):214–24. https://doi.org/10.1053/j.ajkd.2005.05.005. PMID: 16112039.
32. Barr EL, Wong TY, Tapp RJ, Harper CA, Zimmet PZ, Atkins R, Shaw JE, AusDiab Steering Committee. Is peripheral neuropathy associated with retinopathy and albuminuria in individuals with impaired glucose metabolism? The 1999-2000 AusDiab. Diabetes Care. 2006;29(5):1114–6. https://doi.org/10.2337/diacare.2951114. PMID: 16644648.
33. Thiruvoipati T, Kielhorn CE, Armstrong EJ. Peripheral artery disease in patients with diabetes: epidemiology, mechanisms, and outcomes. World J Diabetes. 2015;6(7):961–9. https://doi.org/10.4239/wjd.v6.i7.961. PMID: 26185603; PMCID: PMC4499529.
34. Kralev S, Zimmerer E, Buchholz P, Lin J, Economopoulou M, Lang S, Kälsch T, Süselbeck T, Hammes HP. Microvascular retinal changes in patients presenting with acute coronary syndromes. Microvasc Res. 2010;79(2):150–3. https://doi.org/10.1016/j.mvr.2009.12.007. Epub 2010 Jan 4. PMID: 20053365.
35. Wong TY. Is retinal photography useful in the measurement of stroke risk? Lancet Neurol. 2004;3(3):179–83. https://doi.org/10.1016/s1474-4422(04)00682-9. PMID: 15029894.
36. Garofolo M, Gualdani E, Giannarelli R, Aragona M, Campi F, Lucchesi D, Daniele G, Miccoli R, Francesconi P, Del Prato S, Penno G. Microvascular complications burden (nephropathy, retinopathy and peripheral polyneuropathy) affects risk of major vascular events and all-cause mortality in type 1 diabetes: a 10-year follow-up study. Cardiovasc Diabetol. 2019;18(1):159. https://doi.org/10.1186/s12933-019-0961-7. PMID: 31733651; PMCID: PMC6858978.

2 Retinal Arteriolar Macroaneurysms (RAM)

2.1 Epidemiology

Retinal arteriolar macroaneurysms (RAM) are a rare, acquired malformation of retinal arterioles. In the Beijing eye study, a population-based study of 40 years and older individuals, the study of fundus photographs revealed two macroaneurysms (MAs) in a single 67-year-old woman giving a prevalence rate of 1 in 4500 people) [1]. In a similar study from Central India, three patients (3 eyes; 2 women) of the 4543 patients above the age of 30 years with assessable fundus photographs were found to have RAM with a prevalence rate of 1 in 1500. These authors calculated that 260,000 people in India suffer from retinal MAs [2]. However, there is no racial predilection for RAMs [3].

2.2 Historical Aspects of Retinal Macroaneurysms

Raehlmann [4] described the first two cases of RAM while describing the phenomenon of retinal arteriosclerosis. However, the most detailed clinical description in English literature of RAMs was given by Pringle [5] in a 23-year-old patient with two fusiform pale pink macroaneurysms along the second branch of the upper temporal arteriole. These were filled uniformly with blood and appeared to have thick walls. A third macroaneurysm that appeared to arise from the anterior wall of the same arteriole was saccular in shape, had thin walls, and the blood column was seen deep to this macroaneurysm; the fourth macroaneurysm was the smallest on the same arteriole. When the pressure was applied to the globe, the largest macroaneurysms became pulsatile (Box 2.1).

Box 2.1 Causes of Retinal Arterial Macroaneurysms

Systemic Diseases

1. Most common—hypertension in old women
2. Hypercholesterolemia
3. Atherosclerotic cardiovascular disease
4. Rheumatoid arthritis
5. Sarcoidosis uveitis
6. Polyarteritis nodosa
7. Leukaemia

Ocular Diseases

1. Branch retinal vein occlusion
2. Kyrieleis arteritis in toxoplasma retinochoroiditis
3. Congenital AVM type1
4. Congenital macrovessel
5. Congenital anomalous retinal artery

Abbreviation: *AVM* arteriovenous malformation

A. Gupta et al., *Ophthalmic Signs in Practice of Medicine*,
https://doi.org/10.1007/978-981-99-7923-3_2

2.3 Systemic Associations of RAM

2.3.1 Hypertension

In contrast to microaneurysms that are focal dilatations of retinal capillaries and a hallmark of diabetes retinopathy (DR), RAMs are either fusiform, a circumferential dilation of the arteriole or saccular—a focal outpouching of the retinal arteriolar wall (Figs. 2.1 and 2.2) [6]. These dilatations of the retinal arterioles are typically seen in patients with longstanding hypertension, mostly in older women. While microaneurysms are smaller than 100 μm and are preferentially seen in the upper temporal quadrant of the posterior pole, MAs are 100–250 μm in size and are seen along the secondary branches of the upper or lower temporal retinal arterioles (Fig. 2.3). Rarely, these may also be seen along other retinal arterioles or on the optic disc (Fig. 2.4) [7]. Very rarely, RAM may be bilateral (Fig. 2.5) (Boxes 2.2 and 2.3).

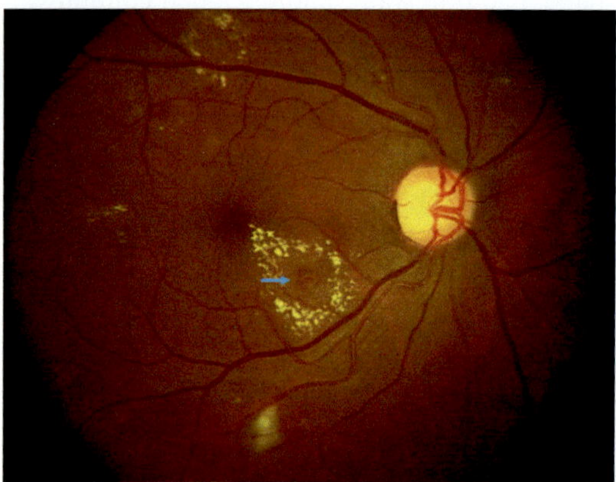

Fig. 2.1 Retinal arteriolar macroaneurysm (RAM) seen near the lower temporal arcade (blue arrow), surrounded by hard exudates, in a 60-year-old male

Box 2.2 How to Measure Blood Pressure

Measure in both upper arms; if consistently >10 mmHg in one arm, use that arm for recording.

1. No smoking, exercise, or coffee for 30 min before the test
2. Record BP after sitting for 3–5 min, back supported, and feet flat on the floor
3. No talking during the recording of the BP
4. Cuff of appropriate size, arm resting on a table at the heart level
5. Take three readings at the 1-min interval and take the mean of the last two readings
6. >20 mmHg needs further evaluation

Source: American Heart Association, Inc.

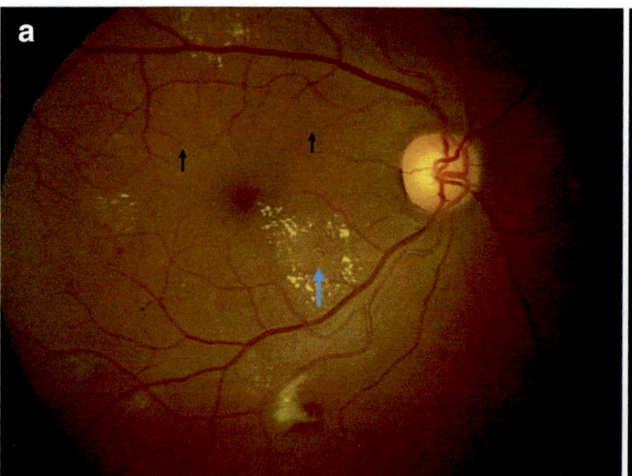

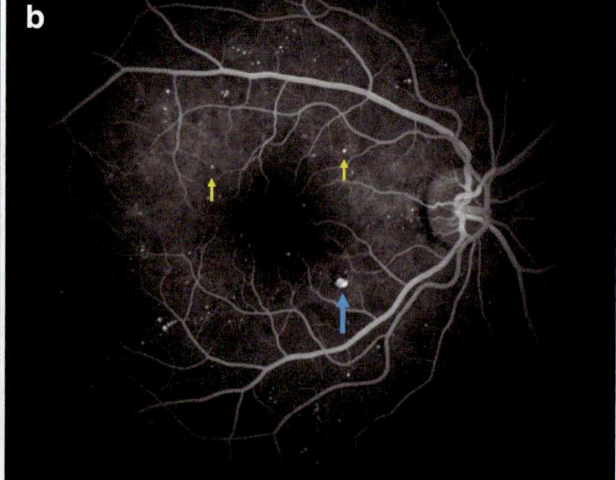

Fig. 2.2 Fundus photograph (**a**) of the same eye (as in Fig. 2.1) after 4 months, with moderate non-proliferative diabetic retinopathy showing microaneurysms (black arrows) and RAM (blue arrow). Fluorescein angiography (**b**) delineates more sharply the microaneurysms (yellow arrows) and RAM (blue arrow)

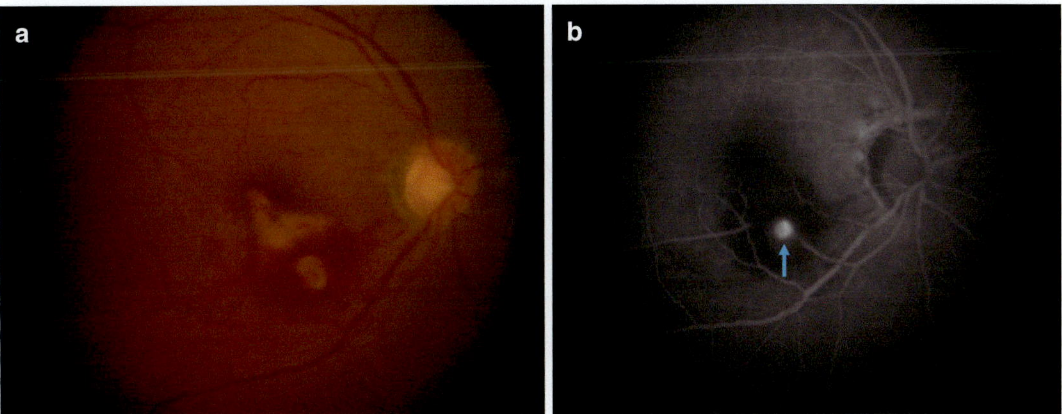

Fig. 2.3 RAM is seen along the lower temporal arcade, causing dense haemorrhage and exudation (**a**), with fundus fluorescein angiography showing the RAM (blue arrow) along the secondary branch of the lower temporal retinal artery (**b**)

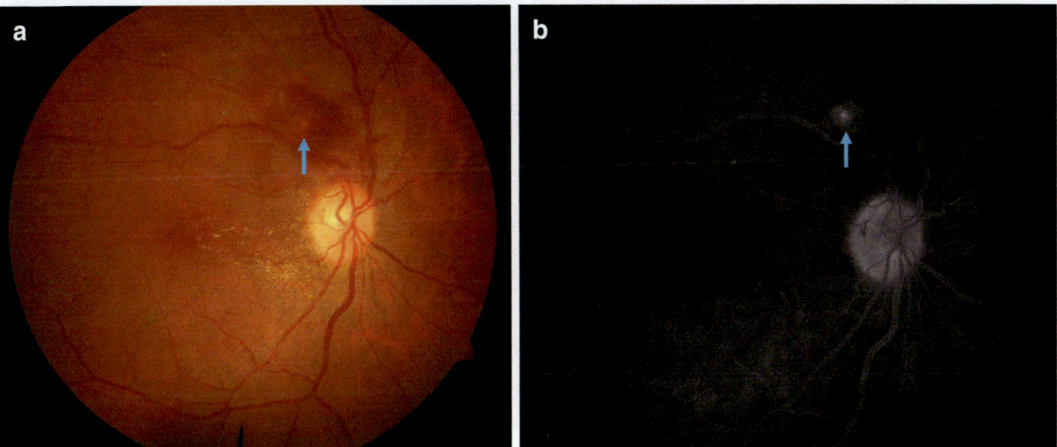

Fig. 2.4 Fundus photograph (**a**) and fluorescein angiogram (**b**) showing the RAM (blue arrow) along the upper temporal retinal artery as it exits the optic disc

Box 2.3 Definition of Hypertension

Hypertension is defined after 2–3 visits at 1–4 weeks intervals depending upon the BP

Hypertension-Clinic recording—SBP ≥ 140 mmHg and/or DBP ≥ 90 mmHg

Hypertension home recording—SBP ≥ 135 mmHg and/or DBP ≥ 85 mmHg

Normal BP—SBP ≤ 130 mmHg and/or DBP ≤ 85 mmHg

Abbreviations: *SBP* systolic blood pressure, *DBP* diastolic blood pressure

Adapted from [8] with permission of the publishers Elsevier Inc.

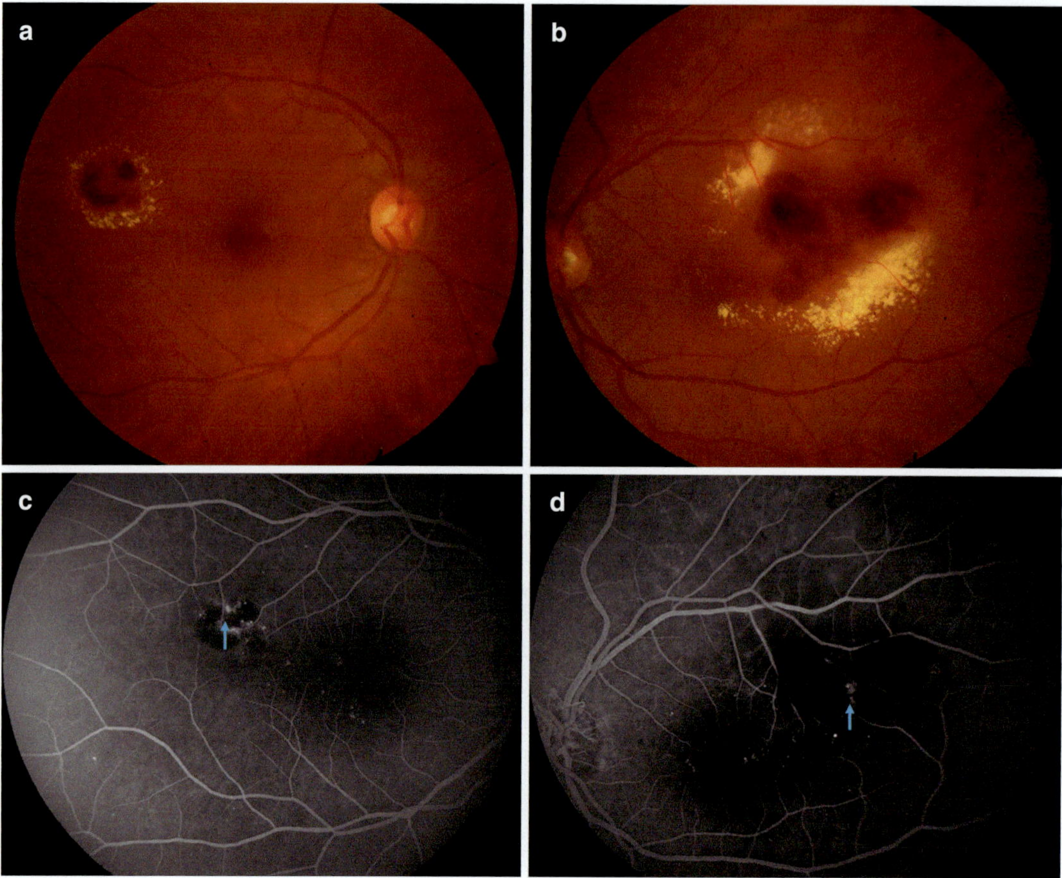

Fig. 2.5 A patient with hypertension presented with RAM in both right (**a**) and left (**b**) eyes. Fluorescein angiography (**c** and **d**) confirmed the location of RAM (blue arrows)

2.3.2 Diabetes Mellitus

Microaneurysms are the hallmark of DR. However, macroaneurysms may also be associated with DR and are termed retinal 'capillary macroaneurysms' [9]. Diabetic capillary macroaneurysms are near the hard exudates, often at the center of the circinate ring (Fig. 2.1). They are also significantly correlated with the severity of diabetic retinopathy [9–11]. Because of their proximity to retinal capillary microaneurysms and similar imaging features in optical coherence tomography (OCT) and indocyanine green angiography, capillary macroaneurysms in DR are thought to originate from microaneurysms. They are likely to be overlooked in eyes with severe diabetic macular edema and should be looked for in all these eyes with fluorescein angiography and OCT [12] (Box 2.4).

Box 2.4 Systemic Workup in Retinal Arterial Macroaneurysm

A. **For atherosclerotic cardiovascular disease (ASCVD)***
   1. Calculate 10-year risk for (ASCVD)
   2. Lp(a) if family history of premature ASCVD
   3. ApoB if S triglycerides are ≥200 mg/dL
   4. Waist circumference and BMI

5. Complete lipid profile including LDL, S cholesterol, and triglycerides
6. Blood sugar level
7. Antiphospholipid antibodies (APLA)
8. C-reactive proteins
9. Ankle-brachial index

*For more detailed information, the readers are advised to read the guidelines on the primary prevention of cardiovascular diseases [13].

B. **For other inflammatory diseases**
   1. Rule out sarcoidosis* if RAM is accompanied by uveitis
      (a) Contrast-enhanced CT chest
      (b) Lymph node histopathology using EBUS
      (c) Complete blood counts (look for anaemia, leukopenia, and lymphopenia)
      (d) Serum markers ACE, lysozyme, soluble Interleukin-2 receptor, S. amyloid A
      (e) S. creatinine
      (f) S alkaline phosphate
      (g) S. calcium or, if possible 24-h urine calcium

*For more detailed information on diagnosing and detecting sarcoidosis, readers are advised to read the American Thoracic Society guidelines [14].

C. If RA and PAN are suspected
   1. Rheumatoid factor
   2. ANCA
   3. CECT abdomen and CT angiography of abdomen
   4. ADA2 gene analysis and ADA2 levels if a monogenic variant of PAN known as DADA2 is suspected

Abbreviations: *ASCVD* Atherosclerotic cardiovascular disease, *Lp(a)* Lipoprotein (a), *ApoB* Apolipoprotein B, *BMI* Body-mass index, *LDL* low-density lipoproteins, *CT* computerized tomography, *EBUS* endoscopic ultrasound bronchoscopy, *ACE* Angiotensin-converting enzyme, *ANCA* Antineutrophil cytoplasmic antibodies, *CECT* contrast-enhanced computerized tomography, *ADA2* adenosine deaminase 2, *PAN* polyarteritis nodosa, *DADA2* deficiency of adenosine deaminase 2

2.3.3 Sarcoidosis and Uveitis

Older women with sarcoidosis, independent of hypertension, may present with RAM in the eye [15]. These patients have other eye inflammation signs, including perivascular candle-wax infiltrates and multifocal choroidal granulomas. Significantly, women with sarcoid RAMs also have a high incidence of cardiovascular disease [15]. It may be noted that RAM is seen in less than 1.5% of patients with uveitis and, if present, is highly suggestive of sarcoidosis. Most RAMs in sarcoidosis are exudative and rarely present with haemorrhage [16]. RAMs in sarcoidosis appear to be related to the formation of sarcoid granuloma in the vessel wall that leads to several changes, including capillary occlusion, duplication of arterioles, irregular focal narrowing, sheathing, segmental beading, comma-shaped kinking, and ectasias that evolve into RAMs [17]. Histopathological studies have shown the presence of epithelioid cell granuloma in the vessel walls and retina of patients presenting with RAM [18, 19]. For more detailed information on diagnosing and detecting sarcoidosis, readers are advised to read the American Thoracic Society guidelines [14].

2.3.3.1 Systemic Arterial Macroaneurysms and Sarcoidosis

Although not directly related to RAM, arterial macroaneurysms have also been described in patients with sarcoidosis's heart, aorta, pulmonary artery, and brain [20–23].

2.3.4 Polyarteritis Nodosa

RAM in the past has led to the diagnosis of periarteritis nodosa (PAN) [24].

2.3.5 Leukaemia

In young people, RAM may occasionally be seen due to leukaemia [25].

2.3.6 Cerebral Macroaneurysms

While most often, the RAMs are solitary, there is a suggestion in the literature that multiple RAMs, if present, may be associated with cerebral macroaneurysms [26]. However, looking at the fundus images of patients previously diagnosed with intracranial macroaneurysms, no such association has been found. Terson's syndrome, a bilateral or less commonly a unilateral vitreous, subhyaloid or retinal haemorrhage is often, apart from head trauma, caused by a subarachnoid haemorrhage due to the rupture of the intracranial aneurysms. None of these patients reported having RAM in their retina [27].

It is unlikely that RAMs in the retina are associated with intracerebral aneurysms.

2.3.7 Other Systemic Associations

While there is a consistent relationship between older women with hypertension, they may also have hypercholesterolaemia, atherosclerotic heart disease, and rheumatoid arthritis [6, 28, 29]. Focal damage to the arterial wall from emboli has been considered in the pathogenesis of RAMs, and patients should be investigated for the source of a possible embolus [30].

2.4 Ocular Associations of RAM

2.4.1 Congenital Retinal Arteriolar Anomalies

Occasionally RAM may be associated with congenital arterio-venous malformations type1 (AVM type1) [31], congenital macrovessels [32], or congenital anomalous retinal artery [33]. High arterial flow rates in these abnormal arteries may lead to RAM formation [34].

2.4.2 Idiopathic Retinal Vasculitis, Aneurysms, and Neuroretinitis (IRVAN) and RAM

The RAMs in IRVAN are multiple and usually located along the major arteries in the posterior pole [35, 36]. They are more commonly seen along the arterial bifurcations and may involve the optic disc also. They may be of various shapes and give the involved artery a 'knot-like' appearance. The RAMs in IRVAN cause extensive exudation due to vessel wall inflammation.

2.4.3 Retinal Vein Occlusion

RAMs are significantly associated with branch retinal vein occlusion in the same quadrant (Fig. 2.6). Although the cause-and-effect relationship is unclear, local factors may play a role [3].

2.4.4 Toxoplasma

The inflammation of the arteriolar wall may contribute to the formation of RAM. Multiple RAMs were reported in a patient with toxoplasmic retinochoroiditis with Kyrieleis arteriolitis [37].

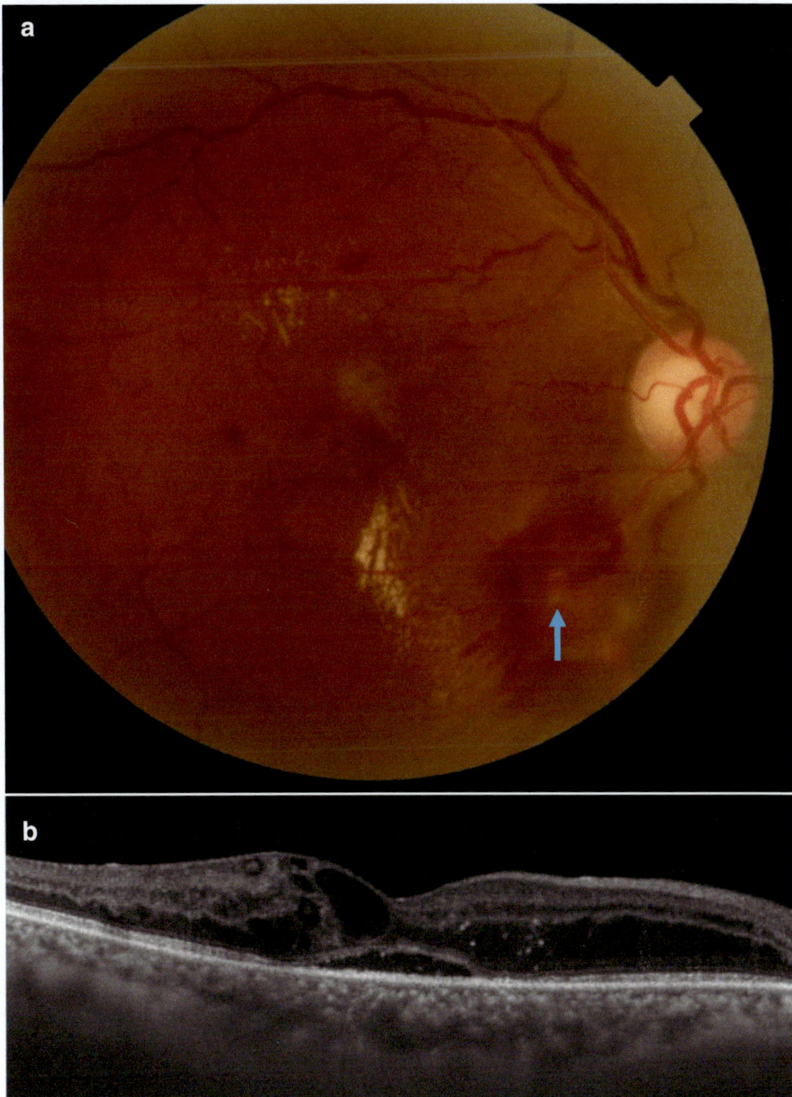

Fig. 2.6 RAM (blue arrow) along the lower temporal mimicking lower temporal branch retinal vein occlusion (**a**). Optical coherence tomography (**b**) shows macular oedema

2.5 Clinical Presentations of RAM

The RAMs are primarily of two types, fusiform and saccular.

2.5.1 Fusiform RAM

Fusiform RAMs often have a halo around them due to the thickening of the wall. These RAMs are more chronic and exudative and lead to the accumulation of perianeurysmal retinal edema and exudates (Fig. 2.7). Exudates may also get deposited in the macula. Fluid leaks diffuse from the RAMs. The fluid leaking from the RAMs at the AV crossing may flow along the perivenous tunnel before diffusing into the retina [38].

2.5.2 Saccular RAM

The saccular forms are more acute and likely to present as intraocular haemorrhages (Fig. 2.8). Depending upon the rupture site, subhyaloid haemorrhage arises from the anterior wall of the

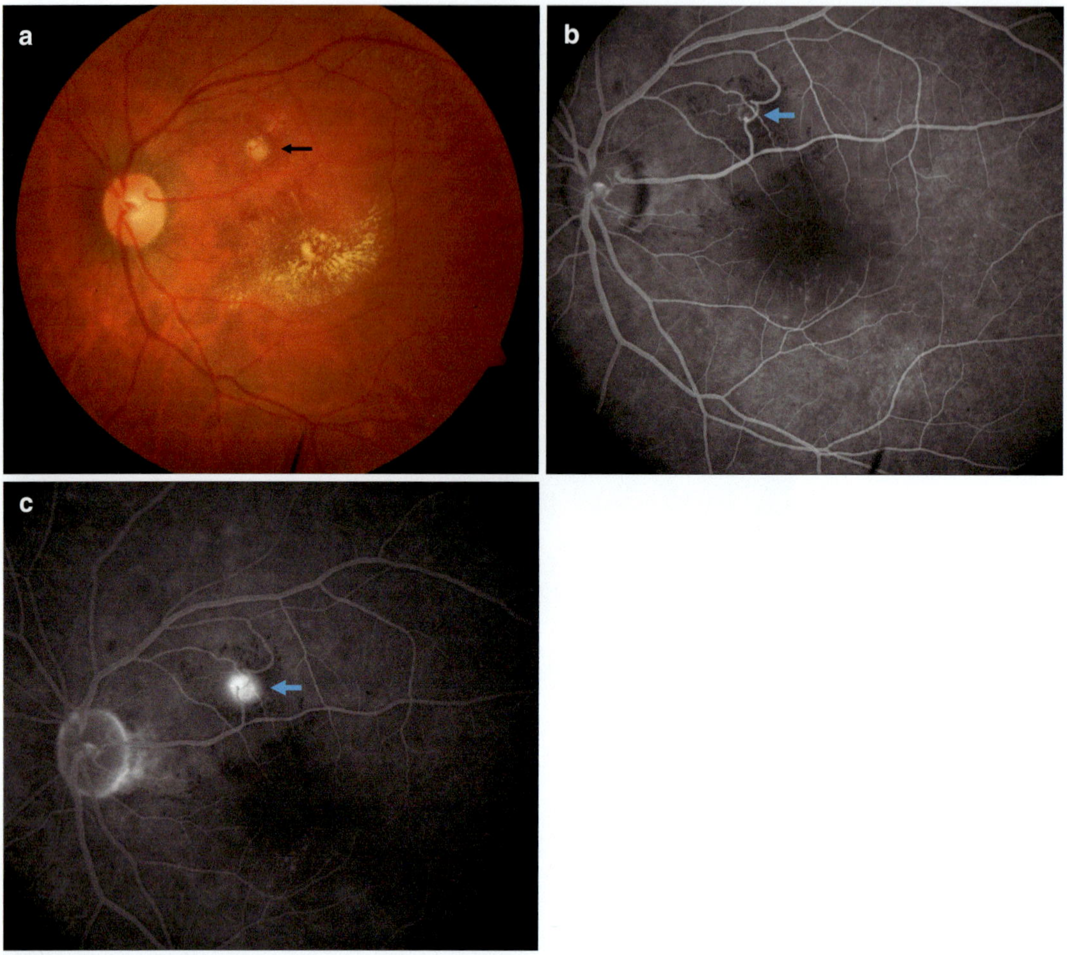

Fig. 2.7 The 'fusiform' type of RAM is more chronic, has a halo around it (black arrow), and causes retinal edema and exudation (**a**). Fluorescein angiography shows the aneurysmal dilatation (blue arrow) along the arteriolar wall in the early phase (**b**) and filling of RAM (blue arrow) in the late phase (**c**)

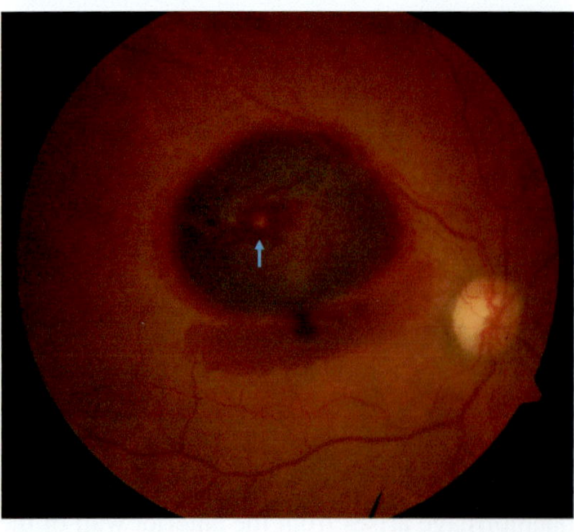

Fig. 2.8 The 'saccular' form of RAM (blue arrow) presenting with a sudden intraocular haemorrhage

aneurysm's thin, stretched wall. Posterior rupture may lead to intraretinal or subretinal haemorrhage [28]. Saccular RAM may show subtle or clinically apparent pulsations during the cardiac cycle when present on the optic disc. SD-OCT may show internal hyporeflectivity, which becomes hyperreflective as it gets thrombosed [7, 39]. It is noted that the bursting of the optic disc macroaneurysm is often associated with branch retinal artery occlusion [40]. Near-infrared reflectance imaging may reveal a circumferential halo around the arteriole years before the actual development of the RAM at that site [41, 42]. Optic disc macroaneurysms undergo spontaneous thrombosis with or without complications [43].

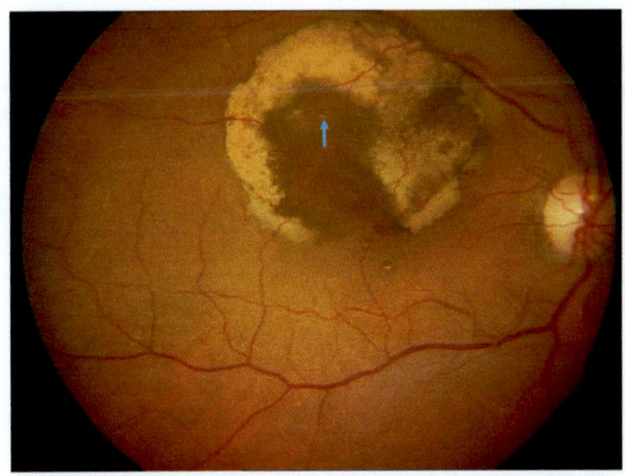

Fig. 2.9 Fundus photograph of the same patient (as in Fig. 2.8) taken 2 months later, showing spontaneous closure of the RAM (blue arrow), with resolving residual subretinal haemorrhage

Intraocular haemorrhages present in the vitreous, preretinal, intraretinal, or subretinal spaces are often caused by RAMs. The ruptured RAMs show spontaneous closure and often leave a Z-shaped kink in the arterial wall as a sequela (Fig. 2.9). Later in life, such aneurysms may go unrecognized [28, 43].

2.5.3 Retinal Capillary Macroaneurysms

Unassociated with either diabetes mellitus or retinal vascular disease, solitary persistent macroaneurysms have been associated with capillaries much larger than the typical microaneurysms seen in the abovementioned diseases. These increase over time and expand, become leaky and develop exudates or haemorrhages [44]. These capillary macroaneurysms are sensitive to anti-VEGF agents. Age-related large microaneurysms have increased expression of matrix-metalloproteinase (MMP)-9, which is responsible for the degradation of the capillary basement membrane, and the increased expression of plasminogen activator inhibitor promotes microthrombi formation in the microaneurysms [45]. It has been proposed that a similar mechanism may be at work to produce isolated large macroaneurysms [44].

2.6 Imaging of RAM

The most common angiography tool for the evaluation of retinal pathology, the fundus fluorescein angiography, may not reveal the presence of a RAM if it is covered by a thick layer of haemorrhage (Fig. 2.10) [46]. RAM fills early during the arterial phase of the angiogram. Nearly 90% of the RAMs show dye flow in the arteriole beyond the RAM [47]. Compared to the blue light in the FFA, the infrared light in indocyanine green angiography/videography has better penetration through the haemorrhage (Fig. 2.11). It can demonstrate the pulsatile nature and contiguity of RAM to the retinal arterioles [48]. The SD-OCT shows a hyperreflective wall of the RAM and a hyporeflective lumen. OCT can be used to monitor the RAM for the development of thrombosis seen as homogenous hyperreflectivity of the lumen [49]. On SD-OCT, the initial hyporeflectivity of the lumen becomes hyperreflective as it gets thrombosed [37]. As the RAM involutes, reduced blood flow can be demonstrated using a laser speckle flowgraph [50].

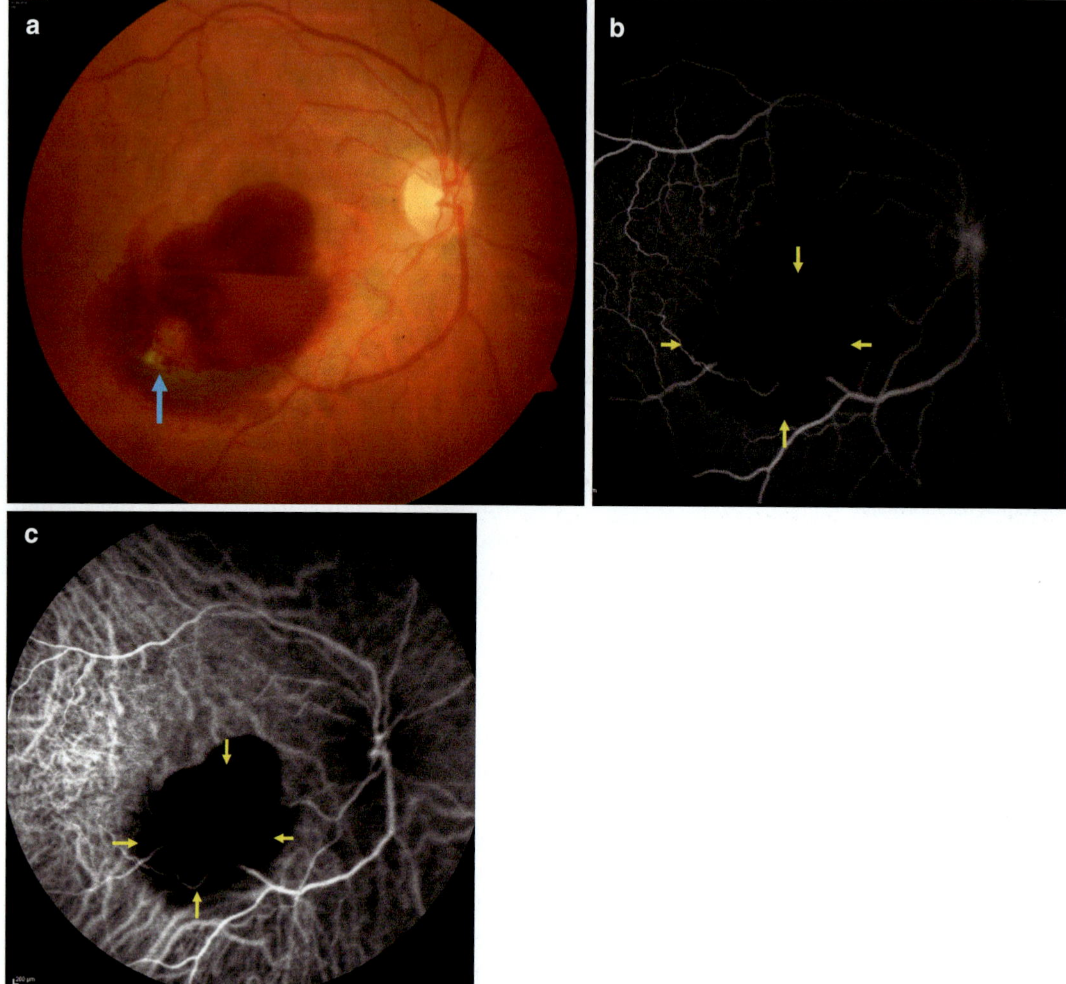

Fig. 2.10 RAM (blue arrow) in a female with hypertension, presenting with massive preretinal, intraretinal and subretinal haemorrhage (**a**), which is not visible in the early phase of fluorescein angiography (**b**) and indocyanine green angiography (**c**) due to dense haemorrhage. A large area of blocked fluorescence (yellow arrows) is seen due to dense retinal haemorrhage

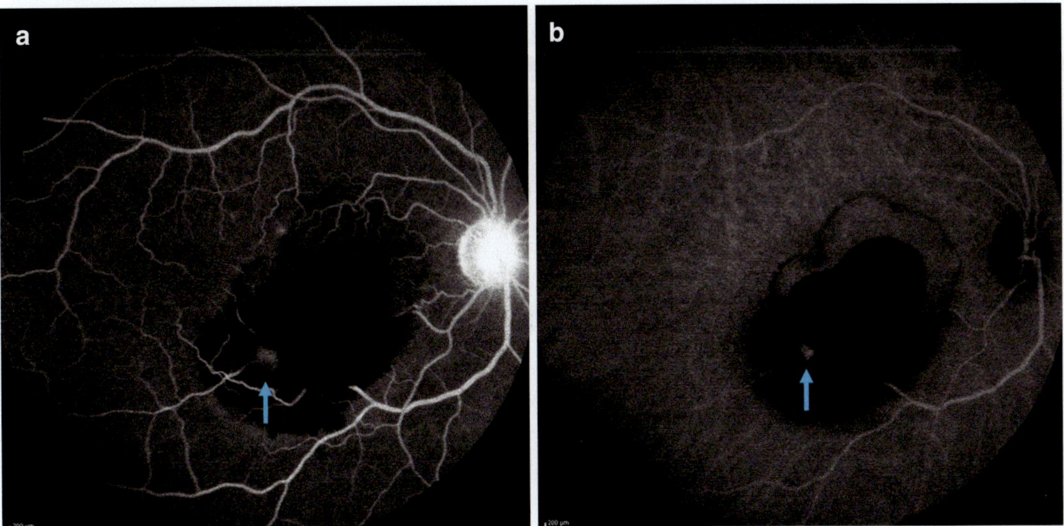

Fig. 2.11 Fluorescein angiography (**a**) and indocyanine green angiography (**b**) of the same patient (as in Fig. 2.10), demonstrating RAM (blue arrow) in the late phase

2.7 Treatment of RAM

Most RAMs, especially haemorrhagic RAMs, undergo spontaneous involution (Fig. 2.12) [3]. If the visual acuity does not improve even after the resolution of the RAM, it may be due to persistent hard exudates or subfoveal haemorrhage in the macula [51].

Significant vitreous haemorrhage, if present, may require pars plana vitreous surgery (PPV) for its clearance. Patients with subretinal haemorrhage may require displacement of blood by injection of tPA and gas tamponade with PPV (Figs. 2.13 and 2.14) [52]. Significant visual improvement has been noted following laser photocoagulation of haemorrhagic RAMs, although no difference was noted in the visual improvement in those observed or laser-treated exudative RAMs [53]. However, exudative RAMs treated with laser photocoagulation carry the risk of branch retinal artery occlusion. In recent years, intravitreal injections of anti-VEGF agents have been used successfully to treat RAMs [54–56]. These agents decrease fluid leakage and exudates from the RAM and faster vision improvement. Instead of the conventional laser, navigated laser photocoagulation may provide a safer approach [57]. However, these strategies only buy time till there is a spontaneous thrombosis in the RAM.

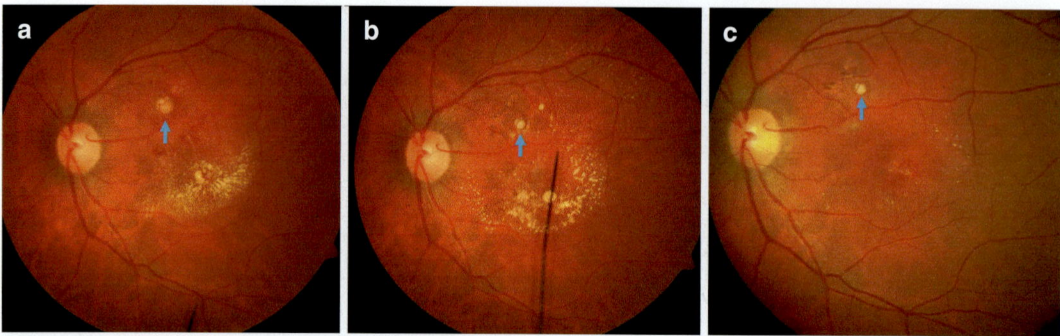

Fig. 2.12 RAM (blue arrow) in the same patient (as in Fig. 2.7) at initial presentation (**a**), showing spontaneous involution at 3 months of follow-up (**b**) and 10 months later (**c**), with a subsequent decrease in retinal oedema and exudation

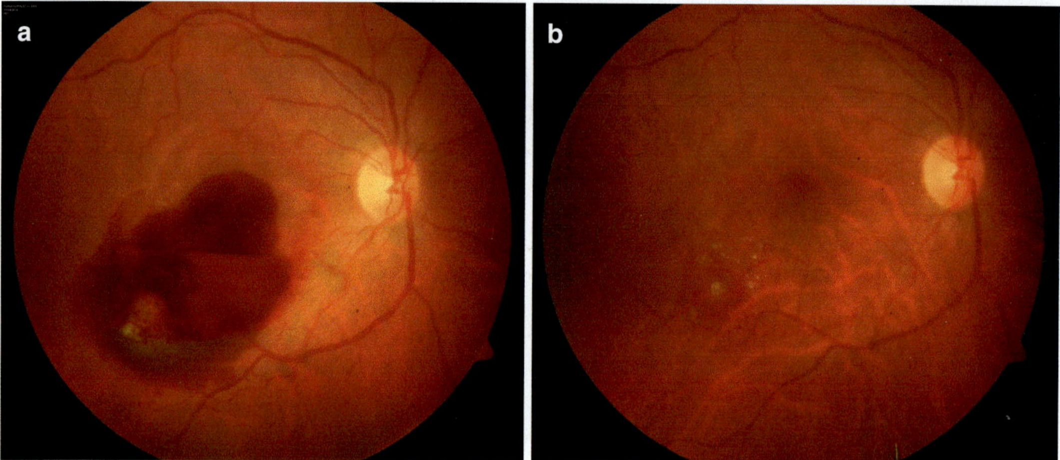

Fig. 2.13 Massive preretinal, intraretinal and subretinal haemorrhage due to RAM in a female (same as in Fig. 2.10) at presentation (**a**), showing resolution after surgical intervention by vitrectomy with tPA injection and intraocular gas tamponade (**b**)

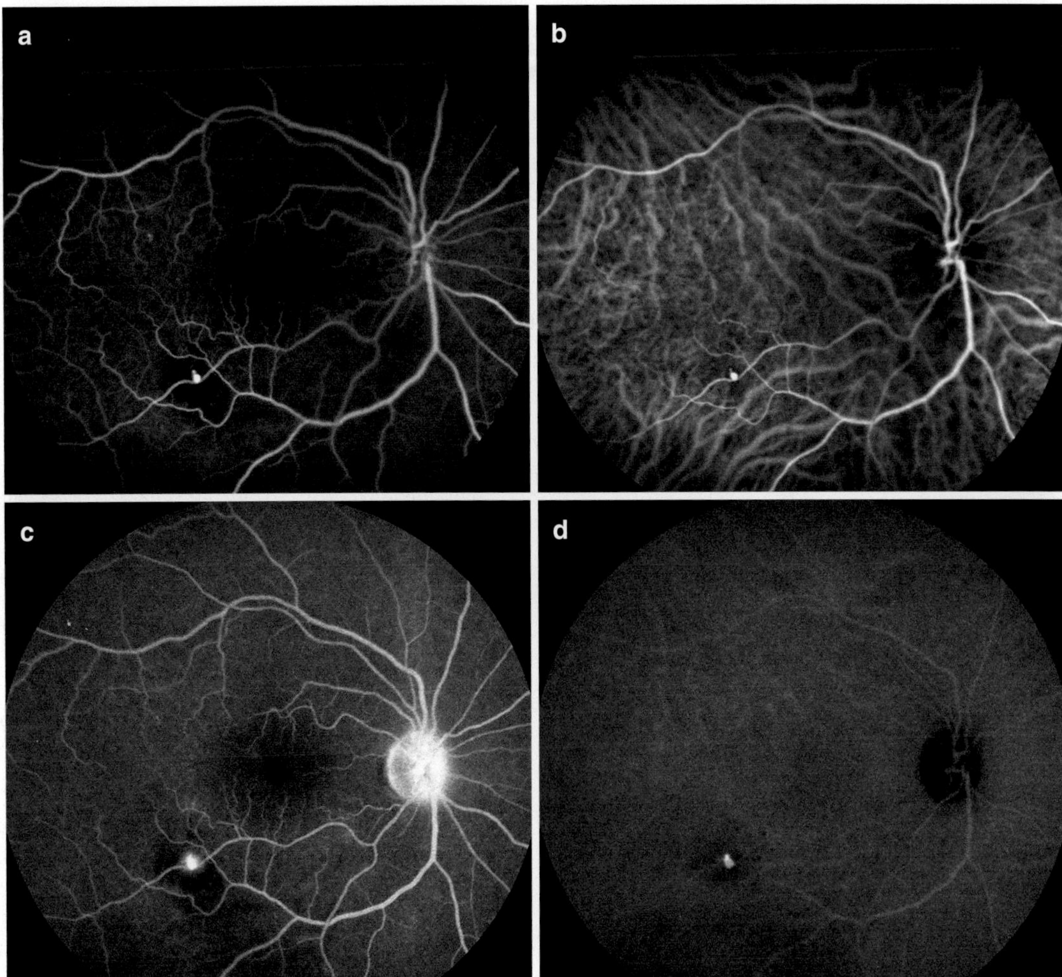

Fig. 2.14 Following surgical treatment in the patient, as in Fig. 2.13, the RAM was seen in the 'Early' phase fluorescein angiography (**a**) and indocyanine green angiography (**b**), as well as in the 'late' phase fluorescein angiography (**c**) and indocyanine green angiography (**d**)

2.8 Pathology of RAM

There are very few pathological studies of RAM. Longstanding RAMs show fibrous encapsulation, lipid-filled macrophages, cholesterol clefts, and hemosiderin. The corresponding vein shows infiltration with inflammatory cells. In the beginning, the wall of RAM stains with Periodic acid-Schiff (PAS) indicative of hyalinization and fibrin deposit in the wall, which splits, followed by outpouching and leakage of RBC and lipids. There are areas of capillary non-perfusion and dilated capillaries near the RAM. Often thrombus is found in the resolved RAM. It is a long-held belief that the retinal arterioles do not have internal elastic lamina except for the central retinal artery. Thus, finding fragments that stain for elastic lamina [58] or finding only a break in the well-formed internal elastic lamina of a RAM [59] cannot be easily explained.

2.9 RAM Versus Intracerebral Arterial Microaneurysms

Ever since intracerebral haemorrhage was ascribed to miliary aneurysms of the brain, the pathogenesis of intracerebral haemorrhage has remained controversial for nearly 150 years [60]. Using a postmortem brain imaging technique first described by [61], Cole and Yates [62] described intracerebral arterial microaneurysms by X-raying 5 mm thick coronal slices after perfusing the arteries of the freshly removed brains with a barium-gelatin radiopaque dye. They found fusiform and saccular arterial microaneurysms varying from 50 to 2000 μm in 46% of the hypertensive patients and only 7% of the gender and age-matched normotensives. Like the RAMs seen in the eye, most of these aneurysms were seen in ages 65–74. Of the 20 brains seen with massive intracerebral haemorrhage, 18 had associated intracerebral arterial aneurysms, most of which were in the brains of hypertensive patients [62]. Whereas the RAMs in the eye are clearly shown to result in either exudation or intraocular haemorrhage, the question remains whether similar aneurysms seen in the brain are incidental.

References

1. Xu L, Wang Y, Jonas JB. Frequency of retinal macroaneurysms in adult Chinese: the Beijing Eye Study. Br J Ophthalmol. 2007;91(6):840–1. https://doi.org/10.1136/bjo.2006.107342. PMID: 17510482; PMCID: PMC1955572.
2. Nangia V, Jonas JB, Khare A, Sinha A, Lambat S. Prevalence of retinal macroaneurysms. The Central India Eye and Medical Study. Acta Ophthalmol. 2013;91(2):e166–7. https://doi.org/10.1111/j.1755--3768.2012.02465.x. Epub 2012 Jun 13. PMID: 22690702.
3. Panton RW, Goldberg MF, Farber MD. Retinal arterial macroaneurysms: risk factors and natural history. Br J Ophthalmol. 1990;74(10):595–600. https://doi.org/10.1136/bjo.74.10.595. PMID: 2285682; PMCID: PMC1042226.
4. Raehlmann E. Ophthalmoscopically visible disease of the retinal vessels during general arterial sclerosis, with special consideration of cerebral vessel sclerosis. Z Klin Med. 1889;16:606.
5. Pringle JA. A case of multiple aneurisms of the retinal arteries (with coloured plate). Br J Ophthalmol. 1917;1(2):87–92. https://doi.org/10.1136/bjo.1.2.87. PMID: 18167657; PMCID: PMC513271.
6. Moosavi RA, Fong KC, Chopdar A. Retinal artery macroaneurysms: clinical and fluorescein angiographic features in 34 patients. Eye (Lond). 2006;20(9):1011–20. https://doi.org/10.1038/sj.eye.6702068. Epub 2005 Sep 2. PMID: 16138114.
7. Yang JF, Kishore K. Recurrent vitreous hemorrhage from an optic nerve retinal arterial macroaneurysm. Case Rep Ophthalmol. 2017;8(3):503–9. https://doi.org/10.1159/000481704. PMID: 29282401; PMCID: PMC5731140.
8. Verdecchia P, Reboldi G, Angeli F. The 2020 International Society of Hypertension global hypertension practice guidelines—key messages and clinical considerations. Eur J Intern Med. 2020;82:1–6. https://doi.org/10.1016/j.ejim.2020.09.001. Epub 2020 Sep 22. PMID: 32972800.
9. Bourhis A, Girmens JF, Boni S, Pecha F, Favard C, Sahel JA, Paques M. Imaging of macroaneurysms occurring during retinal vein occlusion and diabetic retinopathy by indocyanine green angiography and high resolution optical coherence tomography. Graefes Arch Clin Exp Ophthalmol. 2010;248(2):161–6. https://doi.org/10.1007/s00417-009-1175-6. Epub 2009 Aug 25. PMID: 19701812.
10. Castro Farías D, Matsui Serrano R, Bianchi Gancharov J, de Dios CU, Sahel J, Graue Wiechers F, Dupas B, Paques M. Indocyanine green angiography for identifying telangiectatic capillaries in diabetic macular oedema. Br J Ophthalmol. 2020;104(4):509–13. https://doi.org/10.1136/bjophthalmol-2019-314355. Epub 2019 Jul 29. PMID: 31358497.
11. Paques M, Philippakis E, Bonnet C, Falah S, Ayello-Scheer S, Zwillinger S, Girmens JF, Dupas B. Indocyanine-green-guided targeted laser photocoagulation of capillary macroaneurysms in macular oedema: a pilot study. Br J Ophthalmol. 2017;101(2):170–4. https://doi.org/10.1136/bjophthalmol-2015-308142. Epub 2016 Jun 6. PMID: 27267449.
12. Karti O, Ipek SC, Saatci AO. Multimodal imaging characteristics of a large retinal capillary macroaneurysm in an eye with severe diabetic macular edema: a case presentation and literature review. Med Hypothesis Discov Innov Ophthalmol. 2020;9(1):33–7. Epub 2020 Jan 1. PMID: 31976341; PMCID: PMC6969556.
13. Arnett DK, Blumenthal RS, Albert MA, Buroker AB, Goldberger ZD, Hahn EJ, Himmelfarb CD, Khera A, Lloyd-Jones D, McEvoy JW, Michos ED, Miedema MD, Muñoz D, Smith SC Jr, Virani SS, Williams KA Sr, Yeboah J, Ziaeian B. 2019 ACC/AHA guideline on the primary prevention of cardiovascular disease: a report of the American College of Cardiology/American Heart Association task force on clinical practice guidelines. Circulation. 2019;140(11):e596–646.

https://doi.org/10.1161/CIR.0000000000000678. Epub 2019 Mar 17. Erratum in: Circulation. 2019 Sep 10;140(11):e649–e650. Erratum in: Circulation. 2020 Jan 28;141(4):e60. Erratum in: Circulation. 2020 Apr 21;141(16):e774. PMID: 30879355; PMCID: PMC7734661.

14. Crouser ED, Maier LA, Wilson KC, Bonham CA, Morgenthau AS, Patterson KC, Abston E, Bernstein RC, Blankstein R, Chen ES, Culver DA, Drake W, Drent M, Gerke AK, Ghobrial M, Govender P, Hamzeh N, James WE, Judson MA, Kellermeyer L, Knight S, Koth LL, Poletti V, Raman SV, Tukey MH, Westney GE, Baughman RP. Diagnosis and detection of sarcoidosis. An official American Thoracic Society clinical practice guideline. Am J Respir Crit Care Med. 2020;201(8):e26–51. https://doi.org/10.1164/rccm.202002-0251ST. PMID: 32293205; PMCID: PMC7159433.
15. Rothova A, Lardenoye C. Arterial macroaneurysms in peripheral multifocal chorioretinitis associated with sarcoidosis. Ophthalmology. 1998;105(8):1393–7. https://doi.org/10.1016/S0161-6420(98)98018-6. PMID: 9709748.
16. Yamanaka E, Ohguro N, Kubota A, Yamamoto S, Nakagawa Y, Tano Y. Features of retinal arterial macroaneurysms in patients with uveitis. Br J Ophthalmol. 2004;88(7):884–6. https://doi.org/10.1136/bjo.2003.035923. PMID: 15205230; PMCID: PMC1772231.
17. Verougstraete C, Snyers B, Leys A, Caspers-Velu LE. Multiple arterial ectasias in patients with sarcoidosis and uveitis. Am J Ophthalmol. 2001;131(2):223–31. https://doi.org/10.1016/s0002-9394(00)00786-8. PMID: 11228299.
18. Gass JD, Olson CL. Sarcoidosis with optic nerve and retinal involvement. Arch Ophthalmol. 1976;94(6):945–50. https://doi.org/10.1001/archopht.1976.03910030475008. PMID: 938285.
19. Palmer HE, Stanford MR, McCartney AC, Graham EM. Non-caseating granulomas as a cause of ischaemic retinal vasculitis. Br J Ophthalmol. 1997;81(11):1018–9. https://doi.org/10.1136/bjo.81.11.1016c. PMID: 9505832; PMCID: PMC1722047.
20. Gedalia A, Shetty AK, Ward K, Correa H, Venters CL, Loe WA. Abdominal aortic aneurysm associated with childhood sarcoidosis. J Rheumatol. 1996;23(4):757–9. PMID: 8730140.
21. Gerloni R, Merlo M, Vitrella G, Lardieri G, Pinamonti B, Pappalardo A, Cattin L, Sinagra G. Pulmonary artery aneurysm and sarcoidosis. J Cardiovasc Med (Hagerstown). 2015;16 Suppl 2:S77–8. https://doi.org/10.2459/JCM.0b013e328365a04f. PMID: 25635751.
22. Nielsen-Kudsk JE. Ventrikelflimren og kardiale aneurysmer forårsaget af sarkoidose [Ventricular fibrillation and cardiac aneurysms caused by Sarcoidosis]. Ugeskr Laeger. 1993;155(41):3299–301. Danish. PMID: 8256325.
23. Russegger L, Weiser G, Twerdy K, Grunert V. Neurosarcoid reaction in association with a ruptured ACA-aneurysm. Neurochirurgia (Stuttg). 1986;29(1):42–4. https://doi.org/10.1055/s--2008-1053697. PMID: 3960255.
24. Goldsmith J. Periarteritis nodosa with involvement of the choroidal and retinal arteries. Am J Ophthalmol. 1946;29:435–46. https://doi.org/10.1016/0002-9394(46)90526-0. PMID: 21019949.
25. Bekmez S, Eris D. Retinal arterial macroaneurysm in leukemia. Eur J Ophthalmol. 2022;32(4):NP22–5. https://doi.org/10.1177/1120672121993781. Epub 2021 Feb 8. PMID: 33550829.
26. Nalcaci S, Oztas Z, Eraslan C, Akkin C. Are multiple retinal arterial macroaneurysms considered a sign of cerebral aneurysms? Ophthalmic Surg Lasers Imaging Retina. 2017;48(1):79–82. https://doi.org/10.3928/23258160-20161219-12. PMID: 28060399.
27. Stiebel-Kalish H, Turtel LS, Kupersmith MJ. The natural history of nontraumatic subarachnoid hemorrhage-related intraocular hemorrhages. Retina. 2004;24(1):36–40. https://doi.org/10.1097/00006982-200402000-00006. PMID: 15076942.
28. Abdel-Khalek MN, Richardson J. Retinal macroaneurysm: natural history and guidelines for treatment. Br J Ophthalmol. 1986;70(1):2–11. https://doi.org/10.1136/bjo.70.1.2. PMID: 3947596; PMCID: PMC1040895.
29. Ng RJ, Bae S. Retinal artery macroaneurysm without hypertension. Clin Exp Optom. 2021;104(2):250–2. https://doi.org/10.1111/cxo.13098. PMID: 32449215.
30. Lewis RA, Norton EW, Gass JD. Acquired arterial macroaneurysms of the retina. Br J Ophthalmol. 1976;60(1):21–30. https://doi.org/10.1136/bjo.60.1.21. PMID: 1268157; PMCID: PMC1017462.
31. Noble CW, Di Nicola M, Hermanson ME, Williams BK Jr. Retinal arterial macroaneurysm in the setting of type 1 arteriovenous malformation. Retina. 2021;41(2):e15–6. https://doi.org/10.1097/IAE.0000000000003024. PMID: 33323901.
32. Sebrow DB, Cunha de Souza E, Belúcio Neto J, Roizenblatt M, Zett Lobos C, Paulo Bonomo P, Modi Y, Schuman JS, Freund KB. Macroaneurysms associated with congenital retinal macrovessels. Retin Cases Brief Rep. 2020;14(1):61–5. https://doi.org/10.1097/ICB.0000000000000619. PMID: 28799971; PMCID: PMC5807243.
33. Musadiq M, Gibson JM. Spontaneously resolved macroaneurysm associated with a congenital anomalous retinal artery. Retin Cases Brief Rep. 2010;4(1):70–2. https://doi.org/10.1097/ICB.0b013e318196b2c8. PMID: 25390126.
34. Ichibe M, Oya Y, Yoshizawa T, Abe H. Macroaneurysm on the optic disk associated with congenital retinal arterial malformation. Retina. 2004;24(6):985–6. https://doi.org/10.1097/00006982-200412000-00029. PMID: 15580007.

35. Ali Khan H, Ali Khan Q, Shahzad MA, Awan MA, Khan N, Jahangir S, Shaheen F, Wali K, Rodman J, Pizzimenti J, Saatci AO. Comprehensive overview of IRVAN syndrome: a structured review of case reports and case series. Ther Adv Ophthalmol. 2022;14:25158414211070880. https://doi.org/10.1177/25158414211070880. PMID: 35282003; PMCID: PMC8905214.
36. Tripathy K. Pathogenesis of idiopathic retinal vasculitis, aneurysms, and neuroretinitis (IRVAN) or 'idiopathic retinal arteriolar aneurysms (IRAA)' with macular star. Med Hypotheses. 2018;112:65–6. https://doi.org/10.1016/j.mehy.2018.01.016. PMID: 29447942.
37. Huang N, Lee WA, Rivera S, Montezuma SR. Ruptured retinal arterial macroaneurysm secondary to toxoplasmic Kyrieleis arteriolitis: a case report. Case Rep Ophthalmol. 2017;8(2):390–5. https://doi.org/10.1159/000478720. PMID: 28924434; PMCID: PMC5597918.
38. Munch IC, Li XQ, Hansen LH, Larsen M. Retinal macroaneurysm leaking fluid at 0.0018 μl/min through a perivenous tunnel. Acta Ophthalmol. 2012;90(3):e240–2. https://doi.org/10.1111/j.1755--3768.2011.02220.x. Epub 2011 Aug 11. PMID: 21834926.
39. Ozgonul C, Besirli CG. Arterial macroaneurysm of the optic disc. Am J Ophthalmol Case Rep. 2018;10:279–81. https://doi.org/10.1016/j.ajoc.2018.04.001. PMID: 29780952; PMCID: PMC5956723.
40. Mitamura Y, Miyano N, Suzuki Y, Ohtsuka K. Branch retinal artery occlusion associated with rupture of retinal arteriolar macroaneurysm on the optic disc. Jpn J Ophthalmol. 2005;49(5):428–9. https://doi.org/10.1007/s10384-004-0219-z. PMID: 16187050.
41. Das-Bhaumik RG, Lindfield D, Quinn SM, Charles SJ. Optic disc macroaneurysm in evolution: from incidental finding to branch retinal artery occlusion and spontaneous resolution. Br J Ophthalmol. 2011;95(1):145–6, 155. PMID: 21427799. https://doi.org/10.1136/bjo.2008.151928.
42. Zienkiewicz A, Francone A, Cirillo MP, Zompa T, Charles M. Near-infrared reflectance imaging to detect an incipient retinal arterial macroaneurysm. Case Rep Ophthalmol. 2021;12(1):150–3. https://doi.org/10.1159/000513344. PMID: 33976673; PMCID: PMC8077541.
43. Rahimy E, Doyle BC, Brown GC. Ruptured retinal arterial macroaneurysm on the optic disk. Retin Cases Brief Rep. 2017;11(1):12–4. https://doi.org/10.1097/ICB.0000000000000275. PMID: 26829446.
44. Spaide RF, Barquet LA. Retinal capillary macroaneurysms. Retina. 2019;39(10):1889–95. https://doi.org/10.1097/IAE.0000000000002406. PMID: 30489449.
45. López-Luppo M, Nacher V, Ramos D, Catita J, Navarro M, Carretero A, Rodriguez-Baeza A, Mendes-Jorge L, Ruberte J. Blood vessel basement membrane alterations in human retinal microaneurysms during aging. Invest Ophthalmol Vis Sci. 2017;58(2):1116–31. https://doi.org/10.1167/iovs.16-19998. PMID: 28196225.
46. Chew EY. Acquired retinal macroaneurysms. In: Sadda SR, Sarraf D, Freund KB, Schachat AP, Wilkinson CP, Wiedemann P, editors. Ryan's retina. 7th ed. Amsterdam: Elsevier; 2022. p. 1172–6.
47. Hughes EL, Dooley IJ, Kennelly KP, Doyle F, Siah WF, Connell P. Angiographic features and disease outcomes of symptomatic retinal arterial macroaneurysms. Graefes Arch Clin Exp Ophthalmol. 2016;254(11):2203–7. https://doi.org/10.1007/s00417-016-3388-9. Epub 2016 May 25. PMID: 27221656.
48. Schneider U, Wagner AL, Kreissig I. Indocyanine green videoangiography of hemorrhagic retinal arterial macroaneurysms. Ophthalmologica. 1997;211(2):115–8. https://doi.org/10.1159/000310775. PMID: 9097320.
49. Lee EK, Woo SJ, Ahn J, Park KH. Morphologic characteristics of retinal arterial macroaneurysm and its regression pattern on spectral-domain optical coherence tomography. Retina. 2011;31(10):2095–101. https://doi.org/10.1097/IAE.0b013e3182111711. PMID: 21716167.
50. Hanazaki H, Yokota H, Aso H, Yamagami S, Nagaoka T. Evaluation of ocular blood flow over time in a treated retinal arterial macroaneurysm using laser speckle flowgraphy. Am J Ophthalmol Case Rep. 2021;21:101022. https://doi.org/10.1016/j.ajoc.2021.101022. PMID: 33598588; PMCID: PMC7868799.
51. Pitkänen L, Tommila P, Kaarniranta K, Jääskeläinen JE, Kinnunen K. Retinal arterial macroaneurysms. Acta Ophthalmol. 2014;92(2):101–4. https://doi.org/10.1111/aos.12210. Epub 2013 Jun 25. PMID: 23800325.
52. Koinzer S, Heckmann J, Tode J, Roider J. Long-term, therapy-related visual outcome of 49 cases with retinal arterial macroaneurysm: a case series and literature review. Br J Ophthalmol. 2015;99(10):1345–53. https://doi.org/10.1136/bjophthalmol-2014-305884. Epub 2015 Apr 16. PMID: 25883085.
53. Meyer JC, Ahmad BU, Blinder KJ, Shah GK. Laser therapy versus observation for symptomatic retinal artery macroaneurysms. Graefes Arch Clin Exp Ophthalmol. 2015;253(4):537–41. https://doi.org/10.1007/s00417-014-2730-3. Epub 2014 Jul 13. PMID: 25016479.
54. Kishore K. Long-term management of complications of retinal artery macroaneurysms with intravitreal Aflibercept injection. Case Rep Ophthalmol. 2016;7(3):162–71. https://doi.org/10.1159/000449122. PMID: 27790133; PMCID: PMC5075728.
55. Leung EH, Reddy AK, Vedula AS, Flynn HW Jr. Serial bevacizumab injections and laser photocoagulation for macular edema associated with a retinal artery macroaneurysm. Clin Ophthalmol. 2015;9:601–9. https://doi.org/10.2147/OPTH.S80504. PMID: 25897199; PMCID: PMC4396452.

56. Mansour AM, Foster RE, Gallego-Pinazo R, Moschos MM, Sisk RA, Chhablani J, Rojanaporn D, Sujirakul T, Arevalo JF, Lima LH, Wu L, Charbaji A, Saatci AO, Mansour HA, Martinez-Rubio C, Patel Y, Gangakhedkar S. Intravitreal anti-vascular endothelial growth factor injections for exudative retinal arterial macroaneurysms. Retina. 2019;39(6):1133–41. https://doi.org/10.1097/IAE.0000000000002131. PMID: 29505440.
57. Maltsev DS, Kulikov AN, Uplanchiwar B, Lima LH, Chhablani J. Direct navigated laser photocoagulation as primary treatment for retinal arterial macroaneurysms. Int J Retina Vitreous. 2018;4:28. https://doi.org/10.1186/s40942-018-0133-z. PMID: 30151240; PMCID: PMC6104015.
58. Fichte C, Streeten BW, Friedman AH. A histopathologic study of retinal arterial aneurysms. Am J Ophthalmol. 1978;85(4):509–18. https://doi.org/10.1016/s0002-9394(14)75249-3. PMID: 655232.
59. Gold DH, La Piana F, Zimmerman LE. Isolated retinal arterial aneurysms. Am J Ophthalmol. 1976;82(6):848–57. https://doi.org/10.1016/0002-9394(76)90060-x. PMID: 998701.
60. Wijdicks EFM. Charcot-Bouchard dilatations (Anevrysmes Miliaire) and the search for the cause of cerebral hemorrhage. Neurocrit Care. 2021;34(3):1090–3. https://doi.org/10.1007/s12028-020-00924-4. PMID: 31981024.
61. Rossrussell RW. Observations on intracerebral aneurysms. Brain. 1963;86:425–42. https://doi.org/10.1093/brain/86.3.425. PMID: 14063893.
62. Cole FM, Yates PO. The occurrence and significance of intracerebral micro-aneurysms. J Pathol Bacteriol. 1967;93(2):393–411. https://doi.org/10.1002/path.1700930202. PMID: 6054051.

3 Retinal Cotton Wool Spots

3.1 Introduction

Of all the intraocular signs, the presence of cotton wool spots (CWS) is one of the most significant, as even a single such spot indicates an underlying systemic disease with serious import. Cotton wool spots are dull, greyish-white swelling of the usually transparent retinal nerve fibres (RNFs). The CWS are variable in number and oval in shape; they are about one-third disc in size (varying from 0.1 to 0.8) and have highly characteristic, somewhat fuzzy/feathery borders (Figs. 3.1 and 3.2). These are most often clustered around the optic disc. It is due to the anoxic insult to peripapillary RNF by the closure of the radial capillary plexus. Retinal nerve fibres (RNF) are the axons of the retinal ganglion cells and converge from all parts of the retina to the optic nerve head, from where they exit to form the optic nerve carrying visual impulses from the eye to the brain. As these fibres converge from the optic disc, they are several layers thick in the post pole and around the optic disc. Thus, acquired opacification and swelling of the RNF are most prominent in this area. Cotton wool spots last for 4–6 weeks and disappear, returning the transparency of the affected retina (Fig. 3.3). The RNFs, if dead, are replaced by a glial scar. In the past, CWS have also been called the soft exudates to contrast them from the more common 'hard exudates', which arise from lipoproteinous deposits in the retina and have a shiny yellow-white appearance with sharp borders. It is to be noted that CWS are not exudates and result from intracellular swelling and not extracellular exudation that is seen in hard exudates (Fig. 3.4). CWS lead to RNF bundle defects (Fig. 3.5).

A. Gupta et al., *Ophthalmic Signs in Practice of Medicine*,
https://doi.org/10.1007/978-981-99-7923-3_3

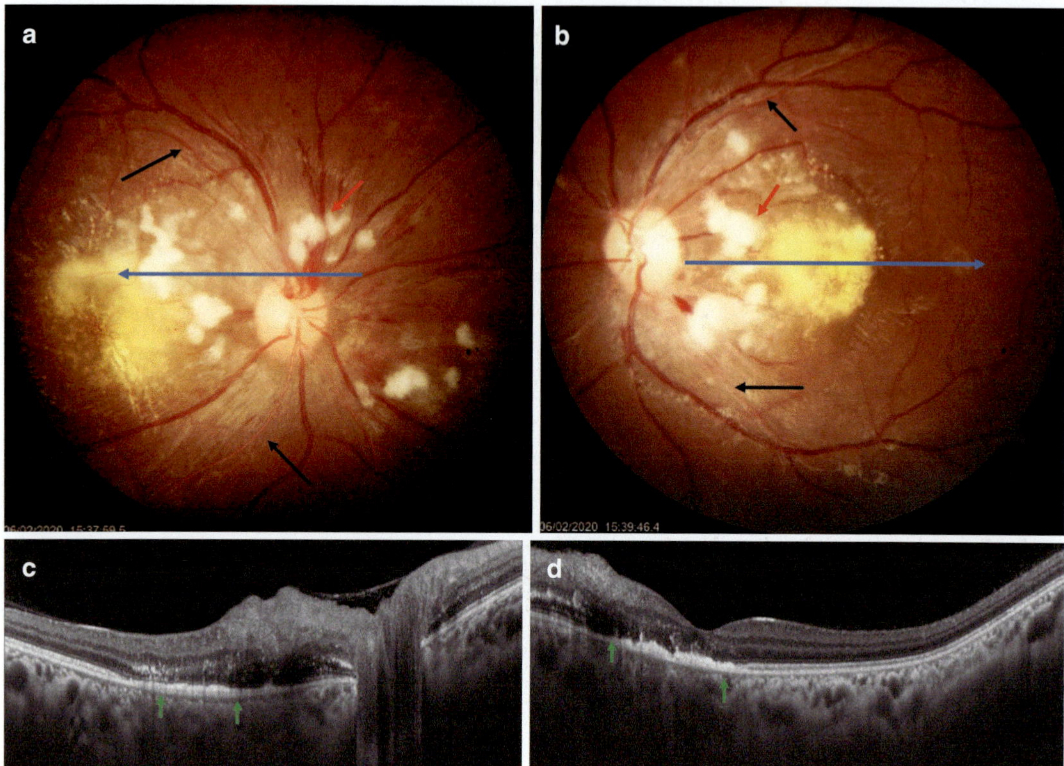

Fig. 3.1 A 17-year-old female with a two-week diminution of vision. Her blood pressure was 220/120. Fundus showed multiple peripapillary cotton wool spots R > L (red arrows) with few splinter haemorrhages R > L and yellowish deposits in the macula (**a**, right eye; **b**, left eye). Note the remarkable attenuation of the retinal arterioles (black arrows). OCT line scan (blue lines) passing through the cotton wool spots shows remarkable thickening of the nerve fibre layer in both eyes (**c**, right eye; **d**, left eye). Hyperreflective dots in the outer retina R > L. There is hyperreflectivity of the interdigitating and ellipsoid zones (green arrows). Retinal architecture temporal to the foveal centre is well maintained. (Images courtesy of Dr. Alok Sen, Sadguru Chikitsa Netralya, Chitrakoot, MP India)

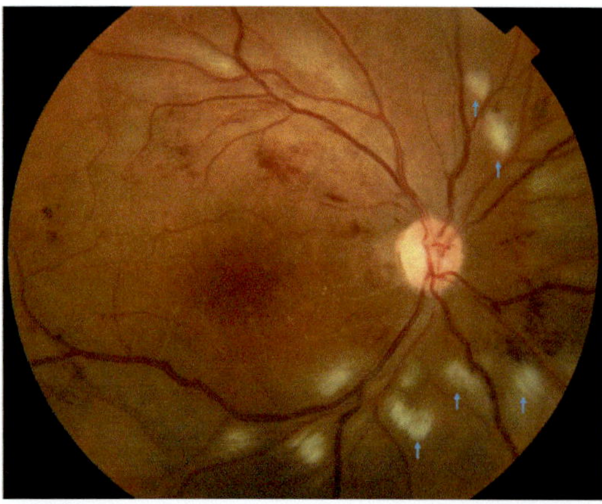

Fig. 3.2 Cotton wool spots (blue arrows), along with retinal haemorrhages, in a patient with diabetes mellitus and hypertension, seen as greyish-white lesions with feathery borders often clustered around the optic disc

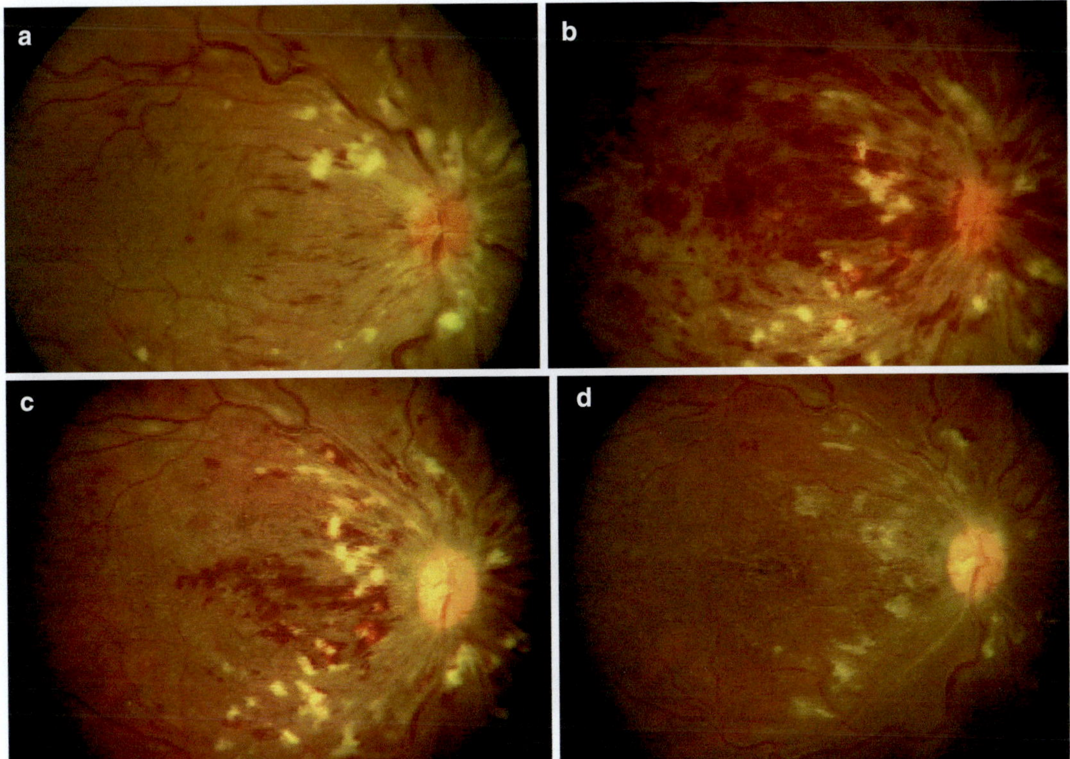

Fig. 3.3 A 30-year-old woman presented with CRVO and cotton wool spots in the right eye (**a**). Within 4 weeks, cotton wool spots and haemorrhages increased (**b**). She was treated with injections of Avastin given every 4 weeks. After the first injection, a dramatic resolution of the haemorrhages is seen, but cotton wool spots persist at 3 weeks (**c**) and 4 months with extensive atrophy of the retina (**d**)

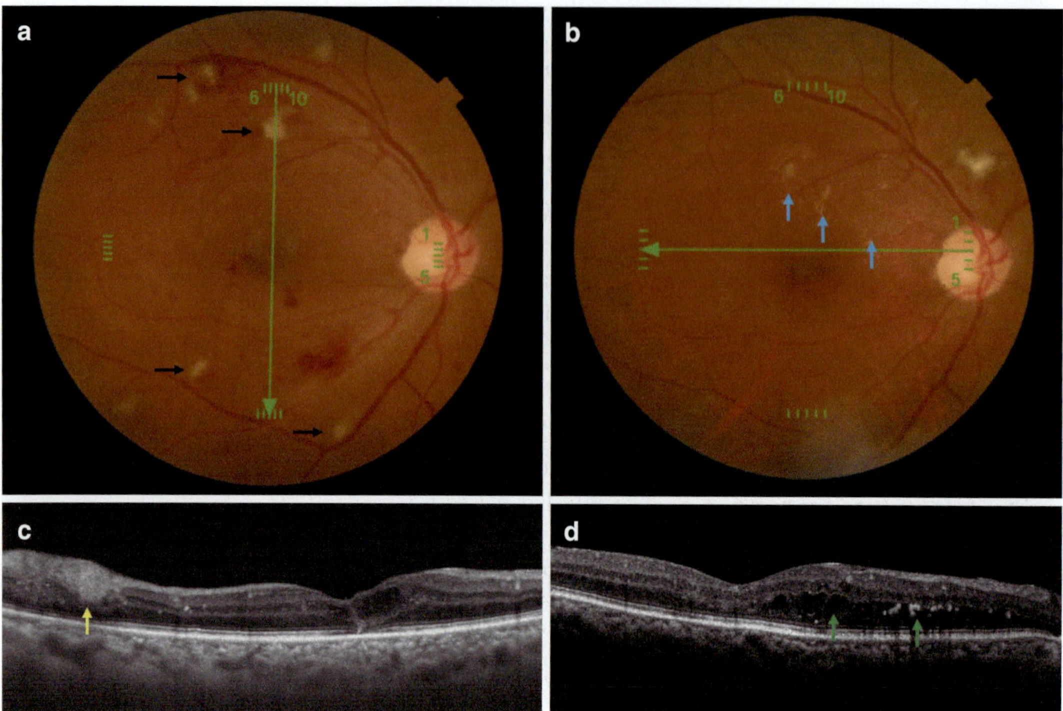

Fig. 3.4 Colour fundus photographs showing cotton wool spots (black arrows) (**a**) and retinal hard exudates (blue arrows) (**b**). The green lines (vertical in 'a' and horizontal in 'b') denote the slice navigators of corresponding OCT scans. Optical coherence tomography shows retinal thickening due to 'intraretinal swelling' (yellow arrow) in the area of cotton wool spot (**c**), while 'extracellular exudation' and 'intraretinal deposits' (green arrow) are associated with hard exudates (**d**)

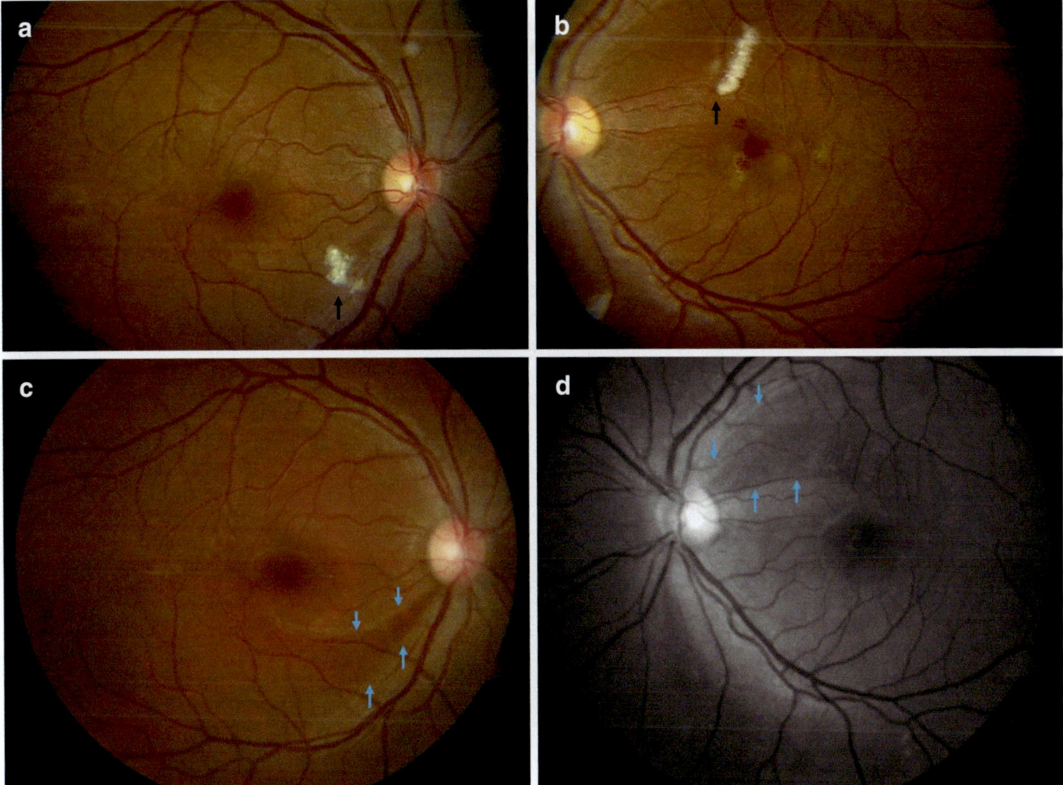

Fig. 3.5 Cotton wool spots (black arrow) in the right (**a**) and left (**b**) eyes of a patient with dengue fever. One year later, there was a loss of the retinal nerve fibre layer (blue arrows) at the site of the cotton wool spot as seen in fundus photograph (**c**) in the right eye and red free photograph (**d**) of the left eye

3.2 Cotton Wool Spots Versus Medullated Nerve Fibres

It should be noted that the RNFs are non-medullated till they exit from the eye. Rarely, the RNFs may become medullated as an anomalous developmental process. These medullated RNFs are opaque and have a broad spectrum of clinical presentation both in extent and severity. Many times, even to the experienced observer, these may be mistaken for the CWS. However, unlike the CWS, the medullated fibres are highly linear, have sharply defined borders and tend to obscure even the large retinal vessels near the optic disc (Figs. 3.6 and 3.7) (Box 3.1).

Box 3.1 Common Causes of Cotton Wool Spots

1. Hypertensive retinopathy	14. IgA nephropathy
2. Diabetic retinopathy	15. Radiation retinopathy
3. Transient CRAO	16. Dengue maculopathy
4. Central retinal vein occlusion	17. Malaria retinopathy
5. Branch retinal vein occlusion	18. Bartonella henselae neuroretintis
6. Polyarteritis nodosa	
7. Giant cell arteritis	
8. SLE	
9. Dermatomyositis	
10. HIV retinopathy	
11. Purtscher's retinopathy	
12. Leukaemic retinopathy	
13. Bone marrow transplant	

Source: Hayreh [1]

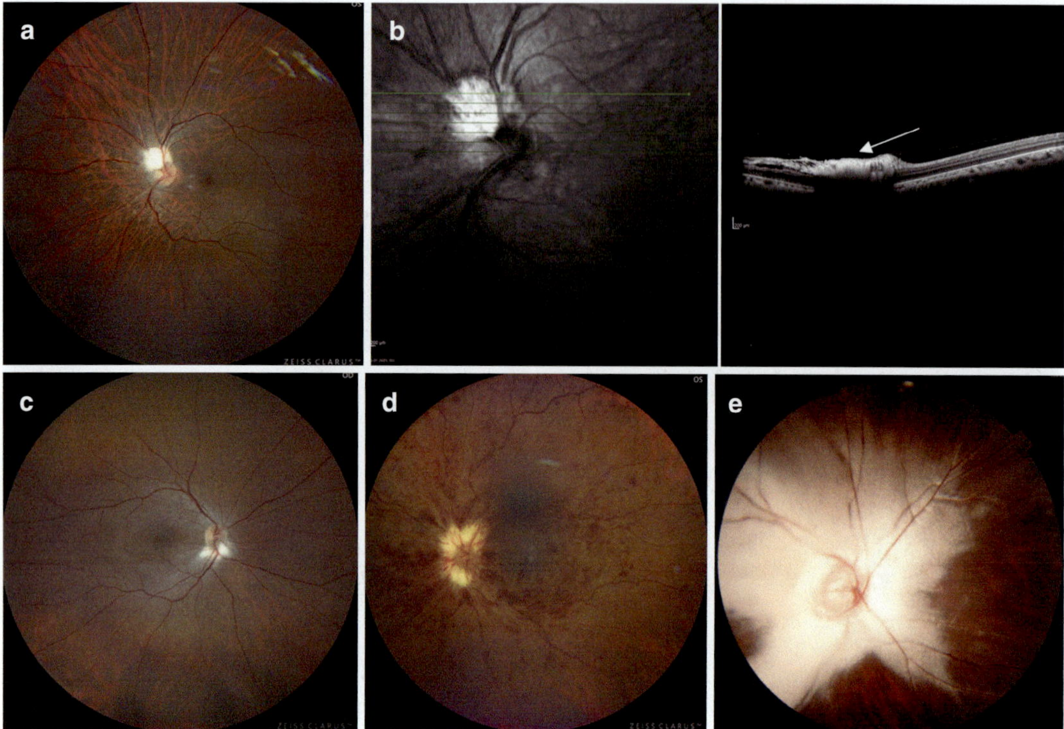

Fig. 3.6 Medullated nerve fibres may vary in severity, follow the distribution of the retinal nerve fibres and have sharply defined borders (**a**) OCT line scan through the medullated nerve fibres shows uniform hyperreflectivity (**b**, arrow). Bilateral myelinated nerve fibres (**c** and **d**). The patient presented with non-ischaemic central retinal vein occlusion in his left eye (**d**). The medullated nerve fibres could be confused with cotton wool spots (**d**). If massive, these are associated with amblyopia and produce corresponding visual field defects (**e**). (Images **a**–**d** courtesy of Dr. Alok Sen, Sadguru Netra Chikitsalya, Chitrakoot, MP, India)

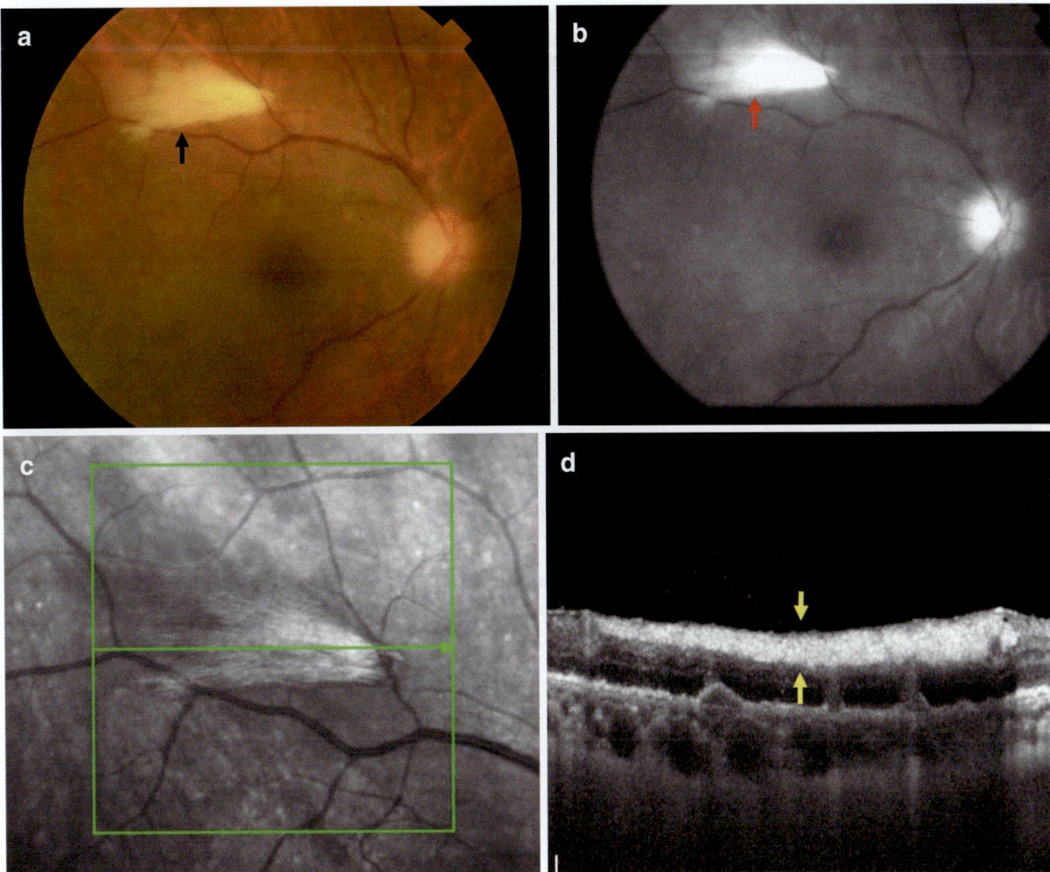

Fig. 3.7 Myelinated nerve fibres (**a**) appear as fluffy patches in the retina with sharply defined borders (black arrows) and are more prominent on red-free fundus photography (**b**). The OCT scan green slice navigator through the the myelinated nerve fibres (**c**) shows thickening of the retinal nerve fibre layer as a white hyper reflective band (yellow arrows) along the inner retina (**d**)

3.3 Causes of Cotton Wool Spots

3.3.1 Cotton Wool Spots in Hypertension

Cotton wool spots are the hallmark of hypertension. Accelerated hypertension in young people is the most common cause of CWS (Figs. 3.1, 3.2, and 3.8). CWS arise because of retinal hypoxia resulting from the occlusion of the retinal precapillary terminal arterioles. Blood supply to the retina is autoregulated, and unlike the other body organs, it is not controlled by the autonomic nervous system. Hence, in accelerated hypertension, there is an abrupt rise in the intravascular hydrostatic pressure due to which the compliant retinal arterioles contract resulting in the occlusion of the terminal arterioles.

Consequently, there is an anoxic/hypoxic insult to the RNFs. Depending upon the severity of hypoxia, there is either an infarction of the RNF if the blood supply is completely cut off or a reversible swelling of the RNF if the blood supply gets restored. Hypoxia leads to a block of orthograde and retrograde axoplasmic flow, which is responsible for the intracellular swelling and collection of organelles. This intracellular swelling, on histopathology, is seen as cytoid bodies. In essential hypertension, on the other hand, the blood pressure rises slowly over a long time, and the arterioles develop a protective arteriolarsclerosis. Arteriolarsclerosis makes the retinal arterioles non-compliant to any future sudden

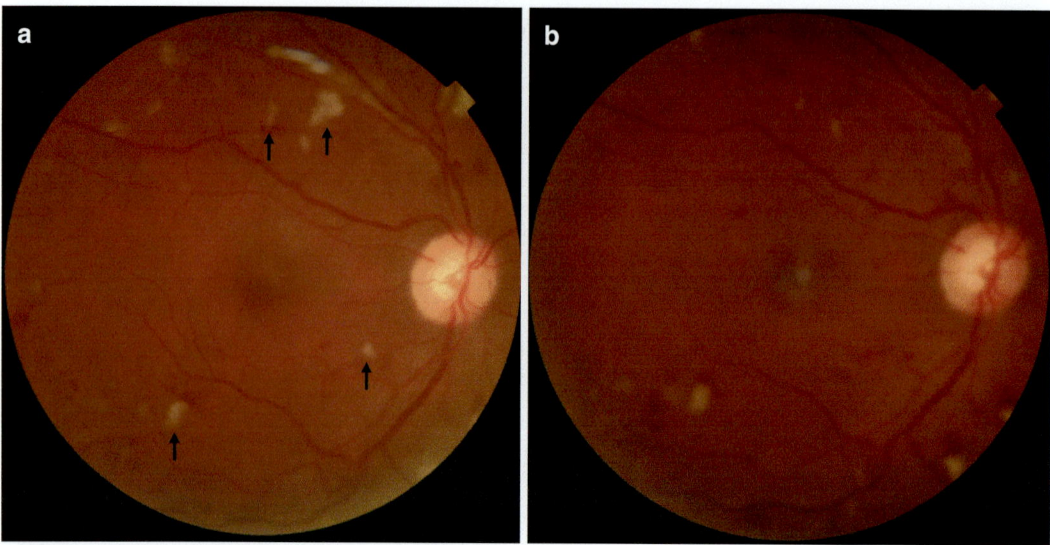

Fig. 3.8 Multiple cotton wool spots (black arrows) in a patient with accelerated hypertension (**a**). Five months later (**b**), many of the cotton wool spots showed resolution

rise in intravascular pressure. Thus, CWS are extremely unlikely in patients with essential hypertension (Boxes 3.2 and 3.3).

Box 3.2 How to Measure Blood Pressure

1. Measure in both upper arms; if consistently >10 mmHg in one arm, use that arm for recording
2. >20 mmHg difference in the two arms needs further evaluation
3. No smoking, exercise, or coffee for 30 min before the test
4. Record sitting for 3–5 min back supported and feet flat on the floor
5. No talking during the recording of the BP
6. Cuff of appropriate size, arm resting on a table at the heart level
7. Take three readings at 1-min intervals and take the mean of the last two readings

Source: American Heart Association, Inc.

Box 3.3 Definition of Hypertension

Hypertension is defined after 2–3 visits at 1–4 weeks intervals depending upon the BP

Hypertension-Clinic recording—SBP ≥ 140 mmHg and/or DBP ≥ 90 mmHg

Hypertension home recording—SBP ≥ 135 mmHg and/or DBP ≥ 85 mmHg

Normal BP—SBP ≤ 130 mmHg and/or DBP ≤ 85 mmHg

Adapted from: Verdecchia et al. [2] with permission of the publishers Elsevier

3.3.2 CWS in Diabetic Retinopathy

CWS, when seen in patients with diabetes mellitus, indicate an abrupt worsening of diabetic retinopathy (Fig. 3.9). Interestingly, uncontrolled type 2 diabetics, when switched to insulin therapy for better control of blood sugar levels, may develop CWS over the next few weeks [3]. A similar phenomenon has been noted in type I diabetic patients in the Oslo study [4], the Kroc

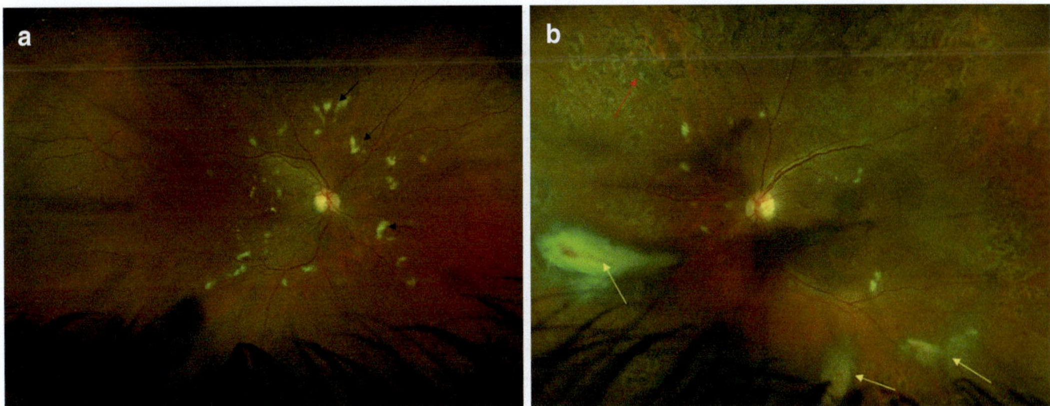

Fig. 3.9 Ultra-wide-field fundus photograph of a patient with moderate non-proliferative diabetic retinopathy in the right eye (**a**) and proliferative diabetic retinopathy in the left eye (**b**) showing extensive peripapillary cotton wool spots in the right eye (black arrows). The left eye of the same patient had developed proliferative diabetic retinopathy, had undergone pan-retinal laser photocoagulation (red arrow) and now shows grey preretinal haemorrhages (yellow arrows)

Study [5], and the Diabetes control and complications trial (DCCT) [6]. The subject has been reviewed recently [7]. Several mechanisms have been proposed on how focal retinal ischaemia resulting in the formation of CWS in diabetics may result from a decreased blood supply to the retina caused by a sudden reduction in the glucose substrate concentration in the retina [8].

Moreover, insulin is known to increase leukocyte-endothelial adhesion via the increased expression of adhesion molecules besides enhancing the breakdown of the blood-retinal barrier via the expression of hypoxia-inducible factor1-α and vascular endothelial growth factor (VEGF). All these mechanisms, singly or in combinations, may be responsible for the appearance of CWS in diabetic retinas during the institution of insulin therapy. In diabetic retinopathy, an increasing number of CWSs are seen with increasing severity in non-proliferative diabetic retinopathy both in the macular and the extramacular areas. Akin to the early worsening of diabetic retinopathy and polyneuropathy [9], a similar worsening of diabetic nephropathy evaluated by a significant decrease in the estimated glomerular filtration rate has been noted [10]. The CWS are smaller in the macular area than in the extramacular area. On fundus fluorescein angiography, these white spots are seen as areas of capillary non-perfusion (Fig. 3.10).

Interestingly, on optical coherence tomography (OCT), the CWSs in the macular area show hyperreflectivity in the RNF layer with corresponding non-perfusion on optical coherence tomography angiography (OCTA). On the other hand, the extramacular white spots show hyperreflectivity spanning from the retinal nerve fibre layer (RNFL) to the outer plexiform layer with a corresponding flow deficit on OCTA (Fig. 3.11) [11]. It has been proposed that in the macular area, the deep capillary plexus (DCP) is seamless and gets its supply from overlapping arterioles and perfusion is not easily compromised compared to the extramacular white spots, which do not have such an arrangement and depend on oxygenation to the choroidal supply [12]. While the macular white spots generally do not expand, the extramacular spots tend to spread toward the optic disc. The non-perfused areas involve both the superficial capillary plexus (SCP) and DCP and the CWS are central to these and mark the junction of non-perfused and perfused areas and are considered a sentinel lesion. The CWS show marked thickening of the RNFL on SD-OCT, impinging on the rest of the retinal layers. Unlike the peripheral non-perfused areas that, on OCTA, show no flow in the SCP and DCP, the area of macular CWS shows a strong decorrelation signal (Figs. 3.11 and 3.12) [13]. CWS on resolution leave behind thinning of the inner retinal layers,

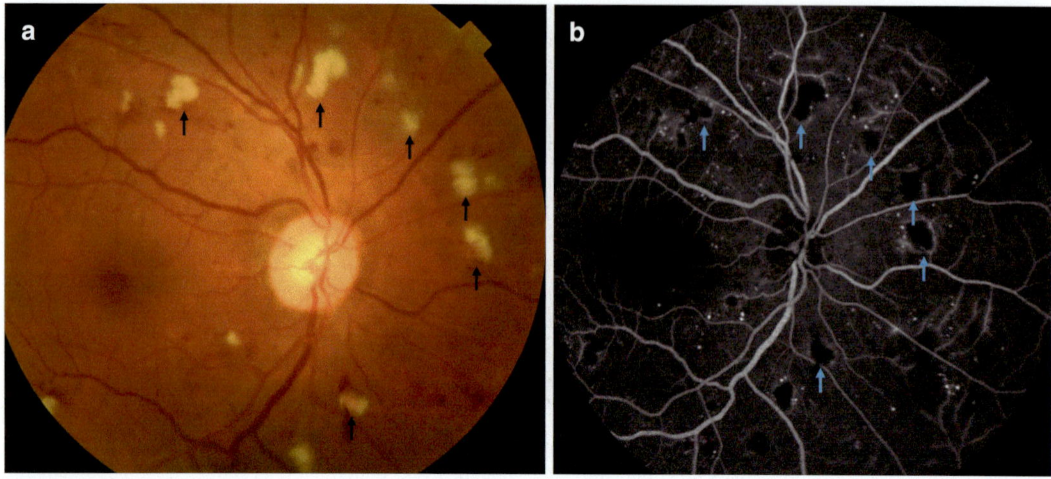

Fig. 3.10 Colour fundus photograph (**a**) showing cotton wool spots (black arrows) in a patient with hypertension and fundus fluorescein angiography (**b**) showing hypofluorescent areas (blue arrows) due to capillary nonperfusion corresponding to cotton wool spots

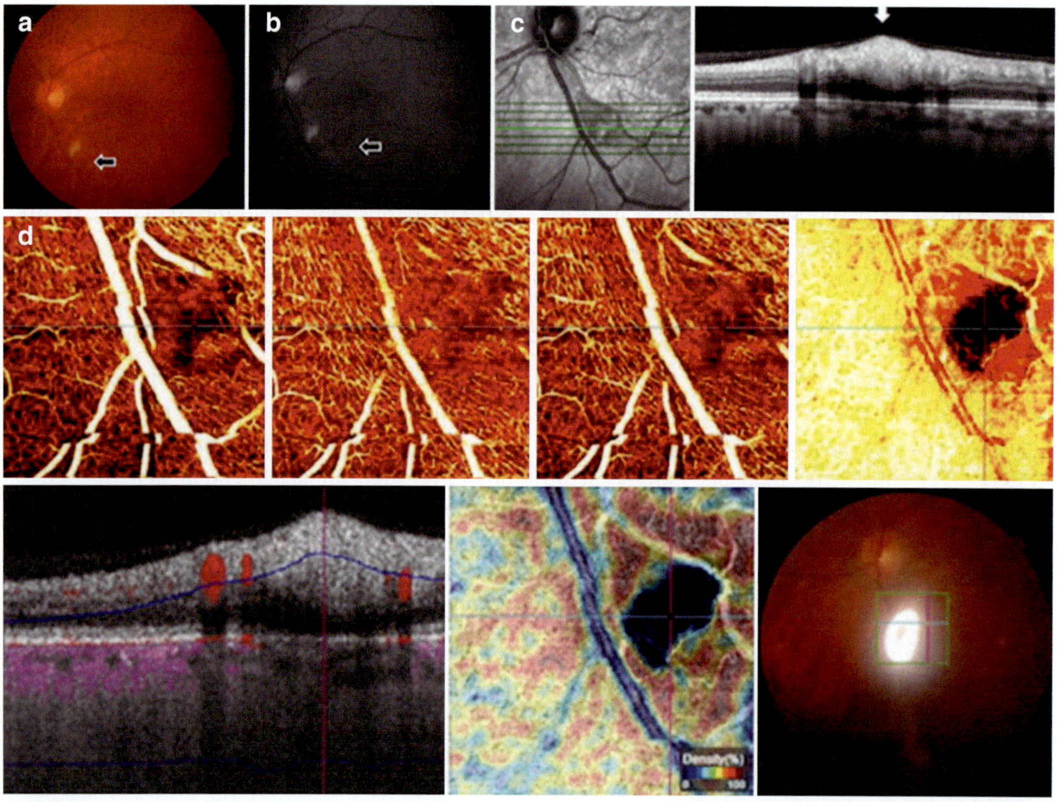

Fig. 3.11 Colour (**a**) and red-free (**b**) fundus photographs of a 57-year-old male patient in the convalescent phase, examined after 22 days of COVID-19 diagnosis, showing a CWS in the left eye. The SD-OCT (**c**) shows retinal nerve fibre layer swelling (arrow) in the region of CWS. The OCTA (**d**) showed an absence of signal (arrows) in all layers at the location of CWS. (Reproduced from Bansal R, Markan A, Gautam N, Guru RR, Lakshmi PVM, Katoch D, Agarwal A, Singh MP, Suri V, Mohindra R, Sahni N, Bhalla A, Malhotra P, Gupta V and Puri GD (2021) Retinal Involvement in COVID-19: Results From a Prospective Retina Screening Program in the Acute and Convalescent Phase. Front. Med. 8:681942. https://doi.org/10.3389/fmed.2021.681942. Under the Creative Commons attribution License (CC-BY)

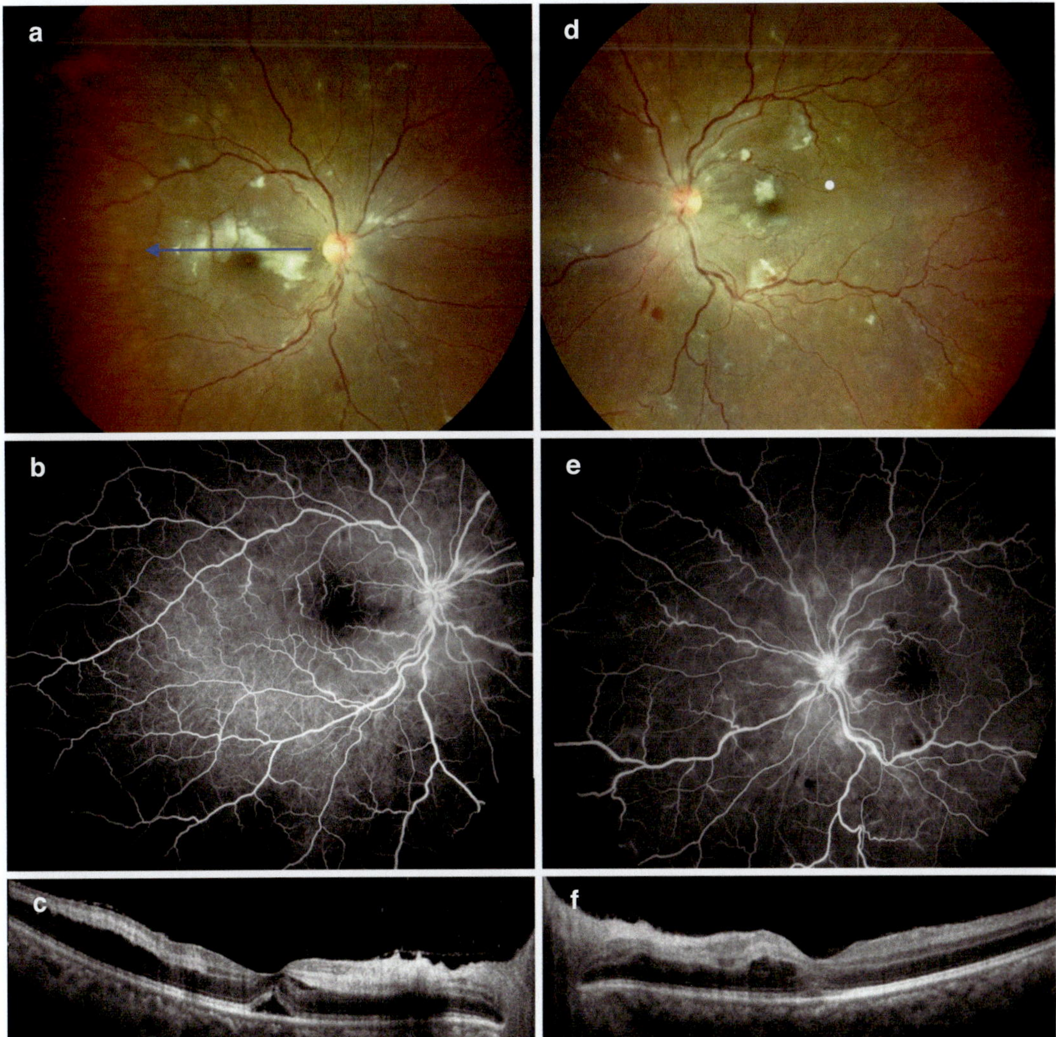

Fig. 3.12 A 30-year-old woman complained of diminution of vision 2 weeks following the COVID-19 vaccine. Visual acuity was 6/18 and 6/12 in the right and left eyes, respectively. The right eye fundus examination showed pale opacification in the macula (**a**). The fluorescein angiography was unremarkable except for a small area of hypofluorescence just above the fovea (**b**). SD-OCT line scan passing through the lesion (scan line indicated in **a**) showed hyperreflectivity in the inner nuclear layer, outer plexiform layer in the macula and nerve fibre layer medial to foveal centre, (**c**). The left eye showed similar changes (**d**–**f**). (Images courtesy of Dr. Alok Sen, Sadguru Netra Chikitsalya, Chitrakoot, MP, India)

middle layers. or the combined inner and middle layers. These focal areas of retinal thinning are significantly related to coronary artery disease, especially in the younger age group, decreasing estimated glomerular filtration rates, increasing serum creatinine, and higher HbA1c. Focal areas of retinal thinning have been proposed as a surrogate biomarker for systemic disease [14].

3.3.3 Cotton Wool Spots and Giant Cell Arteritis

Giant cell arteritis (GCA) is a blinding systemic vasculitis affecting the temporal arteries in elderly individuals. It presents as a sudden loss of vision due to arteritic ischaemic optic neuropathy due to the involvement of the posterior ciliary arteries that innervate the optic nerve. Most patients have at least one or more systemic constitutional symptoms, including jaw claudication, headache, low-grade fever, myalgia, anorexia, loss of weight, and scalp tenderness. Most patients with GCA have transient visual obscurations before developing chalky white arteritic ischaemic optic neuropathy or central retinal artery occlusion. Nearly 20% of the patients with GCA have no systemic symptoms and are labelled as occult GCA [15]. CWS are the presenting sign in one-third of patients with GCA [16]. It should be noted that GCA affects medium to large arteries and has no direct involvement of the terminal arterioles. It is postulated that CWS may arise due to an embolic process if there is incomplete occlusion due to vasculitis of the common trunk of the ophthalmic artery from which the medial ciliary artery and the central retinal artery arise [1].

In an elderly asymptomatic patient, the presence of CWS should alert the physicians to the possibility of GCA as a timely institution of high-dose corticosteroids can save the patient from blindness [17–20].

All patients suspected of arteritic anterior ischemic optic neuropathy (A-AION) should have their ESR and C-reactive proteins (CRP) tested. Elevation of both is highly sensitive for the diagnosis of GCA. Patients with GCA have significantly elevated platelet counts, but the predictability of thrombocytosis alone is not higher than the ESR and CRP [21].

The American College of Rheumatology and the European Alliance of Associations for Rheumatology (EULAR) 2022 gave new classification criteria for diagnosing GCA, the commonest cause of arteritic-AION. The essential criteria were age above 50 and ruling out other causes of medium or large vessel disease. They included a set of symptoms and signs, including morning stiffness in shoulders and neck, sudden onset of visual loss, jaw or tongue claudication, new temporal headache, scalp tenderness, cord-like thickening of the temporal artery, tenderness, and decreased or absent pulsations. Each of these was assigned a score of two. These were combined with information from a set of tests, including ESR > 50 mm/first hour or CRP > 10 mg/L, halo sign on ultrasonography of the temporal artery, a positive temporal artery biopsy, bilateral axillary artery halo sign, stenosis on angiography, or increased FDG uptake on PET CT scan. All criteria were given a score of two except a positive temporal artery biopsy, which was given a score of five, and loss of vision and ESR/CRP were allowed scores of three each. A score of >6 gave a diagnosis of GCA [22].

3.3.4 CWS in Systemic Lupus Erythematosus (SLE)

SLE is an autoimmune inflammatory disorder of the connective tissue and can involve multiple organs, including, among others, the skin, kidney, GI tract, brain, and vessel walls. Women are affected almost nine times more commonly than men [23]. If patients with SLE are screened, the eye is involved in 2–29% of patients with SLE [24].

Besides external eye involvement like keratoconjunctivitis sicca, CWS are a vital clue to the presence of an active SLE and are seen in nearly 50% of patients with ocular involvement (Fig. 3.13) and often accompanied by retinal haemorrhages and vascular occlusions (Fig. 3.14). Retinal vasculopathy is significantly associated with neuropsychiatric SLE [25].

3.3.5 CWS in HIV

Microangiopathy is very common in patients infected with HIV. In the eye, microangiopathy is seen in the conjunctiva, the retina, and the optic nerve. HIV retinopathy comprising CWS, microaneurysms, and retinal haemorrhages is seen in almost 40–100% of HIV-infected patients (Figs. 3.15 and 3.16). Nearly 45% of patients with $CD4^+$ counts less than 50 cells/μL have CWS compared to just 6% with higher counts [26]. HIV retinopathy is a marker for subsequent CMV retinitis. CWS resulting from focal occlusions of the capillaries are believed to provide the portal for entry of CMV into the retina.

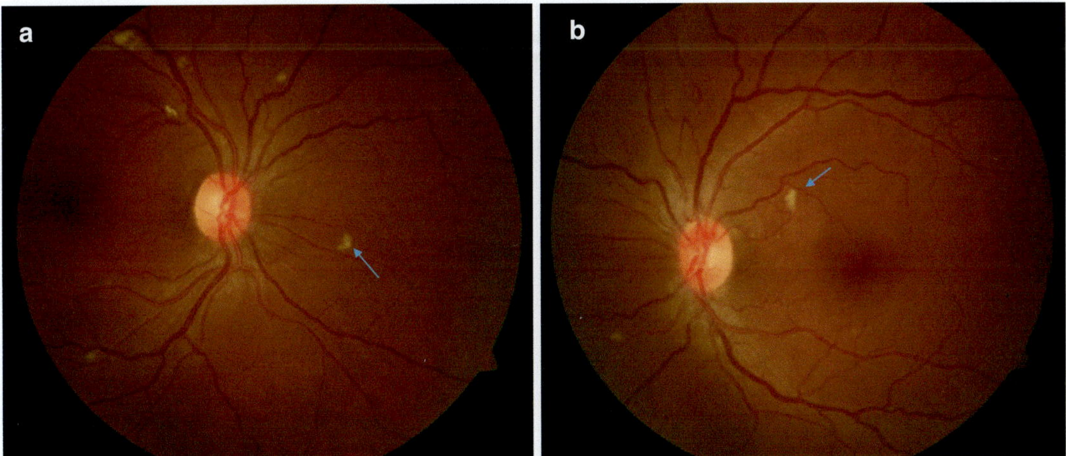

Fig. 3.13 Colour fundus photographs showing cotton wool spots in the right (**a**) and left (**b**) eyes of a patient with systemic lupus erythematosus

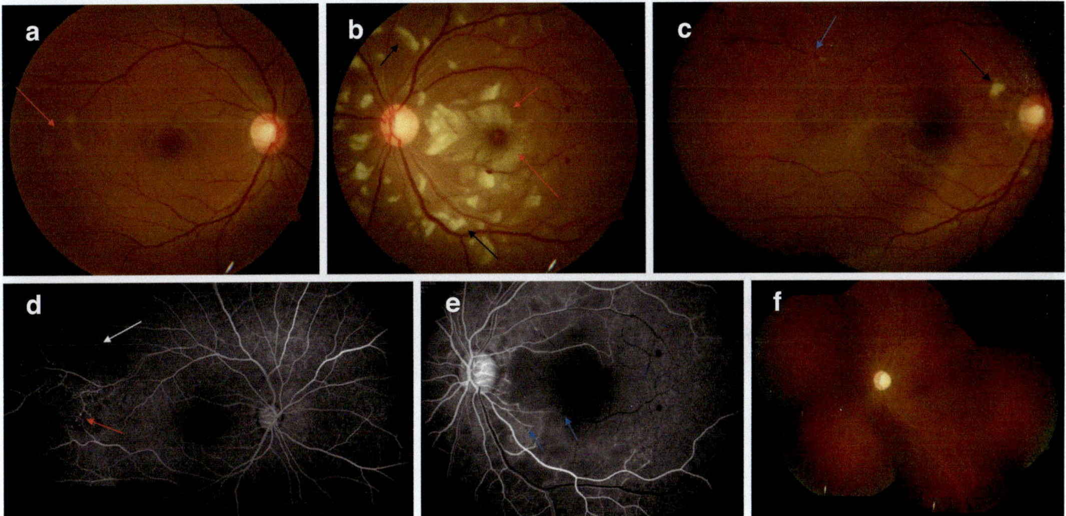

Fig. 3.14 Colour fundus photographs of a patient with systemic lupus erythematosus, with perivascular sheathing along the upper temporal vein in the right eye (**a**) and extensive cotton wool spots with a few retinal haemorrhages in the left eye (**b**), red arrows show pale opacification of the peritoneal retina with cherry-red appearance of the fovea (**b**). Three weeks later, a fresh cotton wool spot (black arrow) and a new retinal vasculitis (blue arrow) appeared in the right eye (**c**). Funds fluorescein angiography into right eye showed an area of capillary non-perfusion (white arrow) and microaneurysms (red arrow) (**d**) and extensive capillary non-perfusion and abrupt stumping of the retinal arterioles (arrow, **e**). On follow up one year later, right eye showed extensive sheathing of the vessels and a pale optic disc (**f**)

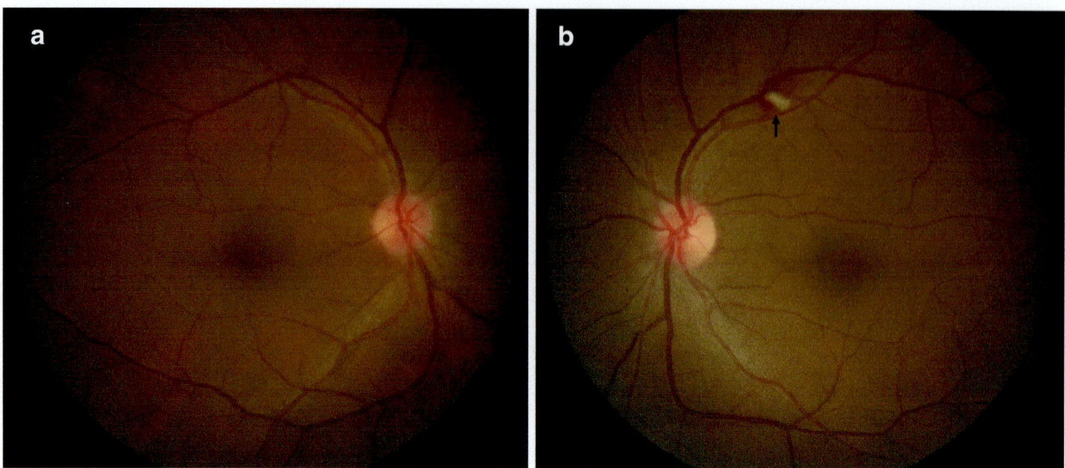

Fig. 3.15 Colour fundus photographs of a patient with HIV, with a normal right eye (**a**) and a single cotton wool spot with retinal haemorrhage (black arrow) in the left eye (**b**)

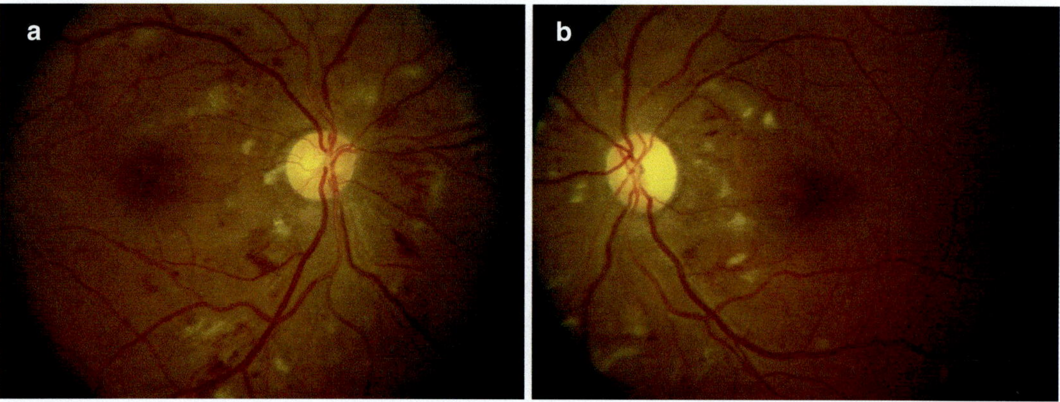

Fig. 3.16 Multiple cotton wool spots and retinal haemorrhages in right (**a**) and left (**b**) eyes of a patient with HIV

3.4 Imaging of the CWS

On fundus fluorescein angiography, the CWS show non-filling of the retinal capillaries in the territory of the occluded vessel. At the junction of the capillary non-perfused areas and the normally perfused capillaries, stumps of the normal capillaries are often mistaken for retinal microaneurysms [1]. On OCT, CWS shows hyperreflectivity, known as the 'Hyperreflectivity sign', which persists even after CWS is resolved [27]. The persistent hyperreflectivity is likely due to the replacement of RNFs with glial scars at the site of the CWS. It is to be noted that the axons passing through the CWS do not transmit signals and show a corresponding relative arcuate scotoma on perimetry. At the same time, the site of the CWS has an absolute scotoma. Some axons passing through the CWS are likely to survive the hypoxic insult [28].

The CWS due to HIV, when followed for several years, show highly significant thinning of the inner retina, which is maximum in the ganglion cell layer, besides significant thinning of the RNFL, the inner plexiform layer, the inner nuclear layer, and the outer plexiform layer [29]. Upon resolution, the CWS in hypertension leave behind localized RNF layer defects (RNFLD). Such RNFLDs in young people have been associated with higher glycated haemoglobin levels

(HbA1c), higher mean and daytime 24-h systolic and diastolic blood pressures, and lower estimated glomerular filtration rates. The RNFLDs are associated with a higher 10-year atherosclerotic heart disease at 9.7% in the middle and 25.6% in the older age group. Thus, any patient with CWS or their remnants—the RNFLD must be evaluated for cardiovascular disease [30]. CWS, superficial linear haemorrhages, and hard exudates characterize hypertensive retinopathy [30]. Uncontrolled accelerated hypertension may also develop characteristic lesions of hypertensive choroidopathy and optic neuropathy. Even though blood pressure in these patients can be successfully controlled with medical treatment, these patients show a significant loss of the RNFL thickness when seen later [31]. Microperimetry studies show permanent relative scotomas, denser in diabetes than hypertension, at the site of CW spots even after their resolution. Interestingly, the uninvolved surrounding retina in diabetic eyes shows lesser sensitivity compared to hypertensive eyes [32].

3.5 Paracentral Acute Middle Maculopathy (PAMM)

The retina's blood supply is organized into three layers. The outermost layer comprising the RPE and the outer nuclear layer get the micronutrients and oxygen from the choriocapillaris, the middle retinal layers comprising the outer plexiform layer, inner nuclear layer, and the inner plexiform layer from the intermediate and DCP of the central retinal arterial (CRA) system, and the innermost retinal layers comprising the ganglion cells and the retinal nerve fibre layer get their vascular supply from the SCP of the CRA [33]. Unlike the CWS, which results from non-perfusion of the SCP and the radial peripapillary capillaries that lie in the RNF layer and the ganglion cell layer, ischaemic insult to the intermediate and DCP that supply the inner nuclear layer and the inner and outer plexiform layers results in the opacification of the middle layers of the retina, namely, the inner nuclear layer and the inner and outer plexiform layers. It is to be noted that these plexuses are downstream in the hierarchy of the blood supply and represent a watershed in the anteroposterior axis of the blood supply of the retina and thus vulnerable to hypoperfusion and hypoxic insult [34]. The availability of advanced imaging techniques in recent years, such as optical coherence tomography (OCT) and OCT angiography, has made it possible to observe paracentral acute middle maculopathy (Figs. 3.17 and 3.18). Clinically, these areas may vary in size and appear to have a very subtle colour change of retina to apparent opacification [35]. On structural OCT, PAMM lesions are seen as a hyperreflective band at the level of the inner nuclear layer

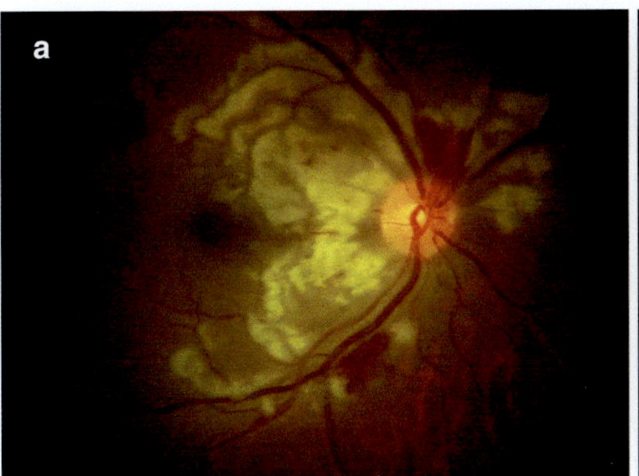

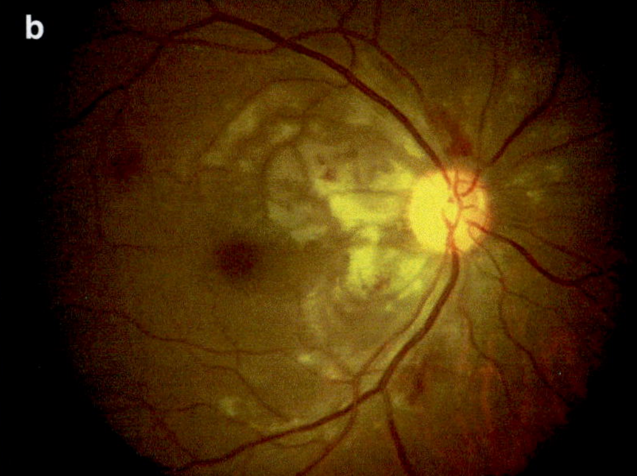

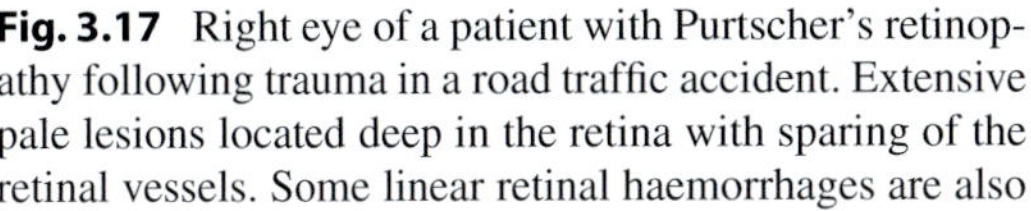

Fig. 3.17 Right eye of a patient with Purtscher's retinopathy following trauma in a road traffic accident. Extensive pale lesions located deep in the retina with sparing of the retinal vessels. Some linear retinal haemorrhages are also seen (**a**) and after 2 months (**b**). Most of these lesions appear to be PAMM lesions. The images are from a pre-OCT era, which were erroneously diagnosed as cotton wool spots in the absence of the OCT

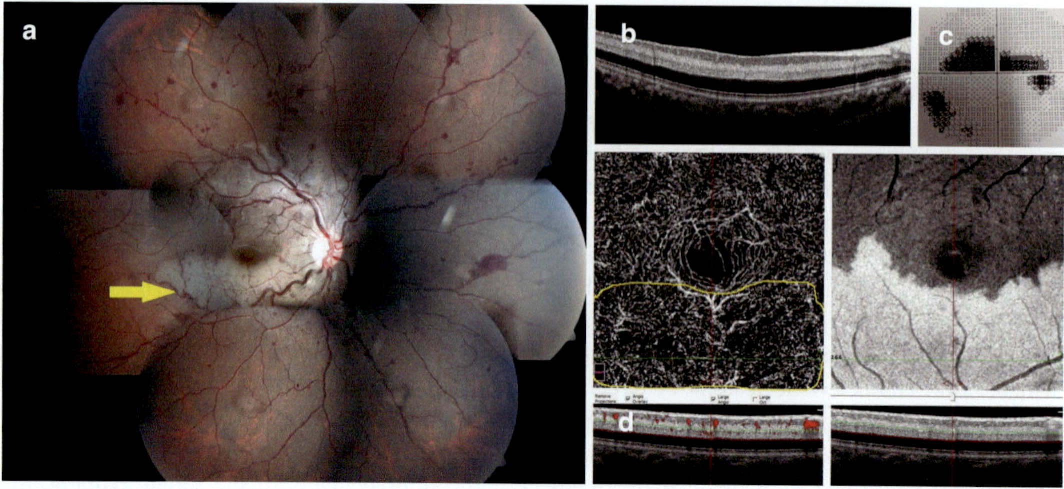

Fig. 3.18 A 19-year-old male presented with non-ischemic central retinal vein occlusion (yellow arrow) in the right eye (**a**). The SD-OCT showed hyperreflectivity of the inner nuclear layer, corresponding to the opacified macula, suggestive of Paracentral Acute Middle Maculopathy (PAMM) (**b**), which corresponded with a superior half scotoma in the macula (**c**). OCT angiography with enface imaging showed disruption of the DCP (**d**) contrasting from the dilated capillary bed in the SCP (**e**). (Images courtesy Dr. Alok Sen, Sadguru Netra Chikitsalya, Chitrakoot, MP, India)

and the inner and outer plexuses. On OCTA, these lesions show non-perfusion of the intermediate and deep capillary plexuses. Very subtle PAMM lesions may be picked up on fundus autofluorescence imaging as hypoautofluorescent. The acute lesions of deep capillary ischaemia that result in PAMM lesions appear as deep opacification of the involved retina, which disappear over the next few weeks and are hard to detect.

In contrast to the CWS, the PAMM lesions appear greyer with a smoother contour [36]. On OCT, in the acute stage, these lesions appear as hyperreflective bands extending from the inner plexiform layer to the outer plexiform layer. On resolution, there is a marked thinning of these layers. These contrast with CWS, which show thinning of the RNFL with the preservation of the middle retinal layers [37]. The PAMM lesions have been seen in sickle cell disease, hypertensive retinopathy, compressive injury of the globe, Purtscher's retinopathy (Fig. 3.13), post H1N1 vaccine, migraine, occlusive retinal vasculitis, following an upper respiratory infection [38], central retinal vein occlusion (Fig. 3.14), and more recently in SARS-CoV-2 infection [39] (Fig. 3.15).

Unfortunately, the PAMM lesions, due to compromised circulation in the deep capillary plexus of the middle retinal layers, are not delineated on fundus fluorescein angiography. Hence, this entity's discovery was delayed until SD-OCT imaging was available.

References

1. Hayreh SS. Cotton-wool spots (inner retinal ischemic spots). In: Ocular vascular occlusive disorders. 2014. pp. 365–377. https://doi.org/10.1007/978-3-319-12781-1_17. © Springer International Publishing Switzerland 2015.
2. Verdecchia P, Reboldi G, Angeli F. The 2020 International Society of Hypertension global hypertension practice guidelines—key messages and clinical considerations. Eur J Intern Med. 2020;82:1–6. https://doi.org/10.1016/j.ejim.2020.09.001. Epub 2020 Sep 22. PMID: 32972800.
3. Roysarkar TK, Gupta A, Dash RJ, Dogra MR. Effect of insulin therapy on progression of retinopathy in noninsulin-dependent diabetes mellitus. Am J Ophthalmol. 1993;115(5):569–74. https://

doi.org/10.1016/s0002-9394(14)71452-7. PMID: 8488908.

4. Dahl-Jørgensen K, Brinchmann-Hansen O, Hanssen KF, Sandvik L, Aagenaes O. Rapid tightening of blood glucose control leads to transient deterioration of retinopathy in insulin dependent diabetes mellitus: the Oslo study. Br Med J (Clin Res Ed). 1985;290(6471):811–5. https://doi.org/10.1136/bmj.290.6471.811. PMID: 3919804; PMCID: PMC1418598.
5. The Kroc Collaborative Study Group. Collaborative studies of the effects of continuous subcutaneous insulin infusion in insulin-dependent diabetes mellitus. Conclusions. Diabetes. 1985;34 Suppl 3:87–9. https://doi.org/10.2337/diab.34.3.s87. PMID: 3894131.
6. Early worsening of diabetic retinopathy in the diabetes control and complications trial. Arch Ophthalmol. 1998;116(7):874–86. https://doi.org/10.1001/archopht.116.7.874.
7. Bain SC, Klufas MA, Ho A, Matthews DR. Worsening of diabetic retinopathy with rapid improvement in systemic glucose control: a review. Diabetes Obes Metab. 2019;21(3):454–66. https://doi.org/10.1111/dom.13538. Epub 2018 Oct 15. PMID: 30226298; PMCID: PMC6587545.
8. Grunwald JE, Riva CE, Martin DB, Quint AR, Epstein PA. Effect of an insulin-induced decrease in blood glucose on the human diabetic retinal circulation. Ophthalmology. 1987;94(12):1614–20. https://doi.org/10.1016/s0161-6420(87)33257-9. PMID: 3323985.
9. Gibbons CH, Freeman R. Treatment-induced neuropathy of diabetes: an acute, iatrogenic complication of diabetes. Brain. 2015;138(Pt 1):43–52. https://doi.org/10.1093/brain/awu307. Epub 2014 Nov 11. PMID: 25392197; PMCID: PMC4285188.
10. Cundy T, Holden A, Stallworthy E. Early worsening of diabetic nephropathy in type 2 diabetes after rapid improvement in chronic severe hyperglycemia. Diabetes Care. 2021;44(3):e55–6. https://doi.org/10.2337/dc20-2646. Epub 2021 Jan 22. PMID: 33483357; PMCID: PMC7896259.
11. Morino K, Murakami T, Dodo Y, Yasukura S, Yoshitake T, Fujimoto M, Tsujikawa A. Characteristics of diabetic capillary nonperfusion in macular and extramacular white spots on optical coherence tomography angiography. Invest Ophthalmol Vis Sci. 2019;60(5):1595–603. https://doi.org/10.1167/iovs.18-26534. PMID: 30995316.
12. Yasukura S, Murakami T, Suzuma K, Yoshitake T, Nakanishi H, Fujimoto M, Oishi M, Tsujikawa A. Diabetic nonperfused areas in macular and extramacular regions on wide-field optical coherence tomography angiography. Invest Ophthalmol Vis Sci. 2018;59(15):5893–903. https://doi.org/10.1167/iovs.18-25108. PMID: 30550612.
13. Mahdjoubi A, Bousnina Y, Barrande G, Bensmaine F, Chahed S, Ghezzaz A. Features of cotton wool spots in diabetic retinopathy: a spectral-domain optical coherence tomography angiography study. Int Ophthalmol. 2020;40(7):1625–40. https://doi.org/10.1007/s10792-020-01330-7. Epub 2020 Mar 21. PMID: 32200508.
14. Preti RC, Iovino C, Abalem MF, Garcia R, Dos Santos HNV, Sakuno G, Au A, Cunha LP, Zacharias LC, Monteiro MLR, Sadda SR, Sarraf D. Prevalence of focal inner, middle, and combined retinal thinning in diabetic patients and its relationship with systemic and ocular parameters. Transl Vis Sci Technol. 2021;10(2):26. https://doi.org/10.1167/tvst.10.2.26. PMID: 34003911; PMCID: PMC7900871.
15. Hayreh SS, Podhajsky PA, Zimmerman B. Occult giant cell arteritis: ocular manifestations. Am J Ophthalmol 1998;125(4):521–6. doi: https://doi.org/10.1016/s0002-9394(99)80193-7. Erratum in: Am J Ophthalmol 1998 Jun;125(6):893. PMID: 9559738.
16. Hayreh SS, Podhajsky PA, Zimmerman B. Ocular manifestations of giant cell arteritis. Am J Ophthalmol. 1998;125(4):509–20. https://doi.org/10.1016/s0002-9394(99)80192-5. PMID: 9559737.
17. Gospe SM 3rd, Walter SD, Bhatti MT. A woman with a spot in her vision. JAMA Ophthalmol. 2017;135(9):997–8. https://doi.org/10.1001/jamaophthalmol.2017.0426. PMID: 28617913.
18. Johnson MC, Lee AG. Giant cell arteritis presenting with cotton wool spots. Semin Ophthalmol. 2008;23(3):141–2. https://doi.org/10.1080/08820530801946903. PMID: 18432539.
19. Rai AS, Freund P, Margolin EA, Micieli JA. Numerous cotton wool spots from giant cell arteritis. J Clin Rheumatol. 2020;26(5):e124. https://doi.org/10.1097/RHU.0000000000000995. PMID: 30664545.
20. Velusami P, Doherty M, Gnanaraj L. A case of occult giant cell arteritis presenting with bilateral cotton wool spots. Eye (Lond). 2006;20(7):863–4. https://doi.org/10.1038/sj.eye.6702038. Epub 2005 Aug 12. PMID: 16096661.
21. Costello F, Zimmerman MB, Podhajsky PA, Hayreh SS. Role of thrombocytosis in diagnosis of giant cell arteritis and differentiation of arteritic from non-arteritic anterior ischemic optic neuropathy. Eur J Ophthalmol. 2004;14(3):245–57. https://doi.org/10.1177/112067210401400310. PMID: 15206651.
22. Szekeres D, Al Othman B. Current developments in the diagnosis and treatment of giant cell arteritis. Front Med (Lausanne). 2022;9:1066503. https://doi.org/10.3389/fmed.2022.1066503. PMID: 36582285; PMCID: PMC9792614.
23. Silpa-archa S, Lee JJ, Foster CS. Ocular manifestations in systemic lupus erythematosus. Br J Ophthalmol. 2016;100(1):135–41. https://doi.org/10.1136/bjophthalmol-2015-306629. Epub 2015 Apr 22. PMID: 25904124.

24. Davies JB, Rao PK. Ocular manifestations of systemic lupus erythematosus. Curr Opin Ophthalmol. 2008;19(6):512–8. https://doi.org/10.1097/icu.0b013e3283126d34. PMID: 18998618.
25. Gao N, Li MT, Li YH, Zhang SH, Dai RP, Zhang SZ, Zhao LD, Wang L, Zhang FC, Zhao Y, Zeng XF. Lupus. 2017;26(11):1182–9. https://doi.org/10.1177/0961203317698050. Epub 2017 Mar 29. PMID: 28355986. Erratum in: Arch Ophthalmol 1998;116(11):1469. PMID: 9682700.
26. Stewart MW. Human immunodeficiency virus and its effects on the visual system. Infect Dis Rep. 2012;4(1):e25. https://doi.org/10.4081/idr.2012.e25. PMID: 24470932; PMCID: PMC3892652.
27. Kozak I, Bartsch DU, Cheng L, Freeman WR. Hyperreflective sign in resolved cotton wool spots using high-resolution optical coherence tomography and optical coherence tomography ophthalmoscopy. Ophthalmology. 2007;114(3):537–43. https://doi.org/10.1016/j.ophtha.2006.06.054. PMID: 17324696.
28. Chui TY, Thibos LN, Bradley A, Burns SA. The mechanisms of vision loss associated with a cotton wool spot. Vision Res. 2009;49(23):2826–34. https://doi.org/10.1016/j.visres.2009.08.017. Epub 2009 Aug 22. PMID: 19703485; PMCID: PMC2783881.
29. Gomez ML, Mojana F, Bartsch DU, Freeman WR. Imaging of long-term retinal damage after resolved cotton wool spots. Ophthalmology. 2009;116(12):2407–14. https://doi.org/10.1016/j.ophtha.2009.05.012. Epub 2009 Oct 7. PMID: 19815278; PMCID: PMC4172325.
30. Shin JY, Lee J, Lee CJ, Park S, Byeon SH. Association between localized retinal nerve fibre layer defects and cardiovascular risk factors. Sci Rep. 2019;9(1):19340. https://doi.org/10.1038/s41598-019-55846-9. PMID: 31852922; PMCID: PMC6920147.
31. Lee HM, Lee WH, Kim KN, Jo YJ, Kim JY. Changes in thickness of central macula and retinal nerve fibre layer in severe hypertensive retinopathy: a 1-year longitudinal study. Acta Ophthalmol. 2018;96(3):e386–92. https://doi.org/10.1111/aos.13521. Epub 2017 Oct 4. PMID: 28975766.
32. Kim JS, Maheshwary AS, Bartsch DG, et al. The microperimetry of resolved cotton-wool spots in eyes of patients with hypertension and diabetes mellitus. Arch Ophthalmol. 2011;129(7):879–84. https://doi.org/10.1001/archophthalmol.2011.51.
33. Scharf J, Freund KB, Sadda S, Sarraf D. Paracentral acute middle maculopathy and the organization of the retinal capillary plexuses. Prog Retin Eye Res. 2021;81:100884. https://doi.org/10.1016/j.preteyeres.2020.100884. Epub 2020 Aug 9. PMID: 32783959.
34. Dansingani KK, Freund KB. Paracentral acute middle maculopathy and acute macular neuroretinopathy: related and distinct entities. Am J Ophthalmol. 2015;160(1):1–3.e2. https://doi.org/10.1016/j.ajo.2015.05.001. PMID: 26054463.
35. Sarraf D, Rahimy E, Fawzi AA, et al. Paracentral acute middle maculopathy: a new variant of acute macular neuroretinopathy associated with retinal capillary ischemia. JAMA Ophthalmol. 2013;131(10):1275–87. https://doi.org/10.1001/jamaophthalmol.2013.4056.
36. Rahimy E, Kuehlewein L, Sadda SR, Sarraf D. Paracentral acute middle maculopathy: what we knew then and what we know now. Retina. 2015;35(10):1921–30. https://doi.org/10.1097/IAE.0000000000000785. PMID: 26360227.
37. Yu S, Wang F, Pang CE, Yannuzzi LA, Freund KB. Multimodal imaging findings in retinal deep capillary ischemia. Retina. 2014;34(4):636–46. https://doi.org/10.1097/IAE.0000000000000048. PMID: 24240565.
38. Chen X, Rahimy E, Sergott RC, Nunes RP, Souza EC, Choudhry N, Cutler NE, Houston SK, Munk MR, Fawzi AA, Mehta S, Hubschman JP, Ho AC, Sarraf D. Spectrum of retinal vascular diseases associated with paracentral acute middle maculopathy. Am J Ophthalmol. 2015;160(1):26–34.e1. https://doi.org/10.1016/j.ajo.2015.04.004. Epub 2015 Apr 4. PMID: 25849522.
39. Padhy SK, Dcruz RP, Kelgaonkar A. Paracentral acute middle maculopathy following SARS-CoV-2 infection: the D-dimer hypothesis. BMJ Case Rep. 2021;14(3):e242043. https://doi.org/10.1136/bcr-2021-242043. PMID: 33664047; PMCID: PMC7934752.

4 Retinal Hard Exudates

4.1 Introduction

The presence of retinal hard exudates is most often a sign of an underlying serious systemic disease. The appearance of hard exudate in a patient with diabetes who, till then, had shown only retinal microaneurysms (MAs), the hallmark of diabetic retinopathy, indicates that the patient has moved to the next level in the severity of diabetic retinopathy (Fig. 4.1). While evaluating fundus images in telemedicine units, it may not be possible to see tiny red microaneurysms, and the retinal hard exudates may be the only visible sign of diabetic retinopathy. To maintain transparency of the retina, the retinal blood vessels are endowed with tight endothelial junctions, which do not allow leakage of fluid or macromolecules into the extravascular space. Retinal hard exudates are almost always accompanied by thickening of the retina. They are seen in any disease that breaks down the tight endothelial junctions allowing the extravasation of fluid and macromolecules into the extravascular space (Fig. 4.2).

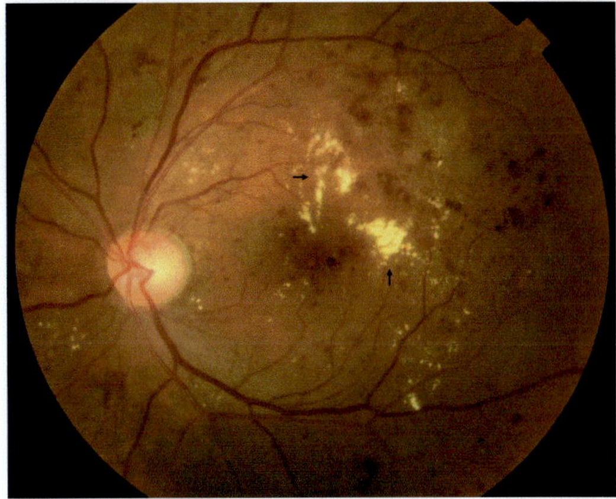

Fig. 4.1 Hard exudates (black arrows), along with microaneurysms and retinal haemorrhages, seen in a patient with diabetes mellitus, indicating the presence of moderate non-proliferative diabetic retinopathy

A. Gupta et al., *Ophthalmic Signs in Practice of Medicine*,
https://doi.org/10.1007/978-981-99-7923-3_4

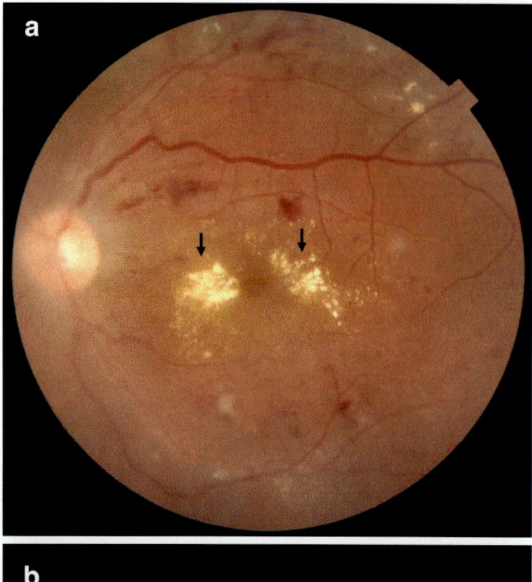

Fig. 4.2 Colour fundus photograph (**a**) showing retinal hard exudates (black arrows) in the macula. Optical coherence tomography (OCT) scan through the macula (**b**) shows thickening of the retina, with hard exudates seen as hyperreflective foci (blue arrows), subretinal fluid (red arrow), and intraretinal fluid (yellow arrows) suggestive of extravasation of fluid due to the breakdown of the blood–retina barrier

4.2 Causes of Retinal Hard Exudates

The common causes of retinal hard exudates include diabetic retinopathy followed by hypertensive retinopathy, branch retinal vein occlusion, central retinal vein occlusion, retinal arterial macroaneurysm (RAM), neuro retinitis, idiopathic retinal vasculitis, aneurysms and neuro retinitis (IRVAN), retinal vasculitis, Coats' disease, retinitis, retinal capillary hemangioblastoma (von Hippel-Lindau's disease), choroidal neovascular membranes, and choroidal hemangiomas to name a few.

4.3 Differential Diagnosis of Retinal Hard Exudates

4.3.1 Hard Exudates Versus Soft Exudates

Retinal hard exudates are yellow-white in colour, have a waxy glistening appearance with sharp margins, and vary in size from a pinpoint to massive mounds measuring several disc diameters. These exudates consist of leaked lipids and lipoproteins or may represent the remnants of the degenerated neural tissue. The retinal hard exudates need to be differentiated from the cotton wool spots, previously called the retinal soft exudates, which are greyish-white, fudgy-bordered swellings of the retinal nerve fibre layer (axons of the retinal ganglion cells) resulting from an ischemic insult to the retinal nerve fibres which results in the blockade of the axoplasmic flow (Fig. 4.3). The cotton wool spots and the hard exudates are seen in the posterior pole of the retina or the peripapillary region. Both may co-exist in diabetic retinopathy and hypertensive retinopathy, although the hard exudates predominate in diabetics and the cotton wool spots dominate in the hypertensives. While the cotton wool spots are in the superficial layers of the inner layers of the neurosensory retina, the retinal hard exudates are present deeper in the retina. Unlike the cotton wool spots with a short life span of 4–6 weeks, the retinal hard exudates often last for months or even years if the pathology that caused these continues to persist. The presence of hard exudates indicates a rather chronic process, while the presence of the cotton wool spots indicates an acute event that calls for urgent attention from the physicians for appropriate intervention.

4.3.2 Hard Exudates Versus Drusen

Apart from the cotton wool spots, hard exudates must be differentiated from drusen bodies, mostly seen in the elderly as a manifestation of age-related macular degeneration. The drusen

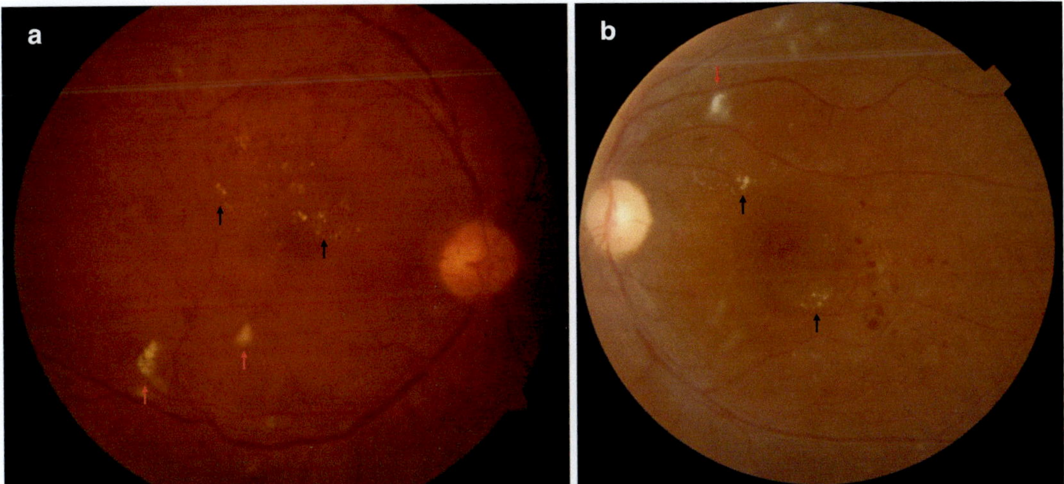

Fig. 4.3 Colour fundus photograph of a patient with non-proliferative diabetic retinopathy (**a**) and another patient with hypertensive retinopathy (**b**) showing co-existing hard exudates (black arrows) and soft exudates (red arrows) in the posterior pole. Hard exudates are seen as yellow-white deposits with a glistening appearance and sharp margins, while soft exudates are seen as greyish-white lesions with fudgy borders

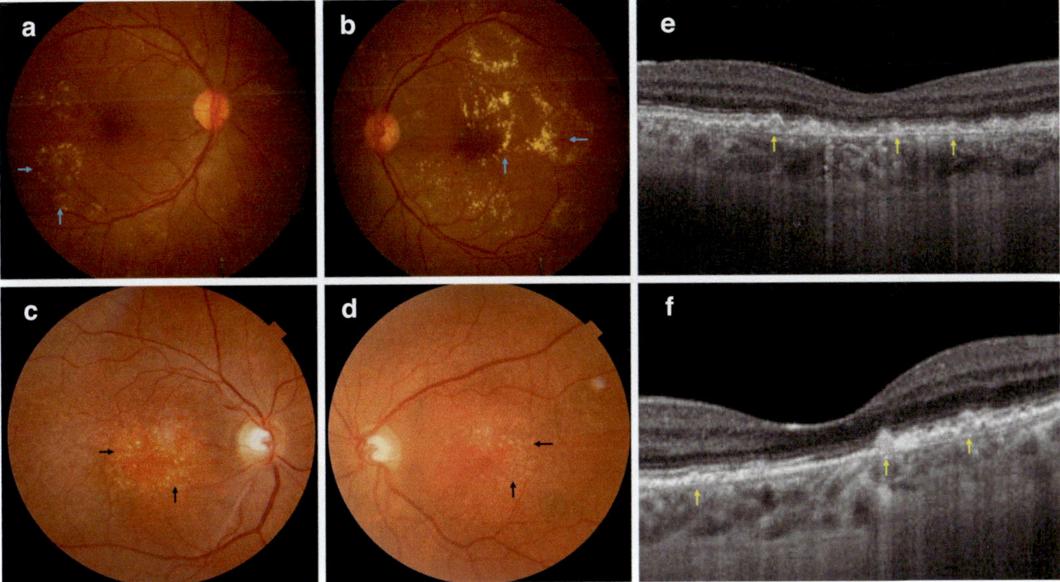

Fig. 4.4 Retinal hard exudates (blue arrows) in a patient with moderate non-proliferative diabetic retinopathy (**a** and **b**), seen as yellow-white deposits, having a waxy glistening appearance and sharp margins. In contrast, the retinal hard drusen (black arrows) in a patient with dry age-related macular degeneration (**c** and **d**) are seen as yellowish nodular lesions, deeper and more discrete than hard exudates. Optical coherence tomography (**e** and **f**) in the patient with dry age-related macular degeneration reveals the location of hard drusen seen as excrescences (yellow arrows) deep to the basal cell membrane of the retinal pigment epithelium (RPE) cells in Bruch's membrane

are seen in clusters deeper into the neurosensory retina and typically arise as excrescences located deep to the basal cell membrane of the retinal pigment epithelial cells in Bruch's membrane. Drusen may be hard or soft. The hard drusen are yellowish nodular lesions less than 63 μm in size. These are discrete, variable in number, and have sharp borders (Fig. 4.4). On the other hand,

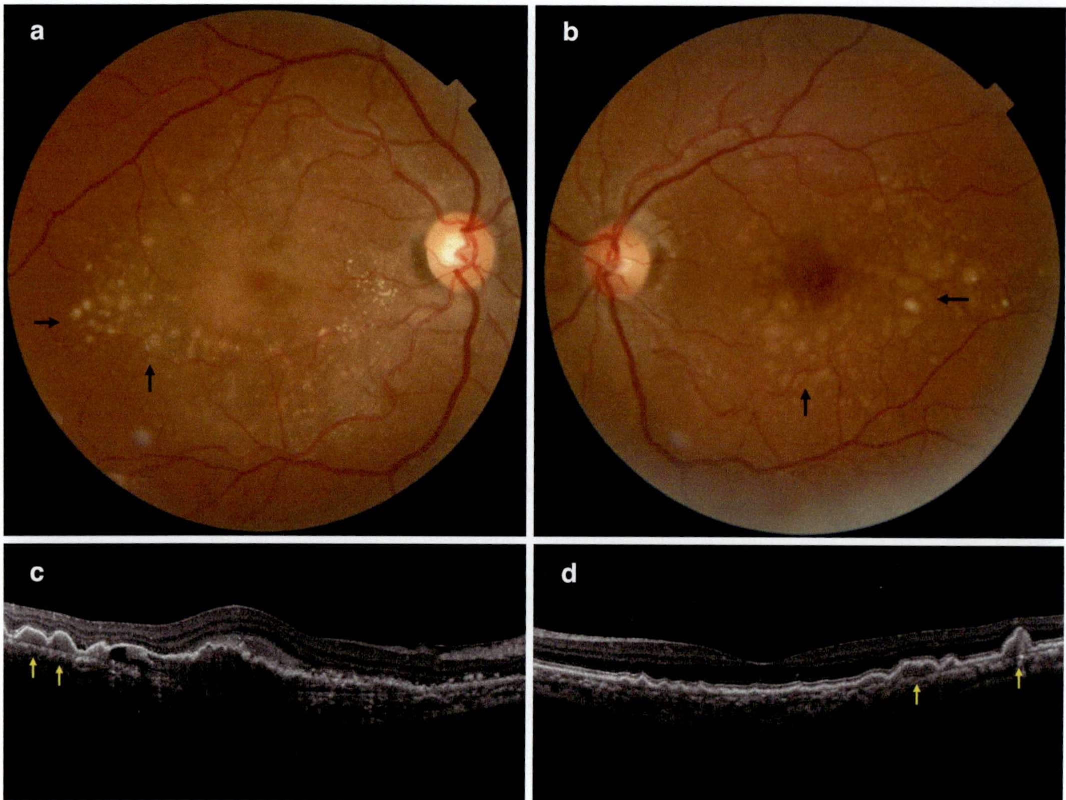

Fig. 4.5 Soft drusen (black arrows) in a patient with right eye neovascular (**a**) and left eye intermediate (**b**) age-related macular degeneration, seen as pale-yellow deposits, larger in size and more confluent than hard drusen, with ill-defined borders. Optical coherence tomography (**c** and **d**) shows them as large excrescences (yellow arrows) under the RPE cells

the soft drusen are larger pale-yellow deposits under the RPE and have an ill-defined border (Fig. 4.5). These may be discrete and tend to become confluent over time. These may be associated with both hypo and hyperpigmentary changes. The hard and the soft drusen increase over time [1].

4.4 Classification of Retinal Hard Exudates [2]

Retinal hard exudates are classified according to the modified Airlie House classification based on standard stereoscopic fundus photographs. The area occupied by hard exudates in the standard fundus photographs 3, 4, and 5 are used for evaluating the severity of hard exudates. Grade 0 = no hard exudates; Grade 1 = questionable hard exudates; Grade 2 = definitive hard exudates but less than those shown in standard fundus photograph #3; Grade 3 = hard exudates equal to or greater than shown in standard photograph # 3 but less than that shown in photograph # 5; Grade 4 = hard exudates equal or more than shown in photograph # 5 but less than shown in photograph # 4; Grade 5 is hard exudates greater or equal to those shown in photograph 4; and Grade 8 = cannot grade.

4.5 Significance of Retinal Hard Exudates

In recent years there has been immense interest in the automated detection of diabetic retinopathy from 2-D retinal photographs using machine learning and artificial intelligence algorithms. While the microaneurysms and dot haemorrhages are coloured red, the hard exudates, cotton wool spots, and the drusen may look similar [3]. Contextual presence of the lesions, e.g., microaneurysms and hard exudates in the context of retinal vessels, may help differentiate them from drusen, which are discrete without any context to the retinal vessels. Semiautomatic algorithms have also been attempted to detect and grade the severity of hard exudates from colour fundus pictures [4].

4.6 Formation of Retinal Hard Exudates

Retinal hard exudates are formed when plasma leaks from the microaneurysms (MAs) and the retinal capillaries with a damaged endothelial barrier. The retina is tightly packed with cells in all its layers except the inner and outer plexiform layers, which have a potential space for fluid collection. Most leaking microaneurysms are located in the inner nuclear layer (INL); hence, the fluid tends to collect in the outer plexiform layer. The leaked fluid can move back into the intravascular compartment of the neighbouring, still normal, capillaries leaving behind the macromolecules consisting of the lipoprotein–cholesterol complex that is seen as yellow-white shiny hard exudates. The area of abnormal leaky MAs thus gets surrounded by incomplete or complete rings of hard exudates called circinate retinopathy (Fig. 4.6). There may be one or many rings of these deposits in the posterior pole of the retina. This appears to be a dynamic process, and as the new exudates are getting deposited, the older ones are getting phagocytosed by the microglia, the retinal macrophages carry these to the vessel walls where their contents may be discharged into the lumen or remain in the vessel walls.

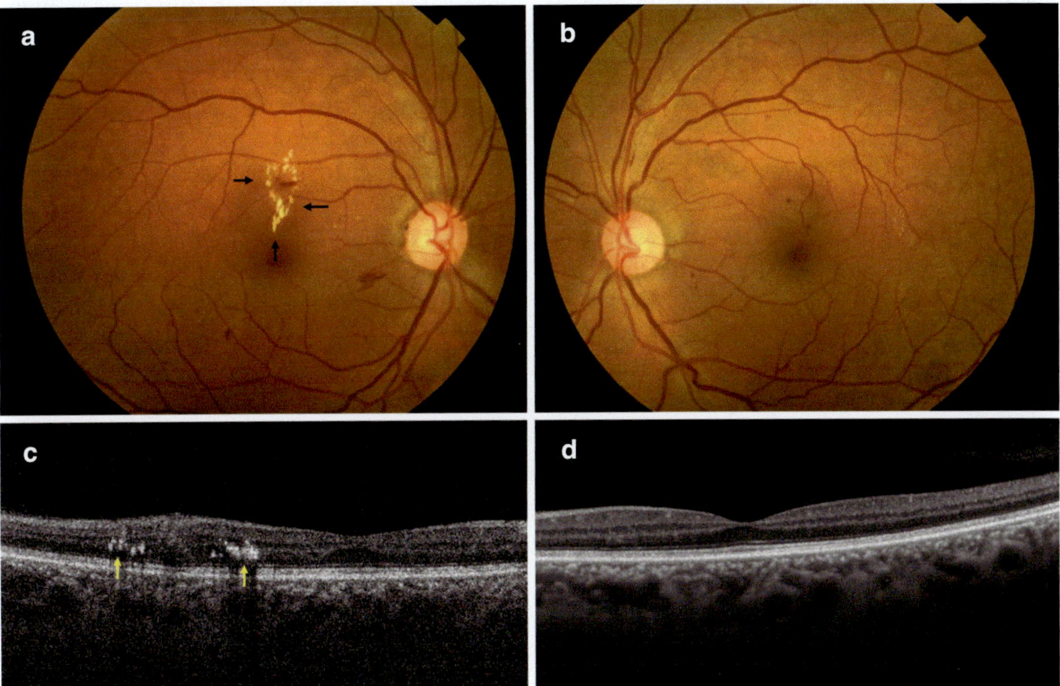

Fig. 4.6 A complete ring of hard exudates, known as circinate retinopathy (black arrows), is seen in the right eye (**a**) of a patient with moderate non-proliferative diabetic retinopathy, The left eye (**b**) shows only microaneurysms and dot haemorrhages. Optical coherence tomography shows the leaked lipoproteins and fluid in the outer plexiform layer as hyper-reflective foci (yellow arrows) in the right eye (**c**), while the left eye scan (**d**) appears normal due to the absence of any leakage so far from the microaneurysms

Ultimately, homeostasis is reached in the retinal microenvironment, which remains static or worsens over time until an intervention to stop fluid leakage from the MAs reverses the pathology. Using a high-resolution real-time camera employing adaptive optics, two patterns of hard exudates can be observed. Those associated with the resolution of macular oedema are associated with the breaking down of aggregates into smaller foci. In persistent macular oedema, smaller exudates get aggregated into larger ones. These changes happen over a short time and are not assessable clinically [5].

4.7 Hyperreflective Foci as Forme Fruste of Retinal Hard Exudates

Using optical coherence tomography (OCT), Bolz et al. [6] described the presence of highly characteristic and well-demarcated hyperreflective foci (HF) in the retina in eyes with diabetic macular oedema. These HF could not be appreciated clinically either on fundoscopy or conventional fundus or infrared imaging and were seen distributed throughout the thickness of the neurosensory retina. These were seen in the walls of the microaneurysms and retinal vessels. These HF had the same hyperreflective character as the hard exudates and correlated well when the hard exudates were present in aggregates. Most of these were plaque lesions in the outer plexiform layer and its junction with the outer nuclear layer. Bolz et al. [6] believed that the HF represented extravasated lipids from microaneurysms. Previously, Cusick et al. [7] using immunofluorescent and lipid histochemistry techniques, had demonstrated a heavy deposition of apolipoprotein B and cholesteryl ester (components of LDL) in the perivascular space in the retina, foam cells, and heavy infiltration by macrophages. It was also proposed that the efflux of lipids by endocytosis by macrophages can overcome the influx of lipids following treatment with lipid-lowering agents and laser photocoagulation [7]. On adaptive optics scanning laser ophthalmoscopy, irrespective of the cause of macular oedema, two types of hard exudates are seen—(1) round and (2) irregular. The round hard exudates are about 27 μm in size (macrophage = 20 μm) and are likely to be swollen macrophages due to endocytosis of lipids. The hyperreflective foci (HF) seen on OCT are likely the round lesions seen on adaptive optics-scanning laser ophthalmoscope (AO-SLO) ophthalmoscopy. Notably, histopathological studies have shown the presence of foam cells in hard exudates, which are lipid-filled macrophages or retinal microglia. The round lesions evolve into the irregular type, likely representing the bursting of macrophages and deposition of extravascular lipids and hyaline material. These extravasated lipids may be responsible for the persistent hard exudates in patients with diabetes, as the macrophages are believed to be dysfunctional in patients with diabetes [8]. After the initial discovery of HF [6], several other reports have confirmed the presence of these HF in the early stages of diabetic retinopathy and diabetic macular oedema [9, 10].

In diabetic macular oedema, HF are nearly always present in the inner retina, but as many as 50% of eyes may have these in the outer retina. The HF in the outer retina are associated with disruptions in the external limiting membrane, IS/OS junction and poorer visual acuity [11]. The absence of HF, intact IS/OS (ellipsoid zone), and the presence of subretinal fluid are OCT biomarkers for the improvement of vision following the use of DEXA implants in patients with naïve or chronic diabetic macular oedema [12]. The HF seen in the diabetic macular oedema get resolved by the DEXA implants and the anti-vascular endothelial growth factor (VEGF) agents (Fig. 4.7) [13]. However, the anti-VEGF agents cause a dynamic shift of these HF from the inner to the outer retinal layers suggesting an inflammatory origin of these HF. These HF may be precursors of hard exudates, microglia-macrophages, degenerated photoreceptors, or migrated RPE cells (in age-related macular degeneration). Some of these HF are visible on fundoscopy as aggregates of hard exudates in the outer retinal layers [14]. On OCT, the HF are also seen in the subretinal fluid, which on resolution of the serous fluid get deposited as hard exudates [15, 16].

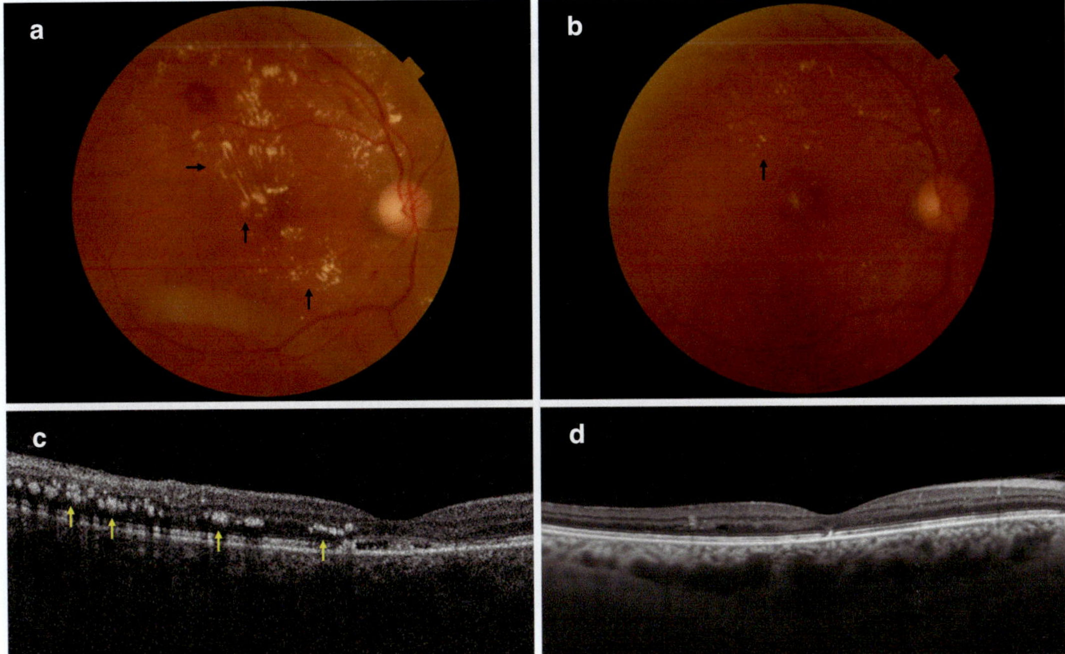

Fig. 4.7 Fundus photograph showing hard exudates (black arrows) in moderate non-proliferative diabetic retinopathy at presentation (**a**). Following intravitreal injections of anti-VEGF therapy, hard exudates (black arrows) are significantly resolved at 6 months (**b**). Optical coherence tomography shows dense hyperreflective foci (yellow arrows) in the outer plexiform layers before treatment (**c**), which resolved almost completely after treatment (**d**)

Contiguous hyperreflective dots lining the cystic cavities in the outer plexiform layer have been called 'Pearl necklace sign'. These HF are believed to be formed by lipid-laden macrophages [17]. Patients with diabetic macular oedema have hyperreflective cystic spaces, most of which have associated HF. On the resolution of hyperreflective cystic spaces, nearly one-third show the deposition of hard exudates in the same area [18].

On OCT angiography, the HF may be seen in intraretinal cysts as non-vascular decorrelation signals representing suspended scattering particles in motion (SSPiM) which may determine the response to treatment. Following treatment with intravitreal corticosteroids, the intraretinal cysts are seen to respond to the treatment. However, the cysts with the SSPiM do not seem to respond, and this sign may serve as a useful treatment response biomarker in diabetic macular oedema [19]. Earlier, it was shown that the SSPiM arise from the intraretinal cysts containing hyperreflective material/HF. Most of which are seen in Henle's fibre layer. These cysts consist of suspended lipid particles in the fluid and produce non-vascular decorrelation signals from the movement of these particles in the cystic fluid. When some of these patients were followed, the resolution of these cysts resulted in the formation of hard exudates [20]. Decorrelation signals in Henle's fibre layer were associated with the HF but not with HF in the INL. On OCTA, HF were seen attached to the capillaries in the INL [21]. Using quantitative data automatically extracted from the colour fundus photographs and SD-OCT, a high degree of correlation between HF and hard exudates was shown for different stages of diabetic retinopathy [22]. Some of the HF in the inner or outer retina are too small to be visible in fundus pictures. Still, the HF are likely to be precursors of the hard exudates.

It has been our experience that following the resolution of diabetic macular oedema, irrespective of the intervention, the hard exudates tend to move posteriorly and centrally, get aggregated, and deposited under the fovea. Concomitant use of statins to decrease the LDL and triglyceride levels in patients with diabetic macular oedema is strongly recommended to prevent this complication [23]. Dramatic resolution of massive retinal hard exudates has been observed following statins [24].

4.8 Histopathology of Hard Exudates

There are hardly any histopathological studies in patients with diabetic retinopathy after the early studies in the 1950–1960s. One of the more recent immunohistochemical studies has shown the presence of oxidized apolipoprotein B100 (ApoB100), a marker for LDL, in the retina of diabetic eyes even without retinopathy but not in eyes from non-diabetic individuals. Moreover, there were increasing amounts of ApoB100 staining with increasing severity of retinopathy. Macrophages were co-localized with ApoB100 only in eyes with proliferative retinopathy. It was proposed that extravasated heavily oxidized-glycated LDL may lead to the apoptotic loss of pericytes even before the onset of clinical retinopathy [25].

4.9 Hard Exudates: A Surrogate for Atherosclerosis

Dyslipidaemia is an independent risk factor for cardiovascular complications of diabetes. It is well known that Apo-B LDL moves across the arterial wall extracellularly and more so in atherosclerotic arteries and sets up inflammation. Macrophage is the major immune cell in all stages of atherosclerosis and is derived from the progenitor cells of bone marrow origin [26]. Macrophages are functionally highly plastic cells capable of producing pro and anti-inflammatory microenvironments in the atheromatous plaque [27]. Lipids get deposited in the subendothelial space and later move into the media and even the adventitia of the arteries. In the early atherpomatous lesions the foam cells (lipid laden cells) are of monocytic origin but in late atheromatous lesions these are of myocytic origin. Macrophages play a role in the deposition of lipids by acting as opsonizers for myocytes and scavenging these deposits [28]. Macrophages carry scavenger receptors on their surface to phagocytose lipoprotein aggregates and modify LDL [26]. The pathology of the hard exudates is similar to atherosclerosis, perhaps the only difference being that atherosclerosis occurs in the artery walls, and hard exudates are deposited in the retina.

4.10 Serum Lipids and Diabetic Retinopathy

Notably, cholesterol and triacylglycerol (commonly called triglyceride) are hydrophobic and carried in the blood plasma in the core of hydrophilic complex proteins called apolipoproteins, making these soluble. Low-density lipoproteins (LDL) carry 70% of the total cholesterol and the remaining 30% is carried by high-density lipoproteins (HDL) [29]. Apolipoproteins act as a ligand to facilitate the entry of lipoproteins into the intracellular compartment of various cells. Apo-A is the structural protein associated with HDL and responsible for the accumulation of lipids in the peripheral tissues. In contrast, Apo-B is the protein of LDL and a predictor of cardiovascular disease. In recent years, the study of apolipoproteins as markers of lipid metabolic metabolism has drawn increasing attention. Serum levels of Apo B and the Apo B/Apo A1 ratio are positively associated with DR [30]. These are also the most significant metabolic risk factors for proliferative diabetic retinopathy (PDR) and clinically significant macular edema (CSME) [31].

4.10.1 Hyperlipidaemia and Diabetic Retinopathy

Hyperlipidaemia is a known risk factor for peripheral neuropathy, a microangiopathic complication of diabetes [32]. In the past, several attempts to explore the role of dyslipidaemia/hyperlipidaemia in the onset and progression of diabetic retinopathy had met with inconsistent results. More recently, however, a large prospective cohort study from Taiwan found a significant increase in the cumulative incidence of diabetic retinopathy and diabetic macular oedema but not the PDR in patients with diabetes and dyslipidaemia. Moreover, statins, the lipid-lowering agents, were protective in preventing the development of non-proliferative diabetic retinopathy [33]. Previously, lowering the cholesterol levels in younger-onset diabetics did not protect either the incidence or progression of diabetic retinopathy and diabetic macular oedema [34]. However, dyslipidaemia has always been associated with the severity of retinal hard exudates in diabetic retinopathy. In a large population-based study, the Wisconsin epidemiologic study diabetic retinopathy (WESDR), increasing cholesterol levels were associated with the severity of hard exudates in diabetic retinopathy in type 1 diabetic patients [35]. In a multicentric landmark trial, the early treatment diabetic retinopathy study (ETDRS), raised cholesterol and LDL levels at the baseline were twice as likely as the normal levels for the presence of hard exudates [36]. Moreover, reducing the lipid levels was associated with a 50% risk reduction in doubling the visual angle [36, 37].

Higher total and LDL cholesterol levels were associated with the severity of hard exudates in African-American patients with type 2 diabetes [38]. A similar association of elevated serum lipid levels with the severity of hard exudates in diabetic retinopathy was seen in the 'Atherosclerosis risk in communities' study wherein the carotid artery intima-medial wall thickness was associated with diabetic retinopathy [39].

Multicolour imaging may be superior to conventional colour fundus pictures for detecting hard exudates in the macula. Using multicolour retinal imaging, serum lipid levels were significantly associated with hard exudates in the macula [40].

4.10.2 Role of Statins in Hard Exudates

Notably, increasing severity of hard exudates is associated with increasing vision impairment. Although limited by small numbers, early trials showed the effectiveness of using either simvastatin [41] or atorvastatin [23] for successfully lowering the LDL levels and improving diabetic macular oedema and/or disappearance of hard exudates (Fig. 4.8). These early studies laid the ground for establishing the role of using statins in lowering cholesterol and LDL in diabetic retinopathy patients. A more recent large-scale study from Taiwan has shown the protective effect of statin in decreasing the incidence of diabetic retinopathy and the need for treatment for vision-threatening retinopathy complications [42]. Similar conclusions were reached in a systematic review and meta-analysis of the use of statins [43]. Combining fenofibrate with simvastatin and tight glycemic control reduced the severity of diabetic retinopathy by 40% compared to the statins alone [44] or the need for laser photocoagulation by 31% [45, 46]. Among the patients with type I diabetes who participated in the diabetes control and complications trial (DCCT) trial, higher serum lipid levels, especially the total cholesterol to HDL ratio, were significantly associated with hard exudates and macular oedema. In the DCCT cohort (type 1 DM), inflammatory markers high sensitivity CRP and circulating levels of inter-cellular adhesion molecules-1 (ICAM-1) were significantly associated with clinically significant macular oedema and the severity of hard exudates [47]. These are well-established markers for coronary artery disease. It is well known that statins lower hs-CRP and ICAM-1, reduce the inflammatory activity of coronary artery atherosclerotic plaques, and improve endothelial dysfunction. [48]. It is recommended that among type 1 diabetics, statins not only decrease the risk of cardiovascular risk but reduce the risk of diabetic macular oedema and improve quality of life as well [49].

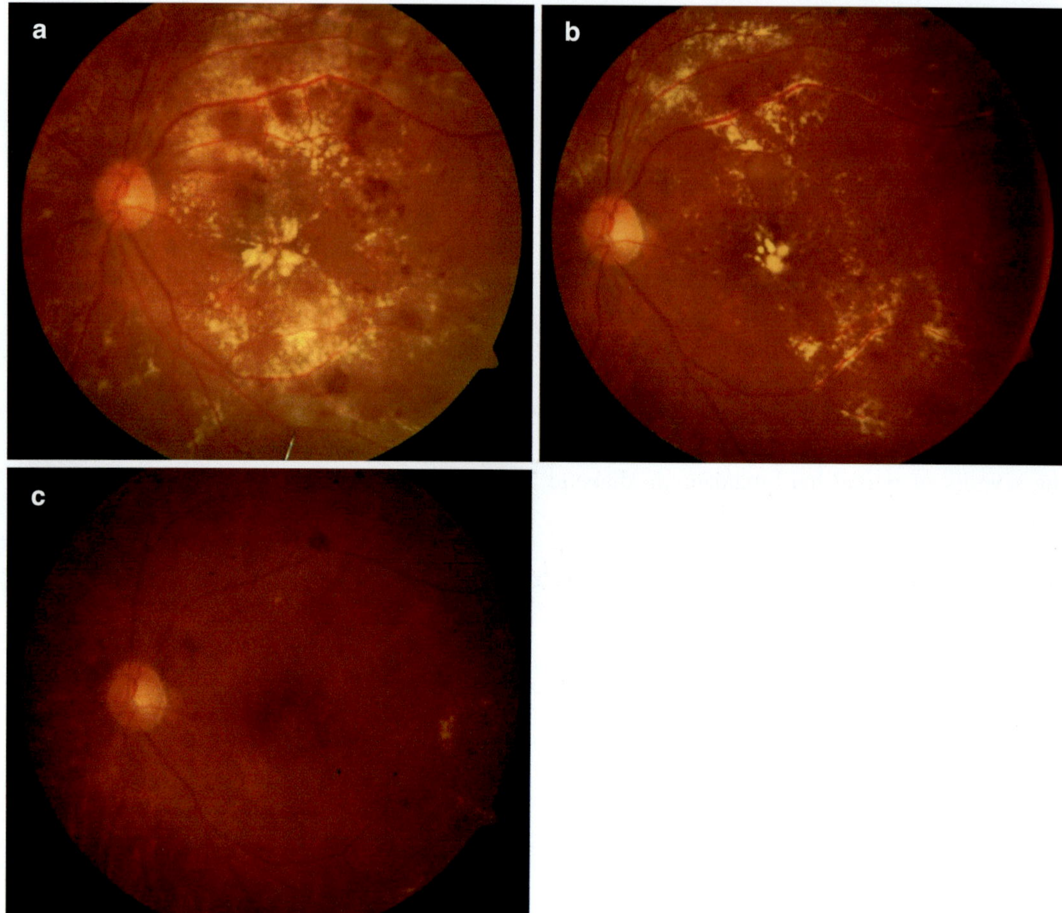

Fig. 4.8 Dense hard exudates (**a**) in a patient with diabetic macular oedema with hyperlipidaemia. Following the initiation of atorvastatin, there was a decrease in the hard exudates at one year (**b**), which resolved almost completely at 27 months (**c**)

4.11 Complications of Retinal Hard Exudates

Currently, the standard of care for managing diabetic macular oedema involves using either anti-VEGF or intravitreal steroids. Both have been found effective in reducing the extent of hard exudates in the macula, although steroids led to a quicker clearance of hard exudates [50]. If subfoveal hard exudates persist, they may develop subretinal fibrosis even following the standard of care intravitreal ranibizumab injections [51]. If under the fovea, these fibrous scars cause irreversible damage to the vision (Fig. 4.9). It should be noted that subretinal fibrosis is extremely uncommon in eyes with clinically significant macular oedema who do not have hard exudates. However, uncommonly, focal laser photocoagulation may also lead to subfoveal fibrosis. The risk factors for subretinal fibrosis noted in the ETDRS study were the extent and severity of hard exudates and elevated levels of serum lipids (total cholesterol and triglyceride). Subretinal fibrosis is a mound-like plaque under the retina [52]. A clinicopathological study of subretinal fibrous plaque in a patient with diabetic retinopathy did not find any break in

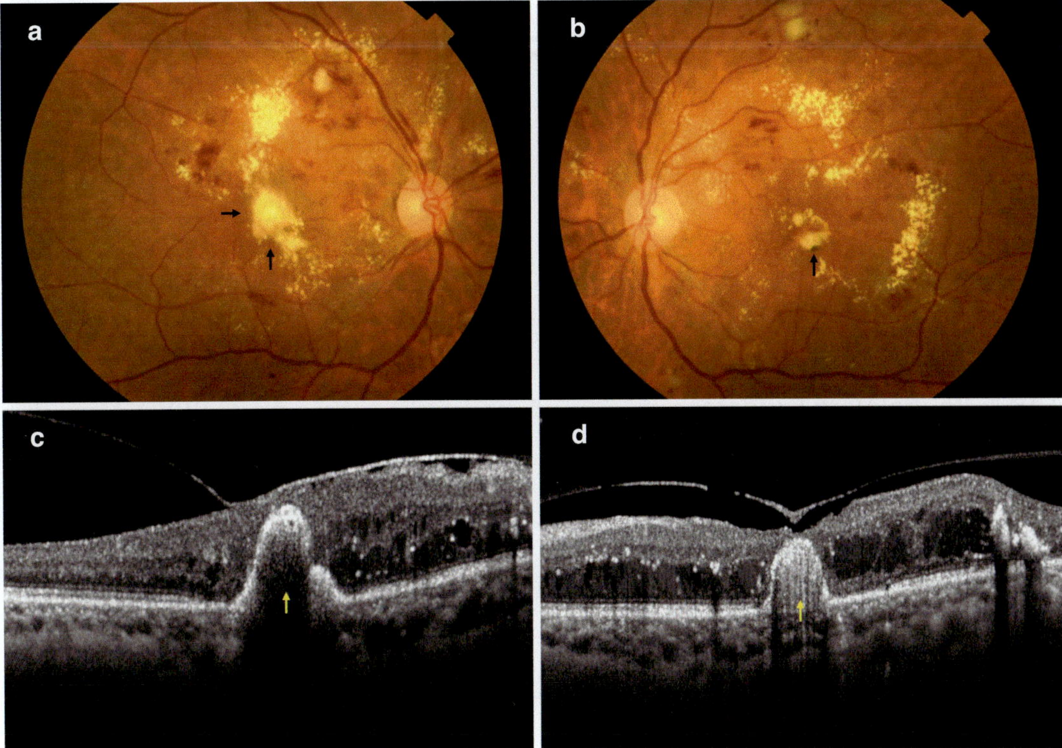

Fig. 4.9 Persistence of hard exudates leads to the development of subfoveal fibrosis (black arrows), which affects vision adversely (**a** and **b**). Optical coherence tomography (**c** and **d**) shows dense mound-like plaque (yellow arrows) under the fovea (**c** and **d**)

Bruch's membrane or the choroidal neovascular membrane, the common causes of subretinal scarring. The presence of the hard exudates itself was responsible for the fibrous plaque [53, 54]. To prevent this complication, attempts have been made to surgically wash out these hard exudates from under the neurosensory retina with a balanced salt solution, using a 38-size cannula through a hole created in the retina in the macular area [55]. These plaque-like hard exudates have also been surgically excised [56].

4.12 Treatment of Retinal Hard Exudates Associated with Macular Oedema

Currently, the standard of care for treating macular oedema associated with either diabetic retinopathy or retinal vascular occlusions involves monthly injections of an anti-VEGF injection. Intravitreal corticosteroids such as long-acting triamcinolone acetonide or slow-release depot steroids like DEXA implants, such as Ozurdex (Allergan, Inc., Irvine, CA, USA) or fluocinolone implants, Iluvien 0.19 mg (Alimera Sciences Ltd., Alpharetta, Georgia, USA) or the Fluocinolone 0.18 mg Yutiq (EyePoint Pharmaceuticals Pvt. Ltd., Watertown, Massachusetts), are used as a second-line treatment for patients who are either non-responders to the anti-VEGF therapy or have a chronic persistent macular oedema. Monthly ranibizumab injections in diabetic macular oedema resulted in the resolution of intraretinal hard exudates in parallel with macular thickness and volume resolution [57]. Likewise, the rapid resolution of hard exudates is seen with intravitreal triamcinolone acetonide [58]. In the RISE and RIDE trials, intravitreal ranibizumab was associated with a significant decrease in hard exudates, albeit more gradual than the retinal oedema. Contrary to expectations, there was no increase in the hard exudates following this treatment [59]. The bevacizumab and DEXA implant effectively reduced the area of hard exudates, although the response was quicker with steroids [50].

4.13 Other Causes of Retinal Hard Exudates

4.13.1 Retinal Hard Exudates in Branch Retinal Vein Occlusion

Next to diabetic retinopathy, branch retinal vein occlusion (BRVO) is the second most common retinal vascular disease. The major risk factors for the development of BRVO include increasing age, hypertension, history of cardiovascular disease, smoking, low HDL levels, high BMI at the age of 20, and focal arteriolar narrowing [60, 61]. The commonest site of BRVO is at the first or the second A-V crossing in the upper temporal quadrant or a little less common in the lower temporal quadrant. The next common is a macular vein occlusion that occurs when a small venous tributary draining the macula gets blocked. BRVO is accompanied by retinal haemorrhages and plasma fluid leakage due to the blood-retinal barrier's breakdown. By 3 months, most of the hemorrhages were absorbed, leaving behind macular oedema. At this time, a fundus fluorescein angiography (FFA) is performed to determine the status of perfusion in the territory of the occluded retinal vein. It may be a perfused or non-perused BRVO. Within 6 weeks to 6 months of BRVO, the retinal capillaries develop collateral channels across the horizontal raphe and start draining the blood/fluid via the venous channels in the opposite quadrant [62]. Nearly 80% of these eyes develop collateral channels to drain away the leaked fluid in the extravascular space [63], most of which are located in the deep capillary plexus of the retina [64]. Many of these collateral channels are leaky and may develop microaneurysms that continue to leak fluid [65] The leaked lipoproteins get deposited in the retina, most often in the macula as circinate rings (Fig. 4.10).

These circinate rings may mimic similar ring like exudates seen in diabetic retinopathy. However, unlike diabetic retinopathy, leaky vessels and microaneurysms in BRVO have a strict quadrantic distribution, although the hard exudates often cross the horizontal raphe. Thus, FFA plays an important role in distinguishing the two pathologies in these patients. In the last 15 years, intravitreal injections of anti-VEGF agents have supplanted gird laser photocoagulation for treating macular oedema due to BRVO. Many such agents have been tested in several controlled trials and have found almost equivalent results with the use of ranibizumab, bevacizumab, or aflibercept that need to be given initially every month for three injections and followed by a PRN (pro re nata) basis.

4.13.2 Retinal Hard Exudates in Adult Coats' Disease

Coats' disease is an uncommon unilateral sporadic disease of young children, mostly boys in the first two decades, characterized by telangiectatic retinal vessels in the periphery or midperiphery of the retina involving one or more quadrants [66]. While the disease is of uncertain origin, fundus fluorescein angiography shows highly characteristic large leaky microaneurysms and macroaneurysms visible as lighted bulbs. Leakage from the microaneurysms and the telangiectatic retinal vessels results in the deposition of the hard exudates in variable amounts on the retina and the subretinal space. Massive exudation may lead to a limited or total exudative retinal detachment. On histopathology, cholesterol crystals, ghost cells (histiocytes), and glial cells are seen in the inner retina. In contrast, the subretinal fibrinous exudates show lipid and pigment-laden macrophages and fibrous scars [67]. Massive mounds of lipids under the macula very often lead to extensive fibrous scar formation.

When seen in adults over 35 years, Coats' disease is more benign and less extensive. Notably, a proportion of these patients may have associ-

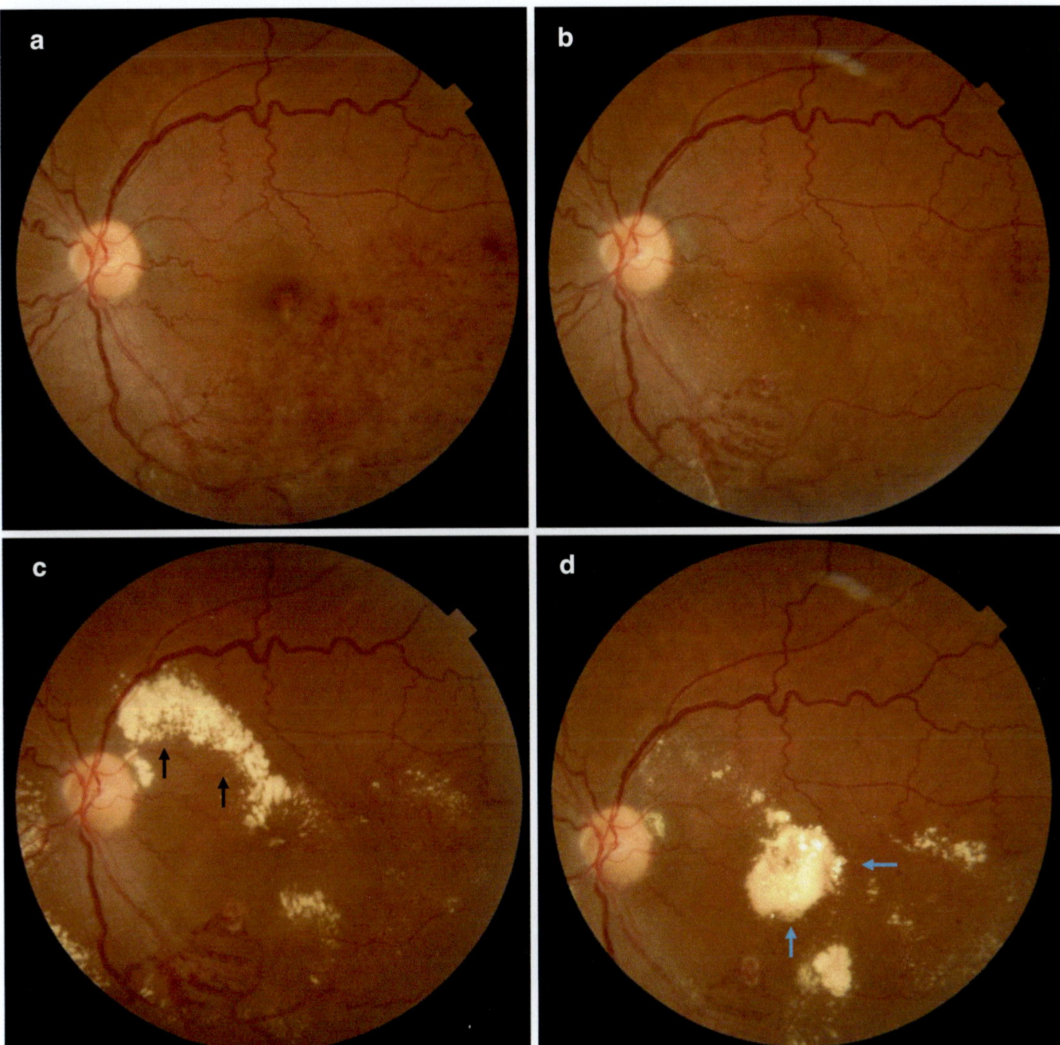

Fig. 4.10 A case with lower temporal branch retinal vein occlusion (**a**), showed resolution of retinal haemorrhages at 18 months (**b**) following intravitreal anti-VEGF therapy. At 30 months, hard exudates (black arrows) developed during the course (**c**), which migrated under the fovea and caused subfoveal fibrosis (blue arrow) at 42 months (**d**)

ated hypertension [68]. In the past patients of Coats' disease have been treated with laser photocoagulation of the retinal periphery and the microaneurysms or cryopexy of the retinal periphery. Significantly high levels of VEGF levels are found in Coats' disease [69]. More recently, anti-VEGF agents have been used in addition to laser photocoagulation to treat these patients [70]. There is evidence that proinflammatory cytokines and VEGF are also at elevated levels in Coats' disease [71], hence an increasing trend to combine laser photocoagulation, anti-VEGF agents, and periocular corticosteroids or even intravitreal DEXA implants. The recent advances in the management of Coats' disease were recently reviewed [72]. Nearly 90% of the patients show adequate response to treatment. The visual outcome is often limited due to submacular fibrosis caused by delays in seeking treatment.

4.13.3 Retinal Hard Exudates in Idiopathic Retinal Vasculitis, Aneurysms and Neuroretinitis (IRVAN)

IRVAN, an idiopathic retinal vasculitis, is a rare retinal disease of young people characterized by bilateral retinal vasculitis, arteriolar macroaneurysms, and neuroretinitis. In addition, usually, there are areas of peripheral capillary nonperfusion and retinal telangiectasia. Macular oedema with dense deposits of hard exudates often compromises vision (Fig. 4.11). The fusiform retinal arteriolar aneurysms at the branching of arterioles and on the optic disc are highly characteristic and best demonstrated in fundus fluorescein angiography (Figs. 4.11 and 4.12) [73]. Late complications involve retinal neovascularization and vitreous haemorrhage or traction retinal detachment. Rarely IRVAN may be complicated by branch retinal artery occlusion [74, 75]. The treatment has included laser photocoagulation of the ischemic peripheral retina and anti-VEGF agents, DEXA implants, and systemic immunosuppressive therapy. The subject was recently reviewed [73].

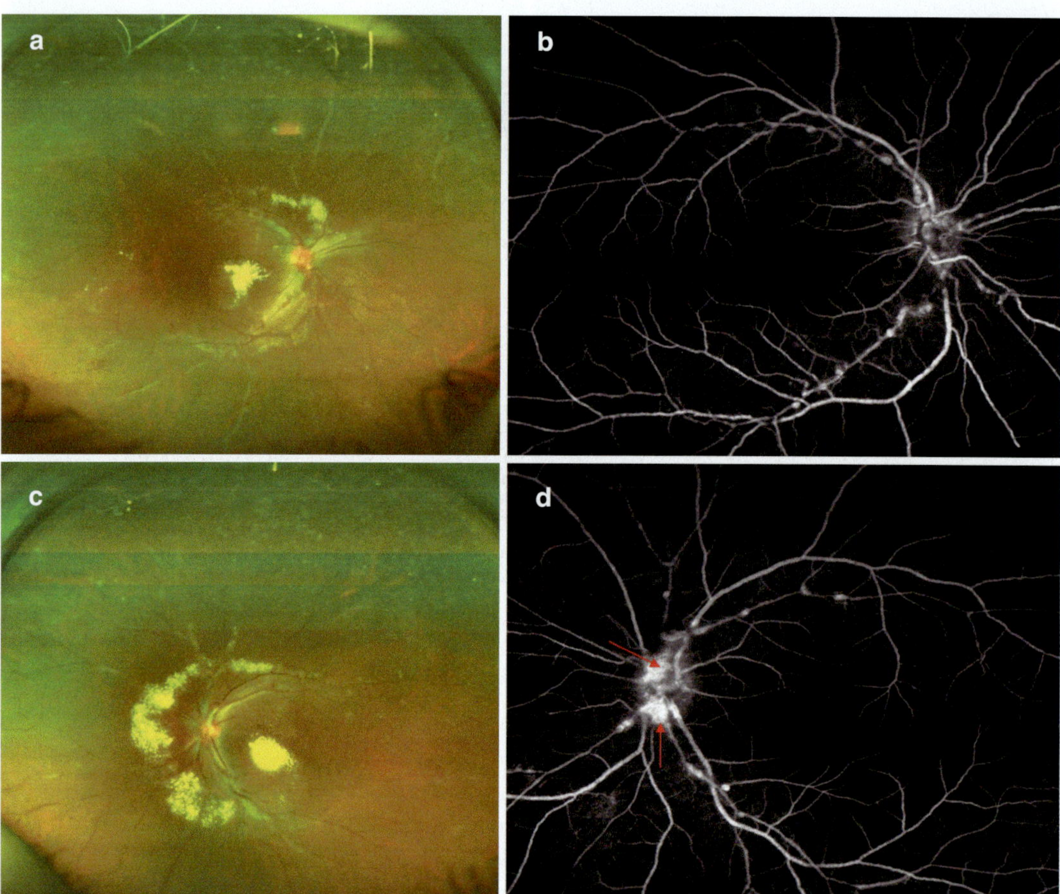

Fig. 4.11 A case of idiopathic retinal vasculitis, aneurysms, and neuroretinitis (IRVAN) shows massive hard exudates in the macula and peripapillary retina L > R (**a**, **c**). The fundus fluorescein angiography during the venous phase shows aneurysmal dilatations along the temporal retinal arterioles in both eyes (**b**, **d**). Note aneurysmal dilatations on the optic disc in the left eye (red arrows)

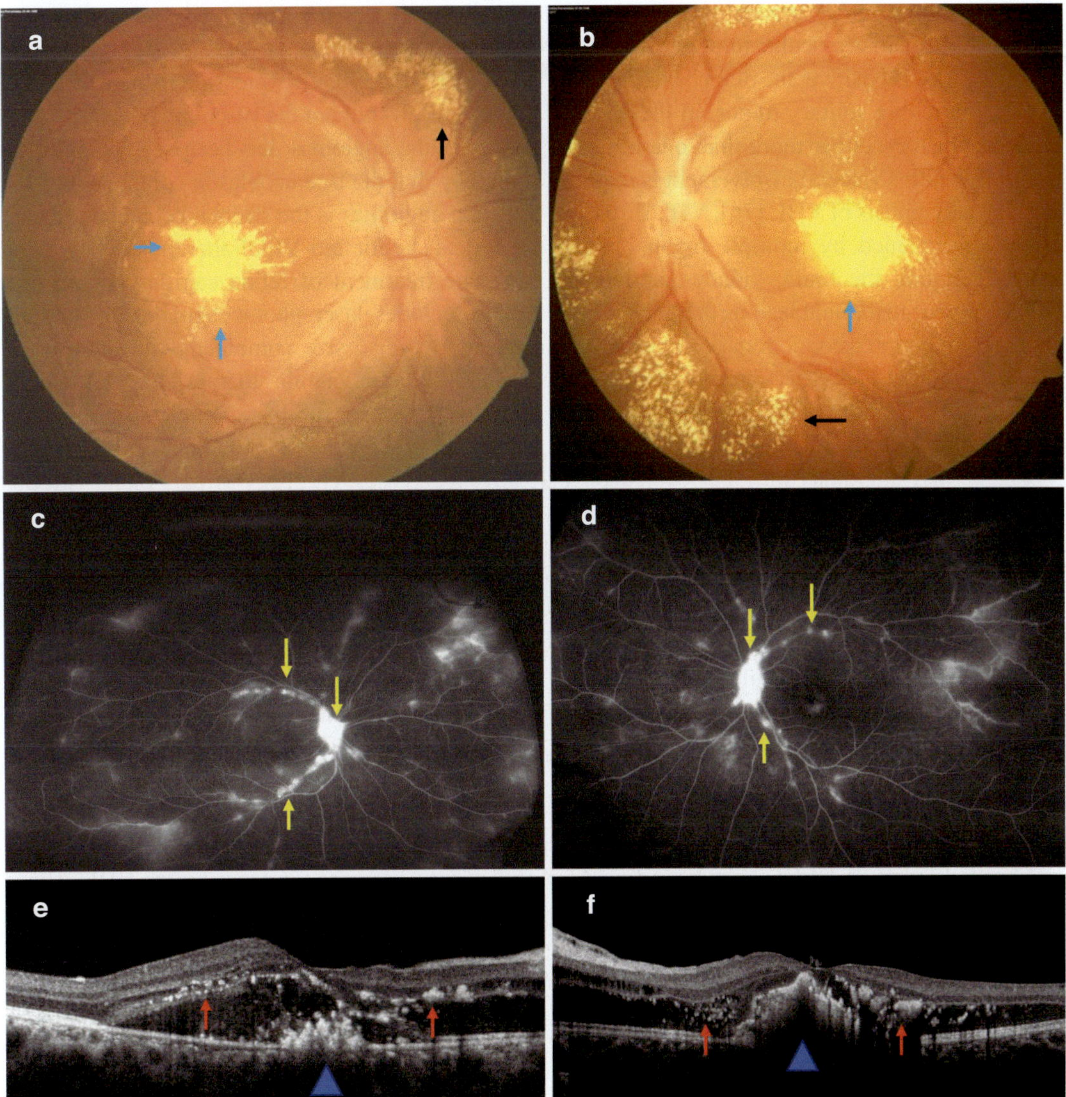

Fig. 4.12 A case of idiopathic retinal vasculitis, aneurysms, and neuroretinitis (IRVAN) having hard exudates (black arrows) and subfoveal fibrosis (blue arrows) in both eyes (**a** and **b**). Fundus fluorescein angiography (**c** and **d**) showed retinal arterial aneurysms along the arterioles and optic disc (yellow arrows). Optical coherence tomography (**e** and **f**) showed hard exudates (red arrows) lining the cavities containing subretinal fluid, and dense mound-like plaque under the fovea (blue arrowheads) corresponding to subfoveal fibrosis

4.13.4 Retinal Hard Exudates in Von Hippel–Lindau Disease

Retinal capillary hemangiomas are a rare retinal disorder of young people presenting either sporadically as a unilateral, monofocal disorder or as von Hippel –Lindau's (VHL) disease, an autosomal dominant disorder characterized by multifocal bilateral retinal capillary hemangiomas/hemangioblastoma. More than half of the retinal capillary hemangiomas/hemangioblastomas are sporadic and present at a median age of 36. If the patients with sporadic disease do not have systemic associations at the diagnosis, they are unlikely to progress to VHL. VHL appears at a median age of 18 years, and this distribution agrees with a two-hit model of the mutation responsible for many ocular tumors [76]. If the family history is positive, the diagnosis of VHL is made even with a solitary tumor; in the absence of family history, either more than one tumor or one tumor with a visceral involvement is required to make a diagnosis of VHL [76]. VHL disease is often accompanied by multiple organ involvement, including the brain, kidneys, and others with benign or malignant lesions that include cerebellar hemangioblastoma, renal cell cysts, renal cell carcinoma, and pheochromocytoma. The VHL gene is a tumor suppressor gene located on chromosome 3p25.5.

The retinal angiomas may be located on or near the optic disc or in the retinal periphery. Most patients with VHL first present to the ophthalmologists with massive hard exudates. The hemangioblastoma/angiomas are small and continue to grow and leak profusely, leading to massive hard exudates in the macula, prompting them to report vision loss (Fig. 4.13). The angiomas have a feeder arteriole and a drainage vein that are dilated. It may be difficult to tell the difference on a clinical exam, but it is readily identified on fundus fluorescein angiography.

Elevated levels of VEGF have been found in 80% of the aqueous humor of the eyes with retinal angiomas [77]. On histopathological studies, loss of heterozygosity of the VHL gene, co-localized with VEGF gene overexpression in the vacuolated stromal cells but not the vascular cells or the glial cells in the angiomas, has been seen, suggesting thereby that the true neoplastic component of the retinal angiomas is the stromal cells and thus are an ideal site for anti-VEGF therapy [78].

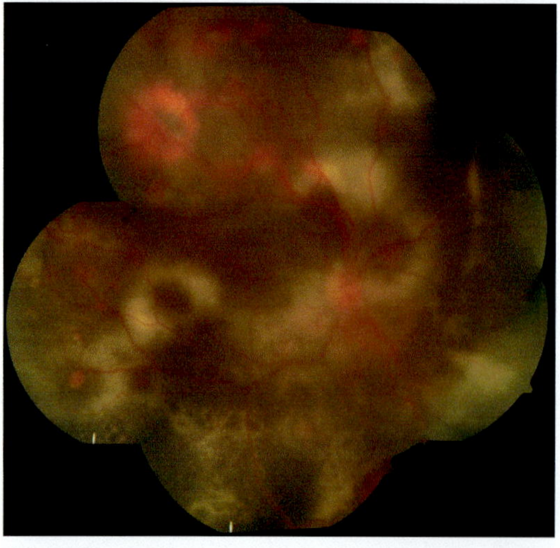

Fig. 4.13 Massive exudation with hard exudates seen with retinal angiomas in a patient with von Hippel–Lindau (VHL) disease

The treatment of retina capillary hemangiomas includes laser photocoagulation of tumors up to two-disc size combined with anti-VEGF agents. Photodynamic therapy has effectively controlled retinal capillary hemangiomas, including the VHL and the sporadic forms [79]. For advanced cases, cryopexy or pars plana vitreous surgery can often be done with poorer results than thermal laser photocoagulation.

4.13.4.1 Screening for VHL

Since VHL is a potentially lethal disease associated with benign lesions in several organs and renal cell carcinoma, it is recommended that patients with a positive family history or those at risk should undergo screening by a multidisciplinary team. Essentially, it consists of offering a DNA test to rule out mutation. A negative test rules out a life-long vigilance for the VHL. Those positive for the VHL mutation should undergo annual ophthalmological, neurological, and neuro-otological exams every 2–3 years starting in infancy. After 16 years, these examinations should be done annually, including checking for blood pressure, a plasma-free metanephrine test, or a 24-hour urine metanephrine test to rule out pheochromocytoma, and ultrasonography of the abdomen. MRI should be done every 2–3 years [80]. The details of screening guidelines can be seen on the website of the VHL Alliance. https://vhl.org/professionals/screening-diagnosis/importance-of-screening/ [80].

References

1. Ding X, Patel M, Chan CC. Molecular pathology of age-related macular degeneration. Prog Retin Eye Res. 2009;28(1):1–18. https://doi.org/10.1016/j.preteyeres.2008.10.001. Epub 2008 Nov 6. PMID: 19026761; PMCID: PMC2715284.

2. Early Treatment Diabetic Retinopathy Study Research Group. Grading diabetic retinopathy from stereoscopic colour fundus photographs—an extension of the modified Airlie House classification. ETDRS report number 10. Ophthalmology. 1991;98(5 Suppl):786–806. PMID: 2062513.
3. Niemeijer M, van Ginneken B, Russell SR, Suttorp-Schulten MS, Abràmoff MD. Automated detection and differentiation of drusen, exudates, and cotton-wool spots in digital color fundus photographs for diabetic retinopathy diagnosis. Invest Ophthalmol Vis Sci. 2007;48(5):2260–7. https://doi.org/10.1167/iovs.06-0996. PMID: 17460289; PMCID: PMC2739583.
4. Marupally AG, Vupparaboina KK, Peguda HK, Richhariya A, Jana S, Chhablani J. Semi-automated quantification of hard exudates in colour fundus photographs diagnosed with diabetic retinopathy. BMC Ophthalmol. 2017;17(1):172. https://doi.org/10.1186/s12886-017-0563-7. PMID: 28931389; PMCID: PMC5607622.
5. Loganadane P, Delbosc B, Saleh M. Short-term progression of diabetic hard exudates monitored with high-resolution camera. Ophthalmic Res. 2019;61(1):3–9. https://doi.org/10.1159/000493858. Epub 2018 Nov 22. PMID: 30466082.
6. Bolz M, Schmidt-Erfurth U, Deak G, Mylonas G, Kriechbaum K, Scholda C, Diabetic Retinopathy Research Group Vienna. Optical coherence tomographic hyperreflective foci: a morphologic sign of lipid extravasation in diabetic macular edema. Ophthalmology. 2009;116(5):914–20. https://doi.org/10.1016/j.ophtha.2008.12.039. PMID: 19410950.
7. Cusick M, Chew EY, Chan CC, Kruth HS, Murphy RP, Ferris FL 3rd. Histopathology and regression of retinal hard exudates in diabetic retinopathy after reduction of elevated serum lipid levels. Ophthalmology. 2003;110(11):2126–33. https://doi.org/10.1016/j.ophtha.2003.01.001. PMID: 14597519.
8. Yamaguchi M, Nakao S, Kaizu Y, Kobayashi Y, Nakama T, Arima M, Yoshida S, Oshima Y, Takeda A, Ikeda Y, Mukai S, Ishibashi T, Sonoda KH. High-resolution imaging by adaptive optics scanning laser ophthalmoscopy reveals two morphologically distinct types of retinal hard exudates. Sci Rep. 2016;6:33574. https://doi.org/10.1038/srep33574. Erratum in: Sci Rep 2016;6:35127. PMID: 27641223; PMCID: PMC5027520.
9. De Benedetto U, Sacconi R, Pierro L, Lattanzio R, Bandello F. Optical coherence tomographic hyperreflective foci in early stages of diabetic retinopathy. Retina. 2015;35(3):449–53. https://doi.org/10.1097/IAE.0000000000000336. PMID: 25170862.
10. Framme C, Schweizer P, Imesch M, Wolf S, Wolf-Schnurrbusch U. Behavior of SD-OCT-detected hyperreflective foci in the retina of anti-VEGF-treated patients with diabetic macular edema. Invest Ophthalmol Vis Sci. 2012;53(9):5814–8. https://doi.org/10.1167/iovs.12-9950. PMID: 22836760.
11. Uji A, Murakami T, Nishijima K, Akagi T, Horii T, Arakawa N, Muraoka Y, Ellabban AA, Yoshimura N. Association between hyperreflective foci in the outer retina, status of photoreceptor layer, and visual acuity in diabetic macular edema. Am J Ophthalmol. 2012;153(4):710–7, 717.e1. Epub 2011 Dec 3. PMID: 22137207. https://doi.org/10.1016/j.ajo.2011.08.041.
12. Zur D, Iglicki M, Busch C, Invernizzi A, Mariussi M, Loewenstein A, International Retina Group. OCT biomarkers as functional outcome predictors in diabetic macular edema treated with dexamethasone implant. Ophthalmology. 2018;125(2):267–75. https://doi.org/10.1016/j.ophtha.2017.08.031. Epub 2017 Sep 19. PMID: 28935399.
13. Schreur V, Altay L, van Asten F, Groenewoud JMM, Fauser S, Klevering BJ, Hoyng CB, de Jong EK. Hyperreflective foci on optical coherence tomography associate with treatment outcome for anti-VEGF in patients with diabetic macular edema. PLoS One. 2018;13(10):e0206482. https://doi.org/10.1371/journal.pone.0206482. PMID: 30379920; PMCID: PMC6209345.
14. Rübsam A, Wernecke L, Rau S, Pohlmann D, Müller B, Zeitz O, Joussen AM. Behavior of SD-OCT detectable hyperreflective foci in diabetic macular edema patients after therapy with anti-VEGF agents and dexamethasone implants. J Diabetes Res. 2021;2021:8820216. https://doi.org/10.1155/2021/8820216. PMID: 33937416; PMCID: PMC8060103.
15. Murakami T, Yoshimura N. Structural changes in individual retinal layers in diabetic macular edema. J Diabetes Res. 2013;2013:920713. https://doi.org/10.1155/2013/920713. Epub 2013 Aug 29. PMID: 24073417; PMCID: PMC3773460.
16. Ota M, Nishijima K, Sakamoto A, Murakami T, Takayama K, Horii T, Yoshimura N. Optical coherence tomographic evaluation of foveal hard exudates in patients with diabetic maculopathy accompanying macular detachment. Ophthalmology. 2010;117(10):1996–2002. https://doi.org/10.1016/j.ophtha.2010.06.019. Epub 2010 Aug 17. PMID: 20723993.
17. Gelman SK, Freund KB, Shah VP, Sarraf D. The pearl necklace sign: a novel spectral domain optical coherence tomography finding in exudative macular disease. Retina. 2014;34(10):2088–95. https://doi.org/10.1097/IAE.0000000000000207. PMID: 25020214.
18. Couturier A, Mane V, Lavia CA, Tadayoni R. Hyperreflective cystoid spaces in diabetic macular oedema: prevalence and clinical implications. Br J Ophthalmol. 2022;106(4):540–6. https://doi.org/10.1136/bjophthalmol-2020-317191. Epub 2020 Dec 1. PMID: 33262106.
19. Ahn J, Han S, Ahn SM, Kim SW, Oh J. Clinical implications of suspended scattering particles in motion observed by optical coherence tomography angiography. Sci Rep. 2020;10(1):15. https://doi.org/10.1038/s41598-019-55606-9. PMID: 31913306; PMCID: PMC6949280.

20. Kashani AH, Green KM, Kwon J, Chu Z, Zhang Q, Wang RK, Garrity S, Sarraf D, Rebhun CB, Waheed NK, Schaal KB, Munk MR, Gattoussi S, Freund KB, Zheng F, Liu G, Rosenfeld PJ. Suspended scattering particles in motion: a novel feature of OCT angiography in exudative maculopathies. Ophthalmol Retina. 2018;2(7):694–702. https://doi.org/10.1016/j.oret.2017.11.004. Epub 2017 Dec 15. PMID: 30221214; PMCID: PMC6133252.
21. Murakami T, Suzuma K, Dodo Y, Yoshitake T, Yasukura S, Nakanishi H, Fujimoto M, Oishi M, Tsujikawa A. Decorrelation signal of diabetic hyperreflective foci on optical coherence tomography angiography. Sci Rep. 2018;8(1):8798. https://doi.org/10.1038/s41598-018-27192-9. PMID: 29892079; PMCID: PMC5995832.
22. Niu S, Yu C, Chen Q, Yuan S, Lin J, Fan W, Liu Q. Multimodality analysis of hyper-reflective foci and hard exudates in patients with diabetic retinopathy. Sci Rep. 2017;7(1):1568. https://doi.org/10.1038/s41598-017-01733-0. PMID: 28484225; PMCID: PMC5431476.
23. Gupta A, Gupta V, Thapar S, Bhansali A. Lipid-lowering drug atorvastatin as an adjunct in the management of diabetic macular edema. Am J Ophthalmol. 2004;137(4):675–82. https://doi.org/10.1016/j.ajo.2003.11.017. PMID: 15059707.
24. Waller S, Thyagarajan S, Kaplan F, Viljoen A. Dramatic resolution of massive retinal hard exudates after correction of extreme dyslipidaemia. Eye (Lond). 2009;23(3):738. https://doi.org/10.1038/eye.2008.109. PMID: 18437181.
25. Wu M, Chen Y, Wilson K, Chirindel A, Ihnat MA, Yu Y, Boulton ME, Szweda LI, Ma JX, Lyons TJ. Intraretinal leakage and oxidation of LDL in diabetic retinopathy. Invest Ophthalmol Vis Sci. 2008;49(6):2679–85. https://doi.org/10.1167/iovs.07-1440. Epub 2008 Mar 24. PMID: 18362112.
26. Tabas I, Bornfeldt KE. Macrophage phenotype and function in different stages of atherosclerosis. Circ Res. 2016;118(4):653–67. https://doi.org/10.1161/CIRCRESAHA.115.306256. PMID: 26892964; PMCID: PMC4762068.
27. Yang D, Yang L, Cai J, Hu X, Li H, Zhang X, Zhang X, Chen X, Dong H, Nie H, Li Y. A sweet spot for macrophages: focusing on polarization. Pharmacol Res. 2021;167:105576. https://doi.org/10.1016/j.phrs.2021.105576. Epub 2021 Mar 24. PMID: 33771700.
28. Wolman M, Gaton E. Reappraisal of the role of macrophages in the pathogenesis of atherosclerosis. Pathobiology. 1991;59(2):92–5. https://doi.org/10.1159/000163622. PMID: 1863356.
29. Lim LS, Wong TY. Lipids and diabetic retinopathy. Expert Opin Biol Ther. 2012;12(1):93–105. https://doi.org/10.1517/14712598.2012.641531.
30. Chang YC, Wu WC. Dyslipidemia and diabetic retinopathy. Rev Diabet Stud. 2013;10(2–3):121–32. https://doi.org/10.1900/RDS.2013.10.121. Epub 2013 Aug 10. PMID: 24380088; PMCID: PMC4063092.
31. Crosby-Nwaobi R, Chatziralli I, Sergentanis T, Dew T, Forbes A, Sivaprasad S. Cross talk between lipid metabolism and inflammatory markers in patients with diabetic retinopathy. J Diabetes Res. 2015;2015:191382. https://doi.org/10.1155/2015/191382. Epub 2015 Jul 29. PMID: 26295054; PMCID: PMC4532932.
32. Vincent AM, Hinder LM, Pop-Busui R, Feldman EL. Hyperlipidemia: a new therapeutic target for diabetic neuropathy. J Peripher Nerv Syst. 2009;14(4):257–67. https://doi.org/10.1111/j.1529--8027.2009.00237.x. PMID: 20021567; PMCID: PMC4239691.
33. Jeng CJ, Hsieh YT, Yang CM, Yang CH, Lin CL, Wang IJ. Diabetic retinopathy in patients with dyslipidemia: development and progression. Ophthalmol Retina. 2018;2(1):38–45. https://doi.org/10.1016/j.oret.2017.05.010. Epub 2017 Aug 9. PMID: 31047300.
34. Klein BE, Klein R, Moss SE. Is serum cholesterol associated with progression of diabetic retinopathy or macular edema in persons with younger-onset diabetes of long duration? Am J Ophthalmol. 1999;128(5):652–4. https://doi.org/10.1016/s0002-9394(99)00222-6. PMID: 10577544.
35. Klein BE, Moss SE, Klein R, Surawicz TS. The Wisconsin Epidemiologic Study of Diabetic Retinopathy. XIII. Relationship of serum cholesterol to retinopathy and hard exudate. Ophthalmology. 1991;98(8):1261–5. https://doi.org/10.1016/s0161-6420(91)32145-6. PMID: 1923364.
36. Chew EY, Klein ML, Ferris FL 3rd, Remaley NA, Murphy RP, Chantry K, Hoogwerf BJ, Miller D. Association of elevated serum lipid levels with retinal hard exudate in diabetic retinopathy. Early Treatment Diabetic Retinopathy Study (ETDRS) Report 22. Arch Ophthalmol. 1996;114(9):1079–84. https://doi.org/10.1001/archopht.1996.01100140281004. PMID: 8790092.
37. Ferris FL 3rd, Chew EY, Hoogwerf BJ. Serum lipids and diabetic retinopathy. Early Treatment Diabetic Retinopathy Study Research Group. Diabetes Care. 1996;19(11):1291–3. https://doi.org/10.2337/diacare.19.11.1291. PMID: 8908399.
38. Papavasileiou E, Davoudi S, Roohipoor R, Cho H, Kudrimoti S, Hancock H, Wilson JG, Andreoli C, Husain D, James M, Penman A, Chen CJ, Sobrin L. Association of serum lipid levels with retinal hard exudate area in African Americans with type 2 diabetes. Graefes Arch Clin Exp Ophthalmol. 2017;255(3):509–17. https://doi.org/10.1007/s00417-016-3493-9. Epub 2016 Sep 15. PMID: 27632216.
39. Klein R, Sharrett AR, Klein BE, Moss SE, Folsom AR, Wong TY, Brancati FL, Hubbard LD, Couper D, ARIC Group. The association of atherosclerosis, vascular risk factors, and retinopathy in adults with diabetes: the atherosclerosis risk in communities study. Ophthalmology. 2002;109(7):1225–34. https://doi.org/10.1016/s0161-6420(02)01074-6. PMID: 12093643.

40. Gong R, Han R, Guo J, Liu W, Xu G. Quantitative evaluation of hard exudates in diabetic macular edema by multicolor imaging and their associations with serum lipid levels. Acta Diabetol. 2021;58(9):1161–7. https://doi.org/10.1007/s00592-021-01697-8. Epub ahead of print. PMID: 33811294.
41. Sen K, Misra A, Kumar A, Pandey RM. Simvastatin retards progression of retinopathy in diabetic patients with hypercholesterolemia. Diabetes Res Clin Pract. 2002;56(1):1–11. https://doi.org/10.1016/s0168-8227(01)00341-2. PMID: 11879715.
42. Kang EY, Chen TH, Garg SJ, Sun CC, Kang JH, Wu WC, Hung MJ, Lai CC, Cherng WJ, Hwang YS. Association of statin therapy with prevention of vision-threatening diabetic retinopathy. JAMA Ophthalmol. 2019;137(4):363–71. https://doi.org/10.1001/jamaophthalmol.2018.6399. PMID: 30629109; PMCID: PMC6459113.
43. Pranata R, Vania R, Victor AA. Statin reduces the incidence of diabetic retinopathy and its need for intervention: a systematic review and meta-analysis. Eur J Ophthalmol. 2021;31(3):1216–24. https://doi.org/10.1177/1120672120922444. Epub ahead of print. PMID: 32530705.
44. ACCORD Study Group; ACCORD Eye Study Group, Chew EY, Ambrosius WT, Davis MD, Danis RP, Gangaputra S, Greven CM, Hubbard L, Esser BA, Lovato JF, Perdue LH, Goff DC Jr, Cushman WC, Ginsberg HN, Elam MB, Genuth S, Gerstein HC, Schubart U, Fine LJ. Effects of medical therapies on retinopathy progression in type 2 diabetes. N Engl J Med. 2010;363(3):233–44. https://doi.org/10.1056/NEJMoa1001288. Epub 2010 Jun 29. Erratum in: N Engl J Med. 2011 Jan 13;364(2):190. Erratum in: N Engl J Med. 2012 Dec 20;367(25):2458. PMID: 20587587; PMCID: PMC4026164.
45. Kawasaki R, Konta T, Nishida K. Lipid-lowering medication is associated with decreased risk of diabetic retinopathy and the need for treatment in patients with type 2 diabetes: a real-world observational analysis of a health claims database. Diabetes Obes Metab. 2018;20(10):2351–60. https://doi.org/10.1111/dom.13372. Epub 2018 Jun 21. PMID: 29790265.
46. Keech AC, Mitchell P, Summanen PA, O'Day J, Davis TM, Moffitt MS, Taskinen MR, Simes RJ, Tse D, Williamson E, Merrifield A, Laatikainen LT, d'Emden MC, Crimet DC, O'Connell RL, Colman PG, FIELD Study Investigators. Effect of fenofibrate on the need for laser treatment for diabetic retinopathy (FIELD study): a randomised controlled trial. Lancet. 2007;370(9600):1687–97. https://doi.org/10.1016/S0140-6736(07)61607-9. Epub 2007 Nov 7. PMID: 17988728.
47. Muni RH, Kohly RP, Lee EQ, Manson JE, Semba RD, Schaumberg DA. Prospective study of inflammatory biomarkers and risk of diabetic retinopathy in the diabetes control and complications trial. JAMA Ophthalmol. 2013;131(4):514–21. https://doi.org/10.1001/jamaophthalmol.2013.2299. PMID: 23392399; PMCID: PMC3625475.
48. Diamantis E, Kyriakos G, Quiles-Sanchez LV, Farmaki P, Troupis T. The anti-inflammatory effects of statins on coronary artery disease: an updated review of the literature. Curr Cardiol Rev. 2017;13(3):209–16. https://doi.org/10.2174/1573403X13666170426104611. PMID: 28462692; PMCID: PMC5633715.
49. Miljanovic B, Glynn RJ, Nathan DM, Manson JE, Schaumberg DA. A prospective study of serum lipids and risk of diabetic macular edema in type 1 diabetes. Diabetes. 2004;53(11):2883–92. https://doi.org/10.2337/diabetes.53.11.2883. PMID: 15504969.
50. Mehta H, Fraser-Bell S, Yeung A, Campain A, Lim LL, Quin GJ, McAllister IL, Keane PA, Gillies MC. Efficacy of dexamethasone versus bevacizumab on regression of hard exudates in diabetic maculopathy: data from the BEVORDEX randomised clinical trial. Br J Ophthalmol. 2016;100(7):1000–4. https://doi.org/10.1136/bjophthalmol-2015-307797. Epub 2015 Nov 4. PMID: 26537156.
51. Chaikitmongkol V, Bressler NM. Intraretinal fibrosis in exudative diabetic macular edema after ranibizumab treatments. Retin Cases Brief Rep 2014;8(4):336-339. doi: https://doi.org/10.1097/ICB.0000000000000063. PMID: 25372542.
52. Fong DS, Segal PP, Myers F, Ferris FL, Hubbard LD, Davis MD. Subretinal fibrosis in diabetic macular edema. ETDRS report 23. Early Treatment Diabetic Retinopathy Study Research Group. Arch Ophthalmol. 1997;115(7):873–7. https://doi.org/10.1001/archopht.1997.01100160043006. PMID: 9230827.
53. Begg IS, Rootman J. Clinico-pathological study of an organized plaque in exudative diabetic maculopathy. Can J Ophthalmol. 1976;11(3):197–202. PMID: 949627.
54. Sigurdsson R, Begg IS. Organised macular plaques in exudative diabetic maculopathy. Br J Ophthalmol. 1980;64(6):392–7. https://doi.org/10.1136/bjo.64.6.392. PMID: 7190023; PMCID: PMC1043715.
55. Kumagai K, Ogino N, Fukami M, Furukawa M. Removal of foveal hard exudates by subretinal balanced salt solution injection using 38-gauge needle in diabetic patients. Graefes Arch Clin Exp Ophthalmol. 2020;258(9):1893–9. https://doi.org/10.1007/s00417-020-04756-y. Epub 2020 May 25. PMID: 32451607.
56. Avci R, Inan UU, Kaderli B. Long-term results of excision of plaque-like foveal hard exudates in patients with chronic diabetic macular oedema. Eye (Lond). 2008;22(9):1099–104. https://doi.org/10.1038/sj.eye.6702877. Epub 2007 Jul 20. PMID: 17641680.
57. Srinivas S, Verma A, Nittala MG, Alagorie AR, Nassisi M, Gasperini J, Sadda SR. Effect of intravitreal Ranibizumab on Intraretinal hard exudates in eyes with diabetic macular edema. Am J Ophthalmol. 2020;211:183–90. https://doi.org/10.1016/j.ajo.2019.11.014. Epub 2019 Nov 20. PMID: 31758926.

58. Larsson J, Kifley A, Zhu M, Wang JJ, Mitchell P, Sutter FK, Gillies MC. Rapid reduction of hard exudates in eyes with diabetic retinopathy after intravitreal triamcinolone: data from a randomized, placebo-controlled, clinical trial. Acta Ophthalmol. 2009;87(3):275–80. https://doi.org/10.1111/j.1755-3768.2008.01245.x. Epub 2008 Sep 10. PMID: 18785964.
59. Domalpally A, Ip MS, Ehrlich JS. Effects of intravitreal ranibizumab on retinal hard exudate in diabetic macular edema: findings from the RIDE and RISE phase III clinical trials. Ophthalmology. 2015;122(4):779–86. https://doi.org/10.1016/j.ophtha.2014.10.028. Epub 2015 Jan 17. PMID: 25601535.
60. Klein R, Klein BE, Moss SE, Meuer SM. The epidemiology of retinal vein occlusion: the Beaver Dam Eye Study. Trans Am Ophthalmol Soc. 2000;98:133–41; discussion 141–3. PMID: 11190017; PMCID: PMC1298220.
61. The Eye Disease Case-control Study Group. Risk factors for branch retinal vein occlusion. Am J Ophthalmol. 1993;116(3):286–96. PMID: 8357052.
62. Christoffersen NL, Larsen M. Pathophysiology and hemodynamics of branch retinal vein occlusion. Ophthalmology. 1999;106(11):2054–62. https://doi.org/10.1016/S0161-6420(99)90483-9. PMID: 10571337.
63. Suzuki N, Hirano Y, Tomiyasu T, Kurobe R, Yasuda Y, Esaki Y, Yasukawa T, Yoshida M, Ogura Y. Collateral vessels on optical coherence tomography angiography in eyes with branch retinal vein occlusion. Br J Ophthalmol. 2019;103(10):1373–9. https://doi.org/10.1136/bjophthalmol-2018-313322. Epub 2018 Nov 22. PMID: 30467130.
64. Freund KB, Sarraf D, Leong BCS, Garrity ST, Vupparaboina KK, Dansingani KK. Association of optical coherence tomography angiography of collaterals in retinal vein occlusion with major venous outflow through the deep vascular complex. JAMA Ophthalmol. 2018;136(11):1262–70. https://doi.org/10.1001/jamaophthalmol.2018.3586. PMID: 30352115; PMCID: PMC6248171.
65. Tomiyasu T, Hirano Y, Yoshida M, Suzuki N, Nishiyama T, Uemura A, Yasukawa T, Ogura Y. Microaneurysms cause refractory macular edema in branch retinal vein occlusion. Sci Rep. 2016;6:29445. https://doi.org/10.1038/srep29445. PMID: 27389770; PMCID: PMC4937381.
66. Shields CL, Udyaver S, Dalvin LA, Lim LS, Atalay HT, Khoo CTL, Mazloumi M, Shields JA. Coats disease in 351 eyes: analysis of features and outcomes over 45 years (by decade) at a single center. Indian J Ophthalmol. 2019;67(6):772–83. https://doi.org/10.4103/ijo.IJO_449_19. PMID: 31124485; PMCID: PMC6552575.
67. Sigler EJ, Randolph JC, Calzada JI, Wilson MW, Haik BG. Current management of Coats disease. Surv Ophthalmol. 2014;59(1):30–46. https://doi.org/10.1016/j.survophthal.2013.03.007. Epub 2013 Oct 15. PMID: 24138893.
68. Rishi E, Rishi P, Appukuttan B, Uparkar M, Sharma T, Gopal L. Coats' disease of adult-onset in 48 eyes. Indian J Ophthalmol. 2016;64(7):518–23. https://doi.org/10.4103/0301-4738.190141. PMID: 27609165; PMCID: PMC5026078.
69. He YG, Wang H, Zhao B, Lee J, Bahl D, McCluskey J. Elevated vascular endothelial growth factor level in Coats' disease and possible therapeutic role of bevacizumab. Graefes Arch Clin Exp Ophthalmol. 2010;248(10):1519–21. https://doi.org/10.1007/s00417-010-1366-1. Epub 2010 Apr 9. PMID: 20379736.
70. Goel N, Kumar V, Seth A, Raina UK, Ghosh B. Role of intravitreal bevacizumab in adult onset Coats' disease. Int Ophthalmol. 2011;31(3):183–90. https://doi.org/10.1007/s10792-011-9436-x. Epub 2011 Mar 25. PMID: 21437759.
71. Feng J, Zheng X, Li B, Jiang Y. Differences in aqueous concentrations of cytokines in paediatric and adult patients with Coats' disease. Acta Ophthalmol. 2017;95(6):608–12. https://doi.org/10.1111/aos.13151. Epub 2016 Jun 30. PMID: 27364629.
72. Yang X, Wang C, Su G. Recent advances in the diagnosis and treatment of Coats' disease. Int Ophthalmol. 2019;39(4):957–70. https://doi.org/10.1007/s10792-019-01095-8. Epub 2019 Mar 20. PMID: 30895419.
73. Bajgai P, Katoch D, Dogra MR, Singh R. Idiopathic retinal vasculitis, aneurysms, and neuroretinitis (IRVAN) syndrome: clinical perspectives. Clin Ophthalmol. 2017;11:1805–17. https://doi.org/10.2147/OPTH.S128506. PMID: 29062224; PMCID: PMC5640394.
74. Parchand S, Bhalekar S, Gupta A, Singh R. Primary branch retinal artery occlusion in idiopathic retinal vasculitis, aneurysms, and neuroretinitis syndrome associated with hyperhomocysteinemia. Retin Cases Brief Rep. 2012;6(4):349–52. https://doi.org/10.1097/ICB.0b013e31823c1289. PMID: 25389928.
75. Zina S, Ksiaa I, Abdelhedi C, Ben Amor H, Attia S, Khochtali S, Khairallah M. Multimodal imaging in IRVAN syndrome presenting with branch retinal artery occlusion. Eur J Ophthalmol. 2020:1120672120965492. https://doi.org/10.1177/1120672120965492. Epub ahead of print. PMID: 33092394.
76. Singh AD, Nouri M, Shields CL, Shields JA, Smith AF. Retinal capillary hemangioma: a comparison of sporadic cases and cases associated with von Hippel-Lindau disease. Ophthalmology. 2001;108(10):1907–11. https://doi.org/10.1016/s0161-6420(01)00758-8. PMID: 11581072.
77. Los M, Aarsman CJ, Terpstra L, Wittebol-Post D, Lips CJ, Blijham GH, Voest EE. Elevated ocular levels of vascular endothelial growth factor in patients with von Hippel-Lindau disease. Ann Oncol. 1997;8(10):1015–22. https://doi.org/10.1023/a:1008213320642. PMID: 9402176.

78. Chan CC, Vortmeyer AO, Chew EY, Green WR, Matteson DM, Shen DF, Linehan WM, Lubensky IA, Zhuang Z. VHL gene deletion and enhanced VEGF gene expression detected in the stromal cells of retinal angioma. Arch Ophthalmol. 1999;117(5):625–30. https://doi.org/10.1001/archopht.117.5.625. PMID: 10326959.
79. Di Nicola M, Williams BK Jr, Hua J, Bekerman VP, Mashayekhi A, Shields JA, Shields CL. Photodynamic therapy for retinal hemangioblastoma: treatment outcomes of 17 consecutive patients. Ophthalmol Retina. 2022;6(1):80–8. https://doi.org/10.1016/j.oret.2021.04.007. S2468-6530(21)00124-X. Epub ahead of print. PMID: 33892136.
80. Aronow ME, Wiley HE, Gaudric A, Krivosic V, Gorin MB, Shields CL, Shields JA, Jonasch EW, Singh AD, Chew EY. Von Hippel-Lindau disease: update on pathogenesis and systemic aspects. Retina. 2019;39(12):2243–53. https://doi.org/10.1097/IAE.0000000000002555. PMID: 31095066.

5 Retinal Haemorrhages

5.1 Introduction

The presence of retinal haemorrhages is one of the most common intraocular signs physicians encounter. Without exception, retinal haemorrhages indicate a breakdown of the retinal vascular homeostasis, which is critical for maintaining retinal transparency and ensuring optimal visual tasks assigned to the retina's photoreceptors. The central area of 500 μm of the retina, called the fovea centralis, has the maximum concentration of the cone photoreceptors and is responsible for the detailed vision required in day-to-day activities like reading, recognition, colour vision, and driving. This area is bereft of blood capillaries to allow unrestricted passage of light to the photoreceptors. The haemorrhages in the retina may remain asymptomatic so long as these do not obscure the central fovea.

5.1.1 Blood Supply of the Retina and the Ocular Barriers

The blood supply of the retina is multitier. The superficial and deep capillary plexus and the interconnecting capillaries arise from the branches of the central retinal artery and supply oxygen and micronutrients to the inner neurosensory retina [from the retinal nerve fibre layer (RNFL) to the inner nuclear layer]. In contrast, the outer neurosensory retina has no blood supply and is served by the choroid, one of the human body's highest blood flow tissues. Tight endothelial junctions in the retinal blood vessels constitute the inner blood-retinal barrier that does not allow the movement of macromolecules and cellular components into the extravascular space in the neurosensory retina. Moreover, the retinal arterial system is autoregulated to maintain a constant blood flow to the inner retina. The retinal pigment epithelium (RPE) is the outermost layer of the retina and separates the neurosensory retina from the choroid. The blood supply in the choroid is multilayered and is under autonomic control. The choroid's innermost layer of blood vessels consists of fenestrated capillaries, known as the choriocapillaris, which lie immediately below the retinal pigment epithelium. The tight gap junctions in the RPE provide the outer blood-retinal barrier and control the movement of micronutrients into the retina.

5.1.2 Role of Physicians

Many systemic and ocular disorders may cause haemorrhages in the eye and, specifically, in the retina. Unless the haemorrhages obscure the macula, patients may remain asymptomatic, thereby delaying the diagnosis of both sight-threatening and life-threatening diseases. Using deep learning algorithms, ultrawide colour fundus photographs taken through an undilated pupil

A. Gupta et al., *Ophthalmic Signs in Practice of Medicine*,
https://doi.org/10.1007/978-981-99-7923-3_5

have shown potential for automated general population screening with remarkably high sensitivity and specificity in diagnosing retinal haemorrhages. The automated detection of retinal haemorrhages was more sensitive than the detection of these haemorrhages by general ophthalmologists. The retinal haemorrhages occupying the macular area call for an immediate referral to a retinal specialist [1]. The physician needs to identify the location and distribution of the haemorrhage, the extent, the shape, the number and specific characteristics, and other accompanying eye signs that help narrow the etiological diagnosis.

5.2 Location of Haemorrhages in the Eye

Haemorrhage may be localized in the anterior chamber (hyphema), vitreous cavity (vitreous haemorrhage), under the post hyaloid membrane (subhyaloid haemorrhage), under the internal limiting membrane but in front of the RNFL (sub-ILM haemorrhage), in the RNFL (superficial, linear or flame-shaped), in the ganglion cell layer, inner plexiform and the inner nuclear layer (dot and blot haemorrhages), in the Henle's layer (petaloid haemorrhage), under the neurosensory retina (sub-retinal haemorrhage), under the RPE (sub-RPE haemorrhage), in the choroid, or in the suprachoroidal space that lies between the sclera and the choroid (suprachoroidal haemorrhage). Clarity of the visual media permitting crossectional line scans on the spectral domain optical coherence tomography can determine the location of the haemorrhages, whether in front of the retina, within, or below the retina.

5.2.1 Haemorrhage in the Anterior Chamber

Hyphema often follows trauma to the eye and is a red-coloured layered collection of RBCs in the anterior chamber. If it covers the pupillary area, vision is obscured. Severe blunt trauma may cause haemorrhage to fill the anterior segment's anterior and posterior chambers, which gets clotted and is dark coloured. Less commonly, RBCs red or grey coloured may move into the anterior chamber from a dissolving blood clot in the vitreous cavity or erosion of the ciliary blood vessels by a misplaced haptic of an intraocular lens implant. It is called microhyphema, is not visible to the naked eye, and requires careful biomicroscopy. In all cases of hyphema, it is mandatory to monitor the intraocular pressure, which is often increased.

5.2.2 Vitreous Haemorrhage

Several ocular or systemic disorders or trauma may result in haemorrhage in the vitreous cavity. Visual symptoms may vary from the sudden onset of cobwebs (floaters) to the complete obscuration of vision, depending upon the severity of the haemorrhage (Figs. 5.1 and 5.2). If it prevents a satisfactory examination of the entire retina, ocular ultrasonography must be done.

5.2.3 Subhyaloid and Sub-ILM Haemorrhages

A characteristic boat shape can recognize these due to the gravitational settling of the RBCs and a horizontal level (Fig. 5.3). The boat shape indicates that there is no blood clot formation. The

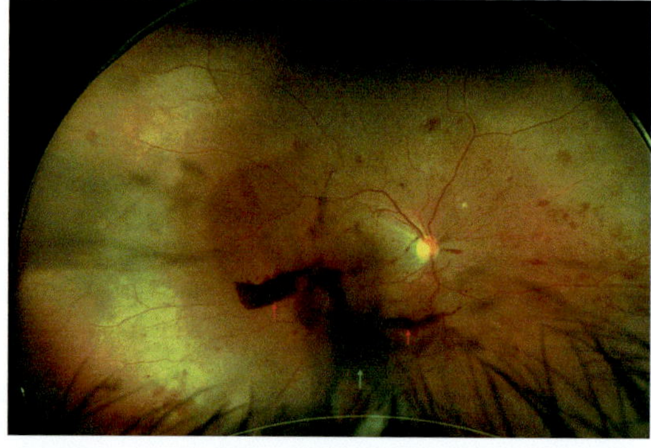

Fig. 5.1 A patient with proliferative diabetic retinopathy (PDR) presented with floaters in the right eye due to vitreous haemorrhage (green arrow) and subhyaloid haemorrhage (red arrows)

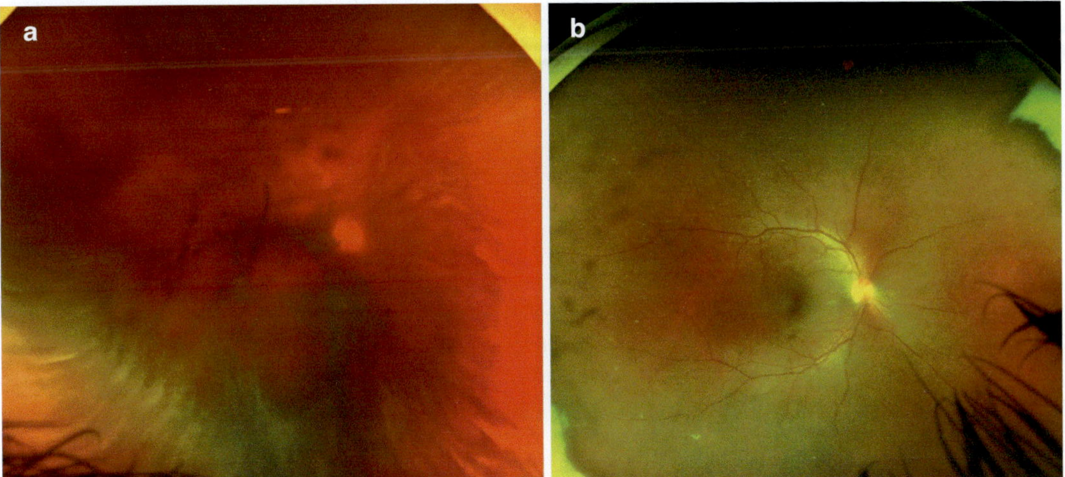

Fig. 5.2 A patient with hypertension presented with sudden onset dimness of vision due to vitreous haemorrhage (**a**). Three months later, there was spontaneous and complete resolution of vitreous haemorrhage (**b**)

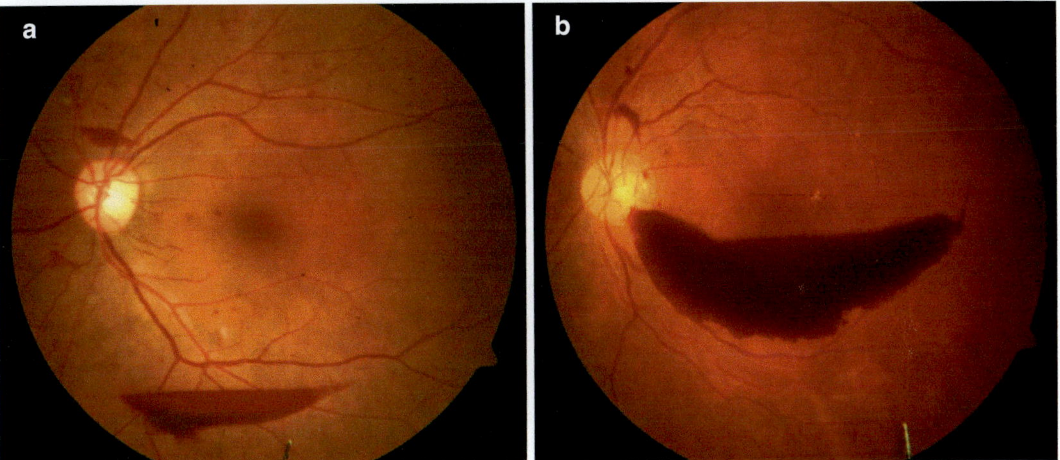

Fig. 5.3 Subhyaloid haemorrhage (boat-shaped) in a 55-year-old male (**a**) and 61-year-old female (**b**) with proliferative diabetic retinopathy

most common cause of subhyaloid haemorrhage is proliferative diabetic retinopathy. The subhyaloid haemorrhage may break into the vitreous cavity obscuring the retina's details and preventing pan-retinal laser photocoagulation (Fig. 5.4). A dense subhyaloid haemorrhage does not resolve spontaneously and may facilitate intense fibrovascular proliferation. Such patients require pars plana vitreous surgery to remove the haemorrhage and also do a pan-retinal laser photocoagulation (Fig. 5.5).

If it obscures the fovea, a simple puncturing of the posterior hyaloid membrane or ILM with a neodymium:YAG laser can release the trapped RBCs from these spaces and trickle into the lower periphery of the retina. Sub-ILM haemorrhage (Fig. 5.6) may unmask underlying pancytopenia due to COVID-19 [2] or megaloblastic anaemia [3].

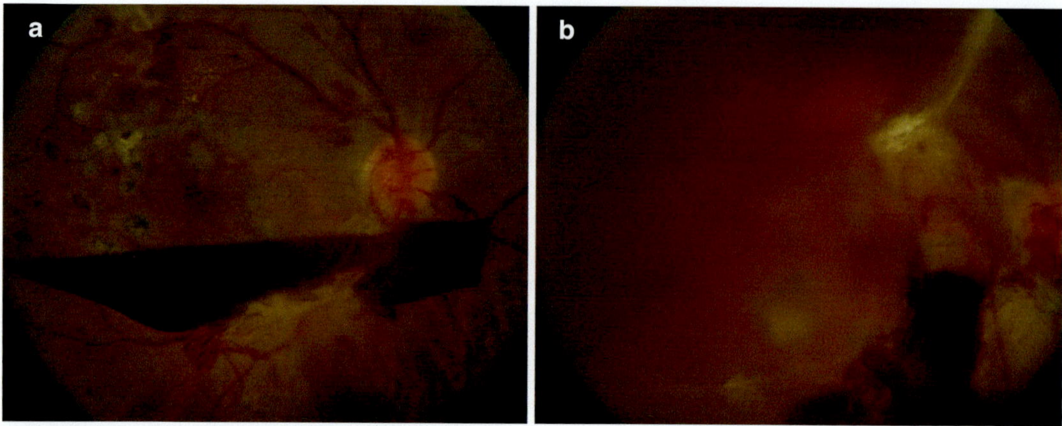

Fig. 5.4 A patient with proliferative diabetic retinopathy (Note new vessels on the optic disc and fibrovascular proliferation along the lower temporal vessels. Laser photocoagulation scars can be seen temporal to the fovea (**a**). While waiting for spontaneous resolution of the subhyaloid haemorrhage, it broke into the vitreous cavity obscuring all details of the retina (**b**)

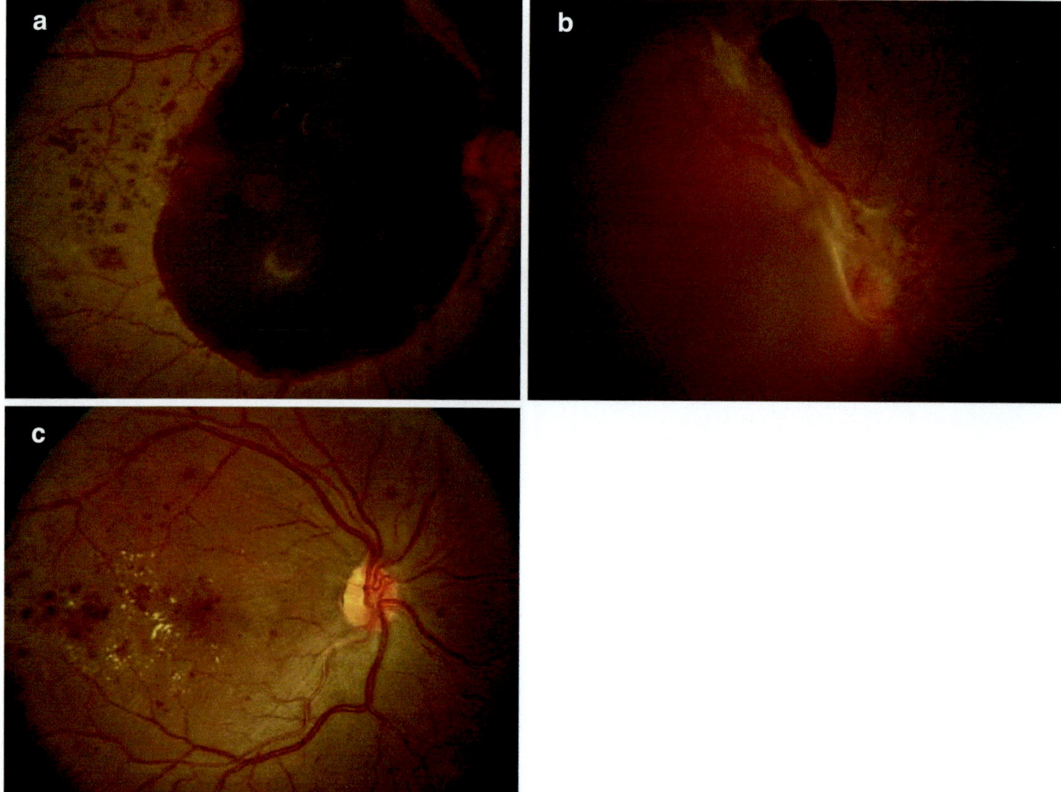

Fig. 5.5 A 22-year-old type 1 diabetic presented with sudden visual loss from the right eye due to a dense subhyaloid haemorrhage over the macula (**a**). Three months later, there was a massive fibrovascular proliferation on the optic disc, and the haemorrhage over the macula persisted (**b**). Six months following pars plana vitreous surgery, the media has cleared, but he required treatment for macular oedema (**c**)

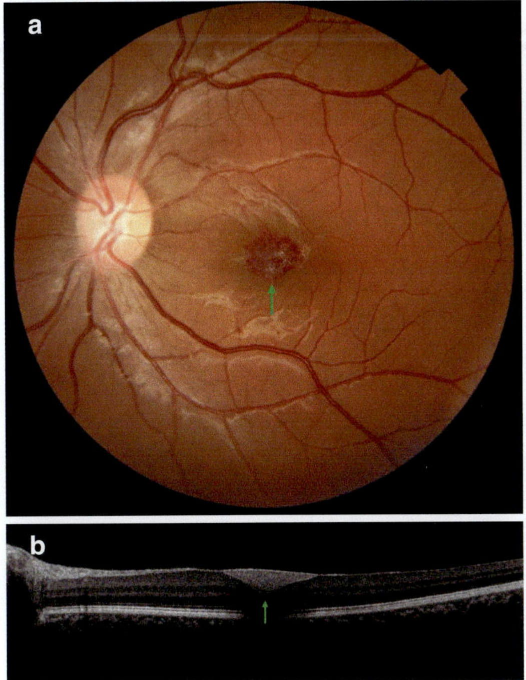

Fig. 5.6 Fundus photograph (**a**) and OCT (**b**) showing sub-internal limiting membrane haemorrhage (green arrow) at the fovea in a patient with iron deficiency anaemia

5.2.4 Superficial Retinal Haemorrhages

These lie within the RNFL and assume a flame shape or linear orientation as the RBCs follow the course of the thick RNFL bundle as they converge onto the optic disc. The flame shape of these superficial haemorrhages is lost beyond the posterior pole due to the thinning of the RNFL bundles, which may appear more like ink blots. The flame-shaped haemorrhages are seen mainly around the optic disc (peripapillary) and the major vascular arcades. These are most commonly seen in patients with hypertensive retinopathy, retinal vein occlusions, and diabetic retinopathy (Fig. 5.7). These haemorrhages arise from a capillary tight endothelial junction breakdown due to hypoxia in accelerated hypertension and diabetic retinopathy and increased hydrostatic pressure in retinal vascular occlusions. Once the blood pressure is controlled, the haemorrhages disappear in a few weeks, never returning if the blood pressure remains controlled. The breakdown in endothelial junctions appears more permanent due to increased intravascular hydrostatic pressure, as seen in retinal vascular occlusions. Predominant flame-shaped retinal haemorrhages in patients with diabetes mellitus indicate a concomitant decompensated hypertension.

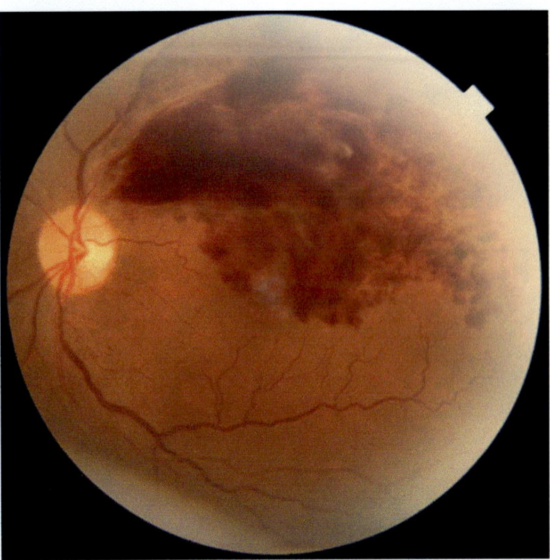

Fig. 5.7 Superficial retinal haemorrhages (flame shaped) in a patient with supero-temporal branch retinal vein occlusion

5.2.5 Dot and Blot Haemorrhages

While microaneurysms are the sine qua non of diabetic retinopathy, dot and blot haemorrhages are the hallmarks of non-proliferative diabetic retinopathy. Most of these arise from the extravasation of RBCs from the retinal microaneurysms and capillary segments. The collections of blood elements from the leaking microaneurysms in the ganglion cell layer and the inner nuclear layer take a dot-like appearance due to the vertical orientation of the tightly packed retinal cells in these layers, while in the inner and outer plexiform layers, these haemorrhages appear larger blot-like due to a comparatively less density of the interstitial tissue and the horizontal orientation of the neural fibres (Fig. 5.8a and b).

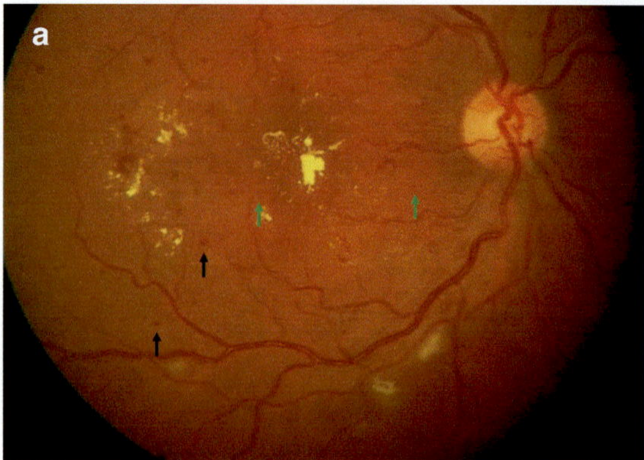

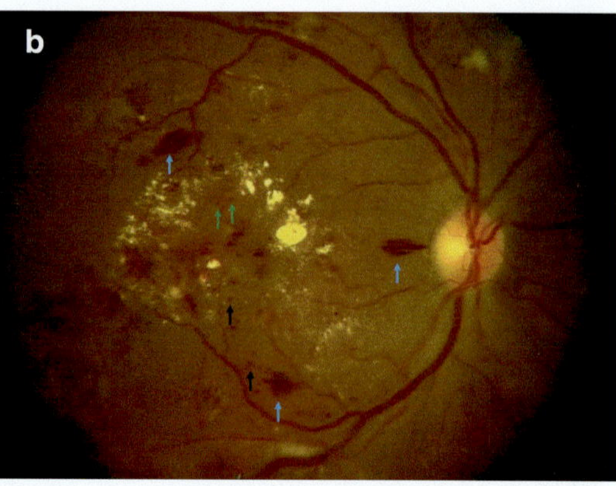

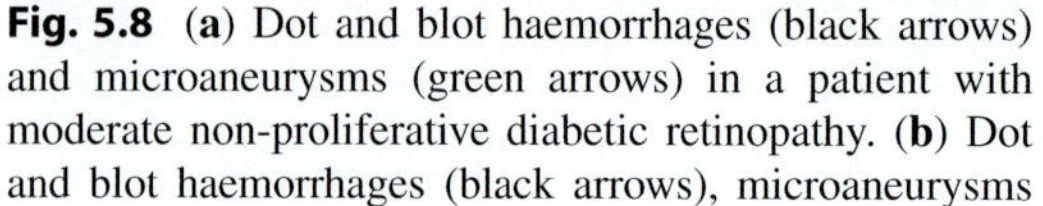

Fig. 5.8 (**a**) Dot and blot haemorrhages (black arrows) and microaneurysms (green arrows) in a patient with moderate non-proliferative diabetic retinopathy. (**b**) Dot and blot haemorrhages (black arrows), microaneurysms (green arrows) and superficial flame-shaped retinal haemorrhages (blue arrows) in a patient with non-proliferative diabetic retinopathy

5.2.6 Petaloid Retinal Haemorrhages (Henle Haemorrhages)

In recent years, the SD-OCT study of the radially oriented deep intraretinal haemorrhages found them localized to the Henle fibre layer. The subfoveal outer plexiform layer fibers are oriented obliquely in the macula; thus, the Henle haemorrhages (HHs) assume a petaloid pattern with feathery margins. Most of these haemorrhages likely arise from the retinal deep capillary plexus in the inner nuclear layer. These may occasionally be accompanied by paracentral acute middle maculopathy (PAMM) or acute macular neuroretinopathy due to ischaemic insult in the deep capillary plexus [4]. Although initially described in eyes with Macular telangiectasia type 2 [5], bilateral HH may be seen in diverse etiologies that cause an increase in central venous pressure, including head trauma or chest compression, subarachnoid haemorrhage, general or epidural anaesthesia, and ruptured intracranial aneurysms. Some of these cases may have subhyaloid or sub-ILM haemorrhages as well. Unilateral cases of HH may be seen in branch or central retinal vein occlusion [4].

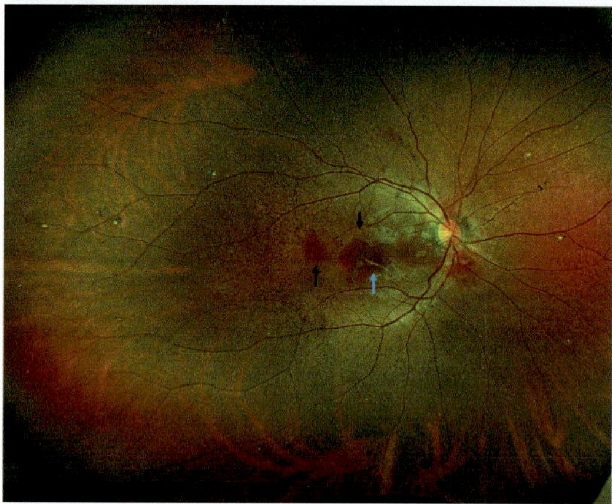

Fig. 5.9 Submacular haemorrhage (black arrows) with rupture of Bruch's membrane (blue arrow) in a young female following trauma

5.2.7 Submacular and Sub-RPE Haemorrhage

Haemorrhage under the submacular area has the potential to cause irreversible damage to the central vision and hence needs urgent attention for diagnosis and appropriate treatment. In young adults, the submacular haemorrhage is most often due to a rupture of the Bruch's membrane sustained during blunt trauma to the eye (Fig. 5.9).

In the elderly, this is due to age-related choroidal neovascular membrane/s (CNVM) or polypoidal choroidal vasculopathy (PCV). Other less common causes of submacular haemorrhages at any age include CNVM complicating myopia, angioid streaks, ocular histoplasmosis, toxoplasmosis retinochoroiditis scars, and tubercular choroiditis. Because of its transparency, blood under the neurosensory retina appears bright red, while that under the RPE appears dark due to the pigmented nature of the RPE. Unlike the boat-shaped sub-ILM or subhyaloid haemorrhage, blood under the neurosensory retina or sub-RPE space is clotted and shows no fluid level. Depending upon its location, fibrin strands pull the photoreceptors or the RPE and cause irreversible damage and the loss of central vision. As most of these haemorrhages are due to abnormal CNVM, the treatment revolves around using only an intravitreal anti-VEGF agent if the haemorrhage is small and thin; however, if it is large and thick, the tissue plasminogen activator (tPA) administered either intravitreal or subretinal (this approach necessitates pars plana vitreous surgery and some surgeons also combine it with a subretinal air bubble) for clot lysis is followed by pneumatic displacement of the blood by injecting a long-acting gas bubble (SF6 or C3F8) into the vitreous cavity or if PPV has been done by doing a fluid gas exchange. The patient lies prone for a few days, so that the lysed blood gets displaced from the macula [6, 7]. Monthly injections of an anti-VEGF agent follow this to keep the CNVM regressed. If thick and large, submacular haemorrhage following blunt trauma may require tPA and pneumatic displacement. The mild and thin haemorrhages resolve spontaneously.

5.2.8 Optic Disc Haemorrhage

Linear haemorrhage on the optic disc margin indicates chronic open glaucoma. It is often seen along the lower temporal margin and extends into the peripapillary area. It marks the junction of healthy and damaged RNFL. For more than 100 years, these haemorrhages were considered a risk factor for glaucoma progression as new visual field defects appeared to coincide with their appearance. More recently, these haemorrhages have been considered an indicator of the presence of glaucoma and not merely a risk factor. These haemorrhages likely arise from a mechanical insult due to structural collapse in the neuroretinal rim or an ischaemic insult, including a capillary rupture or ischaemic infarct of the RNFL. Both mechanisms are likely at play. Systemic diseases like diabetes mellitus, hypertension, hypotension, migraine and the use of antiplatelet agents are associated with these haemorrhages (Figs. 5.10 and 5.11) [8].

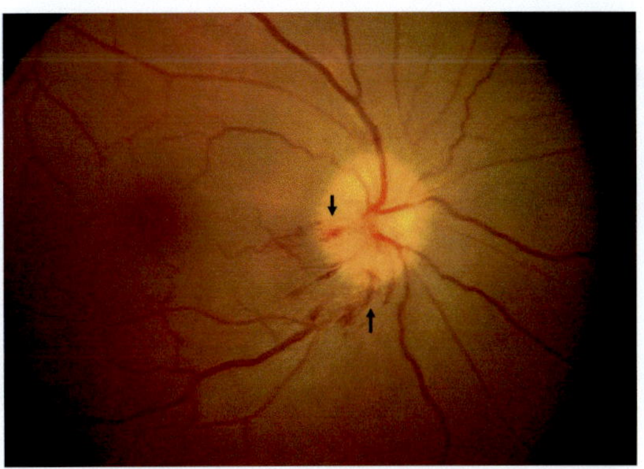

Fig. 5.10 Optic disc haemorrhages (black arrows) in a patient with anterior ischaemic optic neuropathy

5.2.9 Optic Disc and Peripapillary Haemorrhages in Adolescents

Intrapapillary haemorrhage with adjacent peripapillary subretinal haemorrhage may be seen in young myopic women due to a uniquely tilted optic disc with an elevated nasal margin. These resolve spontaneously and carry an excellent prognosis [9]. Most of these haemorrhages are unilateral. These are seen as a crescent nasal to the optic disc. The nasal margin of the disc appears thick, and the disc may be smaller and tilted [10, 11]. Occasionally there may be a small vitreous haemorrhage. These haemorrhages arise from a partial detachment of the posterior vitreous tightly adherent to the optic disc margins

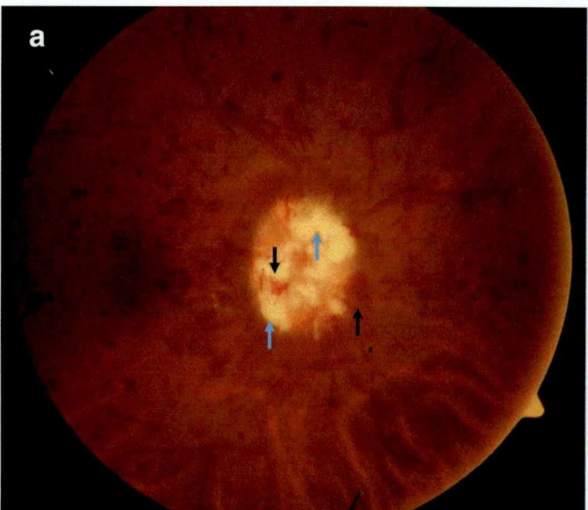

Fig. 5.11 Optic disc haemorrhages (black arrows) and infiltrates (blue arrows) in the right (**a**) and left (**b**) eyes of a 52-year-old female who had received chemotherapy and radiotherapy for carcinoma of breast, suggestive of intra-ocular metastasis

[12]. However, these haemorrhages may remain asymptomatic and discovered on routine ophthalmoscopy [13].

5.3 Retinal Haemorrhages in Childhood

As seen in adults, retinal haemorrhages in infants and young children may also be located in the preretinal space and vitreous cavity, subhyaloid or sub-ILM, superficial retina, intraretinal, subretinal, sub-RPE, choroid, or suprachoroidal spaces. The outcome of these haemorrhages may vary from benign to grave, and in a large majority, the aetiology of these haemorrhages is not the same as in adults [14].

5.3.1 Birth Trauma and Neonatal Retinal Haemorrhages

Retinal haemorrhages, often bilateral, of varying severity are noted in nearly 25% of neonates, most often in the posterior pole, even following a normal vaginal delivery. However, nearly 40–50% of neonates in instrument-assisted deliveries may have these haemorrhages. The haemorrhages are generally superficial flame-shaped, although dot and blot are also seen, albeit less commonly. These haemorrhages are transient and resolve within 2–3 weeks [15]. Prolonged labour, especially if it exceeds 30 h (100%), and the primiparous status of the mother are recognized as significant risk factors. Breech deliveries and the Caesarean section caused negligible retinal haemorrhages [16]. It is believed that an increase in intracranial pressure due to head compression during its passage in the birth canal may result in the obstruction of blood flow in the central retinal vein leading to rupture of the retinal capillaries [17]. In the past, it was believed that some cases of congenital amblyopia might be due to unilateral foveal haemorrhages at birth and those of nystagmus due to bilateral foveal haemorrhage [16]. More recently, however, when neonates with or without retinal haemorrhages were followed for 4 years, there was no difference in the visual acuity in the two groups. However, on OCT, a shallow foveal pit and a thicker outer nuclear layer were noted in children with foveal haemorrhage at birth [18].

5.3.2 Battered Child, Abusive Head Trauma (AHT), and the Retinal Haemorrhages

Unlike the transient nature of retinal haemorrhages that occur during normal childbirth, severe intraocular haemorrhages, including preretinal and vitreous haemorrhage that last very long and are accompanied by evidence of physical trauma, head injury, or fractures, should raise the suspicion of child abuse (battered baby or shaken baby). Soon after the first description of such babies, primarily unwanted, physically battered by the parents or caregivers, the first case of bilateral retinal detachment in a battered baby was reported [19].

In children, spontaneous retinal haemorrhages due to convulsions (0.7%), vomiting (0%), chest compression (2.3%), and severe persistent coughing (0%) are rare. While the incidence of retinal haemorrhages in severe accidental trauma is only 0–10%, it may increase to 53–80% in abusive head trauma. In shaken baby syndrome, the haemorrhages are almost always bilateral. The most vulnerable age group for abusive head trauma (AHT) is less than 5 years [20]. Thus, any retinal haemorrhages in young children beyond the neonatal age should arouse the suspicion of AHT [21].

Nearly 40% of the babies with shaken baby syndrome may not show any external evidence of abuse. In suspected shaken baby syndrome, the presence of retinal haemorrhages, especially if bilateral, is almost always associated with intracranial pathology. In most cases, intracranial pathology is a collection of extracerebral fluid mixed with blood elements indicative of chronicity due to subacute, chronic, or rarely acute subdural haemorrhage [20, 22]. In AHT, the haemorrhages are often multilayered and widespread, and extend into the retina's periphery. These may be associated with retinoschisis (splitting of the retina) with or without blood collection in the schisis cavities [23]. Post-mortem studies in children who did not survive AHT show multilayered haemorrhage in the optic nerve sheath, especially in the subdural space, the extraocular muscles, and the orbit [21]. The severity and extent of the retinal haemorrhages relate to the severity of the abusive head injury and are severest in children who die of this injury. In young children, the vitreous is firmly adherent to the retinal vessels. Acceleration–deceleration injury causes extensive haemorrhages as the baby is repeatedly shaken. On the other hand, very few such haemorrhages are seen in a single event, as in a vehicular accident [24].

5.3.3 Differential Diagnosis of Retinal Haemorrhages in Children

Several disorders, including hypertension, thrombophilia, hypoxia, anaemia, leukaemia, cerebral aneurysms, infections, and meningitis can cause retinal haemorrhages in children. These are much fewer in number and are located most often in the post-pole (Fig. 5.12) [24]. Children who were diagnosed with retinal haemorrhages and cerebral venous thrombosis (CVT) may get mislabeled as having abusive head trauma. In a study of 29 children with CVT, retinal haemorrhages were seen in only five children (17%), and four were located in the peripapillary region. The haemorrhages were both superficial and intraretinal, along with optic disc oedema. Only in one child these were seen in the posterior pole. Optic disc oedema was more common than haemorrhages. The risk factors for CVT included sepsis, meningitis, mastoiditis, etc. [25]. Likewise, children who suffer from thrombophilia and become victims of the shaken baby syndrome run the risk of wrong attribution of retinal haemorrhages to thrombophilia. Retinal haemorrhages are rare in children with thrombophilia. Most infants with protein C or protein S deficiency (Neonatal purpura fulminans), a rare, life-threatening disease, present with retinal vessel thrombosis and large intra, pre and subretinal and vitreous haemorrhage. They suffer from life-threatening disseminated intravascular coagulopathy. Even if the retinal haemorrhages are present these are preceded by highly characteristic purpura fulminans skin lesions that manifest as erythematous lesions that rapidly progress to haemorrhagic necrotic lesions [26].

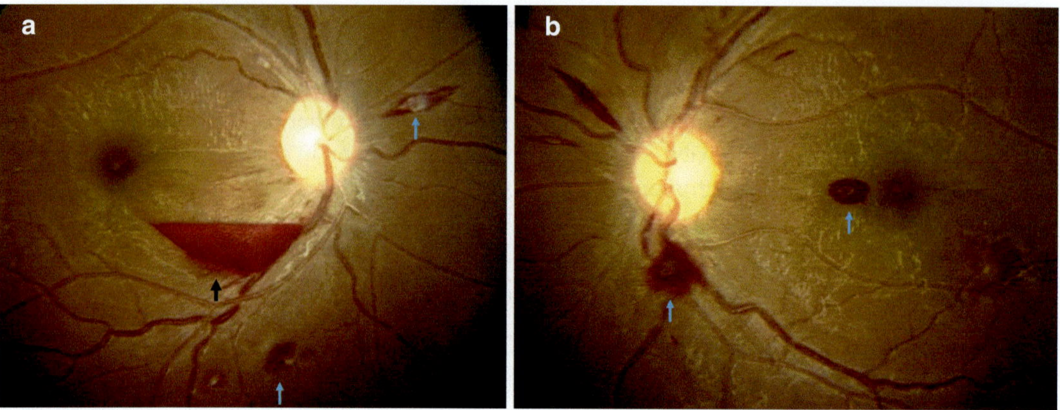

Fig. 5.12 Right (**a**) and left (**b**) eyes of a 13-year-old child with acute lymphoblastic leukaemia, showing white-centred retinal haemorrhages (Roth spots, blue arrows) and subhyaloid haemorrhage (black arrow)

5.4 Retinal Haemorrhages in Hematological Disorders

Diminution of vision due to retinal haemorrhages in the macula of one or both eyes usually prompts the patient to seek medical attention (Fig. 5.13). On the other hand, peripheral retinal haemorrhages are often asymptomatic. Their detection on a routine ophthalmoscopic examination may lead to the discovery of potentially life-threatening or disabling systemic disorders such as von Willebrand disease, one of the common bleeding disorders that may show a high degree of variation in its clinical presentations [27].

5.4.1 Retinal Haemorrhages in Anaemia, Pancytopenia, and Thrombocytopenia

Retinal haemorrhages are frequently (28%) seen in patients with anaemia and thrombocytopenia and 38% if both are present concomitantly (Fig. 5.13).

Haemoglobin less than 8 gm % and platelet count less than 50,000/μL are most often associated with retinal haemorrhages. Most of the haemorrhages are flame shaped and located in the superficial retina; occasionally, these may be white-centred (Fig. 5.12). Rarely haemorrhage may even be preretinal (Fig. 5.13). It is believed that tissue hypoxia is responsible for these haemorrhages. There is no long-term consequence of such retinal haemorrhages on visual functions [28]. Unless accompanied by anaemia or paraproteinaemias, thrombocytopenia usually will not cause retinal haemorrhages. Retinal haemorrhages are exceptional in patients with immune thrombocytopenic purpura, and routine fundus examination is not recommended [29]. However, these cases rarely present with suprachoroidal haemorrhage and pose a major diagnostic challenge [30].

Megaloblastic anaemia is rare and caused by a deficiency of either Vitamin B12 or folic acid but frequently in combined deficiency of both these vitamins. Nearly half of the patients with megaloblastic anaemia may also have pancytopenia. Consumption of a vegetarian diet is a major risk factor [31]. Megaloblastic anaemia may present with bilateral sub-ILM haemorrhage [32]. Sub-ILM haemorrhage in a patient presenting with fever, peripheral neuropathy, drowsiness, and other encephalopathy symptoms may help diagnose megaloblastic anaemia due to Vitamin B12 deficiency, which shows a remarkable response to the parental administration of Vitamin B12.

Optic disc oedema is unusual in iron deficiency anaemia but may be seen along with haemorrhages and cotton wool spots in patients

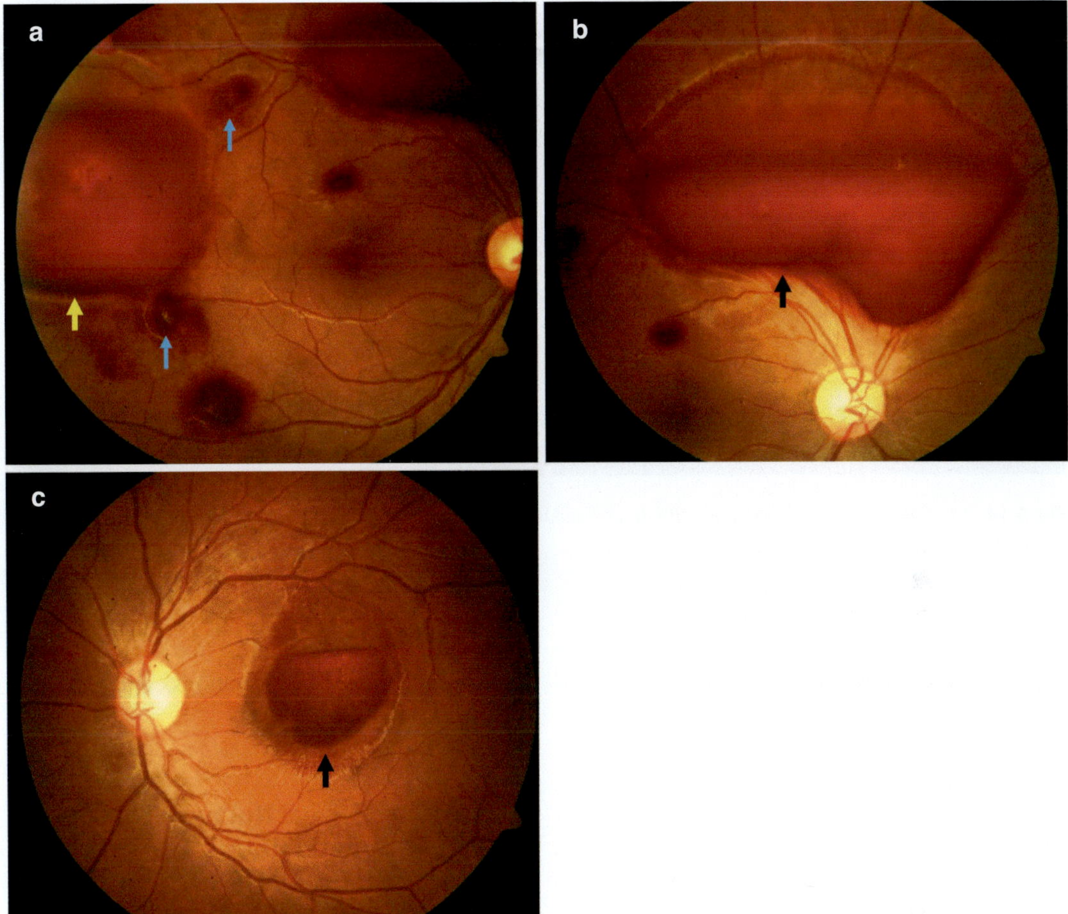

Fig. 5.13 Fundus photographs of right (**a** and **b**) and left (**c**) eyes of a patient who presented with left eye decreased vision. There were white centred retinal haemorrhages (blue arrows), with large pre-retinal (yellow arrow) and sub-ILM (black arrows) haemorrhages in both eyes. The patient was diagnosed with acute lymphoblastic leukaemia (ALL) with anaemia

with aplastic anaemia. The disc oedema in these cases is due to increased intracranial pressure following cortical venous thrombosis [33].

A high index of suspicion for an underlying systemic disorder in a patient with unilateral recurrent optic disc oedema and worsening anaemic retinopathy due to iron deficiency led to the detection of colorectal cancer in an older person. A timely total resection of cancer and correction of anaemia led to the resolution of retinopathy and disc oedema [34].

5.4.2 Retinal Haemorrhages in Leukaemias

Patients with acute leukaemias often present with fever, fatigue, loss of appetite, recurrent infections, and easy bruising. They may present with petechial haemorrhages on their arms and legs. Retinal haemorrhages may be asymptomatic and seen in nearly half the patients with leukaemia who, besides leukocytosis, have anaemia, Thrombocytopenia and cellular hyperviscosity.

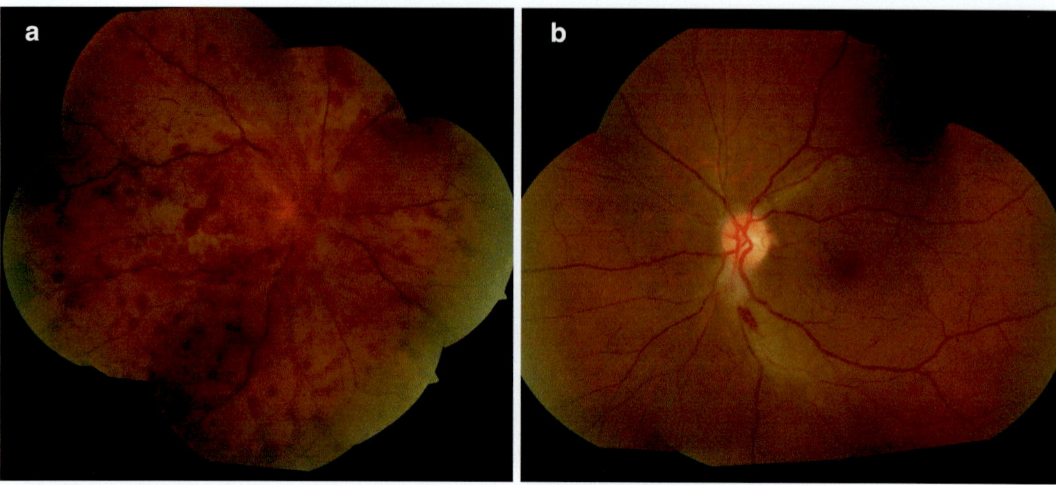

Fig. 5.14 Multiple retinal haemorrhages with dilated and tortuous veins in the right eye (**a**) and a single retinal haemorrhage in the left eye (**b**) of a patient with leukaemia

The retinal veins, thus, are often dilated, may show leukemic infiltration in their walls and are accompanied by intraretinal and preretinal haemorrhages (Fig. 5.14). Haemorrhages may be white-centred due to high white cell counts. Chemotherapy for leukaemia may cause anaemia and thrombocytopenia, which may also present as vitreous or pre-retinal haemorrhage. These changes are reversible, and the haemorrhages resolve within the next few months without leaving any residual microstructural defect in the retina [35–37].

5.4.3 Hyperviscosity Syndromes

Peripheral retinal haemorrhages accompanied by sausage-like venous dilatations, optic disc oedema, and microaneurysms on retinal examination may provide early clinical clues for the presence of hyperviscosity syndromes due to increased blood viscosity, most commonly seen in paraproteinaemias. This life-threatening condition often presents with mucosal bleeding and neurological disturbances. Plasmapheresis may be lifesaving in such patients [38, 39]. Waldenstrom anaemia is a non-Hodgkin lymphoma characterized by blood hyperviscosity due to the overproduction of gamma globulins. It is one of the most common causes of hyperviscosity syndrome. Mobile arterial and venous emboli were documented in one such case with extensive collateral formations and vascular occlusions [40].

5.4.4 Paroxysmal Nocturnal Haemoglobinuria

Paroxysmal nocturnal hematuria (PNH) is a rare acquired life-threatening hematological disorder caused by a mutation in the PIG-A gene in which there is premature rupture of the blood cells due to a lack of expression of CD 55 and CD 59 on their cell surface, making them vulnerable to haemolysis [41].

Abnormal platelets in these patients often lead to devastating thrombotic and haemorrhagic complications. While hepatic vein thrombosis is the most frequent complication of PNH, cortical venous thrombosis (CVT) may complicate PNH, especially in young women. CVT may be the earliest sign of PNH or in some cases, it may follow years after the diagnosis of PNH. Headache is the most consistent complaint in patients of PNH who develop CVT, followed by papilloedema, seizures, hemiparesis, and loss of consciousness [42]. Patients with PNH may first present to the ophthalmologists with papilloedema and extensive peripheral retinal haemorrhages due to CVT

[43] or rarely as multiple retinal vein occlusions in young persons [44]. Notably, in a large series of retinal vein occlusions in the elderly age group, not even a single case of PNH was detected [45]. A high index of suspicion is required to investigate patients of CVT for a possible PNH, as they carry a poor prognosis due to frequent thrombotic complications [42].

5.4.5 Retinal Haemorrhages in COVID-19

In a large prospective cohort with confirmed SARS-CoV-2 infection in Singapore, asymptomatic retinal microhaemorrhages were noted in nearly 8% of patients with controlled blood pressure versus 4% of those with normal blood pressure [46].

5.4.6 High Altitude Retinal Haemorrhages

Unacclimatized mountain climbers who ascend more than 3500 m often develop superficial retinal haemorrhages due to hypobaric hypoxia. They may also concomitantly suffer from acute mountain sickness and pulmonary and cerebral oedema. Optic disc swelling often accompanies these; even a frank branch retinal or central retina vein occlusion may be seen. At this time, it is unclear whether high-altitude retinopathy can predict the development of cerebral oedema [47].

5.5 Retinal Haemorrhages in Neurological Disorders

5.5.1 Subarachnoid Haemorrhage and Preretinal Haemorrhage

A ruptured intracranial aneurysm is the most common cause of a non-traumatic subarachnoid haemorrhage and is life-threatening if not treated promptly. Sudden onset of severe headache with loss of vision due to a sub-ILM haemorrhage in the post pole of the retina (Terson syndrome) is diagnostic of this condition (Fig. 5.15). Subarachnoid haemorrhage and Terson's syndrome may occasionally occur due to cortical venous thrombosis (CVT). While a ruptured aneurysm requires embolization, the CVT needs anticoagulation. Such patients, thus, should undergo imaging studies in an emergency setting to rule out the presence of either a ruptured aneurysm or CVT [48, 49].

5.5.2 Idiopathic Intracranial Hypertension (IIH) and Retinal Haemorrhages

Patients, mostly obese women in their 40s, presenting with headache, pulsatile tinnitus, and transient blurring of vision but without cranial nerve palsies, are suspected of having idiopathic intracranial hypertension [50]. Optic disc oedema (papilloedema) is a highly characteristic feature of IIH. In long-standing cases, it may lead to visual loss (Fig. 5.16). Increased intracranial pressure gets transmitted to the vaginal space in the optic nerve sheath surrounding the optic nerve, leading to axoplasmic stasis and possibly ischaemia of the optic nerve head. In severe cases of IIH, there may be retinal vascular changes, including retinal venous dilation and retinal haemorrhages mimicking a picture of bilateral central retinal vein occlusion. In such cases rarely, a Terson's syndrome-like picture may also be seen [51–53]. Patients with IIH are often associated with CVT. Initiation of anticoagulant therapy in such patients may precipitate peripapillary haemorrhages, however, without any long-term visual consequences [54]. Rarely, patients with IIH may develop a juxtapapillary choroidal neovascular membrane and produce a juxtapapillary subretinal haemorrhage which may or may not be vision threatening. Often, treatment of IIH will cause spontaneous regression of these neovascular membranes. However, if persistent, these will require an intravitreal injection of one of the anti-VEGF agents [55].

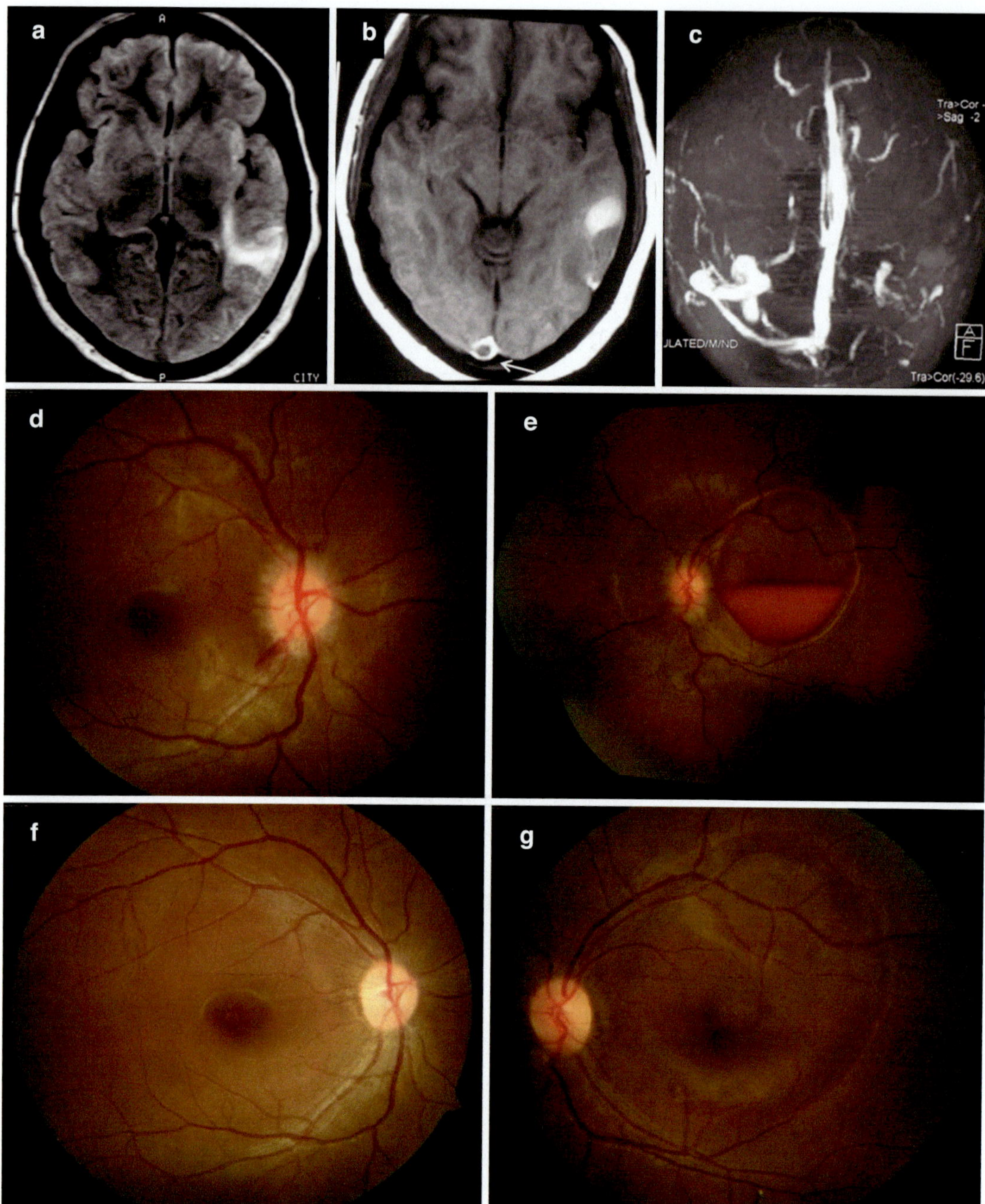

Fig. 5.15 In a patient with Terson Syndrome due to venous sinus thrombosis, (**a**) MRI brain (non-contrast T1 weighted sequence) showing acute left temporal haemorrhagic infarct, and (**b**) filling defect in the superior sagittal sinus (arrow) on Gadolinium-enhanced T1 sequence; (**c**) MR Venography showing left-sided sigmoid and transverse sinus thrombosis. Baseline fundus photograph shows optic disc haemorrhage in the right eye (**d**) and a large premacular sub–internal limiting membrane and subhyaloid bleed in the left eye (**e**). Follow-up fundus photographs (**f**, **g**) show substantial resolution. (Reproduced with permission of the publisher from Takkar A, Kesav P, Lal V, Gupta A. Teaching NeuroImages: Terson syndrome in cortical venous sinus thrombosis. Neurology. 2013 Aug 6;81(6):e40-1. https://doi.org/10.1212/WNL.0b013e31829e6f13. PMID: 23918868)

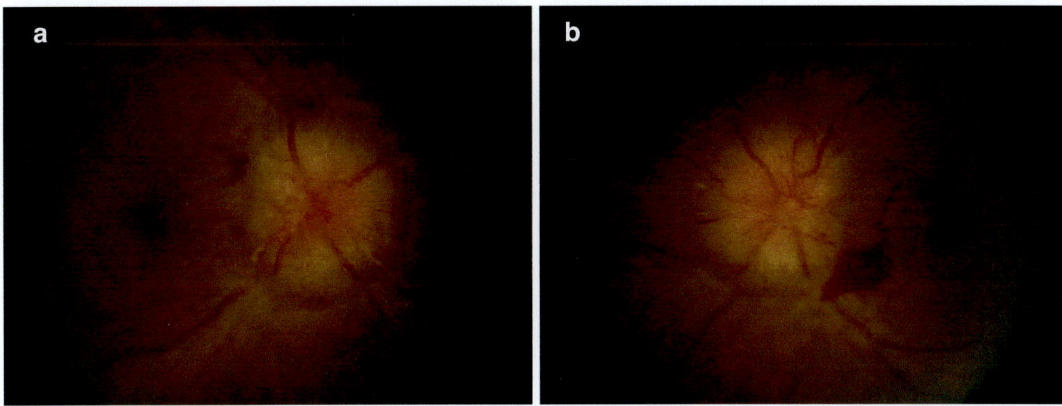

Fig. 5.16 Optic disc oedema and haemorrhages in both eyes (**a**, **b**) of a patient with idiopathic intracranial hypertension

5.5.3 Wernicke's Encephalopathy and Retinal Haemorrhages

Thiamine (Vitamin B1) deficiency may cause a life-threatening condition of central and peripheral neuropathy characterized by confusion, ataxia, and ophthalmoplegia. While Carl Wernicke noted the presence of optic disc swelling and retinal haemorrhages in his initial patients, Cogan and Victor [56] did not find ptosis, pupillary signs, optic disc swelling, or retinal haemorrhages in any of patients with Wernicke's disease [56, 57]. Cogan's study led to a misconception that the presence of retinal haemorrhages ruled out Wernicke's encephalopathy. Physicians should know that Wernicke's encephalopathy has described retinal haemorrhages and optic disc swelling. Their presence should not delay the diagnosis of this rapidly fatal but quickly reversible disease [58–60].

5.5.4 Ocular Ischaemic Syndrome

Midperipheral retinal haemorrhages are seen in a vast majority of patients (more than 80%) with ocular ischaemic syndrome due to severe obstruction of carotid arteries [61, 62].

Patients with carotid artery obstructive disease remain asymptomatic for a long time. Peripheral retinal dot and blot haemorrhages are accompanied by narrow or thread-like retinal arterioles and dilated retinal veins without tortuosity (Fig. 5.17). [63]. Occasionally peripheral retinal haemorrhages may be seen in patients with insulin-dependent diabetes who may show only minimal, or no background retinopathy changes [64].

5.5.5 Retinal Haemorrhages in Increased Intracranial Pressure

Patients with increased intracranial pressure presenting with papilloedema often have superficial retinal haemorrhages in the peripapillary area. In patients with diabetes, hypertension, or central retinal vein occlusion, retinal haemorrhages may be seen even in the far periphery of the retina and pose a diagnostic challenge [65].

5.5.6 Valsalva Retinopathy

Seemingly benign activities such as lifting weights, a bout of forceful coughing, or straining at stools etc., especially against a closed glottis (Valsalva manoeuvre), may cause a sudden increase in the intraabdominal and intrathoracic pressure, which in the absence of valves in the veins located above the heart leads to a spike in the intravenous pressure in the upper part of the body. This sudden increase in pressure gets trans-

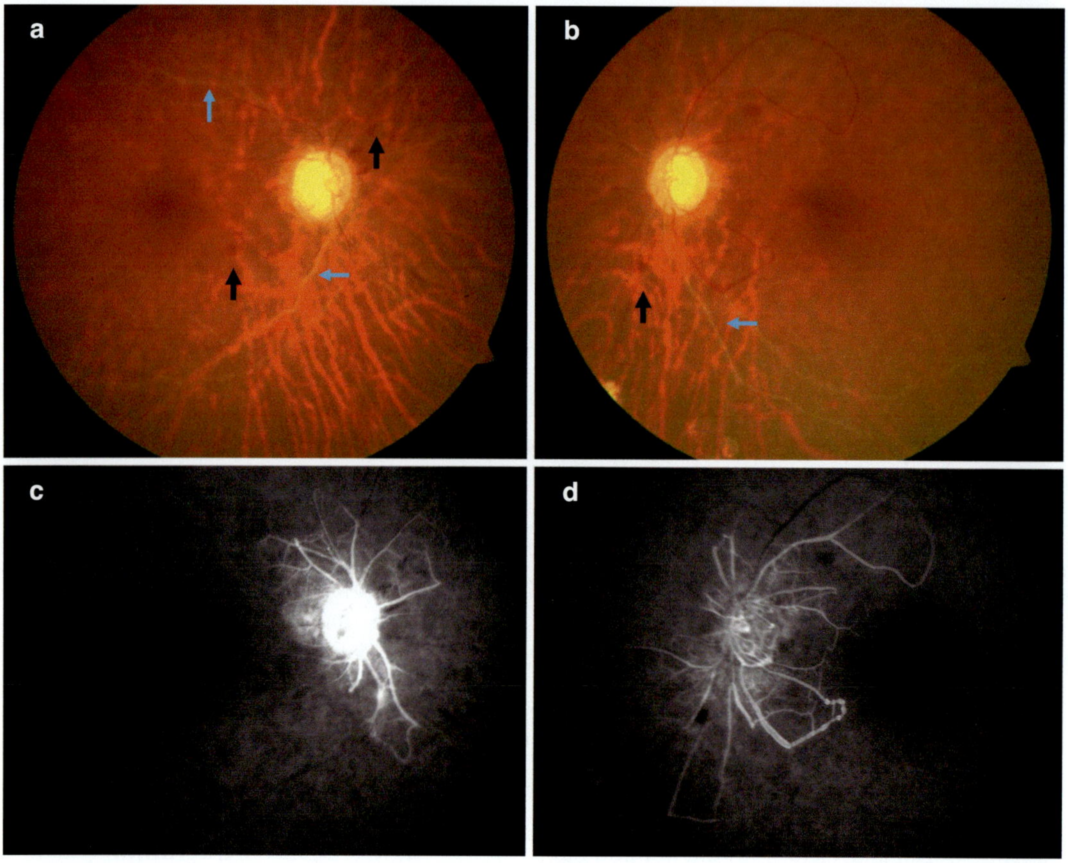

Fig. 5.17 Retinal haemorrhages (black arrows) are accompanied by narrow or even thread-like retinal arterioles (blue arrows) in both eyes (**a**, **b**) of a patient with ocular ischaemic syndrome. Fluorescein angiography (**c**, **d**) showed extensively non-perfused retina

mitted to the retinal veins and capillaries that may rupture, resulting in a haemorrhage in the subhyaloid or sub-ILM space or the retina leading to a sudden loss of vision (Fig. 5.18) [66]. The presence of two rings suggests the presence of both sub-ILM and subhyaloid locations of the blood [67]. The actual site of retinal vein rupture has been documented in a patient who developed preretinal and vitreous haemorrhage following self-induced emesis [68]. Visual disturbances discovered by a patient on waking up following general anaesthesia may be due to the Valsalva retinopathy caused by difficult intubation [69, 70].

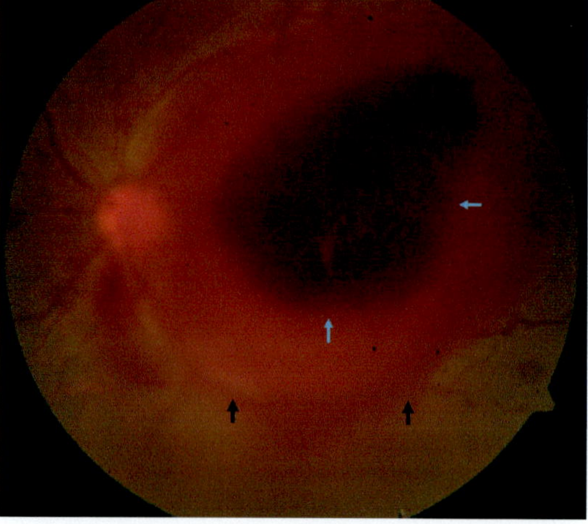

Fig. 5.18 Massive subhyaloid (black arrows) and sub-ILM haemorrhage (blue arrows) following a Valsalva manoeuvre

The Valsalva retinopathy resolves spontaneously in a few days, and the patients who usually report to the emergency department need nothing more than reassurance. The physician looking after the patient needs to be aware of this entity. If the haemorrhage does not resolve spontaneously within 3 weeks, Nd:YAG laser hyaloidotomy may drain the liquefied blood into a more dependent part of the vitreous cavity with immediate improvement in the vision.

By and large, Valsalva retinopathy is unilateral except when there may be an underlying retinal pathology. Bilateral loss of vision due to Valsalva retinopathy in a young woman during a normal vaginal delivery necessitated vitreous surgery in one eye to remove the haemorrhage [71].

While in the past, most of the cases of Valsalva retinopathy were noted in the sub-ILM or sub-hyaloid space, with the availability of spectral domain OCT, these haemorrhages are now reported even in the deeper layers of the retina that may necessitate the use of intravitreal TPA and gas to displace the haemorrhage [72].

References

1. Li Z, Guo C, Nie D, Lin D, Zhu Y, Chen C, Xiang Y, Xu F, Jin C, Zhang X, Yang Y, Zhang K, Zhao L, Zhang P, Han Y, Yun D, Wu X, Yan P, Lin H. Development and evaluation of a deep learning system for screening retinal hemorrhage based on ultra-Widefield fundus images. Transl Vis Sci Technol. 2020;9(2):3. https://doi.org/10.1167/tvst.9.2.3. PMID: 32518708; PMCID: PMC7255628.
2. Kumar A, Kumar P, Singh A, D S, Kaushik J. Bilateral premacular sub-hyaloid hemorrhage-unmasking COVID-19 induced pancytopenia. J Med Virol. 2021;93(5):2576–7. https://doi.org/10.1002/jmv.26752. Epub 2020 Dec 29. PMID: 33368339.
3. Sharma A, Upadhyaya A, Madan S, Singh P, Beri S. Sub-internal limiting membrane haemorrhage following pancytopenia in megaloblastic anemia. Clin Exp Optom. 2021;104(5):653–5. https://doi.org/10.1080/08164622.2021.1878842. Epub 2021 Mar 1. PMID: 33689650.
4. Baumal CR, Sarraf D, Bryant T, Gui W, Muakkassa N, Pichi F, Querques G, Choudhry N, Teke MY, Govetto A, Invernizzi A, Eliott D, Gaudric A, Cunha de Souza E, Naysan J, Lembo A, Lee GC, Freund KB. Henle fibre layer haemorrhage: clinical features and pathogenesis. Br J Ophthalmol. 2021;105(3):374–80. https://doi.org/10.1136/bjophthalmol-2019-315443. Epub 2020 May 6. PMID: 32376610.
5. Au A, Hou K, Baumal CR, Sarraf D. Radial hemorrhage in Henle layer in macular telangiectasia type 2. JAMA Ophthalmol. 2018;136(10):1182–5. https://doi.org/10.1001/jamaophthalmol.2018.2979. PMID: 30054619; PMCID: PMC6233838.
6. Lu AQ, Prensky JG, Baker PS, Scott IU, Mahmoud TH, Todorich B. Update on medical and surgical management of submacular hemorrhage. Expert Rev Ophthalmol. 2020;15(1):43–57. https://doi.org/10.1080/17469899.2020.1725474.
7. Todorich B, Scott IU, Flynn HW Jr, Johnson MW. Evolving strategies in the management of submacular hemorrhage associated with choroidal neovascularization in the anti-vascular endothelial growth factor era. Retina. 2011;31(9):1749–52. https://doi.org/10.1097/IAE.0b013e31821504df. PMID: 21562448.
8. Lee EJ, Kee HJ, Han JC, Kee C. Evidence-based understanding of disc hemorrhage in glaucoma. Surv Ophthalmol. 2021;66(3):412–22. https://doi.org/10.1016/j.survophthal.2020.09.001. Epub 2020 Sep 17. PMID: 32949554.
9. Hwang JF, Lin CJ. Multilayered optic disc hemorrhages in adolescents. J Pediatr Ophthalmol Strabismus. 2014;51(5):313–8. https://doi.org/10.3928/01913913-20140715-01. Epub 2014 Jul 22. PMID: 25036104.
10. Kokame GT, Yamamoto I, Kishi S, Tamura A, Drouilhet JH. Intrapapillary hemorrhage with adjacent peripapillary subretinal hemorrhage. Ophthalamology. 2004;111(5):926–30. https://doi.org/10.1016/j.ophtha.2003.08.040. PMID: 15121370.
11. Zou M, Zhang Y, Huang X, et al. Demographic profile, clinical features, and outcome of peripapillary subretinal hemorrhage: an observational study. BMC Ophthalmol. 2020;20:156. https://doi.org/10.1186/s12886-020-01426-9.
12. Zhang X, Cheng X, Chen B, Sun X. Multimodal imaging characteristics and presumed cause of intrapapillary hemorrhage with adjacent peripapillary subretinal hemorrhage. Clin Ophthalmol. 2021;15:2583–90. https://doi.org/10.2147/OPTH.S304861. PMID: 34177259; PMCID: PMC8219308.
13. Sibony P, Fourman S, Honkanen R, El Baba F. Asymptomatic peripapillary subretinal hemorrhage: a study of 10 cases. J Neuroophthalmol. 2008;28(2):114–9. https://doi.org/10.1097/WNO.0b013e318175cd90. PMID: 18562843.
14. Kaur B, Taylor D. Fundus hemorrhages in infancy. Surv Ophthalmol. 1992;37(1):1–17. https://doi.org/10.1016/0039-6257(92)90002-b. PMID: 1509354.
15. Watts P, Maguire S, Kwok T, Talabani B, Mann M, Wiener J, Lawson Z, Kemp A. Newborn retinal hemorrhages: a systematic review. J AAPOS. 2013;17(1):70–8. https://doi.org/10.1016/j.jaapos.2012.07.012. Epub 2013 Jan 28. Erratum in: J AAPOS. 2013 Jun;17(3):341. PMID: 23363882.
16. Duke-Elder S, Dobree JH, editors. System of ophthalmology, diseases of the retina, vol. X. London: Henry Kimpton; 1967. p. 140.

17. Cho IH, Kim MS, Heo NH, Kim SY. Birth-related retinal hemorrhages: the Soonchunhyang University Cheonan Hospital universal newborn eye screening (SUCH-NES) study. PLoS One. 2021;16(11):e0259378. https://doi.org/10.1371/journal.pone.0259378. PMID: 34752467; PMCID: PMC8577753.
18. Sun L, Jiang Z, Li S, Liu J, Su M, Lu Y, Li Z, Ding X. What is left after resolution of neonatal retinal hemorrhage: the longitudinal long-term outcome in foveal structure and visual function. Am J Ophthalmol. 2021;226:182–90. https://doi.org/10.1016/j.ajo.2021.01.028. Epub 2021 Feb 5. PMID: 33556380.
19. Kiffney GT Jr. The eye of the "battered child". Arch Ophthalmol. 1964;72:231–3. https://doi.org/10.1001/archopht.1964.00970020231016. PMID: 14162948.
20. Togioka BM, Arnold MA, Bathurst MA, Ziegfeld SM, Nabaweesi R, Colombani PM, Chang DC, Abdullah F. Retinal hemorrhages and shaken baby syndrome: an evidence-based review. J Emerg Med. 2009;37(1):98–106. https://doi.org/10.1016/j.jemermed.2008.06.022. Epub 2008 Dec 11. PMID: 19081701.
21. Binenbaum G, Forbes BJ. The eye in child abuse: key points on retinal hemorrhages and abusive head trauma. Pediatr Radiol. 2014;44 Suppl 4:S571–7. https://doi.org/10.1007/s00247-014-3107-9. Epub 2014 Dec 14. PMID: 25501729.
22. Thiblin I, Andersson J, Wester K, Högberg G, Högberg U. Retinal haemorrhage in infants investigated for suspected maltreatment is strongly correlated with intracranial pathology. Acta Paediatr. 2022;111(4):800–8. https://doi.org/10.1111/apa.16139. Epub 2021 Oct 28. PMID: 34617346.
23. Hansen JB, Killough EF, Moffatt ME, Knapp JF. Retinal hemorrhages: abusive head trauma or not? Pediatr Emerg Care. 2018;34(9):665–70. https://doi.org/10.1097/PEC.0000000000001605. PMID: 30180101.
24. Levin AV. Retinal hemorrhages: advances in understanding. Pediatr Clin North Am. 2009;56(2):333–44. https://doi.org/10.1016/j.pcl.2009.02.003. PMID: 19358919.
25. Binenbaum G, Reid JE, Rogers DL, Jensen AK, Billinghurst LL, Forbes BJ. Patterns of retinal hemorrhage associated with pediatric cerebral sinovenous thrombosis. J AAPOS. 2017;21(1):23–7. https://doi.org/10.1016/j.jaapos.2016.10.004. Epub 2017 Jan 11. PMID: 28087346.
26. Thau A, Saffren B, Anderst JD, Carpenter SL, Levin AV. A review on clotting disorders and retinal hemorrhages: can they mimic abuse? Child Abuse Negl. 2021;118:105070. https://doi.org/10.1016/j.chiabu.2021.105070. Epub 2021 May 25. PMID: 34049052.
27. Quan SC, Skondra D. Case report: peripheral retinal ischemia and retinal neovascularization in von Willebrand disease. Optim Vis Sci. 2021;98(4):418–24. https://doi.org/10.1097/OPX.0000000000001670. PMID: 33828041.
28. Carraro MC, Rossetti L, Gerli GC. Prevalence of retinopathy in patients with anemia or thrombocytopenia. Eur J Haematol. 2001;67(4):238–44. https://doi.org/10.1034/j.1600-0609.2001.00539.x. PMID: 11860445.
29. Capua T, Cohen N, Anafy A, Greisman D, Levin D, Rimon A. Routine funduscopy in immune thrombocytopenic purpura—is it really necessary? Eur J Pediatr. 2019;178(6):957–60. https://doi.org/10.1007/s00431-019-03371-2. Epub 2019 Apr 2. PMID: 30937605.
30. Honig SE, Srinivasan A, Shields CL. Suprachoroidal hemorrhage simulating melanoma in idiopathic thrombocytopenic purpura. Ocul Oncol Pathol. 2019;5(3):162–6. https://doi.org/10.1159/000490390. Epub 2018 Oct 11. PMID: 31049321; PMCID: PMC6489043.
31. Kaur N, Nair V, Sharma S, Dudeja P, Puri P. A descriptive study of clinico-hematological profile of megaloblastic anemia in a tertiary care hospital. Med J Armed Forces India. 2018;74(4):365–70. https://doi.org/10.1016/j.mjafi.2017.11.005. Epub 2017 Dec 27. PMID: 30449923; PMCID: PMC6224687.
32. Vaggu SK, Bhogadi P. Bilateral macular hemorrhage due to megaloblastic anemia: a rare case report. Indian J Ophthalmol. 2016;64(2):157–9. https://doi.org/10.4103/0301-4738.179720. PMID: 27050355; PMCID: PMC4850815.
33. Mansour AM, Salti HI, Han DP, Khoury A, Friedman SM, Salem Z, Ibrahim K, Bazerbachi A, Saghir N. Ocular findings in aplastic anemia. Ophthalmologica. 2000;214(6):399–402. https://doi.org/10.1159/000027532. PMID: 11053999.
34. Toh ZH, Chin CF, Gan NY. Case of unilateral anaemic retinopathy unmasking colorectal carcinoma. BMJ Case Rep. 2022;15(2):e248029. https://doi.org/10.1136/bcr-2021-248029. PMID: 35228244; PMCID: PMC8886398.
35. Liu TYA, Johnson TV, Barnett BP, Scott AW. Evolution of leukemic retinal hemorrhages documented by spectral-domain OCT and color fundus photography. Ophthalmol Retina. 2018;2(5):494–501. https://doi.org/10.1016/j.oret.2017.08.014. Epub 2017 Oct 18. PMID: 31047332.
36. Rodrigues GR, Mendonca TM. Retinal hemorrhages in leukemia. N Engl J Med. 2022;386(19):e50. https://doi.org/10.1056/NEJMicm2116866. Epub 2022 May 7. PMID: 35522023.
37. Zhuang I, Gupta I, Weng CY. Retinal hemorrhages in a patient with petechiae. JAMA Ophthalmol. 2019;137(4):459–60. https://doi.org/10.1001/jamaophthalmol.2018.6220. Erratum in: JAMA Ophthalmol. 2020;138(2):223. PMID: 30763438.
38. Dobberstein H, Solbach U, Weinberger A, Wolf S. Correlation between retinal microcirculation and blood viscosity in patients with hyperviscosity syndrome. Clin Hemorheol Microcirc. 1999;20(1):31–5. PMID: 11185681.
39. da Cruz NFS, Milhomens Filho JAP, Ferraro DMN, Polizelli MU, de Moraes Ambrogini

NSB. Hyperviscosity retinopathy and immunogammopathy maculopahy as new onset of multiple myeloma. Case Rep Ophthalmol. 2021;12(2):578–84. https://doi.org/10.1159/000514695. PMID: 34326757; PMCID: PMC8299375.
40. Choi RY, Jacoby R, Shakoor A. Multimodality ocular imaging in a case report of hyperviscosity syndrome associated with lymphoplasmacytic leukemia: the images tell the story. Retin Cases Brief Rep. 2019;13(3):238–40. https://doi.org/10.1097/ICB.0000000000000565. PMID: 28333850.
41. Rachidi S, Musallam KM, Taher AT. A closer look at paroxysmal nocturnal hemoglobinuria. Eur J Intern Med. 2010;21(4):260–7. https://doi.org/10.1016/j.ejim.2010.04.002. Epub 2010 May 13. PMID: 20603032.
42. Meppiel E, Crassard I, Latour RP, de Guibert S, Terriou L, Chabriat H, Socié G, Bousser MG. Cerebral venous thrombosis in paroxysmal nocturnal hemoglobinuria: a series of 15 cases and review of the literature. Medicine (Baltimore). 2015;94(1):e362. https://doi.org/10.1097/MD.0000000000000362. PMID: 25569655; PMCID: PMC4602837.
43. Hauser D, Barzilai N, Zalish M, Oliver M, Pollack A. Bilateral papilledema with retinal hemorrhages in association with cerebral venous sinus thrombosis and paroxysmal nocturnal hemoglobinuria. Am J Ophthalmol. 1996;122(4):592–3. https://doi.org/10.1016/s0002-9394(14)72130-0. PMID: 8862066.
44. Scheuerle AF, Serbecic N, Beutelspacher SC. Paroxysmal nocturnal hemoglobinuria may cause retinal vascular occlusions. Int Ophthalmol. 2009;29(3):187–90. https://doi.org/10.1007/s10792-007-9188-9. Epub 2008 Apr 24. PMID: 18437293.
45. Sorigue M, Juncà J, Orna E, Romanic N, Sarrate E, Castellvi J, Soler M, Rodríguez-Hernandez I, Feliu E, Ruiz S. Retinal vein occlusion and paroxysmal nocturnal hemoglobinuria. J Thromb Thrombolysis. 2017;44(1):63–6. https://doi.org/10.1007/s11239-017-1502-4. PMID: 28447244.
46. Sim R, Cheung G, Ting D, Wong E, Wong TY, Yeo I, Wong CW. Retinal microvascular signs in COVID-19. Br J Ophthalmol. 2022;106(9):1308–12. https://doi.org/10.1136/bjophthalmol-2020-318236. Epub ahead of print. PMID: 33741583; PMCID: PMC7985973.
47. Bosch MM, Barthelmes D, Landau K. High altitude retinal hemorrhages—an update. High Alt Med Biol. 2012;13(4):240–4. https://doi.org/10.1089/ham.2012.1077. PMID: 23270439.
48. Takkar A, Kesav P, Lal V, Gupta A. Teaching neuroimages: Terson syndrome in cortical venous sinus thrombosis. Neurology. 2013;81(6):e40–1. https://doi.org/10.1212/WNL.0b013e31829e6f13. PMID: 23918868.
49. Verma R, Sahu R, Lalla R. Subarachnoid haemorrhage as the initial manifestation of cortical venous thrombosis. BMJ Case Rep. 2012;2012:bcr2012006498. https://doi.org/10.1136/bcr-2012-006498. PMID: 22914236; PMCID: PMC4543949.
50. Wall M. Idiopathic intracranial hypertension. Neurol Clin. 2010;28(3):593–617. https://doi.org/10.1016/j.ncl.2010.03.003. PMID: 20637991; PMCID: PMC2908600.
51. Raevis J, Elmalem VI. Pseudotumor cerebri syndrome causing a terson like syndrome. Am J Ophthalmol Case Rep. 2020;20:100993. https://doi.org/10.1016/j.ajoc.2020.100993. PMID: 33305067; PMCID: PMC7710506.
52. Voldman A, Durbin B, Nguyen J, Ellis B, Leys M. Fulminant idiopathic intracranial hypertension and venous stasis retinopathy resulting in severe bilateral visual impairment. Eur J Ophthalmol. 2017;27(2):e25–7. https://doi.org/10.5301/ejo.5000918. PMID: 28009405.
53. Younus O, Savides P. Papilloedema with retinal haemorrhages in idiopathic intracranial hypertension. BMJ Case Rep. 2022;15(2):e248912. https://doi.org/10.1136/bcr-2022-248912. PMID: 35228253; PMCID: PMC8886392.
54. Brodsky MC, Biousse V. A bloody mess! Sur Ophthalmol. 2018;63(2):268–74. https://doi.org/10.1016/j.survophthal.2017.05.004. Epub 2017 May 18. PMID: 28527856.
55. Ozgonul C, Moinuddin O, Munie M, Lee MS, Bhatti MT, Landau K, Van Stavern GP, Mackay DD, Lebas M, DeLott LB, Cornblath WT, Besirli CG. Management of peripapillary choroidal neovascular membrane in patients with idiopathic intracranial hypertension. J Neuroophthalmol. 2019;39(4):451–7. https://doi.org/10.1097/WNO.0000000000000781. PMID: 30951011; PMCID: PMC8063500.
56. Cogan DG, Victor M. Ocular signs of Wernicke's disease. AMA Arch Ophthalmol. 1954;51(2):204–11. https://doi.org/10.1001/archopht.1954.00920040206007. PMID: 13123606.
57. Thomson AD, Cook CC, Guerrini I, Sheedy D, Harper C, Marshall EJ. Wernicke's encephalopathy revisited. Translation of the case history section of the original manuscript by Carl Wernicke 'Lehrbuch der Gehirnkrankheiten fur Aerzte and Studirende' (1881) with a commentary. Alcohol Alcohol. 2008;43(2):174–9. https://doi.org/10.1093/alcalc/agm144. Epub 2007 Dec 4. PMID: 18056751.
58. Bohnsack BL, Patel SS. Peripapillary nerve fiber layer thickening, telangiectasia, and retinal hemorrhages in wernicke encephalopathy. J Neuroophthalmol. 2010;30(1):54–8. https://doi.org/10.1097/WNO.0b013e3181ceb4d0. PMID: 20182209.
59. Mumford CJ. Papilloedema delaying diagnosis of Wernicke's encephalopathy in a comatose patient. Postgrad Med J. 1989;65(764):371–3. https://doi.org/10.1136/pgmj.65.764.371. PMID: 2608577; PMCID: PMC2429353.
60. Pereira FB, Soares Dutra Oliveira H, Lima VC, Lima LH, Balaratnasingam C, Pulido JS, de Souza EC. Retinal hemorrhages in a patient with acute ataxia. Retin Cases Brief Rep. 2021;15(Suppl 1):S32–4. https://doi.org/10.1097/ICB.0000000000001149. PMID: 34171899.

61. Brown GC, Magargal LE. The ocular ischemic syndrome. Clinical, fluorescein angiographic and carotid angiographic features. Int Ophthalmol. 1988;11(4):239–51. https://doi.org/10.1007/BF00131023. PMID: 3182177.
62. Vazirani JA, Zadeng Z, Dogra MR, Gupta A. Ocular ischemic syndrome. Indian J Ophthalmol. 2014;62(5):658–60. https://doi.org/10.4103/0301-4738.97083.
63. Hussain N, Falali S, Kaul S. Carotid artery disease and ocular vascular disorders. Indian J Ophthalmol. 2001;49(1):5–14. Erratum in: Indian J Ophthalmol. 2001;49(3):150. PMID: 15887709.
64. Roy MS, McCulloch JC. Peripheral retinal hemorrhages in long-duration insulin-dependent diabetes with minimal background retinopathy. Br J Ophthalmol. 1982;66(5):286–9. https://doi.org/10.1136/bjo.66.5.286. PMID: 7074003; PMCID: PMC1039781.
65. Galvin R, Sanders MD. Peripheral retinal haemorrhages with papilloedema. Br J Ophthalmol. 1980;64(4):262–6. https://doi.org/10.1136/bjo.64.4.262. PMID: 7387960; PMCID: PMC1043666.
66. Duane TD. Valsalva hemorrhagic retinopathy. Trans Am Ophthalmol Soc. 1972;70:298–313. PMID: 4663671; PMCID: PMC1310456.
67. Mathew DJ, Sarma SK. Valsalva retinopathy with double ring sign: laser membranotomy for twin bleeds. Saudi J Ophthalmol. 2016;30(1):68–70. https://doi.org/10.1016/j.sjopt.2015.10.003. Epub 2015 Oct 30. PMID: 26949364; PMCID: PMC4759518.
68. Kadrmas EF, Pach JM. Vitreous hemorrhage and retinal vein rupture. Am J Ophthalmol. 1995;120(1):114–5. https://doi.org/10.1016/s0002-9394(14)73769-9. PMID: 7611317.
69. Flikier S, Flikier D, Flikier B, Wu L. Multimodal imaging of valsalva petaloid maculopathy secondary to acute laryngospasm and endotracheal intubation. Eur J Ophthalmol. 2022;32(2):NP6–NP10. https://doi.org/10.1177/11206721211032515.
70. Patane PS, Krummenacher TK, Rao RC. Valsalva hemorrhagic retinopathy presenting as a rare cause of impaired vision after a general anesthetic—a case report and review of the literature. J Clin Anesth. 2015;27(4):341–6. https://doi.org/10.1016/j.jclinane.2015.03.013. Epub 2015 Apr 9. PMID: 25865821.
71. Mutha V, Narde HK, Chandra P, Kumar A. Valsalva retinopathy following normal vaginal delivery: 'bilaterality a rarity'. BMJ Case Rep. 2018;2018:bcr2018224781. https://doi.org/10.1136/bcr-2018-224781. PMID: 29666102; PMCID: PMC5905816.
72. Leisser C, Huemer JC, Findl O. Henle fibre layer haemorrhage after a valsalva manoeuvre. Case Rep Ophthalmol. 2021;12(1):105–9. https://doi.org/10.1159/000511373. PMID: 33976665; PMCID: PMC8077655.

6 New Vessels on the Optic Disc and Elsewhere in the Retina

6.1 Introduction

Development of pathological new vessels on the optic disc (NVD), new vessels elsewhere in the retina (NVE), and uncommonly, the anterior segment of the eye is the most significant and sight-threatening complication of diabetes mellitus (DM) and the common cause of severe visual loss in the developed world. According to the International Diabetes Federation, in 2021, 537 million people worldwide were living with diabetes, estimated to go up to 783 million by 2045. Moreover, 541 million people will have impaired glucose tests in 2021. It is anticipated that nearly 6.7 million people will die from diabetes and its related complications in 2021, making it one of the fastest-growing public health emergencies [1]. Diabetes is also the most common cause of blindness or severe visual impairment in the working-age group in the developed world. Given the critical role that physicians and ophthalmologists play in avoiding this unnecessary blindness, we discuss in some detail the pathophysiological mechanisms that lead to blindness in DM.

The severest form of symmetrical bilateral pathological neovascularization, the bane of middle- and low-income regions of the world, termed retinopathy of prematurity (ROP), is seen in preterm babies and, if not recognized and timely treated in an extremely narrow window of opportunity, leads to irreversible blindness. Autosomal dominant familial exudative vitreoretinopathy (FEVR) is a rare cause of peripheral pathological fibrovascular proliferation, almost similar to ROP in appearance, bilateral but highly asymmetric, and without a history of prematurity or oxygen therapy. The other, not uncommon, causes include ischaemic branch retinal vein occlusion, ischaemic central retinal vein occlusion, inflammatory occlusion of the retinal veins, sickle cell retinopathies, and atherosclerotic and inflammatory carotid artery diseases (see Box 6.1). The development of abnormal vessels in the retina is a highly complex phenomenon and, in the last several decades, has continued to be a subject of intense research to unravel the mystery of the highly orchestrated biological interactions that underpin the development of abnormal vasculature. We shall briefly discuss the pathophysiological mechanisms underlying abnormal retinal vascularization development.

Box 6.1 Common Causes of Retinal New Vessels

1	Proliferative diabetic retinopathy
2	Ischaemic retinal venous occlusion
3	Retinopathy of prematurity
4	Ischaemic retinal periphlebitis
5	Sickle cell anemia
6	Familial exudative vitreoretinopathy
7	Ocular ischaemic syndrome

A. Gupta et al., *Ophthalmic Signs in Practice of Medicine*,
https://doi.org/10.1007/978-981-99-7923-3_6

6.1.1 Blood Supply of the Retina

The retina is metabolically one of the most active tissues of the body. While the photoreceptors in the outer retina get their oxygen supply from the choroid, the inner retina gets its oxygen and micronutrient requirements through a 3-tiered capillary distribution network of the central retinal artery. Like other natural phenomena, such as the branches of a tree or the bronchial tree, the blood supply in the human body and the retinal blood supply follows a complex fractal geometry (cf. Euclidean geometry that follows straight lines) to maximize the distribution of blood supply in a confined space. Quantifying the various aspects of retinal vessel geometry, including their fractal dimensions, is now possible using digital images or digitizing them. The fractal dimension, a measure of the complexity of the retinal vessels, has been calculated as 1.7 [2]. While the choroidal blood vessels that supply the oxygen and micronutrients to the photoreceptors are under autonomic control, autoregulation at the level of the neuro-glial-vascular unit controls the blood supply to meet the metabolic requirements of the neural elements in the inner retina. The fractal geometry of the retinal vessels ensures a uniform blood flow and supply and removal of the metabolites from the inner retina.

6.1.2 Development of Normal Retinal Vessels

Normal retinal vasculature develops initially as capillary plexuses around the optic disc that extends peripherally, the first to start is the superficial capillary plexus (SCP) in the retinal nerve fibre layer and the ganglion cells beginning at about 14–16 weeks of gestation and the deep capillary plexus (DCP) on either side of the inner nuclear layer about 8 weeks later. The DCP always lags behind the SCP. Even at full term, the temporal SCP is yet to develop. The retinal arterioles and veins differentiate from these plexuses [3]. The capillaries are believed to grow in retinal tissue planes that offer the least resistance, namely the nerve fibre layer, the inner plexiform, and the outer plexiform layer that lies on either side of the inner nuclear layer. The perifoveal area always remains avascular. In the past, it has been debated whether the retinal vasculature develops by vasculogenesis or angiogenesis. In Ang-2 deficient transgenic mice, the hyaloid vessels being vasculogenic in origin were present. However, the retina remained avascular, settling the issue of retinal vasculature development in favour of angiogenesis. VEGF-A and Ang-1 play a significant role in the embryonic development of retinal vasculature, but Ang-2 is necessary for post-natal remodelling of the retinal vessels [4]. It is currently believed that cellular interactions between the retinal ganglion cells (RGC), retinal astrocytes (derived from the optic nerve head; these migrate into the nerve fibre layer), and the endothelial cells lead to the development of normal retinal vessels. The development of the retinal vasculature is mediated by the platelet-derived growth factor A from the RGC, the platelet-derived growth factor B from the endothelial cells, and the VEGF gradient that exists due to hypoxia in the retinal tissue [5].

6.2 Pathophysiology of Diabetic Retinopathy

6.2.1 Muller Cells

Each retinal capillary cell shares a very intimate relationship with the processes of the Muller cells, the macroglia cells, and the resident macrophages, the microglial cells. The non-activated microglia lie in the inner and outer plexiform layers. Once activated, they assume the functions of a macrophage, move throughout the retina, and produce inflammatory cytokines. The Muller cell processes extend throughout the thickness of the neurosensory retina, and their footplates form the internal elastic lamina (ILM). The outer limiting membrane is formed by the contact of the Muller cell processes with the photoreceptors at the junction of their inner and outer segments. These processes maintain intimate contact with the capillary endothelial cells, retinal ganglion cells, bipolar cells, horizontal cells, amacrine cells, and the photoreceptors to form a neuro-glia-vascular unit, commonly called a neurovascular unit. The primary function of this unit is to maintain metabolic homeostasis in the retina by controlling glucose metabolism. The Muller cells remove the toxic glutamate, prevent oxidative damage, and recycle neurotrophic factors critical for cell survival [6].

The hypoxic milieu in the retina, as in diabetic retinopathy, leads to the overexpression of hypoxia-inducible factor 1-α (HIF-1α) in the endothelial cells and the Muller cells. Hypoxic Muller cells also produce VEGF, leading to overexpression of the matrix metallic proteinase-2 (MMP-2) by the endothelial cells. Typically, the tissue inhibitors of matrix metalloproteinase (TIMP-2) are in a strict balance with the MMP-2, but in a diseased state, this balance is disturbed. While HIF-1α is a regulator of vascular endothelial growth factor (VEGF) that promotes neovascular budding, MMP-2 leads to proteolysis of the extracellular matrix essential for the growth of new vessels outside the retina [7]. It is to be noted that VEGF is involved in both the hypoxia-induced physiological as well as pathological development of retinal vessels. In a mouse model, $VEGF_{164}$ was overexpressed in the pathological development of new vessels compared to their physiological development [8].

6.2.2 Pericytes-Endothelial Cell Interaction

Pericytes are intimately connected with the endothelial cells of the capillaries in all organs and play a significant role in the control of microcirculation because of their contractile properties. Relaxation of pericytes causes increased capillary blood flow, and contraction does the opposite [9]. Electron microscopic studies in the human retina have shown that pericytes cover more than 85% of the endothelial cells, much greater coverage than seen in the cerebral cortex or any other organ [10]. A basement membrane surrounds the endothelial cells, and another surrounds the pericyte-endothelial cell complex. Pericytes appear buried in the basement of the endothelial cells. Pericytes play a significant role in checking endothelial cell proliferation. Furthermore, the pericytes regulate the expression of tight junction proteins that maintain the inner blood-retinal barrier. Pores (gap junctions) in the extracellular matrix (ECM) of the basement membrane (BM) allow for the cell-to-cell crosstalk between the pericytes and the endothelial cells [11]. It is to be noted that pericytes do not have the potential to regenerate, while endothelial cells can proliferate. The vascular endothelial cells and pericytes share similar insulin receptors. One of the significant characteristics of diabetic microvascular disease is insulin resistance by the endothelial cells and impaired endothelial repair by the endothelial progenitor cells [12]. Recently, a decrease in insulin-stimulated Angiopoetin-1 (Ang-1) secretion in a pericyte insulin receptor knock-out mice model led to reduced angiopoietin-Tie2 signalling. It caused excessive vascular abnormalities mimicking diabetic retinopathy [13]. The authors proposed that Insulin signalling controls Ang-1 secretion from the pericytes in a healthy state.

Ang-1, in turn, interacts with the Tie-2 receptors, the transmembrane tyrosine kinase receptors on the endothelial cells, and ensures vascular stability by preventing transcription of the Ang-2. In diabetes, lack of insulin signalling results in decreased Ang-1 release to interact with the Tie-2 receptors and leads to overexpression of Ang-2, a factor in angiogenic sprouting [13]. Ang-2 expression increases in several diseases, such as cancer, sepsis, and diabetes. Ang-2 blocking agents restore the normalcy of sprouting vessels [14]. Moreover, Ang-2, a competitive antagonist of Ang-1, also turns off the Tie-2 receptor, setting the stage for increased endothelial permeability and angiogenesis [15]. Simultaneous use of a bispecific Ang-2 and VEGF-A blocking agent, Faricimab, has shown promising results in treating diabetic macular oedema [16]. This drug is currently FDA-approved for treating diabetic macular oedema and neovascular AMD.

6.2.3 Thickening of Basement Membrane in Diabetes Mellitus

One of the earliest pathological changes noted in the capillaries all over the body is the thickening of the basement membrane (BM) surrounding the endothelial cells, which is most profound in the retinal capillaries. The thickening occurs because of the deposition of the extracellular matrix (ECM) proteins in the basement membrane of the capillaries due to the non-enzymatic glycation of proteins (advanced glycation end products—AGE) in the presence of long-term hyperglycemia. At least 17 proteins, including collagen IV and fibronectin, were found overexpressed and four under-expressed in the diabetic basement membranes compared to those from the non-diabetic human donor eye specimens. Diabetes-related proteins were found to be more abundant in the area of microaneurysms. The deposition of these ECM proteins caused a doubling of the thickness of the BM. Two components of the complement family, C4 and C9, were also exclusively detected in the diabetic BM, suggesting a role for complement-mediated chronic inflammation in diabetic retinopathy.

Contrary to the belief that thick BM in people with diabetes is stiffer, atomic force microscopy revealed the BM in diabetics to be softer. Additionally, norrin—a growth factor protein associated with vascular proliferation—was upregulated in the BM [17]. Apart from providing structural support to the vascular endothelial cells, the BM plays a significant role in maintaining homeostasis, provides an additional blood-retinal permeability barrier, controls pericyte contraction, promotes cell-to-cell communication, plays a role in apoptosis, and is a repository of growth factors that promote new vessel growth [18]. Research is going on to regulate the genetic mechanisms that lead to the deposition of the ECM in the basement membrane as a strategy to prevent the development of diabetic retinopathy [18].

6.2.4 Consequences of the Basement Membrane Thickening

One of the consequences of the thickened BM is the loss of pericytes due to poor cell-matrix adhesions. It is one of the earliest pathological lesions in diabetic retinopathy [19, 20].

It is likely that a thickened BM also causes a breakdown in the cell-to-cell communication between the Muller cells, pericytes, and endothelial cells, leading to a loss of the auto-regulatory control by this neurovascular unit leading to a state of hypoxia, which also leads to activation of the microglia, and the Muller cells throughout the thickness of the retina [11]. Once activated, the microglia assume phagocytic activity and release proinflammatory cytokines.

6.2.5 Formation of Acellular Retinal Capillaries

Loss of the endothelial cells and the pericytes leads to forming acellular capillaries seen in trypsin digest studies as BM-bound hollow tubes. These hollow tubes lie next to the retinal arterioles. The activated microglia assume the role of macrophages to phagocytose the cellular debris. These are visible as capillary non-perfusion (CNP) areas on fundus fluorescein angiography (Figs. 6.1 and 6.2). The CNP areas are the hallmark of retinal ischaemia and mark the beginning of clinical manifestations of diabetic retinopathy, ultimately leading to abnormal vessels that grow into the vitreous cavity. Several mechanisms may be responsible for the loss of pericytes. Upregulation of Ang-2 (discussed in Sect. 6.1.4) in the presence of high blood glucose leads to apoptosis or migration of the pericytes. Advanced glycation end products are accumulated in the pericytes; inflammatory pathways via retinal autoantibodies against the pericytes through complement activation or accumulation of oxidative LDL products may also play a role. Activation

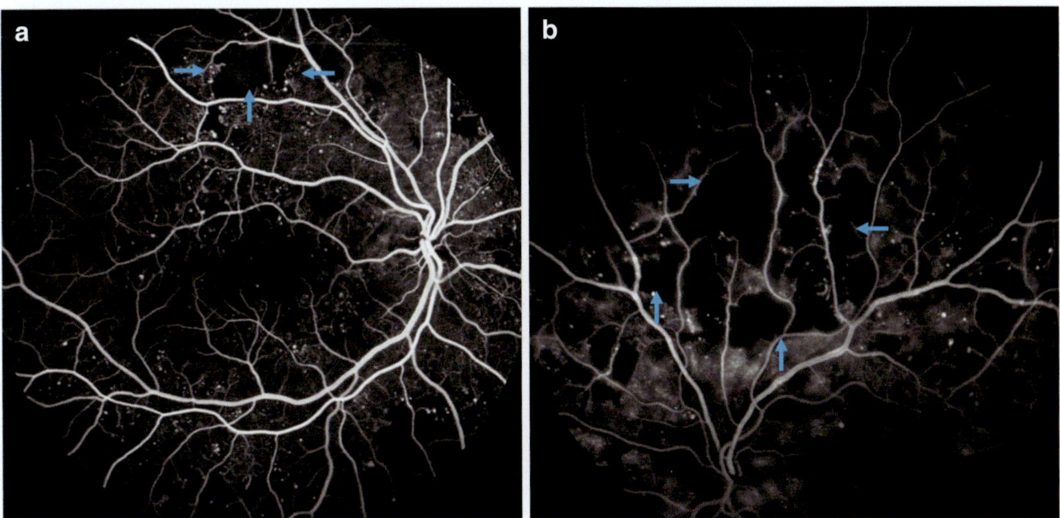

Fig. 6.1 Fundus fluorescein angiography showing areas of capillary non-perfusion (CNP) (blue arrows) in the mid periphery of the retina in the right (**a**) and the left (**b**) eyes of a patient with diabetic retinopathy

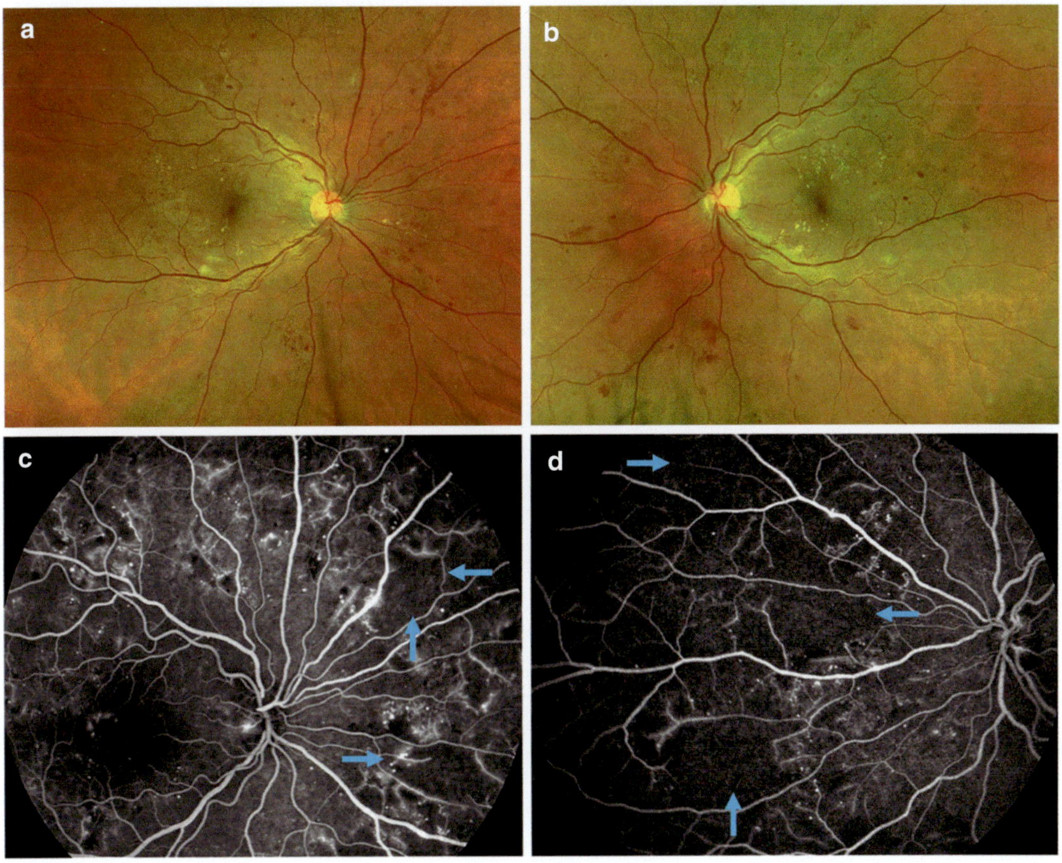

Fig. 6.2 Fundus photographs showing moderate non-proliferative diabetic retinopathy (**a**, **b**). Fluorescein angiography shows areas of capillary non-perfusion (CNP) in the nasal retina in the right and left eyes of the patient (**c**, **d**)

of multiple biochemical pathways, including the NF-kB activation by the reactive oxygen species, protein kinase C activation, and dephosphorylation of the platelet-derived growth factor receptor-β (PDGFR-β)ultimately lead to the apoptosis of the pericytes [21].

In the endothelial cells, a number of biochemical mechanisms get activated in the hyperglycemic state, including the activation of polyol and hexosamine pathways. Accumulation of AGE products and activation of the PKC lead to the induction of the enzyme, the inducible nitric oxide synthase (iNOS). Overproduction of the highly cytotoxic nitric oxide (NO) and release of the reactive oxygen species ultimately lead to the loss of endothelial cells [21]. Additionally, the capillary endothelial cells express adhesion molecules in response to the inflammatory cytokines released by the activation of microglia, which cause leukostasis and occlusion of the capillaries. Furthermore, there are significant rheological changes in the blood flow in patients with diabetes. The release of oxygen from the RBC is deficient, especially if the HbA1C is high, as oxygen binds more strongly with the glycated Hb. The RBCs are swollen, lose their biconcave shape, and hence lose their deformability and ability to negotiate through the normal capillaries efficiently. All these factors also contribute to retinal capillaries' occlusion [22]. Another major challenge in diabetes is the inability of the circulating endothelial progenitor cells to repair the dysfunctional endothelial cells. Progressive capillary non-perfusion leads to the release of VEGF from the neurovascular unit, the most potent growth factor for angiogenesis and the development of abnormal new vessels in the retina and the optic disc [11]. A significant increase in the aqueous humour levels of inflammatory cytokines, including IL1β, IL-6, IL-8, IL-10, TNF-α, MCP-1, and the VEGF, have been noted to correlate with the severity of peripheral retinal capillary non-perfusions areas in patients with PDR. These proinflammatory cytokines may be responsible for the progression of diabetic retinopathy changes [23].

6.2.6 Retinal Capillary Non-Perfusion and Severity of Diabetic Retinopathy

In the last 50 years, the areas of acellular retinal capillaries, as discussed above, have been demonstrated in diabetic retinopathy using fundus fluorescein angiography (FFA). These capillary/retinal non-perfusion/non-perfused regions or areas (CNP/RNP/NPR/NPA) are not uniformly distributed in the retina. Generally, the retinal area within a circle of radius 10 mm from the foveal centre is considered central, between 10–15 mm as midperipheral and beyond 15 mm as the peripheral retina [24]. In the early stages of diabetic retinopathy, CNP areas are most commonly distributed in the midperipheral retina and are often accompanied by retinal haemorrhages, cotton wool spots, and dilated retinal vessels (Figs. 6.1 and 6.2). The CNP areas may be less often seen in the central retina, especially nasal to the optic disc, and least common in the peripheral retina. When located in the extreme periphery, several microaneurysms may be seen around these CNP areas without cotton wool spots or blot haemorrhages [25]. Optical coherence tomography angiography (OCTA) studies have shown that smaller areas of CNP are seen next to the retinal arterioles. However, larger areas are near the retinal veins [26]. Eyes with non-proliferative diabetic retinopathy with a threshold of a 107-disc area of CNP, especially in the midperiphery, are at a high risk of developing retinal new vessels (NVE). The greater the area of CNP in the retinal midperiphery and the central retina, the higher the chance of developing new vessels on the optic disc (Fig. 6.3) [27].

Eyes that show dye leakage with a nonperfused retina (NPR) in the central retina are associated with diabetic macular oedema (DME) (Fig. 6.4). The NPR in the peripheral areas is usually not associated with dye leakage and correlates negatively with the occurrence of the DME [28]. Recent years have seen increasing use of wide-field- swept-source optical coherence tomography angiography (SS-OCTA) to quantify

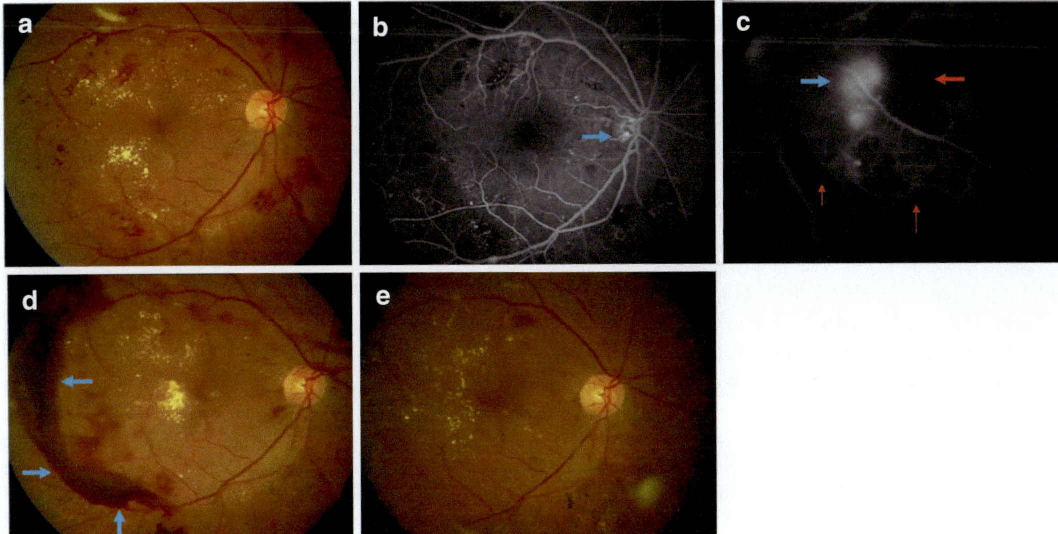

Fig. 6.3 A 60-year-old man with type 2 diabetes mellitus presented with clinically apparent non-proliferative diabetic retinopathy in the posterior pole (**a**). Most microaneurysms were seen away from the fovea on Fundus fluorescein angiography of the posterior pole. A doubtful new vessel was on the optic disc (**b**, blue arrow). However, there was extensive capillary non-perfusion in the nasal retina (red arrows) with new vessels (blue arrow) (**c**). Five months later, despite laser pan-retinal photocoagulation, he developed vitreous and subhyaloid haemorrhage (**d**, blue arrows) A supplemental laser photocoagulation led to resolution (**e**)

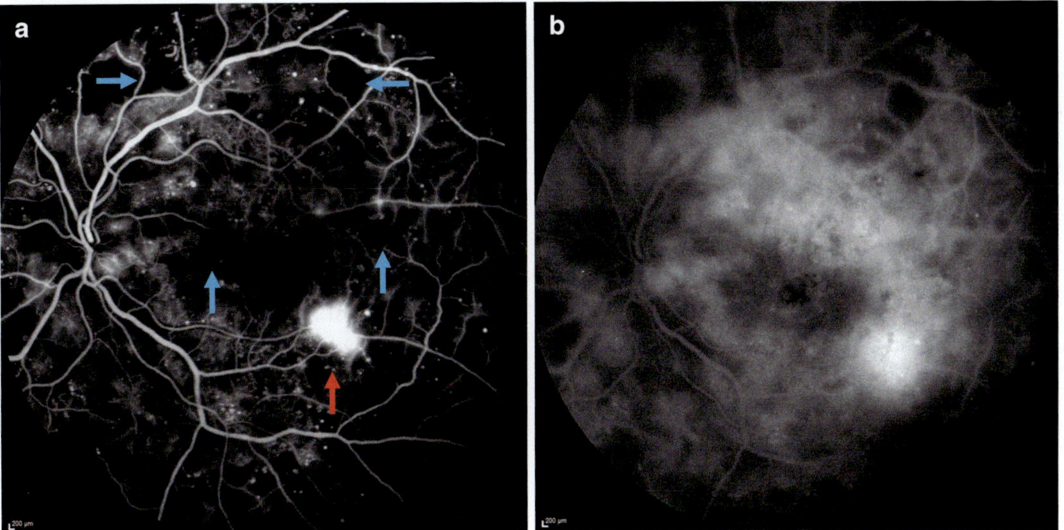

Fig. 6.4 Fundus fluorescein angiography showing areas of the non-perfused retina (blue arrows) in the central retina (**a**) with retinal neovascularization (red arrow). Late phase (**b**) shows diffuse dye leakage with diabetic macular edema (DME)

and analyse the retinal microvascular parameters using semi-automated software algorithms. Unlike the ultrawide-angle FFA that can simultaneously visualize almost 200 degrees of the retina, SS-OCTA is limited by the maximum scan area of 12 × 12 mm^2 at a time. The SS-OCTA, however, is a non-invasive technique without using any dye. The DCP cannot be separately

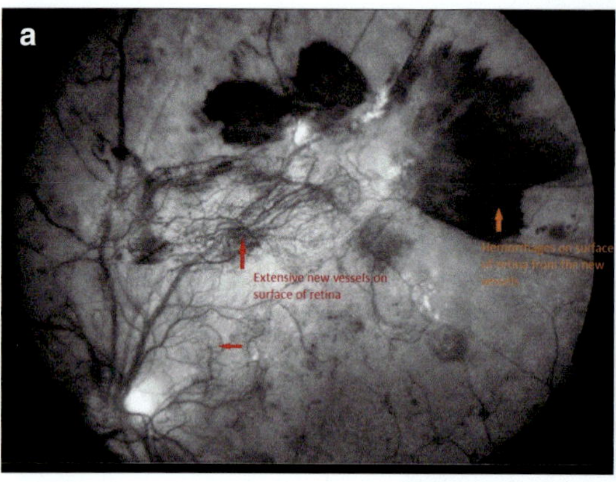

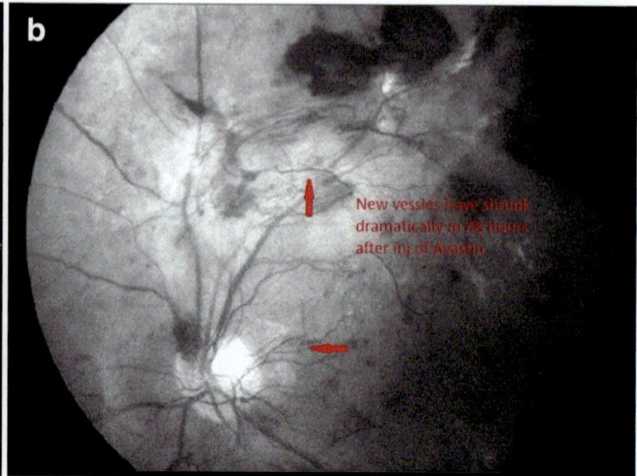

Fig. 6.5 Left eye retina of a patient with PDR (**a**). Note the extensive network of abnormal vessels (thin red arrows) that have started bleeding (thin orange arrows). He was the Author's (AG) first patient to receive an intravitreal injection of 2.5 mg of Avastin in early 2006. The same eye, as shown in (**a**), after 48 h of Avastin injection into the vitreous cavity, shows a dramatic disappearance of most abnormal retinal vessels(thick red arrows) (**b**). The abnormal retinal vessels need a continuous supply of VEGF to sustain them. Anti-VEGF antibodies like Avastin, Lucentis, or Eylea block the free VEGF leading to the disappearance of the vessels. However, the effect of one injection lasts for only 4 weeks or so. (Reproduced from Gupta, A. (2022). Bench-to-Bedside Research in Ophthalmology. In: Sobti, R., Ganju, A.K. (eds) Biomedical Translational Research. Springer, Singapore. https://doi.org/10.1007/978-981-16-8845-4_5. With permission of the publishers)

appreciated with the dye-based FFA, and dye leakage from the permeable retinal capillaries obscures the CNP areas. These areas cannot be accurately quantitated.

Using wide-field SS-OCTA, increasing RNP areas in the peripheral retina was associated with increasing the severity of diabetic retinopathy. Therefore, effective is the SS-OCTA technique that in the future, the severity of retinopathy grading is likely to be done by using an objective assessment of the RNP areas [29]. Intravitreal injections of anti-VEGF agents, such as Lucentis, Eylea, or bevacizumab, have become the standard of care for eyes with diabetic macular oedema, PDR, or even the NPDR (Fig. 6.5). While using these agents slows down the progression of the CNP areas, these agents fail to revascularize the ischaemic areas. The apparent revascularization of the CNP noted in some instances after using anti-VEGF agents may be due to the unplugging of the retinal capillaries blocked by the leukostasis. However, the capillaries that have lost their endothelial cells to apoptosis cannot be vascularized [24]. Even after 3 months of the pan-retinal photocoagulation (PRP) for the PDR, no change in the RNP areas was observed either on the UWF-FA or on the WF SS-OCTA [30, 31].

6.2.7 Development of Retinal New Vessels

In response to chronic hypoxia in diabetic retinopathy and retinal vein occlusions, several growth factors are produced by the neural and glial elements of the hypoxic retina, the most abundant of which is the vascular endothelial growth factor (VEGF). Michaelson, in 1948, had first hypothesized the presence of such a diffusible factor in the eyes that developed pathological new vessels either in the retina or in the anterior segment of the eye. He called it 'factor X' [32]. Only after four decades, this factor was identified as VEGF [33–35].

The VEGF is the gene involved in normal organogenesis, embryogenesis, and development of normal blood vessels. After the embryogenesis is over, the role of the growth factors is limited to menstruation and the heart and skeletal muscles during strenuous exercise. Another growth factor from the VEGF family was discovered in

1991[36], called the placental growth factor (PlGF), which also plays a significant role in pathological angiogenesis.

Soon after the discovery of VEGF, it was detected in the eyes of a primate model of diabetic retinopathy [37] and the ocular fluids of patients with diabetic retinopathy [38]. Injecting VEGF into non-human primate eyes led to a clinical picture mimicking diabetic retinopathy [39], establishing VEGF as the primary growth factor in the pathogenesis of diabetic retinopathy.

6.2.8 Intraretinal Microvascular Abnormalities (IRMA)

VEGF released from a hypoxic retina is responsible for developing intraretinal microvascular abnormalities (IRMA) and is an attempt to revascularize the ischaemic area. Muraoka and Shimizu [40] followed their patients of the NPDR and PDR eyes on FFA for up to 4 years and demonstrated attempts to form zigzag or hairpin loops in a single area of CNP and called this intraretinal neovascularization (IRNV) (Fig. 6.6). These dilated capillary segments always arose from the retinal veins and did not leak fluorescein. On average, 2–3 such IRNV were seen per eye, but as many as 12 lesions have been seen. The concept of IRMA as collateral vessels was initially based on fundus pictures [40]. In any case, the term IRMA continues to be the preferred term.

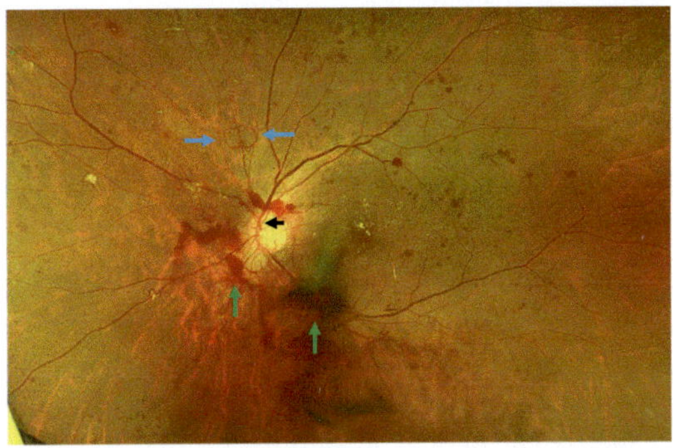

Fig. 6.6 Intraretinal neovascularisation (IRNV) or intraretinal microvascular abnormalities (IRMAs) seen as hairpin loops (blue arrows) are formed as an attempt to revascularize the ischaemic retina in diabetic retinopathy. Also seen are neovascularisation of the optic disc (black arrow) and vitreous and subhyaloid haemorrhages (green arrows)

Increasing retinal hypoxia results in more retinal haemorrhages, venous dilatation, and the formation of IRMAs. The early treatment diabetic retinopathy study (ETDRS) group classified the presence of more than 20 retinal haemorrhages in all four quadrants of the retina, the venous dilation and beading in two quadrants or the presence of IRMA in one quadrant as severe non-proliferative diabetic retinopathy (NPDR), the rule of 4-2-1 [41, 42]. All of these signs are strong risk factors for the development of proliferative diabetic retinopathy. The simultaneous presence of two or more signs was classified as moderately severe NPDR and portended an imminent development of proliferative diabetic retinopathy (PDR). IRMAs are much better delineated on the depth-resolved OCTA than on the 2-D FFA. The IRMAs are dilated capillary segments that arise from the retinal vein and loop back into the vein. These are located on the border of the non-perfused area; on OCTA, most of the IRMAs are seen to arise in the inner plexiform layer or sometime in the ganglion cell layer or the nerve fibre layer. These remain within the retina and only breach the ILM once they develop into NVE. On FFA, these generally do not leak except occasionally at the tips (Fig. 6.7) [43].

Recently, the behaviour of the IRMAs before and 3 months after laser pan-retinal photocoagulation (PRP) prompted a further characterization of these vessels as unchanged, tufting, reperfusion, mixed, and worsening types. Some of these IRMAs did not change or even showed reperfusion of the NPAs. Most interesting was the tuft type, wherein the tips of the irregularly dividing capillary network were twice the calibre of the capillaries, had a bulbous ending, and were seen to elevate the ILM (outpouching of ILM). Following the laser PRP, the tufts seemed to regress, and IRMAs appeared like pruned branches of a tree. The tuft-like IRMA appears to be the precursor of the NVE [44]. Prospectively followed on the OCTA, IRMA has been shown to develop into NVE [30, 31]. Interestingly, post hoc analysis of the CLARITY trial (comparing

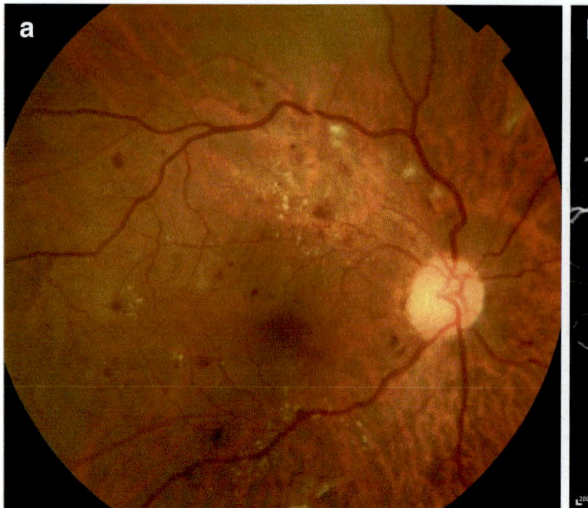

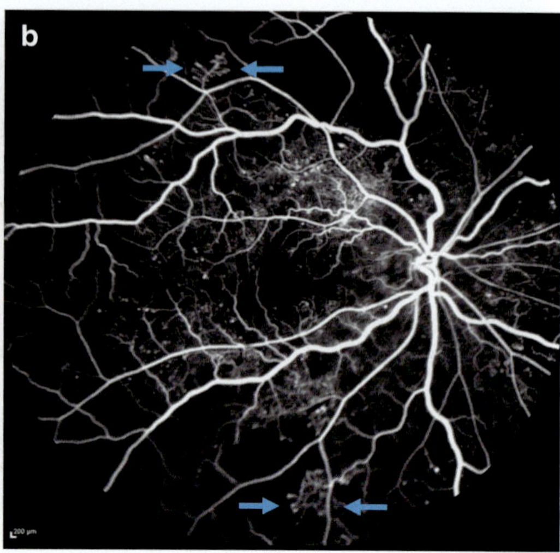

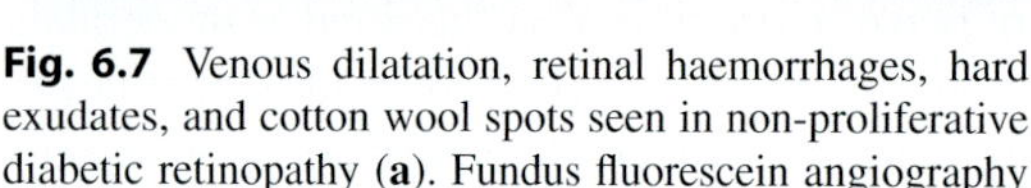

Fig. 6.7 Venous dilatation, retinal haemorrhages, hard exudates, and cotton wool spots seen in non-proliferative diabetic retinopathy (**a**). Fundus fluorescein angiography (**b**) showing IRMAs (blue arrows) at the border of the non-perfused retina and no dye leakage

PRP vs Intravitreal aflibercept in severe NPDR) found that while intravitreal aflibercept injections led to improvement in the severity score of the diabetic retinopathy in 75% of the eyes, including the deep retinal haemorrhages and the IRMA, there was no change in the venous beading [45]. It is likely that while anti-VEGF agents lead to a cosmetic improvement in the appearance of diabetic retinopathy, there is no reversal of hypoxia or decrease in the area of RNA.

6.2.9 Retinal Veins Dilatation, Beading, and Risk of Progression

In the early treatment diabetic retinopathy study (ETDRS) report #12, the group identified the severity of haemorrhages/microaneurysms, IRMA, and venous beading as the most significant risk factors for the progression of retinopathy [41, 42]. In prospective studies, a 10 μm increase in the central retinal vein equivalent over 4 years predicted the progression of diabetic retinopathy development of PDR and DME. However, such an association was not seen with a change in the calibre of the central retinal arterioles [46].

More recently, using UWF-FFA, while confirming the above observations, it was suggested that venous dilatation in the peripheral retina (outer zone), although not related to the retinal non-perfusion area, is perhaps more sensitive in predicting the progression of diabetic retinopathy. Moreover, the narrowing of the retinal arterioles in the outer zone, but not in the inner zone, was related to the retinal non-perfusion area and the progression of the retinopathy [47]. The retinal venous dilatation/ beading reflects the degree of retinal hypoxia in the retinal periphery and is a strong predictor of the development of PDR (Figs. 6.3 and 6.8). Almost 50% of the eyes with PDR show venous beading, while less than 10% with NPDR show such abnormality (Fig. 6.8). These are seen more often in the temporal half of the retina and the secondary branches rather than in the primary, tertiary, or smaller branches [48]. There may be ethnic differences as in a Chinese population, venous beading in >2 quadrants was seen in only 6% and 2% of eyes with moderately severe and severe NPDR, respectively, and none in the NPDR eyes. The authors felt that >2 quadrants of venous beading is too strict a criteria to diagnose severe NPDR [49]. While the retinal loops may be seen in 25% of the eyes with PDR, duplication of the veins is uncommon. If a venous loop is seen clinically, it is almost always suggestive of PDR, and a thorough search is done to locate new vessels using FFA (Fig. 6.9) [48]. The

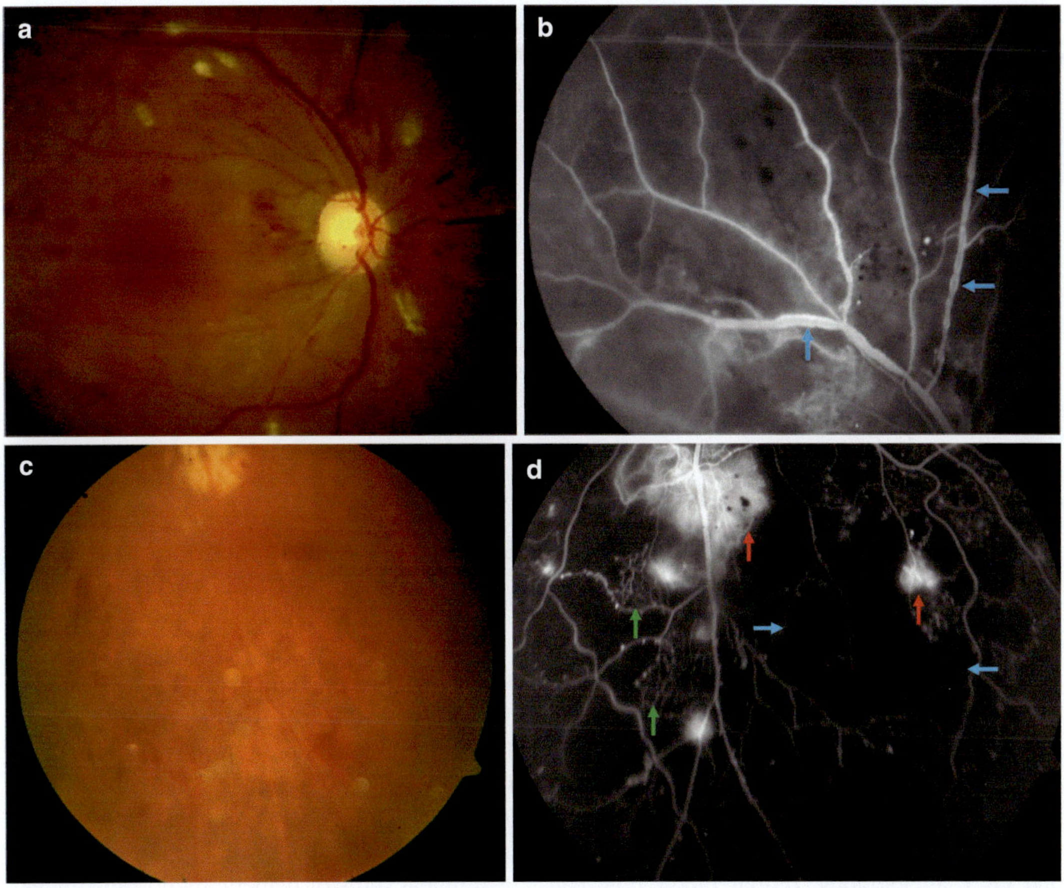

Fig. 6.8 (**a**, **b**) Venous fullness and beading in the retinal veins with retinal haemorrhages and a few cotton wool spots (**a**) in a patient with moderate NPDR. Funds fluorescein angiography (**b**) shows extensive capillary non-perfusion and venous beading (blue arrows). (**c**, **d**) Peripheral retina as seen on fundus photography (**c**) and fluorescein angiography (**d**). Note the IRMAs (green arrows), neovascularization of the retina elsewhere (NVE, red arrows), and vast areas of capillary non-perfusion (blue arrows)

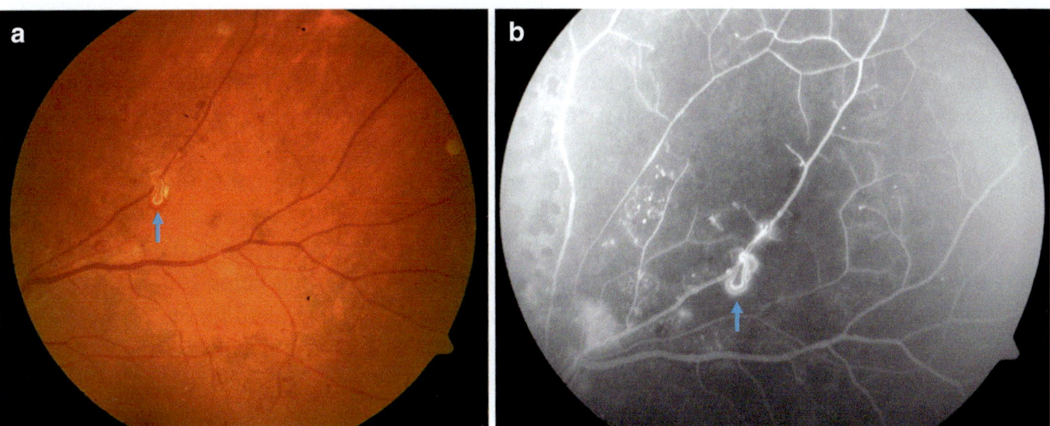

Fig. 6.9 The presence of a venous loop (blue arrows) seen clinically (**a**) is almost always suggestive of proliferative diabetic retinopathy, as confirmed by fluorescein angiography (**b**)

venous loops and duplication are proposed to result from a non-thrombotic occlusion of the large retinal vein and the opening of the collateral channels [50]. The availability of wide-field fundus imaging may show nearly 40% more lesions that are not captured on the standard 7-field fundus photographs [51]. Eyes with diabetic retinopathy that predominantly show peripheral lesions have an increased risk of retinopathy progression, and the progression of these peripheral lesions enhances the risk of the development of PDR [52].

In the past, there have been contradictory reports on the blood flow in patients with diabetic retinopathy. An increase in the flow due in the early stages of diabetic retinopathy may be due to autoregulatory control, the failure of which in the late stages of retinopathy may account for reduced flow in the retina. Previously, blood flow measurements could not be done in smaller vessels. Using more current techniques like multi-plane Doppler spectral domain OCT, the blood flow in the early stages of diabetic retinopathy was comparable to the normal population but was reduced in patients with PDR [53, 54]. Using adaptive optics scanning laser ophthalmoscopy and OCT angiography, retinal blood flow can now be measured in SCP, DCP, and across major retinal vessels. This technique showed that in a normal population, there is an increase in the blood flow and velocity with the increasing size of the blood vessels. There is an increase in the blood flow in vessels up to 60 μm size in patients with diabetes with no retinopathy and a decreased flow in those with retinopathy. It was hypothesized that increased blood flow and velocity in retinal vessels coupled with increased shear rate before the onset of diabetic retinopathy led to capillary endothelial damage resulting in capillary closure and hence the decreased flow and velocity once the retinopathy had set in [55]. At 3 months following laser photocoagulation, there was a significant increase in the oxygen saturation of both the retinal arterioles and retinal veins. There was a reduction in the calibre and the blood flow in the retinal arterioles and the veins. However, this reduction in calibre was more significant in the retinal veins. Reduced flow in the post-PRP eyes does not appear from the restoration of the normal autoregulatory mechanisms but is likely due to the elimination of hypoxic areas [56]. Using adaptive optics technology, it is now possible to measure the thickness of the wall of retinal arterioles and the diameter of their lumen. Following pan-retinal photocoagulation, while the external diameter of the retinal arterioles remained the same, a significant increase in the wall-to-lumen ratio (WLR) in eyes with PDR compared to that in the normal, no diabetic retinopathy or NPDR may be responsible for the decreased flow rate in these eyes. The increased WLR was also associated with hypertension [57].

6.2.10 New Vessels on the Retina Elsewhere (NVE) and the Optic Disc (NVD)

New vessels on the retina or/and optic disc mark the proliferative stage of diabetic retinopathy. The NVE is seen more frequently than the NVD, although the NVD signifies a more severe PDR (Fig. 6.10). The NVE accompanies NVD in the majority of eyes. The ETDRS report #10 defined the clinical signs of diabetic retinopathy, including the NVE and NVD. On stereoscopic fundus photograph examination, the NVE (irregularly arborizing vessels) should lie on the retina's surface or into the posterior vitreous.

In contrast, those on the optic disc surface or growing into the vitreous or within one disc diameter of the optic disc margin were defined as NVD. If vessels grow on the retina elsewhere and reach within 1/2 to 1 DD of the optic disc margin and no new vessels grow on the optic disc, these would be labelled as NVE. The severity of the NVE was further graded into five levels based on the absence, doubtful presence, or definitive presence and the area covered by the NVE (scale of 1/2 DA) in the retinal fields 1, 3–8, and severity graded as per the standard fundus photograph 7A [41, 42]. Likewise, the new vessels on the optic disc (NVD) were evaluated in field 1, standard photographs 10A and C (which are centred on the optic disc of the fundus), and five severity grades were defined based on the presence/absence and

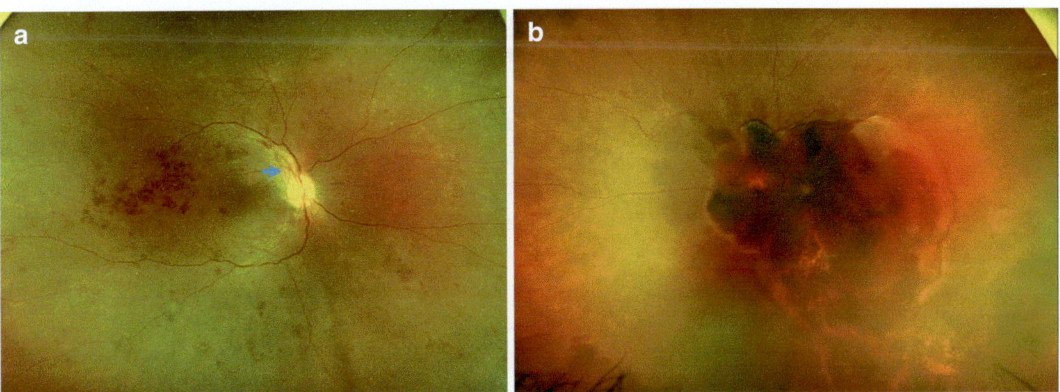

Fig. 6.10 The neovascularization of the optic disc (NVD, blue arrow) in the right (**a**) eye of a patient with insulin-dependent diabetes mellitus. The NVD in the left eye (**b**) is obscured by the large subhyaloid haemorrhage

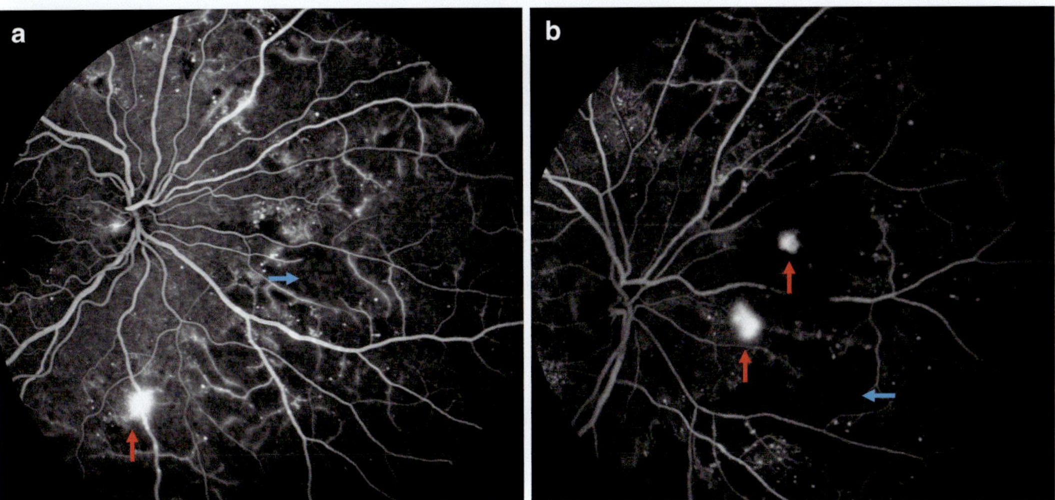

Fig. 6.11 Neovascularization of the retina elsewhere (NVE, red arrows) seen nasal to the optic disc in left eyes of two different patients (**a**, **b**), along with areas of capillary non-perfusion (blue arrows) as seen on fundus fluorescein angiography

the area of the new vessels. Grade 0 was no NVD, grade 1 questionable NVD, and grade 2 NVD less than that shown in standard photograph 10A. NVD in the standard photograph 10A was one third of the disc area. Grade 3 NVD was equal to or more than the NVD shown in standard photograph 10A but less than the NVD shown in standard photograph 10C, and grade 4 was equal to or larger than the NVD shown in standard photograph 10C. New vessels within the one disc diameter were also defined as NVD [41, 42].

The NVE is most often seen nasal to the optic disc or along the vascular arcades in the temporal retina (Fig. 6.11). NVE is not seen in the foveal area. They are seen farther from the fovea and are larger and more in number in type 1 DM compared to type 2 DM. NVD may be seen in up to one third of the eyes with PDR, and the new vessels are distributed most frequently along the upper temporal region of the neuroretinal rim of the optic disc. New vessels over the optic disc cup are highly unusual [58]. The NVE and the NVD are often accompanied by supporting fibrous tissue seen as strands or sheets of opaque scar tissue on the posterior hyaloid surface (Fig. 6.12).

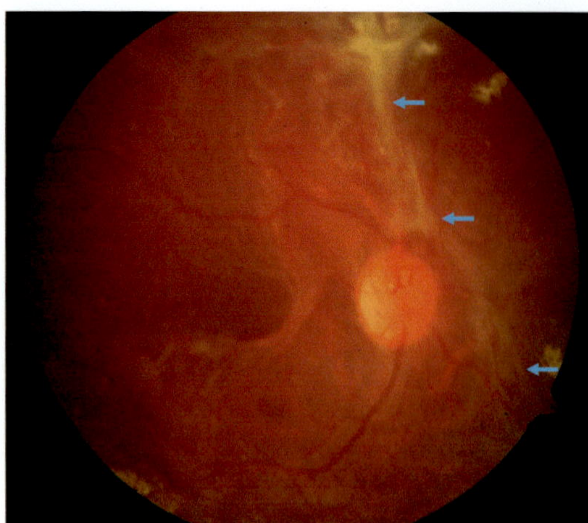

Fig. 6.12 Supporting fibrous tissue seen as strands or sheets of opaque scar tissue (blue arrows) on the posterior hyaloid surface, accompanying the NVE and NVD

Fluorescein angiography provides definitive evidence of the NVE and NVD that leak fluorescein dye (Figs. 6.3, 6.4, 6.8, and 6.11). However, the dye obscures the abnormal leaking vessels and the surrounding area, making it difficult to assess the exact size of the area occupied by the new vessels. The IRMA's growing tips (tufts) may occasionally leak fluorescein, adding to the confusion. Lee et al. [59] used OCT to differentiate NVE from IRMA. While ILM pouching and inner retina hyperreflective dots were almost exclusively seen in IRMA, ILM breach, posterior hyaloid breach, and vitreous hyperreflective dots were significantly common in NVE [59].

On structural SD-OCT, the NVD appears as hyperreflective tissue on the optic disc with either an attached or a detaching posterior hyaloid. The posterior hyaloid surface is a scaffold on which the new vessels grow. The NVE on SD-OCT appears as homogenous hyperreflective tissue seen breaching the ILM, growing forward onto the posterior hyaloid or into the vitreous cavity. These may be seen pulling the retina anteriorly while still attached to the retina, causing a tabletop detachment of the retina [60]. Taking B scan OCT as the standard for diagnosis of NVD, B Scan OCTA was more sensitive to detect NVD than the vitreoretinal slab on en face OCTA [61]. Ophthalmologists are able to detect new vessels in PDR with equal facility in both the FFA scans and the OCTA, making the latter a helpful noninvasive tool to study the new vessels [62]. On the en face OCTA, the new vessels on the optic nerve head appear as fine arborizing vessels-the exuberant vessel proliferation or as non-exuberant or pruned loops of abnormal vessels (Fig. 6.13).

Following PRP, the original NVD assumes the appearance of a large-trunk and branches appear pruned, while the growing tips of any new NVD appear more exuberant [63]. One may have to differentiate between optic disc collateral vessels from the NVD. The former is seen commonly in retinal vein occlusions and only occasionally in diabetic retinopathy. The collateral vessels form from the existing capillary network and may vary in size depending on the size of the obstructed vessel. Collaterals bypass the obstructed segment in a vein or an artery. Blood flow in these collaterals appears to be slow. These lie in the plane of the retina. While the NVD leaks profusely on FFA, the collateral vessels do not leak dye [64]. On the OCTA, the collateral vessels appear as dilated looping vessels in the radial peripapillary segment slab (Fig. 6.14).

In contrast, the NVD appears as a fine meshlike vessel in the VRI slab (Fig. 6.13) [65]. It has been suggested that the NVD shows a higher oxygen saturation than the collateral vessels that typically arise from the venous end of the circulation, unlike the NVD that seems to arise from the arterial end of the blood supply [66]. Study of the en-face vitreoretinal slab on SS-OCTA is a sensitive technique to non-invasively detect and monitor the progress of NVD and NVE [67–69] and is as sensitive as the FFA to detect new vessels [70]. In the vitreoretinal slabs of the SS-OCTA, NVE has predominantly two morphological patterns, namely the round pattern and the ramified pattern. The former type is associated with more severe retinal non-perfusion areas. On OCTA, the area of the NVE can be measured, and the progression rates calculated. The vessel density of the NVE decreases as the NVE increases in size [71].

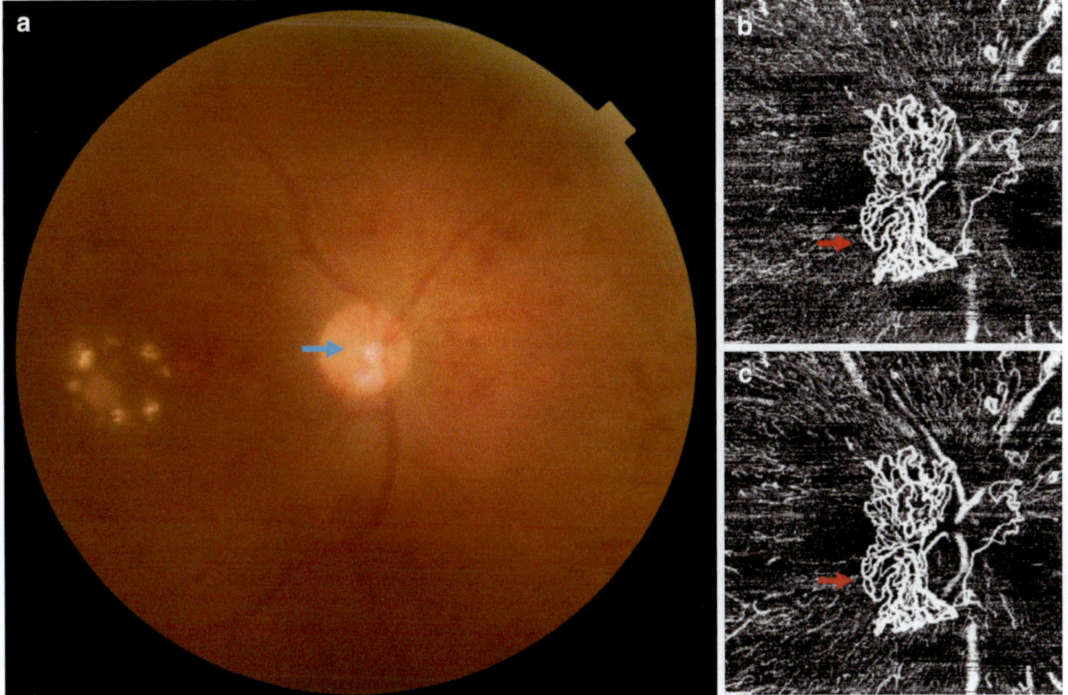

Fig. 6.13 Fundus photograph of a patient with diabetic retinopathy, with suspected NVD (**a**, blue arrow). On the en-face optical coherence tomography angiography (OCTA), the new vessels on the optic nerve head appear as fine arborizing vessels (red arrows), at the level of deep capillary plexus (**b**) as well as the outer retina (**c**)

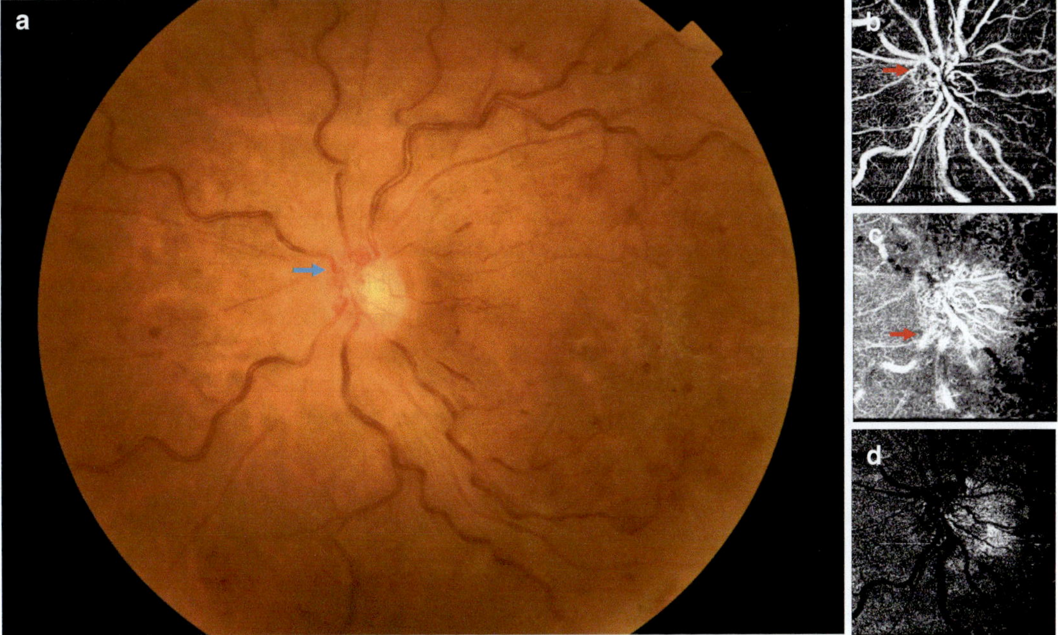

Fig. 6.14 Fundus photograph showing old central retinal vein occlusion with collaterals on the optic disc (**a**, blue arrow). On the en-face optical coherence tomography angiography (OCTA), the collaterals on the optic nerve head appear as dilated looping vessels (red arrows) at the level of superficial (**b**) and deep (**c**) capillary plexus. They are not appreciated at the level of the choriocapillaris (**d**)

The S-OCTA is a non-invasive tool to monitor the regression of new vessels. These are seen to start regressing as early as 1 week after the first session of pan-retinal photocoagulation [72]. Following the en-face OCTA, intravitreal injection of bevacizumab was seen to decrease the blood flow area and cause progressive regression of NVD starting within 24 h that was maintained for at least 1 month [73]. The presence of NVE of more than four-disc diameters and the forward-located NVE growing into the vitreous on the SS OCTA can predict the occurrence of vitreous haemorrhage. However, NVE that lie flat on the retina and do not grow into the vitreous had a low risk of such haemorrhages [74]. For patients less than 45 years of age, increasing blood urea nitrogen and smoking are independent risk factors for the progression of fibrovascular proliferation in PDR [75].

6.2.11 Automated Detection of New Vessels in Diabetic Retinopathy

There are two main mechanisms by which vision may be lost in patients with diabetes, the most common being collection of fluid in/or under the neurosensory retina, causing a swelling of the macular area called diabetic macular oedema, which is responsible for moderate visual loss. The second, although less common, is the development of NVE that ruptures to cause preretinal haemorrhages or the NVD that causes vitreous haemorrhage. Both may cause sudden and severe loss of vision. Till the patient loses vision, diabetic retinopathy remains asymptomatic. Fundus screening has been practiced for several decades, either manually by ophthalmologists or using tele screening using non-mydriatic cameras. However, it has not significantly reduced unnecessary blindness from diabetic retinopathy. In the last 15 years or so, there has been intense focus on the development of artificial intelligent strategies to automatically detect lesions of diabetic retinopathy, such as retinal microaneurysms/dot hemorrhages, retinal vessel calibre changes, or detection of NVE/NVD for prompt referral of the patient for detailed evaluation and timely treatment. Several features of the new vessels on the optic disc, such as the number, thin calibre, convoluted, irregular, and randomly directed, have low contrast and, if elevated above the surface, may be blurred, have been used to develop an automated detector [76].

6.2.12 Chronic Kidney Disease and Diabetic Retinopathy

Diabetes affects the micro and macro vessels of all organs. Besides affecting the eyes, diabetes targets the kidneys, peripheral nerves, and cardiovascular system. Nearly one third of patients with diabetes will develop chronic kidney disease (CKD) that begins as asymptomatic albuminuria, shows a progressive decline in the glomerular filtration rates, and finally turns into an end-stage kidney disease (ESRD) requiring renal replacement therapy. Diabetes is the most common cause of ESRD. The glomerular capillary changes in the kidneys mimic the changes happening in the retinal capillaries, as discussed above, including the deposition of extracellular matrix proteins leading to the thickening of the endothelial basement membrane and loss of foot plates of the podocytes. These highly specialized pericytes wrap around the endothelial cells on the side of the urinary pole. Thickening of the basement membrane leads to a breach in the cell-to-cell communication between the endothelial cells and the podocytes. The podocytes expressing VEGF are responsible for endothelial turnover and normal functioning. The endothelial cells in the kidney are fenestrated (unlike in the retinal capillaries) and provide for the glomerular filtration barrier that usually prevents the passage of proteins into the filtrate. Changes due to diabetes lead to progressive apoptosis of the podocytes and the endothelial cells leading to albumin excretion [77]. There is an increased deposition of extracellular matrix from the mesangial cells due to non-enzymatic glycation of proteins leading to nodular glomerular sclerosis, the pathology defining lesions of the diabetic kidney disease (Kimmelstiel-Wilson disease) [78].

There is strong evidence that patients with diabetic retinopathy have concurrent diabetic kidney disease [79, 80]. On the other hand, patients with DM and CKD also show a strong association with diabetic retinopathy [81]. In a prospective 8-year study, high baseline ACR (>30 mg/g), low eGFR (<60 mL/min/1.73 m^2), and serum creatinine were associated with the development of PDR. At the same time, high ACR was also associated with the development of diabetic macular oedema [82]. Abnormal renal functions predict the presence of significant non-perfusion of the retina and vice-versa [83]. Retinal non-perfusion areas on ultra-wide FA in patients with type 2 DM were associated with the high urinary albumin creatinine ratio, creatinine levels, and the estimated glomerular filtration rate (eGFR). As imaged on the OCTA, retinal non-perfusion areas also showed a negative correlation with the eGFR [84]. Extensive capillary non-perfusion is also associated with the progression of CKD [85, 86] and may also define the outcomes of CKD [87].

6.3 Other Causes of New Vessels on the Retina

While diabetic retinopathy is the most significant and the most common cause of the development of pathological retinal new vessels on the retina, several other retinal diseases may lead to blindness from the development of pathological new vessels on the retina, including the retinopathy of prematurity, sickle cell retinopathy, retinal vein occlusions (Fig. 6.15), and inflammations of the retinal veins (Fig. 6.16).

6.3.1 Retinopathy of Prematurity (ROP)

6.3.1.1 Historical Perspective

More than 75 years ago, an ever-increasing number of surviving babies born prematurely led to the recognition of a bilateral blinding condition called retrolental fibroplasia (RLF), so named because of a white reflex behind the crystalline lens caused by massive intraocular fibrosis. Terry saw this in 12% of preterm babies with a birth weight of 1360 g or less. He also observed no white reflex in some babies up to 8 weeks after birth, discounting the prevalent theory that the RLF represented the persistence of the hyaloid artery and persistent tunica vasculosa lentis. At times, the eyes even got enucleated for an incorrect diagnosis of retinoblastoma [88–91].

Owens and Owens [92] followed babies with birth weights less than 2000 g and described in detail for the first time the earliest retinal changes that led to RLF. The earliest change was retinal vein dilatation, tortuosity of both retinal veins

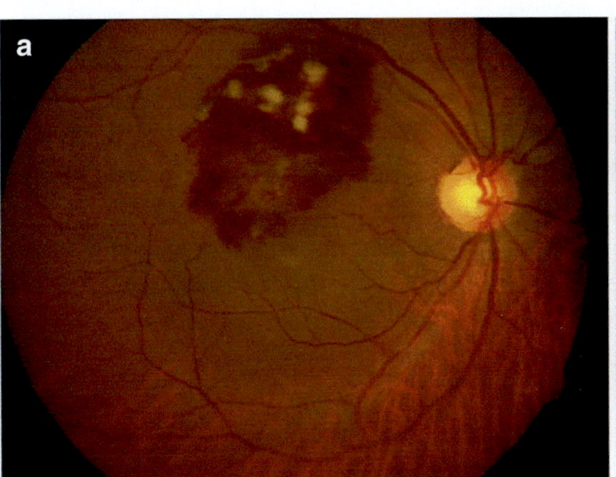

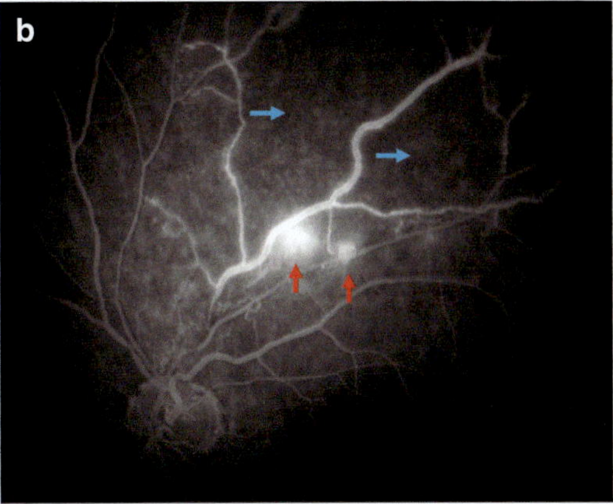

Fig. 6.15 Fundus photograph (**a**) showing macular branch retinal vein occlusion. Fluorescein angiography from another patient with upper temporal retinal vein occlusion showing NVEs (red arrows) and areas of capillary non-perfusion (blue arrows) (**b**)

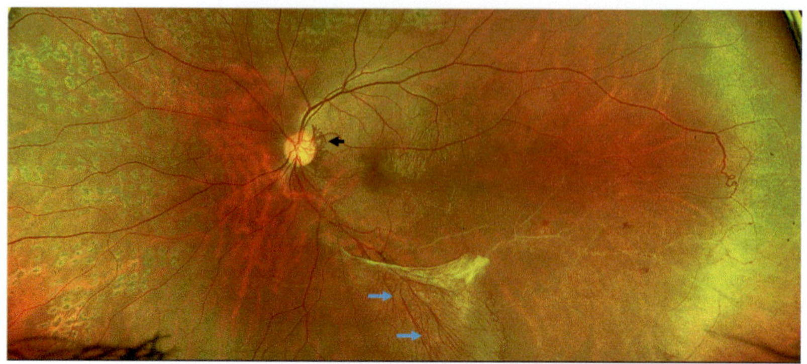

Fig. 6.16 NVD (black arrow) and NVE (blue arrows) in a case of retinal vasculitis

and arteries, followed soon by the appearance of a grey membrane with numerous vessels that, between the second and the fifth month of birth, ended up with a picture consistent with RLF [92].

6.3.1.2 Role of Oxygen Supplementation

The turn of the twentieth century had seen increasing use of oxygen supplementation to deal with acute respiratory distress that was common in preterm babies. The use of oxygen supplementation undoubtedly led to increased survival of premature babies. However, it coincided with an ever-increasing number of bilateral blind infants due to massive fibrovascular proliferation behind the crystalline lens, termed retrolental fibroplasia (RLF). In the early 1950s, diametrically, opposite views were held of whether the over or the underuse of oxygen was responsible for the RLF till Ashton [93], through his experiments on kittens up to 12 days of age, demonstrated complete obliteration of the retinal blood vessels on exposure to high concentration (70–80%) of oxygen. Notably, retinal vascularization in human babies is only complete once they attain a weight of 2000 g. Unlike human full-term newborn babies, the kitten does not develop complete retinal vascularization till 3 weeks of age and mimics the retina of preterm human babies [93]. On being shifted to the ambient air, the obliterative phase was followed by a disorderly and profuse proliferative phase of the retinal vessels that grew into the vitreous cavity. Ashton speculated that the release of a hypoxic factor from the anoxic retina is responsible for the vasoproliferative phase [94]. Simultaneously, similar conclusions were reached by Patz [95], who showed on histopathology the development of endothelial proliferation, budding of the new vessels through the ILM, and retinal haemorrhages in several animal models of oxygen toxicity. Patz recommended monitored use of oxygen with frequent measurements of oxygen tension [95]. Patz [96], after an extensive review of the clinical and experimental evidence, concluded that long-duration unmonitored high concentration of oxygen was the significant risk factor for the development of RLF.

6.3.1.3 Classification of ROP

Nearly 35 years after, Owens and Owens [92] first described the clinical stages of the disease that ultimately caused RLF an international classification of retinopathy of prematurity (IC ROP) was developed with an intent to bring about uniformity in reporting epidemiological data and treatment outcomes in various stages of the ROP [62]. The term ROP was preferred over the RLF that had been used previously but represented only stage 5 of the ROP. The retina was divided into three zones to indicate the location of the ROP changes. The innermost zone, zone I, was the area within a circle, centred on the optic disc, with a radius twice the distance between the centre of the optic disc and the centre of the macula; zone II was the retina between the outer boundary of zone I and a circle tangent to the nasal ora serrata and the zone III was the temporal crescent beyond the outer limit of zone II (Later a poste-

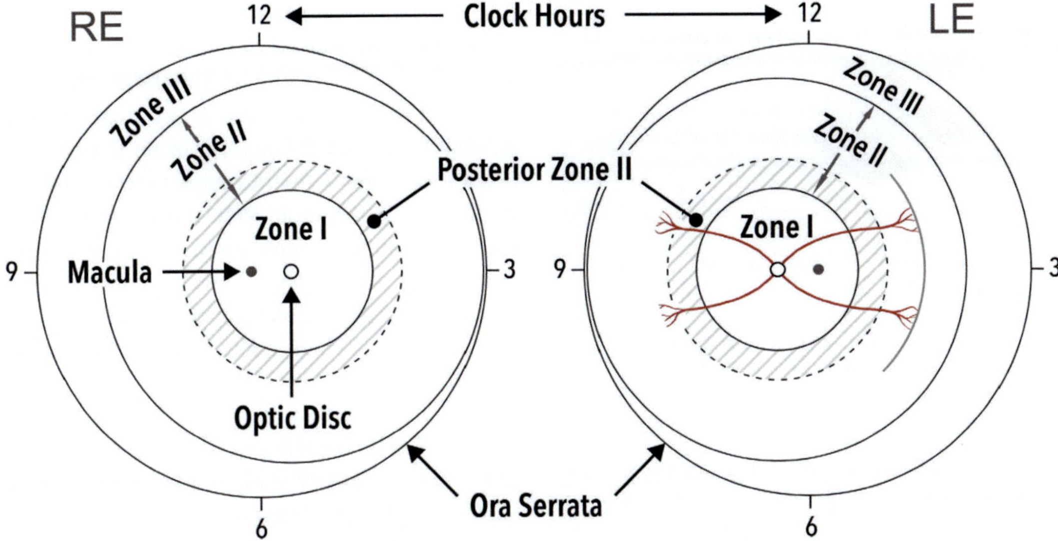

Fig. 6.17 Schema of the right eye (RE) and left eye (LE) showing zone borders and clock hour sectors used to describe the location of vascularization and extent of the retinopathy. Solid circles represent borders of zones I through III, and dotted circles represent borders of posterior zone II (2-disc diameters beyond zone I). A hypothetical example of examination findings is shown in LE, representing approximately three clock hours of stage 1 disease in zone II (note single line on drawing to document the presence of stage 1 disease). (Reproduced with publishers' permission from Chiang et al. International Classification of Retinopathy of Prematurity, Third Edition. Ophthalmology. 2021 Oct;128(10):e51-e68. https://doi.org/10.1016/j.ophtha.2021.05.031. Epub 2021 Jul 8. PMID: 34247850)

rior zone II was added that lay two-disc diameter beyond the outer boundary of zone I). Each zone was further divided into 12 clock hours (30° each) to show the circumferential spread of the pathology (Fig. 6.17). Stage 1 was defined as a demarcation line marking the junction of the vascularized and avascular retina. In stage 2, this demarcation line developed a volume and was seen as a ridge. Stage 3 was defined by the development of pathological extra-retinal fibrovascular proliferation on the ridge that lay perpendicular to the retina. Initially, stage 4 was defined as the development of any retinal detachment, either tractional or exudative. More recently, in the third edition of the IC-ROP, stage 4 was modified into Stage 4A, a peripheral retinal detachment not involving the fovea, and Stage 4B, when involving the fovea. In stage 5, there is a total tractional retinal detachment; if the optic disc is visible, it is stage 5A, and if the optic disc is not visible due to the retrolental fibrous membrane, it is stage 5B.

Furthermore, if there was a significant dilatation and tortuosity of the retinal vessels, it is labelled a Plus disease. The pre-plus disease is only vascular dilation without sufficient tortuosity. The plus disease should be assessed only in zone I vessels. Plus disease often has vascular dilation on the iris, rigid iris, and vitreous haze ([97]; see Box 6.2).

Box 6.2 Classification of Retinopathy of Prematurity

Zone I Retinal area within a circle centred on the optic disc and of a diameter twice the distance between the optic disc's centre and the macula's centre

Zone II Retinal area between the boundary of zone I in a circle tangent to the nasal ora serrata
Posterior Zone II Two-disc diameters beyond the boundary of zone 1

Zone III Temporal crescent

The circumferential extent of retinopathy is measured in clock hours. Each clock hour is 30°. The cumulative clock hours mean the total of the clock hours

Stage 1: Demarcation line between the vascularized and non-vascularized retina

Stage 2: The demarcation line has a volume and is seen as a ridge

Stage 3: Pathological extraretinal new vessels perpendicular to the ridge

Stage 4A: Tractional or exudative retinal detachment not involving the macula
Stage 4B: Retinal detachment involving the macula

Stage 5A: Total retinal detachment, but the optic disc is visible
Stage 5B: Total retinal detachment, the optic disc is not visible

Preplus disease: Dilatation of retinal vessels in zone I
Plus disease: Dilatation and tortuosity of retinal vessels in zone I

Chiang et al. [97]

6.3.1.4 Threshold ROP

Given the uncertainty of the progression or a spontaneous regression of the ROP, the pre-threshold ROP was defined as any stage of ROP in zone I, or stage 2 (ridge) in zone II with plus disease or stage 3 (extra retinal new vessels) in Zone III. The threshold ROP was considered the stage that, if left untreated, had a 50% risk of developing blindness. Threshold ROP was defined as stage 3 disease in eight cumulative or five contiguous clock hours in zone 1 or 2 with plus disease [98] (Figs. 6.18).

6.3.1.5 Early Treatment of ROP

In the natural history study of the CRYO-ROP, it was seen that pre-threshold eyes with specific characteristics progressed in 66.4% versus 15.5% in eyes without those features. The treatment strategy was revised to treat (mostly laser photocoagulation, but even cryotherapy was allowed) the high-risk pre-threshold eyes designated as type 1 ROP. These characteristics were zone I, any stage with plus disease or stage 3 without plus disease; zone II, stage 2 or 3 with plus disease. Disease severity less than type 1 was labelled type 2, and careful follow-up of these eyes was recommended. With the early treatment of the type 1 ROP, the 9-month unfavourable

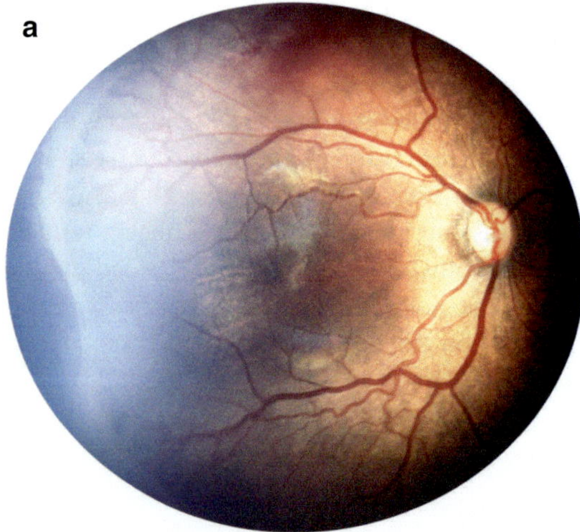

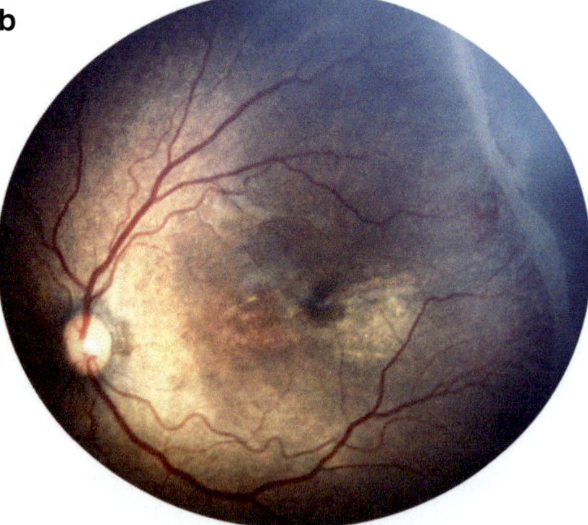

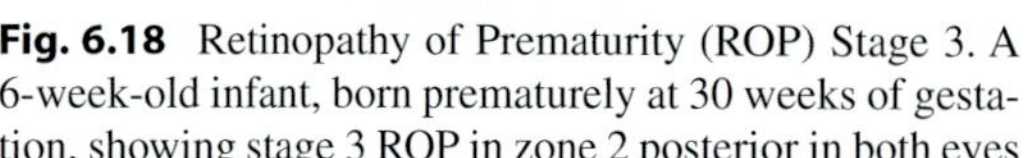

Fig. 6.18 Retinopathy of Prematurity (ROP) Stage 3. A 6-week-old infant, born prematurely at 30 weeks of gestation, showing stage 3 ROP in zone 2 posterior in both eyes (**a** and **b**). (Images courtesy of Dr. Simar Rajan Singh. Post Graduate Institute of Medical Education and Research, Chandigarh)

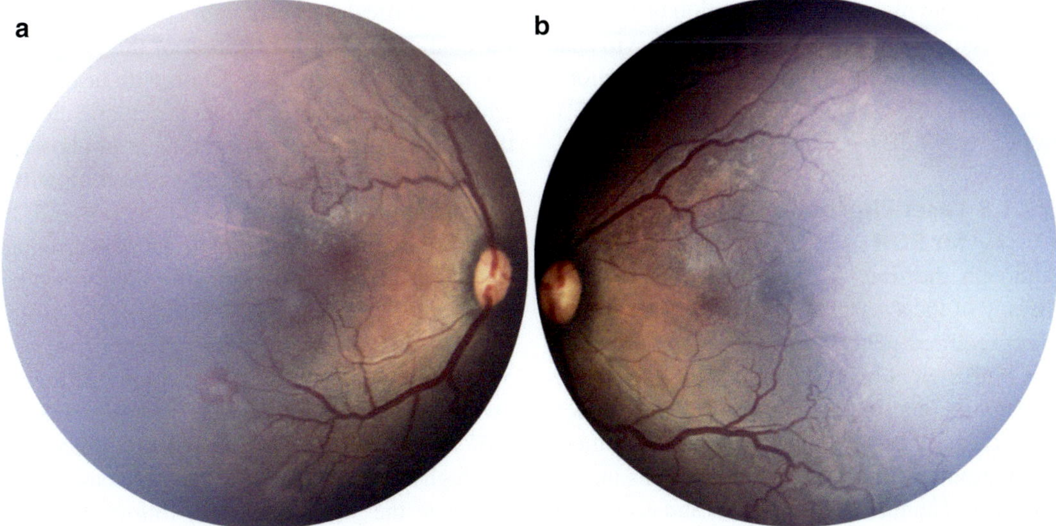

Fig. 6.19 Aggressive Retinopathy of Prematurity (AROP). A 4-week-old infant, born prematurely at 28 weeks of gestation, showed features of AROP in Zone 1 with avascular loops and flat neovascularization in both eyes (**a** and **b**). (Images courtesy of Dr. Simar Rajan Singh. Post Graduate Institute of Medical Education and Research, Chandigarh)

structural outcomes reduced from 15.6 to 9.1% [99]. At 6 years, the type 1 ROP-treated eye had significantly better visual (25.1% vs 32.8%) and structural outcomes (8.9% vs 15.2%). However, there was no benefit of treatment on visual and structural outcomes in type 2 ROP eyes. Notably, 52% of the untreated eyes with type 2 ROP showed spontaneous regression.

6.3.1.6 Aggressive ROP (A-ROP)

Previously defined as Aggressive posterior ROP (AP-ROP), Infants <1000 g birth weight or <28 weeks GA risk developing an aggressive disease seen in zone I or posterior zone II and do not follow the usual stages of progression. Clinically, it is characterized by forming vascular loops at the junction of the vascular and avascular retina rather than having a line or a ridge. There are no retinal capillaries in between the vascular loops. It is accompanied by a significant plus disease. These eyes tend to develop flat new vessels along the retina's surface and are frequently associated with preretinal and vitreous haemorrhages. The blood vessels may have a brush fire appearance and quickly progress into stages 4 and 5 [100]. Recognizing that the rapidly progressive ROP may not always be limited only to the posterior zones I and II and may also be seen in infants much higher in weight or GA, the nomenclature of AP-ROP has been revised to Aggressive-ROP (A-ROP) in the third edition of IC-ROP [97] (Fig. 6.19).

6.3.1.7 Cryoablation of ROP

In Japan, ROP had been treated with cryotherapy for more than a decade before it prompted a randomized multicentric trial named 'CRYO-ROP' to evaluate the efficacy of cryotherapy of the non-vascularized peripheral retina in eyes with threshold ROP. The preliminary results reported at 3 months of the treatment were highly promising and showed an unfavourable outcome in 21.8% of the treated eyes compared to 43% of the untreated eyes, firmly establishing the role of cryoablation [98]). The 15-year results of the CRYO-ROP trial (2005) demonstrated that the beneficial effects in the treated eyes were maintained for at least 15 years. Following cryoablation of the non-vascularized peripheral retina in eyes with threshold ROP, 52% of the untreated versus 30% of the treated eyes had adverse structural outcomes (partial or total retinal detachment involving the macula, or obscuration of the macula by retinal fold or media opacities due to cataract or corneal opacity) and adverse functional outcomes (VA < 20/200) in 64.3% and 44.7%, respectively [101].

6.3.1.8 Laser Photocoagulation for ROP

Although the trans-scleral application of cryotherapy of the avascular retina was efficacious, it often required general anaesthesia in extremely low birth weight babies, the procedure was time-consuming, and the babies had spells of apnea, bradycardia, or arrhythmias during the treatment. In addition, too many local complications including marked conjunctival chemosis and even vitreous haemorrhage [102]. By then, laser photocoagulation had already been established as the standard of care for proliferative diabetic retinopathy. The availability of laser delivery through indirect binocular ophthalmoscopes prompted preliminary studies comparing the outcomes of argon laser photocoagulation with the then-standard-of-care cryotherapy. Laser ablation of the peripheral avascular retina had a favourable outcome in 94% of the eyes versus 75% with cryoablation [102]. Soon after, Capone Jr et al. [103] reported successfully using diode laser photocoagulation in the zone I threshold ROP. Since then, it has been realized that there is more damage to the photoreceptor layer with the diode laser and higher chances of over-treatment because of less visible photocoagulation marks. The majority of ophthalmologists, in any case, possess a green laser. The odds of a favourable outcome in the long term were almost seven times higher with the laser compared to the cryotherapy. It firmly established laser photoablation of the avascular retina as the standard of care in threshold ROP [104–106].

6.3.1.9 Anti-VEGF Therapy for ROP

As the role of the VEGF in the pathogenesis of pathological neovascularization in ROP became clearer, initial anecdotal cases were followed by more extensive studies, including prospective studies comparing the outcomes of the laser vs the intravitreal anti-VEGF therapy [107, 108]. The intravitreal bevacizumab treatment allowed for continued revascularization of the peripheral retina, unlike the retinal ablation with laser/cryo, which did not allow for further vascularization of the peripheral retina. Furthermore, laser photocoagulation resulted in a lifelong contraction of the peripheral visual fields [109]. In the beat—ROP group study comparing intravitreal bevacizumab (0.625 mg in 0.025 mL) with laser photocoagulation for zone I, stage 3 + ROP and zone II posterior, stage 3 + ROP, the recurrence rates at 54 weeks postmenstrual age (PMA) were highly favourable for the intravitreal group at 6% vs 26% in the laser group and the difference was still higher 6% vs 42% in the zone I disease [109]. However, the patients must be followed closely until the peripheral retina is vascularized. In a multicentric controlled trial, intravitreal ranibizumab (0.2 mg) was also found to be better than laser photoablation, with 80% of the eyes receiving ranibizumab 0.2 mg till 24 weeks of follow-up were alive, with no active disease, no any unfavorable structural abnormality, or no need for any retreatment [110]. In type 1 zone I ROP, combining laser photocoagulation (outside zone I) with intravitreal bevacizumab resulted in better anatomical results and fewer chances of myopia [111]. However, unlike the classic cases of ROP in zone I, aggressive posterior ROP (AP-ROP), now re-defined as A-ROP treated alone with intravitreal bevacizumab, had larger peripheral non-perfusion areas on FA and higher recurrence rates. Lower birthweight, prolonged hospitalization, and AP-ROP are significant risk factors for recurrence (~8% of patients) of fibrovascular proliferation and disease in eyes treated with a single injection of bevacizumab [112]. Prophylactic laser photocoagulation following intravitreal injection in AP-ROP eyes minimized the adverse anatomical outcomes [113]. There are several advantages of using anti-VEGF therapy in type 1 ROP as the time to treat is much shorter (these babies have very low birth weight), there is no difference in the efficacy compared to the laser photoablation, and there is no tissue destruction or restriction of peripheral visual fields and fewer chances of developing myopia. While there are conflicting results on the recurrence rates of fibrovascular proliferation and the need to retreat, the delay in vascularization of the retina, especially in the zone I disease, requires these babies to be closely followed up for as long as 70 weeks PMA till the vascularization is complete [114]. Plasma VEGF levels were reduced one day following intravitreal ranibizumab therapy for ROP, but this effect was not seen after one week [115]. In a dose de-escalation study, intravitreal bevacizumab as low as 0.002 mg led to reduced plasma VEGF levels, and this effect was still evident at 2 and 4 weeks after the injection [116]. Recent studies also suggest that most babies receiving bevacizumab developed new-onset systemic hypertension within a month of the treatment [117].

Moreover, the long-term adverse impact of VEGF suppression on organ development, primarily neurodevelopment, is unknown. Therefore, this treatment may be restricted to type 1 ROP in zone I or the posterior zone II [114]. Nearly 8% of the ROP eyes, especially those with a plus disease receiving anti-VEGF therapy, may develop retinal detachment requiring pars plana vitreous surgery [118]. Informed consent from the parents should be taken before considering anti-VEGF therapy for these infants. Advances in understanding the pathogenesis and management have been recently reviewed, and readers seeking greater details may refer to these publications [119–121].

6.3.1.10 Screening Strategies for ROP

Many treatment options that are now available can achieve favourable and stable anatomical and functional outcomes in more than 90% of ROP babies. However, the window of opportunity to treat them efficaciously is extremely narrow. Hence, the key to success lies in the timely detection and recognition of babies at high risk of developing ROP. Neonatal care has been relatively standardized in western countries but shows wide variations across the world's middle and low-income regions. The major risk factors besides preterm birth and low birth weight include prolonged hospital stay due to comorbidities like infections, haemorrhages and the need for blood transfusion, as well as notably unmonitored oxygen ventilation.

In three of the most advanced countries with well-developed neonatal care, preterm babies with a mean gestational age (GA) of <26 weeks and a mean birth weight of <800 g developed threshold 3+ or higher ROP whereas in the middle-income and low-income countries where the neonatal care may be less than optimal, babies with 34 weeks GA and birth weight of even 2000 g may develop it [122]. In most advanced countries, the screening criteria are birth weight <1500 g and gestational age <34 weeks [122]. In the three multicentric trials of ROP in the US from 1986 to 2013, there was a progressive decline in the GA (28–27 weeks) and birth weight (954–864 g) of preterm babies with ROP while the prevalence remained stable. During this time, there has been a steady improvement in obstetrical care, the use of antenatal corticosteroids, human milk feeding, surfactants, and better oxygen monitoring, resulting in increased survival of these babies [123]. In sharp contrast, in a retrospective study of 275 ROP eyes seen over 10 years in an Indian tertiary care centre, the mean birth weight was 1534 g (range 1251–2750 g), and the mean gestation period was 31 weeks (range 26–35). Applying the US or the UK screening criteria to this cohort would have missed 17.6% and 22.6% of babies with threshold or worse ROP [124]. Similar conclusions were reached in a prospective study in a South India referral centre [125]. Thus, all countries must develop criteria to include all ROP babies. The current screening guidelines by the American Academy of Pediatrics and Ophthalmology suggest that all infants born with a birth weight of <1500 g or GA of <30 weeks or any infant with birth weight between 1500 and 2000 g or GA of >30 weeks who have received oxygen even for more than a few days or unmonitored oxygen or received ionotropic support for hypotension should be screened for ROP at postmenstrual age of 31–34 weeks [126]. Monitoring oxygen saturation (SpO_2) using pulse monitors, setting low and high saturation level alarms, maintaining high levels of hygiene, washing the hands by the staff, and avoiding unnecessary blood transfusions are some measures that can help reduce the incidence of ROP. All babies born in India with gestational age < 34 weeks or birth weight < 2000 g or babies with even higher birth weight who have comorbidities, such as sepsis, respiratory distress, intraventricular hemorrhages, and requiring cardiopulmonary support, should be screened by an Ophthalmologist who is trained to use binocular indirect ophthalmoscope and well versed with the identification, classification, and documentation of the ROP [127]. It can be supplanted with a Ret cam or a similar ultra-wide angle fundus imaging camera, which can be used by a trained nurse/non-physician and use teleophthalmology to submit the images to a remote centre for interpretation and decision for treatment [128, 129]. By and large digital imaging is as sensitive as the clinical retinal examination; the latter may, however, have an edge in evaluating for a zone 3 disease and ROP stage 3 disease [130]. However, digital imaging is a permanent record and can objectively document any ROP progression [131]. It is recommended that screening should be done from 25 to 30 days of birth or at discharge, whichever is earlier. If the babies have comorbid conditions or receive unmonitored oxygen, they should be screened earlier. Most preterm babies are still in the hospital at this time, and if they are discharged, they should be called to the outpatient clinic for screening. They should be monitored weekly or even two weekly depending upon the development and maturation of retinal vessels, and their progress should be documented on the fundus imaging and the paper charts [126]. The follow-up screening should be done for all babies who have been treated irrespective of either the laser photocoagulation or with an intravitreal injection of bevacizumab till there is complete regression of ROP lesions or retinal vascularization has reached the temporal periphery. As mentioned earlier, the babies receiving bevacizumab or incomplete ablation with laser photocoagulation may develop recurrence of plus disease or fibrovascular proliferation later and must be monitored closely. Babies need periodic visual rehabilitation examinations and monitoring of cognitive and other neural development milestones until at least 5 years of age [127].

6.3.2 Familial Exudative Vitreoretinopathy (FEVR)

FEVR is a rare genetic disorder seen in children with a high level of heterogeneity both in hereditary patterns and in clinical manifestations. The clinical spectrum of the disease may vary from asymptomatic family members who may show only peripheral avascular retina to peripheral retinal neovascularization and fibrous proliferation, prominent temporal retinal fold, vitreous hemorrhage, and exudative, tractional or rhegmatogenous retinal detachment. Compared to the normal population, more non-branching vessels radiate from the optic disc [132]. Narrowing the temporal vascular arcades with multiple branching and straightening of the peripheral vessels gives it a broom-like appearance. Temporal dragging of the optic disc vasculature is highly characteristic. The retinal periphery may show abnormal arteriovenous loops and a V-shaped avascular area in the temporal meridian [133].

FEVR is classified into five stages. Stage 1 is avascular peripheral retina seen on FFA; stage 2 is avascular retina with peripheral neovascularization without exudation (2A) or with exudation (2B); stage 3 is extramacular retinal detachment without exudation (3A) or with exudation (3B), stage 4 is retinal detachment involving macula without exudation (4A) or with exudation (4B), and stage 5 is total retinal detachment [134] (Fig. 6.20).

Mutations are known in at least five genes that play a critical role in the development of the retina and are detectable in nearly half of the patients. The genes are NDP, an X-linked gene, FZD4, LRP, TSPAN12 (all three autosomal dominant and recessive), and ZNF 408, an autosomal dominant gene [135]. Most of the clinical features of FEVR may also be seen in ROP, and the diagnosis gets compounded as some of the children with FEVR may have been born prematurely and have low birth weight. However, ROP is a highly symmetric and aggressive disease

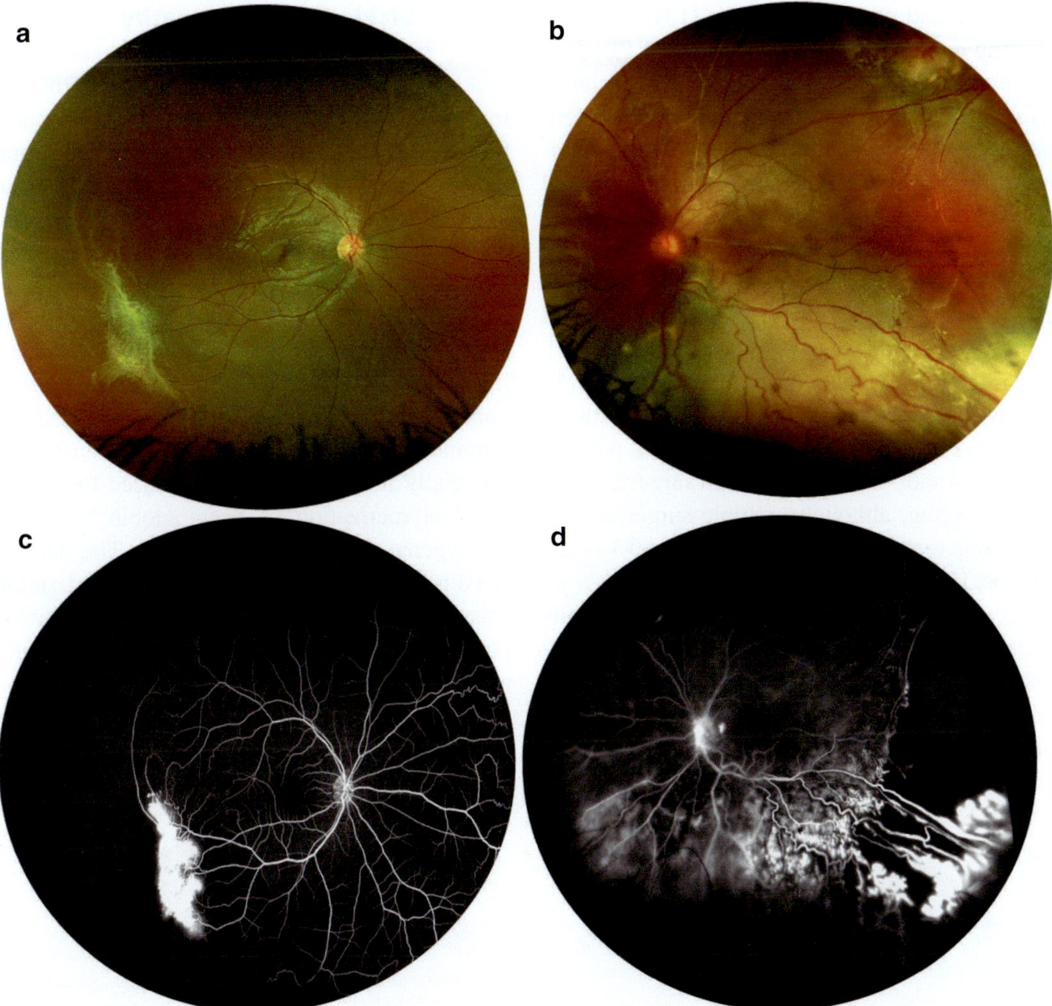

Fig. 6.20 Familial Exudative Vitreoretinopathy (FEVR). A 12-year-old female patient with FEVR Stage 2A in the right eye (**a**) and Stage 4B in the left eye (**b**). Ultra-wide field fundus fluorescein angiography documents the presence of extra-retinal neovascularisation with a large area of temporal capillary non-perfusion (**c** and **d**). (Images courtesy of Dr. Simar Rajan Singh, Advanced Eye Centre, Post Graduate Institute of Medical Education and Research, Chandigarh)

with no genetic background and a consistent history of prematurity, low birth weight, and history of oxygen therapy at birth. Family history may be available in less than 20% of the FEVR patients.

Examination of the parents often reveals features consistent with FEVR [136]. Most of the family members have stage 1 or 2 lesions which are asymptomatic stages of the disease, while 3/4 of the patients show stage 3–5 lesions [137, 138]. Ultra-wide scanning laser ophthalmoscopy of the asymptomatic family members can be highly sensitive to detect early stages [139], and a temporal midperipheral vitreoretinal interface abnormality, prominent in the green channel may be detected in the majority of the early stages of FEVR [140]. Peripheral avascular retina on FFA is one of the most consistent features of FEVR and is seen in both the patients and the family members.

Besides the non-perfused retina, wide-angle FFA may show circumferential vessels, venous anastomosis, telangiectasia, and leakage from the optic disc and peripheral vessels [137, 138]. On spectral domain OCT, a key feature of FEVR is the presence of the thickening of the posterior hyaloid, causing a varying amount of vitreoretinal and vitreopapillary traction. The other important element of OCT is the persistence of the fetal microstructures in the foveal centre, such as the ganglion cell layer, inner plexiform layer, inner nuclear layer, and outer plexiform layer. Other changes include cystoid macular oedema, and intraretinal or subretinal lipid exudation [141]. The role of laser photocoagulation of the peripheral avascular retina is controversial as the course of the disease is unpredictable. However, patients in stages 4 and 5 need vitreoretinal surgery, which is challenging, although multiple surgeries may ultimately reattach the retina in nearly 80% of the patients [142] (Fig. 6.21).

Genetic testing and counselling of the patients and their family members of childbearing age are essential to look for genetic mutations. The progression of this disease is unpredictable, and they need a lifelong follow-up.

6.3.3 Sickle Cell Retinopathy

Sickle cell disease (SCD) is a generic term that includes, among other genotypes, the commonest form, sickle cell anaemia, which is an autosomal recessive disorder caused by a point mutation in the β-globin chain of haemoglobin [143]. The disease is characterized by episodes of severe pain and affects practically all body organs due to an occlusive microvascular disease. Microvascular occlusion is best appreciated clinically in the retina. Proliferative sickle cell retinopathy is one of the most common causes of blindness in young people in Sub-Saharan Africa, especially in Jamaica. SCD is caused by abnormal polymerization of haemoglobin S during deoxygenation, leading to sickling. The disease is named after the peculiar crescent and sickle shape of the RBCs first observed by Herrick [144], who also noted anaemia and many nucleated RBCs in the peripheral blood of a young black student originally from Grenada (West Indies) who suffered multiorgan involve-

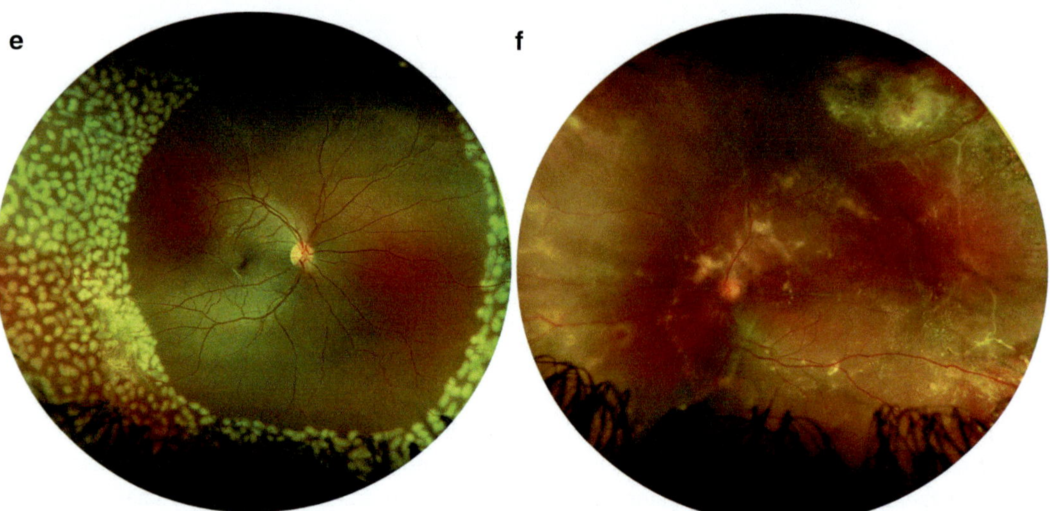

Fig. 6.21 The same patient as in Fig. 6.20 was managed with laser photocoagulation of the avascular retina in the right eye (**e**) and scleral buckling with external drainage of subretinal fluid with cryotherapy in the left eye (**f**). (Images courtesy of Dr. Simar Rajan Singh, Advanced Eye Centre, Post Graduate Institute of Medical Education and Research, Chandigarh)

ment following the occurrence of episodes of skin and ear infection [144].

6.3.3.1 Genetics of Sickle Cell Disease

The disease severity depends upon the genetic variants. The most common allele is homozygous β^s responsible for the severest form of sickle cell anaemia (HbSS) in nearly 70% of African SCD patients. The next common variant is heterozygous β^s β^C alleles that cause less severe systemic disease (HbSC). The third common is coinheritance with the β-thalassemia allele resulting in HbS/ β-thalassemia disease [145].

6.3.3.2 Pathophysiology of Sickle Cell Disease

The rigidity of RBCs is caused by the amount of HbS available for polymerizing its β globin chains that fill the RBC. Patients co-inheriting genes that allow fetal Hb to persist have less severe disease as the quantum of HbS available for polymerization is reduced. Recent years have seen the application of CRISPR/Cas9 gene editing tools to induce fetal haemoglobin expression in these patients [146]. Initial clinical results have been encouraging [147, 148]. The two primary components of the disease are recurrent episodes of occlusion of post-capillary veins and haemolytic anaemia precipitated by infections. Each episode of infection leads to exacerbation of ischaemic events in different organs of the body. Unlike 120 days as the life span of normal RBCs, the life span of RBCs is reduced to just 14 days in SCD, causing hemolysis and release of free haemoglobin [149] The free haemoglobin is toxic as it leads to the generation of oxy free radicals, which quench endothelial nitric oxide, a critical molecule that controls vasodilatation. Oxidative stress is also brought about by reperfusion injury as the blood flow stops and restarts intermittently in the capillaries. Apart from occlusion of the post-capillary venules by the sickled RBCs, activation of endothelial cell adhesion molecules VCAM by the oxidative stress and the inflammatory cytokines contribute to the vascular occlusion by adhesion of RBCs and leucocytes.

6.3.3.3 Clinical Manifestations of Sickle Cell Disease

While the HbSS disease has the severest forms of systemic complications, the ocular complications are severest in the HbSC variant [150].

While some of the earliest cases reported vitreous hemorrhage in patients with SCD, definitive ocular changes and their correlation with the type of SCD were given by Welch and Goldberg in [151]. Nearly 3/4 of the patients with HbSS and HbSC show retinal changes. In general, no retinal signs are seen in patients with Sickle cell trait (HbAS).

Nearly half of the patients with HbSS disease show tortuosity of the retinal veins, a stellate, and speculated pigmented scar with feeder arterioles and arteriolar occlusions, the so-called 'black sunburst sign'. These are accompanied by peripheral non-perfusion and arteriolar infarction. Proliferative retinopathy is seen only occasionally. On the other hand, in the HbSC disease, nearly 3/4th of the patients have abnormal arteriovenous proliferation into the vitreous cavity, which has been described as 'sea-fan vascularization' along with arteriolar and venous segment occlusions. All the sea-fan new vessels have peripheral retinal capillary non-perfusion [151].

6.3.3.4 Classification of Proliferative Sickle Cell Retinopathy

Goldberg [152] first described five stages of proliferative SCR in HbSC disease based primarily on clinical and FFA studies of the retinal vascular changes at the equatorial or post-equatorial retina. These were Stage I, peripheral arteriolar occlusion; Stage II, arteriovenous anastomosis; Stage III, sea fan neovascular and fibrous proliferation; Stage IV, vitreous hemorrhage, and Stage V, retinal detachment. Each stage was further sub-classified based on circumferential involvement [152]. Based on a prospective study of the Jamaican Sickle cohort, a classification based on the qualitative assessment of the vascular border into type I and type II was proposed, limited, however, by the inability of the then FFA technology to study the extreme peripheral vascular bed in all eyes. However, this study showed that the retinopathy's severity was more in the SC variant than in the SS variant [153].

6.3.3.5 Fundus Imaging Studies in Sickle Cell Disease

In some of the earliest studies using FFA, a dynamic remodelling of the retinal vessels, equatorial or post-equatorial venous segment dilations, dilated capillaries, capillary occlusion, hairpin loops, A-V shunts, and capillary budding had been noted. In a 3-year prospective study, a continuous remodelling of the macular capillaries was noted [154]. This dramatic phenomenon of intermittent flow cessation and reperfusion was recently demonstrated on OCT angiography of the retina by taking sequential OCTA images every minute for 10 min and then repeating these after an hour at the same site. As the images were stacked, the capillaries that showed intermittent flow deficit or started reperfusion could be identified and quantified [155]. Availability of the ultra-wide-field (UWF) FFA revealed more extensive peripheral vascular changes than were possible with the 7-standard field fundus imaging in SCR [156]. More recently, using UWF FFA, 100% of the pediatric age group patients with SCD were shown to have at least stage I of the Goldberg classification [157]. Even for screening SCD patients, UWF color imaging is more sensitive than the dilated fundus examination [158]. UWF imaging can monitor SCR patients for progression, tele-screening, and machine learning development [150]. Using a deep learning classifier, UWF imaging can accurately distinguish between various proliferative retinopathies in up to 90% of the cases [159].

References

1. International Diabetes Federation. IDF diabetes atlas. 10th ed. Brussels: International Diabetes Federation; 2021.
2. Mainster MA. The fractal properties of retinal vessels: embryological and clinical implications. Eye (Lond). 1990;4(Pt 1):235–41. https://doi.org/10.1038/eye.1990.33. PMID: 2323476.
3. Gariano RF. Cellular mechanisms in retinal vascular development. Prog Retin Eye Res. 2003;22(3):295–306. https://doi.org/10.1016/s1350-9462(02)00062-9. PMID: 12852488.
4. Gale NW, Thurston G, Hackett SF, Renard R, Wang Q, McClain J, Martin C, Witte C, Witte MH, Jackson D, Suri C, Campochiaro PA, Wiegand SJ, Yancopoulos GD. Angiopoietin-2 is required for postnatal angiogenesis and lymphatic patterning, and only the latter role is rescued by angiopoietin-1. Dev Cell. 2002;3(3):411–23. https://doi.org/10.1016/s1534-5807(02)00217-4. PMID: 12361603.
5. Selvam S, Kumar T, Fruttiger M. Retinal vasculature development in health and disease. Prog Retin Eye Res. 2018;63:1–19. https://doi.org/10.1016/j.preteyeres.2017.11.001. Epub 2017 Nov 10. PMID: 29129724.
6. Jayaram H, Jones MF, Eastlake K, Cottrill PB, Becker S, Wiseman J, Khaw PT, Limb GA. Transplantation of photoreceptors derived from human Muller glia restore rod function in the P23H rat. Stem Cells Transl Med. 2014;3(3):323–33. https://doi.org/10.5966/sctm.2013-0112. Epub 2014 Jan 29. PMID: 24477073; PMCID: PMC3952927.
7. Rodrigues M, Xin X, Jee K, Babapoor-Farrokhran S, Kashiwabuchi F, Ma T, Bhutto I, Hassan SJ, Daoud Y, Baranano D, Solomon S, Lutty G, Semenza GL, Montaner S, Sodhi A. VEGF secreted by hypoxic Müller cells induces MMP-2 expression and activity in endothelial cells to promote retinal neovascularization in proliferative diabetic retinopathy. Diabetes. 2013;62(11):3863–73. https://doi.org/10.2337/db13-0014. Epub 2013 Jul 24. PMID: 23884892; PMCID: PMC3806594.
8. Ishida S, Usui T, Yamashiro K, Kaji Y, Amano S, Ogura Y, Hida T, Oguchi Y, Ambati J, Miller JW, Gragoudas ES, Ng YS, D'Amore PA, Shima DT, Adamis AP. VEGF164-mediated inflammation is required for pathological, but not physiological, ischemia-induced retinal neovascularization. J Exp Med. 2003;198(3):483–9. https://doi.org/10.1084/jem.20022027. PMID: 12900522; PMCID: PMC2194095.
9. Trost A, Lange S, Schroedl F, Bruckner D, Motloch KA, Bogner B, Kaser-Eichberger A, Strohmaier C, Runge C, Aigner L, Rivera FJ, Reitsamer HA. Brain and retinal pericytes: origin, function and role. Front Cell Neurosci. 2016;10:20. https://doi.org/10.3389/fncel.2016.00020. PMID: 26869887; PMCID: PMC4740376.
10. Frank RN, Turczyn TJ, Das A. Pericyte coverage of retinal and cerebral capillaries. Invest Ophthalmol Vis Sci. 1990;31(6):999–1007. PMID: 2354923.
11. Lechner J, O'Leary OE, Stitt AW. The pathology associated with diabetic retinopathy. Vision Res. 2017;139:7–14. https://doi.org/10.1016/j.visres.2017.04.003. Epub 2017 Apr 29. PMID: 28412095.

12. Cubbon RM, Ali N, Sengupta A, Kearney MT. Insulin- and growth factor-resistance impairs vascular regeneration in diabetes mellitus. Curr Vasc Pharmacol. 2012;10(3):271–84. https://doi.org/10.2174/157016112799959305. PMID: 22239629.
13. Warmke N, Platt F, Bruns AF, Ozber CH, Haywood NJ, Abudushalamu Y, Slater C, Palin V, Sukumar P, Wheatcroft SB, Yuldasheva NY, Kearney MT, Griffin KJ, Cubbon RM. Pericyte insulin receptors modulate retinal vascular remodeling and endothelial angiopoietin signaling. Endocrinology. 2021;162(11):bqab182. https://doi.org/10.1210/endocr/bqab182. PMID: 34460911; PMCID: PMC8462386.
14. Saharinen P, Leppänen VM, Alitalo K. SnapShot: angiopoietins and their functions. Cell. 2017;171(3):724–724.e1. https://doi.org/10.1016/j.cell.2017.10.009. PMID: 29053972.
15. Ciulla LM, Patel NA, Yannuzzi NA, Hussain RM. Angiopoietins as targets for diabetic retinopathy treatment. In: Giudice GL, editor. Diabetic eye disease—from therapeutic pipeline to the real world [internet]. London: IntechOpen; 2021 [cited 2022 Jun 14]. https://www.intechopen.com/chapters/78191. https://doi.org/10.5772/intechopen.99749.
16. Sahni J, Patel SS, Dugel PU, Khanani AM, Jhaveri CD, Wykoff CC, Hershberger VS, Pauly-Evers M, Sadikhov S, Szczesny P, Schwab D, Nogoceke E, Osborne A, Weikert R, Fauser S. Simultaneous inhibition of angiopoietin-2 and vascular endothelial growth factor-A with Faricimab in diabetic macular edema: BOULEVARD phase 2 randomized trial. Ophthalmology. 2019;126(8):1155–70. https://doi.org/10.1016/j.ophtha.2019.03.023. Epub 2019 Mar 21. PMID: 30905643.
17. Halfter W, Moes S, Asgeirsson DO, Halfter K, Oertle P, Melo Herraiz E, Plodinec M, Jenoe P, Henrich PB. Diabetes-related changes in the protein composition and the biomechanical properties of human retinal vascular basement membranes. PLoS One. 2017;12(12):e0189857. https://doi.org/10.1371/journal.pone.0189857. Erratum in: PLoS One. 2018 Apr 6;13(4):e0195772. PMID: 29284024; PMCID: PMC5746242.
18. Roy S, Kim D. Retinal capillary basement membrane thickening: Role in the pathogenesis of diabetic retinopathy. Prog Retin Eye Res. 2021;82:100903. https://doi.org/10.1016/j.preteyeres.2020.100903. Epub 2020 Sep 18. PMID: 32950677; PMCID: PMC8590904.
19. Beltramo E, Buttiglieri S, Pomero F, Allione A, D'Alù F, Ponte E, Porta M. A study of capillary pericyte viability on extracellular matrix produced by endothelial cells in high glucose. Diabetologia. 2003;46(3):409–15.https://doi.org/10.1007/s00125--003-1043-6. Epub 2003 Feb 26. PMID: 12687340.
20. Beltramo E, Pomero F, Allione A, D'Alù F, Ponte E, Porta M. Pericyte adhesion is impaired on extracellular matrix produced by endothelial cells in high hexose concentrations. Diabetologia. 2002;45(3):416–9. https://doi.org/10.1007/s00125-001-0761-x. PMID: 11914747.
21. Stitt AW, Curtis TM, Chen M, Medina RJ, McKay GJ, Jenkins A, Gardiner TA, Lyons TJ, Hammes HP, Simó R, Lois N. The progress in understanding and treatment of diabetic retinopathy. Prog Retin Eye Res. 2016;51:156–86. https://doi.org/10.1016/j.preteyeres.2015.08.001. Epub 2015 Aug 18. PMID: 26297071.
22. Little HL. The role of abnormal hemorrheodynamics in the pathogenesis of diabetic retinopathy. Trans Am Ophthalmol Soc. 1976;74:573–636. PMID: 867639; PMCID: PMC1311529.
23. Lee MY, Park S, Song JY, Ra H, Baek JU, Baek J. Inflammatory cytokines and retinal nonperfusion area in quiescent proliferative diabetic retinopathy. Cytokine. 2022;154:155774. https://doi.org/10.1016/j.cyto.2021.155774. Epub 2022 Apr 26. PMID: 35487091.
24. Wykoff CC, Yu HJ, Avery RL, Ehlers JP, Tadayoni R, Sadda SR. Retinal non-perfusion in diabetic retinopathy. Eye (Lond). 2022;36(2):249–56. https://doi.org/10.1038/s41433-021-01649-0. Epub 2022 Jan 11. PMID: 35017700; PMCID: PMC8807828.
25. Niki T, Muraoka K, Shimizu K. Distribution of capillary nonperfusion in early-stage diabetic retinopathy. Ophthalmology. 1984;91(12):1431–9. https://doi.org/10.1016/s0161-6420(84)34126-4. PMID: 6084212.
26. Ishibazawa A, De Pretto LR, Alibhai AY, Moult EM, Arya M, Sorour O, Mehta N, Baumal CR, Witkin AJ, Yoshida A, Duker JS, Fujimoto JG, Waheed NK. Retinal nonperfusion relationship to arteries or veins observed on widefield optical coherence tomography angiography in diabetic retinopathy. Invest Ophthalmol Vis Sci. 2019;60(13):4310–8. https://doi.org/10.1167/iovs.19-26653. PMID: 31622467; PMCID: PMC6996665.
27. Nicholson L, Ramu J, Chan EW, Bainbridge JW, Hykin PG, Talks SJ, Sivaprasad S. Retinal nonperfusion characteristics on ultra-Widefield angiography in eyes with severe nonproliferative diabetic retinopathy and proliferative diabetic retinopathy. JAMA Ophthalmol. 2019;137(6):626–31. https://doi.org/10.1001/jamaophthalmol.2019.0440. Erratum in: JAMA Ophthalmol 2019 Jun 1;137(6):721. PMID: 30973596; PMCID: PMC6567981.
28. Fang M, Fan W, Shi Y, Ip MS, Wykoff CC, Wang K, Falavarjani KG, Brown DM, van Hemert J, Sadda SR. Classification of regions of nonperfusion on ultra-widefield fluorescein angiography in patients with diabetic macular edema. Am J Ophthalmol. 2019;206:74–81. https://doi.org/10.1016/j.ajo.2019.03.030. Epub 2019 Apr 6. PMID: 30959003.
29. Kim K, In You J, Park JR, Kim ES, Oh WY, Yu SY. Quantification of retinal microvascular parameters by severity of diabetic retinopathy using widefield swept-source optical coherence tomography

angiography. Graefes Arch Clin Exp Ophthalmol. 2021;259(8):2103–11. https://doi.org/10.1007/s00417-021-05099-y. Epub 2021 Feb 2. PMID: 33528650.

30. Russell JF, Al-Khersan H, Shi Y, Scott NL, Hinkle JW, Fan KC, Lyu C, Feuer WJ, Gregori G, Rosenfeld PJ. Retinal nonperfusion in proliferative diabetic retinopathy before and after panretinal photocoagulation assessed by Widefield OCT angiography. Am J Ophthalmol. 2020;213:177–85. https://doi.org/10.1016/j.ajo.2020.01.024. Epub 2020 Mar 13. PMID: 32006481; PMCID: PMC7962743.
31. Russell JF, Shi Y, Scott NL, Gregori G, Rosenfeld PJ. Longitudinal angiographic evidence that intraretinal microvascular abnormalities can evolve into neovascularization. Ophthalmol Retina. 2020;4(12):1146–50. https://doi.org/10.1016/j.oret.2020.06.010. Epub 2020 Jun 13. PMID: 32544625.
32. Patz A. Retinal neovascularisation: early contributions of Professor Michaelson and recent observations. Br J Ophthalmol. 1984;68(1):42–6. https://doi.org/10.1136/bjo.68.1.42. PMID: 6197084; PMCID: PMC1040236
33. Connolly DT, Olander JV, Heuvelman D, Nelson R, Monsell R, Siegel N, Haymore BL, Leimgruber R, Feder J. Human vascular permeability factor. Isolation from U937 cells. J Biol Chem. 1989;264:20017–24.
34. Ferrara N, Henzel WJ. Pituitary follicular cells secrete a novel heparin-binding growth factor specific for vascular endothelial cells. Biochem Biophys Res Commun. 1989;161(2):851–8. https://doi.org/10.1016/0006-291x(89)92678-8. PMID: 2735925.
35. Leung DW, Cachianes G, Kuang WJ, Goeddel DV, Ferrara N. Vascular endothelial growth factor is a secreted angiogenic mitogen. Science. 1989;246(4935):1306–9. https://doi.org/10.1126/science.2479986. PMID: 2479986.
36. De Falco S. The discovery of placenta growth factor and its biological activity. Exp Mol Med. 2012;44(1):1–9. https://doi.org/10.3858/emm.2012.44.1.025. PMID: 22228176; PMCID: PMC3277892.
37. Miller JW, Adamis AP, Shima DT, D'Amore PA, Moulton RS, O'Reilly MS, Folkman J, Dvorak HF, Brown LF, Berse B, et al. Vascular endothelial growth factor/vascular permeability factor is temporally and spatially correlated with ocular angiogenesis in a primate model. Am J Pathol. 1994;145(3):574–84. PMID: 7521577; PMCID: PMC1890317.
38. Aiello LP, Avery RL, Arrigg PG, Keyt BA, Jampel HD, Shah ST, Pasquale LR, Thieme H, Iwamoto MA, Park JE, et al. Vascular endothelial growth factor in ocular fluid of patients with diabetic retinopathy and other retinal disorders. N Engl J Med. 1994;331(22):1480–7. https://doi.org/10.1056/NEJM199412013312203. PMID: 7526212.
39. Tolentino MJ, McLeod DS, Taomoto M, Otsuji T, Adamis AP, Lutty GA. Pathologic features of vascular endothelial growth factor-induced retinopathy in the nonhuman primate. Am J Ophthalmol. 2002;133(3):373–85.https://doi.org/10.1016/s0002--9394(01)01381-2. PMID: 1186097.
40. Muraoka K, Shimizu K. Intraretinal neovascularization in diabetic retinopathy. Ophthalmology. 1984;91(12):1440–6.https://doi.org/10.1016/s0161--6420(84)34125-2. PMID: 6084213.
41. Early Treatment Diabetic Retinopathy Study Research Group. Grading diabetic retinopathy from stereoscopic color fundus photographs—an extension of the modified Airlie House classification. ETDRS report number 10. Ophthalmology. 1991;98(5 Suppl):786–806. PMID: 2062513.
42. Early Treatment Diabetic Retinopathy Study Research Group. Fundus photographic risk factors for progression of diabetic retinopathy. ETDRS report number 12. Ophthalmology. 1991;98(5 Suppl):823–33. PMID: 2062515.
43. Pan J, Chen D, Yang X, Zou R, Zhao K, Cheng D, Huang S, Zhou T, Yang Y, Chen F. Characteristics of neovascularization in early stages of proliferative diabetic retinopathy by optical coherence tomography angiography. Am J Ophthalmol. 2018;192:146–56. https://doi.org/10.1016/j.ajo.2018.05.018. Epub 2018 May 26. PMID: 29806991.
44. Shimouchi A, Ishibazawa A, Ishiko S, Omae T, Ro-Mase T, Yanagi Y, Yoshida A. A proposed classification of intraretinal microvascular abnormalities in diabetic retinopathy following panretinal photocoagulation. Invest Ophthalmol Vis Sci. 2020;61(3):34. https://doi.org/10.1167/iovs.61.3.34. PMID: 32191287; PMCID: PMC7401423.
45. Pearce E, Chong V, Sivaprasad S. Aflibercept reduces retinal hemorrhages and intravitreal microvascular abnormalities but not venous beading: secondary analysis of the CLARITY study. Ophthalmol Retina. 2020;4(7):689–94. https://doi.org/10.1016/j.oret.2020.02.003. Epub 2020 Feb 11. PMID: 32473901.
46. Klein R, Myers CE, Lee KE, Gangnon R, Klein BE. Changes in retinal vessel diameter and incidence and progression of diabetic retinopathy. Arch Ophthalmol. 2012;130(6):749–55. https://doi.org/10.1001/archophthalmol.2011.2560. PMID: 22332203; PMCID: PMC3357449.
47. Ashraf M, Shokrollahi S, Pisig AU, Sampani K, Abdelal O, Cavallerano JD, Robertson G, Fleming A, van Hemert J, Pitoc CM, Sun JK, Aiello LP, Silva PS. Retinal vascular caliber association with nonperfusion and diabetic retinopathy severity depends on vascular caliber measurement location. Ophthalmol Retina. 2021;5(6):571–9. https://doi.org/10.1016/j.oret.2020.09.003. Epub 2020 Sep 11. PMID: 32927151.
48. Sato Y, Kamata A, Matsui M. Clinical study of venous abnormalities in diabetic retinopathy. Jpn J Ophthalmol. 1993;37(2):136–42. PMID: 8230837.

49. Chen L, Zhang X, Wen F. Venous beading in two or more quadrants might not be a sensitive grading criterion for severe nonproliferative diabetic retinopathy. Graefes Arch Clin Exp Ophthalmol. 2018;256(6):1059–65. https://doi.org/10.1007/s00417-018-3971-3. Epub 2018 Apr 6. PMID: 29626228; PMCID: PMC5956090.
50. Bek T. Venous loops and reduplications in diabetic retinopathy. Prevalence, distribution, and pattern of development. Acta Ophthalmol Scand. 1999;77(2):130–4. https://doi.org/10.1034/j.1600--0420.1999.770202.x. PMID: 10321524.
51. Aiello LP, Odia I, Glassman AR, Melia M, Jampol LM, Bressler NM, Kiss S, Silva PS, Wykoff CC, Sun JK, Diabetic Retinopathy Clinical Research Network. Comparison of early treatment diabetic retinopathy study standard 7-field imaging with ultrawide-field imaging for determining severity of diabetic retinopathy. JAMA Ophthalmol. 2019;137(1):65–73. https://doi.org/10.1001/jamaophthalmol.2018.4982. PMID: 30347105; PMCID: PMC6439787.
52. Silva PS, Cavallerano JD, Haddad NM, Kwak H, Dyer KH, Omar AF, Shikari H, Aiello LM, Sun JK, Aiello LP. Peripheral lesions identified on ultrawide field imaging predict increased risk of diabetic retinopathy progression over 4 years. Ophthalmology. 2015;122(5):949–56. https://doi.org/10.1016/j.ophtha.2015.01.008. Epub 2015 Feb 19. PMID: 25704318.
53. Pechauer AD, Hwang TS, Hagag AM, Liu L, Tan O, Zhang X, Parker M, Huang D, Wilson DJ, Jia Y. Assessing total retinal blood flow in diabetic retinopathy using multiplane en face Doppler optical coherence tomography. Br J Ophthalmol. 2018;102(1):126–30. https://doi.org/10.1136/bjophthalmol-2016-310042. Epub 2017 May 11. PMID: 28495904; PMCID: PMC5800769.
54. Srinivas S, Tan O, Nittala MG, Wu JL, Fawzi AA, Huang D, Sadda SR. Assessment of retinal blood flow in diabetic retinopathy using Doppler Fourier-domain optical coherence tomography. Retina. 2017;37(11):2001–7. https://doi.org/10.1097/IAE.0000000000001479. PMID: 28098726; PMCID: PMC6581777.
55. Palochak CMA, Lee HE, Song J, Geng A, Linsenmeier RA, Burns SA, Fawzi AA. Retinal blood velocity and flow in early diabetes and diabetic retinopathy using adaptive optics scanning laser ophthalmoscopy. J Clin Med. 2019;8(8):1165. https://doi.org/10.3390/jcm8081165. PMID: 31382617; PMCID: PMC6723736.
56. Jørgensen C, Bek T. Increasing oxygen saturation in larger retinal vessels after photocoagulation for diabetic retinopathy. Invest Ophthalmol Vis Sci. 2014;55(8):5365–9. https://doi.org/10.1167/iovs.14-14811. PMID: 25097242.
57. Ueno Y, Iwase T, Goto K, Tomita R, Ra E, Yamamoto K, Terasaki H. Association of changes of retinal vessels diameter with ocular blood flow in eyes with diabetic retinopathy. Sci Rep. 2021;11(1):4653. https://doi.org/10.1038/s41598-021-84067-2. PMID: 33633255; PMCID: PMC7907275.
58. Jansson RW, Frøystein T, Krohn J. Topographical distribution of retinal and optic disc neovascularization in early stages of proliferative diabetic retinopathy. Invest Ophthalmol Vis Sci. 2012;53(13):8246–52. https://doi.org/10.1167/iovs.12-10918. PMID: 23169887.
59. Lee CS, Lee AY, Sim DA, Keane PA, Mehta H, Zarranz-Ventura J, Fruttiger M, Egan CA, Tufail A. Reevaluating the definition of intraretinal microvascular abnormalities and neovascularization elsewhere in diabetic retinopathy using optical coherence tomography and fluorescein angiography. Am J Ophthalmol. 2015;159(1):101–10.e1. https://doi.org/10.1016/j.ajo.2014.09.041. Epub 2014 Oct 25. PMID: 25284762; PMCID: PMC5006953.
60. Vaz-Pereira S, Morais-Sarmento T, Esteves Marques R. Optical coherence tomography features of neovascularization in proliferative diabetic retinopathy: a systematic review. Int J Retina Vitreous. 2020;6:26. https://doi.org/10.1186/s40942-020-00230-3. PMID: 32612851; PMCID: PMC7322867.
61. Wang XN, Zhou J, Cai X, Li T, Long D, Wu Q. Optical coherence tomography angiography for the detection and evaluation of ptic disc neovascularization: a retrospective, observational study. BMC Ophthalmol. 2022;22(1):125. https://doi.org/10.1186/s12886-022-02351-9. PMID: 35296271; PMCID: PMC8928692.
62. Al-Khersan H, Russell JF, Lazzarini TA, Scott NL, Hinkle JW, Patel NA, Yannuzzi NA, Fowler BJ, Hussain RM, Barikian A, Sridhar J, Russell SR, Haddock LJ, Smiddy WE, Hariprasad SM, Shi Y, Wang L, Feuer W, Gregori G. An international classification of retinopathy of prematurity. Prepared by an international committee. Br J Ophthalmol. 1984;68(10):690–7. https://doi.org/10.1136/bjo.68.10.690. PMID: 6548150; PMCID: PMC1040449.
63. Ishibazawa A, Nagaoka T, Yokota H, Takahashi A, Omae T, Song YS, Takahashi T, Yoshida A. Characteristics of retinal neovascularization in proliferative diabetic retinopathy imaged by optical coherence tomography angiography. Invest Ophthalmol Vis Sci. 2016;57(14):6247–55. https://doi.org/10.1167/iovs.16-20210. PMID: 27849310.
64. Henkind P. Retinal blood vessels. Neovascularization, collaterals, and shunts. Aust J Ophthalmol. 1981;9(4):273–7. https://doi.org/10.1111/j.1442-9071.1981.tb00921.x. PMID: 6177308.
65. Singh A, Agarwal A, Mahajan S, Karkhur S, Singh R, Bansal R, Dogra MR, Gupta V. Morphological differences between optic disc collaterals and neovascularization on optical coherence tomography angiography. Graefes Arch Clin Exp Ophthalmol. 2017;255(4):753–9.https://doi.org/10.1007/s00417--016-3565-x. Epub 2016 Dec 9. PMID: 27942950.
66. Nicholson L, Sivapathasuntharam C, Zola M, Hykin P, Bainbridge JW, Sivaprasad S. Retinal

oximetry differences between optic disc collateral vessels and new vessels. JAMA Ophthalmol. 2017;135(9):1003–4. https://doi.org/10.1001/jamaophthalmol.2017.2624. PMID: 28772311; PMCID: PMC6583255.

67. Khalid H, Schwartz R, Nicholson L, Huemer J, El-Bradey MH, Sim DA, Patel PJ, Balaskas K, Hamilton RD, Keane PA, Rajendram R. Widefield optical coherence tomography angiography for early detection and objective evaluation of proliferative diabetic retinopathy. Br J Ophthalmol. 2021;105(1):118–23. https://doi.org/10.1136/bjophthalmol-2019-315365. Epub 2020 Mar 19. PMID: 32193221.
68. Lu ES, Cui Y, Le R, Zhu Y, Wang JC, Laíns I, Katz R, Lu Y, Zeng R, Garg I, Wu DM, Eliott D, Vavvas DG, Husain D, Miller JW, Kim LA, Miller JB. Detection of neovascularisation in the vitreoretinal interface slab using widefield swept-source optical coherence tomography angiography in diabetic retinopathy. Br J Ophthalmol. 2022;106(4):534–9. https://doi.org/10.1136/bjophthalmol-2020-317983. Epub 2020 Dec 21. PMID: 33355148; PMCID: PMC9092312.
69. Russell JF, Shi Y, Hinkle JW, Scott NL, Fan KC, Lyu C, Gregori G, Rosenfeld PJ. Longitudinal wide-field swept-source OCT angiography of neovascularization in proliferative diabetic retinopathy after panretinal photocoagulation. Ophthalmol Retina. 2019;3(4):350–61. https://doi.org/10.1016/j.oret.2018.11.008. Epub 2018 Nov 24. PMID: 31014688; PMCID: PMC6482856.
70. Hirano T, Hoshiyama K, Hirabayashi K, Wakabayashi M, Toriyama Y, Tokimitsu M, Murata T. Vitreoretinal interface slab in OCT angiography for detecting diabetic retinal neovascularization. Ophthalmol Retina. 2020;4(6):588–94. https://doi.org/10.1016/j.oret.2020.01.004. Epub 2020 Jan 10. PMID: 32107187.
71. Shiraki A, Sakimoto S, Eguchi M, Kanai M, Hara C, Fukushima Y, Nishida K, Kawasaki R, Sakaguchi H, Nishida K. Analysis of progressive neovascularization in diabetic retinopathy using Widefield OCT angiography. Ophthalmol Retina. 2022;6(2):153–60. https://doi.org/10.1016/j.oret.2021.05.011. Epub 2021 May 26. PMID: 34051418.
72. Feng HE, Weihong YU, Dong F. Observation of retinal neovascularization using optical coherence tomography angiography after panretinal photocoagulation for proliferative diabetic retinopathy. BMC Ophthalmol. 2021;21(1):252. https://doi.org/10.1186/s12886-021-01964-w. PMID: 34098891; PMCID: PMC8182899.
73. Falavarjani KG, Habibi A, Khorasani MA, Anvari P, Sadda SR. Time course of changes in optic disk neovascularization after a single intravitreal bevacizumab injection. Retina. 2019;39(6):1149–53. https://doi.org/10.1097/IAE.0000000000002107. PMID: 29466258.
74. Cui Y, Zhu Y, Lu ES, Le R, Laíns I, Katz R, Wang JC, Garg I, Lu Y, Zeng R, Eliott D, Vavvas DG, Husain D, Miller JW, Kim LA, Wu DM, Miller JB. Widefield swept-source OCT angiography metrics associated with the development of diabetic vitreous hemorrhage: a prospective study. Ophthalmology. 2021;128(9):1312–24. https://doi.org/10.1016/j.ophtha.2021.02.020. Epub 2021 Feb 26. PMID: 33647282; PMCID: PMC9055532.
75. Wu YB, Wang CG, Xu LX, Chen C, Zhou XB, Su GF. Analysis of risk factors for progressive fibrovascular proliferation in proliferative diabetic retinopathy. Int Ophthalmol. 2020;40(10):2495–502. https://doi.org/10.1007/s10792-020-01428-y. Epub 2020 May 28. PMID: 32468429.
76. Goatman KA, Fleming AD, Philip S, Williams GJ, Olson JA, Sharp PF. Detection of new vessels on the optic disc using retinal photographs. IEEE Trans Med Imaging. 2011;30(4):972–9. https://doi.org/10.1109/TMI.2010.2099236. Epub 2010 Dec 13. PMID: 21156389.
77. Mahtal N, Lenoir O, Tharaux PL. Glomerular endothelial cell crosstalk with podocytes in diabetic kidney disease. Front Med (Lausanne). 2021;8:659013. https://doi.org/10.3389/fmed.2021.659013. PMID: 33842514; PMCID: PMC8024520.
78. Tervaert TW, Mooyaart AL, Amann K, Cohen AH, Cook HT, Drachenberg CB, Ferrario F, Fogo AB, Haas M, de Heer E, Joh K, Noël LH, Radhakrishnan J, Seshan SV, Bajema IM, Bruijn JA, Renal Pathology Society. Pathologic classification of diabetic nephropathy. J Am Soc Nephrol. 2010;21(4):556–63. https://doi.org/10.1681/ASN.2010010010. Epub 2010 Feb 18. PMID: 20167701.
79. Aronov M, Allon R, Stave D, Belkin M, Margalit E, Fabian ID, Rosenzweig B. Retinal vascular signs as screening and prognostic factors for chronic kidney disease: a systematic review and meta-analysis of current evidence. J Pers Med. 2021;11(7):665. https://doi.org/10.3390/jpm11070665. PMID: 34357132; PMCID: PMC8307097.
80. Edwards MS, Wilson DB, Craven TE, Stafford J, Fried LF, Wong TY, Klein R, Burke GL, Hansen KJ. Associations between retinal microvascular abnormalities and declining renal function in the elderly population: the Cardiovascular Health Study. Am J Kidney Dis. 2005;46(2):214–24. https://doi.org/10.1053/j.ajkd.2005.05.005. PMID: 16112039.
81. Rodríguez-Poncelas A, Mundet-Tudurí X, Miravet-Jiménez S, Casellas A, Barrot-De la Puente JF, Franch-Nadal J, Coll-de Tuero G. Chronic kidney disease and diabetic retinopathy in patients with type 2 diabetes. PLoS One. 2016;11(2):e0149448. https://doi.org/10.1371/journal.pone.0149448. PMID: 26886129; PMCID: PMC4757564.
82. Hsieh YT, Tsai MJ, Tu ST, Hsieh MC. Association of abnormal renal profiles and proliferative diabetic retinopathy and diabetic macular edema in an Asian population with type 2 diabetes. JAMA Ophthalmol. 2018;136(1):68–74. https://doi.org/10.1001/jamaophthalmol.2017.5202. Erratum in: JAMA

Ophthalmol. 2019 Feb 1;137(2):233. PMID: 29167896; PMCID: PMC5833599.

83. Min JW, Kim HD, Park SY, Lee JH, Park JH, Lee A, Ra H, Baek J. Relationship between retinal capillary nonperfusion area and renal function in patients with type 2 diabetes. Invest Ophthalmol Vis Sci. 2020;61(14):14. https://doi.org/10.1167/iovs.61.14.14. PMID: 33315053; PMCID: PMC7735947.
84. Tom ES, Saraf SS, Wang F, Zhang Q, Vangipuram G, Limonte CP, de Boer IH, Wang RK, Rezaei KA. Retinal capillary nonperfusion on OCT-angiography and its relationship to kidney function in patients with diabetes. J Ophthalmol. 2020;2020:2473949. https://doi.org/10.1155/2020/2473949. PMID: 33763237; PMCID: PMC7949871.
85. Gupta M, Rao IR, Nagaraju SP, Bhandary SV, Gupta J, Babu GTC. Diabetic retinopathy is a predictor of progression of diabetic kidney disease: a systematic review and meta-analysis. Int J Nephrol. 2022;2022:3922398. https://doi.org/10.1155/2022/3922398. PMID: 35531467; PMCID: PMC9076335.
86. Lee WJ, Sobrin L, Kang MH, Seong M, Kim YJ, Yi JH, Miller JW, Cho HY. Ischemic diabetic retinopathy as a possible prognostic factor for chronic kidney disease progression. Eye (Lond). 2014;28(9):1119–25. https://doi.org/10.1038/eye.2014.130. Epub 2014 Jul 4. PMID: 24993319; PMCID: PMC4166629.
87. Zhang J, Wang Y, Li L, Zhang R, Guo R, Li H, Han Q, Teng G, Liu F. Diabetic retinopathy may predict the renal outcomes of patients with diabetic nephropathy. Ren Fail. 2018;40(1):243–51. https://doi.org/10.1080/0886022X.2018.1456453. PMID: 29633887; PMCID: PMC6014304.
88. Sitchevaska O. Retrolental fibroplasia in premature infants; Terry's syndrome. Arch Ophthalmol. 1946;36:362. PMID: 20999242.
89. Terry TL. Fibroblastic overgrowth of persistent tunica vasculosa lentis in infants born prematurely: II. Report of cases-clinical aspects. Trans Am Ophthalmol Soc. 1942;40:262–84. PMID: 16693285; PMCID: PMC1315050.
90. Terry TL. Retrolental fibroplasia in the premature infant: V. Further studies on fibroplastic overgrowth of the persistent tunica vasculosa lentis. Trans Am Ophthalmol Soc. 1944;42:383–96. PMID: 16693360; PMCID: PMC1315141.
91. Terry TL. Retrolental fibroplasia. J Pediatr. 1946;29(6):770–3. https://doi.org/10.1016/s0022-3476(46)80009-x. PMID: 20277990.
92. Owens WC, Owens EU. Retrolental fibroplasia in premature infants. Am J Ophthalmol. 1949;32(1):1–21. https://doi.org/10.1016/0002-9394(49)91102-2. PMID: 18106909.
93. Ashton N, Ward B, Serpell G. Role of oxygen in the genesis of retrolental fibroplasia; a preliminary report. Br J Ophthalmol. 1953;37(9):513–20. https://doi.org/10.1136/bjo.37.9.513. PMID: 13081949; PMCID: PMC1324188.
94. Ashton N, Ward B, Serpell G. Effect of oxygen on developing retinal vessels with particular reference to the problem of retrolental fibroplasia. Br J Ophthalmol. 1954;38(7):397–432. https://doi.org/10.1136/bjo.38.7.397. PMID: 13172417; PMCID: PMC1324374.
95. Patz A, Eastham A, Higginbotham DH, Kleh T. Oxygen studies in retrolental fibroplasia. II. The production of the microscopic changes of retrolental fibroplasia in experimental animals. Am J Ophthalmol. 1953;36(11):1511–22. PMID: 13104558.
96. Patz A. The role of oxygen in retrolental fibroplasia. Trans Am Ophthalmol Soc. 1968;66:940–85. PMID: 4888959; PMCID: PMC1310320.
97. Chiang MF, Quinn GE, Fielder AR, Ostmo SR, Paul Chan RV, Berrocal A, Binenbaum G, Blair M, Peter Campbell J, Capone A Jr, Chen Y, Dai S, Ells A, Fleck BW, Good WV, Elizabeth Hartnett M, Holmstrom G, Kusaka S, Kychenthal A, Lepore D, Lorenz B, Martinez-Castellanos MA, Özdek Ş, Ademola-Popoola D, Reynolds JD, Shah PK, Shapiro M, Stahl A, Toth C, Vinekar A, Visser L, Wallace DK, Wu WC, Zhao P, Zin A. International classification of retinopathy of prematurity, third edition. Ophthalmology. 2021;128(10):e51–68. https://doi.org/10.1016/j.ophtha.2021.05.031. Epub 2021 Jul 8. PMID: 34247850.
98. Cryotherapy for Retinopathy of Prematurity Cooperative Group. Multicenter trial of cryotherapy for retinopathy of prematurity. Preliminary results. Arch Ophthalmol. 1988;106(4):471–9. https://doi.org/10.1001/archopht.1988.01060130517027. PMID: 2895630.
99. Early Treatment For Retinopathy of Prematurity Cooperative Group. Revised indications for the treatment of retinopathy of prematurity: results of the early treatment for retinopathy of prematurity randomized trial. Arch Ophthalmol. 2003;121(12):1684–94. https://doi.org/10.1001/archopht.121.12.1684. PMID: 14662586.
100. Kumawat D, Sachan A, Shah P, Chawla R, Chandra P. Aggressive posterior retinopathy of prematurity: a review on current understanding. Eye (Lond). 2021;35(4):1140–58. https://doi.org/10.1038/s41433-021-01392-6. Epub 2021 Jan 29. PMID: 33514899; PMCID: PMC8115681.
101. Palmer EA, Hardy RJ, Dobson V, Phelps DL, Quinn GE, Summers CG, Krom CP, Tung B, Cryotherapy for Retinopathy of Prematurity Cooperative Group. 15-year outcomes following threshold retinopathy of prematurity: final results from the multicenter trial of cryotherapy for retinopathy of prematurity. Arch Ophthalmol. 2005;123(3):311–8. https://doi.org/10.1001/archopht.123.3.311. PMID: 15767472.
102. McNamara JA, Tasman W, Brown GC, Federman JL. Laser photocoagulation for stage 3+ retinopathy of prematurity. Ophthalmology. 1991;98(5):576–80. https://doi.org/10.1016/s0161-6420(91)32247-4. PMID: 2062488.

103. Capone A Jr, Diaz-Rohena R, Sternberg P Jr, Mandell B, Lambert HM, Lopez PF. Diode-laser photocoagulation for zone 1 threshold retinopathy of prematurity. Am J Ophthalmol. 1993;116(4):444–50. https://doi.org/10.1016/s0002-9394(14)71402-3. PMID: 8213974.
104. Connolly BP, McNamara JA, Sharma S, Regillo CD, Tasman W. A comparison of laser photocoagulation with trans-scleral cryotherapy in the treatment of threshold retinopathy of prematurity. Ophthalmology. 1998;105(9):1628–31. https://doi.org/10.1016/S0161-6420(98)99029-7. PMID: 9754168.
105. Laser ROP Study Group. Laser therapy for retinopathy of prematurity. Arch Ophthalmol. 1994;112(2):154–6. https://doi.org/10.1001/archopht.1994.01090140028007. PMID: 8311759.
106. Ng EY, Connolly BP, McNamara JA, Regillo CD, Vander JF, Tasman W. A comparison of laser photocoagulation with cryotherapy for threshold retinopathy of prematurity at 10 years: part 1. Visual function and structural outcome. Ophthalmology. 2002;109(5):928–34; discussion 935. PMID: 11986099. https://doi.org/10.1016/s0161-6420(01)01017-x.
107. Hwang CK, Hubbard GB, Hutchinson AK, Lambert SR. Outcomes after intravitreal bevacizumab versus laser photocoagulation for retinopathy of prematurity: a 5-year retrospective analysis. Ophthalmology. 2015;122(5):1008–15. https://doi.org/10.1016/j.ophtha.2014.12.017. Epub 2015 Feb 14. PMID: 25687024; PMCID: PMC4414677.
108. Sternberg P Jr, Durrani AK. Evolving concepts in the management of retinopathy of prematurity. Am J Ophthalmol. 2018;186:xxiii–xii. https://doi.org/10.1016/j.ajo.2017.10.027. Epub 2017 Nov 3. PMID: 29109051.
109. Mintz-Hittner HA, Kennedy KA, Chuang AZ, BEAT-ROP Cooperative Group. Efficacy of intravitreal bevacizumab for stage 3+ retinopathy of prematurity. N Engl J Med. 2011;364(7):603–15. https://doi.org/10.1056/NEJMoa1007374. PMID: 21323540; PMCID: PMC3119530.
110. Stahl A, Lepore D, Fielder A, Fleck B, Reynolds JD, Chiang MF, Li J, Liew M, Maier R, Zhu Q, Marlow N. Ranibizumab versus laser therapy for the treatment of very low birthweight infants with retinopathy of prematurity (RAINBOW): an open-label randomised controlled trial. Lancet. 2019;394(10208):1551–9. https://doi.org/10.1016/S0140-6736(19)31344-3. Epub 2019 Sep 12. PMID: 31522845.
111. Yoon JM, Shin DH, Kim SJ, Ham DI, Kang SW, Chang YS, Park WS. Outcomes after laser versus combined laser and bevacizumab treatment for type 1 retinopathy of prematurity in zone I. Retina. 2017;37(1):88–96. https://doi.org/10.1097/IAE.0000000000001125. PMID: 27347645.
112. Mintz-Hittner HA, Geloneck MM, Chuang AZ. Clinical management of recurrent retinopathy of prematurity after intravitreal bevacizumab monotherapy. Ophthalmology. 2016;123(9):1845–55. https://doi.org/10.1016/j.ophtha.2016.04.028. Epub 2016 May 27. PMID: 27241619; PMCID: PMC4995132.
113. Garcia Gonzalez JM, Snyder L, Blair M, Rohr A, Shapiro M, Greenwald M. Prophylactic peripheral laser and fluorescein angiography after bevacizumab for retinopathy of prematurity. Retina. 2018;38(4):764–72. https://doi.org/10.1097/IAE.0000000000001581. PMID: 28267112.
114. VanderVeen DK, Melia M, Yang MB, Hutchinson AK, Wilson LB, Lambert SR. Anti-vascular endothelial growth factor therapy for primary treatment of type 1 retinopathy of prematurity: a report by the American Academy of Ophthalmology. Ophthalmology. 2017;124(5):619–33. https://doi.org/10.1016/j.ophtha.2016.12.025. Epub 2017 Mar 22. PMID: 28341474.
115. Zhou Y, Jiang Y, Bai Y, Wen J, Chen L. Vascular endothelial growth factor plasma levels before and after treatment of retinopathy of prematurity with ranibizumab. Graefes Arch Clin Exp Ophthalmol. 2016;254(1):31–6. https://doi.org/10.1007/s00417--015-2996-0. Epub 2015 Apr 9. PMID: 25851862.
116. Writing Committee for the Pediatric Eye Disease Investigator Group, Hartnett ME, Wallace DK, Dean TW, Li Z, Boente CS, Dosunmu EO, Freedman SF, Golden RP, Kong L, Prakalapakorn SG, Repka MX, Smith LE, Wang H, Kraker RT, Cotter SA, Holmes JM. Plasma levels of bevacizumab and vascular endothelial growth factor after low-dose bevacizumab treatment for retinopathy of prematurity in infants. JAMA Ophthalmol. 2022;140(4):337–44. https://doi.org/10.1001/jamaophthalmol.2022.0030. Erratum in: JAMA Ophthalmol. 2022 Apr 1;140(4):441. PMID: 35446359; PMCID: PMC8895318.
117. Twitty G, Weiss M, Bazacliu C, O'Mara K, Mowitz ME. Hypertension in neonates treated with intravitreal bevacizumab for retinopathy of prematurity. J Perinatol. 2021;41(6):1426–31. https://doi.org/10.1038/s41372-021-01021-w. Epub 2021 Mar 8. PMID: 33686120.
118. Kondo C, Iwahashi C, Utamura S, Kuniyoshi K, Konishi Y, Wada N, Kawasaki R, Kusaka S. Characteristics of eyes developing retinal detachment after anti-vascular endothelial growth factor therapy for retinopathy of prematurity. Front Pediatr. 2022;10:785292. https://doi.org/10.3389/fped.2022.785292. PMID: 35463897; PMCID: PMC9021749.
119. Hansen ED, Hartnett ME. A review of treatment for retinopathy of prematurity. Expert Rev Ophthalmol. 2019;14(2):73–87. https://doi.org/10.1080/17469899.2019.1596026. Epub 2019 Mar 29. PMID: 31762784; PMCID: PMC6874220.

120. Hartnett ME. Advances in understanding and management of retinopathy of prematurity. Surv Ophthalmol. 2017;62(3):257–76. https://doi.org/10.1016/j.survophthal.2016.12.004. Epub 2016 Dec 22. PMID: 28012875; PMCID: PMC5401801.
121. Ramshekar A, Hartnett ME. Vascular endothelial growth factor signaling in models of oxygen-induced retinopathy: insights into mechanisms of pathology in retinopathy of prematurity. Front Pediatr. 2021;9:796143. https://doi.org/10.3389/fped.2021.796143. PMID: 34956992; PMCID: PMC8696159.
122. Gilbert C, Fielder A, Gordillo L, Quinn G, Semiglia R, Visintin P, Zin A, International NO-ROP Group. Characteristics of infants with severe retinopathy of prematurity in countries with low, moderate, and high levels of development: implications for screening programs. Pediatrics. 2005;115(5):e518–25. https://doi.org/10.1542/peds.2004-1180. Epub 2005 Apr 1. PMID: 15805336.
123. Quinn GE, Barr C, Bremer D, Fellows R, Gong A, Hoffman R, Repka MX, Shepard J, Siatkowski RM, Wade K, Ying GS. Changes in course of retinopathy of prematurity from 1986 to 2013: comparison of three studies in the United States. Ophthalmology. 2016;123(7):1595–600. https://doi.org/10.1016/j.ophtha.2016.03.026. Epub 2016 Apr 12. PMID: 27084562; PMCID: PMC4921295.
124. Vinekar A, Dogra MR, Sangtam T, Narang A, Gupta A. Retinopathy of prematurity in Asian Indian babies weighing greater than 1250 grams at birth: ten year data from a tertiary care center in a developing country. Indian J Ophthalmol. 2007;55(5):331–6. https://doi.org/10.4103/0301-4738.33817. PMID: 17699940; PMCID: PMC2636032.
125. Jalali S, Matalia J, Hussain A, Anand R. Modification of screening criteria for retinopathy of prematurity in India and other middle-income countries. Am J Ophthalmol. 2006;141(5):966–8. https://doi.org/10.1016/j.ajo.2005.12.016. PMID: 16678524.
126. Fierson WM, American Academy of Pediatrics Section on Ophthalmology; American Academy of Ophthalmology; American Association for Pediatric Ophthalmology and Strabismus; American Association of Certified Orthoptists. Screening examination of premature infants for retinopathy of prematurity. Pediatrics. 2018;142(6):e20183061. https://doi.org/10.1542/peds.2018-3061. Erratum in: Pediatrics. 2019 Mar;143(3): PMID: 30478242.
127. Shukla R, Murthy GVS, Gilbert C, Vidyadhar B, Mukpalkar S. Operational guidelines for ROP in India: a summary. Indian J Ophthalmol. 2020;68(Suppl 1):S108–14. https://doi.org/10.4103/ijo.IJO_1827_19. PMID: 31937744; PMCID: PMC7001189.
128. Quinn GE, Ying GS, Daniel E, Hildebrand PL, Ells A, Baumritter A, Kemper AR, Schron EB, Wade K, e-ROP Cooperative Group. Validity of a telemedicine system for the evaluation of acute-phase retinopathy of prematurity. JAMA Ophthalmol. 2014;132(10):1178–84. https://doi.org/10.1001/jamaophthalmol.2014.1604. PMID: 24970095; PMCID: PMC4861044.
129. Vinekar A, Jayadev C, Mangalesh S, Shetty B, Vidyasagar D. Role of tele-medicine in retinopathy of prematurity screening in rural outreach centers in India—a report of 20,214 imaging sessions in the KIDROP program. Semin Fetal Neonatal Med. 2015;20(5):335–45. https://doi.org/10.1016/j.siny.2015.05.002. Epub 2015 Jun 17. PMID: 26092301.
130. Biten H, Redd TK, Moleta C, Campbell JP, Ostmo S, Jonas K, Chan RVP, Chiang MF, Imaging & Informatics in Retinopathy of Prematurity (ROP) Research Consortium. Diagnostic accuracy of ophthalmoscopy vs telemedicine in examinations for retinopathy of prematurity. JAMA Ophthalmol. 2018;136(5):498–504. https://doi.org/10.1001/jamaophthalmol.2018.0649. PMID: 29621387; PMCID: PMC6036899.
131. Chiang MF, Melia M, Buffenn AN, Lambert SR, Recchia FM, Simpson JL, Yang MB. Detection of clinically significant retinopathy of prematurity using wide-angle digital retinal photography: a report by the American Academy of Ophthalmology. Ophthalmology. 2012;119(6):1272–80. https://doi.org/10.1016/j.ophtha.2012.01.002. Epub 2012 Apr 27. PMID: 22541632; PMCID: PMC3637992.
132. Yuan M, Yang Y, Yan H, Li J, Liu R, Li T, Li Y, Liang X, Ding X, Lu L. Increased posterior retinal vessels in mild asymptomatic familial exudative vitreoretinopathy eyes. Retina. 2016;36(6):1209–15. https://doi.org/10.1097/IAE.0000000000000830. PMID: 26655609.
133. Miyakubo H, Hashimoto K, Miyakubo S. Retinal vascular pattern in familial exudative vitreoretinopathy. Ophthalmology. 1984;91(12):1524–30. https://doi.org/10.1016/s0161-6420(84)34119-7. PMID: 6084219.
134. Pendergast SD, Trese MT. Familial exudative vitreoretinopathy. Results of surgical management. Ophthalmology. 1998;105(6):1015–23. https://doi.org/10.1016/S0161-6420(98)96002-X. PMID: 9627651.
135. Gilmour DF. Familial exudative vitreoretinopathy and related retinopathies. Eye (Lond). 2015;29(1):1–14. https://doi.org/10.1038/eye.2014.70. Epub 2014 Oct 17. PMID: 25323851; PMCID: PMC4289842.
136. Ranchod TM, Ho LY, Drenser KA, Capone A Jr, Trese MT. Clinical presentation of familial exudative vitreoretinopathy. Ophthalmology. 2011;118(10):2070–5. https://doi.org/10.1016/j.ophtha.2011.06.020. Epub 2011 Aug 25. PMID: 21868098.
137. Kashani AH, Brown KT, Chang E, Drenser KA, Capone A, Trese MT. Diversity of retinal vascular anomalies in patients with familial exudative vitreoretinopathy. Ophthalmology. 2014;121(11):2220–7.

https://doi.org/10.1016/j.ophtha.2014.05.029. Epub 2014 Jul 5. PMID: 25005911.
138. Kashani AH, Learned D, Nudleman E, Drenser KA, Capone A, Trese MT. High prevalence of peripheral retinal vascular anomalies in family members of patients with familial exudative vitreoretinopathy. Ophthalmology. 2014;121(1):262–8. https://doi.org/10.1016/j.ophtha.2013.08.010. Epub 2013 Sep 29. PMID: 24084499.
139. Lyu J, Zhang Q, Wang SY, Chen YY, Xu Y, Zhao PQ. Ultra-wide-field scanning laser ophthalmoscopy assists in the clinical detection and evaluation of asymptomatic early-stage familial exudative vitreoretinopathy. Graefes Arch Clin Exp Ophthalmol. 2017;255(1):39–47.https://doi.org/10.1007/s00417--016-3415-x. Epub 2016 Jul 14. PMID: 27416933.
140. Zhang T, Wang Z, Sun L, Li S, Huang L, Liu C, Chen C, Luo X, Yu B, Ding X. Ultra-wide-field scanning laser ophthalmoscopy and optical coherence tomography in FEVR: findings and its diagnostic ability. Br J Ophthalmol. 2021;105(7):995–1001. https://doi.org/10.1136/bjophthalmol-2020-316226. Epub 2020 Aug 11. PMID: 32788330.
141. Yonekawa Y, Thomas BJ, Drenser KA, Trese MT, Capone A Jr. Familial exudative vitreoretinopathy: spectral-domain optical coherence tomography of the vitreoretinal interface, retina, and choroid. Ophthalmology. 2015;122(11):2270–7. https://doi.org/10.1016/j.ophtha.2015.07.024. Epub 2015 Aug 20. PMID: 26299697.
142. Sen P, Singh N, Rishi E, Bhende P, Rao C, Rishi P, Bhende M, Sharma T, Gopal L. Outcomes of surgery in eyes with familial exudative vitreoretinopathyassociated retinal detachment. Can J Ophthalmol. 2020;55(3):253–62. https://doi.org/10.1016/j.jcjo.2019.11.001. Epub 2020 Jan 13. PMID: 31941588.
143. Bain BJ, Littlewood T, Rees DC. What does the term 'sickle cell disease' mean? Br J Haematol. 2022;197(3):381–2. https://doi.org/10.1111/bjh.18024. Epub 2021 Dec 28. PMID: 34961949.
144. Herrick JB. Peculiar elongated and sickle-shaped red blood corpuscles in a case of severe anemia. Arch Intern Med (Chic). 1910;VI(5):517–21. https://doi.org/10.1001/archinte.1910.00050330050003.
145. Rees DC, Williams TN, Gladwin MT. Sickle-cell disease. Lancet. 2010;376(9757):2018–31. https://doi.org/10.1016/S0140-6736(10)61029-X. Epub 2010 Dec 3. PMID: 21131035.
146. Demirci S, Leonard A, Haro-Mora JJ, Uchida N, Tisdale JF. CRISPR/Cas9 for sickle cell disease: applications, future possibilities, and challenges. Adv Exp Med Biol. 2019;1144:37–52. https://doi.org/10.1007/5584_2018_331.
147. Esrick EB, Lehmann LE, Biffi A, et al. Post-transcriptional genetic silencing of *BCL11A* to treat sickle cell disease. N Engl J Med. 2021;384(3):205–15. https://doi.org/10.1056/NEJMoa2029392.
148. Quintana-Bustamante O, Fañanas-Baquero S, Dessy-Rodriguez M, Ojeda-Pérez I, Segovia JC. Gene editing for inherited red blood cell diseases. Front Physiol. 2022;13:848261. Published 2022 Mar 28. https://doi.org/10.3389/fphys.2022.848261.
149. Kavanagh PL, Fasipe TA, Wun T. Sickle cell disease: a review. JAMA. 2022;328(1):57–68. https://doi.org/10.1001/jama.2022.10233. PMID: 35788790.
150. Linz MO, Scott AW. Wide-field imaging of sickle retinopathy. Int J Retina Vitreous. 2019;5(Suppl 1):27. https://doi.org/10.1186/s40942-019-0177-8. PMID: 31890287; PMCID: PMC6907105.
151. Welch RB, Goldberg MF. Sickle-cell hemoglobin and its relation to fundus abnormality. Arch Ophthalmol. 1966;75(3):353–62. https://doi.org/10.1001/archopht.1966.00970050355008. PMID: 5903820.
152. Goldberg MF. Classification and pathogenesis of proliferative sickle retinopathy. Am J Ophthalmol. 1971;71(3):649–65. https://doi.org/10.1016/0002--9394(71)90429-6. PMID: 5546311.
153. Penman AD, Talbot JF, Chuang EL, Thomas P, Serjeant GR, Bird AC. New classification of peripheral retinal vascular changes in sickle cell disease. Br J Ophthalmol. 1994;78(9):681–9. https://doi.org/10.1136/bjo.78.9.681. PMID: 7947547; PMCID: PMC504905.
154. Asdourian GK, Nagpal KC, Busse B, Goldbaum M, Patriankos D, Rabb MF, Goldberg MF. Macular and perimacular vascular remodelling sickling haemoglobinopathies. Br J Ophthalmol. 1976;60(6):431–53. https://doi.org/10.1136/bjo.60.6.431. PMID: 952816; PMCID: PMC1017523.
155. Zhou DB, Castanos MV, Pinhas A, Gillette P, Migacz JV, Rosen RB, Glassberg J, Chui TYP. Quantification of intermittent retinal capillary perfusion in sickle cell disease. Biomed Opt Express. 2021;12(5):2825–40. https://doi.org/10.1364/BOE.418874. PMID: 34123506; PMCID: PMC8176806.
156. Cho M, Kiss S. Detection and monitoring of sickle cell retinopathy using ultra wide-field color photography and fluorescein angiography. Retina. 2011;31(4):738–47. https://doi.org/10.1097/IAE.0b013e3181f049ec. PMID: 21836403.
157. Pahl DA, Green NS, Bhatia M, Lee MT, Chang JS, Licursi M, Briamonte C, Smilow E, Chen RWS. Optical coherence tomography angiography and ultra-widefield fluorescein angiography for early detection of adolescent sickle retinopathy. Am J Ophthalmol. 2017;183:91–8. https://doi.org/10.1016/j.ajo.2017.08.010. Epub 2017 Aug 30. PMID: 28860042; PMCID: PMC5660939.
158. Alabduljalil T, Cheung CS, VandenHoven C, Mackeen LD, Kirby-Allen M, Kertes PJ, Lam

WC. Retinal ultra-wide-field colour imaging versus dilated fundus examination to screen for sickle cell retinopathy. Br J Ophthalmol. 2021;105(8):1121–6. https://doi.org/10.1136/bjophthalmol-2020-316779. Epub 2020 Aug 19. PMID: 32816790.

159. Abitbol E, Miere A, Excoffier JB, Mehanna CJ, Amoroso F, Kerr S, Ortala M, Souied EH. Deep learning-based classification of retinal vascular diseases using ultra-widefield colour fundus photographs. BMJ Open Ophthalmol. 2022;7(1):e000924. https://doi.org/10.1136/bmjophth-2021-000924. PMID: 35141420; PMCID: PMC8819815.

7 Subretinal/Submacular Haemorrhage

7.1 Introduction

Haemorrhage under the retina, especially the macula, portends an underlying serious ocular disease and occasionally a life-threatening systemic disease. If not treated urgently, itmay lead to irreversible loss of central vision. Submacular haemorrhages may occur at all ages under the retinal pigment epithelium (RPE) or the neurosensory retina, varying from a small thin blood film to extensive and massive mounds of blood clots. When unilateral and small, these often go unnoticed by the patient. When discovered, the symptoms may vary from distortion of objects to more significant vision loss. This central dark spot moves with the eye or causes a complete loss of central vision, including the ability to read, recognize people, or identify colours from the affected eye. Ambulatory vision is often preserved if the haemorrhage remains limited to the macula. It is important to distinguish the location of the blood. It appears bright red when under the neurosensory retina (transparent) and dark when under the RPE (pigmented). Unlike superficial retinal haemorrhages that obscure the retinal vessels, submacular haemorrhages do not obscure the overlying retinal structures and the vessels are seen running normally over the blood. It may be challengingto clinically distinguish between the intraretinal haemorrhages in the Henle's layer (often assumes a petaloid pattern) and the submacular location, which can be easily solved with a structural OCT scan.

Submacular haemorrhages are commonly seen in old age and result from the rupture of abnormal new vessels from the choroid (choroidal neovascular membrane, or CNVM) that develop in nearly 10% of people with age-related macular degeneration (AMD). It is commonly designated as the wet form of AMD or neovascular age-related macular degeneration (nAMD). Notably, nearly 190 million people across the world suffer from AMD. In the Asia-Pacific region, massive submacular haemorrhages may occur from a specific variant ofnAMD known as polypoidal choroidal vasculopathy (PCV). In young people, blunt trauma may cause rupture of the choroid resulting in submacular haemorrhage. Rupture of retinal macroaneurysms, seen more often in older women with hypertension, may cause intraocular haemorrhage that may dissect below the retina. Several posterior uveitis entities include toxoplasmic retinochoroiditis, Vogt-Koyanagi-Harada's (VKH) disease, tubercular choroiditis, punctate inner choroidopathy, and multifocal choroiditis with panuveitis may get complicated by the development of CNVM and present with a submacular haemorrhage. Less commonly, degenerative myopia, angioid streaks, choroidal osteoma, choroidal melanoma, metastatic lesions, and leukaemia also present with subretinal haemorrhages.

A. Gupta et al., *Ophthalmic Signs in Practice of Medicine*,
https://doi.org/10.1007/978-981-99-7923-3_7

7.2 Age-Related Macular Degeneration

Age-related macular degeneration (AMD) is the most common cause of visual disability in old age (>50 years) inWestern countries. It is fast emerging as a challenge in the ageing population of developing countries. AMD is mainly of two types:the non-exudative or the dry type, characterized by the formation of soft drusen and pigmentary changes that progress to geographic atrophy in the macula, and the exudative or the wet type, the neovascular stage, a sight-threatening complication marked by the development of abnormal macular neovascularization (MNV) in the macula that causes exudation, haemorrhage, and sometimes deposition of hard exudates. If untreated, the nAMD results in extensive fibrosis in the macula. The late stage of non-exudative AMD is remarkable for atrophy of the choriocapillaris, RPE and the overlying photoreceptors in the macula, known as geographic atrophy (GA) (Fig. 7.1). There is no known treatment to prevent or reverse this late stage of dry AMD. Even the exudative AMD, whether treated or not, ultimately progresses to geographic atrophy.

The most characteristic feature of the AMD that distinguishes it from other causes of CNVM is the deposition of extracellular debris between the plasma membrane and the basement membrane of the RPE (basal laminar deposit) or between the basement membrane of the RPE and the inner collagenous layer of the Bruch's membrane called a basal linear deposit that is responsible for drusen formation [1]. Drusen, the

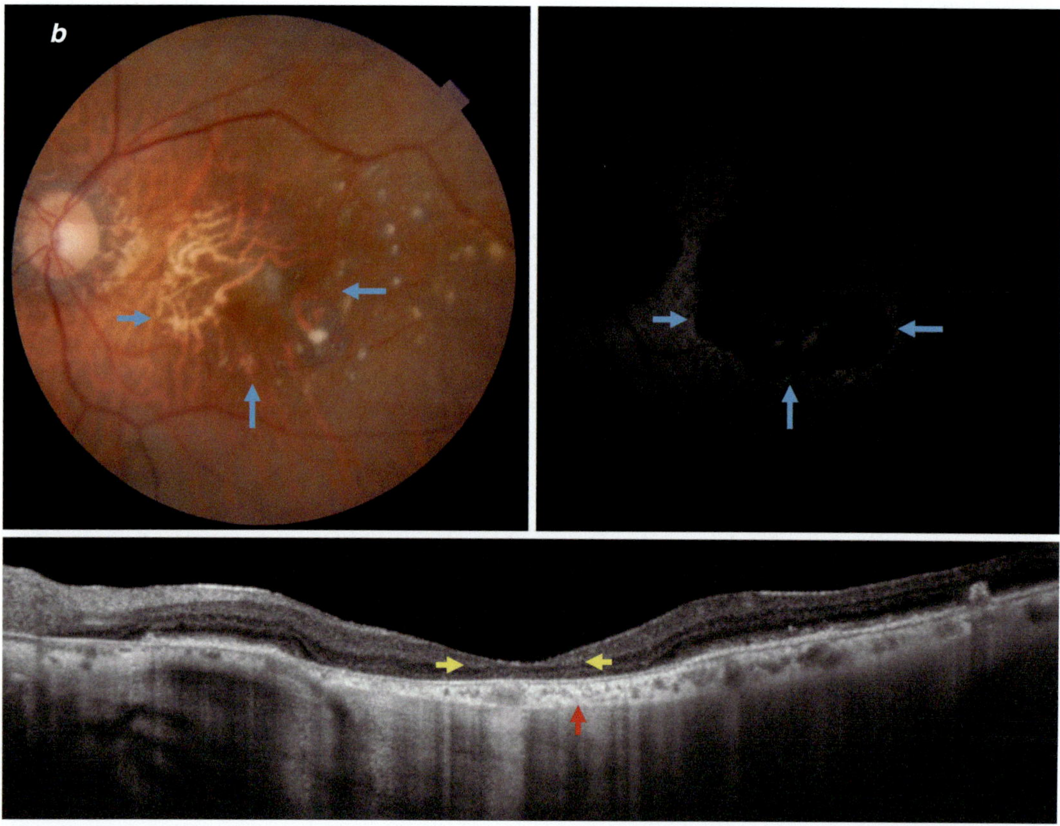

Fig. 7.1 A sharply demarcated area of RPE atrophy (blue arrows) with baring of the large choroidal vessels (**a**), seen as a dark hypoautofluorescent area on fundus autofluorescence (**b**). OCT (**c**) shows loss of outer retinal layers with atrophy of inner retina (yellow arrows) and the choroid (red arrow)

hallmark of AMD, is extracellular deposits between the basement membrane of the RPE and Bruch's membrane.

For epidemiological studies, many classifications have been used. In one such classification based oncolourdigital fundus images of the macula, AMD was classified as: Stage 0a, no evidence of AMD, 0b, hard drusen <63 μ in size; 1a, soft drusen with distinct borders ≥63 μ; 1b, no drusen and only pigmentary changes; 2a, soft drusen ≥125 μ with indistinct borders or reticular drusen; 2b, soft drusen ≥63 μ and ≤ to 125 μ with pigmentary changes; 3, soft drusen ≥125 μ with indistinct borders or reticular drusen with pigmentary changes; 4, geographic atrophy; and 5, neovascular AMD [2]. Stages 2 and 3 are classified as early AMD and stages 4 and 5 as late AMD. Data based on this classification from ten European countries showed the prevalence of early AMD varying from 3.5% in the youngest population (55–59 years) to 17.5% in the oldest population (≥85 years). The late AMD (Stage 4) was seen in nearly 10% of the oldest group (≥85 years) [3]. Until the introduction of anti-VEGF therapy in 2006 for nAMD, no effective therapyeither improved or prevented further loss of vision in such eyes. Following the availability of this treatment,while there has been a significant decrease in the prevalence of late AMD, early AMD continues to show a rising prevalence [3]. These numbers are expected to rise further in the coming decades [4].

7.3 Risk Factors for AMD

AMD is a complex multifactorial disease with significant genetic and environmental risk factors. Interestingly, besides ageing, several common and preventable risk factors are shared between AMD and cardiovascular disease (CVD). See Boxes 7.1 and 7.2. All these factors, namely family history, hypertension, smoking, obesity, and sedentary lifestyle, are well known to cause chronic systemic inflammation and increase oxidative stress [5]. The Mediterranean diet recommended for preventing CVD, consisting of leafy vegetables, fruits, fish, and legumes, has also been shown to reduce the incidence of late AMD by almost 40% [6]. Additionally, prospective population-based cohorts have shown beneficial effects of high levels of physical activity in preventing the occurrence of early AMD [7].

Box 7.1 Systemic Associations of Age-Related Macular Degeneration

1. 10-year progression of coronary artery calcium (CAC) [8].
2. Persons with AMD shares risk factors with atherosclerosis. These patients have a high incidence of CVD
3. Persons with AMD have a higher risk of stroke-intracerebral hemorrhage than cerebral infarction [9].

Box 7.2 Systemic Risk Factors for AMD and PCV

1. Aging
2. Smoking
3. High blood pressure
4. Obesity/High Body mass index
5. Sedentary lifestyle
6. Nutritional lack of vegetables/fruits
7. Genetic factors—single nucleotide polymorphisms in inflammation, lipid metabolism, and oxidative stress pathways

7.4 Pathogenesis of AMD

As stated above, drusen are extracellular deposits between the basement membrane of RPE and Bruch's membrane. Detection of some components of the alternate complement system in these deposits indicates a low-grade inflammation [10]. Complement factor H encodes for a protein that is vital in controlling inflammation. A single-point mutation in the genes coding for this protein first pointed out the role of genetics in the causation of AMD [11–13].

Obesity and smoking in people who show SNPs CFH Y402H and ARMS 2 (LOC387715 A69S) genes raise the risk of progressive AMD by 19-fold [14].

Since the original studies in 2005, although more than 30 more loci have been discovered in genome-wide association studies,there is still a dearth of information on the exact transcriptome-wide associations or the gene expressions directly responsible for the causation of AMD pathology [15]. However, most of the loci discovered in AMDare involved in either complement-mediated inflammation or lipid metabolism.

ARMS2 gene located on chromosome 10 plays an essential role in the complement pathway by opsonization of the necrotic cells. Single nucleotide point mutation rs10490924 in this gene interferes with the normal apoptotic mechanisms and the complement-mediated clearance ofthe cellular debris. A deficiency of the normal ARMS2 protein may be responsible for drusen formation [16]. It is proposed that environmental factors with defective innate and adaptive immune mechanisms in aged peopledue to their genetic predisposition lead to low-gradesystemic inflammation,which in the eye leads to AMD. The same factors also lead to systemic atherosclerosis, which explains the high risk of CVD in patients with AMD.

Further, ageing decreases the choroidal blood flow and thinning of the choroid, interfering with the normal debris-clearing mechanisms from the outer retina. This subject has been extensively reviewed by Rozing et al. [17]. The cellular debris is deposited under the retina in the Bruch's membrane as well-defined hard drusen, ill-defined soft drusen, or densely packed small reticular drusen. On the other hand, subretinal drusenoid deposits (SDD), earlier known as pseudo reticular drusen, are deposited under the neurosensory retina. The latter differs from the classic drusen in their location and lipid composition. The SDD may breach the ellipsoid zone and extend into the retina. The SDD is associated with type 3 new vessels and geographic atrophy [18]. The site where the drusen will appear does not appear to be a random phenomenon but relates to the areas of choroidal ischemia. Although histopathological studies in the past had shown thinning of choriocapillaris in the AMD eyes, more recently, imaging studies using OCT angiography have shown significant flow deficits in choriocapillaris underlying the existing drusen, expanding drusen or even those that will appear in future suggesting that choroidal ischemia is a critical event in the development of AMD [19]. Age-related thickening of Bruch's membrane, deposition of advanced glycosylated end products (AGE) and extracellular debris as basal laminar deposits, and increased expression of VEGF from the RPE and microglia in an ischemic microenvironment lead to the formation of pathological new vessels that grow most commonly under the RPE (type1), less commonly under the neurosensory retina (type 2) or even into the retina (type 3). These vessels do not have tight endothelial junctions and leak fluid or rupture to cause blood under the macula (submacular haemorrhage).

7.5 Clinical Signs of Age-Related Macular Degeneration

The non-exudative AMD in early and intermediate stages is asymptomatic and gets diagnosed in patients who may visit an ophthalmology/optometry clinic for a routine examination/screening for cataracts and glaucoma. By and large non-exudative AMD is symmetric bilateral disease, and 90% of patients do not progress to an exudative stage. Drusen are the hallmark of AMD and vary in size from <63 μ to nearly 1000 μ (Fig. 7.2). Small drusen, <63 μ, are seen in the macula as yellow-white discrete dot lesions and are commonly seen in older people. These are called hard drusen and usually are not seen on fundus fluorescein angiography (FFA). These stay unaltered for several years and may show mineralization. They appear as tiny nodular elevations over Bruch's membrane on structural OCT and do not progress further to the GA or predispose to CNV formation (Fig. 7.2). Soft drusen are made ofsimilar lipoproteins debris but are larger than 63 μ, are pale yellow, and have indistinct borders. The presence of soft drusen <125 μ is labelled as early AMD. These may become confluent over time and increase in

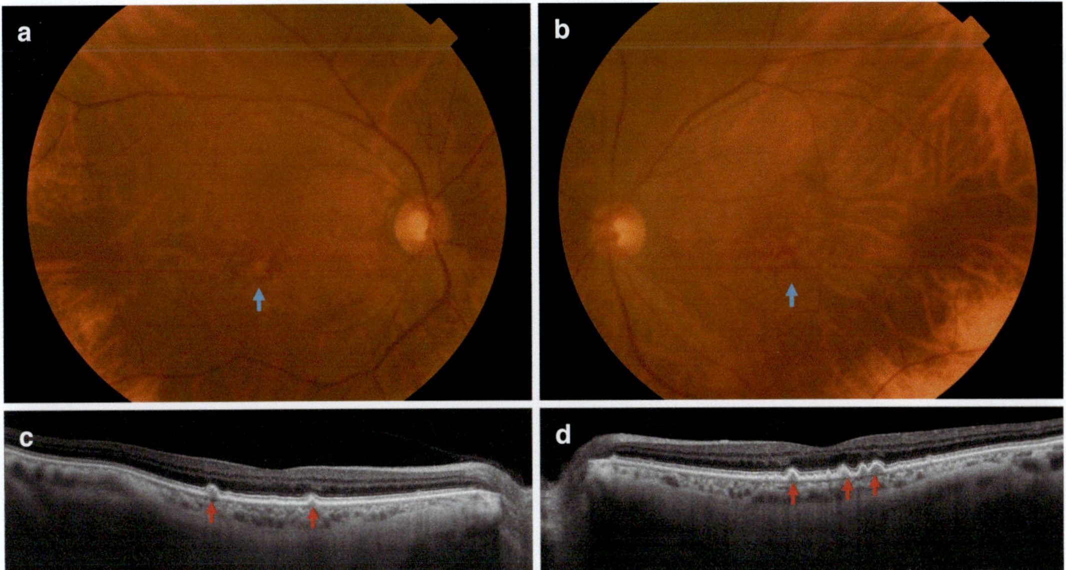

Fig. 7.2 Drusen, the hallmark of AMD, are seen in the macula as yellow-white discrete dot lesions on clinical examination (**a**, **b**). They appear as tiny nodular elevations over Bruch's membrane on structural OCT (**c**, **d**)

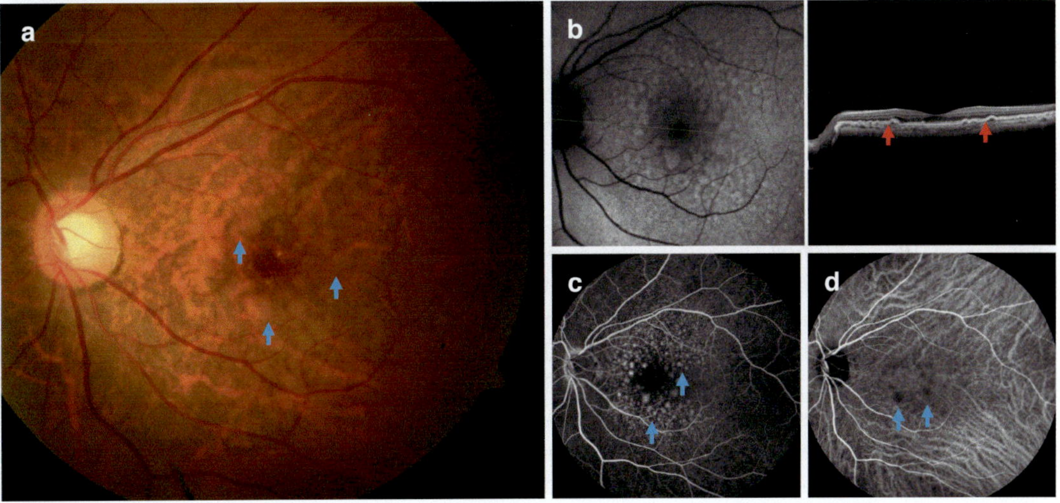

Fig. 7.3 Soft drusen indicate intermediate AMD, are larger than 63 μ, and appear as pale-yellow lesions (blue arrows) with indistinct borders (**a**). OCT shows RPE elevations (red arrows) (**b**). Fluorescein angiography (**c**) shows hyperfluorescent lesions (blue arrows), and ICGA (**d**) shows subtle hypocyanescent lesions (blue arrows)

numbers. More than 20 soft drusen >63–124 μ or multiple small with a single large soft druse >125 μ is classified as an intermediate stage of AMD. Pigmentary changes may accompany the soft drusen, and both hyper and hypopigmentation may be seen. The soft drusen are mound-like deposits on structural OCT between the RPE and Bruch's membrane. On autofluorescence, some of these may show a central hypoautofluorescence with a ring of hyperautofluorescence (Fig. 7.3). A thin layer of basal linear deposits may connect the soft drusen. The most significant type of drusen isthe subretinal drusenoid deposits (previously termed reticular pseudo drusen) under the neurosensory retina and overlie the RPE. These were correctly localized only after the availability of

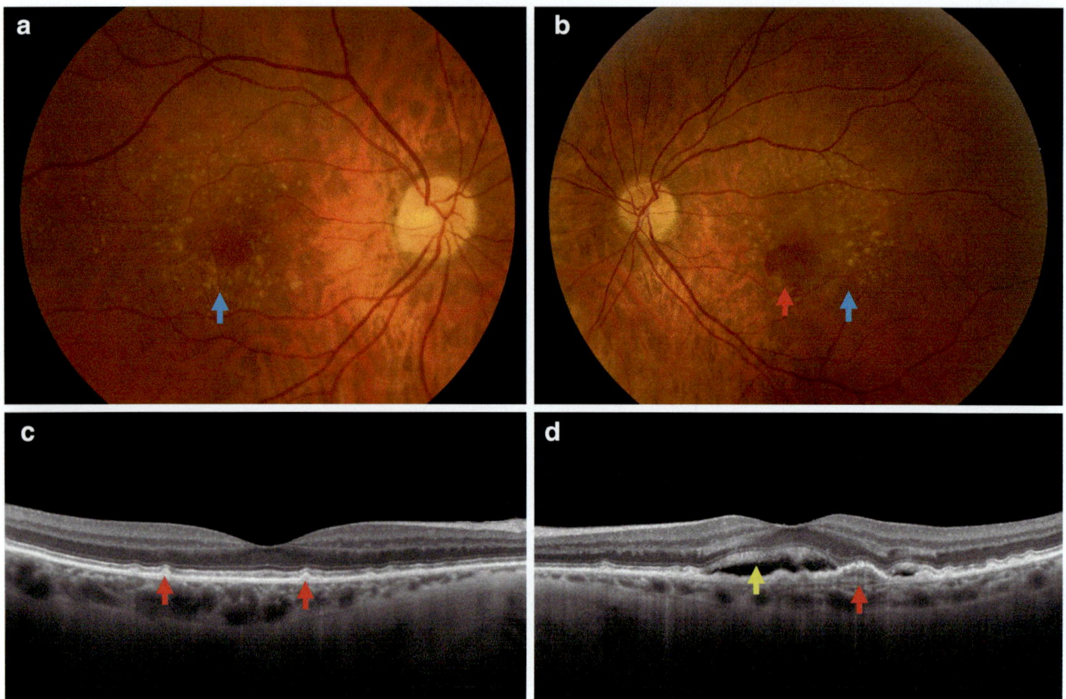

Fig. 7.4 Right eye (**a**) shows hard drusen (blue arrows), and the left eye shows hard drusen (blue arrows) along with a subretinal haemorrhage (red arrow) suggestive of a CNVM (**b**). OCT (**c**) shows sub-RPE drusenoid deposits in the right eye (red arrows) and a CNV complex (red arrow) with subretinal fluid (yellow arrow) in the left eye (**d**). (Images courtesy of Dr. Anita Agarwal, West Coast Medical Retina Group, San Francisco, USA)

structural OCT. These may be best seen in blue light rather than colour fundus or IR reflectance images [18]. Gass [20] first showed the development of nAMD in 18% of eyes with drusen at an average age of 75 years and an average follow-up of nearly 5 years. These eyes were characterized by the development of sub-RPE and subretinal exudation through either an intact Bruch's membrane or the growth of new vessels through breaks in the Bruch's membrane causing exudative and haemorrhagic detachment of the RPE and the neurosensory retina (Fig. 7.4) [20].

7.6 Current Nomenclature for AMD Lesions [1]

Development of advanced retinal imaging tools in recent years has led to the recognitionthat new vessels may also arise from the neurosensory retina prompting the abandonment of the term CNVM (choroidal neovascular membrane) in favour of macular neovascularization (MNV). Further, the nomenclature for the nAMD has been standardized. Type 1 MNV is the growth of new vessels from choriocapillaris that stay under the RPE and cause pigment epithelium detachments (PED). In contrast, the type 2 MNV arise from the choriocapillaris and traverses through breaks in the Bruch's membrane and the RPE to grow under the neurosensory retina (Fig. 7.5). Type 3 new vessels arise from the retina's deep capillary plexus, grow towards the outer retina, and communicate with vessels arising from the choriocapillaris. In the past, based on fundus fluorescein angiography studies, type 1 MNV were called occult CNVM, while type 2 MNV were called classic CNVM. Type 3 MNV was called occult chorioretinal anastomosis [21, 22] or retinal angiomatous proliferation [23] and was characterized by intraretinal hyperfluorescence.

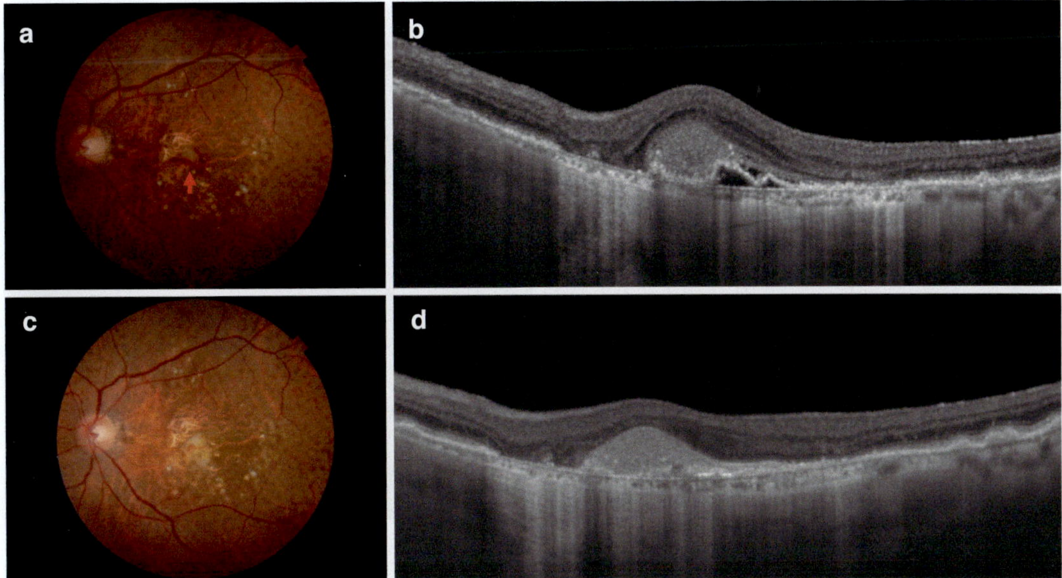

Fig. 7.5 A subretinal haemorrhage (red arrow) along with drusen and area of geographic atrophy seen at baseline (**a**). OCT shows Type 2 CNVM with a breach in RPE and Bruch's membrane (**b**). Following intravitreal injection of anti-VEGF therapy, the subretinal haemorrhage resolved (**c**), and OCT shows the resolution of subretinal fluid (**d**)

Leakage of fluid from the new vessels more than what can be absorbed by the normal mechanisms in the retina leads to the accumulation of intraretinal fluid. In contrast, the collection of such fluid under the retina results in subretinal fluid. The collection of serum, fibrin, and inflammatory cells under the neurosensory retina, based on characteristic reflectivity seen on structural OCT, is called subretinal hyperreflective material (SHRM). PED may occur due to the collection of serous fluid, drusenoid material, or haemorrhage under the pigment epithelium. Serous PEDs in AMD are usually associated with new vessels at their margins. Haemorrhage may collect in the sub-RPE, subretinal, or intraretinal space. The RPE layer may rip due to contractile forces of the fibrovascular tissue under the RPE that scrolls on itself, leading to the baring of the choroid. Persistent subretinal fluid, large drusen, or regression of subretinal drusenoid deposits may lead to outer retinal atrophy and is seen on OCT as loss of ellipsoid, interdigitating zones and thinning of the outer nuclear layerand loss of RPE [1].

7.7 Imaging Studies in Macular New Vessels (MNV)

Decades before the advent of OCT technology, fundus fluorescein angiography (FFA) and indocyanine green (ICG) angiography werethe standard imaging tools to study the presence of CNVM, now rechristened as macular new vessels (MNV). Type 1 MNV, earlier labelled as 'occult CNVM', could not bevisualized on FFA because of the masking effect of the RPE. However, these were visible in the late frames of FFA as ill-defined diffuse/punctate hyperfluorescence. As theexact site of this hyperfluorescence could not be ascertained, thiswaslabelled as hyperfluorescence of uncertain origin. In the late frames of ICG angiography, however, these occult CNVM were often seen as well-defined plaque-like hyperfluorescence and nearly 40% of these got reclassified as classic CNVM [24].

The ICG angiography also predicted the development of exudative AMD by demonstrating hyperfluorescent plaques associated with soft

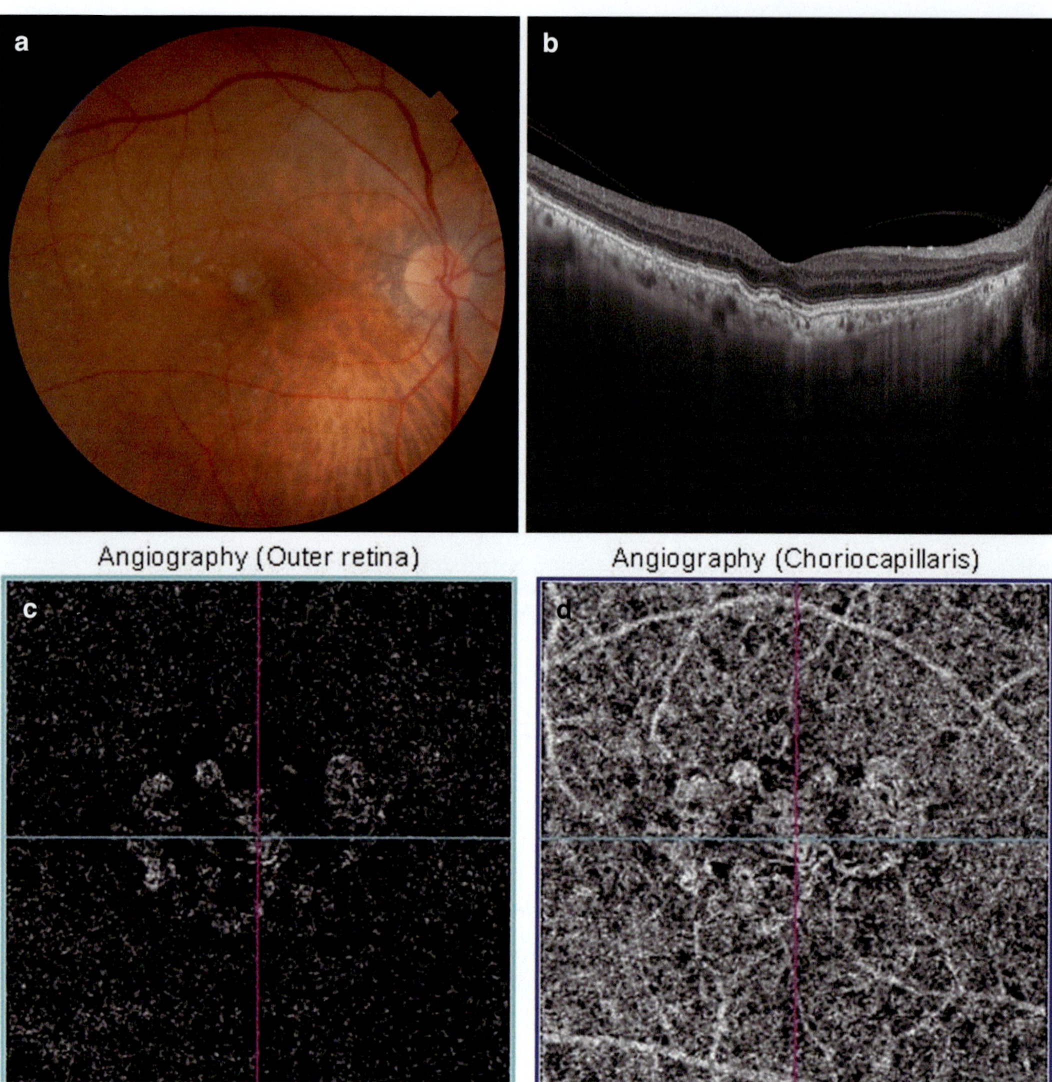

Fig. 7.6 Drusen appear as yellow, discrete lesions in the macula (**a**), and are seen as focal RPE elevations on OCT (**b**). OCT angiography reveals an underlying CNV complex in the outer retina (**c**) and choriocapillaris (**d**) (non-exudative AMD)

drusen even when clinically, these eyes were seen as non-exudative AMD [25]. On the structural OCT, the type 1 MNV is seen as a heterogeneous hyperreflective lesion under an elevated RPE, while the OCTA additionally shows flow within this heterogeneous material. The enface OCTA images of the RPE-choriocapillaris slab clearly show the presence of these so-called occult new vessels. Interestingly, SS-OCT angiography can also detect the non-exudative type of MNV previouslyreported only with ICG angiography (Fig. 7.6). A high number of such eyes go on to develop the exudative AMD [26]. The type 2 MNV, earlier labelled 'classical CNVM' on the other hand, being under the transparent neurosensory retina, is seen as well-defined hyperfluorescent lesionsin the early frames of FFA and shows profuse leakage in the late frames. In many patients,variable components of both type 1 and type 2 MNV may be seen, one being more predominant than the other. On OCT angiography, the type 2 MNV appears as a well-defined cartwheel-like lesion above the RPE. However, a mixed type 1 and 2 MNV mayalso show a similar lesion below the RPE slab [1]. B-scan OCT can show the type 2 MNV breaching the RPE layer and proliferating in the subretinal space, accumulating fluid, blood, and lipids. Fluid may extend into the outer retina as well. The presence of submacular haemorrhage, in either case, blocks fluorescence. Fundus autofluorescence studies can help to distinguish fresh submacular haemorrhage from the old. The red blood is hypoautofluorescent, but the old grey submacular haemorrhage is hyperautofluorescent. MNV type 1 is most commonly seen in nAMD, while MNV type 2 is more common in pathologies other than nAMD, such as myopia, multifocal choroiditis, and Angioid streaks. Type 3 MNV, earlier called RAP (retinal angiomatous proliferation), arises from the deep capillary plexus and extends into the outer retinal layer. It is often associated with SDD. It is characterized by small haemorrhages in the inner retinal layers, likely due to higher pressure in the retinal circulation causing bleeds from the fragile new vessels. Early lesions show tiny dot-like hyperfluorescence on the FFA and the ICG angiography. In addition, feeding and draining vessels may be seen on ICG angiography. Type 3 MNV is a hyperreflective lesion extending from the inner nuclear layer to the outer retina on the B-scan OCT. It ismore often associated with intraretinal cystic spaces than the other two types. OCT angiography detects these new vessels in the outer retina [1].

Type 3 MNV progress through 3 stages. In the earliest stage A, it does not breach the external limiting membrane/ellipsoid zone; in stage B, the new vessels breach the ELM/ellipsoid zone, and in stage C, they breach the RPE layer. The stage of the type 3 MNV determines the location of the fluid collection. In stage A, fluid is seen in the intraretinal space on B-scan OCT as hyporeflective cavities. Stage A of type 3 MNV carries the best visual outcome following treatment with anti-VEGF agents. In stages B and C, the fluid collects in the subretinal and the sub-RPE space, respectively. However,if intraretinal fluid is collected in type 1or 2 MNV, the visual outcome following treatment seems poor [27].

7.8 Polypoidal Choroidal Vasculopathy

Polypoidal choroidal vasculopathy (PCV), a variant of type 1 MNV, is characterized by the presence of a network of branching vessels (BVN) under the RPE withsingle or multiple aneurysmal dilatations called polyps at the ends of the branching vascular network. Both the BVN and the polyps are variable in size and location. The polyps may be clinically visible as orange nodular lesions under the retina. While PCV lesions are rare in Caucasians, nearly half of the AMD patients in the Asian population may show PCV. The PCV remains asymptomatic till the polyps show exudation or rupture to cause, often, a massive haemorrhagic pigment epithelial detachment which may break through into the subretinal space and even cause a vitreous haemorrhage (Figs. 7.7, 7.8, and 7.9). The serosanguinous collection under the retina and the RPE was initially labelled a posterior uveal bleeding syndrome [28]. However, these lesions were characterized as idiopathic PCV, a distinct clinical entity different from AMD [29]. Patients with PCV lack tell-tale signs of AMD, such as soft drusen, pigmentary changes, and RPE atrophy. Unlike the nAMD, the submacular haemorrhages show spontaneous resolution with minimal scarring. Nearly 50% of the PCV eyes may have a favourable outcome. At the same time, there may be recurrent episodes of exudation and haemorrhages that finally lead to visual loss from the degenerative changes in the macula and subretinal fibrosis (Fig. 7.10) [30]. In the Asian population, more than 90% of the patients with PCV have unilateral disease,which is seen predominately in men [31].

On the other hand, PCV in the US was seen as bilateral, more often in the peripapillary and predominantly in women of black and Asian origin [32]. More recent data have shown significant ethnic differences in the clinical presentations of PCV in the Caucasian versus the Asian population. While Asian patients present with more frequent and significantly larger subretinal haemorrhages, more eyes have thick (pachy) choroidal vessels, choroidal hyperpermeability,

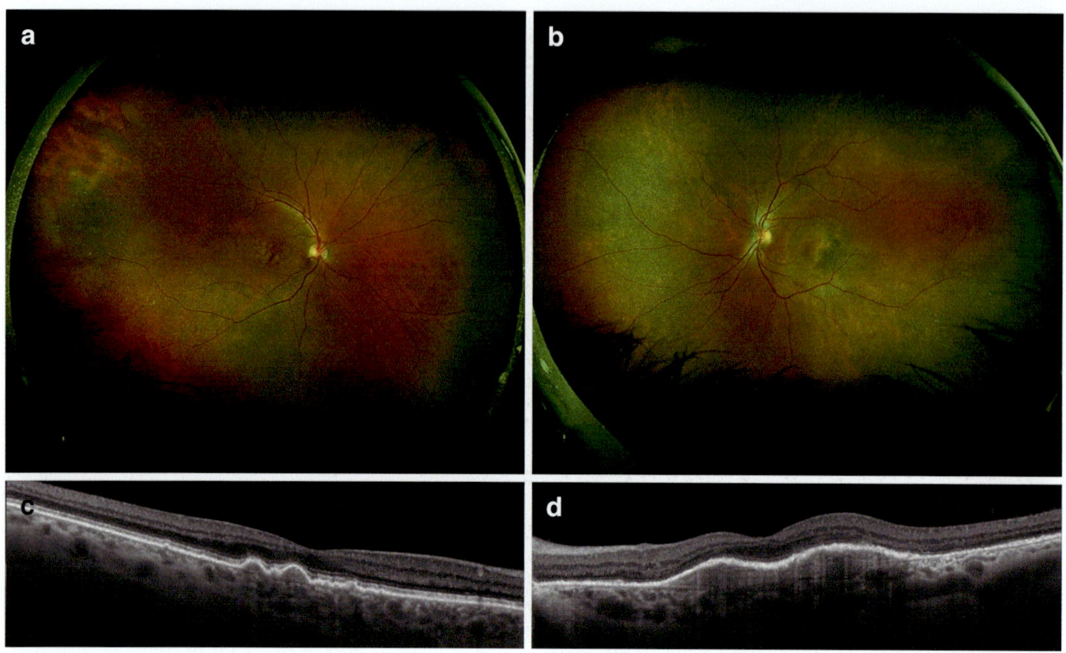

Fig. 7.7 (**a–d**): A 74-year-old man presented with drusen in the right eye (**a**) and PED in the left eye (**b**). OCT showed mound-like RPE elevations in the right eye (**c**) and a hyperreflective PED in the left eye (**d**)

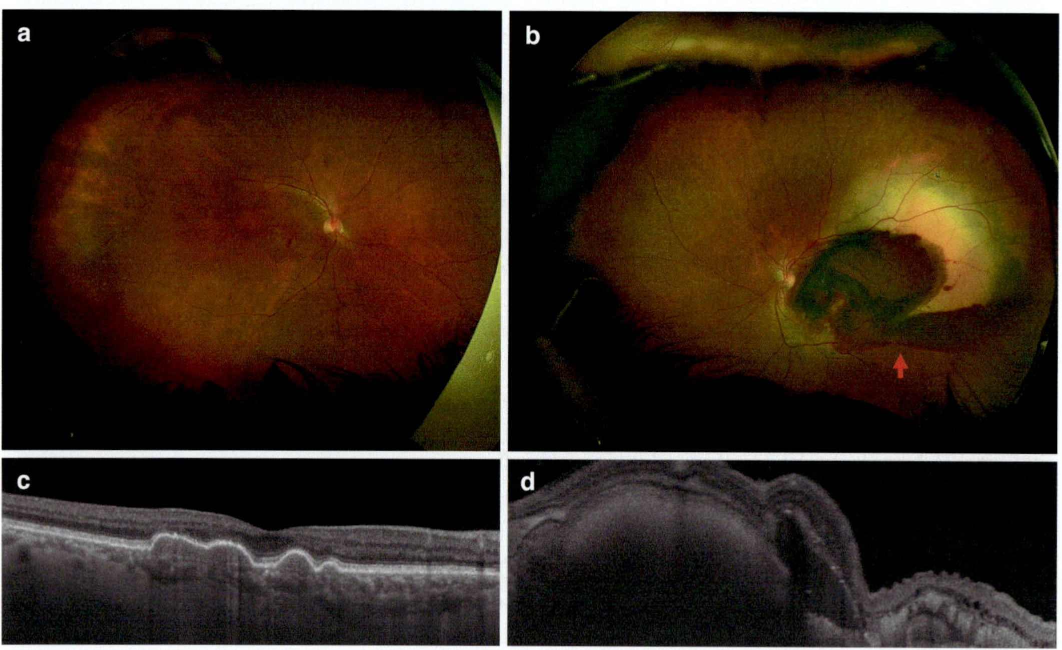

Fig. 7.8 (**a–d**): 7 months later, while the patient was asymptomatic in the right eye with almost similar drusen (**a**), he complained of a sudden loss of vision in the left eye due to a large submacular haemorrhage (**b**). OCT showed an increase in the size of drusen (**c**) in the right eye, while left eye OCT (**d**) massive subretinal and sub-RPE hyperreflectivity due to haemorrhage (**d**)

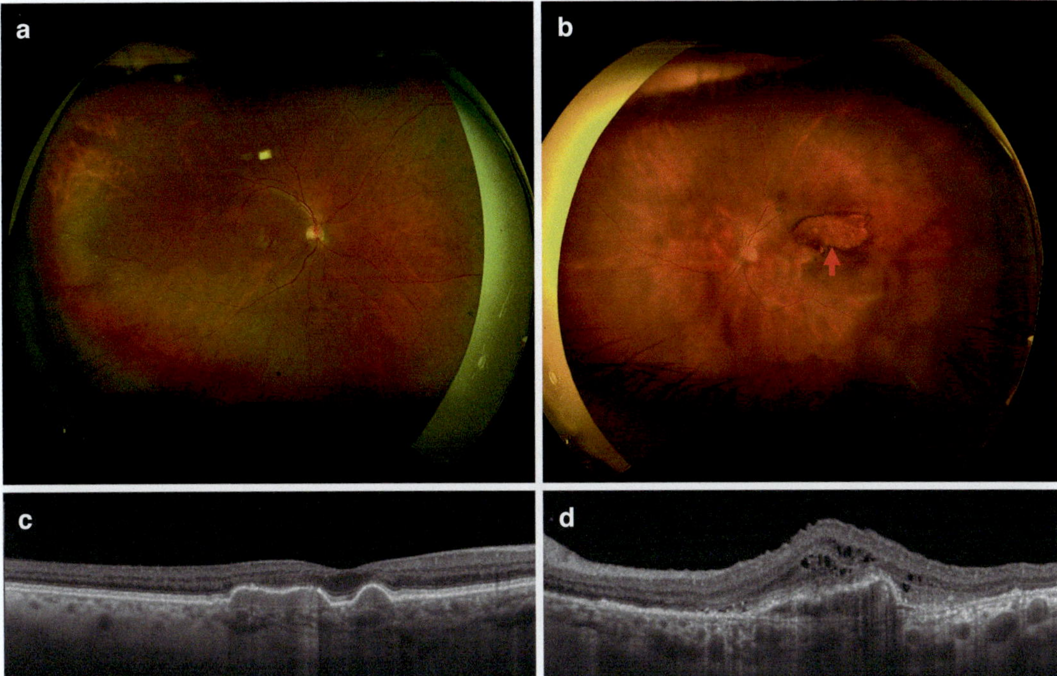

Fig. 7.9 (**a–d**): 2 months after undergoing vitreous surgery in the left eye, the right eye (**a**) drusen were the same. The left eye showed a small residual subretinal haemorrhage (red arrow) (**b**). Right eye OCT remained stable (**c**), and the left eye showed significant resolution of subretinal haemorrhage with a few residual cystoid spaces (**d**)

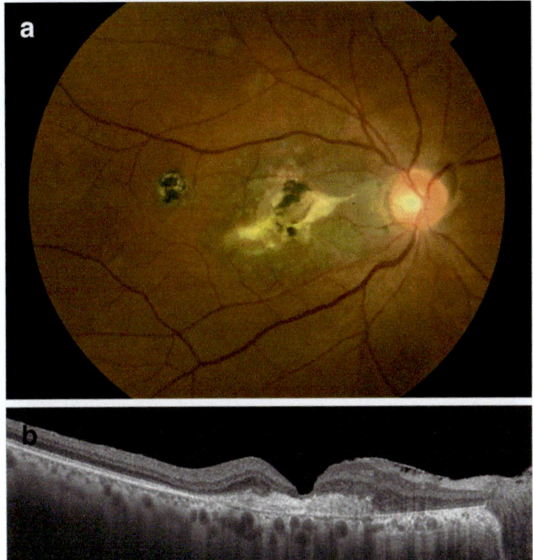

Fig. 7.10 Subretinal fibrosis (**a**) resulting from a CNVM leading to visual loss. OCT (**b**) shows foveal atrophy with a dense underlying scar

and polyps; Caucasian eyes havemore often drusen [33]. The PCV lesions are located at the PED's margin, creating a notch visible clinically and angiographically as a 'notched PED'. As the PCV exudes serosanguinous fluid, these lesions detach from Bruch's membrane and lie under the pigment epithelium [34]. ICG better defines new vessels located under the subretinal haemorrhage than FFA [35]. While the FFA is of little help except for showing leakage of dye in the exudative phase of PCV, suggesting at best the presence of an occult CNVM, the ICG angiography is highly diagnostic. ICG angiography, however, may only be available in some places. Specific FFA characteristics, including hyperfluorescence of the nodule, blocked fluorescence from subretinal haemorrhage, a notched PED, and a pattern suggestive of occult CNVM, highly suggests PCV rather than nAMD (Fig. 7.11) [36]. The ICG angiography shows well-defined

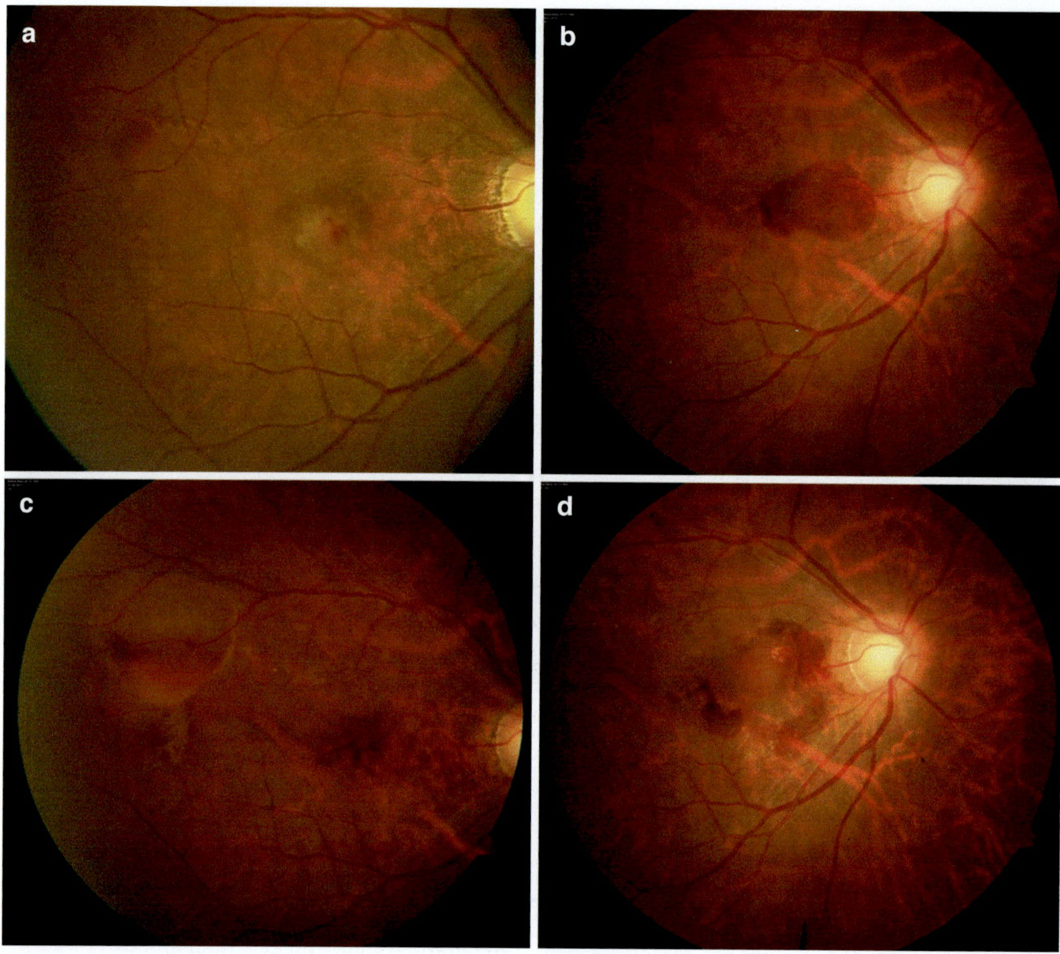

Fig. 7.11 A 40-year-old woman presented with a sudden decrease in vision in the right eye with a foveal haemorrhage and a haemorrhagic PED in the superotemporal-quadrant (**a**). Ten months later, there was a significant increase in the size of the foveal haemorrhage (**b**). At 11 months, while the subfoveal haemorrhage was resolving, the haemorrhage beneath the PED in the superotemporal quadrant increased (**c**). At 16 months, more subretinal haemorrhage was seen in the macula (**d**)

BVN and the polyps in the early frames that empty in the late frames. The polyps do not show any hyperfluorescence unless there is a rupture of the polyp, sharply contrasting these from the nAMD. The ICG angiography may also reveal the pulsatile nature of the polyps. On the B-scan OCT, the PCV lesions show characteristic multiple PEDs with a sharp notch, finger-like peaks, and hyporeflective lumen. Further, a double layer sign can be appreciated on the SS-OCT because the type1 MNV in PCV develops in Bruch's membrane. On the enface OCT, polyps appear as hyperreflective RPE rings and closely correlate with the polyps seen on the ICGA [37]. The presence of intraretinal and subretinal fluid on the OCT indicates an active exudative phase of the PCV. Compared to ICG angiography, the role of OCT angiography in making a firm diagnosis of PCV is limited. Although the OCT angiography can demonstrate more BVN under the RPE, it may not show all the polyps, possibly due to the low blood flow. Compared to larger polyps, smaller polypoidal lesions may be seen on OCT angiography [38]. OCT angiography of the PCV in eyes, which show subretinal hyperreflective material on B-scan OCT and a classic CNVM on the FFA, reveals the presence of type 1 MNV [39].

On ICG angiography, three distinct types of BVN can be identified; type 1 shows a trunk with branching vessels, type 2 shows an anastomosing branching network without an identifiable feeder trunk, and type 3 has a small stick-like tangled vessel. Compared to types 2 and 3, type 1 BVN are large and associated with poorer initial vision and a poor visual outcome following therapy [40]. The fundus autofluorescence images show confluent hypoautofluorescence surrounded by a ring of hyperautofluorescence at the site of polyps, whereas the site of the BVN shows granular hypoautofluorescent spots [41]. Histopathology of naïve early stage PCV, in autopsy eyes, has shown thinning of the choriocapillaris, a thickened choroid, and arteriosclerotic arterioles in the Sattler layer intertwined with dilated choroidal veins in the post pole. The dilated veins showed sloughing of the endothelial cells and were filled with a fibrinous material. Dilated nodular new vessels were seen under the RPE [42]. However, histopathological studies of the excised polyps obtained during retinal surgery have shown these polyps to be located within the schitic Bruch's membrane and filled with a serosanguinous fluid. Sometimes, a neovascular complex may be associated with polyps [43, 44]. Immunohistochemistry study of the surgically removed PCV lesions shows strong immunoreactivity for both pigment epithelium-derived factor (inhibitor of angiogenesis) and the VEGF (promotor of angiogenesis) in the vascular endothelial cells and the RPE [45]. Interestingly, once they rupture and cause a subretinal haemorrhage, some polyps may not be seen on ICG angiography again [46].

7.9 Pathogenesis and Risk Factors for Polypoidal Choroidal Vasculopathy

While AMD is associated with a thinner choroid, PCV is often associated with a thick choroid suggesting a different pathogenic mechanism for PCV [47]. The choroidal thickness is due to expansion from hyperpermeability of the outermost large choroidal veins (pachyvessels) in the Haller layer, which compress the middle Sattler layer and the choriocapillaris. The PCV appears to be a part of the spectrum of thick choroid disorders (pachychoroid), pachychoroid pigment epitheliopathy, chronic central serous chorioretinopathy, and the pachychoroid neovasculopathy [48–50]. Detection of type 1 MNV on OCT angiography under the shallow irregular PEDs in the pachychoroid spectrum disorders appears more sensitive than the ICG angiography for diagnosing PCV [51]. The anti-VEGF therapy (aflibercept) leads to a significant reduction in the volume andor the resolution of the PEDs, a decrease in the mean choroidal thickness and an increased choroidal vascularity index leading to speculation that PCV may represent high flow arteriovenous shunts in the large choroidal vessels that cause transudation into the choroidal stroma [52]. Although the pathogenic mechanisms of PCV may differ from AMD, the two share several risk factors-most notably the history of smoking, higher body mass index, coronary artery disease, and inflammatory risk factors such as C-reactive proteins [37]. Genetic studies have shown a significant association of at least 31 SNPs in 10 ARMS2, HTRA1, CFH, and CETP gene loci. Twelve polymorphisms in the ARMS2 and HTRA1 genes were found to be different in patients with AMD and PCV and likely play a role in the clinical manifestation of the two different phenotypes [53].

7.10 Treatment of Polypoidal Choroidal Vasculopathy

The endpoint for any treatment strategy for PCV includes improvement of visual acuity, reduction/regression of the polyps and stoppage of leakage with the restoration of choroidal thickness and prevention of recurrences. In the past, extrafoveal polyps of PCV were treated with thermal laser photocoagulation. However, it led to extensive scarring if BVN was also included in the treatment. Moreover, it did not prevent recurrences of exudation or haemorrhages. A selective combination of laser photocoagulation of extrafoveal polyps combined with anti-VEGF therapy hasimproved visual acuity and choroidal thickness [54]. Before the advent of anti-VEGF therapy, photodynamic therapy (PDT) with intravenous verteporfin for PCV was a popular treatment modality. However, the initial promising results could not be sustained in the long-term studies, and nearly half of the eyes had a recurrence by the third year of follow-up. Recurrences led to poorer outcomes [55]. Complications of PDT such as the RPE rip, even with half fluence PDT [56] and choroidal infarction, although rare, were a cause of concern, especially if the initial visual acuity was good [57]. Although the anti-VEGF therapy alone can close the polyps in less than 40% of eyes and needs multiple injections, it is much safer than PDT and thermal laser. Several randomized controlled trials have compared intravitreal anti-VEGF agents such as ranibizumab or aflibercept alone versus only PDT or anti-VEGF agents alone vs anti-VEGF agents combined with rescue therapy with PDT [54]. In the Planet trial, 85% of patients treated with intravitreal aflibercept did not need rescue therapy with PDT [58]. However, the significant advantage of combining PDT with intravitreal ranibizumab is a very high closure rate of the polyps as well as a reduction in the number of injections. Despite the higher incidence of inflammation with intravitreal brolucizumab, compared to the aflibercept, it yielded better visual outcomes in Japanese eyes with PCV. More than 2/3 of the eyes that were given brolucizumab monotherapy did not require more frequent injections than every 12 weeks [59]. Choroidal vascular hyperpermeability, as seen in ICG studies, rather than the choroidal thickness, as measured on SS-OCT, appears to be a better predictor of the outcome of both the anti-VEGF monotherapy andthe combination therapy [60], in sharp contrast to an earlier observation that a lower subfoveal choroidal thickness was a better predictor than the choroidal vascular permeability [61].

7.11 Treatment of Massive Submacular Haemorrhage

Massive submacular haemorrhage (MSH) is at least three times more common in PCV eyes than in nAMD eyes [62]. When followed for up to 10 years, nearly 30% of eyes with PCV, especially those with multiple grape-like polyps, may develop MSH causing immediate and severe loss of the central vision (Fig. 7.12). They also defined any submacular haemorrhage as significant if its largest diameter was >1-optic disc diameter (DD) but <4 DD and massive if it was >4 DD [63]. The anti-VEGF therapy alone or in combination with PDT is protective of MSH compared to when PDT alone is used for treating PCV (Fig. 7.13). Apart from the PCV and the AMD, rupture of the retinal arterial macroaneurysms and trauma may also result in sub-macular haemorrhage. The prolonged presence of blood under the retina may have toxic effects (iron toxicity) on the photoreceptors besides the tractionexerted by the shear forces of the contracting fibrin content of the clot that limit the visual outcome of SMH in its natural course. Earlier attempts to surgically remove the AMD fibrovascular complex and the blood clots stripped the overlying RPE resulting in photoreceptor degeneration and permanent loss of central vision. Heriot first demonstrated the successful clinical use of intravitreal tissue plasminogen activator (tPA) and long-acting expansile perfluoropropane (C3 F8) gas injection, followed by prone positioning to displace the blood clot from the submacular space [64]. Earlier, experimental studies on subretinal blood had shown that intravitreal tPA led to clot lysis within 24 h [65] albeit partially [66, 67]. In one of the earliest clinical studies, complete displacement of SMH was seen when intravitreal tPA was combined with pneumatic displacement of the submacular blood by prone positioning [68]. Given its potentialfor toxicity, the dose of intravitreal tPA was suggested to be limited to 50 mcg [69]. Currently, however, most surgeons use 25 mcg of tPA. To facilitate a

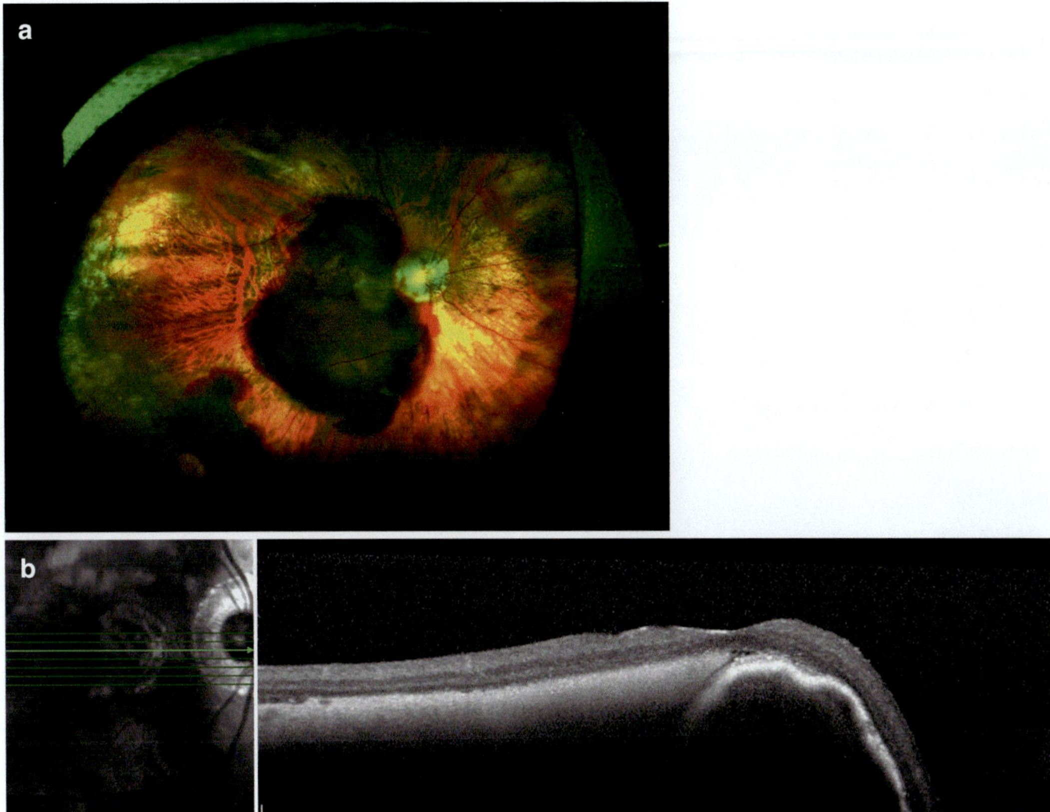

Fig. 7.12 Massive submacular haemorrhage (**a**) from a PCV causing immediate and severe loss of central vision in an 88-year-old man. OCT showed a dense hyperreflectivity in the subretinal and sub-RPE layers (**b**)

quicker displacement of the blood clot,subretinal tPA (25 mcg) and air (0.4 mL) with a microneedle combined with small gauge vitreous surgeryfollowed by overnight prone positioning led to 100% displacement of the blood clot [70, 71]. Since the primary cause of the SMH is either a PCV or nAMD, compared to the expansile gas and intravitreal rtPA (recombinant tissue plasminogen activator), better outcomes were seen if simultaneous anti-VEGF was also used [72, 73]. The initial fears that bevacizumab may get cleaved or get functionally inactivated by the action of tPA were unfounded [74].

Although the initial studies had used intravitreal tPA [68], there were unfounded concerns that intravitreal tPA may not cross the retina, and a trendto perform small gauge vitreous surgery and deliver subretinal tPA began. While subretinal rtPA may be more effective in the complete displacement of the clot, serious complications such as vitreous haemorrhage and retinal detachment are higher with the PPV approach [75–77]. Moreover, a small, randomized study that compared the efficacy of intravitreal tPA vs PPV with subretinal tPA combined with intravitreal bevacizumab and expansile gas found both techniques to be equally effective [78]. Similar results were found in a more recent study where three techniques were compared: intravitreal bevacizumab and expansile gas with intravitreal rtPA vs PPV with subretinal tPA or intravitreal rtPA combined with bevacizumab and expansile gas (Fig. 7.14) [79]. Combining PPV with subretinal rtPA, aflibercept, and intraocular air yields better outcomes regardingthe subsequentlyreduced frequency of the need for anti-VEGF agents [80]. A novel approach may be to perform PPV, subretinal rtPA, and intravitreal anti-VEGF, followed by positioning the patient to ensure a gravitational settlement of the blood [81]. Vitreous haemor-

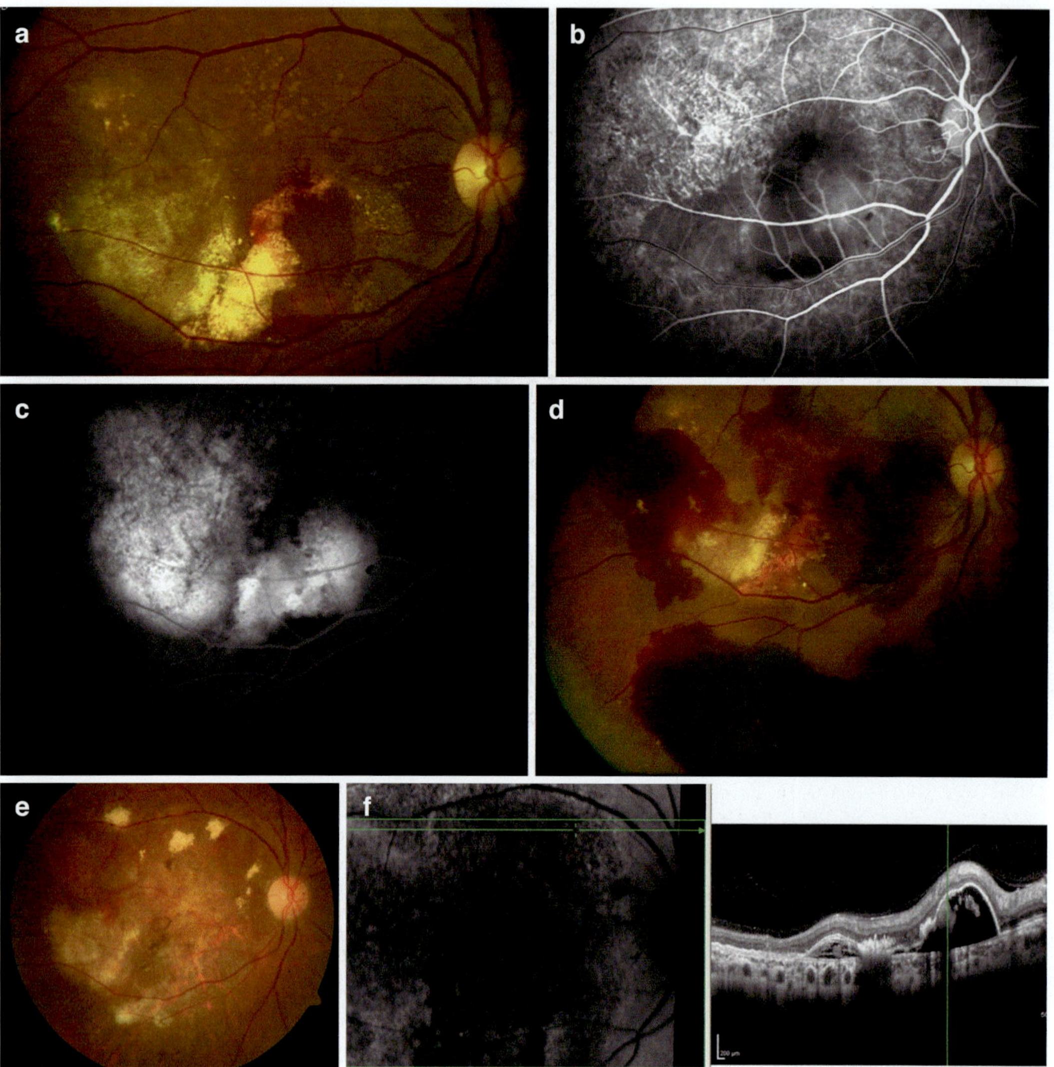

Fig. 7.13 (**a–d**): A 47-year-old woman presented with recurrent massive subretinal haemorrhages in both eyes. She was diagnosed with PCV and underwent photodynamic therapy (PDT) with Visudyne elsewhere. The right eye at presentation showed extensive retina atrophy due to PDT, residual hard exudates, large PED and residual blood (**a**). FFA showed transmission defects due to retinal atrophy and a large PED (**b**, **c**). Shortly thereafter, she presented with a fresh massive submacular haemorrhage (**d**), for which she received intravitreal bevacizumab. (**e**, **f**): She was followed for several years with intravitreal anti-VEGF therapy as and when required. Six years after the presentation, she resolved most of the haemorrhages (**e**). OCT shows a thumb-like PED with hyperreflectivity in its lumen with a shadow effect (a residual sub-RPE haemorrhage) and residual hard exudate (**f**)

rhage as a major complication was seen in nearly 18% of eyes following the use of rtPA and gas injection for extensive MSH, especially in eyes with PCV [82]. The incidence of this break-through haemorrhage may go up to 30% in patients who are smokers, have a larger area, and have a thicker MSH [83].

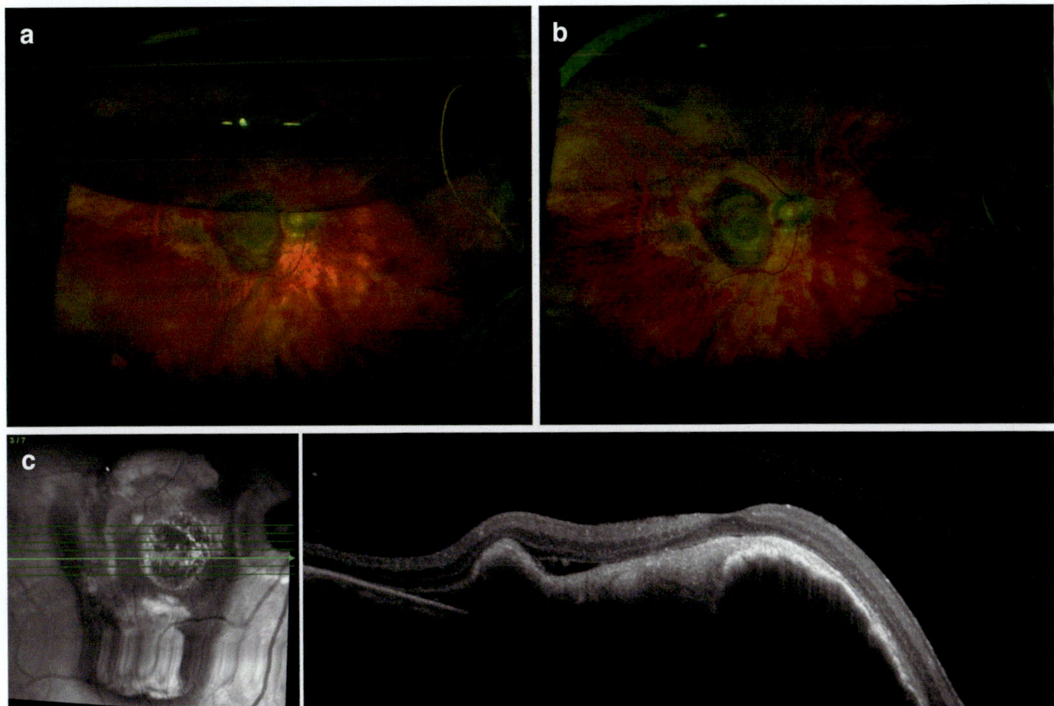

Fig. 7.14 Same patient as in Fig. 7.12 shows a partially gas-filled eye one week (**a**) and 2 weeks (**b**) after undergoing vitreous surgery with subretinal tPA combined with ranibizumab and expansile gas. OCT showed partial resolution of the submacular haemorrhage (**c**)

7.12 Other Causes of Submacular Haemorrhage

Apart from the common causes of submacular haemorrhages discussed above, some severe systemic or local diseases may present as submacular haemorrhage. See Boxes 7.3 and 7.4.

Box 7.3 Systemic Associations of Submacular Haemorrhage

1. Acute promyelocytic leukaemia may present with intraretinal haemorrhages and choroidal effusions [84] but at times, may present as haemorrhagic retinal detachment [85].
2. Spontaneous occurrence of subretinal haemorrhage may be the presenting sign of very high blood pressure in young patients [86].
3. Metastatic choroidal lesions especially renal cell carcinoma.

Box 7.4 Ocular Causes of Submacular/Subretinal Haemorrhages

1. Age-related macular degeneration
2. Polypoidal choroidal vasculopathy
3. Rupture of retinal arteriolar macroaneurysm [87].

4. Blunt trauma with choroidal rupture [88].
5. Degenerative myopia
6. Inflammatory choroidal neovascular membranes
   (a) Toxoplasmic retinochoroiditis
   (b) Tubercular serpiginous like choroiditis
   (c) VKH disease
   (d) Sarcoid uveitis
   (e) Multifocal choroidites with panuveitis
   (f) Punctate inner choroidopathy
   (g) Presumed ocular histoplasmosis syndrome (POHS)
7. Angioid streaks
8. Choroidal osteoma
9. Choroidal melanoma
10. Globe perforation during retrobulbar anaesthesia injection [89].

References

1. Spaide RF, Jaffe GJ, Sarraf D, Freund KB, Sadda SR, Staurenghi G, Waheed NK, Chakravarthy U, Rosenfeld PJ, Holz FG, Souied EH, Cohen SY, Querques G, Ohno-Matsui K, Boyer D, Gaudric A, Blodi B, Baumal CR, Li X, Coscas GJ, Brucker A, Singerman L, Luthert P, Schmitz-Valckenberg S, Schmidt-Erfurth U, Grossniklaus HE, Wilson DJ, Guymer R, Yannuzzi LA, Chew EY, Csaky K, Monés JM, Pauleikhoff D, Tadayoni R, Fujimoto J. Consensus nomenclature for reporting neovascular age-related macular degeneration data: consensus on Neovascular Age-Related Macular Degeneration Nomenclature Study Group. Ophthalmology. 2020;127(5):616–36. https://doi.org/10.1016/j.ophtha.2019.11.004. Epub 2019 Nov 14. Erratum in: Ophthalmology. 2020 Oct;127(10):1434-1435. PMID: 31864668.
2. van Leeuwen R, Chakravarthy U, Vingerling JR, Brussee C, Hooghart AJ, Mulder PG, de Jong PT. Grading of age-related maculopathy for epidemiological studies: is digital imaging as good as 35-mm film? Ophthalmology. 2003;110(8):1540–4. https://doi.org/10.1016/S0161-6420(03)00501-3. PMID: 12917169.
3. Colijn JM, Buitendijk GHS, Prokofyeva E, Alves D, Cachulo ML, Khawaja AP, Cougnard-Gregoire A, Merle BMJ, Korb C, Erke MG, Bron A, Anastasopoulos E, Meester-Smoor MA, Segato T, Piermarocchi S, de Jong PTVM, Vingerling JR, Topouzis F, Creuzot-Garcher C, Bertelsen G, Pfeiffer N, Fletcher AE, Foster PJ, Silva R, Korobelnik JF, Delcourt C, Klaver CCW, EYE-RISK Consortium; European Eye Epidemiology (E3) Consortium. Prevalence of age-related macular degeneration in Europe: the past and the future. Ophthalmology. 2017;124(12):1753–63. https://doi.org/10.1016/j.ophtha.2017.05.035. Epub 2017 Jul 14. PMID: 28712657; PMCID: PMC5755466.
4. Li JQ, Welchowski T, Schmid M, Mauschitz MM, Holz FG, Finger RP. Prevalence and incidence of age-related macular degeneration in Europe: a systematic review and meta-analysis. Br J Ophthalmol. 2020;104(8):1077–84. https://doi.org/10.1136/bjophthalmol-2019-314422. Epub 2019 Nov 11. PMID: 31712255.
5. Mauschitz MM, Finger RP. Age-related macular degeneration and cardiovascular diseases: revisiting the common soil theory. Asia Pac J Ophthalmol (Phila). 2022;11(2):94–9. https://doi.org/10.1097/APO.0000000000000496. Epub 2022 Feb 23. PMID: 35213420.
6. Merle BMJ, Colijn JM, Cougnard-Grégoire A, de Koning-Backus APM, Delyfer MN, Kiefte-de Jong JC, Meester-Smoor M, Féart C, Verzijden T, Samieri C, Franco OH, Korobelnik JF, Klaver CCW, Delcourt C, EYE-RISK Consortium. Mediterranean diet and incidence of advanced age-related macular degeneration: the EYE-RISK consortium. Ophthalmology. 2019;126(3):381–90. https://doi.org/10.1016/j.ophtha.2018.08.006. Epub 2018 Aug 13. PMID: 30114418.
7. Mauschitz MM, Schmitz MT, Verzijden T, Schmid M, Thee EF, Colijn JM, Delcourt C, Cougnard-Grégoire A, Merle BMJ, Korobelnik JF, Gopinath B, Mitchell P, Elbaz H, Schuster AK, Wild PS, Brandl C, Stark KJ, Heid IM, Günther F, Peters A, Klaver CCW, Finger RP, European Eye Epidemiology (E3) Consortium. Physical activity, incidence, and progression of age-related macular degeneration: a multicohort study. Am J Ophthalmol. 2022;236:99–106. https://doi.org/10.1016/j.ajo.2021.10.008. Epub 2021 Oct 22. PMID: 34695401.
8. Fernandez AB, Ballard KD, Wong TY, Guo M, McClelland RL, Burke G, Cotch MF, Klein B, Allison M, Klein R. Age-related macular degeneration and progression of coronary artery calcium: the multi-ethnic study of atherosclerosis. PLoS One. 2018;13(7):e0201000. https://doi.org/10.1371/journal.pone.0201000. PMID: 30020999; PMCID: PMC6051657.
9. Ikram MK, Mitchell P, Klein R, Sharrett AR, Couper DJ, Wong TY. Age-related macular degeneration and long-term risk of stroke subtypes. Stroke. 2012;43(6):1681–3. https://doi.org/10.1161/STROKEAHA.112.654632. Epub 2012 Apr 24. PMID: 22535267; PMCID: PMC3361598.
10. Anderson DH, Radeke MJ, Gallo NB, Chapin EA, Johnson PT, Curletti CR, Hancox LS, Hu J, Ebright JN, Malek G, Hauser MA, Rickman CB, Bok D,

Hageman GS, Johnson LV. The pivotal role of the complement system in ageing and age-related macular degeneration: hypothesis re-visited. Prog Retin Eye Res. 2010;29(2):95–112. https://doi.org/10.1016/j.preteyeres.2009.11.003. Epub 2009 Dec 2. PMID: 19961953; PMCID: PMC3641842.

11. Edwards AO, Ritter R 3rd, Abel KJ, Manning A, Panhuysen C, Farrer LA. Complement factor H polymorphism and age-related macular degeneration. Science. 2005;308(5720):421–4. https://doi.org/10.1126/science.1110189. Epub 2005 Mar 10. PMID: 15761121.
12. Haines JL, Hauser MA, Schmidt S, Scott WK, Olson LM, Gallins P, Spencer KL, Kwan SY, Noureddine M, Gilbert JR, Schnetz-Boutaud N, Agarwal A, Postel EA, Pericak-Vance MA. Complement factor H variant increases the risk of age-related macular degeneration. Science. 2005;308(5720):419–21. https://doi.org/10.1126/science.1110359. Epub 2005 Mar 10. PMID: 1576112.
13. Klein RJ, Zeiss C, Chew EY, Tsai JY, Sackler RS, Haynes C, Henning AK, SanGiovanni JP, Mane SM, Mayne ST, Bracken MB, Ferris FL, Ott J, Barnstable C, Hoh J. Complement factor H polymorphism in age-related macular degeneration. Science. 2005;308(5720):385–9. https://doi.org/10.1126/science.1109557. Epub 2005 Mar 10. PMID: 15761122; PMCID: PMC1512523.
14. Seddon JM, Francis PJ, George S, Schultz DW, Rosner B, Klein ML. Association of CFH Y402H and LOC387715 A69S with progression of age-related macular degeneration. JAMA. 2007;297(16):1793–800. https://doi.org/10.1001/jama.297.16.1793. Erratum in: JAMA (2007) 297(23):2585. PMID: 1745682.
15. Strunz T, Kiel C, Sauerbeck BL, Weber BHF. Learning from fifteen years of genome-wide association studies in age-related macular degeneration. Cells. 2020;9(10):2267. https://doi.org/10.3390/cells9102267. PMID: 33050425; PMCID: PMC7650698.
16. Micklisch S, Lin Y, Jacob S, et al. Age-related macular degeneration associated polymorphism rs10490924 in ARMS2 results in deficiency of a complement activator. J Neuroinflammation. 2017;14:4. https://doi.org/10.1186/s12974-016-0776-3.
17. Rozing MP, Durhuus JA, Krogh Nielsen M, Subhi Y, Kirkwood TB, Westendorp RG, Sørensen TL. Age-related macular degeneration: a two-level model hypothesis. Prog Retin Eye Res. 2020;76:100825. https://doi.org/10.1016/j.preteyeres.2019.100825. Epub 2019 Dec 30. PMID: 31899290.
18. Spaide RF, Ooto S, Curcio CA. Subretinal drusenoid deposits AKA pseudodrusen. Surv Ophthalmol. 2018;63(6):782–815. https://doi.org/10.1016/j.survophthal.2018.05.005. Epub 2018 May 31. PMID: 29859199.
19. Nassisi M, Tepelus T, Nittala MG, Sadda SR. Choriocapillaris flow impairment predicts the development and enlargement of drusen. Graefes Arch Clin Exp Ophthalmol. 2019;257(10):2079–85. https://doi.org/10.1007/s00417-019-04403-1. Epub 2019 Jul 1. PMID: 31263948.
20. Gass JD. Drusen and disciform macular detachment and degeneration. Trans Am Ophthalmol Soc. 1972;70:409–36. PMID: 4663679; PMCID: PMC1310465.
21. Gass JD, Agarwal A, Lavina AM, Tawansy KA. Focal inner retinal hemorrhages in patients with drusen: an early sign of occult choroidal neovascularization and chorioretinal anastomosis. Retina. 2003;23(6):741–51. https://doi.org/10.1097/00006982-200312000-00001. PMID: 14707822.
22. Soubrane G, Coscas G. Discussion. Ophthalmology. 2000;107(4):753–4. https://doi.org/10.1016/S0161-6420(00)00010-5.
23. Yannuzzi LA, Negrão S, Iida T, Carvalho C, Rodriguez-Coleman H, Slakter J, Freund KB, Sorenson J, Orlock D, Borodoker N. Retinal angiomatous proliferation in age-related macular degeneration. Retina. 2001;21(5):416–34. https://doi.org/10.1097/00006982-200110000-00003. PMID: 11642370.
24. Yannuzzi LA, Slakter JS, Sorenson JA, Guyer DR, Orlock DA. Digital indocyanine green videoangiography and choroidal neovascularization. Retina. 1992;12(3):191–223. PMID: 1384094.
25. Hanutsaha P, Guyer DR, Yannuzzi LA, Naing A, Slakter JS, Sorenson JS, Spaide RF, Freund KB, Feinsod M, Orlock DA. Indocyanine-green videoangiography of drusen as a possible predictive indicator of exudative maculopathy. Ophthalmology. 1998;105(9):1632–6. https://doi.org/10.1016/S0161-6420(98)99030-3. PMID: 9754169.
26. de Oliveira Dias JR, Zhang Q, Garcia JMB, Zheng F, Motulsky EH, Roisman L, Miller A, Chen CL, Kubach S, de Sisternes L, Durbin MK, Feuer W, Wang RK, Gregori G, Rosenfeld PJ. Natural history of subclinical neovascularization in nonexudative age-related macular degeneration using swept-source OCT angiography. Ophthalmology. 2018;125(2):255–66. https://doi.org/10.1016/j.ophtha.2017.08.030. Epub 2017 Sep 28. PMID: 28964581.
27. Sharma A, Cheung CMG, Arias-Barquet L, Ozdek S, Parachuri N, Kumar N, Hilely A, Zur D, Loewenstein A, Vella G, Bandello F, Querques G. Fluid-based visual prognostication in type 3 macular neovascularization-flip-3 study. Retina. 2022;42(1):107–13. https://doi.org/10.1097/IAE.0000000000003261. PMID: 34255761.
28. Kleiner RC, Brucker AJ, Johnston RL. The posterior uveal bleeding syndrome. Retina. 1990;10(1):9–17. PMID: 2343198.
29. Yannuzzi LA, Sorenson J, Spaide RF, Lipson B. Idiopathic polypoidal choroidal vasculopathy (IPCV). Retina. 1990;10(1):1–8. PMID: 1693009.
30. Uyama M, Wada M, Nagai Y, Matsubara T, Matsunaga H, Fukushima I, Takahashi K, Matsumura M. Polypoidal choroidal vasculopathy: natural his-

tory. Am J Ophthalmol. 2002;133(5):639–48. https://doi.org/10.1016/s0002-9394(02)01404-6. PMID: 11992861.

31. Sho K, Takahashi K, Yamada H, Wada M, Nagai Y, Otsuji T, Nishikawa M, Mitsuma Y, Yamazaki Y, Matsumura M, Uyama M. Polypoidal choroidal vasculopathy: incidence, demographic features, and clinical characteristics. Arch Ophthalmol. 2003;121(10):1392–6. https://doi.org/10.1001/archopht.121.10.1392. PMID: 14557174.
32. Yannuzzi LA, Ciardella A, Spaide RF, Rabb M, Freund KB, Orlock DA. The expanding clinical spectrum of idiopathic polypoidal choroidal vasculopathy. Arch Ophthalmol. 1997;115(4):478–85. https://doi.org/10.1001/archopht.1997.01100150480005. PMID: 9109756.
33. Corvi F, Chandra S, Invernizzi A, Pace L, Viola F, Sivaprasad S, Staurenghi G, Cheung CMG, Teo KYC. Multimodal imaging comparison of polypoidal choroidal vasculopathy between Asian and Caucasian populations. Am J Ophthalmol. 2022;234:108–16. https://doi.org/10.1016/j.ajo.2021.08.006. Epub 2021 Aug 24. PMID: 34450112.
34. Tsujikawa A, Sasahara M, Otani A, Gotoh N, Kameda T, Iwama D, Yodoi Y, Tamura H, Mandai M, Yoshimura N. Pigment epithelial detachment in polypoidal choroidal vasculopathy. Am J Ophthalmol. 2007;143(1):102–11. https://doi.org/10.1016/j.ajo.2006.08.025. Epub 2006 Sep 28. PMID: 17101112.
35. Kramer M, Mimouni K, Priel E, Yassur Y, Weinberger D. Comparison of fluorescein angiography and indocyanine green angiography for imaging of choroidal neovascularization in hemorrhagic age-related macular degeneration. Am J Ophthalmol. 2000;129(4):495–500. https://doi.org/10.1016/s0002-9394(99)00388-8. PMID: 10764859.
36. Tan CS, Ngo WK, Lim LW, Tan NW, Lim TH. EVEREST study report 4: fluorescein angiography features predictive of polypoidal choroidal vasculopathy. Clin Exp Ophthalmol. 2019;47(5):614–20. https://doi.org/10.1111/ceo.13464. Epub 2019 Feb 10. PMID: 30652395; PMCID: PMC6767036.
37. Cheung CMG, Lai TYY, Ruamviboonsuk P, Chen SJ, Chen Y, Freund KB, Gomi F, Koh AH, Lee WK, Wong TY. Polypoidal choroidal vasculopathy: definition, pathogenesis, diagnosis, and management. Ophthalmology. 2018;125(5):708–24. https://doi.org/10.1016/j.ophtha.2017.11.019. Epub 2018 Jan 10. PMID: 29331556.
38. Takayama K, Ito Y, Kaneko H, Kataoka K, Sugita T, Maruko R, Hattori K, Ra E, Haga F, Terasaki H. Comparison of indocyanine green angiography and optical coherence tomographic angiography in polypoidal choroidal vasculopathy. Eye (Lond). 2017;31(1):45–52. https://doi.org/10.1038/eye.2016.232. Epub 2016 Nov 4. PMID: 27813526; PMCID: PMC5233943.
39. Izumi T, Koizumi H, Maruko I, Hasegawa T, Iida T. Optical coherence tomography angiography findings of classic choroidal neovascularization in polypoidal choroidal vasculopathy. Retina. 2022;42(1):123–8. https://doi.org/10.1097/IAE.0000000000003264. PMID: 34292224.
40. Ma ST, Huang CH, Chang YC, Lai TT, Hsieh YT, Ho TC, Yang CM, Cheng CG, Yang CH. Clinical features and prognosis of polypoidal choroidal vasculopathy with different morphologies of branching vascular network on optical coherence tomography angiography. Sci Rep. 2021;11(1):17848. https://doi.org/10.1038/s41598-021-97340-1. PMID: 34497317; PMCID: PMC8426494.
41. Yamagishi T, Koizumi H, Yamazaki T, Kinoshita S. Fundus autofluorescence in polypoidal choroidal vasculopathy. Ophthalmology. 2012;119(8):1650–7. https://doi.org/10.1016/j.ophtha.2012.02.016. Epub 2012 Apr 17. PMID: 22512987.
42. Tso MOM, Suarez MJ, Eberhart CG. Pathologic study of early manifestations of polypoidal choroidal vasculopathy and pathogenesis of choroidal neo-vascularization. Am J Ophthalmol Case Rep. 2017;11:176–80. https://doi.org/10.1016/j.ajoc.2017.10.012. PMID: 30128371; PMCID: PMC6097175.
43. Lafaut BA, Aisenbrey S, Van den Broecke C, Bartz-Schmidt KU, Heimann K. Polypoidal choroidal vasculopathy pattern in age-related macular degeneration: a clinicopathologic correlation. Retina. 2000;20(6):650–4. https://doi.org/10.1097/00006982-200011000-00010. PMID: 11131419.
44. Liu G, Han L, Lu Y, Wang C, Ma L, Zhang P, Liu C, Lu X, Ma Z. Clinicopathological study of the polypoidal lesions of polypoidal choroidal vasculopathy. Graefes Arch Clin Exp Ophthalmol. 2022;260(7):2369–77. https://doi.org/10.1007/s00417-021-05525-1. Epub 2022 Feb 11. PMID: 35147748.
45. Matsuoka M, Ogata N, Otsuji T, Nishimura T, Takahashi K, Matsumura M. Expression of pigment epithelium derived factor and vascular endothelial growth factor in choroidal neovascular membranes and polypoidal choroidal vasculopathy. Br J Ophthalmol. 2004;88(6):809–15. https://doi.org/10.1136/bjo.2003.032466. PMID: 15148217; PMCID: PMC1772169.
46. Baek J, Kim JH, Lee MY, Lee WK. Disease activity after development of large subretinal hemorrhage in polypoidal choroidal vasculopathy. Retina. 2018;38(10):1993–2000. https://doi.org/10.1097/IAE.0000000000001817. PMID: 28834950.
47. Chung SE, Kang SW, Lee JH, Kim YT. Choroidal thickness in polypoidal choroidal vasculopathy and exudative age-related macular degeneration. Ophthalmology. 2011;118(5):840–5. https://doi.org/10.1016/j.ophtha.2010.09.012. Epub 2011 Jan 6. PMID: 21211846.
48. Pang CE, Freund KB. Pachychoroid neovasculopathy. Retina. 2015;35(1):1–9. https://doi.org/10.1097/IAE.0000000000000331. PMID: 25158945.
49. Wang TA, Chan WC, Tsai SH, et al. Clinical features of pachyvessels associated with polypoidal choroidal

vasculopathy in chronic central serous chorioretinopathy. Sci Rep. 2021;11:13867. https://doi.org/10.1038/s41598-021-93476-2.

50. Warrow DJ, Hoang QV, Freund KB. Pachychoroid pigment epitheliopathy. Retina. 2013;33(8):1659–72. https://doi.org/10.1097/IAE.0b013e3182953df4. PMID: 23751942.
51. Dansingani KK, Balaratnasingam C, Klufas MA, Sarraf D, Freund KB. Optical coherence tomography angiography of shallow irregular pigment epithelial detachments in pachychoroid spectrum disease. Am J Ophthalmol. 2015;160(6):1243–1254.e2. https://doi.org/10.1016/j.ajo.2015.08.028. Epub 2015 Aug 28. PMID: 26319161.
52. Shen M, Zhou H, Kim K, Bo Q, Lu J, Laiginhas R, Jiang X, Yan Q, Iyer P, Trivizki O, Shi Y, de Sisternes L, Durbin MK, Feuer W, Gregori G, Wang RK, Sun X, Wang F, Yu SY, Rosenfeld PJ. Choroidal changes in eyes with polypoidal choroidal vasculopathy after anti-VEGF therapy imaged with swept-source OCT angiography. Invest Ophthalmol Vis Sci. 2021;62(15):5. https://doi.org/10.1167/iovs.62.15.5. PMID: 34860239; PMCID: PMC8648060.
53. Ma L, Li Z, Liu K, Rong SS, Brelen ME, Young AL, Kumaramanickavel G, Pang CP, Chen H, Chen LJ. Association of genetic variants with polypoidal choroidal vasculopathy: a systematic review and updated meta-analysis. Ophthalmology. 2015;122(9):1854–65. https://doi.org/10.1016/j.ophtha.2015.05.012. Epub 2015 Jun 13. PMID: 26081444.
54. Gemmy Cheung CM, Yeo I, Li X, Mathur R, Lee SY, Chan CM, Wong D, Wong TY. Argon laser with and without anti-vascular endothelial growth factor therapy for extrafoveal polypoidal choroidal vasculopathy. Am J Ophthalmol. 2013;155(2):295–304.e1. https://doi.org/10.1016/j.ajo.2012.08.002. Epub 2012 Oct 27. PMID: 23111181.
55. Wong CW, Cheung CM, Mathur R, Li X, Chan CM, Yeo I, Wong E, Lee SY, Wong D, Wong TY. Three-year results of polypoidal choroidal vasculopathy treated with photodynamic therapy: retrospective study and systematic review. Retina. 2015;35(8):1577–93. https://doi.org/10.1097/IAE.0000000000000499. PMID: 25719986.
56. Kim SW, Oh J, Oh IK, Huh K. Retinal pigment epithelial tear after half fluence PDT for serous pigment epithelial detachment in central serous chorioretinopathy. Ophthalmic Surg Lasers Imaging. 2009;40(3):300–3. https://doi.org/10.3928/15428877-20090430-14. PMID: 19485297.
57. Klais CM, Ober MD, Freund KB, Ginsburg LH, Luckie A, Mauget-Faÿsse M, Coscas G, Gross NE, Yannuzzi LA. Choroidal infarction following photodynamic therapy with verteporfin. Arch Ophthalmol. 2005;123(8):1149–53. https://doi.org/10.1001/archopht.123.8.1149. PMID: 16087856.
58. Lee WK, Iida T, Ogura Y, Chen SJ, Wong TY, Mitchell P, Cheung GCM, Zhang Z, Leal S, Ishibashi T, PLANET Investigators. Efficacy and safety of intravitreal aflibercept for polypoidal choroidal vasculopathy in the PLANET study: a randomized clinical trial. JAMA Ophthalmol. 2018;136(7):786–93. https://doi.org/10.1001/jamaophthalmol.2018.1804. Erratum in: JAMA Ophthalmol. 2018 Jul 1;136(7):840. PMID: 29801063; PMCID: PMC6136040.
59. Ogura Y, Jaffe GJ, Cheung CMG, Kokame GT, Iida T, Takahashi K, Lee WK, Chang AA, Monés J, D'Souza D, Weissgerber G, Gedif K, Koh A. Efficacy and safety of brolucizumab versus aflibercept in eyes with polypoidal choroidal vasculopathy in Japanese participants of HAWK. Br J Ophthalmol. 2022;106(7):994–9. https://doi.org/10.1136/bjophthalmol-2021-319090. Epub 2021 Jul 22. PMID: 34301613; PMCID: PMC9234403.
60. Yanagi Y, Ting DSW, Ng WY, Lee SY, Mathur R, Chan CM, Yeo I, Wong TY, Cheung GCM. Choroidal vascular hyperpermeability as a predictor of treatment response for polypoidal choroidal vasculopathy. Retina. 2018;38(8):1509–17. https://doi.org/10.1097/IAE.0000000000001758. PMID: 28704255.
61. Kim H, Lee SC, Kwon KY, Lee JH, Koh HJ, Byeon SH, Kim SS, Kim M, Lee CS. Subfoveal choroidal thickness as a predictor of treatment response to anti-vascular endothelial growth factor therapy for polypoidal choroidal vasculopathy. Graefes Arch Clin Exp Ophthalmol. 2016;254(8):1497–503. https://doi.org/10.1007/s00417-015-3221-x. Epub 2015 Dec 1. PMID: 26626772.
62. Cho SC, Cho J, Park KH, Woo SJ. Massive submacular hemorrhage in polypoidal choroidal vasculopathy versus typical neovascular age-related macular degeneration. Acta Ophthalmol. 2021;99(5):e706–14. https://doi.org/10.1111/aos.14676. Epub 2020 Dec 2. PMID: 33289345.
63. Cho JH, Ryoo NK, Cho KH, Park SJ, Park KH, Woo SJ. Incidence rate of massive submacular hemorrhage and its risk factors in polypoidal choroidal vasculopathy. Am J Ophthalmol. 2016;169:79–88. https://doi.org/10.1016/j.ajo.2016.06.014. Epub 2016 Jun 16. PMID: 27318076.
64. Heriot W. Intravitreal gas and tPA: an outpatient procedure for subretinal haemorrhage. In: Vail vitrectomy meeting; 1996; Vail, CO.
65. Coll GE, Sparrow JR, Marinovic A, Chang S. Effect of intravitreal tissue plasminogen activator on experimental subretinal hemorrhage. Retina. 1995;15(4):319–26. https://doi.org/10.1097/00006982-199515040-00009. PMID: 8545578.
66. Boone DE, Boldt HC, Ross RD, Folk JC, Kimura AE. The use of intravitreal tissue plasminogen activator in the treatment of experimental subretinal hemorrhage in the pig model. Retina. 1996;16(6):518–24. https://doi.org/10.1097/00006982-199616060-00009. PMID: 9002136.
67. Johnson MW, Olsen KR, Hernandez E. Tissue plasminogen activator treatment of experimental subretinal hemorrhage. Retina. 1991;11(2):250–8. https://

doi.org/10.1097/00006982-199111020-00011. PMID: 1925092.

68. Hassan AS, Johnson MW, Schneiderman TE, Regillo CD, Tornambe PE, Poliner LS, Blodi BA, Elner SG. Management of submacular hemorrhage with intravitreous tissue plasminogen activator injection and pneumatic displacement. Ophthalmology. 1999;106(10):1900–6; discussion 1906–7. PMID: 10519583. https://doi.org/10.1016/S0161-6420(99)90399-8.
69. Chen CY, Hooper C, Chiu D, Chamberlain M, Karia N, Heriot WJ. Management of submacular hemorrhage with intravitreal injection of tissue plasminogen activator and expansile gas. Retina. 2007;27(3):321–8. https://doi.org/10.1097/01.iae.0000237586.48231.75. PMID: 17460587.
70. Kadonosono K, Arakawa A, Yamane S, Inoue M, Yamakawa T, Uchio E, Yanagi Y. Displacement of submacular hemorrhages in age-related macular degeneration with subretinal tissue plasminogen activator and air. Ophthalmology. 2015;122(1):123–8. https://doi.org/10.1016/j.ophtha.2014.07.027. Epub 2014 Sep 4. PMID: 25200400.
71. Sharma S, Kumar JB, Kim JE, Thordsen J, Dayani P, Ober M, Mahmoud TH. Pneumatic displacement of submacular hemorrhage with subretinal air and tissue plasminogen activator: initial United States experience. Ophthalmol Retina. 2018;2(3):180–6. https://doi.org/10.1016/j.oret.2017.07.012. Epub 2017 Sep 28. PMID: 31047581.
72. Chakraborty D, Sheth JU, Mondal S, Boral S. Role of intravitreal brolucizumab with intravitreal rtPA and pneumatic displacement for submacular hemorrhage: a case series. Am J Ophthalmol Case Rep. 2022;25:101390. https://doi.org/10.1016/j.ajoc.2022.101390. PMID: 35198814; PMCID: PMC8841994.
73. Guthoff R, Guthoff T, Meigen T, Goebel W. Intravitreous injection of bevacizumab, tissue plasminogen activator, and gas in the treatment of submacular hemorrhage in age-related macular degeneration. Retina. 2011;31(1):36–40. https://doi.org/10.1097/IAE.0b013e3181e37884. PMID: 20921929.
74. Klettner A, Puls S, Treumer F, Roider J, Hillenkamp J. Compatibility of recombinant tissue plasminogen activator and bevacizumab co-applied for neovascular age-related macular degeneration with submacular hemorrhage. Arch Ophthalmol. 2012;130(7):875–81. https://doi.org/10.1001/archophthalmol.2012.120. PMID: 22410628.
75. Hillenkamp J, Surguch V, Framme C, Gabel VP, Sachs HG. Management of submacular hemorrhage with intravitreal versus subretinal injection of recombinant tissue plasminogen activator. Graefes Arch Clin Exp Ophthalmol. 2010;248(1):5–11. https://doi.org/10.1007/s00417-009-1158-7. Epub 2009 Aug 11. PMID: 19669780.
76. Kimura S, Morizane Y, Hosokawa M, Shiode Y, Kawata T, Doi S, Matoba R, Hosogi M, Fujiwara A, Inoue Y, Shiraga F. Submacular hemorrhage in polypoidal choroidal vasculopathy treated by vitrectomy and subretinal tissue plasminogen activator. Am J Ophthalmol. 2015;159(4):683–9. https://doi.org/10.1016/j.ajo.2014.12.020. Epub 2014 Dec 30. PMID: 25555798.
77. van Zeeburg EJ, van Meurs JC. Literature review of recombinant tissue plasminogen activator used for recent-onset submacular hemorrhage displacement in age-related macular degeneration. Ophthalmologica. 2013;229(1):1–14. https://doi.org/10.1159/000343066. Epub 2012 Oct 12. PMID: 23075629.
78. de Jong JH, van Zeeburg EJ, Cereda MG, van Velthoven ME, Faridpooya K, Vermeer KA, van Meurs JC. Intravitreal versus subretinal administration of recombinant tissue plasminogen activator combined with gas for acute submacular hemorrhages due to age-related macular degeneration: an exploratory prospective study. Retina. 2016;36(5):914–25. https://doi.org/10.1097/IAE.0000000000000954. PMID: 26807631.
79. Grohmann C, Dimopoulos S, Bartz-Schmidt KU, Schindler P, Katz T, Spitzer MS, Skevas C. Surgical management of submacular hemorrhage due to n-AMD: a comparison of three surgical methods. Int J Retina Vitreous. 2020;6:27. https://doi.org/10.1186/s40942-020-00228-x. PMID: 32637155; PMCID: PMC7331168.
80. Iglicki M, Khoury M, Melamud JI, Donato L, Barak A, Quispe DJ, Zur D, Loewenstein A. Naïve subretinal haemorrhage due to neovascular age-related macular degeneration. Pneumatic displacement, subretinal air, and tissue plasminogen activator: subretinal vs intravitreal aflibercept-the native study. Eye (Lond). 2023;37:1659. https://doi.org/10.1038/s41433-022-02222-z. Epub ahead of print. PMID: 36038720.
81. Erdogan G, Kirmaci A, Perente I, Artunay O. Gravitational displacement of submacular haemorrhage in patients with age-related macular disease. Eye (Lond). 2020;34(6):1136–41. https://doi.org/10.1038/s41433-019-0720-8. Epub 2019 Dec 2. PMID: 31792350; PMCID: PMC7253466.
82. Wu TT, Kung YH, Hong MC. Vitreous hemorrhage complicating intravitreal tissue plasminogen activator and pneumatic displacement of submacular hemorrhage. Retina. 2011;31(10):2071–7. https://doi.org/10.1097/IAE.0b013e31822528c8. PMID: 21817964.
83. Lim JH, Han YS, Lee SJ, Nam KY. Risk factors for breakthrough vitreous hemorrhage after intravitreal tissue plasminogen activator and gas injection for submacular hemorrhage associated with age related macular degeneration. PLoS One. 2020;15(12):e0243201. https://doi.org/10.1371/journal.pone.0243201. PMID: 33270725; PMCID: PMC7714180.
84. Hua HU, Rayess N, Moshfeghi AA. Acute promyelocytic leukemia with sudden vision loss. JAMA Ophthalmol. 2020;138(2):206–7. https://doi.org/10.1001/jamaophthalmol.2019.4838. PMID: 31804661.

85. Lee C, Hwang Y-S. Hemorrhagic retinal detachment in acute promyelocytic leukemia. Taiwan J Ophthalmol. 2013;3:123–5. https://doi.org/10.1016/j.tjo.2012.12.006.
86. Hu HH, Zhu XY, Xie ZG, Chen F. Multimodal imaging of spontaneous subretinal hemorrhage in a young male: a case report. BMC Ophthalmol. 2020;20(1):374. https://doi.org/10.1186/s12886-020-01634-3. PMID: 32962682; PMCID: PMC7510117.
87. Sakaguchi S, Muraoka Y, Kadomoto S, Ooto S, Murakami T, Nishigori N, Ishikura M, Miyake M, Miyata M, Uji A, Tsujikawa A. Three-dimensional locations of ruptured retinal arterial macroaneurysms and their associations with the visual prognosis. Sci Rep. 2022;12(1):503. https://doi.org/10.1038/s41598-021-04500-4. PMID: 35017582; PMCID: PMC8752622.
88. Chen KJ, Sun MH, Sun CC, Wang NK, Hou CH, Wu AL, Wu WC, Lai CC. Traumatic maculopathy with massive subretinal hemorrhage after closed-globe injuries: associated findings, management, and visual outcomes. Ophthalmol Retina. 2019;3(1):53–60. https://doi.org/10.1016/j.oret.2018.08.007. Epub 2018 Aug 25. PMID: 30935658.
89. Dai Y, Sun T, Gong JF. Inadvertent globe penetration during retrobulbar anesthesia: a case report. World J Clin Cases. 2021;9(8):2001–7. https://doi.org/10.12998/wjcc.v9.i8.2001. PMID: 33748253; PMCID: PMC7953384.

8 Retinal Arteriolar Changes in Hypertension and Arteriolosclerosis

8.1 Structural Considerations of the Blood Vessels

The cardiovascular system in the body is highly organized into the arteries, the capillaries, and the veins. The largest of the arteries is the aorta and its branches that carry oxygenated blood from the left ventricle of the heart (except the pulmonary vein that carries oxygenated blood from the lungs to the left atrium), the medium size arteries carry the blood to various parts and organs of the body. The small arteries distribute it further to every part of the target organs and tissues by subdividing it into arterioles. Diffusion of oxygen and micronutrients occurs at the level of the arteriolar end of the capillaries; the waste products enter the intravascular space at the venous end of the capillaries, which further organize into the progressively increasing size and finally drain into the right atrium via the superior and inferior vena cava. The veins carry the deoxygenated blood except for the pulmonary artery, which carries the deoxygenated blood from the right ventricle to the lungs.

The arteries and the veins, irrespective of their size, share the same structure: the outer tunica adventitia, a tunica media, and a tunica intima. The large arteries nearer the heart, such as the aorta and the common carotid artery, have more elastin per unit area than the muscular arteries. It helps smoothen the high-pressure wave of blood flow from the heart. The medium and small arteries, called muscular arteries, have more smooth muscle cells than elastin because these arteries have contractile properties, which help regulate the blood supply to the target organ. There are many functional and anatomical differences in the elastic and muscular arteries, and the readers are referred to an extensive discussion on the subject [1]. Muscular arteries also have internal and external elastic lamina on either side of the tunica media. The veins distinctly lack the elastic lamina and very few smooth muscle cells but have unidirectional valves, especially in the leg veins, as they carry blood against gravity.

The tunica intima consists of endothelial cells. In the arteries, the endothelial cells are longer and oriented toward the blood flow, while in the veins, these are rounder. The essential difference between the endothelial cells of the arteries and veins is that the former controls the vascular tone. At the same time, the latter is the site for adherence and migration of phagocytes and lymphocytes into the organs. The endothelial cells in the large and medium arteries are also the primary site of atherosclerosis. The tunica media consists of smooth muscle cells and elastic fibres. The tunica media is much thicker in the arteries than the veins and is responsible for the thickness of the wall of the vessels. The tunica adventitia consists essentially of supporting fibrous tissue [2].

A. Gupta et al., *Ophthalmic Signs in Practice of Medicine*,
https://doi.org/10.1007/978-981-99-7923-3_8

8.1.1 Anatomical Considerations of the Central Retinal Artery and the Blood Supply of the Retina

Our current understanding of the central retinal artery (CRA) anatomy is based on extensive dissections and studies by Dr. S. S. Hayreh [3]. The CRA, often the first branch of the ophthalmic artery, is the primary source of blood supply to the inner retina. It first traverses in orbit and enters the optic nerve dural sheath to run in the vaginal space before penetrating the optic nerve about 10 mm behind the globe to emerge as a single artery in the centre of the optic nerve head. As it emerges from the optic nerve head, it divides into a superior and an inferior division, subdividing further to supply all four quadrants of the retina. The retinal arterial system is end-arterial, and thus occlusion of any branch of the arteriolar system will lead to retina ischaemia in the arteriole's supply area. The CRA is responsible for the supply to the inner retina up to the outer limit of the inner nuclear layer and accounts for only 20% of the blood supply of the retina, the outer retina meeting its oxygen and micronutrient requirements from the choroid, which is fed by the posterior ciliary arteries. The posterior ciliary arteries are also branches of the ophthalmic artery. In nearly one third of the eyes, bilateral in nearly 15% of people, there may be an additional small artery, the cilioretinal artery, a branch of a posterior ciliary artery or the peripapillary choroid that supplies a variable area of the entire thickness of the macula. Rarely, a minor arterial branch may arise from the CRA in the optic nerve head before it emerges into the eye and resembles a cilioretinal artery. The origin of the cilioretinal artery is best demonstrated on the fundus fluorescein angiography as the dye fills the cilioretinal artery synchronously with the choroid a short while before the dye reaches the CRA [4]. In the retina, only the CRA is structurally a muscular artery, and like all such arteries, the purpose of the CRA is to distribute blood to the retina. These arteries are pulsatile; even in the retina, the CRA pulsates synchronously with the cardiac rhythm. Pulsations of the CRA at the optic disc before it divides are an excellent sign and rule out raised intracranial pressure.

Once the CRA divides into branches, they lose their internal elastic lamina and thus anatomically are 'arterioles' [5]. The tunica media in the human retinal arterioles near the optic disc consists of 5–7 layers of circumferentially oriented smooth muscle cells, which in the peripheral retina get reduced to just 1–2 layers [6]. The arterioles cross the veins anteriorly in the retina, and at the arteriovenous crossing (AV crossing), they share a common adventitial sheath. The blood supply of the retina is multitier. The central 500 μm of the retina, the fovea centralis, is bereft of any blood capillaries to allow unrestricted passage of light to the photoreceptors. The superficial and deep capillary plexus and the interconnecting capillaries arise from the branches of the CRA and supply oxygen and micronutrients to the inner neurosensory retina [from the retinal nerve fibre layer (RNFL) to the outer limit of the inner nuclear layer]. In contrast, the outer neurosensory retina does not have any blood supply of its own and is served by the choroid, one of the human body's highest blood flow tissues. Tight endothelial junctions in the retinal blood vessels constitute the inner blood-retinal barrier that does not allow the movement of macromolecules and cellular components into the extravascular space in the neurosensory retina.

Moreover, the retinal arterial system is autoregulated to maintain a constant blood flow to the inner retina. It can maintain perfusion of the inner retina even if the intraocular pressure rises to 40–50 mm of Hg [5]. The autoregulation of blood flow at the level of the neuro-glial-vascular unit controls the blood supply to meet the metabolic requirements of the neural elements in the inner retina. The fractal geometry of the retinal vessels ensures a uniform blood flow and supply and removal of the metabolites from the inner retina.

The retinal pigment epithelium (RPE), the outermost layer of the retina, separates the neurosensory retina from the choroid. The blood supply in the choroid is multilayered and is under autonomic control. The innermost layer of blood vessels in the choroid consists of fenestrated capillaries, known as the choriocapillaris, a layer which lies immediately below the RPE. The tight gap junctions in the RPE provide the outer blood-retinal barrier and control the movement of micronutrients into the retina. The choriocapillaris is fed by the middle Sattler and the outermost Haller layer of blood vessels that are branches of the ciliary vessels.

8.1.2 Diameter of the Retinal Arterioles and Their Fractal Dimensions

The blood supply in the medium and small arteries and arterioles is diffusion limited. Therefore, the diameter of these arteries and their branches are governed by Murray's principle of the cube root of the blood flow these arteries are supposed to convey to allow the principle of the optimal use of space [7]. Thus, like the other natural phenomenon such as the branches of a tree or the bronchial tree, the blood supply in the human body and so also the retinal blood supply follow a complex fractal geometry (cf. Euclidean geometry that follows straight lines) to maximize the distribution of blood supply in a confined space.

Quantifying the various aspects of retinal vessel geometry, including their fractal dimensions, is now possible using digital images or digitizing them. The fractal dimension, a measure of the complexity of the retinal vessels, has been calculated as 1.7 [8, 9]. Patients with Alzheimer's disease have been found to show decreased arteriolar and venular fractal dimensions [10] and, in future, may become an important biomarker to predict the onset of Alzheimer's disease.

The diameter of the CRA in the optic nerve is ~200 μm [4]. In recent years, retinal vessel size and their fractal complexities have been studied in the context of several systemic disorders, including atherosclerosis, inflammation, hypertension, coronary heart disease, and renal disease [11]. Notably, the retinal blood vessel walls are transparent in young people. Thus, on funduscopic examination/fundus imaging, only the central red column is visible and documented. Any measurement of the vessel diameter precludes the thickness of the peripheral clear plasma flow and the wall of the vessel. The vessels appear thicker on fundus fluorescein angiography (FFA) because the dye occupies the entire lumen of the vessels. Several platforms are available to analyze fundus pictures, and vessel diameter measurements may vary with each of these. Most reliable, although not commonly available everywhere, are adaptive optics camera systems which yield high-resolution images by eliminating optical errors [12]. Adaptive optics photography has been used to measure the retinal arteriolar wall thickness. It has been measured as 24.3 ± 4.8 μm [11]. It should be noted that the retinal vessel diameter, especially of the retinal arterioles, changes with the cardiac cycle, increasing by almost 3.4% during the mid-cycle and late systole and reducing back during the diastole [11].

For a long time, increase in peripheral resistance from the narrowing of the peripheral arterioles has been speculated as a leading cause of primary hypertension. This phenomenon has been demonstrated in experimental models [13]. As the retinal arterioles share similar properties with the peripheral arterioles, studying the retinal arterioles' diameter may provide clues to the development of incident hypertension. Indeed, that was the case in a prospective study of more than 5000 middle-aged non-hypertensive patients who were followed up, 14.4% (it varied from 8.9 to 22.3% in the lowest to the highest quintiles of AV ratio) of patients who had narrowing of retinal arterioles at the start of the study developed incident hypertension (≥140 systolic or ≥90 mm of Hg). The incidence of hypertension went up to 23% in those who also had focal narrowing of the retinal arterioles, thus establishing the diffuse narrowing and focal narrowing as important biomarkers that can predict the development of overt hypertension in the near future [14]. However, it is likely that the narrowing of the peripheral arterioles is a consequence of undiagnosed hypertension [15] and that at the time of recruitment to the study, the patients already had hypertension that was missed by the then criteria used for its diagnosis [14]. The criteria for diagnosing hypertension have changed since then. In patients with stroke, hypertension-induced retinal microvascular changes, namely the diffuse or severe focal narrowing of the retinal arterioles, severe arteriovenous nicking, and venous dilation, provide valuable clues to the presence of cerebral micro-angiopathy that results in deep intracerebral haemorrhage and lacunar infarcts [16].

8.2 Causes of Hypertension

The cause of hypertension varies depending upon the age of the patients. Patients younger than 18 usually have an underlying renal parenchymal disease or Coarctation of the aorta. Those from 19 to 40 may have thyroid dysfunction or Takayasu's arteritis. Patients above 40 but below 65 may have Polyarteritis nodosa or pheochromocytoma, Cushing's syndrome, hyperaldosteronism or even obstructive sleep apnoea. Patients above 65 should be suspected of atherosclerotic renal artery stenosis, renal failure or hypothyroidism [17].

8.3 Measuring Blood Pressure

Many physicians and trainees are unaware of the correct technique for measuring blood pressure in the clinic. All physicians must follow the guidelines of the American Heart Association (See Box 8.1). The definition of blood pressure is changed from time to time as new evidence becomes available. The current (as of 2020) definition and classification of hypertension are provided in Boxes 8.2 and 8.3.

Box 8.1 How to Measure Blood Pressure

1. Measure in both upper arms; if consistently ≥10 mmHg in one arm, use that arm for recording
2. >20 mmHg needs further evaluation
3. No smoking, exercise or coffee for 30 min before the test
4. Record sitting for 3–5 min, back supported and feet flat on the floor
5. No talking during the recording of the BP
6. Cuff of appropriate size, arm resting on a table at heart level
7. Take three readings at the 1-min interval and take a mean of the last two readings

Reference: American Heart Association Inc.

Box 8.2 Definition of Hypertension

Hypertension is defined after 2–3 visits at 1–4 weeks intervals depending upon the BP
Hypertension-clinic recording—
SBP ≥ 140 mmHg and/or DBP ≥ 90 mmHg
Hypertension home recording—
SBP ≥ 135 mmHg and/or DBP ≥ 85 mmHg
Normal BP—SBP ≤ 130 mmHg and/or DBP ≤ 85 mmHg

Adapted from Verdecchia et al. [18] with permission of the publishers

Box 8.3 Classification of Blood Pressure for Adults

Classification BP	Systolic BP (mmHg) Diastolic BP (mmHg)
Normal	<130 and <85
High normal	130–139 and/or 85–89
Stage 1 hypertension	140–159 and/or 90–99
Stage 2 hypertension	≥160 or ≥100
Isolated systolic hypertension	≥ 140 and <90

Source: Verdecchia et al. [18], with permission of the publishers

8.4 Arteriosclerosis and Arteriolosclerosis

Arteriosclerosis is a generic term for stiffness of the wall of the arteries and is a leading cause of mortality worldwide. It is currently classified into three types—(1) Atherosclerosis (Fig. 8.1), (2) Monckeberg calcific medial sclerosis, and (3) Arteriolosclerosis [19]. The large elastic and medium muscular arteries are prone to develop atherosclerosis and Monckeberg calcific medial sclerosis (Internal elastic lamina calcification), and discussion on these is beyond the scope of this chapter. Arteriolosclerosis is seen at the level of small arteries and arterioles. With advancing age, the arterial walls lose elasticity and contractibility. The arteries become stiff due to increasing fibromuscular thickening or intimal hyalinosis [19]. The resulting peripheral resistance is responsible for hypertension and may be seen in

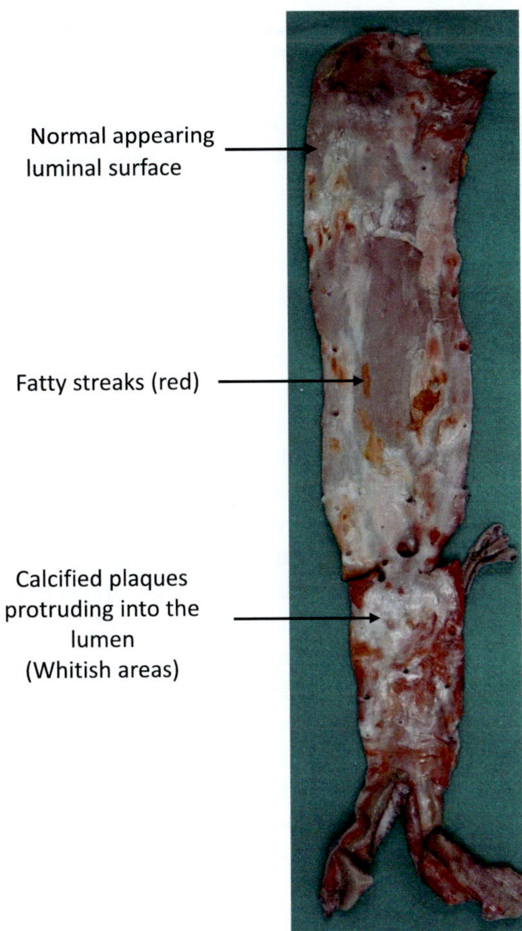

Fig. 8.1 Luminal surface of human abdominal aorta stained with Sudan IV (fat stain) showing patchy atherosclerotic lesions. Red staining indicates fatty streaks and atherosclerotic plaques, and shiny whitish patches are calcified plaques. (Image courtesy of Prof Anjali Agarwal, Department of Anatomy, Postgraduate Institute of Medical Education and Research, Chandigarh and Prof Daisy Sahni, Ex-Professor, Department of Anatomy, Postgraduate Institute of Medical Education and Research, Chandigarh)

up to 2/3 of people above the age of 65 years. Nearly 90% of the patients with hypertension are due to arteriolosclerosis changes in the arterioles. The retinal arteries and arterioles also become increasingly non-compliant to the variations in blood pressure [20]. Once patients develop chronically elevated blood pressure (Primary or essential hypertension), the process gets accelerated, retinal arteriolar walls thicken, lose transparency, and show an increasing wall-to-lumen ratio. Apart from ageing and hypertension, there are several other preventable risk factors, such as diabetes, smoking, obesity, and sedentary life, that accelerate all types of arteriolosclerosis.

8.5 Fundus Signs of Arteriolosclerosis and Hypertension

Since the retinal vessels could have been seen with the direct ophthalmoscope more than 160 years ago, the retinal arterioles have fascinated physicians to see if the retinal arterioles reflected the changes due to elevated blood pressure among other systemic vascular diseases. There is strong evidence that in patients with long-standing hypertension, the retinal arterioles undergo similar arteriolosclerotic changes as elsewhere in the body and the brain. Before effective pharmacotherapy for hypertension, retinal changes in high uncontrolled hypertension were used as a prognostic tool for the survival of the patients [21, 22]. See Box 8.4. To date, arteriolosclerosis is clinically best studied in the retinal arterioles. Using various digital fundus imaging tools, it is now possible to objectively record and document the retinal arteriolar changes and blood flow non-invasively and repetitively over the long term. Semiautomatic soft wares and artificial intelligence-based microvascular analysis tools

Box 8.4 Keith, Wagener, and Barker Classification of Hypertensive Retinopathy

Grade of retinopathy	Fundus signs
1	Mild to moderate diffuse arteriolar narrowing
2	Definitive focal arteriolar narrowing and AV nicking
3	Signs in grade 2 with retinal haemorrhages, cotton wool spots, hard exudates
4	All the signs in grade 3 with papilloedema ± retinal detachment

Reference: Chen et al. [24]

have been developed to measure with great accuracy the changes reflected in the eye that, in the near future, could predict the end-organ damage before it manifests clinically and gets incorporated into the algorithms for cardiovascular risk assessment [23]. See Box 8.5.

Box 8.5 Systemic Consequences of Uncontrolled Hypertension

Classification of hypertension		
Wong and Mitchell	Keith-Wagner-Barker	Target organ damage
Mild	1–2	Microalbuminuria; increased media to lumen ratio in arterioles; TIA; LVH; RAM; BRVO; RAO Carotid stiffness and carotid wall thickness in <55 years of age[!] Untreated five-year survival 70% in grade 1 and 50% in grade 2[*] Seven-year incident chronic heart failure 8%[**]
Moderate	3	Aortic arch calcification[#] Lunar infarcts, chronic/ESRD[*] Stroke[^] Increased carotid intima-media thickness in <60 years[$] Untreated 5-year survival 20%[**] Seven-year incident chronic heart failure 18%[***]
Severe	4	Acute renal failure, encephalopathy, blindness, death Untreated five-year survival 1%[*]

TIA transient ischaemic attacks, *LVH* left ventricular hypertrophy, *RAM* retinal artery macroaneurysms, *BRVO* branch retinal vein occlusion, *RAO* retinal artery occlusion, *ESRD* end-stage renal disease

Source of information: [*] Unger et al. [25, 26], [**] Cuspidi et al. [27], [***] Wong et al. [28], [!] Aissopou et al. [29], [#] Adar et al. [30], [^] Wong and Mitchell [31], [$] Zhang et al. [32]

8.5.1 Enhanced Central Light Reflex

Arteriolosclerosis is visible on ophthalmoscopy as a widening of the light reflex on the retinal arterioles. The increased central light reflex on ophthalmoscopy is a simple clinical clue to the possible underlying hypertension. In a Japanese non-diabetic population above the age of 35 years, the enhanced arterial reflex was seen in 18.7% [33]. Interestingly, the prevalence of the enhanced central light reflex was seen to decrease with increasing age, from 36% in the youngest (<60 years) to ~19% in the oldest (>80 years); however, the markedly increased light reflex when noted was associated with higher mean blood pressure, glucose, and alcohol intake, all well-known risk factors for arteriolosclerosis [34]. Compared to the retinal veins, the central light reflex is of higher intensity in the retinal arterioles and more intense in the larger than, the smaller arterioles [35]. In the late nineteenth century, much debate and experimentation centred on the possible mechanisms involved in this phenomenon, concluding that the light reflected from the vessel walls is responsible for the central light reflex in both the retinal arteries and the veins [36]. More recently, Adaptive optics scanning laser ophthalmoscopy has revealed the arterial light reflex to arise from three components, namely, the peripheral smooth plasma flow, the structural irregularity of the arterial wall, and the irregularities of the RBCs flowing in the centre of the blood column [37]. Semiautomatic software has been developed to reliably measure the ratio of retinal arteriolar diameter and central light reflex to study the associations of retinal arterioles with systemic diseases [38].

8.5.2 Arterial Wall-to-Lumen Ratio

As stated above, hypertension leads to vascular remodelling resulting in hypertrophy of the tunica media's fibromuscular layer, increasing the width of the arterial wall, thus increasing the wall-to-lumen ratio of the arterioles (Fig. 8.2). Small decreases in the lumen of the peripheral arteries are responsible for the increased periph-

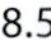

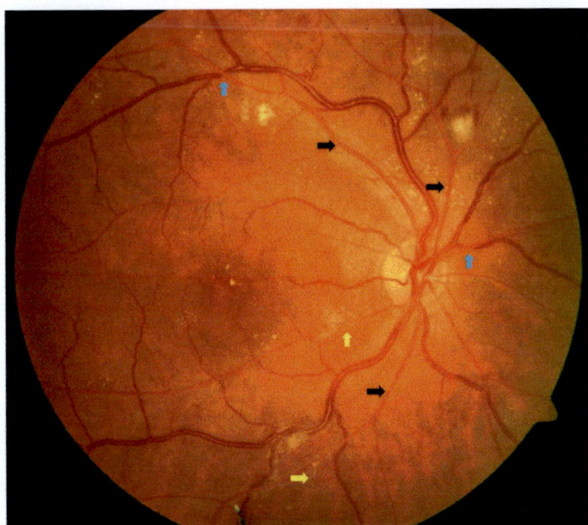

Fig. 8.2 Fundus of the right eye of a patient with hypertension, showing an increased wall-to-lumen ratio in the arteries (black arrows), tapering of blood column on either side of the crossing (Gunn's sign, blue arrows), copper wiring (arterioles appear 'orange or yellow' instead of 'red') (black arrows) due to increased reflectance of light caused by wall thickening, and silver wiring (arterioles appear white as they become occluded) (yellow arrows)

eral resistance and have long-term cardiovascular consequences. Antihypertensive therapy may reverse some of these changes in small arteries and arterioles [39]. Using Doppler scanning flowmeter and automatic full-field perfusion image analysis, patients with a history of past cerebrovascular events showed the highest wall-to-lumen ratio (0.46 ± 0.08), followed by patients with poor blood pressure control (0.40 ± 0.13) that was significantly higher than the normal controls (0.35 ± 0.12) and successfully controlled hypertensive patients (0.31 ± 0.13). Measuring the wall-to-lumen ratio is thus emerging as an interesting tool to see the efficacy of antihypertensive treatment and predict the long-term consequences of continued or inadequately treated hypertension [40].

8.5.3 Arteriovenous Nicking (AVN)

In the retina, the retinal arterioles cross the retinal veins and share a common adventitial sheath at the crossing site. These crossings are most common in the temporal retina and are more frequent in the superior than the inferior retina. As the vessel walls are transparent in healthy young persons, the arterioles do not obscure the venous blood column. However, as the retinal arterioles start developing arteriolosclerosis due to chronically elevated blood pressure, the arteriolar walls progressively lose their transparency, get opacified, and may be seen as a copper or a silver wire (Figs. 8.2 and 8.3). In chronic hypertension, the hardened arterioles progressively compress the underlying vein, which may show tapering of the blood column on either side of the crossing (Gunn's sign) (Figs. 8.2 and 8.4). In more severe cases, the arterioles show an 'S-shaped' deflection in their course (Salus sign) (Figs. 8.2, 8.4, and 8.5). The AVN and opacification of the arterioles have been long predictors of terminal organ damage and cardiovascular disease [41]. Notably, the AVN and opacification of the retinal arterioles are a legacy of past elevated blood pressure and represent the cumulative damage sustained over a long time. These changes do not regress with the control of hypertension and do not refer to the current control status [41, 42].

8.5.4 Focal and Diffuse Narrowing of the Retinal Arterioles

Whenever there is an elevation of blood pressure, the autoregulatory response of the retinal arterioles dictates the narrowing of the retinal arterioles by the contraction of the circumferentially oriented smooth muscle cells in the tunica media. Clinically, the diffuse narrowing of the arterioles is compared with the neighbouring retinal veins, which, lacking a robust tunica media, do not show any alterations in their calibre in patients with hypertension (Figs. 8.4 and 8.5). The normal retinal arteriole to the corresponding vein ratio is 2:3. More discernible is the focal narrowing of the arterioles. Once the hypertension is controlled, focal narrowing may show a reversal in more than 40% of the patients [42]. The compensated arteriolar wall changes, such as diffuse and focal narrowing of arterioles, AV nicking, and copper wire appearances, are classified as 'Mild hypertensive retinopathy' [43].

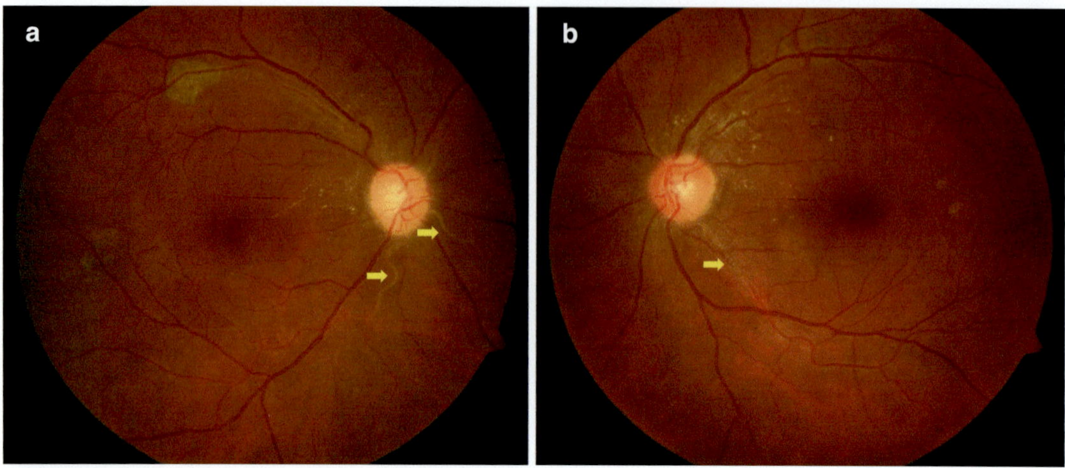

Fig. 8.3 Silver wiring of arteries (yellow arrows) as they appear occluded in hypertensive retinopathy (**a**, **b**)

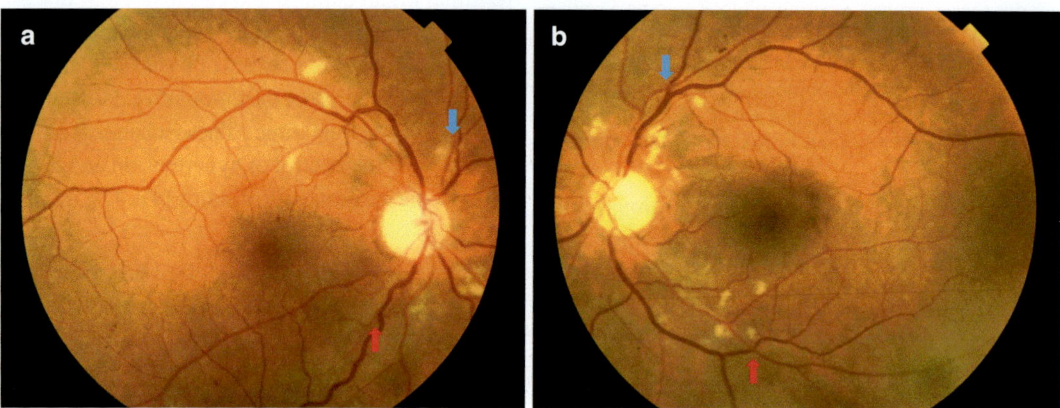

Fig. 8.4 Generalized arterial attenuation, cotton wool spots, Gunn's sign (blue arrow) and Salus sign (red arrow) seen in right (**a**) and left (**b**) eyes of a patient with hypertension

8.5.5 Retinal Haemorrhages, Cotton Wool Spots, and Microaneurysms

Retinal arterioles in acute hypertension may get overwhelmed, resulting in occlusion of the precapillary arterioles manifesting as superficial flame-shaped and dot and blot haemorrhages, exudation, and cotton wool spots (Figs. 8.2 and 8.5). This is classified as 'Moderate hypertensive retinopathy' [43]. Hypertensive retinopathy is a hallmark of decompensated acute hypertension. It is significantly associated with damage to the kidneys, heart, and brain. The narrowing of the retinal arterioles and AVN may be associated with lacunar infarcts, and retinal haemorrhages and microangiopathy due to diabetes mellitus are associated with cerebral haemorrhage [44]. The exudative fluid collects in the Henle's layer, and the lipid deposits form a macular fan (Fig. 8.6). Once the blood pressure is controlled, the retinopathy lesions regress over some time (Fig. 8.7). Current imaging tools such as optical coherence tomography (OCT) angiography have revealed a state of chronic paracentral acute middle maculopathy (PAMM) by demonstrating a thinner inner nuclear layer and disruption of the outer plexiform layer even before the appearance of

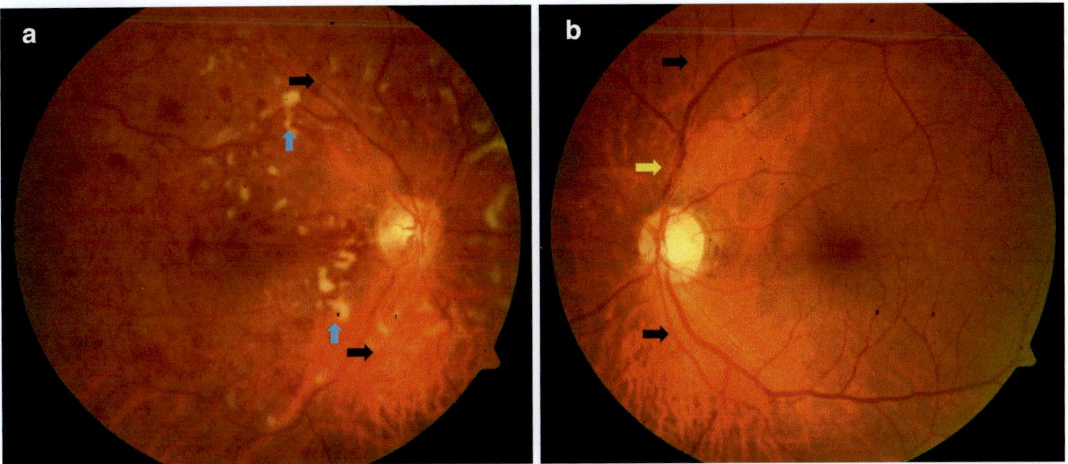

Fig. 8.5 Arterial attenuation (black arrows) in both eyes (**a**, **b**), cotton wool spots (blue arrows) in right eye (**a**), and Salus sign (yellow arrow) in left eye (**b**)

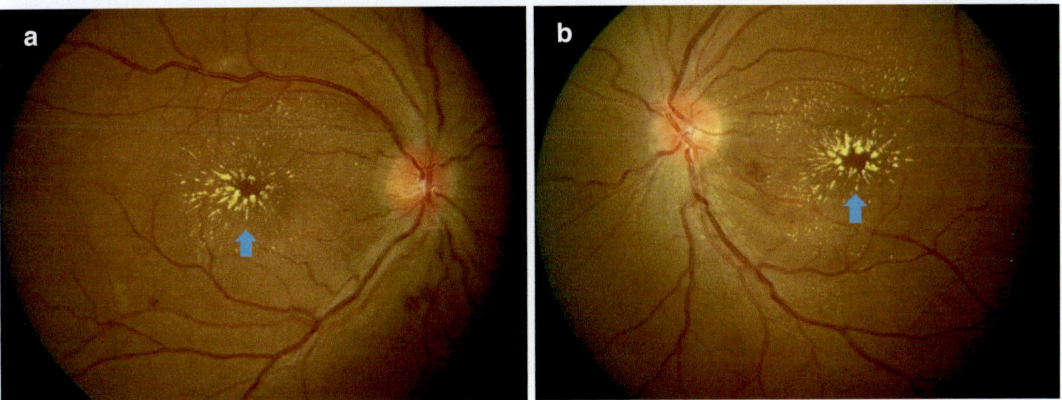

Fig. 8.6 Macular star (blue arrows) formed by the shape taken by lipid deposits in the Henle's layer due to collection of exudative fluid on this layer in both eyes (**a**, **b**)

overt clinical signs of retinopathy or capillary closure in nearly 90% of a small set of patients with mild hypertension [45].

8.5.6 Optic Neuropathy and Choroidopathy in Malignant Hypertension

The patients who develop an acute and severe rise in blood pressure (accelerated hypertension) (Systolic BP ≥180 mm of Hg or diastolic BP of >110 mm of Hg or, by some definitions, diastolic BP ≥130 mm of Hg) who in addition to extensive retinopathy changes also develop papilloedema (optic disc oedema) are labelled as malignant hypertension (Fig. 8.8). Malignant hypertension may occur in poorly controlled patients with primary hypertension or de novo in nearly half of the patients. Hypertension complicates nearly 10% of pregnancies, and less than 2% may get complicated by pre-eclampsia/eclampsia characterized by albuminuria and seizures. These patients have a lower blood pressure threshold for developing malignant hypertension than non-pregnant women. Eclampsia during pregnancy is a leading cause of maternal mortality [46]. Although papilloedema's exact cause is unknown, ischaemia of the optic nerve head, raised intracranial pres-

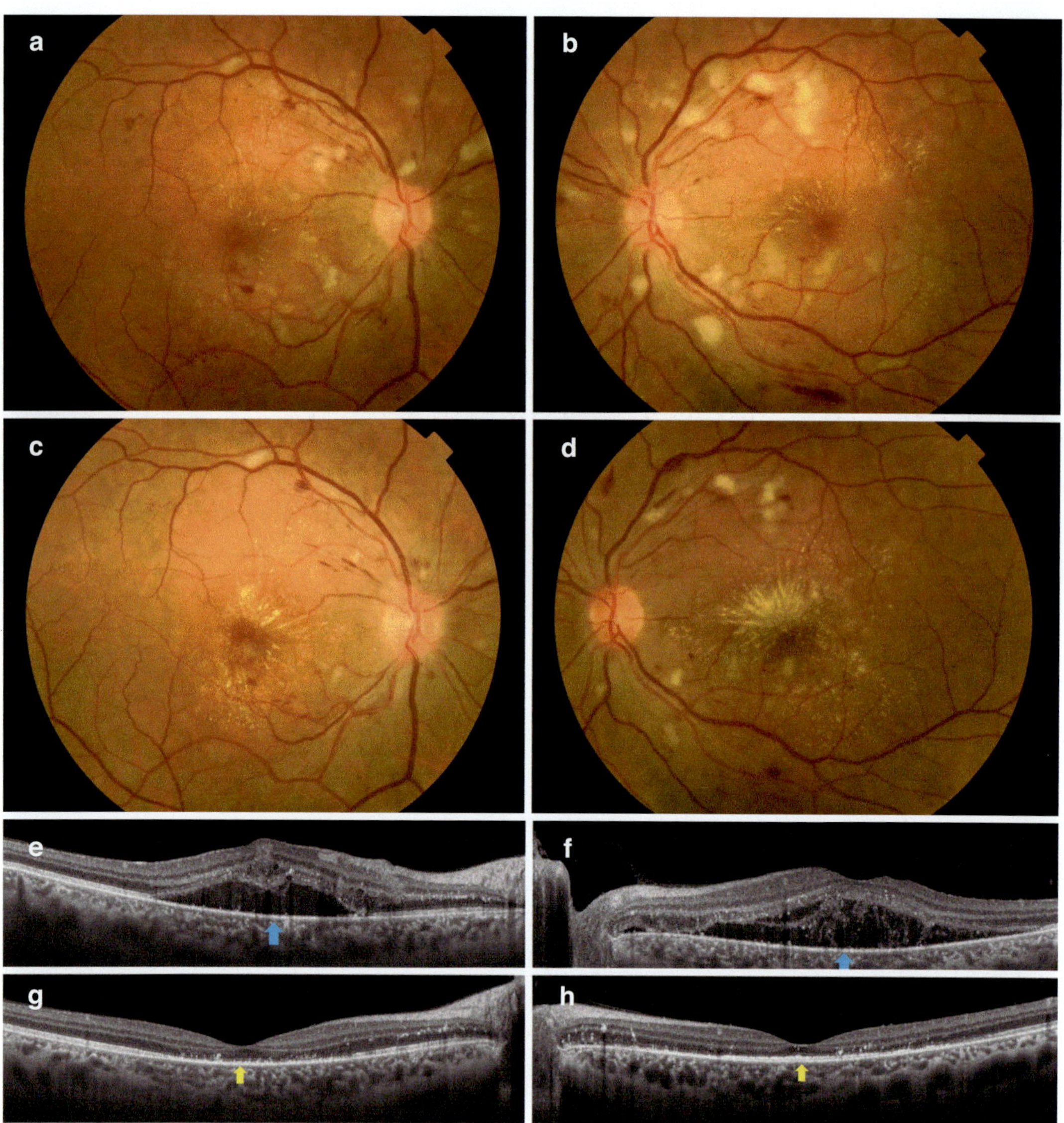

Fig. 8.7 (**a–d**) A 48-year-old male with BP 200/120 mmHg presented with bilateral cotton wool spots, retinal haemorrhages, and arterial changes (**a**, **b**). At 2 weeks, following control of hypertension (BP 160/90 mmHg), there was partial reversal of fundus changes as seen by a decrease in the cotton wool spots, and exudative subretinal fluid leading to macular star formation (**c**, **d**). Optical coherence tomography (OCT) images of the same 48-year-old male patient (as in **a–d**) with BP 200/120 mmHg showing subretinal fluid (blue arrows) in right (**e**) and left (**f**) eyes at initial presentation. At 2 weeks, following control of hypertension (BP 160/90 mmHg), the OCT showed resolution of subretinal fluid (yellow arrows; **g**, **h**)

sure, and hypertensive encephalopathy may all be contributory factors. It is a life-threatening condition and needs emergency care as untreated. It leads to multiple organ failures, including the kidneys, the heart, and the brain, ultimately leading to death. The blood pressure must be lowered slowly under direct supervision in the emergency ward (lower BP by 10–20% in the first hour and 5–15% in the next 24 h) as sudden lowering may lead to infarction of the optic nerve head and lead to ischaemia-reperfusion injury in the target end organs.

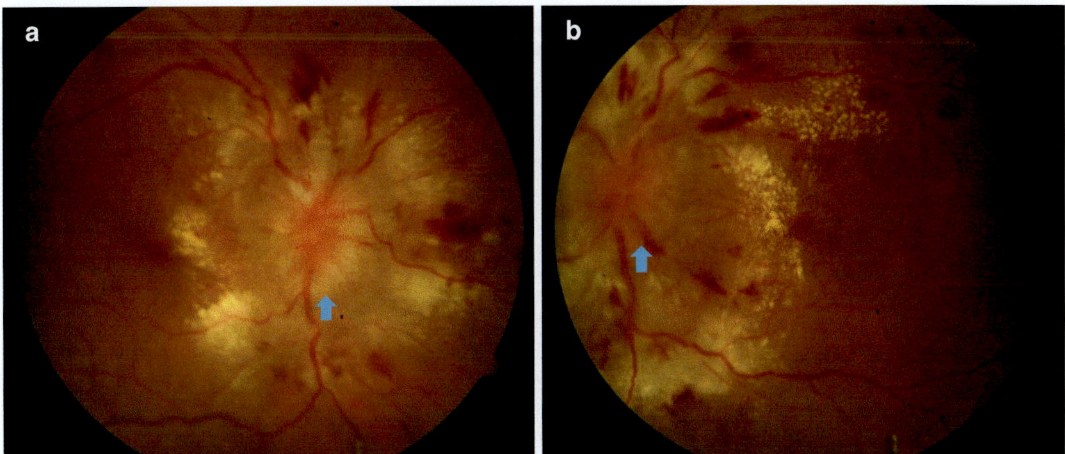

Fig. 8.8 A patient with malignant hypertension presented with extensive retinopathy changes along with optic disc oedema (papilloedema, blue arrows) in both eyes (**a**, **b**)

The term malignant hypertension was coined by Dr. Norman Keith almost 100 years ago, who, besides 'terminal renal insufficiency', also noted on autopsy, diffuse involvement of the arterioles practically in all the organs [47]. For the first time, he defined the critical role of fundus examination in detecting optic disc oedema in diagnosing malignant hypertension. Despite the availability of effective pharmacotherapy to control hypertension, malignant hypertension incidence is not showing a downward trend in certain underdeveloped regions where access to care may be limited [48]. Several events occur during the malignant phase of hypertension, some of which contribute to and others the consequences of malignant hypertension. These include remarkable activation of the renin-angiotensin system, platelet activation, and elevation of fibrinogen levels, endothelial dysfunction, fibrinoid necrosis of arterioles, thrombocytopenia, haemolytic anaemia, cerebral encephalopathy, heart failure [48]. In the eye, malignant hypertension leads to acute ischaemic events due to arteriolar fibroid necrosis in the retinal arterioles (Cotton wool spots) and choroidal arteries (infarction of the choriocapillaris and overlying RPE), resulting in the breakdown of the outer blood-retinal barrier [49]. These ischaemic infarcts in the choriocapillaris are seen primarily on the temporal macula and appear as pale focal areas deep into the retina. These are called acute Elschnig's spots. Fluid leakage from these spots results in the subretinal fluid collection as multiloculated or more extensive as exudative retinal detachment (Fig. 8.9a, b). On FFA, these appear hypofluorescent in the early frames that show late staining. Most retinopathy changes reverse quickly once the blood pressure is controlled (Fig. 8.9c, d). However, pigmented target lesions (central pigmentation with a clear halo) called chronic Elschnig's spots and Linear pigmented lines oriented along the choroidal arteries, the Siegrist's streaks are left behind as a legacy of the past hypertensive choroidopathy. Diabetes mellitus is often a comorbidity in patients with hypertension and requires careful management and monitoring for blood pressure control. See Box 8.6.

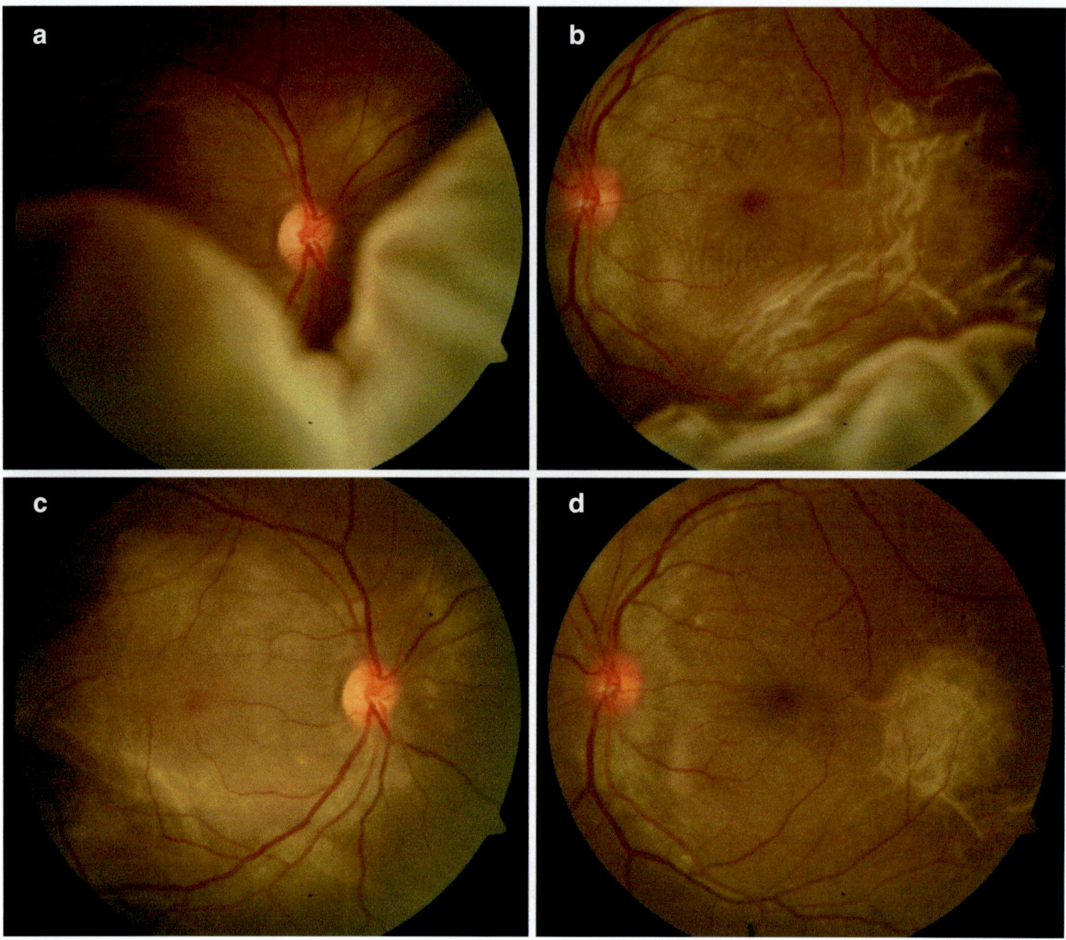

Fig. 8.9 Exudative retinal detachment (**a**, **b**) in a patient with malignant hypertension. After 4 days, with control of hypertension, there was reversal of retinal detachment (**c**, **d**)

Box 8.6 Screening and Targets for Blood Pressure Control in Patients with Hypertension and Diabetes Mellitus

Blood pressure if ≥140/90 mmHg, repeat measurements on same/separate day. Single reading BP ≥ 180/110 with CVD treat the same day BP recording at each visit Home monitoring of BP for all	Target BP < 130/80 mmHg
Existing ASCVD or 10-year ASCVD risk[a] ≥15%	Target BP < 130/80 mmHg if attainable safely
Ten-year ASCVD risk <15%	Target BP < 140/90 mmHg
BP > 120/80 mmHg	Weight control Reduce sodium, increase potassium Alcohol intake moderation Physical activity
BP > 140/90 mmHg	Lifestyle changes Pharmacotherapy

Office recorded BP ≥ 160/100 mmHg, patient has CAD	In addition to lifestyle changes, prompt 2-drug pharmacotherapy, including an ACE inhibitor/ARB Annual eGFR and serum K

Reference: American Diabetes Association [50]

Abbreviations: *CVD* cardiovascular disease, *CAD* coronary artery disease, *ASCVD* atherosclerotic cardiovascular disease

[a] tools.acc.org/ASCVD-Risk-Estimator-Plus

References

1. Leloup AJ, Van Hove CE, Heykers A, Schrijvers DM, De Meyer GR, Fransen P. Elastic and muscular arteries differ in structure, basal NO production and voltage-gated Ca(2+)-channels. Front Physiol. 2015;6:375. https://doi.org/10.3389/fphys.2015.00375. PMID: 26696904; PMCID: PMC4678217.
2. dela Paz NG, D'Amore PA. Arterial versus venous endothelial cells. Cell Tissue Res. 2009;335(1):5–16. https://doi.org/10.1007/s00441-008-0706-5. Epub 2008 Oct 30. PMID: 18972135; PMCID: PMC4105978.
3. Singh S, Dass R. The central artery of the retina. I. Origin and course. Br J Ophthalmol. 1960;44(4):193–212. https://doi.org/10.1136/bjo.44.4.193. PMID: 14447102; PMCID: PMC509919.
4. Hayreh SS. The central retinal artery. In: Ocular vascular occlusive disorders. Cham: Springer; 2015. https://doi.org/10.1007/978-3-319-12781-1_2.
5. Archer DB, Gardiner TA, Stitt AW. Functional anatomy, fine structure and basic pathology of the retinal vasculature. In: Joussen AM, Gardner TW, Kirchhof B, Ryan SJ, editors. Retinal vascular disease. Berlin, Heidelberg: Springer; 2007. https://doi.org/10.1007/978-3-540-29542-6_1.
6. Kur J, Newman EA, Chan-Ling T. Cellular and physiological mechanisms underlying blood flow regulation in the retina and choroid in health and disease. Prog Retin Eye Res. 2012;31(5):377–406. https://doi.org/10.1016/j.preteyeres.2012.04.004. Epub 2012 May 3. PMID: 22580107; PMCID: PMC3418965.
7. Zamir M, Medeiros JA, Cunningham TK. Arterial bifurcations in the human retina. J Gen Physiol. 1979;74(4):537–48. https://doi.org/10.1085/jgp.74.4.537. PMID: 512630; PMCID: PMC2228563.
8. Mainster MA. The fractal properties of retinal vessels: embryological and clinical implications. Eye (Lond). 1990;4(Pt 1):235–41. https://doi.org/10.1038/eye.1990.33. PMID: 2323476.
9. Masters BR. Fractal analysis of the vascular tree in the human retina. Annu Rev Biomed Eng. 2004;6:427–52. https://doi.org/10.1146/annurev.bioeng.6.040803.140100. PMID: 15255776.
10. Cheung CY, Ong YT, Ikram MK, Ong SY, Li X, Hilal S, Catindig JA, Venketasubramanian N, Yap P, Seow D, Chen CP, Wong TY. Microvascular network alterations in the retina of patients with Alzheimer's disease. Alzheimers Dement. 2014;10(2):135–42. https://doi.org/10.1016/j.jalz.2013.06.009. Epub 2014 Jan 15. PMID: 24439169.
11. Mautuit T, Semecas R, Hogg S, Daien V, Gavard O, Chateau N, MacGillivray T, Trucco E, Chiquet C. Comparing measurements of vascular diameter using adaptative optics imaging and conventional fundus imaging. Diagnostics (Basel). 2022;12(3):705. https://doi.org/10.3390/diagnostics12030705. PMID: 35328258; PMCID: PMC8947285.
12. Hampson KM, Turcotte R, Miller DT, Kurokawa K, Males JR, Ji N, Booth MJ. Adaptive optics for high-resolution imaging. Nat Rev Methods Primers. 2021;1:68. https://doi.org/10.1038/s43586-021-00066-7. Epub 2021 Oct 14. PMID: 35252878; PMCID: PMC8892592.
13. Nørrelund H, Christensen KL, Samani NJ, Kimber P, Mulvany MJ, Korsgaard N. Early narrowed afferent arteriole is a contributor to the development of hypertension. Hypertension. 1994;24(3):301–8. https://doi.org/10.1161/01.hyp.24.3.301. PMID: 8082936.
14. Wong TY, Klein R, Sharrett AR, Duncan BB, Couper DJ, Klein BE, Hubbard LD, Nieto FJ, Atherosclerosis Risk in Communities Study. Retinal arteriolar diameter and risk for hypertension. Ann Intern Med. 2004;140(4):248–55. https://doi.org/10.7326/0003-4819-140-4-200402170-00006. PMID: 14970147.
15. Mulvany MJ. Are vascular abnormalities a primary cause or secondary consequence of hypertension? Hypertension. 1991;18(3 Suppl):I52–7. https://doi.org/10.1161/01.hyp.18.3_suppl.i52. PMID: 1889858.
16. Baker ML, Hand PJ, Liew G, Wong TY, Rochtchina E, Mitchell P, Lindley RI, Hankey GJ, Wang JJ, Multi-Centre Retinal Stroke Study Group. Retinal microvascular signs may provide clues to the underlying vasculopathy in patients with deep intracerebral hemorrhage. Stroke. 2010;41(4):618–23. https://doi.org/10.1161/STROKEAHA.109.569764. Epub 2010 Feb 18. PMID: 20167920.
17. Charles L, Triscott J, Dobbs B. Secondary hypertension: discovering the underlying cause. Am Fam Physician. 2017;96(7):453–61. PMID: 29094913.
18. Verdecchia P, Reboldi G, Angeli F. The 2020 International Society of Hypertension global hypertension practice guidelines—key messages and clinical considerations. Eur J Intern Med. 2020;82:1–6. https://doi.org/10.1016/j.ejim.2020.09.001. Epub 2020 Sep 22. PMID: 32972800.

19. Fishbein GA, Fishbein MC. Arteriosclerosis: rethinking the current classification. Arch Pathol Lab Med. 2009;133(8):1309–16. https://doi.org/10.5858/133.8.1309. PMID: 19653731.
20. Dos Santos VP, Pozzan G, Castelli V, Caffaro RA. Arteriosclerosis, atherosclerosis, arteriolosclerosis, and Monckeberg medial calcific sclerosis: what is the difference? J Vasc Bras. 2021;20:e20200211. https://doi.org/10.1590/1677-5449.200211. PMID: 34290756; PMCID: PMC8276643.
21. Keith NM, Wagener HP, Barker NW. Some different types of essential hypertension: their course and prognosis. Am J Med Sci. 1974;268(6):336–45. https://doi.org/10.1097/00000441-197412000-00004. PMID: 4616627.
22. Ritt M, Schmieder RE. Wall-to-lumen ratio of retinal arterioles as a tool to assess vascular changes. Hypertension. 2009;54(2):384–7. https://doi.org/10.1161/HYPERTENSIONAHA.109.133025. Epub 2009 May 18. PMID: 19451413.
23. Wong DYL, Lam MC, Ran A, Cheung CY. Artificial intelligence in retinal imaging for cardiovascular disease prediction: current trends and future directions. Curr Opin Ophthalmol. 2022;33(5):440–6. https://doi.org/10.1097/ICU.0000000000000886. Epub 2022 Jul 19. PMID: 35916571.
24. Chen X, Liu L, Liu M, Huang X, Meng Y, She H, Zhao L, Zhang J, Zhang Y, Gu X, Qin X, Zhang Y, Li J, Xu X, Wang B, Hou FF, Tang G, Liao R, Huo Y, Li J, Yang L. Hypertensive retinopathy and the risk of stroke among hypertensive adults in China. Invest Ophthalmol Vis Sci. 2021;62(9):28. https://doi.org/10.1167/iovs.62.9.28. PMID: 34283210; PMCID: PMC8300046.9094913.
25. Unger T, Borghi C, Charchar F, Khan NA, Poulter NR, Prabhakaran D, Ramirez A, Schlaich M, Stergiou GS, Tomaszewski M, Wainford RD, Williams B, Schutte AE. 2020 International Society of Hypertension global hypertension practice guidelines. J Hypertens. 2020a;38(6):982–1004. https://doi.org/10.1097/HJH.0000000000002453. PMID: 32371787.
26. Unger T, Borghi C, Charchar F, Khan NA, Poulter NR, Prabhakaran D, Ramirez A, Schlaich M, Stergiou GS, Tomaszewski M, Wainford RD, Williams B, Schutte AE. 2020 International Society of Hypertension Global hypertension practice guidelines. Hypertension. 2020b;75(6):1334–57. https://doi.org/10.1161/HYPERTENSIONAHA.120.15026. Epub 2020 May 6. PMID: 32370572.
27. Cuspidi C, Sala C, Grassi G. Updated classification of hypertensive retinopathy: which role for cardiovascular risk stratification? J Hypertens. 2015;33(11):2204–6. https://doi.org/10.1097/HJH.0000000000000733. PMID: 26425835.
28. Wong TY, Rosamond W, Chang PP, Couper DJ, Sharrett AR, Hubbard LD, Folsom AR, Klein R. Retinopathy and risk of congestive heart failure. JAMA. 2005;293(1):63–9. https://doi.org/10.1001/jama.293.1.63. PMID: 15632337.
29. Aissopou EK, Papathanassiou M, Nasothimiou EG, Konstantonis GD, Tentolouris N, Theodossiadis PG, Papaioannou TG, Sfikakis PP, Protogerou AD. The Keith-Wagener-Barker and Mitchell-Wong grading systems for hypertensive retinopathy: association with target organ damage in individuals below 55 years. J Hypertens. 2015;33(11):2303–9. https://doi.org/10.1097/HJH.0000000000000702. PMID: 26335430.
30. Adar A, Onalan O, Sevik O, Turgut Y, Cakan F. Could aortic arch calcification help in detection of hypertensive retinopathy? Blood Press Monit. 2021;26(2):118–23. https://doi.org/10.1097/MBP.0000000000000498. PMID: 33234808.
31. Wong TY, Mitchell P. The eye in hypertension. Lancet. 2007;369(9559):425–35. https://doi.org/10.1016/S0140-6736(07)60198-6. Erratum in: Lancet 2007 Jun 23;369(9579):2078. Wong, Tien [corrected to Wong, Tien Yin]. PMID: 17276782.
32. Zhang W, Li J, Zhao L, Zhang J, She H, Meng Y, Peng Y, Shang K, Zhang Y, Gu X, Chen X, Zhang Y, Yang Y, Sun P, Qin X, Wang B, Xu X, Hou F, Tang G, Liao R, Lin T, Jiang C, Huo Y, Yang L. Positive relationship of hypertensive retinopathy with carotid intima—media thickness in hypertensive patients. J Hypertens. 2020;38(10):2028–35. https://doi.org/10.1097/HJH.0000000000002509. PMID: 32890279.
33. Kawasaki R, Wang JJ, Rochtchina E, Taylor B, Wong TY, Tominaga M, Kato T, Daimon M, Oizumi T, Kawata S, Kayama T, Yamashita H, Mitchell P. Cardiovascular risk factors and retinal microvascular signs in an adult Japanese population: the Funagata Study. Ophthalmology. 2006;113(8):1378–84. https://doi.org/10.1016/j.ophtha.2006.02.052. PMID: 16877076.
34. Kaushik S, Tan AG, Mitchell P, Wang JJ. Prevalence and associations of enhanced retinal arteriolar light reflex: a new look at an old sign. Ophthalmology. 2007;114(1):113–20. https://doi.org/10.1016/j.ophtha.2006.06.046. Epub 2006 Oct 27. PMID: 17070582.
35. Brinchmann-Hansen O, Sandvik L. The intensity of the light reflex on retinal arteries and veins. Acta Ophthalmol (Copenh). 1986;64(5):547–52. https://doi.org/10.1111/j.1755-3768.1986.tb06971.x. PMID: 3811866.
36. Story JB. The light reflex on the retinal vessels. Dublin J Med Sci. 1892;94:313–9. https://doi.org/10.1007/BF02967690.
37. Gast T, Hillard J, Huang J, Burns SA. The optical components of the arteriolar light reflex as analyzed by adaptive optics scanning laser ophthalmoscopy. Invest Ophthalmol Vis Sci. 2014;55(13):4331.
38. Bhuiyan A, Cheung CY, Frost S, Lamoureux E, Mitchell P, Kanagasingam Y, Wong TY. Development and reliability of retinal arteriolar central light reflex quantification system: a new approach for severity grading. Invest Ophthalmol Vis Sci. 2014;55(12):7975–81. https://doi.org/10.1167/iovs.14-14125. PMID: 25358734.

39. Schiffrin EL. Remodeling of resistance arteries in essential hypertension and effects of antihypertensive treatment. Am J Hypertens. 2004;17(12 Pt 1):1192–200. https://doi.org/10.1016/j.amjhyper.2004.05.023. PMID: 15607629.
40. Harazny JM, Ritt M, Baleanu D, Ott C, Heckmann J, Schlaich MP, Michelson G, Schmieder RE. Increased wall:lumen ratio of retinal arterioles in male patients with a history of a cerebrovascular event. Hypertension. 2007;50(4):623–9. https://doi.org/10.1161/HYPERTENSIONAHA.107.090779. Epub 2007 Aug 13. PMID: 17698722.
41. Cheung CY, Biousse V, Keane PA, Schiffrin EL, Wong TY. Hypertensive eye disease. Nat Rev Dis Primers. 2022;8(1):14. https://doi.org/10.1038/s41572-022-00342-0. PMID: 35273180.
42. Wang S, Xu L, Jonas JB, Wang YS, Wang YX, You QS, Yang H, Zhou JQ. Five-year incidence of retinal microvascular abnormalities and associations with arterial hypertension: the Beijing Eye Study 2001/2006. Ophthalmology. 2012;119(12):2592–9. https://doi.org/10.1016/j.ophtha.2012.06.031. Epub 2012 Aug 20. PMID: 22917887.
43. Wong TY, Mitchell P. Hypertensive retinopathy. N Engl J Med. 2004;351(22):2310–7. https://doi.org/10.1056/NEJMra032865. PMID: 15564546.
44. Yatsuya H, Folsom AR, Wong TY, Klein R, Klein BE, Sharrett AR, ARIC Study Investigators. Retinal microvascular abnormalities and risk of lacunar stroke: Atherosclerosis Risk in Communities Study. Stroke. 2010;41(7):1349–55. https://doi.org/10.1161/STROKEAHA.110.580837. Epub 2010 Jun 3. PMID: 20522816; PMCID: PMC2894269.
45. Burnasheva MA, Maltsev DS, Kulikov AN, Sherbakova KA, Barsukov AV. Association of chronic paracentral acute middle maculopathy lesions with hypertension. Ophthalmol Retina. 2020;4(5):504–9. https://doi.org/10.1016/j.oret.2019.12.001. Epub 2019 Dec 16. PMID: 31948908.
46. Too GT, Hill JB. Hypertensive crisis during pregnancy and postpartum period. Semin Perinatol. 2013;37(4):280–7. https://doi.org/10.1053/j.semperi.2013.04.007. PMID: 23916027.
47. Keith NM. Classification of hypertension and clinical differentiation of the malignant type. Am Heart J. 1927;2:597–608. https://doi.org/10.1016/S0002-8703(27)90207-5.
48. Shantsila A, Lip GYH. Malignant hypertension revisited-does this still exist? Am J Hypertens. 2017;30(6):543–9. https://doi.org/10.1093/ajh/hpx008. PMID: 28200072.
49. Hayreh SS, Servais GE, Virdi PS. Fundus lesions in malignant hypertension. VI. Hypertensive choroidopathy. Ophthalmology. 1986;93(11):1383–400. https://doi.org/10.1016/s0161-6420(86)33554-1. PMID: 3808599.
50. American Diabetes Association. Standards of Medical Care in Diabetes—2022 abridged for primary care providers. Clin Diabetes. 2022;40(1):10–38. https://doi.org/10.2337/cd22-as01. PMID: 35221470; PMCID: PMC8865785.

Retinal Vascular Occlusions 9

9.1 Introduction

Retinal vascular occlusions are often associated with life-threatening cardiovascular and cerebrovascular disorders and should initiate a search for either genetic or acquired prothrombotic factors. The incidence of retinal arterial occlusions varies from 1:100,000 in the US population [1] to 1.4–10:100,000 in the Korean population [2]. Major systemic risk factors include type 2 diabetes mellitus, smoking, arteriolosclerosis, carotid atherosclerosis, hypertension, high-serum lipid levels, high body mass index, coagulopathy, and atrial fibrillation [3]. See Box 9.1.

Box 9.1 Systemic Associations of Central/Branch Retinal Artery Occlusion

1	Atherosclerosis of carotid arteries; aortic arch
2	Hypertension; diabetes mellitus; dyslipidaemia
3	Rheumatic heart disease
4	Giant cell arteritis; polyarteritis nodosa including its monogenic variant DADA2; granulomatosis with polyangiitis (Wegener's syndrome); Takayasu's arteritis; Susac's syndrome
5	Systemic lupus erythematosus; antiphospholipid antibodies syndrome
6	Hypercoagulable state; hyperhomocysteinemia; oral contraceptives

Reference: Recchia and Brown (2007)

There is a significant risk for stroke immediately before or within a week to a month following retinal artery occlusion (RAO). All such patients need to be evaluated by a stroke unit [3, 4]. Rarely, giant cell arteritis, systemic vasculitis of large vessels, may first present as an arteritic central retinal artery occlusion (CRAO) [5]. Involvement of the retinal circulation may be the first manifestation of Takayasu's arteritis, another large vessel systemic vasculitis that preferentially affects the arch of the aorta and its branches [6, 7]. Polyarteritis nodosa, another systemic vasculitis affecting the medium and small arteries, may rarely involve the posterior ciliary arteries and cause infarction of the choroid [8, 9]. Immune complex deposition may block peripheral retinal arterioles in systemic lupus erythematosus (SLE). There is an extensive and diffuse inflammation of retinal vessels with Bechet's disease. Several inflammatory disorders may cause retinal vascular occlusions and are summarized in Box 9.2. In TB-endemic countries, occlusive peripheral retinal periphlebitis is not an uncommon cause of vision loss. The vascular occlusions in the eye often lead to irreversible vision loss (arterial occlusions) and, even if reversible (non-ischaemic branch and central retinal vein occlusions), lead to high-visual morbidity. Although the branch and the central retinal artery (CRA) occlusions are less common than the branch retinal vein occlusions (BRVO) and the central retinal vein occlusion (CRVO), these portend systemic severe health issues and are discussed first.

A. Gupta et al., *Ophthalmic Signs in Practice of Medicine*,
https://doi.org/10.1007/978-981-99-7923-3_9

Box 9.2 Retinal Vasculopathy in Autoimmune Systemic Vasculitis, Inflammatory, Infectious, and Demyelinating Diseases

Systemic disease	Key systemic signs and symptoms	Ocular signs	Key labs
Giant cell arteritis	Age > 50 years; extracranial branches of carotid; temporal headache; low-grade fever; malaise; jaw claudication; temporal artery tenderness, and occlusion	Arteritic- AION CRAO; BRAO; OAO; CLRAO	ESR; CRP; TA ultrasonography; TA biopsy; PET-FDG axillary arteries
Takayasu's arteritis	Women <40 years; myalgia; low-grade fever; limb claudication; fainting spells; absent peripheral pulses; amaurosis fugax; carotid bruit; asymmetric BP in various limbs	Hypotensive retinopathy; microaneurysms; anastomotic vessels on optic disc, arteriolar dilatation; iris neovessels; low IOP; hypertensive retinopathy in type 3 (renal artery involvement); rarely BRAO	MR/CT angiography; CRP; ESR; PET-FDG FFA
Poly arteritis nodosa (small- and medium-sized arteries)	Weight loss; myalgia; testicular pain; cardiac systolic dysfunction; peripheral gangrene; mono/ polyneuropathy; elevated diastolic BP; strokes (especially in monogenic variant DADA2)	PCA occlusion	HBV serology; LFT; ANCA-ve; CRP; renal functions; CT/MR arteriography to detect microaneurysms and focal narrowing of medium arteries; biopsy. ADA2 gene mutation and ADA2 levels in monogenic variant DADA2
Granulomatosis with polyangiitis	Upper and lower respiratory symptoms; epistaxis; nasal crusting; cough; haemoptysis; renal involvement; palpable purpura and arthralgia; myalgia	Necrotizing scleritis; orbital inflammation and proptosis; diplopia; retinal haemorrhages; vision loss	PR3 and MPO ANCA; CRP; ESR; TLC; urine analysis; CT chest
SLE	Women >30 years; malar rash; fever; fatigue; weight loss; alopecia; hypertension; renal failure; thrombosis; abdominal pain; encephalopathy	Peripheral branch retinal arteriolar occlusion; cotton wool spots; retinal haemorrhages; retinal neovessels	CBC; APTT; ESR; CRP; ANA; dsDNA; RFT; urine analysis; chest X-ray; ECG; FFA
Sarcoidosis	Low-grade fever; cough; dyspnoea; fatigue; lupus pernio; Erythema nodosum; facial palsy	Panuveitis, vitritis; nodular perivenous infiltrates, arteriolar macroaneurysms; choroidal granuloma	X-ray/CT chest; ACE; RFT; PFT; lysozyme; lymphocytosis Tuberculin skin test
Behcet's disease	Multiorgan thrombotic and necrotizing vasculitis; recurrent oral and genital ulceration; pseudofolliculitis; deep vein thrombosis; recurrent diarrhoea; arthritis; encephalopathy; thromboembolism; IHD	Recurrent hypopyon; vitritis; retinitis; retinal vasculopathy-(capillaries, veins, and arteries); retinal neovessels; retinal vessel occlusion; ION	HLA B5101; pathergy test serum homocysteine; ESR; C-reactive proteins; ASO; neopterin; α-1trypsin; α-2 macroglobulin; FFA
Toxoplasmosis	Fever; lymphadenopathy; abortion; encephalopathy in HIV+	Retinochoroiditis; Kyrieleis arteritis	Toxo serology; HIV serology in bilateral and severe cases
Syphilis	Primary chancre on genitalia; maculopapular rash; rash in oral cavity and palm; dementia	Vitritis; retinal vasculitis; placoid retinopathy; choroidopathy	TPHA; VDRL; HIV

Systemic disease	Key systemic signs and symptoms	Ocular signs	Key labs
Herpes simplex virus (HSV)	Unrecognized primary disease	ARN; occlusive vasculopathy	PCR; HIV; IgM; IgG FFA
Varicella- Zoster virus (VZV)	Acute VZV infection—chickenpox in childhood; herpes zoster in adults and immunocompromised	Progressive outer retinal necrosis; retinal vessel sparing	HIV; IgM; IgG FFA
Cytomegalovirus infection (CMV)	In immunocompetent-asymptomatic or fever lymphadenopathy, lymphocytosis	Retinitis; vasculopathy	CMV qPCR; CD4+ FFA
Leptospira	Rural; flooding; asymptomatic in most; fever; respiratory failure; haemoptysis; high mortality	Hypopyon; panuveitis; retinal vasculopathy	CBC; PCR; urine test; IgM; microscopic agglutination test
Dengue fever (Vector: aedes aegypti and aedes albopictus)	Fever; with retro-ocular pain; myalgia; arthralgia; rash; coagulopathy; haemorrhages of varying severity; respiratory distress; pleural effusion; hepatomegaly; second infection severe with high mortality	Retinopathy, cotton wool spots; vasculopathy; macular oedema; foveolitis	Dengue serology (DEN-1-4); ns-1 antigen RT-PCR; platelet counts; TLC; LFT; serum proteins FFA; OCT: OCTA
Chikungunya (Vector: aedes aegypti and aedes albopictus)	Fever; myalgia; rash; polyarthritis; polyarthralgia; encephalopathy; myocarditis; pericarditis; nephritis; bleeding; pneumonia	Retinopathy, retinal haemorrhages, cotton wool spots, retinal opacification	Chikungunya serology (IgM, IgG); RT-PCR; TLC; platelets; FFA
Rift valley fever	Asymptomatic in the majority; fever	Retinopathy; retinal vasculopathy; retinal haemorrhages; cotton wool spots	RT-PCR; serology; CBC; LFT
Lyme disease	Erythema migrans; fever; arthralgia; myalgia	Vitritis	Immunofluorescence test; Lyme serology; PCR
Cat scratch disease	Fever; maculopapular skin rash lymphadenopathy	Neuroretinitis; multifocal retinitis; BRAO; BRVO	Bartonella serology
Multiple sclerosis	Women 20–40 years; temporary loss of vision, sensory loss	Peripheral retinal vasculopathy; vitritis	MRI brain; spinal cord; AQP4 antibodies; MOG antibodies

Abbreviations: *ESR* erythrocyte sedimentation rate, *CRP* c-reactive proteins, *TA* temporal artery, *RFT* renal function test, *PET-FDG* positron emission tomography-fluorodeoxyglucose, *MR* magnetic resonance, *CT* computerized tomography, *FFA* fundus fluorescein angiography, *HBV* hepatitis B virus, *LFT* liver function tests, *ANCA* antineutrophil cytoplasmic antibodies, *DADA2* deficiency of adenosine deaminase 2, *ADA* adenosine deaminase 2, *ANCA-PR3* anti-neutrophil cytoplasmic antibody-proteinase 3, *ANCA-MPO* anti-neutrophil cytoplasmic antibody-myeloperoxidase, *TLC* total leukocyte counts, *CBC* complete blood counts, *APTT* activated partial thromboplastin time, *ANA* antinuclear antibody, *dsDNA* double-stranded DNA, *ECG* electrocardiograph, *PFT* pulmonary function tests, *ASO* antistreptolysin O tires, *Toxo* toxoplasmosis, *HIV* human immunodeficiency virus, *TPHA* treponemal haemagglutination test, *VDRL* venereal disease research laboratory test, *PCR* polymerase chain reaction, *IgM* immunoglobulin M, *IgG* immunoglobulin G, *CMV* cytomegalovirus, *qPCR* quantitative polymerase chain reaction, *CD4+* clusters of differentiation 4+ cells, *ACE* angiotensin-converting enzyme, *RT-PCR* reverse transcriptase polymerase chain reaction, *OCT* optical coherence tomography, *OCTA* optical coherence tomography angiography, *AQP4* aquaporin 4 antibody, *MOG* anti-myelin oligodendrocyte glycoprotein antibodies

9.2 Non-arteritic Central and Branch Retinal Artery Occlusion

The most common cause of a non-arteritic central or branch retinal artery occlusion (BRAO) is emboli that arise from a thrombus developing on an ulcerated atheromatous plaque in the internal carotid artery and, depending on the size of the emboli may occlude the CRA or pass down any of the branches and usually get stuck at the bifurcation of the arterioles. The patients may report episodes of transient visual loss due to very small emboli, which may finally lodge into the peripheral retinal arterioles. A thorough retinal examination should be done to detect any visible emboli. See Box 9.3.

Asymptomatic retinal emboli may be seen in up to 1.4% of the general population [11], with the prevalence rising in people above the age of 70–75 years [11, 12]. All such patients need to be thoroughly assessed for any risk factors listed above as they are at a higher risk of dying from stroke than those who do not show asymptomatic emboli. The CRA and its branches supply the inner retina up to the outer border of the inner nuclear layer. Complete occlusion of the CRA leads to an immediate loss of vision from the affected eye. Fundus examination reveals a pale opacification of the inner retina with a cherry red spot in the macula (Fig. 9.1). The absence of the inner retinal elements in the fovea centralis (retinal ganglion cells, inner plexiform layer, and the inner nuclear layer) ensures that there is no retinal opacification in the centre of the fovea and no obscuration of the choroidal circulation and hence the cherry red spot. The possibility of an ophthalmic artery occlusion should be seriously considered in the absence of the cherry red spot. In acute CRAO, the retinal arterioles may show 'Box-carring'. The fundus fluorescein angiography (FFA), if done early enough after the onset of CRAO, may show a leading edge of the dye in the retinal arterioles due to the slow filling of the arterioles (Fig. 9.1). In patients who have intermittent CRAO, there may be patchy opacification of the retina. In the event of BRAO, there is sectoral opacification of the retina and loss of vision in the corresponding visual field (Fig. 9.1). If the affected arterioles are the blood supply to the fovea, there may be a complete loss of central vision. The cilioretinal artery, a branch of the posterior ciliary artery, is present in nearly one third of people and may save the central vision in these fortunate patients. On the contrary, an embolus in the cilioretinal artery may lead to central vision loss. Although the experimental studies show a retina survival time of 90–240 min, the survival time of the brain tissue is only 12–15 min. Beyond this time, there will likely be a complete infarction of the retinal ganglion cells as well [13]. However, complete cessation of the blood flow in the CRA is uncommon, which may prolong the retina's survival time. The emboli may be visible in about 20% of the patients with CRAO, and these patients carry the worst visual outcome (Fig. 9.2) [14]. However, irrespective of the visibility of the embolus, all patients with either CRAO or BRAO should undergo evaluation of the internal carotid artery (ICA) for haemodynamically unstable carotid artery stenosis (>60% stenosis) [15] and transthoracic echocardiography to rule out a cardiac source of emboli [16]. Echocardiography can reveal the source of emboli in nearly 60% of patients with CRAO and 50% with BRAO [17]. The Doppler scan/catheter angiography of the carotid artery revealed significant stenosis (>50%) in nearly 30% of both the CRAO and the BRAO eyes on the same side as the occlusion [17]. Simultaneous embolization in both eyes is uncommon [14]. At least three

Box 9.3 Common Causes of Retinal Emboli

1	Atheromatous internal carotid artery; aortic arch; common carotid artery; ophthalmic artery atherosclerosis
2	Valvular heart disease; mitral valve prolapse atrial myxoma; atrial fibrillation
3	Dissection of the aorta; ventral septal defect may allow thromboembolism from deep vein thrombosis
4	Talc emboli in drug addicts; triamcinolone acetonide /methylprednisolone injection for lid or nasal haemangiomas

Reference: [10]

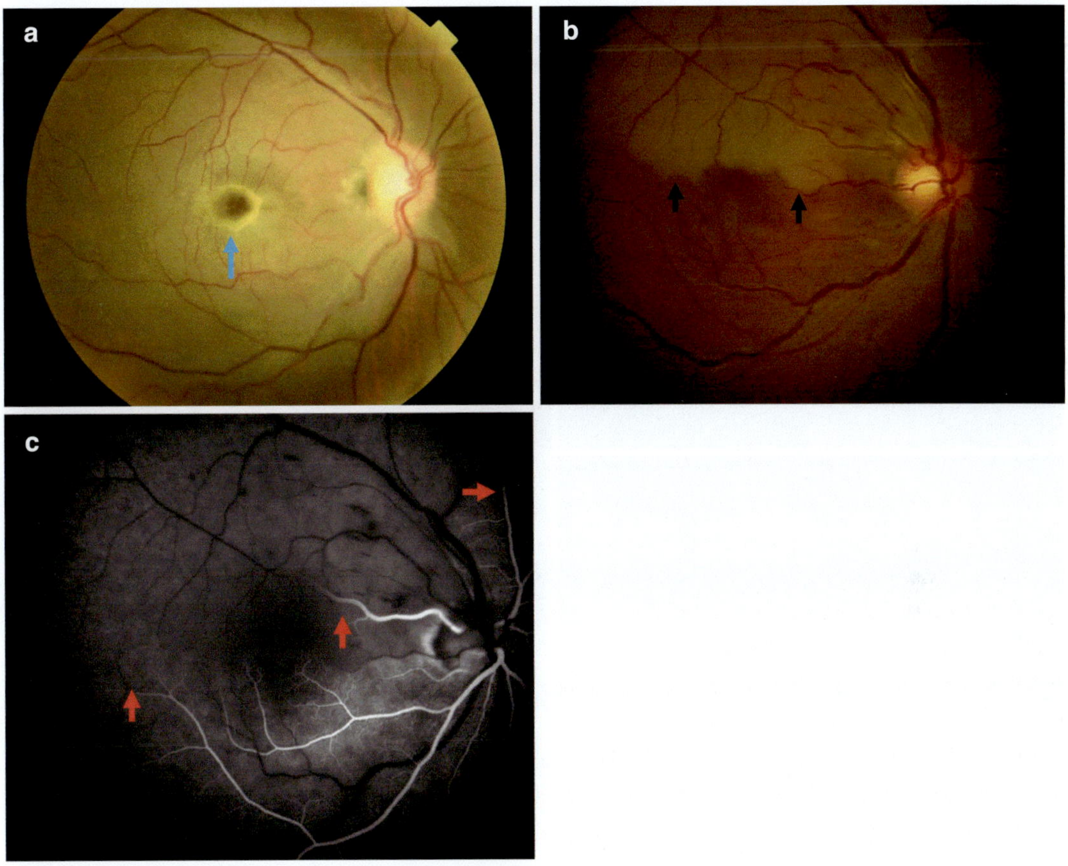

Fig. 9.1 Central retinal artery occlusion (CRAO) is seen as a diffuse pale opacification of the inner retina of the entire fundus with a cherry red spot (blue arrow) in the macula (**a**). Branch retinal artery occlusion (BRAO) is seen as a partial pale opacification (black arrows) of the retina (**b**). Fundus fluorescein angiography shows a leading edge of the dye in the retinal arteries (red arrows) due to the slow filling of the arteries (**c**)

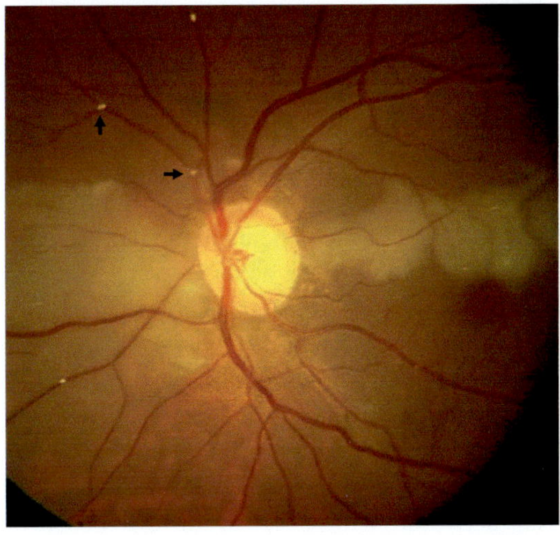

Fig. 9.2 Multiple emboli (black arrows) seen as shiny refractile cholesterol emboli embedded at the bifurcation of arterioles in a patient with BRAO

types of retinal emboli can be recognized. The commonest type of emboli (~70%) are shiny refractile cholesterol emboli that are seen embedded at the bifurcation of arterioles (Fig. 9.2) and arise from ICA atherosclerosis. These are often multiple, and this author has seen a shower of these refractile emboli that shoot down the arterioles to be caught at the bifurcation of the peripheral arterioles. The next common is platelet-fibrin emboli which arise from the ulcerated atheromatous plaque in the ICA or the heart valves. These are dull white, rather soft, and take an elongated shape in alignment with the course of the obstructed arteriole and often cause only transient arterial occlusion (Fig. 9.3). The largest of the emboli is a chalky white irregular-shaped calcific embolus that is stuck in the CRA just before its division and arises from calcified mitral valves

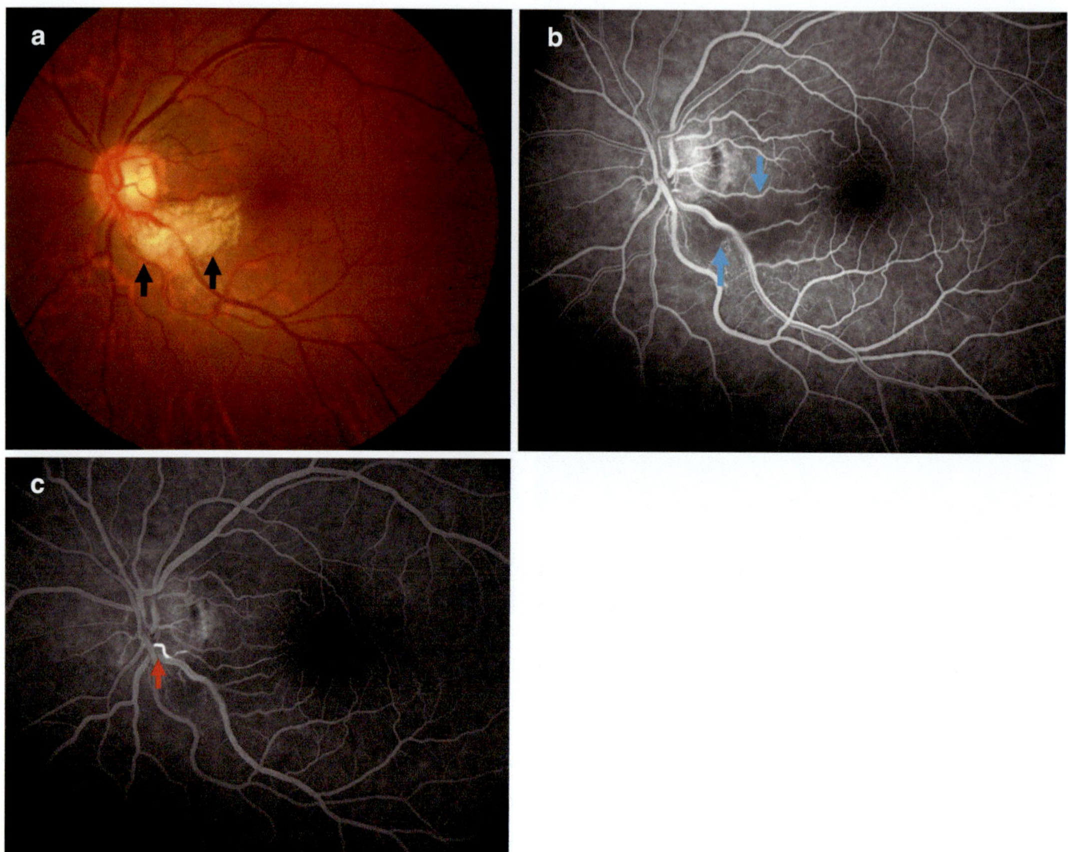

Fig. 9.3 A 44-year-old man presented with blurring of vision in the left eye. There was an opacification of the retina (black arrows) just below and temporal to the optic disc margin (**a**). FFA showed delayed perfusion (blue arrows) of this area (**b**). Late frames revealed a localized hyperfluorescence of the wall of one of the small arterioles (red arrow) feeding the macula (**c**). Note the shape of the embolus characteristic of a soft fibrin-platelet embolus

[10, 18]. Patients who develop CRAO need an emergency evaluation by the hospital stroke team for possible thrombolytic therapy. Unfortunately, due to widespread ignorance about CRAO, there are significantly more delays in symptoms-to-door time for CRAO patients than those with stroke. Compared to stroke patients, less than half (~15%) get the intravenous thrombolytic therapy of CRAO [19].

Some conservative measures commonly used include ocular massage as the most typical strategy, followed by paracentesis, timolol, hyperventilation, oxygen therapy, acetazolamide infusion, and pentoxifylline. However, none of the strategies, including the thrombolytic therapy, if applied after 6 h of the acute onset, seems to effectively change the course of the arterial occlusion [20, 21]. In a controlled multicentric trial, there was no outcome difference between the conservative treatment and intra-arterial thrombolytic therapy in acute CRAO presenting up to 20 h of onset. Visual acuity improved in nearly 60% of the eyes in both groups. More than one third of the patients in the intra-arterial therapy had significant adverse events, including cerebral and cerebellar haemorrhages [22]. Based on the opinion of the experts and a review of the current literature, the American Heart Association has recommended that patients with CRAO be evaluated by a stroke unit and consider the use of an intravenous tissue plasminogen activator within 4.5 h of the onset of symptoms as it seems to be an effective strategy. However, a need is felt for conducting controlled trials [23]. Currently, a few placebo-controlled multicentric trials are evaluating this strategy.

9.3 Branch Retinal Vein Occlusion

9.3.1 Epidemiology of Branch Retinal Vein Occlusion (BRVO)

Next to diabetic retinopathy, branch retinal vein occlusion (BRVO) is the second most common retinal vascular disease. In a population-based study (the Beaver dam eye study), the prevalence and 5-year incidence of BRVO were 0.6% each [24]. When the same population was revisited, the 15-year incidence of BRVO was 1.8%. Retinal vascular occlusions (RVO) accounted for 12% of the causes of severe vision loss (<20/200) over 15 years in this population [25]. In pooled data from different regions of the world, the estimated prevalence of BRVO in persons above the age of 30 years was seen to vary with ethnicity, from 2.82 in Whites to 3.53 in Black, 4.96 in Asians, and 5.98 per 1000 population in the Hispanic population. It is estimated that nearly 14 million people worldwide suffer from BRVO [26, 27]. Patients between the ages of 43–69 years who develop retinal vein occlusions (BRVO and CRVO) have a twofold increased risk of dying from cardiovascular diseases. In contrast, men at any age have a similar twofold, although the non-significant risk of dying from cerebrovascular disorders [28].

9.3.2 Risk Factors for BRVO

The significant risk factors for developing BRVO include increasing age, hypertension, history of cardiovascular disease, smoking, low HDL levels, high BMI at the age of 20, and focal arteriolar narrowing [24, 29, 30]. It was recommended to diagnose and treat hypertension, stop smoking, reduce weight, increase physical activity, and take measures to increase HDL levels.

9.3.3 Pathogenesis of BRVO

The upper temporal quadrant of the retina is the most common site for the occlusion of the branch retinal veins, followed by the lower temporal and least common in the nasal quadrant as there are far more AV crossings in the upper temporal retina compared to the lower temporal and the nasal retina. The eyes that develop BRVO have significantly more AV crossing than those that do not develop BRVO. In eyes with BRVO, the retinal arterioles cross anterior to the retinal vein (AV crossing) in nearly 98% at the occlusion site compared to 67% in normal persons [31]. Notably, the retinal arterioles share a common adventitial sheath with the retinal vein. There is progressive hardening of the arterioles due to fibroplasia in the tunica media and intimal thickening due to arteriolosclerosis, aggravated by hypertension in ageing persons [32]. It leads to progressive nicking at the AV crossing site (Gunn sign and Salus sign). It is believed that endothelial injury caused by turbulence of the blood flow proximal to the site of the AV nicking leads to venous thrombosis [32]. Depending upon whether the occlusion is complete or incomplete, the eye may have an ischaemic (non-perfused) or a non-ischaemic (perfused) type of vein occlusion.

9.3.4 Clinical Presentations of BRVO

The patients may complain of acute loss of vision in the corresponding field of vision, blurring of vision or even remain asymptomatic depending upon the anatomical site of the occlusion and involvement of the macula. There are at least four anatomical sites where BRVO may occur. The commonest is a major vein occlusion near the optic disc either at the first or the second AV crossing in the upper temporal quadrant or a little less common in the lower temporal quadrant (Fig. 9.4). The next common is a macular vein occlusion which occurs when a small venous tributary draining the macula gets blocked (Fig. 9.5). The least common is the peripheral and the nasal sites. The BRVO in the nasal retinal and

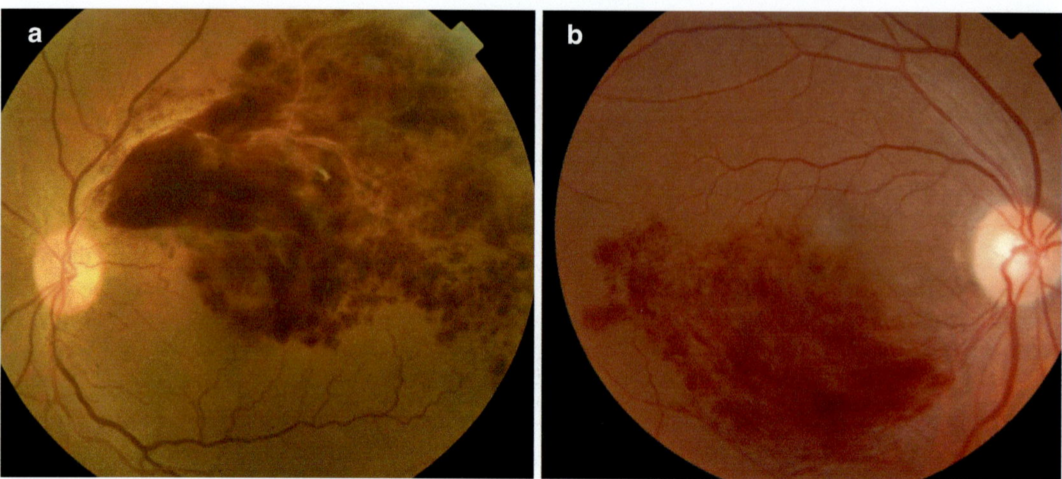

Fig. 9.4 Branch retinal vein occlusion (BRVO) in the upper temporal quadrant (**a**) or lower temporal quadrant (**b**) as the commonest sites

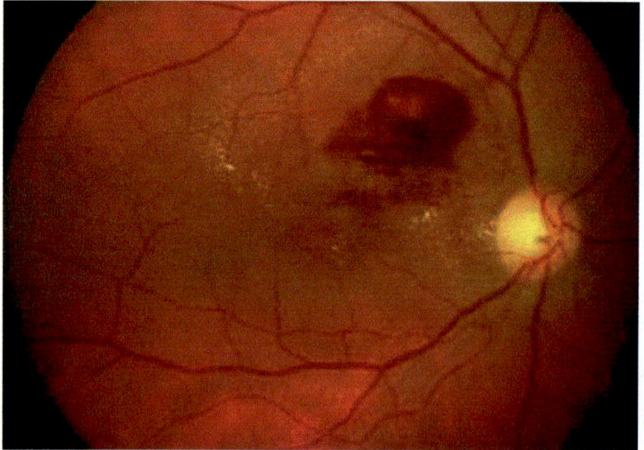

Fig. 9.5 Macular retinal vein occlusion occurs when a small venous tributary draining the macula gets blocked

the peripheral retina often remain asymptomatic as the macula is not affected and is detected either by chance on routine examination or much later if the patient develops either a new BRVO or develops vitreous haemorrhage from neovascular complications that arise typically several months after the acute episode. Acute retinal vein occlusions are characterized by dilatation and tortuosity of the obstructed vein and flame-shaped and dot and blot retinal haemorrhages in the drainage area of the blocked vein. The major and macular vein occlusions often accompany macular oedema (Fig. 9.6). There may be cotton wool spots due to occlusion of the precapillary arterioles supplying blood in the territory of the obstructed retinal vein and are suggestive of the ischaemic type of BRVO. At presentation, nearly one fourth of the patients with major

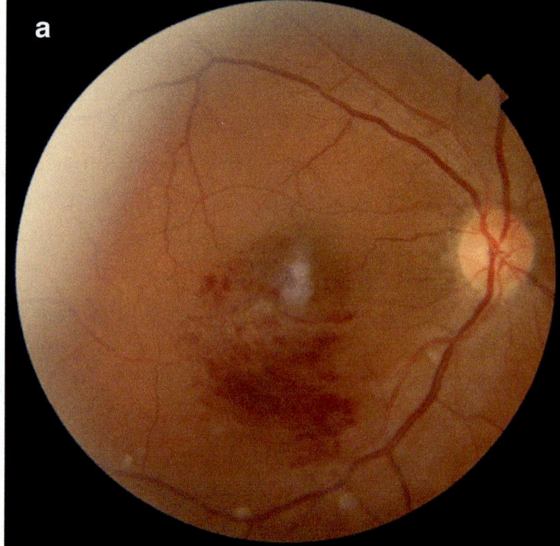

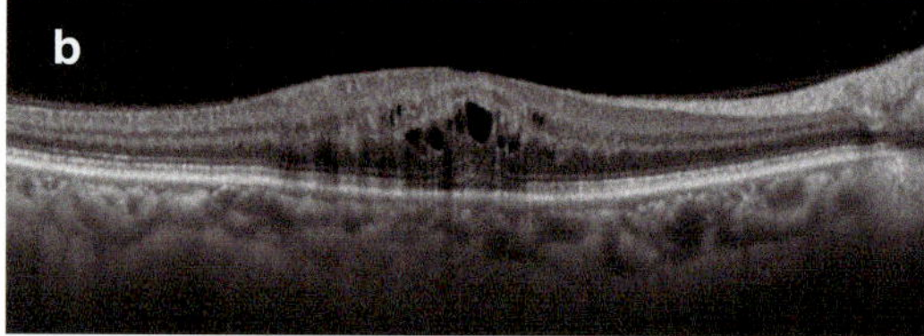

Fig. 9.6 Macular retinal vein occlusion (**a**) with cystoid macular oedema as seen on OCT (**b**)

vein occlusion and a little less than 50% of the macular vein occlusion eyes may have visual acuity of 20/30 or better [33]. Within 6 weeks to 6 months, the retinal capillaries develop collateral channels across the horizontal raphe and start draining the blood/fluid via the venous channels in the opposite

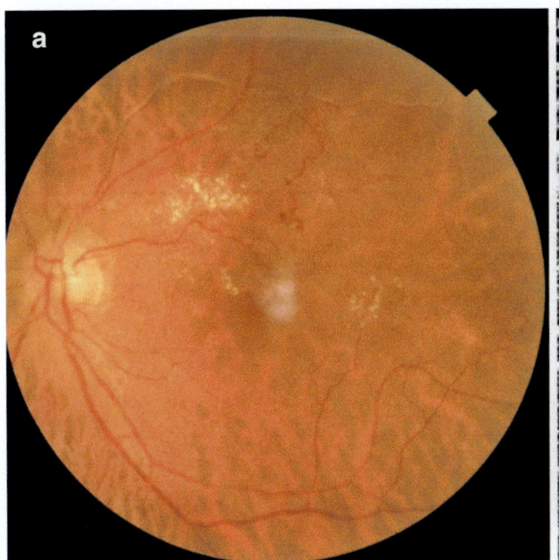

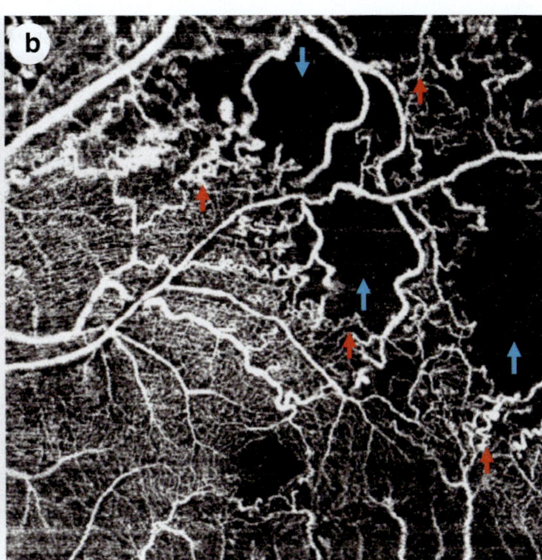

Fig. 9.7 A case of upper temporal BRVO (**a**) at 6 months follow-up, showing the formation of collaterals (red arrows) as seen on OCT angiography (**b**). Areas of capillary non-perfusion are seen as non-perfused areas (blue arrows) on OCT angiography (**b**)

quadrant [32]. These collateral channels help drain the leaky fluid and help reduce the tissue pressure in the extravascular space, thereby helping resolve the macular oedema. Retinal haemorrhages may prevent visualization of the collateral channels in the acute phase. Recently using optical coherence tomography angiography (OCTA), more than 80% of the eyes were shown to have developed collaterals in the macula (Fig. 9.7). However, some of these collaterals also developed microaneurysms responsible for macular oedema's persistence [34]. Further, it has been shown that these collaterals develop in the deep vascular plexus rather than the superficial plexus [35].

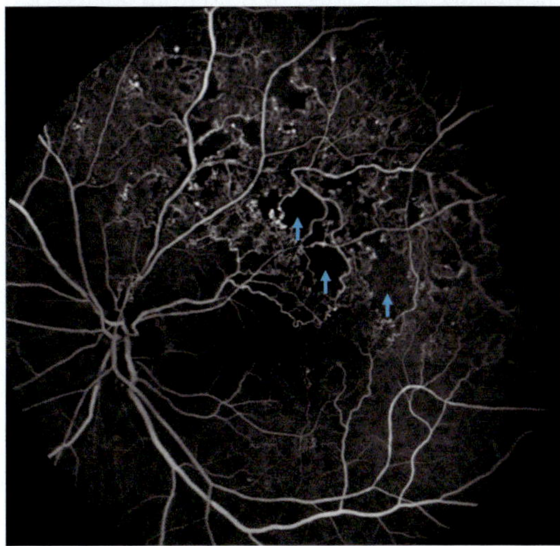

Fig. 9.8 Fundus fluorescein angiography in a case of BRVO showing areas of capillary non-perfusion (blue arrows)

9.3.5 Role of Fundus Fluorescein Angiography

Extensive retinal haemorrhages in the acute phase of BRVO show blocked fluorescence on fundus fluorescein angiography (FFA). However, the staining of the vessel walls of the obstructed vein and its tributaries, fluid in the extravascular spaces in the affected sector of the retina, and cystoid macular oedema can still be appreciated. There are three main causes of diminution of vision in the acute stage of BRVO—the retinal haemorrhage in the foveal centre blocking the transmission of light, ischaemia or macular oedema. Since the absorption of haemorrhages may take up to 3 months for spontaneous resolution, FFA in the acute stage does not help determine the cause of the diminution of vision. However, when most of the haemorrhages have resolved, FFA helps to determine whether it is a perfused or a non-perfused (ischaemic) BRVO (Figs. 9.8 and 9.9), perfusion/non-perfusion of

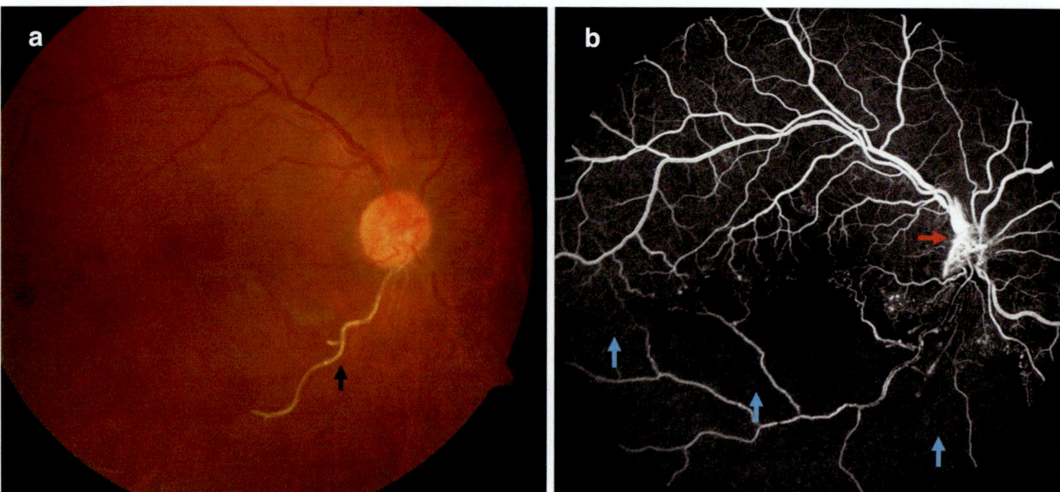

Fig. 9.9 Complete occlusion of a major (lower temporal) branch retinal vein (**a**) seen as a sheathed (black arrow) vessel (**a**). Fluorescein angiography (**b**) shows extensive areas of retinal capillary non-perfusion (blue arrows) and neovascularization of the optic disc (NVD, red arrow)

the macula, and leakage of fluid from dilated (telangiectatic) capillary bed and/ microaneurysms and the presence of the cystoid macular oedema (CME).

9.3.6 Consequences and Complications of BRVO

9.3.6.1 Macular Oedema in BRVO and Treatment Strategies

By 3 months of the onset, most of the retinal haemorrhages get absorbed by the usual phagocytic mechanisms and depending upon the amount of fluid leakage from the broken/decompensated endothelial cell barrier and the capacity of the collateral vessels to drain it, the macular oedema may resolve or continue to persist. By and large, visual acuity improves spontaneously in BRVO eyes without any intervention, but improvement beyond 20/40 visual acuity is uncommon [26, 27]. In the natural course, the median time to resolve macular oedema was 18 months in the macular vein occlusion and 21 months for the major BRVO [33]. In terms of visual improvement, in the branch vein occlusion study, a multicentric controlled trial, there was spontaneous improvement >20/40 in 34% of the untreated eyes versus 60% who had undergone a grid laser photocoagulation in the area of macular oedema [36]. The persisting macular oedema does not follow a zonal distribution and collects in the centre of the macula. Spontaneous resolution in up to 40% of the affected eyes may restore near-normal visual acuity [33]. Clinical diagnosis of macular vein occlusion, especially if the patient presents late, may pose a challenge to differentiate it from diabetic retinopathy. Notably, the veins follow a strict quadrantic pattern, and the haemorrhages and the microaneurysms, unlike the macular oedema, are strictly limited to the affected quadrant above or below the horizontal raphe, as the case may be. In diabetic retinopathy, the microaneurysms and haemorrhages do not follow this rule and are seen across the horizontal raphe. One notable exception is the formation of hard exudates in the BRVO. If the oedema persists, hard exudates may be seen deposited in a circinate pattern around the site of persisting retinal oedema from the decompensated capillary bed and microaneurysms and cross the horizontal raphe. The formation of microaneurysms is a risk factor for the development of refractory macula oedema [37]. In the BRVO eyes with macular oedema and increased subfoveal choroidal thickness, elevated levels of VEGF and IL-8 were seen as predictors of good outcomes following anti-VEGF therapy [38]. Optical coherence tomography (OCT) is used to diagnose and monitor macular oedema (Central retinal thickness, CRT). Additionally, the OCT may show some structural alterations, including disorganization of the internal retinal layers (DRIL) and disruptive changes in the photoreceptors and the external limiting membrane that may limit visual improvement following therapeutic interventions.

In the last 15 years, intravitreal injections of anti-VEGF agents have supplanted gird laser photocoagulation for treating macular oedema due to BRVO. Many such agents have been tested in several controlled trials. They have found almost equivalent results with the use of ranibizumab, bevacizumab or aflibercept that need to be given initially every month for three injections and followed by a PRN (pro re nata) basis. Visual improvement and reduction in CRT, the usual parameters to monitor the response, have shown more significant results with the use of pharmacotherapy compared to laser gird therapy [39, 40]. A more recent Cochrane review of randomized controlled trials has endorsed the recommendations of the earlier studies that compared to no treatment or treatment with grid laser photocoagulation, treatment with any of the anti-VEGF agents or depot corticosteroids was more effective in improving visual acuity, the CRT, and quality of life up to 12 months. Compared to corticosteroids, anti-VEGF agents are more effective. However, there is evidence that steroids lead to high intraocular pressure and cataract formation [41]. Although highly effective, these injections have increased the burden on patients and care providers. Macular laser photocoagulation can reduce the number of intravitreal injections [42].

9.3.6.2 Retinal Neovascularization of Retina and Vitreous Haemorrhage in BRVO

In patients with BRVO, one of the major vision-threatening complications is the development of the retinal new vessels (RNV) and subsequent leakage from these to cause vitreous haemorrhage. Complete occlusion of a major branch retinal vein is complicated by the development of variable areas of retinal capillary non-perfusion that lead to overexpression of vascular endothelial growth factor (VEGF) (Fig. 9.9). There is no strict definition of how much area of non-perfusion area (NPA) will lead to the formation of new vessels and when these new vessels will develop. Such patients must be followed regularly to look for these RNV over several months. The presence of retinal haemorrhages in the acute stage of BRVO does not allow precise estimation of the NPA. Performing FFA, a somewhat invasive technique, has been a standard technique for detecting NPA upon resolution of retinal haemorrhages. More recently, artificial intelligence (AI) techniques using deep learning algorithms have shown that AI can accurately measure the NPA [43]. In a prospective natural history study, new vessels elsewhere (NVE) and new vessels on the optic disc (NVD) were seen to develop at 9% and 8% by 12 months and 15% and 10% by 36 months, respectively [44]. In a multicentric controlled trial (BVOS) study, 22% of the untreated eyes with BRVO developed RNV compared to 12% of those that underwent prophylactic laser scatter argon laser photocoagulation. Most of those who developed either RNV or vitreous haemorrhage had at least a 5-disc area of capillary non-perfusion. In the untreated BRVO, 37% of the non-perfused versus 11% of the perfused and in the laser-treated group, 19.2% of the non-perfused versus 6.7% of the perfused retina developed either RNV or vitreous haemorrhage (Fig. 9.10). Re-evaluation of the perfused cases, which developed these complications, revealed that these patients had developed non-perfusion in the course of follow-up, or the non-perfusion was present but missed on evaluation of the photographs. The study strongly recommended that BRVO eyes should be treated after they develop RNV, as 12% of those prophylactically treated versus only 9% of those treated after the development of RNV went on to develop vitreous haemorrhage [45]. A severe contraction of the visual fields corresponding to the Laser photocoagulation treated sector led to a strong recommendation that laser photocoagulation is done after the development of the RNV [46].

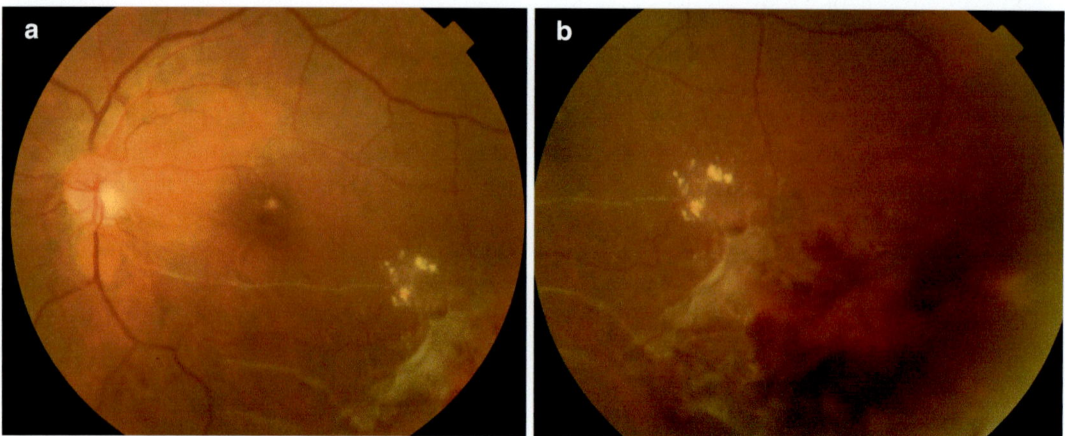

Fig. 9.10 A case of untreated lower temporal BRVO (**a**) developed vitreous haemorrhage and fibrovascular proliferation as a complication (**b**)

9.4 Epidemiology of Central Retinal Vein Occlusion (CRVO)

The prevalence and incidence of CRVO in the population is at least 1/sixth that of the BRVO. In a population-based study (the Beaver Dam eye study), the prevalence of CRVO was 0.1%, and the five-year incidence was 0.2%, respectively [24]. When the same population was revisited, the 15-year incidence of CRVO was 0.5%. Retinal vascular occlusions (RVO) accounted for 12% of the causes of severe vision loss (<20/200) over 15 years in this population [25]. In pooled data from different regions of the world, the estimated prevalence of CRVO in persons above the age of 30 years was seen to vary with ethnicity, from 0.88 in Whites, 0.37 in Black, 0.74 in Asians, and 1.01 per 1000 population in the Hispanic population. It is estimated that nearly two million people worldwide suffer from CRVO [26, 27].

9.4.1 Risk Factors for CRVO

In the 15-year incidence and prevalence study of RVO (The Beaver dam eye study), the significant risk factors for CRVO, apart from age, included glaucoma, history of diabetes, and use of digoxin and barbiturates. Other risk factors include diabetes, lipid abnormalities, smoking, and hyperhomocysteinemia. Resistance of activated protein C, factor 5 Leiden mutation, and a genetic mutation in prothrombin has been reported mainly in younger patients with CRVO. However, inconsistent results do not merit any tests for screening these factors [47, 48].

9.4.2 Pathogenesis of CRVO

The central retinal vein (CRV) exits the eye through the optic nerve head, which shares the adventitial sheath with the central retinal artery. A morphometric study has shown that compared to the CRA, the CRV has a reduced perimeter and lumen and acquires a 'D' shape compared to the circular shape of the CRA [49]. Because of these notable anatomical limitations, the CRV gets narrower in the lamina cribrosa and has a higher flow. Higher intraocular pressure also leads to further compression of the RV in the lamina cribrosa. Further, in patients with arteriolosclerosis, hardening of the central retinal artery wall compresses the CRV leading to turbulence and endothelial injury and the formation of a thrombus just posterior to the lamina cribrosa [50, 51]. Histopathological studies of the eyes with CRVO removed within a week to 10 years after the occlusion have shown a fresh thrombus to a recanalized thrombus along with endothelial cell proliferation in nearly half of the eyes and evidence of chronic inflammation in the other half of the eyes [52]. FFA studies show that blood flow is present in the CRVO eyes by opening pre-existing retinociliary channels. A more posterior site of thrombus formation means the availability of more channels to drain the blood resulting in a non-ischaemic CRVO (ni-CRVO). However, fewer collaterals are available if the thrombus extends anteriorly, leading to an ischaemic CRVO (iCRVO) [53]. According to Hayreh, most iCRVOs begin as non-ischaemic and progress to the ischaemic type. Even the Central Vein Occlusion Study reported that many CRVO eyes initially labelled indeterminate progressed to the iCRVO, emphasizing the need for a thorough and frequent examination, including the slit-lamp, within the first 4 months after onset [29, 30].

9.4.3 Clinical Presentation and Classification of CRVO

Occlusion of the CRV leads to a highly variable clinical picture in the acute phase, the consistent feature being venous dilatation and tortuosity in all four quadrants. The increased hydrostatic pressure in the veins causes loss of the blood-retinal barrier resulting in fluid leakage and varying severity of haemorrhages from a few scattered ones to massive haemorrhages in all the quadrants of the retina (Fig. 9.11). These may be accompanied by optic disc oedema, macular oedema, and cotton wool spots. Hayreh first classified CRVO into two distinct entities, venous stasis retinopathy (non-ischaemic) and haemorrhagic (ischaemic) CRVO, with altogether different outcomes (Fig. 9.12) [54]. According to Hayreh, most of the iCRVOs begin as non-ischaemic and progress to the ischaemic type [53]. Even the Central Vein Occlusion Study reported that many CRVO eyes that were initially labelled indeterminate progressed to the ischaemic type emphasizing the need for a thorough and frequent examination, including the slit-lamp within the first 4 months after onset [29, 30]. Patients with iCRVO present with four highly sensitive and specific functional tests, namely the relative afferent pupillary defect in the affected eye, visual acuity <20/400, contracted visual fields on the kinetic perimeter, and subnormal amplitude (<60%) of the B wave on ERG [55]. The two tests, namely the visual acuity and the subnormal ERG, have 97% sensitivity in the diagnosis of iCRVO. The two morphological tests, the severity of retinal haemorrhages in all four quadrants on the fundus examination and FFA, are less sensitive in the acute stage to differentiate the ischaemic from the ni-CRVO. In the acute stage of CRVO, blockage of the fluorescence by retinal haemorrhages assesses capillary non-perfusion areas misleading [53]. The presenting visual acuity (VA) in the acute ni-CRVO presenting within 3 months of the onset is >20/30 in 40% of eyes and >20/60 in nearly 2/3 of eyes, whereas in the iCRVO VA is <20/400 in 80% of eyes, and none having >20/200. The field defects in non-ischaemic CRVO are only mildly affected in >90 of eyes versus moderate to severe visual field defects in ischaemic CRVO [53]. In a significant number of eyes, haemorrhages and macular oedema will resolve spontaneously in ni-CRVO. However, a cilioretinal artery occlusion may rarely complicate the non-ischaemic more than the iCRVO. Persistent macular oedema is another sight-threatening complication. On the other hand, ischaemic CRVO is complicated by the development of anterior segment neovascularization with consequent neovascular glaucoma.

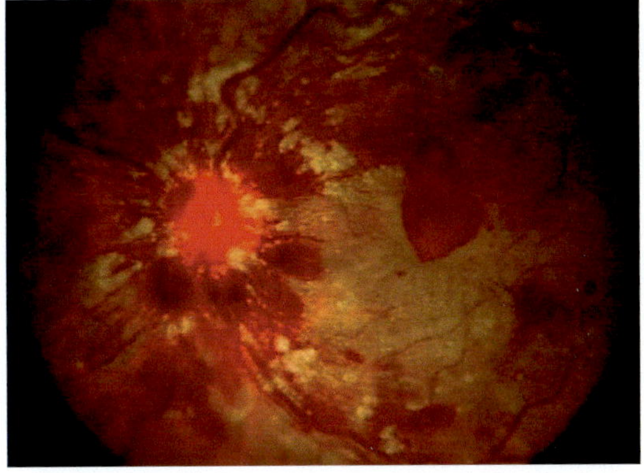

Fig. 9.11 Extensive retinal haemorrhages are seen in all four quadrants in central retinal vein occlusion (CRVO)

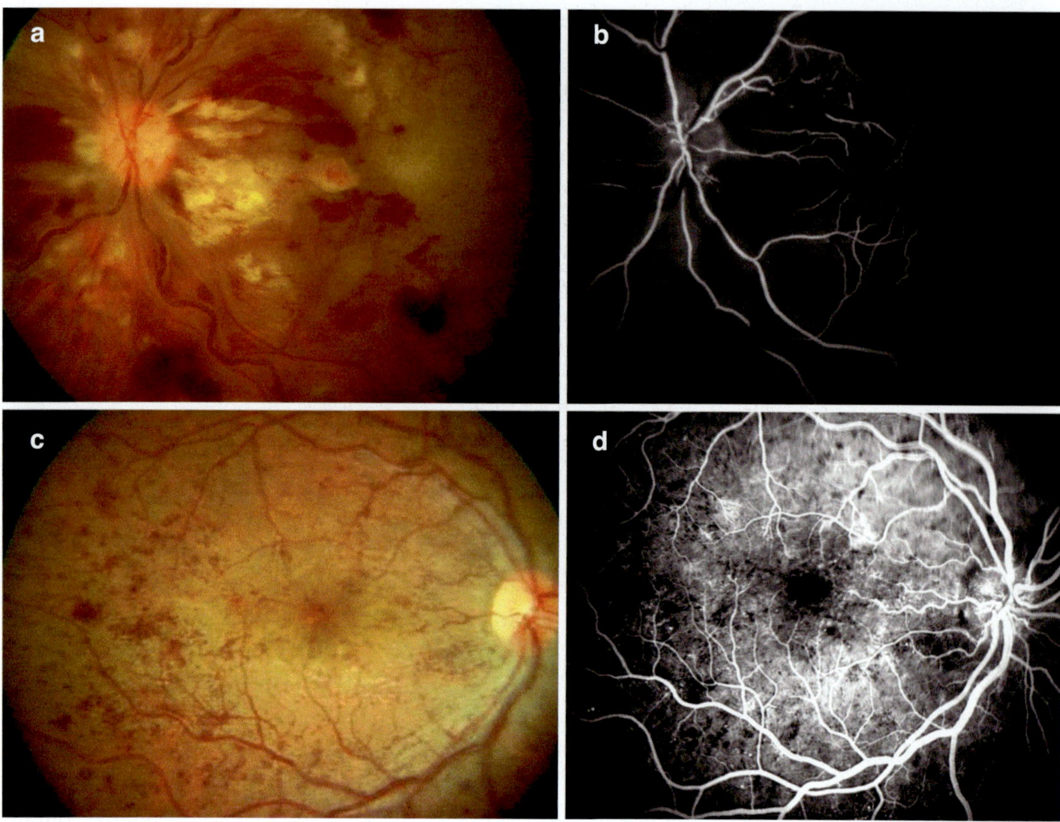

Fig. 9.12 Fundus photographs and fluorescein angiography of ischaemic CRVO (**a**, **b**) and non-ischaemic CRVO (**c**, **d**)

9.4.3.1 Complications of CRVO: Occlusion of the Cilioretinal Artery (CLRA)

Retinal circulation is autoregulated, and therefore whenever there is a rise in the intravascular hydrostatic pressure in the central retinal vein and its tributaries, there is an automatic drop in the high-pressure central retinal artery supply system compared to the non-autoregulated, but a low-pressure ciliary supply system of which the cilioretinal artery (CLRA) is a branch. It is of note that the venous drainage of the CLRA is through the draining capillaries of the retinal veins, and these are met with a raised intracapillary pressure of the retinal venous system. Nearly one third of normal people possess one or sometimes more CLRAs. During autonomic system-controlled nocturnal lowering of blood pressure, a significant drop in the blood pressure in the CLRA may fail to overcome the raised intracapillary pressure (caused by the CRVO), thereby causing either a haemodynamic or permanent cessation of the blood supply via the CLRA (Fig. 9.13). These patients may complain either of transient attacks of blurring of vision or may find their vision diminished on waking up in the morning [56].

Haemodynamic occlusion of this phenomenon can be demonstrated on the FFA, as the bolus of the dye moves back and forth in the cilioretinal artery—a phenomenon given the name of 'dye front reciprocation' [57, 58]. Notably, whether isolated or associated with CRVO, cilioretinal artery occlusion is nearly always associated with paracentral acute middle maculopathy lesions [59].

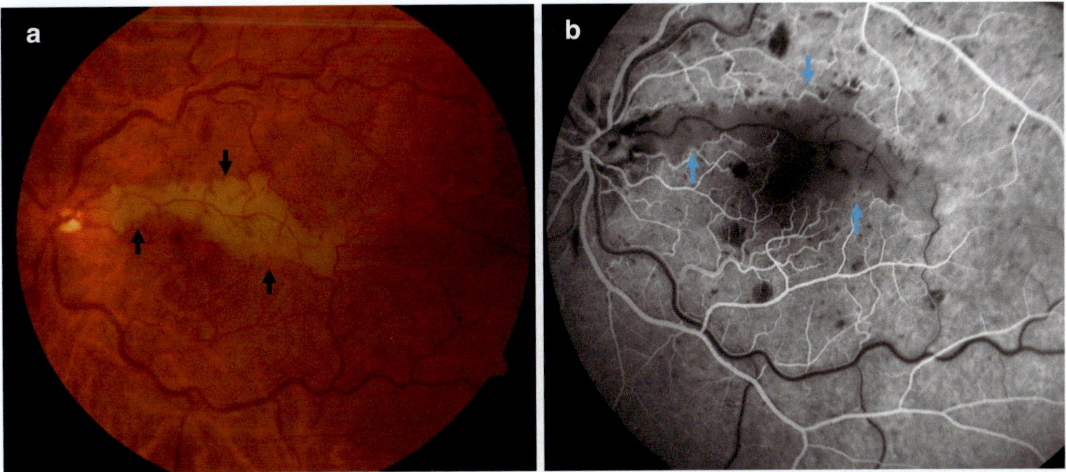

Fig. 9.13 CRVO with cilioretinal artery occlusion seen as a pale island of opacification (black arrows) in the macula (**a**). Fluorescein angiography shows the corresponding area (blue arrows) of non-perfusion (**b**)

9.4.3.2 Complications of CRVO: Paracentral Acute Middle Maculopathy

Paracentral acute middle maculopathy (PAMM) lesions caused by capillary ischaemia in the intermediate and deep capillary plexus can be seen in ~5% of the cases with non-ischaemic CRVO. This area of the retina is a watershed of the oxygen and micronutrient supply between the retinal and the choroidal circulation. It is thus vulnerable to raised interstitial pressure in this zone caused by the non-ischaemic CRVO [60]. A plaque-like hyperreflective band in the inner nuclear layer on the spectral domain OCT characterizes the PAMM lesions (Fig. 9.14). On en face OCT, the PAMM lesions due to CRVO appear as areas of perivenular hyperreflectivity [60]. On fundus examination, these are seen as perivenular opacification of the retina which appears dark on near-infrared reflectance imaging. While the cotton wool spots are white-striated superficial lesions that follow the retinal nerve fibres course, the PAMM lesions are dull grey and located deep in the retina [61]. It is important to note that the perivenular fern pattern of PAMM that starts in the deep capillary plexus may be a harbinger of a branch or central retinal artery occlusion requiring a stroke evaluation [62]. Once the PAMM lesions resolve, they leave behind thinning of the inner nuclear layer.

9.4.3.3 Complications of CRVO: Persistent Macular Oedema

Raised intravascular pressure in the CRVO leads to a breakdown of the blood-retinal barrier and increased fluid leakage into the retina's interstitial tissues. The increased pressure interferes with the perfusion in the retinal tissues and leads to a state of hypoxia and release of hypoxia-inducible factor 1-alpha causing overexpression of the vascular endothelial growth factor (VEGF). Discovered in 1989, the VEGF is expressed in response to hypoxia and is a potent endothelial cell-specific stimulant that causes increased vascular permeability, endothelial cell proliferation, formation of new vessels, and recruitment of leucocytes [63]. Vascular endothelial growth factor (VEGF) was found elevated in the ocular fluids in the patients with proliferative diabetic retinopathy and CRVO [64, 65] and related with the severity of the retinal vein occlusion [66]. Although initial reports had found elevated VEGF levels in the RVOs, it was unknown how much of the fluid in the interstitial fluid is contributed by the increased hydrostatic pressure or the cytokines in the retina. The discovery of VEGF led to the development of an antigen-binding protein against VEGF (bevacizumab) and later a unique antigen-binding fragment (ranibizumab), especially for intraocular use [67, 68]. Initial small

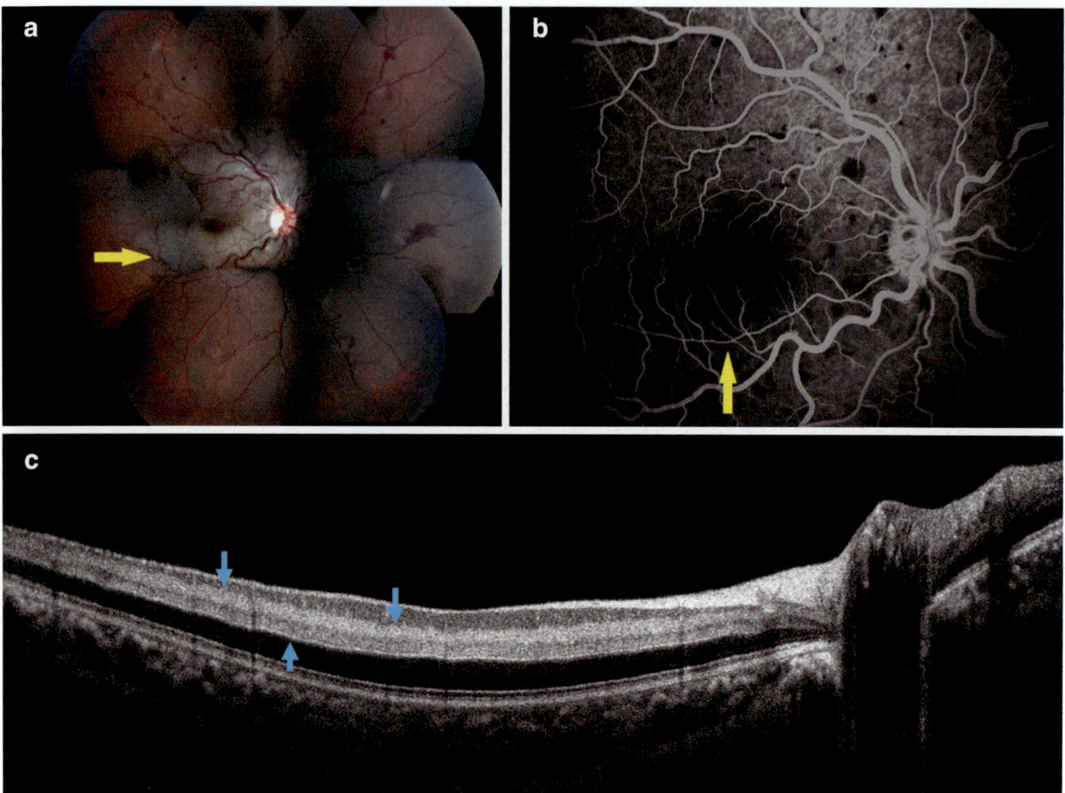

Fig. 9.14 A case of non-ischaemic CRVO with perivenular opacification of the retina (yellow arrow) suggestive of paracentral acute middle maculopathy (PAMM), as seen on fundus photograph (**a**) and fluorescein angiography (**b**). OCT shows a plaque-like hyperreflective band (blue arrows) in the inner nuclear layer characterizing the PAMM lesions (**c**)

controlled trials with 3-monthly injections of an anti-VEGF agent, ranibizumab, led to remarkable improvement in the vision and the reduction in central retinal thickness irrespective of the duration of the RVO (Fig. 9.15).

Moreover, there was some correlation with the decreasing VEGF levels in the aqueous humour [69], suggesting that VEGF was a major driver of macular oedema and laid grounds for establishing the role of anti-VEGF therapy for the resolution of macular oedema, albeit for a short duration (~1 month) in both the BRVO and the CRVOs. It has now been shown that anti-VEGF therapy leads to decreased retinal venous pressure in eyes with CRVO [70]. Several controlled clinical trials have been done both with anti-VEGF agents, that last about one month and intravitreal injections of depot steroids (triamcinolone acetonide, 1 mg Kenalog) or sustained-release dexamethasone implants (Ozurdex) to overcome the increased burden of the monthly injections [71] (Fig. 9.16). There is a significant risk of cataract formation and raised intraocular pressure with intravitreal depot steroids. The anti-VEGF agents remain the first line of therapy for persistent macular oedema in RVOs, with depot steroids being reserved only for patients resistant to the anti-VEGF agents [72]. Strong evidence for a treat and extend strategy has found favours as only ~8 injections were required by 12 months and 13 by the end of

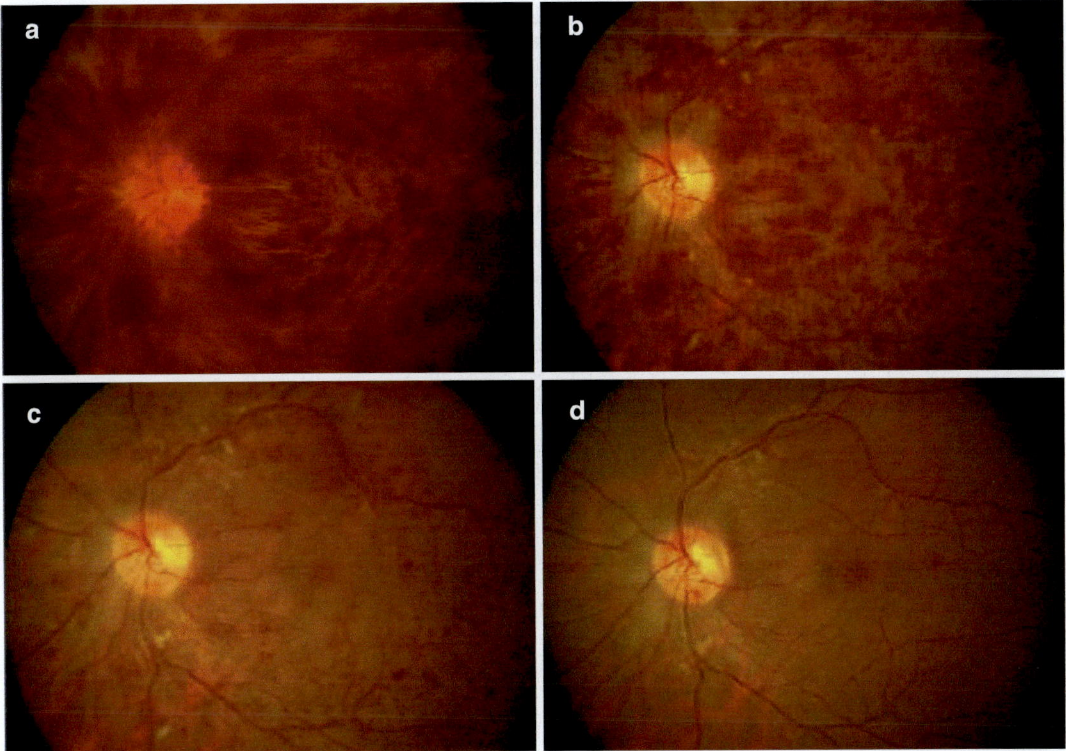

Fig. 9.15 A 51-year-old man presented with sudden visual loss in the left eye due to CRVO (**a**). He received intravitreal injections of bevacizumab every four weeks. Note resolution of retinal hemorrhages at six weeks (**b**), four months (**c**) and eight months (**d**)

24 months [73]. However, most patients continue to receive injections even after 5 years [74] and still require at least four injections per year at the end of 8 years [75]. However, the search for innovative drug delivery systems continues in an attempt to reduce the treatment burden.

9.4.3.4 Complications of CRVO: Ocular Neovascularization

Besides the irreversible loss of central vision, the major complication of iCRVO is the development of neovessels in the iris (INV) and the angle of the anterior chamber (ANV), ultimately leading to a painful blind eye due to neovascular glaucoma. Patients with CRVO have to be followed up regularly to look for early signs of INV as a substantial number of even the ni-CRVO may develop ischaemic CRVO when followed for a long time. There is a sharp rise in the development of INV in the iCRVO eyes within 6 months of the onset. Likewise, NVG, if it has to develop, does so within 12 months in 90% of the cases [76]. The anti-VEGF agents, if used, may delay the onset of INV in iCRVO but do not eliminate the occurrence of this complication [77]. The definitive treatment is pan-retinal photocoagulation to eliminate the hypoxic retina. It is recommended that pan-retinal photocoagulation be done after the development of INV since prophylactic photocoagulation does not prevent the

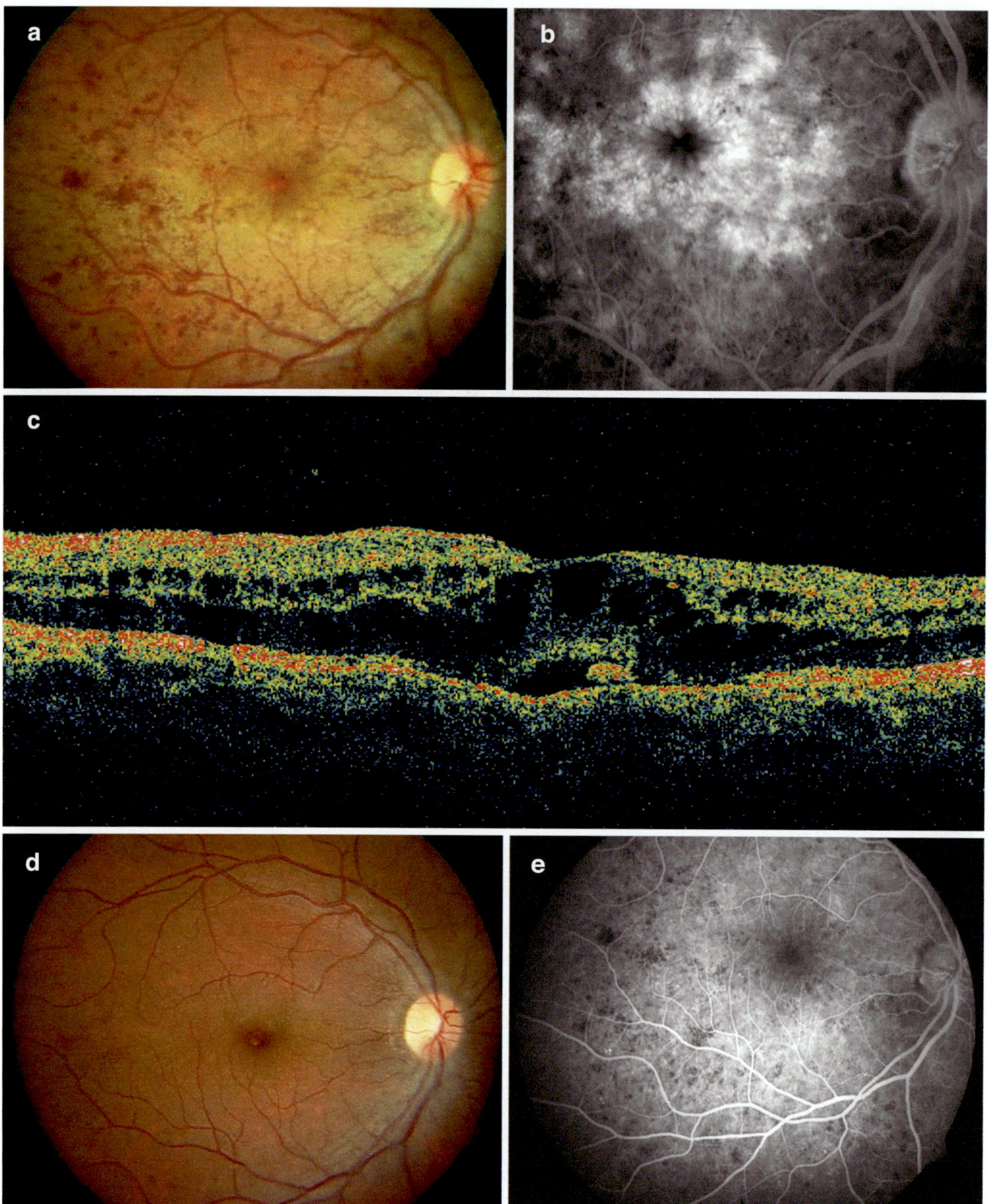

Fig. 9.16 Nonischemic CRVO (**a**) in a 35-year-old woman with macular edema on fluorescein angiography (**b**) and spectral domain OCT (**c**). She received intravitreal triamcinolone 4mg. At the 18-week follow-up, there were no retinal hemorrhages and visual acuity had improved to 6/6 (**a**), there was a significant reduction in perifoveal leakage (**e**) and no macular edema on OCT (**f**)

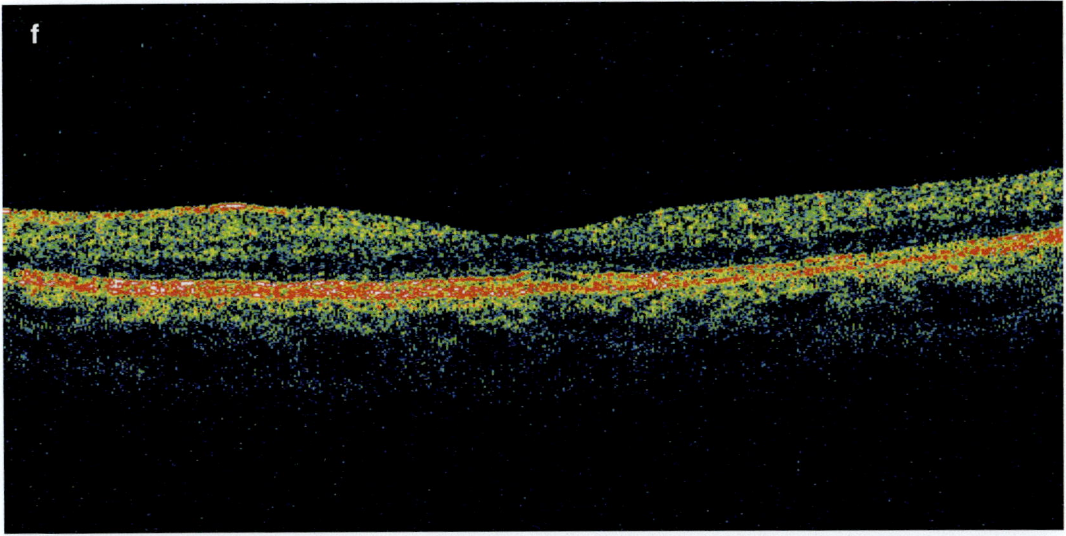

Fig. 9.16 (continued)

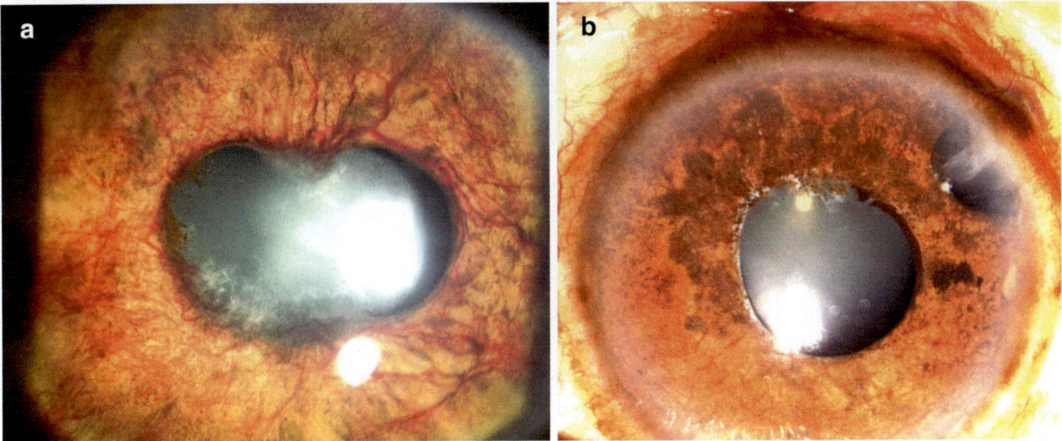

Fig. 9.17 Massive iris neovascularization (INV) with neovascular glaucoma in ischaemic CRVO (**a**). Five months following antiglaucoma surgery and pan-retinal photocoagulation, there was complete regression of INV with control of intraocular pressure (**b**)

occurrence of neovessels on the iris (Fig. 9.17) [76, 78].

As most patients with iCRVO have already lost their central vision, whatever is left of the peripheral field of vision required for ambulation also gets lost due to photocoagulation.

9.5 Inflammatory Retinal Vein Occlusions

Several inflammatory disorders may present with inflammatory occlusion of single or multiple retinal vein occlusions. In TB-endemic

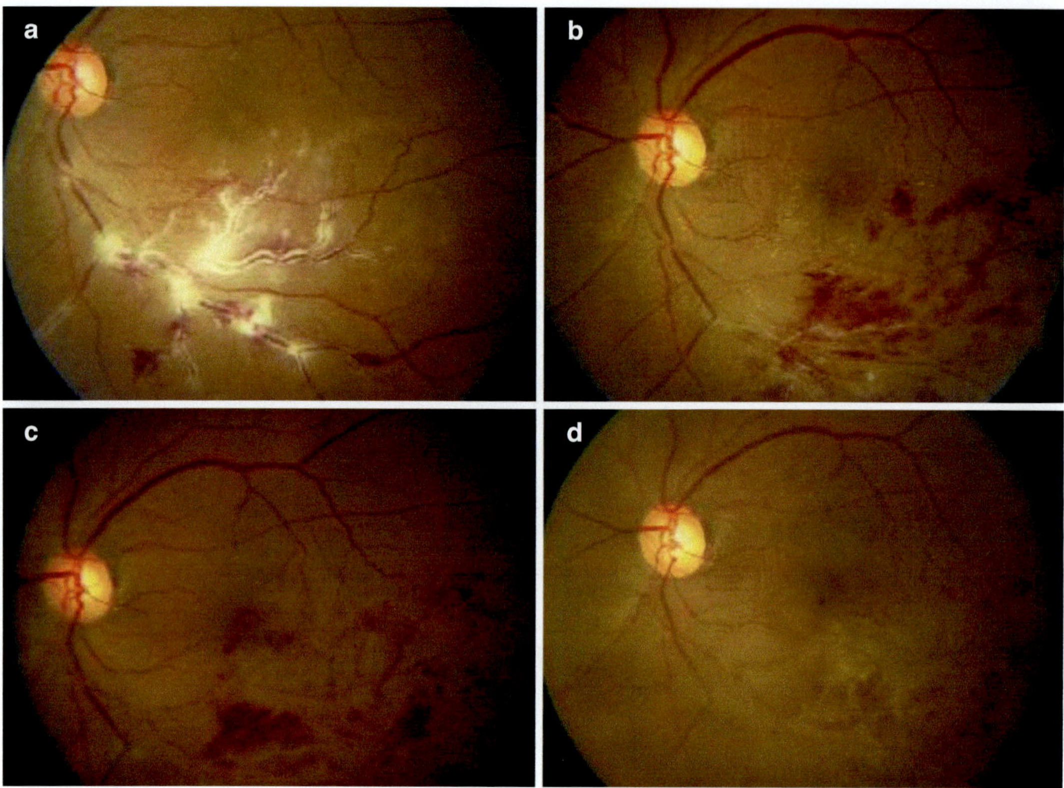

Fig. 9.18 Inflammatory BRVO of lower temporal vein showing exuberant perivenous inflammatory exudates (**a**). Following treatment, the haemorrhages started resolving at 6 weeks (**b**), 4 months (**c**), and 9 months (**d**)

countries, the most common cause is tubercular retinal periphlebitis, which was until recently labelled as Eales' disease. Peripheral retinal veins are often affected, which may show exuberant perivenous inflammatory exudates (Fig. 9.18). Tubercular retinal periphlebitis is often associated with healed or actively inflamed chorioretinal lesions. See Box 9.4. On FFA, there is extensive capillary non-perfusion which leads to retinal neovascularization. They may remain asymptomatic or have floaters or a diminution of vision. When presenting late, they may have total obscuration of vision due to vitreous haemorrhage and still later develop tractional or combined retinal detachments. Other causes of retinal vasculitis/periphlebitis include Behcet's disease, sarcoidosis, Syphilis, Lyme disease, leptospira, toxoplasmosis, cat scratch disease, HSV retinitis, CMV retinitis, leukaemias, multiple sclerosis, and many others [79].

Box 9.4 Idiopathic Retinal Periphlebitis (Eales' Disease; Tubercular Retinal Periphlebitis)

1	Young men > women, often systemically asymptomatic, seen in TB-endemic countries
2	Acute -vitritis; snowballs; vitreous haemorrhage in quiescent stage
3	Acute -segmental periphlebitis (vessel wall exudates, thrombosis)
4	Acute -retinal haemorrhages; macular oedema
5	Acute/healed -perivenular chorioretinitis lesions/scars
6	Healed stage-pipe stem sheathing in healed stage
7	On FFA, extensive capillary non-perfusion, neovessels on optic disc or elsewhere on retina
8	Tractional retinal detachment (TRD) in neglected cases

9	Lab tests in acute stage-tuberculin skin test; CT chest; RT-PCR from ocular fluids; exclude other causes of inflammation Healed stage—no labs
10	In acute stage standard 4-drug anti-TB therapy for 9 months with oral corticosteroids; in healed stage-laser photocoagulation if neovessels; pars plana vitrectomy for vitreous haemorrhage and TRD

References: [80–82]

References

1. Brown GC, Magargal LE, Shields JA, Goldberg RE, Walsh PN. Retinal arterial obstruction in children and young adults. Ophthalmology. 1981;88(1):18–25. https://doi.org/10.1016/s0161-6420(81)35080-5. PMID: 7243224.
2. Park SJ, Choi NK, Seo KH, Park KH, Woo SJ. Nationwide incidence of clinically diagnosed central retinal artery occlusion in Korea, 2008 to 2011. Ophthalmology. 2014;121(10):1933–8. https://doi.org/10.1016/j.ophtha.2014.04.029. Epub 2014 Jun 7. PMID: 24913283.
3. Flaxel CJ, Adelman RA, Bailey ST, Fawzi A, Lim JI, Vemulakonda GA, Ying GS. Retinal and ophthalmic artery occlusions preferred practice pattern®. Ophthalmology. 2020;127(2):259–87. https://doi.org/10.1016/j.ophtha.2019.09.028. Epub 2019 Sep 25. Erratum in: Ophthalmology. 2020 Sep;127(9):1280. PMID: 31757501.
4. Scoles D, McGeehan B, VanderBeek BL. The association of stroke with central and branch retinal arterial occlusion. Eye (Lond). 2022;36(4):835–43. https://doi.org/10.1038/s41433-021-01546-6. Epub 2021 Apr 28. PMID: 33911211; PMCID: PMC8956663.
5. Lee WA, Liao IC. Giant cell arteritis presenting as central retinal artery occlusion. QJM. 2022;115(1):32–3. https://doi.org/10.1093/qjmed/hcab196. PMID: 34264347.
6. Guclu H, Gurlu VP, Ozal SA, Guclu O. Central retinal artery occlusion in Takayasu's arteritis as the first presentation of the disease. Case Rep Ophthalmol Med. 2016;2016:6492513. https://doi.org/10.1155/2016/6492513. Epub 2016 Oct 27. PMID: 27867673; PMCID: PMC5102719.
7. Kaushik S, Gupta A, Gupta V, Jain S, Lal V. Retinal arterial occlusion in Takayasu's arteritis. Indian J Ophthalmol. 2005;53(3):194–6. https://doi.org/10.4103/0301-4738.16680. PMID: 16137966.
8. Emad Y, Basaffar S, Ragab Y, Zeinhom F, Gheita T. A case of polyarteritis nodosa complicated by left central retinal artery occlusion, ischemic optic neuropathy, and retinal vasculitis. Clin Rheumatol. 2007;26(5):814–6. https://doi.org/10.1007/s10067-006-0270-x. Epub 2006 Mar 31. PMID: 16575492.
9. Hsu CT, Kerrison JB, Miller NR, Goldberg MF. Choroidal infarction, anterior ischemic optic neuropathy, and central retinal artery occlusion from polyarteritis nodosa. Retina. 2001;21(4):348–51. https://doi.org/10.1097/00006982-200108000-00009. PMID: 11508881.
10. Thurtell MJ, Rucker JC. Transient visual loss. Int Ophthalmol Clin. 2009;49(3):147–66. https://doi.org/10.1097/IIO.0b013e3181a8d41f. PMID: 19584627.
11. Mitchell P, Wang JJ, Smith W. Risk factors and significance of finding asymptomatic retinal emboli. Clin Exp Ophthalmol. 2000;28(1):13–7. https://doi.org/10.1046/j.1442-9071.2000.00218.x. PMID: 11345337.
12. Klein R, Klein BE, Jensen SC, Moss SE, Meuer SM. Retinal emboli and stroke: the Beaver Dam Eye Study. Arch Ophthalmol. 1999;117(8):1063–8. https://doi.org/10.1001/archopht.117.8.1063. PMID: 10448750.
13. Tobalem S, Schutz JS, Chronopoulos A. Central retinal artery occlusion—rethinking retinal survival time. BMC Ophthalmol. 2018;18(1):101. https://doi.org/10.1186/s12886-018-0768-4. PMID: 29669523; PMCID: PMC5907384.
14. Brown GC, Magargal LE. Central retinal artery obstruction and visual acuity. Ophthalmology. 1982;89(1):14–9. https://doi.org/10.1016/s0161-6420(82)34853-8. PMID: 7070767.
15. Sharma S, Brown GC, Pater JL, Cruess AF. Does a visible retinal embolus increase the likelihood of hemodynamically significant carotid artery stenosis in patients with acute retinal arterial occlusion? Arch Ophthalmol. 1998;116(12):1602–6. https://doi.org/10.1001/archopht.116.12.1602. PMID: 9869788.
16. Sharma S, Naqvi A, Sharma SM, Cruess AF, Brown GC. Transthoracic echocardiographic findings in patients with acute retinal arterial obstruction. A retrospective review. Retinal Emboli of Cardiac Origin Group. Arch Ophthalmol. 1996;114(10):1189–92. https://doi.org/10.1001/archopht.1996.01100140389004. PMID: 8859076.
17. Hayreh SS, Zimmerman MB. Ocular arterial occlusive disorders and carotid artery disease. Ophthalmol Retina. 2017;1(1):12–8. https://doi.org/10.1016/j.oret.2016.08.003. PMID: 28547004; PMCID: PMC5439962.
18. Arruga J, Sanders MD. Ophthalmologic findings in 70 patients with evidence of retinal embolism. Ophthalmology. 1982;89(12):1336–47. https://doi.org/10.1016/s0161-6420(82)34626-6. PMID: 7162779.
19. Ardila Jurado E, Sturm V, Brugger F, Nedeltchev K, Arnold M, Bonati LH, Carrera E, Michel P, Cereda CW, Bolognese M, Albert S, Medlin F, Berger C, Schelosky L, Renaud S, Niederhauser J, Bonvin C, Mono ML, Rodic B, Tarnutzer AA, Schwegler G,

Salmen S, Luft AR, Peters N, Vehoff J, Kägi G, Swiss Stroke Registry Investigators. Central retinal artery occlusion: current practice, awareness and prehospital delays in Switzerland. Front Neurol. 2022;13:888456. https://doi.org/10.3389/fneur.2022.888456. PMID: 35677327; PMCID: PMC9167925.

20. Cugati S, Varma DD, Chen CS, Lee AW. Treatment options for central retinal artery occlusion. Curr Treat Options Neurol. 2013;15(1):63–77. https://doi.org/10.1007/s11940-012-0202-9. PMID: 23070637; PMCID: PMC3553407.
21. Thangamathesvaran L, Miller SC, Tsou B, Fliotsos MJ, Yonekawa Y, Chen A, Hoskin AK, Blanch RJ, Cavuoto K, Meeralakshmi P, Low R, Gardiner M, Alvin Liu TY, Agrawal R, Justin GA, Woreta FA, International Globe and Adnexal Trauma Epidemiology Study (IGATES)(18) Group. Global current practice patterns for the management of central retinal artery occlusion. Ophthalmol Retina. 2022;6(5):429–31. https://doi.org/10.1016/j.oret.2022.01.014. Epub 2022 Jan 31. PMID: 35101631.
22. Schumacher M, Schmidt D, Jurklies B, Gall C, Wanke I, Schmoor C, Maier-Lenz H, Solymosi L, Brueckmann H, Neubauer AS, Wolf A, Feltgen N, EAGLE-Study Group. Central retinal artery occlusion: local intra-arterial fibrinolysis versus conservative treatment, a multicenter randomized trial. Ophthalmology. 2010;117(7):1367–75.e1. https://doi.org/10.1016/j.ophtha.2010.03.061. PMID: 20609991.
23. Mac Grory B, Schrag M, Biousse V, Furie KL, Gerhard-Herman M, Lavin PJ, Sobrin L, Tjoumakaris SI, Weyand CM, Yaghi S, American Heart Association Stroke Council; Council on Arteriosclerosis, Thrombosis and Vascular Biology; Council on Hypertension; and Council on Peripheral Vascular Disease. Management of central retinal artery occlusion: a scientific statement from the American Heart Association. Stroke. 2021;52(6):e282–94. https://doi.org/10.1161/STR.0000000000000366. Epub 2021 Mar 8. Erratum in: Stroke 2021 Jun;52(6):e309. PMID: 33677974.
24. Klein R, Klein BE, Moss SE, Meuer SM. The epidemiology of retinal vein occlusion: the Beaver Dam Eye Study. Trans Am Ophthalmol Soc. 2000;98:133–41; discussion 141–3. PMID: 11190017; PMCID: PMC1298220.
25. Klein R, Moss SE, Meuer SM, Klein BE. The 15-year cumulative incidence of retinal vein occlusion: the Beaver Dam Eye Study. Arch Ophthalmol. 2008;126(4):513–8. https://doi.org/10.1001/archopht.126.4.513. PMID: 18413521.
26. Rogers S, McIntosh RL, Cheung N, Lim L, Wang JJ, Mitchell P, Kowalski JW, Nguyen H, Wong TY, International Eye Disease Consortium. The prevalence of retinal vein occlusion: pooled data from population studies from the United States, Europe, Asia, and Australia. Ophthalmology. 2010;117(2):313–9.e1. https://doi.org/10.1016/j.ophtha.2009.07.017. PMID: 20022117; PMCID: PMC2945292.
27. Rogers SL, McIntosh RL, Lim L, Mitchell P, Cheung N, Kowalski JW, Nguyen HP, Wang JJ, Wong TY. Natural history of branch retinal vein occlusion: an evidence-based systematic review. Ophthalmology. 2010;117(6):1094–1101.e5. https://doi.org/10.1016/j.ophtha.2010.01.058. PMID: 20430447.
28. Cugati S, Wang JJ, Knudtson MD, Rochtchina E, Klein R, Klein BE, Wong TY, Mitchell P. Retinal vein occlusion and vascular mortality: pooled data analysis of 2 population-based cohorts. Ophthalmology. 2007;114(3):520–4. https://doi.org/10.1016/j.ophtha.2006.06.061. Epub 2006 Nov 30. PMID: 17141315.
29. Group. Baseline and early natural history report. The central vein occlusion study. Arch Ophthalmol. 1993;111(8):1087–95. https://doi.org/10.1001/archopht.1993.01090080083022. PMID: 7688950.
30. Group. Risk factors for branch retinal vein occlusion. The Eye Disease Case-control Study Group. Am J Ophthalmol. 1993;116(3):286–96. PMID: 8357052.
31. Weinberg D, Dodwell DG, Fern SA. Anatomy of arteriovenous crossings in branch retinal vein occlusion. Am J Ophthalmol. 1990;109(3):298–302. https://doi.org/10.1016/s0002-9394(14)74554-4. PMID: 2309862.
32. Christoffersen NL, Larsen M. Pathophysiology and hemodynamics of branch retinal vein occlusion. Ophthalmology. 1999;106(11):2054–62. https://doi.org/10.1016/S0161-6420(99)90483-9. PMID: 10571337.
33. Hayreh SS, Zimmerman MB. Branch retinal vein occlusion: natural history of visual outcome. JAMA Ophthalmol. 2014;132(1):13–22. https://doi.org/10.1001/jamaophthalmol.2013.5515. PMID: 24158729.
34. Suzuki N, Hirano Y, Tomiyasu T, Kurobe R, Yasuda Y, Esaki Y, Yasukawa T, Yoshida M, Ogura Y. Collateral vessels on optical coherence tomography angiography in eyes with branch retinal vein occlusion. Br J Ophthalmol. 2019;103(10):1373–9. https://doi.org/10.1136/bjophthalmol-2018-313322. Epub 2018 Nov 22. PMID: 30467130.
35. Freund KB, Sarraf D, Leong BCS, Garrity ST, Vupparaboina KK, Dansingani KK. Association of optical coherence tomography angiography of collaterals in retinal vein occlusion with major venous outflow through the deep vascular complex. JAMA Ophthalmol. 2018;136(11):1262–70. https://doi.org/10.1001/jamaophthalmol.2018.3586. PMID: 30352115; PMCID: PMC6248171.
36. Group. Argon laser photocoagulation for macular edema in branch vein occlusion. The Branch Vein Occlusion Study Group. Am J Ophthalmol. 1984;98(3):271–82. https://doi.org/10.1016/0002-9394(84)90316-7. PMID: 6383055.
37. Tomiyasu T, Hirano Y, Yoshida M, Suzuki N, Nishiyama T, Uemura A, Yasukawa T, Ogura Y. Microaneurysms cause refractory macular edema in branch retinal vein occlusion. Sci Rep. 2016;6:29445.

https://doi.org/10.1038/srep29445. PMID: 27389770; PMCID: PMC4937381.
38. An Y, Park SP, Kim YK. Aqueous humour inflammatory cytokine levels and choroidal thickness in patients with macular edema associated with branch retinal vein occlusion. Int Ophthalmol. 2021;41(7):2433–44. https://doi.org/10.1007/s10792-021-01798-x. Epub 2021 Mar 19. PMID: 33740201.
39. Schmidt-Erfurth U, Garcia-Arumi J, Gerendas BS, Midena E, Sivaprasad S, Tadayoni R, Wolf S, Loewenstein A. Guidelines for the management of retinal vein occlusion by the European Society of Retina Specialists (EURETINA). Ophthalmologica. 2019;242(3):123–62. https://doi.org/10.1159/000502041. Epub 2019 Aug 14. PMID: 31412332.
40. Tan MH, McAllister IL, Gillies ME, Verma N, Banerjee G, Smithies LA, Wong WL, Wong TY. Randomized controlled trial of intravitreal ranibizumab versus standard grid laser for macular edema following branch retinal vein occlusion. Am J Ophthalmol. 2014;157(1):237–247.e1. https://doi.org/10.1016/j.ajo.2013.08.013. Epub 2013 Oct 7. PMID: 24112635.
41. Shalchi Z, Mahroo O, Bunce C, Mitry D. Anti-vascular endothelial growth factor for macular oedema secondary to branch retinal vein occlusion. Cochrane Database Syst Rev. 2020;7(7):CD009510. https://doi.org/10.1002/14651858.CD009510.pub3. PMID: 32633861; PMCID: PMC7388176.
42. Zou W, Du Y, Ji X, Zhang J, Ding H, Chen J, Wang T, Ji F, Huang J. Comparison of the efficiency of anti-VEGF drugs intravitreal injections treatment with or without retinal laser photocoagulation for macular edema secondary to retinal vein occlusion: a systematic review and meta-analysis. Front Pharmacol. 2022;13:948852. https://doi.org/10.3389/fphar.2022.948852. PMID: 35935843; PMCID: PMC9355043.
43. Miao J, Yu J, Zou W, Su N, Peng Z, Wu X, Huang J, Fang Y, Yuan S, Xie P, Huang K, Chen Q, Hu Z, Liu Q. Deep learning models for segmenting non-perfusion area of color fundus photographs in patients with branch retinal vein occlusion. Front Med (Lausanne). 2022;9:794045. https://doi.org/10.3389/fmed.2022.794045. PMID: 35847781; PMCID: PMC9279621.
44. Hayreh SS, Zimmerman MB. Fundus changes in branch retinal vein occlusion. Retina. 2015;35(5):1016–27. https://doi.org/10.1097/IAE.0000000000000418. PMID: 25574785; PMCID: PMC4408204.
45. Group. Argon laser scatter photocoagulation for prevention of neovascularization and vitreous hemorrhage in branch vein occlusion. A randomized clinical trial. Branch Vein Occlusion Study Group. Arch Ophthalmol. 1986;104(1):34–41. https://doi.org/10.1001/archopht.1986.01050130044017. PMID: 2417579.
46. Hayreh SS, Rubenstein L, Podhajsky P. Argon laser scatter photocoagulation in treatment of branch retinal vein occlusion. A prospective clinical trial. Ophthalmologica. 1993;206(1):1–14. https://doi.org/10.1159/000310354. PMID: 7506400.
47. Recchia FM, Brown GC. Systemic disorders associated with retinal vascular occlusion. Curr Opin Ophthalmol. 2000;11(6):462–7. https://doi.org/10.1097/00055735-200012000-00013. PMID: 11141642.
48. Romiti GF, Corica B, Borgi M, Visioli G, Pacella E, Cangemi R, Proietti M, Basili S, Raparelli V. Inherited and acquired thrombophilia in adults with retinal vascular occlusion: a systematic review and meta-analysis. J Thromb Haemost. 2020;18(12):3249–66. https://doi.org/10.1111/jth.15068. Epub 2020 Oct 6. PMID: 32805772.
49. Taylor AW, Sehu W, Williamson TH, Lee WR. Morphometric assessment of the central retinal artery and vein in the optic nerve head. Can J Ophthalmol. 1993;28(7):320–4. PMID: 8313218.
50. McAllister IL. Central retinal vein occlusion: a review. Clin Exp Ophthalmol. 2012;40(1):48–58. https://doi.org/10.1111/j.1442-9071.2011.02713.x. Epub 2011 Dec 6. PMID: 22003973.
51. Scott IU, Campochiaro PA, Newman NJ, Biousse V. Retinal vascular occlusions. Lancet. 2020;396(10266):1927–40. https://doi.org/10.1016/S0140-6736(20)31559-2. PMID: 33308475.
52. Green WR, Chan CC, Hutchins GM, Terry JM. Central retinal vein occlusion: a prospective histopathologic study of 29 eyes in 28 cases. Trans Am Ophthalmol Soc. 1981;79:371–422. PMID: 7342407; PMCID: PMC1312193.
53. Hayreh SS, Podhajsky PA, Zimmerman MB. Natural history of visual outcome in central retinal vein occlusion. Ophthalmology. 2011;118(1):119–133.e1–2. https://doi.org/10.1016/j.ophtha.2010.04.019. Epub 2010 Aug 17. PMID: 20723991; PMCID: PMC2989417.
54. Hayreh SS. Classification of central retinal vein occlusion. Ophthalmology. 1983;90(5):458–74. https://doi.org/10.1016/s0161-6420(83)34530-9. PMID: 6877778.
55. Hayreh SS, Klugman MR, Podhajsky P, Kolder HE. Electroretinography in central retinal vein occlusion. Correlation of electroretinographic changes with pupillary abnormalities. Graefes Arch Clin Exp Ophthalmol. 1989;227(6):549–61. https://doi.org/10.1007/BF02169451. PMID: 2483144.
56. Hayreh SS, Fraterrigo L, Jonas J. Central retinal vein occlusion associated with cilioretinal artery occlusion. Retina. 2008;28(4):581–94. https://doi.org/10.1097/IAE.0b013e31815ec29b. PMID: 18398361.
57. McLeod D. Central retinal vein occlusion with cilioretinal infarction from branch flow exclusion and choroidal arterial steal. Retina. 2009;29(10):1381–95. https://doi.org/10.1097/IAE.0b013e3181b85f41. PMID: 19898176.

58. Ravani R, Chawla R, Jain S, Kumar A. "Dye front reciprocation" in combined central retinal vein occlusion with cilioretinal artery infarction. Indian J Ophthalmol. 2017;65(11):1211–2. https://doi.org/10.4103/ijo.IJO_552_17. PMID: 29133654; PMCID: PMC5700596.
59. Pichi F, Fragiotta S, Freund KB, Au A, Lembo A, Nucci P, Sebastiani S, Gutierrez Hernandez JC, Interlandi E, Pellegrini F, Dolz-Marco R, Gallego-Pinazo R, Orellana-Rios J, Adatia FA, Munro M, Abboud EB, Ghazi N, Cunha Souza E, Amer R, Neri P, Sarraf D. Cilioretinal artery hypoperfusion and its association with paracentral acute middle maculopathy. Br J Ophthalmol. 2019;103(8):1137–45. https://doi.org/10.1136/bjophthalmol-2018-312774. Epub 2018 Sep 26. PMID: 30257961.
60. Antaki F, Milad D, Sahyoun JY, Coussa RG. Paracentral acute middle maculopathy in non-ischaemic central retinal vein occlusion: the role of en face optical coherence tomography. BMJ Case Rep. 2021;14(11):e246842. https://doi.org/10.1136/bcr-2021-246842. PMID: 34764101; PMCID: PMC8587704.
61. Rahimy E, Sarraf D, Dollin ML, Pitcher JD, Ho AC. Paracentral acute middle maculopathy in non-ischemic central retinal vein occlusion. Am J Ophthalmol. 2014;158(2):372–380.e1. https://doi.org/10.1016/j.ajo.2014.04.024. Epub 2014 May 1. PMID: 24794089.
62. Iyer PG, Swaminathan SS, Trivizki O, Shi Y, Shen M, Kansora M, Gregori G, Rosenfeld PJ. Widefield *en face* optical coherence tomography monitoring of the peri-venular fern-like pattern of paracentral acute middle maculopathy. Am J Ophthalmol Case Rep. 2021;22:101047. https://doi.org/10.1016/j.ajoc.2021.101047. PMID: 33763621; PMCID: PMC7973291.
63. Ferrara N. Vascular endothelial growth factor: basic science and clinical progress. Endocr Rev. 2004;25(4):581–611. https://doi.org/10.1210/er.2003-0027. PMID: 15294883.
64. Aiello LP, Avery RL, Arrigg PG, Keyt BA, Jampel HD, Shah ST, Pasquale LR, Thieme H, Iwamoto MA, Park JE, et al. Vascular endothelial growth factor in ocular fluid of patients with diabetic retinopathy and other retinal disorders. N Engl J Med. 1994;331(22):1480–7. https://doi.org/10.1056/NEJM199412013312203. PMID: 7526212.
65. Funk M, Kriechbaum K, Prager F, Benesch T, Georgopoulos M, Zlabinger GJ, Schmidt-Erfurth U. Intraocular concentrations of growth factors and cytokines in retinal vein occlusion and the effect of therapy with bevacizumab. Invest Ophthalmol Vis Sci. 2009;50(3):1025–32. https://doi.org/10.1167/iovs.08-2510. Epub 2008 Dec 5. PMID: 19060280.
66. Ehlken C, Rennel ES, Michels D, Grundel B, Pielen A, Junker B, Stahl A, Hansen LL, Feltgen N, Agostini HT, Martin G. Levels of VEGF but not VEGF(165b) are increased in the vitreous of patients with retinal vein occlusion. Am J Ophthalmol. 2011;152(2):298–303.e1. https://doi.org/10.1016/j.ajo.2011.01.040. Epub 2011 May 28. PMID: 21621189.
67. Ferrara N. From the discovery of vascular endothelial growth factor to the introduction of avastin in clinical trials—an interview with Napoleone Ferrara by Domenico Ribatti. Int J Dev Biol. 2011;55(4–5):383–8. https://doi.org/10.1387/ijdb.103216dr. PMID: 21858763.
68. Ferrara N, Damico L, Shams N, Lowman H, Kim R. Development of ranibizumab, an anti-vascular endothelial growth factor antigen binding fragment, as therapy for neovascular age-related macular degeneration. Retina. 2006;26(8):859–70. https://doi.org/10.1097/01.iae.0000242842.14624.e7. PMID: 17031284.
69. Campochiaro PA, Hafiz G, Shah SM, Nguyen QD, Ying H, Do DV, Quinlan E, Zimmer-Galler I, Haller JA, Solomon SD, Sung JU, Hadi Y, Janjua KA, Jawed N, Choy DF, Arron JR. Ranibizumab for macular edema due to retinal vein occlusions: implication of VEGF as a critical stimulator. Mol Ther. 2008;16(4):791–9. https://doi.org/10.1038/mt.2008.10. Epub 2008 Feb 5. PMID: 18362932.
70. Kida T, Flammer J, Konieczka K, Ikeda T. Retinal venous pressure is decreased after anti-VEGF therapy in patients with retinal vein occlusion-related macular edema. Graefes Arch Clin Exp Ophthalmol. 2021;259(7):1853–8. https://doi.org/10.1007/s00417-020-05068-x. Epub 2021 Jan 15. PMID: 33447857; PMCID: PMC8277612.
71. Gale R, Gill C, Pikoula M, Lee AY, Hanson RLW, Denaxas S, Egan C, Tufail A, Taylor P, UK EMR Database Users Group. Multicentre study of 4626 patients assesses the effectiveness, safety and burden of two categories of treatments for central retinal vein occlusion: intravitreal anti-vascular endothelial growth factor injections and intravitreal Ozurdex injections. Br J Ophthalmol. 2021;105(11):1571–6. https://doi.org/10.1136/bjophthalmol-2020-317306. Epub 2020 Sep 22. PMID: 32962992; PMCID: PMC8140590.
72. Qian T, Zhao M, Xu X. Comparison between anti-VEGF therapy and corticosteroid or laser therapy for macular oedema secondary to retinal vein occlusion: a meta-analysis. J Clin Pharm Ther. 2017;42(5):519–29. https://doi.org/10.1111/jcpt.12551. Epub 2017 Jun 22. PMID: 28639290.
73. Nanji K, Khan M, Khalid MF, Xie JS, Sarohia GS, Phillips M, Thabane L, Garg SJ, Kaiser P, Sivaprasad S, Wykoff CC, Chaudhary V. Treat-and-extend regimens of anti-vascular endothelial growth factor therapy for retinal vein occlusions: a systematic review and meta-analysis. Acta Ophthalmol. 2022;100(6):e1199–208. https://doi.org/10.1111/aos.15068. Epub 2021 Nov 29. PMID: 34845830.
74. Scott IU, VanVeldhuisen PC, Oden NL, Ip MS, Blodi BA, SCORE2 Investigator Group. Month 60 outcomes after treatment initiation with anti-vascular endothelial growth factor therapy for macular edema due to central retinal or hemiretinal vein occlusion.

Am J Ophthalmol. 2022;240:330–41. https://doi.org/10.1016/j.ajo.2022.04.001. Epub 2022 Apr 21. PMID: 35461831.

75. Spooner KL, Fraser-Bell S, Hong T, Wong JG, Chang AA. Long-term outcomes of anti-VEGF treatment of retinal vein occlusion. Eye (Lond). 2022;36(6):1194–201. https://doi.org/10.1038/s41433-021-01620-z. Epub 2021 Jun 11. PMID: 34117379; PMCID: PMC9151794.
76. Hayreh SS. Photocoagulation for retinal vein occlusion. Prog Retin Eye Res. 2021;85:100964. https://doi.org/10.1016/j.preteyeres.2021.100964. Epub 2021 Mar 11. PMID: 33713810.
77. Brown DM, Wykoff CC, Wong TP, Mariani AF, Croft DE, Schuetzle KL, RAVE Study Group. Ranibizumab in preproliferative (ischemic) central retinal vein occlusion: the rubeosis anti-VEGF (RAVE) trial. Retina. 2014;34(9):1728–35. https://doi.org/10.1097/IAE.0000000000000191. PMID: 24914476.
78. Khayat M, Williams M, Lois N. Ischemic retinal vein occlusion: characterizing the more severe spectrum of retinal vein occlusion. Surv Ophthalmol. 2018;63(6):816–50. https://doi.org/10.1016/j.survophthal.2018.04.005. Epub 2018 Apr 27. PMID: 29705175.
79. Abu El-Asrar AM, Herbort CP, Tabbara KF. Differential diagnosis of retinal vasculitis. Middle East Afr J Ophthalmol. 2009;16(4):202–18. https://doi.org/10.4103/0974-9233.58423. PMID: 20404987; PMCID: PMC2855661.
80. Bansal R, Moharana B, Katoch D, Gupta V, Dogra MR, Gupta A. Outcome of pars plana vitrectomy in patients with retinal detachments secondary to retinal vasculitis. Indian J Ophthalmol. 2020;68(9):1905–11. https://doi.org/10.4103/ijo.IJO_551_20. PMID: 32823412; PMCID: PMC7690542.
81. Gupta A, Gupta V, Arora S, Dogra MR, Bambery P. PCR-positive tubercular retinal vasculitis: clinical characteristics and management. Retina. 2001;21(5):435–44. https://doi.org/10.1097/00006982-200110000-00004. PMID: 11642371.
82. Gupta A, Bansal R, Gupta V, Sharma A, Bambery P. Ocular signs predictive of tubercular uveitis. Am J Ophthalmol. 2010;149(4):562–70. https://doi.org/10.1016/j.ajo.2009.11.020. Epub 2010 Feb 10. PMID: 20149341.

Retinal and Choroidal Infections and Inflammation

10

10.1 Anatomical Considerations

Anatomically, the eye is divided into an anterior chamber (AC), a posterior chamber (PC), and a posterior segment consisting of the vitreous cavity, retina, and choroid. The cornea, iris, and anterior part of the ciliary body enclose the AC. The PC is bound anteriorly by the iris, laterally by the pars ciliaris, and posteriorly by the crystalline lens and the zonular fibres. The AC and PC are filled with a transparent fluid, the aqueous humour, which is continuously secreted by the ciliary epithelium into the PC, and a pressure gradient its movement through the pupil into the AC and exits the eye through trabecular meshwork in the angle of the anterior chamber. The cornea is lined with a single layer of hexagonal cells, the endothelial cells arranged in a honeycomb pattern. Like the brain and testes, the eye is an immune-privileged site. The privilege is maintained via an outer retinal barrier by the retinal pigment epithelium cells between the choroid and the retina, the pigmented epithelial cells that line the iris and ciliary body, and a blood-retinal barrier by the tight endothelial cell junctions in the retinal vessels.

One of the major strategies to maintain the eye's immune privilege is the phenomenon of anterior chamber-associated immune deviation (ACAID). The ocular barriers allow only the exchange of oxygen, fluid, and micronutrients within the eye. These barriers also ensure that no noxious agents or cellular elements can enter the retina, vitreous cavity, AC, or PC under normal circumstances. The neurosensory retina consists of three post-mitotic retinal cell layers, namely the photoreceptors (rods and cones, first neuron), bipolar cells (second neuron), and retinal ganglion cells (third neuron) and their connecting fibres, the outer and the inner plexiform layers. Muller cells, the macroglia, extend through the entire thickness of the retina. Their footplates form the inner limiting membrane, and their processes contact the photoreceptors at the junction of the inner and outer segments to form an external limiting membrane.

Along with the microglia, the resident macrophages, Muller cell processes form very intimate contact with photoreceptors, bipolar cells, horizontal cells, amacrine cells, ganglion cells, and the retinal capillary endothelial cells and form a neurovascular complex that controls the retinal microenvironment and homeostasis. The microglia are found in the retina's inner and outer plexiform layers in their inactivated state. Once activated by any insult, they become activated macrophages, move through the retina, and produce cytokines. Notably, there are no progenitor cells in the retina; once the cells die or undergo apoptosis, there is no replacement.

A. Gupta et al., *Ophthalmic Signs in Practice of Medicine*,
https://doi.org/10.1007/978-981-99-7923-3_10

10.2 Mediators of Inflammation

A revolution in cell biology was heralded by the discovery of interferons by Issacs and Lindenmann in 1957 [1]. These molecules blocked and interfered with the replication of viruses. It was followed by the discovery of interleukins (ILs) and a host of similar molecules called cytokines that were abbreviated IL. As more of these were discovered, they were sequentially numbered as IL-1 and onwards [2]. Cytokines are short-lived cell surface proteins that cannot enter the cells but dictate the activation of a host of intracellular signalling pathways involved in normal physiological and pathological pathways. The cells interact with each other via cytokines. The cytokines control the behaviour of cells, including their activation, differentiation, and proliferation, and even decide if the cells should die or produce more cytokines. Cytokines are further subdivided into interferons (prevent viral replication), interleukins (the largest cytokine family for cell-to-cell talking), chemokines (proteins that control trafficking and migration of cells), and tumour necrosis factor-α (TNF-α, a cytokine produced by macrophages, lymphocytes, granulocytes responsible for acute inflammation, cell death, and apoptosis).

The macrophages and B lymphocytes produce IL-1, a pro-inflammatory cytokine that activates the T-helper cells. The IL-2, also a pro-inflammatory cytokine, activates Th-1 helper cells and furthers the proliferation of T cells. IL-6 helps differentiate B lymphocytes into plasma cells and produce antibodies, hence a critical player in inflammation. There is a lot of redundancy and pleiotropy in the functioning of the cytokines. More than one cell type can produce multiple cytokines, which can interact with several different cells. [3].

Briefly, IL-1 is produced by macrophages and B cells, stimulates T-helper cells, and plays a role in inflammation; IL-2 is produced by the Th1 cells and causes proliferation and differentiation of T cells; IL-6 is produced by a variety of cells such as B cells, Th2 cells, macrophages, and endothelial cells and helps in differentiation of B cells into plasma cells and antibody production. It is a key regulator of inflammation; IL-17 is secreted by the Th17 cells. TNF-α, an acute phase reactant, is produced by macrophages, monocytes, lymphocytes, and granulocytes and is responsible for acute inflammation [3].

In their functions, the cytokines are either pro-inflammatory or anti-inflammatory, e.g. in acute inflammation, IL-1 and TNF-α act together to worsen the inflammatory response. Once the infection is controlled, these stop expressing themselves, and the inflammation dies. The IL-10 and TGF-β are anti-inflammatory and get upregulated in the ocular fluids once the inflammation is controlled. In people predisposed to autoimmune disorders, the genes expressing the pro-inflammatory cytokines never shut down entirely, thus perpetuating the autoimmune inflammatory response [4]. Among the cytokines detected in the intraocular fluids and serum of patients with endogenous uveitis include TNF-α, IL-1β, IL-6, IL-10, and IL-17 [5–7]. Developing antibodies to block these cytokines has revolutionized the treatment of systemic autoimmune disorders, including endogenous uveitis [8], and will be discussed in a later section.

10.3 Retinal and Choroidal Infections and Inflammations: Definition

As defined by the Standardization of Uveitis Nomenclature (SUN) working group, the term posterior uveitis includes all intraocular infections and inflammations wherein the primary anatomical site, as determined by clinical examination, is either in the retina, in the choroid, or both [9]. It includes all cases of focal, multifocal, diffuse choroiditis, chorioretinitis, retinochoroiditis, retinitis, and neuroretinitis. Some of the inflammatory disorders that may involve the anterior chamber and vitreous, besides the retina and choroid, defined as panuveitis, will also be discussed in this chapter.

10.4 Introduction

While nearly 40–50% of the uveitis entities remain uncharacterized even today, physicians must differentiate infectious uveitis from the more commonly occurring and perhaps better-characterized immune-mediated non-infectious uveitis. Diagnosis of non-infectious uveitis is definitive due to well-characterized ocular phenotypes often associated with systemic autoinflammatory/autoimmune disorders. However, frequent recurrences of inflammation in these patients pose a major management challenge as they often require long-term anti-inflammatory and/or immunosuppressive therapy. However, a large majority of infectious organisms that manage to break the blood-ocular barrier to set up infection/uveitis in the eye, although they can be controlled with highly effective antibiotics and other chemotherapeutic agents, the tendency for these organisms to sequestrate/hibernate or assume latency in the ocular tissues often results in recurrences. The subject of intensive studies is what triggers these organisms' latency and reactivation to cause recurrent inflammation. Detecting organisms responsible for infectious uveitis has also remained a major challenge. Moreover, their phenotypic expression largely depends upon the host's immune status, the organism's infectious dose, and the possibility of multiple simultaneous infections, especially in patients with HIV. Their diagnosis often requires invasive procedures for obtaining ocular fluid samples to reach a definitive diagnosis.

10.5 Differentiating Retinitis from Choroiditis

It is critical to differentiate retinitis from choroiditis clinically. In general, retinitis is infectious in origin and needs specific antimicrobial therapy. An exception to this statement includes Behcet's autoinflammatory multiorgan disease and immune-mediated retinitis caused by vector-borne viral fevers. Infectious retinitis includes toxoplasma gondii, the herpes viruses, syphilis, and other spirochetes like Borrelia burgdorferi (Lyme) and nematodes. The use of corticosteroids in patients with infectious retinitis can be disastrous for the eye. Most of the inflammations in the choroid are primarily immune-mediated (except for cases of the infectious endogenous endophthalmitis) and require corticosteroids for initial control of inflammation and long-term steroid-sparing therapy with immunosuppressive agents. As the focus of infection is set up in the retina, many inflammatory cells, cytokines, and protein-rich exudates are released into the vitreous gel. These accumulate and cause media haze with a spillover into the AC. The inflammatory response is generally dictated by the patient's immune status, being robust in patients with a normal immune system and muted in immunocompromised patients. The inflammatory exudates in the vitreous cavity are far more in patients with retinitis than in choroiditis, and thus, media haze is more in the former than the latter. The retinal vessels coursing through a retinitis lesion are generally obscured in the retinitis lesion but run a normal course over a choroiditis lesion (Fig. 10.1a, b). On FFA, the retinitis lesions show initial hypofluorescence, staining of the retinal vessel walls running through the lesion, and in the late frames, intense hyperfluorescence of the retinal lesion with indistinct borders (Fig. 10.1c, e).

However, on FFA, the choroiditis lesions show discrete areas of initial hypofluorescence and late hyperfluorescence (Fig. 10.1d, f), which is much less exuberant than the retinitis lesions. In general, the retinal vessels overlying a choroiditis lesion remain normal. Choroiditis lesions are more often associated with exudative subretinal fluid than retinitis lesions (Fig. 10.2). Often, the inflammatory lesion in retinitis extends into the choroid, e.g. toxoplasma retinochoroiditis, and a choroiditis lesion may extend into the retina when labelled as chorioretinitis (Figs. 10.1b, d, f and 10.2b). If the retinitis lesions remain confined to the retina, it may result in only minimum pigmentary changes upon healing, whereas the choroiditis lesions heal with heavily pigmented scars (Fig. 10.3). Structural optical coherence

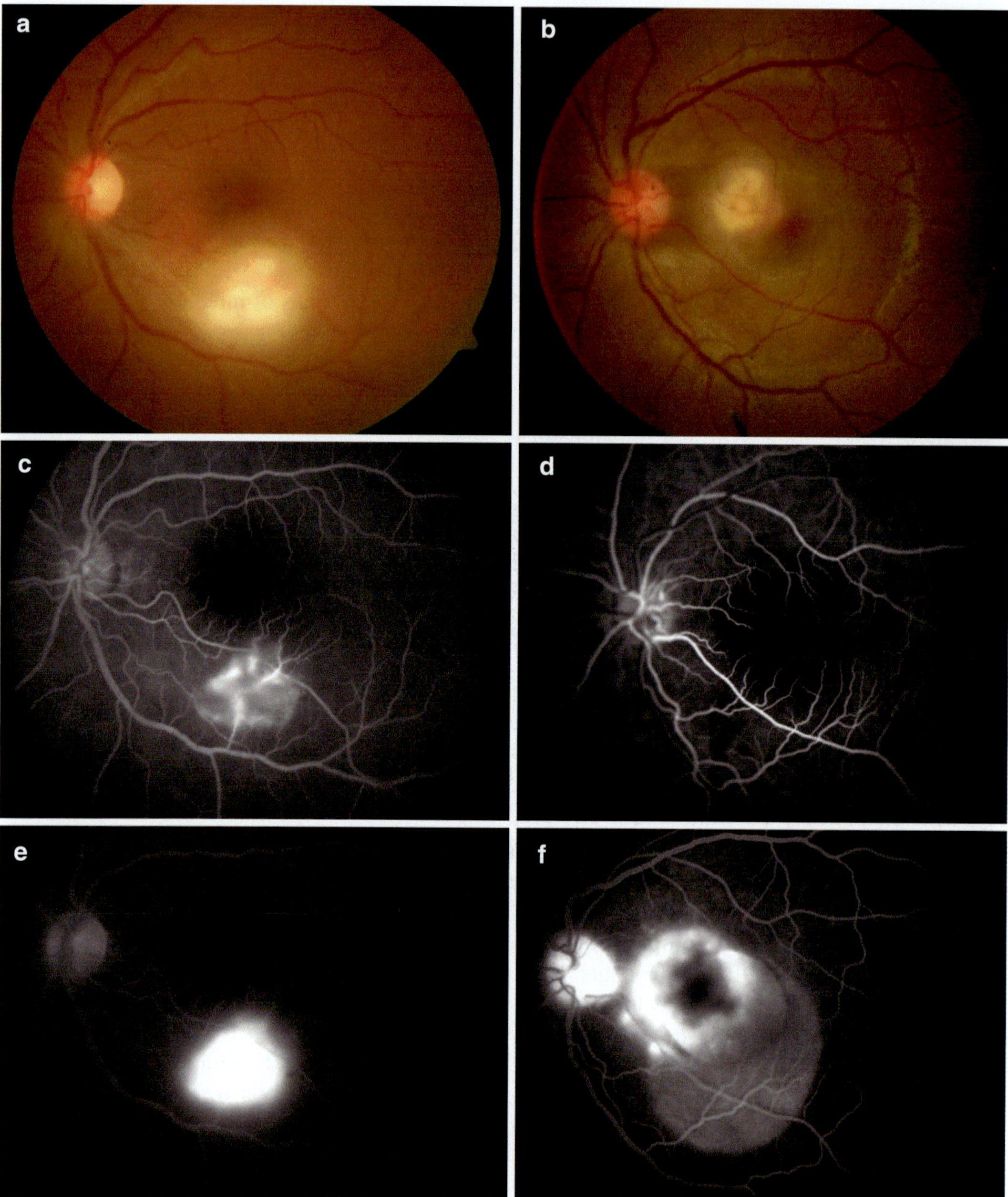

Fig. 10.1 Retinal vessels over a retinitis lesion (**a**) are generally obscured, while they run a normal course over a choroidal lesion (**b**). On FFA, the retinitis lesions show staining of the retinal vessel walls running through the lesion (**c**), while the choroidal lesion shows initial hypofluorescence (**d**). In the late frames of FFA, extensive hyperfluorescence of the retinal lesion with indistinct borders (**e**) is seen, and the choroidal lesion shows hyperfluorescence not as intense as retinitis with dye pooling in the area of exudation (**f**). Note that the example in (**b**, **d**, and **f**) represents a case of chorioretinitis. The intense staining in (**f**) is due to retinal inflammation. (**a**, **c**, and **e** reproduced with permission from *EyeNet Magazine,* Gupta AK, et al., Infectious uveitis-New challenges emerge. September 2014)

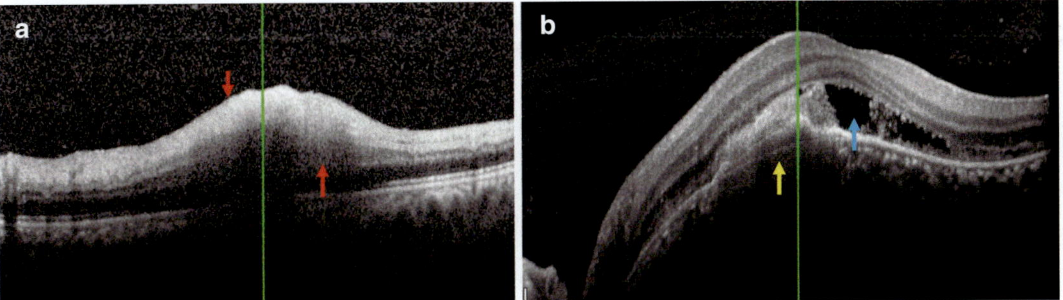

Fig. 10.2 On OCT, the retinitis lesion shows the retinal layers' hyperreflectivity and disorganization (red arrows) (**a**). Choroiditis lesions (granulomas) are associated with exudative subretinal fluid (blue arrow) with a bumpy elevation of the (yellow arrow) of the RPE-Bruch's complex (**b**). Note infiltration of the outer retina from the choroidal granuloma in (**b**)

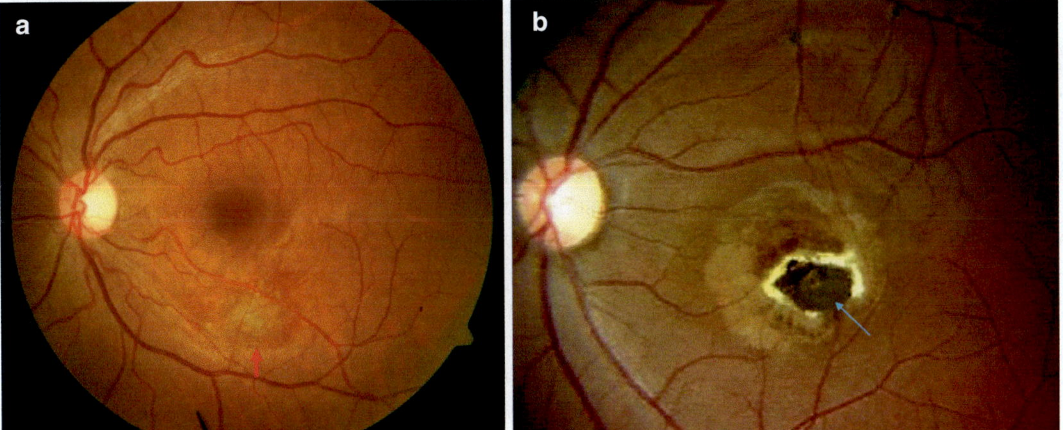

Fig. 10.3 Retinitis lesions (**a**) heal with only minimum pigmentary changes, whereas the choroiditis lesions (**b**) heal with heavily pigmented scars (blue arrow)

tomography (OCT) can easily differentiate between retinitis, retinochoroiditis, choroiditis, and chorioretinitis.

10.6 Infectious Uveitis

10.6.1 Toxoplasmic Retinochoroiditis

10.6.1.1 Prevalence

Toxoplasmosis, a zoonotic disease, is acquired by humans by consumption of raw/undercooked meat or contamination of food with oocysts passed in the cats' litter box. Contaminated municipal water supplies have led to an outbreak of toxoplasmosis epidemic [10]. The infection may also be acquired via the transplacental route from the mothers who get infected during pregnancy or rarely through organ transplants. Contrary to the long-held popular belief that toxoplasmosis is a congenital infection, most cases are now believed to be acquired after birth.

This obligate unicellular parasite poses a global challenge, with nearly 25–30% of the world's population seropositive for toxoplasmosis. It remains the most common cause of infectious uveitis in Brazil, France, and most of the Western world [11]. It is one infection that is preventable by taking appropriate hygienic measures while handling cats' litter, not eating raw meat, and ensuring clean drinking water. Its prevalence in uveitis clinic patients in different regions and periods in the USA has shown a declining trend from 10 to 2.8% [12–16]. It is estimated to cause nearly 20,000 cases of ocular infection in the US population yearly [17]. In European and certain Asian countries, toxoplasma rates have varied from a high of 39% [18] to a low of 2. 3% [19], while the majority have reported the prevalence of toxoplasmic retinochoroiditis in the uveitis clinic to vary from 6 to 10% ([20–30].

From India, the rates have varied from 12% in East India [31] and 8.6–2.5% in South India [32, 33]. In single-centre prevalence studies, a significant decline has been noted in both South India (8.6–5.12%; [34]) and North India (1.69–0.66%; [35, 36]). Very low toxoplasmic retinochoroiditis was also noted in New Delhi, India (0.91%; [37]).

10.6.1.2 Mechanisms of Toxoplasma gondii Infection

Toxoplasma gondii is the subject of intensive studies to address some of the most fundamental questions—how does it reach the eyes, what cells play host to the parasite, how does it remain sequestrated in the retina and other organs, and what leads to egress of the parasites from the host cells to cause inflammation. Following ingestion, the oocysts (from the faeces) or the tissue cysts, the bradyzoites (undercooked meat), and the sporozoites (highly infectious dormant forms of T. gondii) are released from the oocysts that invade the epithelial lining of the intestines and multiply to form the motile tachyzoites (fast replicating). Once released from the tissue cysts (bradyzoites), the tachyzoites enter the circulation either as free or riding in the leucocytes and get widely disseminated to various tissues (muscles, brain, and heart), including the retina [38]. Recently, the pathogenesis of ocular toxoplasmosis was extensively reviewed [39]. The tachyzoites released in the gut must breach the gut epithelial barrier, where they first adhere and then transmigrate through the epithelium into the lamina propria [40]. The *T. gondii* release nanoparticle-sized exosomes containing HSP 70, a chaperone protein, and CD63 protein along with surface marker protein, the P30, and induce expression of IL-12 and TNF-α, which leads to macrophage activation [41]. In the eye, *T. gondii* primarily attacks the retina, where it first adheres and traverses the retinal capillary endothelium through a transcellular or an intercellular path [42]. Unlike in the brain, where the neurons are the preferred host, in the retina, the most preferred cell for sequestration is Muller glial cells. It also infects the RPE cells and leads to the proliferation of the uninfected RPE cells [39].

10.6.1.3 Clinical Diagnosis of Toxoplasma Retinochoroiditis

Of all the infectious uveitis, diagnosis of toxoplasma retinochoroiditis is the least challenging when presenting in immunocompetent patients. The retinal lesion in such patients is characterized by intense focal retinitis, usually smaller than one-disc size, with an overlying intense vitreous reaction leading to the 'lamp in the fog' appearance (Fig. 10.1a). There have been recent developments that facilitate making a clinical diagnosis of this infection. The unique focal vitreous reaction seen in toxoplasma retinochoroiditis can be appreciated by structural OCT that shows the hyperreflective dots in front of the retinitis lesion. There is complete disorganization and thickening of the affected neurosensory retinal layers (Fig. 10.2) and choroidal swelling with hyporeflective spaces under the retinal lesion. The presence of hyporeflective spaces in the retina due to liquefactive necrosis, if present, suggests a poor visual outcome [43]. Coagulative necrosis is a hallmark of the pathology of toxoplasmic retinitis. In fulminant cases, there may be complete necrosis of the neurosensory retina with sparing of the ILM, as is also observed in cases of subacute sclerosing panencephalitis (SSPE) [44, 45]. Even the retinal arterioles away from the lesion may show highly characteristic peri-arterial plaques called the Kyrieleis (Fig. 10.4). On FFA, the retinal vessels within the retinitis lesion tend to show intense staining (Fig. 10.1b). These lesions may be isolated when acquired, but the recurrences are often seen next to a healed pigmented atrophic chorioretinal scar (Fig. 10.5) [46]. In patients with HIV infection, the toxoplasmosis lesions are often bilateral, multifocal, and extensive and may mimic other retinal infections caused by the herpes viruses [47].

10.6.1.4 Laboratory Diagnosis of Toxoplasmic Retinochoroiditis

Laboratory diagnosis of toxoplasmic retinochoroiditis has remained clinical, aided by a positive serology for IgG or IgM antibodies. A negative serology helps to rule out the toxoplasmic aetiology of focal retinitis. Circulating tachyzoites of the T. gondii have been detected in the blood of patients with acute or chronically infected patients with or without toxoplasmic retinochoroiditis, suggesting that they may be responsible for the reactivation of the retinal lesions [48]. In immunocompetent individuals, the sensitivity of PCR for detecting *T. gondii* from the ocular fluids (24%) and blood samples (1.4–16%) has remained unacceptably low and is not recommended. However, it may be valuable in immunocompromised patients where PCR may be positive up to 61.5% from the ocular fluids and 16–45% from the blood. Goldmann-Witmer coefficient to demonstrate a threefold increase in the ocular fluids in immunocompetent patients has remained the standard diagnostic criteria with a sensitivity of nearly 70% irrespective of the immune status [49].

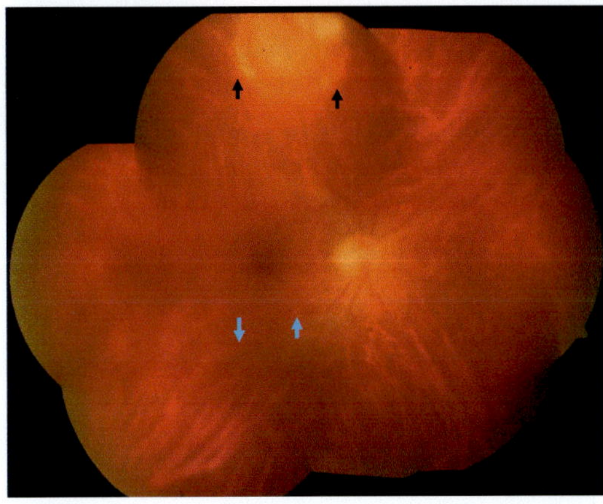

Fig. 10.4 In toxoplasmic retinal infection, the retinal arterioles (blue arrows) away from the retinitis lesion (black arrow) show highly characteristic peri-arterial plaques called the Kyrieleis plaques

10.6.1.5 The Standard of Care for Toxoplasmic Retinochoroiditis

For several decades, the standard of care for toxoplasmic retinochoroiditis has remained oral pyrimethamine, sulphadiazine, and leucovorin, which is highly effective in reducing the size of the toxoplasmic retinochoroiditis lesions compared to the intravitreal clindamycin but cannot be administered in pregnant women due to potential teratogenicity of pyrimethamine besides the risk of myelosuppression, haematological disturbances, and Stevens-Johnson syndrome. Acute toxoplasmic infection, if detected during preg-

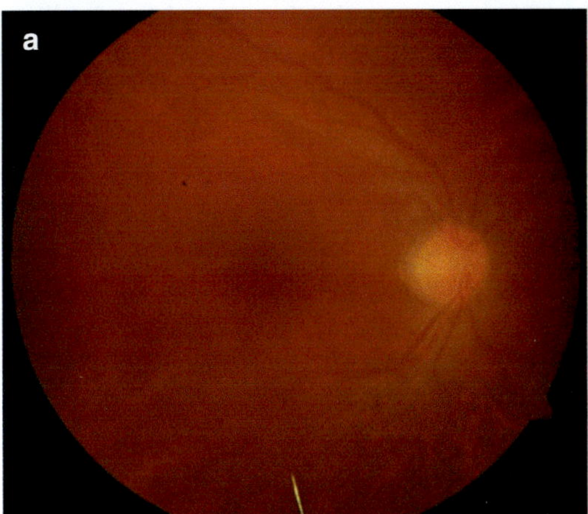

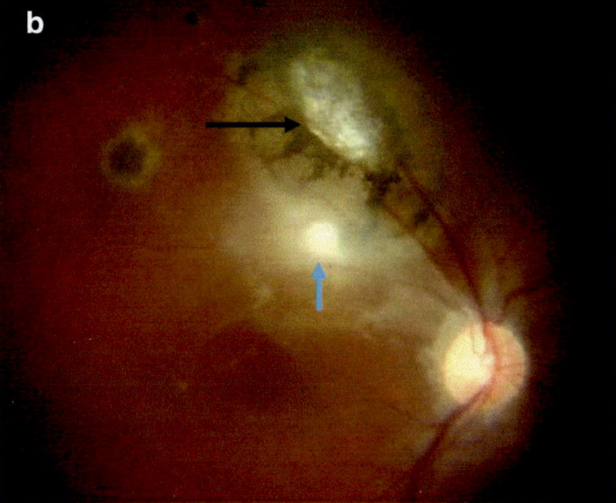

Fig. 10.5 Right eye fundus photograph showing vitreous haze (**a**). Another patient showing a recurrence of retinitis lesion (blue arrow) next to a healed pigmented atrophic chorioretinal scar (black arrow) (**b**)

nancy and managed with oral anti-toxoplasma drugs, prevents the transplacental migration of the infection to the foetus. Spiramycin, a potent macrolide, can be used for a suspected or confirmed toxoplasma infection in pregnancy as it gets concentrated in the placenta but is not transmitted. So far, no antimicrobial agents are available that target the bradyzoites, the tissue cysts of *toxoplasma gondii.* While extensive research is underway to identify or repurpose drugs that target tachyzoites, the search is still on for a strategy to eliminate the cystic stage of toxoplasma [50]. There is a ray of hope from animal experiments following observations that orally bioavailable endochin-like quinolones, especially the ELQ-316 administered as ELQ-334, were effective against both the acute and latent toxoplasma infection and showed a significant reduction in the brain cysts in a mouse model [51].

10.6.1.6 Mechanism of Latency in Toxoplasma gondii Infection

Tachyzoites of *T gondii* are surrounded by a membranous vacuole and convert easily within the nucleated cells into an impenetrable tissue cyst (Bradyzoites), allowing for their latency and persistence. Given an opportunity, these cysts rupture and release numerous tachyzoites, creating another cycle of active inflammation. Recently, the mechanisms that make the toxoplasma hibernate and evade the host's innate immunity have been explored. It was shown that while invading the cell, the parasite injects rhoptry and microneme proteins into the host cell that traffic to the parasitophorous vacuole membrane, nucleus, and cytoplasm [52]. Additionally, once the tachyzoites enter the cell, it transports an inhibitory protein (IST), an inhibitor of the STAT1 transcription, to the host cell to suppress immune signals. It turns off type 1 interferon signalling on the infected cell and is thus successful in evading the innate immune response of the host [53]. As the tachyzoites differentiate into bradyzoites, a change in the transcriptional profile prevents host cell death via apoptotic or necroptotic pathways. Under what conditions the tachyzoites leave the host cell to infect other permissive host cells is probably not a simple cell wall rupture. Still, highly intricate mechanisms facilitate the egress of the tachyzoites from the infected host cell [54].

10.6.2 Infectious Herpes Simplex and Varicella Zoster Virus Retinitis

10.6.2.1 Clinical Signs

The prevalence of anterior and posterior herpes uveitis is rising in clinics worldwide. Unlike tuberculosis, recognized more than 150 years ago, and toxoplasmosis retinochoroiditis more than 70 years ago, acute retinal necrosis (ARN) by the herpes viruses was first reported over 50 years ago in the Japanese literature. In the English literature, Young and Bird [55] described four elderly patients with dense bilateral opacification of the peripheral retina and macula, retinal haemorrhages, and occlusion of vessels in the area of the sloughing retinitis. They called it bilateral acute retinal necrosis [55]. Five of the eight eyes ended up with retinal detachment. The lesions that healed left behind an atrophic retina with sheathed vessels. They suspected it to be caused by the herpes virus, as a similar picture had been described in infants who suffered from herpes viral fever. Using electron microscopy and immunocytopathology techniques, VZV was demonstrated in eyes blinded by ARN [56]. Since then, ARN has been increasingly reported from across the world. In a population-based survey in the UK, the incidence of ARN was reported as 1 case per 1.6 to 2 million population per year [57], and 56% of all those tested were positive for VZV.

In HIV-negative patients, two-thirds of the ARN cases are caused by VZV and less than 25% by HSV [58]. Next to toxoplasmosis, herpes viruses are the commonest cause of infectious uveitis in most parts of the world. Herpes viruses may cause anterior uveitis or necrotizing retinitis. In the posterior segment, varicella zoster virus (VZV), more commonly in the older and the herpes simplex virus (HSV) in the younger individuals, causes blinding necrotizing retinitis irrespective of the immune status. The immunocompetent and the immunocompromised individuals often present with tongue-like areas of necrotic retinal opacification in the periphery that rapidly advance posteriorly and circumferentially (Fig. 10.6). The vitreous reaction is contingent on the immune status of the person being very aggressive in immunocompetent persons but practically shows no reaction in patients living with HIV infection. It remains one of the rare uveitis emergencies that necessitate intravenous acyclovir. Till recently, the diagnosis of ARN was made using the diagnostic criteria by the American Uveitis Society (Box 10.1) [59]. More recently, using machine learning tools from a large database of infectious posterior/pan uveitis (803 cases including 186 of ARN), a fresh set of classification criteria for diagnosis of ARN was developed with an overall accuracy of ~90% (Box 10.2) [60–63]. A distinctive form of highly aggressive ARN, progressive outer retinal necrosis, was described in patients with acquired immune deficiency syndrome, malignancy, or organ transplants. The vitreous inflammatory reaction in these eyes can vary from almost minimum to moderate depending upon the severity of the immunosuppression. They have extensive multifocal deep retinal necrosis and absent retinal haemorrhages, and the retina's characteristic perivenous sparing gives it a mud crack appearance (Fig. 10.7). There appears to be no involvement of the retinal

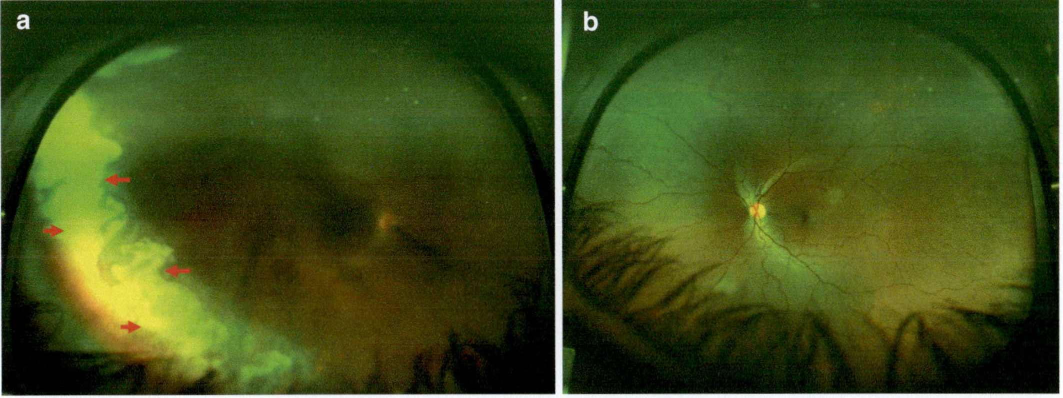

Fig. 10.6 Tongue-like areas (red arrows) of necrotic retinal opacification in the periphery of right eye (**a**) with vitreous haze, suggestive of acute retinal necrosis (ARN). Fellow (left) eye is normal (**b**)

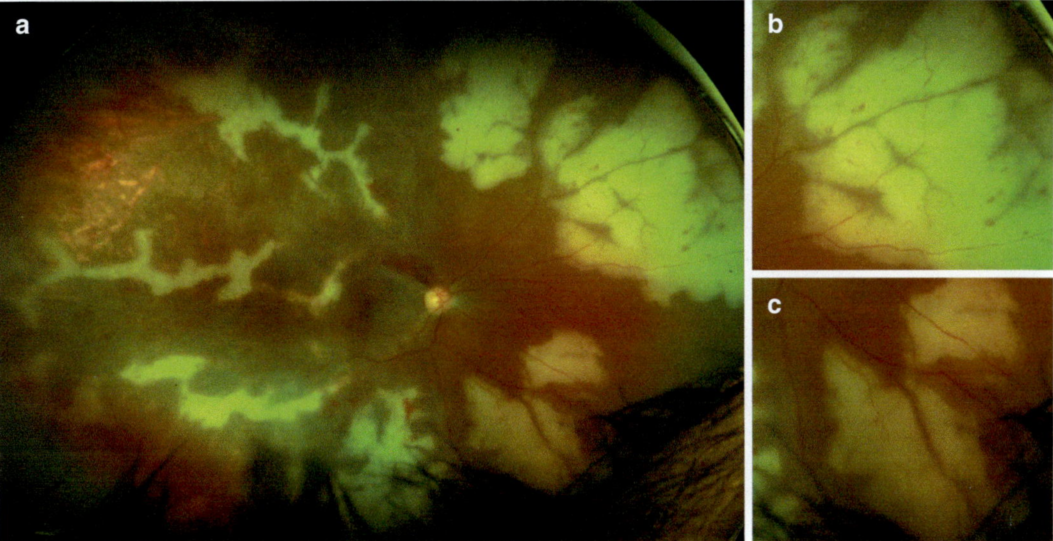

Fig. 10.7 Progressive outer retinal necrosis (in a patient with renal transplant) characterized by multifocal deep retinal necrosis lesions and absent retinal haemorrhages (**a**). The retina's characteristic perivenous sparing gives it a mud crack appearance (**b**, **c**)

Box 10.1 American Uveitis Society Criteria for Diagnosis of Acute Retinal Necrosis

A. Umbrella term necrotizing herpetic retinopathies be used when the involvement of HSV, VZV, or CMV is suspected but not proven	
B. Diagnosis of ARN is clinical. All the following criteria must be met	
(a) Lesions and location	One or more areas of retinal necrosis beyond the temporal retinal vascular arcades. Involvement of macular does not rule out ARN
(b) Spread	Circumferential and posterior
(c) Progression	Rapid
(d) Vessels	Occlusive vasculopathy, especially the arterioles
(e) Vitreous	Prominent inflammatory reaction in the vitreous and AC
Supportive evidence is not essential for diagnosing ARN (a) Optic neuropathy/atrophy (b) Scleritis (c) Pain	
Note: Diagnosis of ARN does not depend upon the age, gender, or immune status or isolation of the offending virus	

HSV herpes simplex virus, *VZV* varicella zoster virus, *CMV* cytomegalovirus, *ARN* acute retinal necrosis, *AC* anterior chamber

Adapted from Holland [59] with permission of the publishers

Box 10.2 Classification Criteria for Acute Retinal Necrosis Standardization of Uveitis Nomenclature (SUN) Working Group

Criteria	Clinical characteristics or laboratory test
1.	Peripheral necrotizing retinitis
2.	PCR from intraocular fluids positive for HSV, VZV
3.	Characteristic clinical appearance of circumferential or confluent necrotizing retinitis, retinal vascular sheathing, and/or occlusion and more than minimum vitritis
Diagnosis of ARN is made if criteria 1 and either 2 or 3 are met	

PCR polymerase chain reaction, *HSV* herpes simplex virus, *VZV* varicella zoster virus, *ARN* acute retinal necrosis

Adapted from Standardization of Uveitis Nomenclature (SUN) Working Group. Classification Criteria for Acute Retinal Necrosis Syndrome 2021.With permission of the publishers

vessels. The macula and the optic disc get affected early in the course. All of them have antecedent or concomitant skin zoster lesions [64–67]. Scanning laser ophthalmoscope (SLO) ultra-wide-filed fundus imaging is a valuable tool for detecting and characterizing the extent of peripheral necrotizing retinitis and associated vascular occlusions, retinal haemorrhages even in the presence of media haze [68]. Retinal detachment is present in 2% of the cases of ARN at presentation, but by the time they finish the course of the disease, it may be seen in up to 47% of the eyes [69]. More than one quadrant involvement in ARN is significantly associated with the development of retinal detachment and consequent poor visual outcome. Retinal detachment develops due to sieve-like retinal breaks that develop in the necrotic retina after about 3 weeks of the onset of the ARN and is prompted by the development of posterior vitreous detachment [58]. All eyes with >2 quadrants of retinal involvement had associated optic disc involvement [70]. Systemic antiviral therapy and prophylactic vitreous surgery may substantially reduce the incidence of retinal detachment from 67 to 43% and 45 to 22%, respectively [69, 71]. While in the past, laser photocoagulation had been used to prevent the occurrence of retinal detachment, there appears to be no advantage of this procedure [69]. The second eye gets involved in nearly one-third of the patients within several weeks, although there may be a delay of years between the involvements of the second eye.

Interestingly, PCR reveals the same virus (most often HSV-1) in the two affected eyes [72].

10.6.2.2 Recurrences and Latency in HSV and VZV Retinitis

Recurrences of herpes zoster in immunocompetent individuals, unlike herpes simplex, are rarely reported, and of those reported cases, the clinical diagnosis may have been mistaken [73]. More than 30 cases of ARN have been reported weeks to years following herpes simplex encephalitis (HSE) [74]. More often, ARN develops within 2 years of HSE. Hence, there is a need for increased awareness among both neurologists and ophthalmologists [75]. Rarely, recurrences of ARN in the same eye may be spread over several years following HSV encephalitis [76]. Herpes virus encephalitis following ARN is a rarity [77]. In any case, oral corticosteroids administered to control inflammation in the treatment of ARN must be stopped before discontinuing antiviral therapy. Recurrence of the ARN in the same eye due to VZV is rare [78]. However, ARN due to HSV may reactivate in the same eye years later [79, 80].

The Herpesviridae family consists of at least nine viruses that infect humans and are further subdivided into three subgroups, α-herpesvirus (HSV-1, HSV-2, and VZV); β-herpesvirus (CMV, HHV-6, HHV-7, and HHV-8); and γ-herpesvirus (EBV and Kaposi sarcoma herpes virus). Almost all people worldwide are infected with at least one of these viruses. The primary target of both the HSV and VZV are the epithelial cells exploited to replicate and spread the virus. The HSV and the VZV are unique as they establish a life-long presence/latency in the cranial nerve ganglia's neuronal cells and get activated occasionally. The viral DNA in these cells is stored as circular episomes in the nucleus of the infected cells. The viral proteins help the episomes tether to the chromosomes enabling the viral episomes to pass onto the daughter cells. The CMV targets monocytes and lymphocytes, where this virus can establish latency [81].

The herpes viruses evade immune recognition by producing non-coding microRNA that suppresses lytic gene expression and limits the expression of proteins, thus disabling the host's innate immune mechanisms to eliminate the infected host cells. While the VZV reactivates only once, the HSV shows frequent reactivation and shedding of the virus. However, since not all the infected cells show activation simultaneously, clinical disease may not become apparent every time the virus is shed [82]. HSV predominantly causes frequent recurrences of epithelial keratitis and anterior uveitis. However, acute retinal necrosis (ARN) caused by the VZV most often does not show recurrences. Extensive basic science research in the last 30 years is focused on the mechanism of latency and reactivation to develop effective strategies [82, 83].

10.6.2.3 Treatment of HSV and VZV Retinitis

Acyclovir is the drug of choice, which is highly effective for the reactivated virus but does not target the latent virus and thus cannot prevent reactivation. However, there is a role for long-term antiviral therapy to prevent the involvement of the other eye, especially if the first eye has had a poor visual outcome. However, for preventing the recurrence of ARN in the same eye, the risks certainly outweigh the advantages, especially since long-term antiviral therapy is fraught with acyclovir-resistant strains of HSV. The virus-specific IFN-γ producing CD8+ T lymphocytes keep the HSV in check. Glutamine, a non-essential amino acid, is an essential ingredient for the proliferation of lymphocytes. Oral glutamine supplements effectively upregulate several IFN-γ producing genes in the ganglia of HSV-1-infected mice and HSV-2-infected guinea pigs. Oral use of glutamine appears to be a promising strategy to prevent the recurrence of HSV infection [84].

10.6.3 CMV Retinitis

10.6.3.1 Risk Factors for CMV Retinitis

CMV retinitis (CMV-R) is one of the 20 life-threatening or opportunistic severe infections that are listed by WHO as defined as an advanced stage of HIV infection when it is labelled as acquired immune deficiency syndrome (AIDS). These opportunistic infections usually occur when the CD4⁺ T-cell counts go below 200 per μL. There is minimal risk of developing CMV-R until CD4⁺ T-cell count 100/μL. Before the advent of highly active antiretroviral drugs (HAART) in the 1990s, the median time to survival after developing CMV retinitis was 10 months. After first developing CD4⁺ T-cell count <100/μL, the incidence of CMV-R rose from 9% by the end of first year to 25% by the end of the fourth year. The risk of CMV-R rose by 3× after the CD4⁺ T-cell count fell <50/μL. By the fourth year, two-thirds of the patients had died [85].

With the universal availability of HAART therapy, CMV-R has become highly uncommon in people living with HIV. Its incidence was noted to be 0.36/100 person-years, the single most risk factor being CD4⁺ T-cell count <50/μL in the immediately prior visit. The CMV-R in patients with HIV may be asymptomatic and is usually detected on fundus examination of these patients. There are two types of retinitis lesions, (1) chronic indolent granular and peripheral perivascular lesions and perivenous infiltrate with fewer retinal haemorrhages or (2) more fulminant haemorrhagic necrotizing retinitis. In HIV patients, there is either minimal or no vitreous reaction. However, once the patients are put on HAART therapy, a severe vitreous inflammatory reaction may occur due to immune reconstitution. The lesions heal with atrophy of the retina and may develop sieve-like retinal holes. Currently, CMV-R is increasingly reported in patients with organ transplants, bone marrow transplants, leukaemias, lymphomas, or connective tissue disorders who are on immunosuppressive therapy. Intraocular and periocular corticosteroids may account for nearly 20% of all CMV retinitis in non-HIV patients [86]. Without any of these non-HIV risk factors, diabetes should be ruled out.

The patients who develop CMV-R without HIV infection tend to be older, all have significant vitreous inflammation and, besides the necrotizing haemorrhagic retinitis, have retinal vasculitis, especially the retinal arteriolar occlusions (Fig. 10.8) [87, 88]. It contrasts sharply with HIV+ patients with CMV-R, in which retinal vascular involvement is limited to only non-occlusive perivenous sheathing [89]. The arteriolar occlusion may be much larger than suspected by the size of the retinitis lesion. Extensive capillary non-perfusion areas exist [87, 89]. Moreover, if a PCR test for detecting CMV DNA from the intraocular fluids has not been done, the CMV-R in non-HIV patients may be mistaken for ARN [90, 91]. Notably, CMV-R in non-HIV patients is unilateral. Also, the favourite sites for CMV infection include the gastrointestinal tract, the brain, and the eyes. See Box 10.3 for the diagnostic criteria of CMV-R.

On optical coherence tomography, the CMV-R shows posterior hyaloid thickening, retinal swelling, retinal hyperreflectivity, retinal disruption, interruption of the IS/OS junction, and hyporeflective spaces (empty spaces) in the outer nuclear layer. Hyperreflective vertical strips (bridges) are seen in the outer nuclear layer [92, 93].

10.6.3.2 Pathogenesis and Pathology of CMV Retinitis

The CMV is latent in the bone marrow CD34+ progenitor cells, the precursors of the monocytes. The monocytes get released into the peripheral blood and have a short life span of 1–3 days. In patients with HIV microangiopathy, the blood-retinal barrier breakdown allows the CMV to infect the retinal cells. In immunocompetent individuals, the circulating pro-inflammatory cytokines (TNF-α and IL-1β) cause endothelial cells to express adhesion molecules (V-CAM, CD106), letting the virus-infected monocytes adhere and enter the capillary endothelial cells. It is recognized that the CMV-R starts near the retinal vessels. Ultrastructural and immunohistochemical studies of CMV-R have shown the presence of viral particles in the Muller cells and the perivascular glial cells in the necrotic retina. These were also seen in the neuronal cells and the RPE cells. In the area of necrosis, there was a complete loss

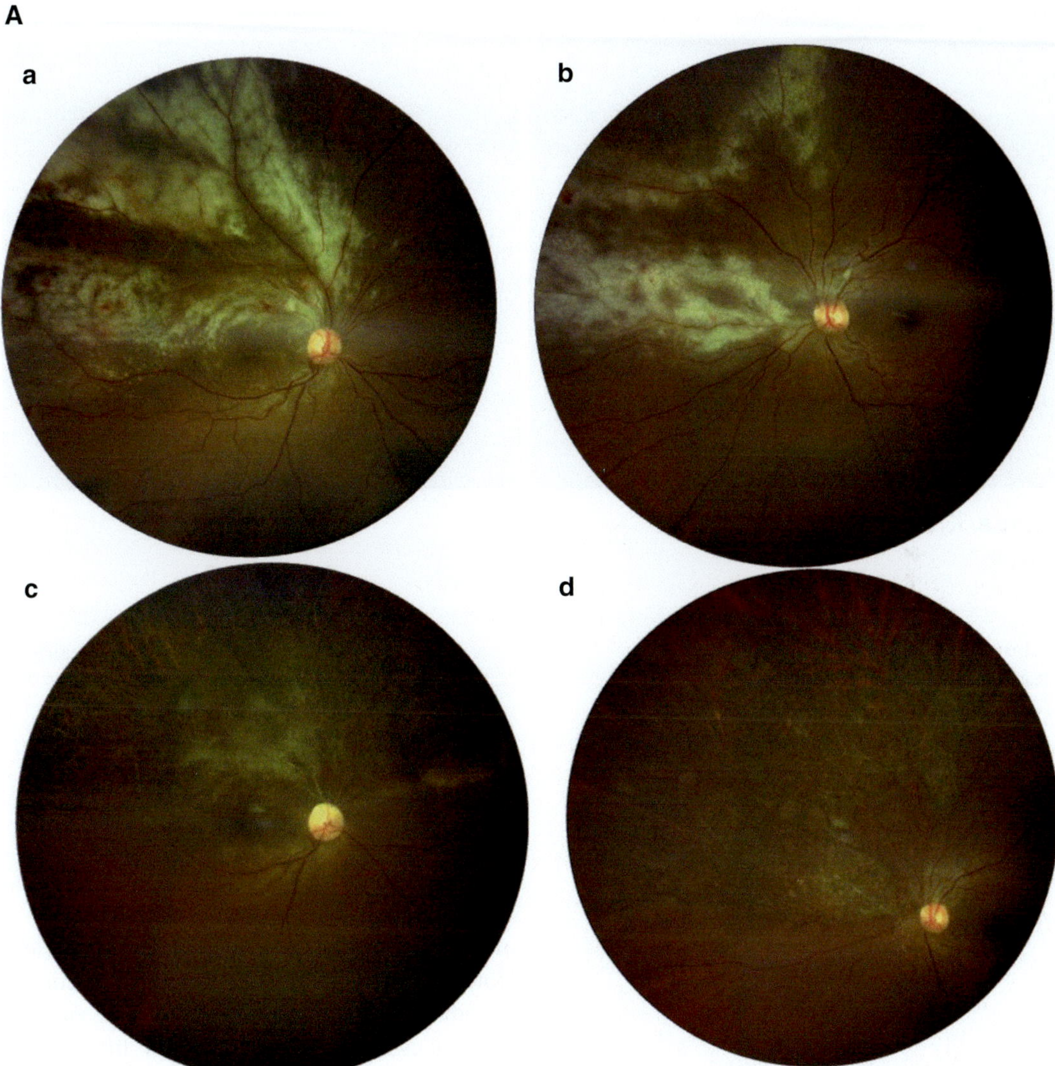

Fig. 10.8 (**A**) A 36-year-old woman presented with bilateral CMV retinitis (**a**). She had pancytopenia and had been diagnosed 9 months earlier dyskeratosis congenita, although without conclusive evidence of the disease. Her white cell counts were 1620/mL. Quantitative PCR for CMV was positive. She was treated with intravitreal and oral ganciclovir. Lesions started healing at follow-up (**b**, **c**) and at 3 months (**d**). (Images courtesy of Dr. Anuradha V. K., Head of uveitis Services, Aravind Eye Hospital, Coimbatore. India). (**B**) A 38-year-old woman with HIV+ with a CD4+ count of 48 mm^3 presented as frosted branch angiitis in the right eye. She had light perception (LP) vision in this eye (**a**). On HAART and systemic ganciclovir, the retinitis and vasculitis improved, but she remained LP+ vision 3 months later (**b**). (Images courtesy of Prof Ramandeep Singh, Advanced Eye Centre, Post Graduate Institute of Medical Education and Research, Chandigarh, India)

B

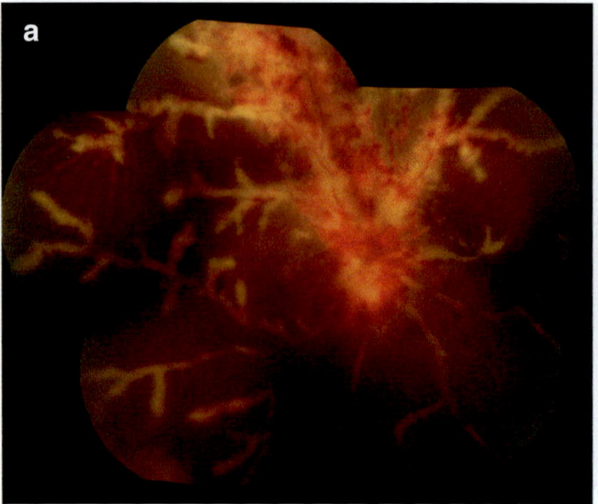

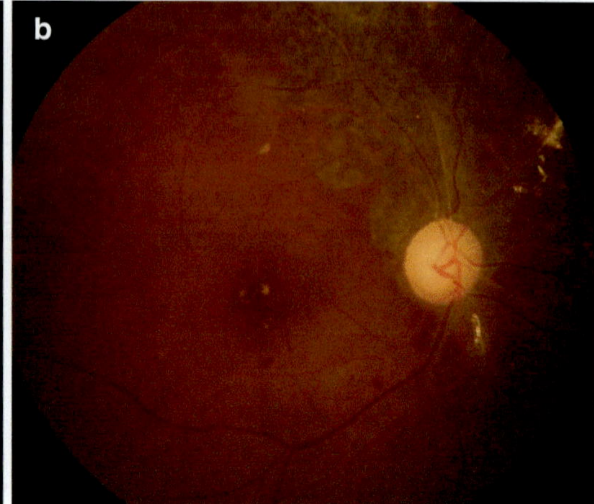

Fig. 10.8 (continued)

Box 10.3 Classification Criteria for CMV Retinitis Standardization of Uveitis Nomenclature (SUN) Working Group

1. Necrotizing retinitis with indistinct borders
2a. Systemic immune compromise due to AIDS, organ or bone marrow transplant, IMT for CTD
2b. Ocular immunosuppression due to periocular or intraocular depot corticosteroids
3. Clinical characteristics: a. Wedge-shaped retinitis or b. Haemorrhagic retinitis or c. Granular retinitis AND d. Absent or minimal vitritis[a]
4. PCR+ from intraocular fluid
Diagnosis of CMV-R requires criteria 1, 2, and either 3 or 4
Exclusion Criteria[b]: Tests for syphilis +; PCR + for HSV or VZV or toxoplasma from the intraocular fluid

Adapted from Standardization of Uveitis Nomenclature (SUN) Working Group. Classification Criteria for Cytomegalovirus Retinitis, 2021. With permission of the publishers

CMV cytomegalovirus, *AIDS* acquired immune deficiency syndrome, *IMT* immunosuppressive therapy, *CTD* connective tissue disorders, *PCR* polymerase chain reaction, *HSV* herpes simplex virus, *VZV* varicella zoster virus, *CMV-R* cytomegalovirus retinitis

[a] In non-HIV patients, the vitreous reaction is severe

[b] In immunocompromised patients, more than two infections may co-exist in the eye

of the endothelial lining of the retinal vessels. However, at the advancing edge of the retinitis, endothelial cells showed the presence of viral proteins establishing that the CMV first spreads to the endothelial cells and then spreads to the other retina cells [94].

10.6.3.3 Treatment of CMV Retinitis

Systemic therapy is preferred in HIV+ CMV-R as it frequently involves both eyes. The standard therapy is intravenous ganciclovir (5 mg/kg body weight to be modified in renal pathology). Induction therapy is given twice daily for 2–3 weeks, followed by maintenance therapy once a week. The treatment is continued till, following the HAART therapy, the CD4+ T-cell count rises >100/μL. Ganciclovir has a broad range of activity against CMV, HSV, VZV, and HHV-6 to HHV-8. Acyclovir, the drug most effective against HSV and VZV, needs thymidine kinase for its phosphorylation which the human

CMV lacks; hence, acyclovir is ineffective in treating CMV-R. The CMV UL-97 protein phosphorylates ganciclovir to its active triphosphate form, a competitive analogue of the viral DNA polymerase, and thus blocks the multiplication of the CMV. The intravenous use of ganciclovir can lead to resistance. Mutations in the UL97 gene make the CMV resistant to ganciclovir. Oral valganciclovir, a prodrug of ganciclovir, is equally effective compared to intravenous ganciclovir in treating CMV-R [95]. Significant side effects of ganciclovir include skin rash, diarrhoea, and haematogenic. Intravitreal ganciclovir inserts have not been available since 2013. The oral valganciclovir 900 mg is equivalent to 5 mg/kg body weight of intravenous ganciclovir. Intravitreal ganciclovir (2 mg/0.1 mL) is effective in non-HIV CMV-R as the disease is most often unilateral. The induction dose is given twice a week and maintained with a once-a-week intravitreal injection [96].

10.6.3.4 Prophylaxis for CMV Retinitis

Valganciclovir prophylaxis is given to all transplant patients as up to 75% of such patients may develop CMV infection, and up to 30% may develop a CMV disease. Recently, letermovir, a CMV terminase inhibitor, has been used effectively as primary prophylaxis in high-risk patients with allogeneic haematopoietic cell transplantation [97]. The high-risk patients are CMV-positive donors/CMV-negative recipients. Positive CMV PCR from blood, pp 65 antigenemia, and positive serology are some markers for prophylactic treatment initiation.

10.6.3.5 Alternate Drugs for the Treatment of CMV-R

For patients who develop ganciclovir-resistant CMV disease and resistant HSV, intravenous foscarnet 90 mg/kg twice daily for 2 weeks, followed by 120 mg/kg daily for maintenance, can be given. It is a highly nephrotoxic drug. The patient must be hydrated well. Other adverse reactions include anaemia, nausea, and neurological side effects.

The intravitreal dose of foscarnet is 1.2–2.4 mg once or twice a week for induction and 1.2 mg weekly for maintenance. Resistance may develop if there is a mutation in the viral DNA polymerase. Unlike ganciclovir, cidofovir does not need viral kinases for activation and hence can also be used in ganciclovir-resistant cases of CMV-R. Cidofovir is given intravenously at 5 mg/kg weekly for 3 weeks and a maintenance dose of 5 mg/kg every 2 weeks. The intravitreal dose of cidofovir is 20 μg every 6 weeks. However, its intravitreal use is limited by severe adverse events like uveitis, cystoid macular oedema, and irreversible hypotony [98]. Other therapies include CMV immune globulin therapy for systemic CMV pneumonia. Progressive cases of CMV retinitis have been treated with donor-derived CMV pp65-specific T cells [99–102].

10.6.3.6 When to Stop the Antiviral Therapy in CMV-R

The guidelines are clear in patients with HIV infection; once the $CD4^+$ T-cell counts reach 100–150 cells per μL, lesions of CMV-R resolve spontaneously and do not need any other antiviral therapy. In patients on immunosuppressive therapy, the dose of IMT is decreased to the level where the absolute neutrophil count is maintained above 1000 per μL. However, in non-HIV CMV-R, the guidelines are not clear. It may help to do PCR for CMV from the blood.

10.6.4 Emerging Viral Infections and Retinitis

In recent years, arthropod-borne seasonal epidemics of viral fever have increasingly become a major public health challenge in several regions of the world, especially South Asia and South America [103]. Most of these are caused by single-stranded RNA viruses like dengue, chikungunya, West Nile, Zika, and Ebola that follow an insect bite from mosquitos of the Aedes species (aegypti or albopictus) that thrive in the tropical and subtropical climate. The severity of uveitis from the anterior to the posterior segment may follow days to months following these infections. The diagnosis is based on the detection of IgM antibodies. Conventional RT-PCR techniques have shown the presence of the chikungunya, Zika, and Ebola virus in the aqueous humour in patients with uveitis even after the systemic symptoms have resolved [104–106].

Dengue is the most common mosquito-borne viral infection that has become endemic in more than 100 countries and is characterized by fever, headache, myalgia, and arthralgia. Haemorrhagic dengue infection may be fatal. Ocular manifestations result from ischaemic, inflammatory, or thrombocytopenic mechanisms that manifest as maculopathy, optic neuropathy, vasculitis, retinal haemorrhages, and multifocal retinitis,

Intensive basic science research is currently focused on elaborating on the pathogenic mechanism of these viral infections. Zika virus infection may be asymptomatic or mild, but it gained widespread recognition upon realizing that in utero infection was associated with microcephaly in the newborn. Zika virus-associated anterior uveitis was described only recently [107]. Furthermore, nearly half of the patients who develop redness of the eyes during fever may develop hypertensive anterior uveitis [108]. RT-PCR can demonstrate the Zika virus RNA. The Zika virus possibly enters the eye riding in myeloid cells. In a human cell line model of iris pigment epithelium, the Zika virus was shown to mount an active type 1 interferon recognition and molecular defence response to limit the ocular inflammatory response in most individuals [106].

West Nile fever is caused by a positive single-stranded neurotropic RNA virus that remains asymptomatic in most people. However, ~20% of cases may develop a self-limiting flu-like illness. Less than 1% may develop meningitis, encephalitis, or a polio-like illness, of which 80% develop self-limiting bilateral multifocal chorioretinitis lesions [109].

10.6.4.1 Treatment of Post-Fever Retinitis

Most of these infections are self-limiting; currently, no antiviral treatment is available. Many of these patients may require supportive treatment during their systemic illness. While systemic corticosteroids are widely used for controlling the immune-mediated inflammatory reaction, controlled studies to prove their efficacy are lacking.

Preventive strategies remain the mainstay, including public health measures to control mosquito breeding and wearing long-sleeved protective clothing. Several vaccines, including those for Ebola, Zika, chikungunya, and dengue, have shown promise in animal models and are either approved or in the process of approval for use in humans. Waxing and waning epidemics of these infections and uncertainty of cost-efficacy of human trials and uptake remain a public health challenge [110].

10.6.5 Bacterial Infectious Uveitis-Spirochetal Infections

Treponema, Borrelia, and leptospira are three of the most common gram-negative spirochetal infections that cause uveitis. *Treponema pallidum* and *Borrelia burgdorferi* are among the most invasive bacteria. These bacteria can easily move through the skin and other body surfaces freely in and out of the blood vessels. *Treponema pallidum* can cross the blood-brain barrier and even the placenta to cause congenital syphilis. Leptospira is also highly mobile in water but needs a skin abrasion or a cut to enter the body. Although it causes a multiorgan disease, it is mainly localized in the kidneys and excreted in the urine of infected mammals [111]. All three infections can be prevented with appropriate measures.

10.6.5.1 Syphilis

In the last two decades, there has been a steady rise in the incidence of primary and secondary syphilis from 2.1/100,000 to 9.5/100,000 population in the USA, mainly because of men having sex with men. HIV commonly accompanies syphilis, and all patients with syphilis must be tested for HIV infection. In our clinic studies, there was no syphilitic uveitis in our 2004 study

[36], but in the 2017 study, 8 of the 507 infectious uveitis cases were due to syphilis [35]. For a long time, syphilis has been known as a great mimic and may manifest as anterior uveitis, intermediate uveitis, retinal vasculitis (Fig. 10.9), neuro-retinitis, optic neuritis, or placoid chorioretinopathy. Posterior uveitis accounts for nearly 50% of the cases. In recent years, multimodal imaging studies have provided clues to a possible syphilis aetiology. Fundus autofluorescence studies show a speckled or well-demarcated hyperautofluorescence. Structural OCT changes are characterized by loss of the external lining membrane and patchy disturbances of the ellipsoid zone, which are reversible. The RPE layer shows granular/nodular hyperreflective projections into the outer retina. Preretinal dots seen on OCT as hyperreflective dots suggest a syphilitic infection.

Diagnosis is based on treponema tests such as fluorescent treponema antibody or the syphilis IgG, treponema haemagglutination, and non-treponemal tests such as VDRL or RPR. Since nearly half of the patients with ocular syphilis may have CNS involvement, it is recommended that CSF be tested, and all ocular syphilis be treated as neuro-syphilis. The treatment includes three to four million units of penicillin G administered intravenously every 4 h for 2 weeks. Alternately, IV or IM ceftriaxone, oral doxycycline (not advised in pregnant women), and amoxicillin or erythromycin may be used. Interestingly, following primary chancre, there is a latent phase during which there is only serological evidence of infection. Most of the ocular involvement is seen in the primary or secondary stage of the infection. Once fully treated, the organism *Treponema pallidum* is eliminated from the body. This infectious cause of uveitis is curable, so it must be ruled out in all patients with uveitis. The subject has been recently reviewed [112].

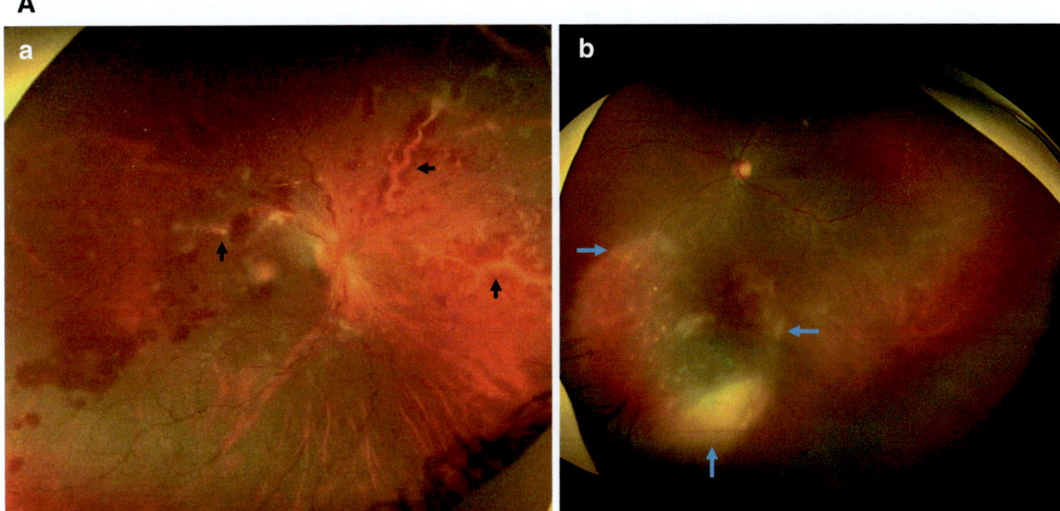

Fig. 10.9 (**A**) A 24-year-old man (**a**) presented with retinal vasculitis (frosted branch angiitis, black arrows). He revealed a history of high-risk behaviour and tested positive for syphilis. Syphilitic retinitis (blue arrows) was seen in a 31-year-old man (**b**). (**B**) A 38-year-old man with metamorphopsia left eye. Visual acuity was 6/6. Two-month history of penile painless sore. Translucent well-demarcated outer placoid chorioretinitis placoid lesion (a, black arrows). Subretinal precipitate-like lesions (a, blue arrow) and focal perivascular lesions (**a**, red arrow). Fundus autofluorescence shows punctate hyperautofluorescent lesions (**b**). Fundus fluorescein angiography in the late frame shows mild staining of the optic disc and posterior pole with hypofluorescent punctate lesions that correspond to the hyperautofluorescent lesions seen in b (**c**). Treponema pallidum haemagglutination and venereal disease research laboratory tests were positive. The placoid lesion resolved one month following intravenous ceftriaxone 1 g twice daily for 14 days (**d**). OCT at presentation shows highly characteristic nodular lesions of the RPE (**e**), which disappear following treatment (**f**). (Images courtesy of Dr. Alok Sen, Sadguru Chikitsa Nethralya, Chitrakoot, MP, India)

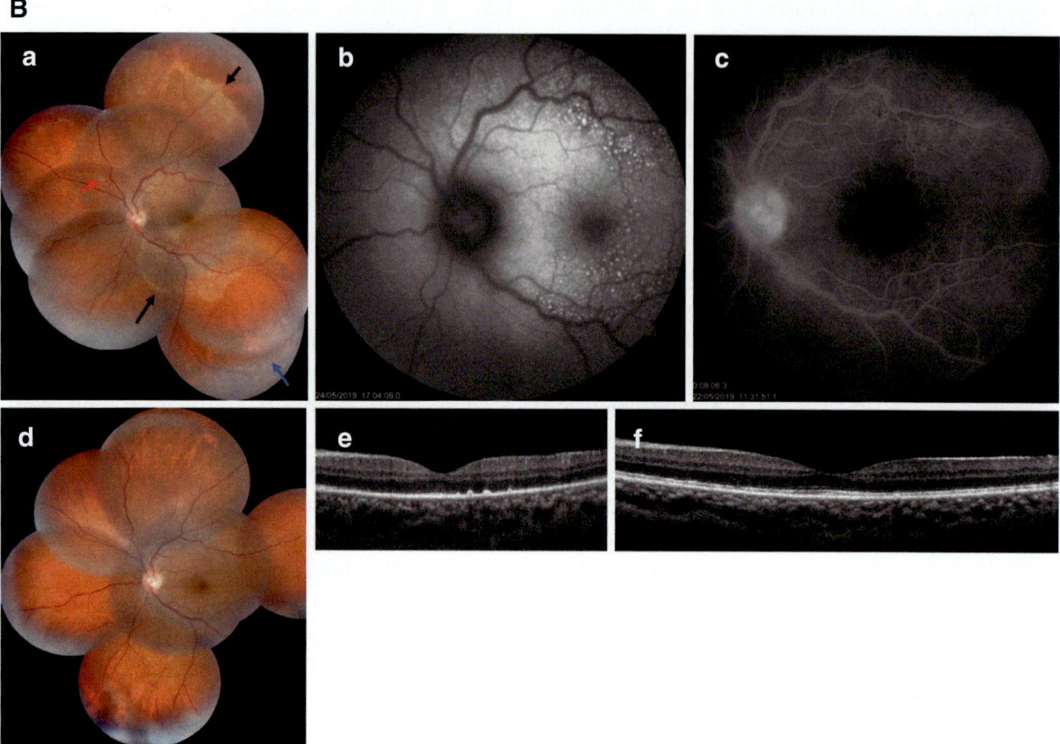

Fig. 10.9 (continued)

10.6.5.2 Lyme borreliosis

While the vector (black-legged tick)-borne Lyme borreliosis caused by *Borrelia Burgdorferi* is showing an upward trend in the endemic areas of several countries of Europe and North America, the ocular Lyme borreliosis is uncommon or perhaps underdiagnosed because of the non-availability of serological tests in many parts of the world. Ocular Lyme borreliosis manifests in the late stages of infection as intermediate uveitis or retinal vasculitis and should be considered in the differential diagnosis, especially in people with a history of erythema migrans (red skin rash spreading in a ring fashion), following a tick bite and those who come from Lyme-endemic areas. Unlike syphilis, routine screening for Lyme borreliosis is not recommended in patients with uveitis [113].

10.6.5.3 Leptospiral Uveitis

Leptospirosis is another spirochetal disease seen in subtropics and tropics, the regions with a humid climate. The organism *Leptospira interrogans* resides in the kidneys of many animals and rodents. The soil gets contaminated from the urine of infected animals, where the organisms can survive for months. Epidemics follow heavy rainfall and flooding of agricultural fields. The organisms enter humans through broken skin or mucosa. Unlike other spirochetal infections that produce skin lesions at the portal of entry, this infection does not leave any trace of entry. People engaged in agricultural activities or water sports are more prone to contract this infection. While most infected patients present with mild disease, nearly 10% develop severe disease and show evidence of cytokine storm, including acute fever, headache, and severe haemorrhagic multiorgan involvement. Like all spirochetal infections, Leptospira is susceptible to penicillin, ampicillin, ceftriaxone, and doxycycline and needs aggressive supportive therapy during acute infection. The microscopic agglutination test is the gold standard but requires dealing with live organisms and is thus not commonly available. The other tests are ELISA, macroscopic agglutination, and

PCR. The circulating spirochetes disappear with the development of antibodies, but the bacteria may survive in the immune-privileged sites, including the eyes. Uveitis is a late complication seen in the convalescent phase of the disease, and nearly half develop hypopyon, panuveitis, and rapidly developing white cataracts. PCR from the aqueous humour is positive for leptospira DNA in nearly 80% of the patients with uveitis [114]. The treatment at this stage requires aggressive corticosteroid therapy. It is still unclear if systemic antibiotic therapy in the acute phase will prevent the occurrence of uveitis [115].

10.6.6 Other Bacterial Uveitis: *Mycobacterium tuberculosis*

The pathology of uveitis caused by *Mycobacterium Tuberculosis* (MTB) from the enucleated globes was known long before the discovery of the MTB in 1882 by Robert Koch [116]. However, the diagnosis of tubercular uveitis (TBU) in the clinic remains a major challenge even today. The cornerstone of the diagnosis of the MTB infection (Koch's postulates), namely the demonstration of the presence of the acid-fast bacilli (AFB) either on smear examination or a positive culture from the TB-affected tissues, can hardly be ever possible from the fluids or tissues of a seeing eye. Thus, the diagnosis of TB uveitis (TBU) to date is based on corroborative evidence rather than fulfilling Koch's postulates.

10.6.6.1 Lessons from the Past-TB or No TB

More than 100 years ago, when tuberculosis infection of the lungs was rampant across the world, most patients with uveitis were attributed to tuberculosis more as a reflection of faith rather than evidence. Before the advent of chemotherapy for treating TB, Woods, in many of his publications on the aetiology of uveitis, reported a steady decline in uveitis attributed to TB from 80% in 1941 to 20% in 1960 [117, 118]. Because of the wide variation in the clinical phenotypes of TBU, some of the cases due to sarcoidosis, brucellosis, toxoplasma, and histoplasmosis, aetiologies that were yet to be discovered, may have been earlier labelled as TBU. In one such telling example, Verhoeff diagnosed a case of TB necrotizing retinitis on histopathology but 25 years later admitted that the reported case had the pathological features of toxoplasmosis retinitis [119] and not TB [120].

10.6.6.2 Endemicity of TB and Tubercular Uveitis

Before Dr. Woods, several authors who sought definitive evidence of TB reported its prevalence from 2 to 11%, while those who applied less stringent criteria estimated the prevalence of TBU in their clinic to vary from 40 to 48% [117, 118]. Undoubtedly, with an incidence of TB at 250–300/100,000 population in that era, the true prevalence may have been between 10 and 40%. As seen in the discussion below, high-burden countries show a high prevalence of TBU in their clinics.

Several measures taken 100 years ago, including the declaration of TB as a notifiable disease, identification of crowded dwellings, poor hygiene, and poor nutrition as possible risk factors, and the availability of anti-TB drugs in the 1950s, have dramatically reduced the incidence of TB from 250–300/100,000 population to 2–10/100,000 in the Western countries. However, it continues to be a hyperendemic and a major public health problem in several regions of the world, including India, China, Indonesia, Philippines, Pakistan, Nigeria, Bangladesh, and S. Africa, where the incidence continues to be higher than 200/per 100,000 population. Although TBU data from the uveitis clinics are not available from all such places, where available, it shows a significant prevalence of TBU in India (19.85–22.8%), Myanmar (32.37%), Vietnam (8.95%), Thailand (8.5%), Singapore (6.7%), and Sri Lanka (6.2%). However, some of the developed countries, Australia (4.2%), New Zealand (3.1%), and S. Korea (1.66%), show a low prevalence of TBU. In the last 30 years, TBU prevalence has consistently been 0.2–0.6% of all cases of uveitis in the USA [121]. It is to be noted that the incidence of TB in the US population is one of the lowest in the world at 2/100,000 population, most of it in foreign-born persons.

10.6.6.3 Clinical Phenotypes of Tubercular Uveitis

The TBU manifests in various phenotypes, most commonly as multifocal serpiginous-like choroiditis, retinal periphlebitis, choroidal granuloma, panuveitis, anterior uveitis, and even intermediate uveitis [122–125]. The diagnosis is often made by recognizing the clinical phenotype in vulnerable populations (high-burden TB countries) who show immunological or radiological evidence of tuberculosis. Recently, a systematic review and meta-analysis on the global prevalence of TBU found a 7% prevalence in TB high-burden countries and 3% in low-burden countries, peaking at 11% in sub-Saharan Africa [126]. However, the authors found a high degree of heterogeneity among the studies because of the need for standard diagnostic criteria that pose a major question of the validity of any figures given for TBU.

Serpiginous-like Choroiditis

Tubercular serpiginous-like choroiditis (TB-SLC) is the most common phenotype of TBU, first reported in 2003 [127] from India, a TB-endemic country. It is characterized by multifocal lesions (>90%) that show actively advancing greyish-white lesions (Fig. 10.10). Focal lesions appear in crops. As some of these are healing, new ones may appear elsewhere in the retina. Uncommonly, the TB-SLC may be a single placoid lesion. The lesions heal centrally and expand centrifugally and become confluent. TB-SLC is predominantly seen in young men

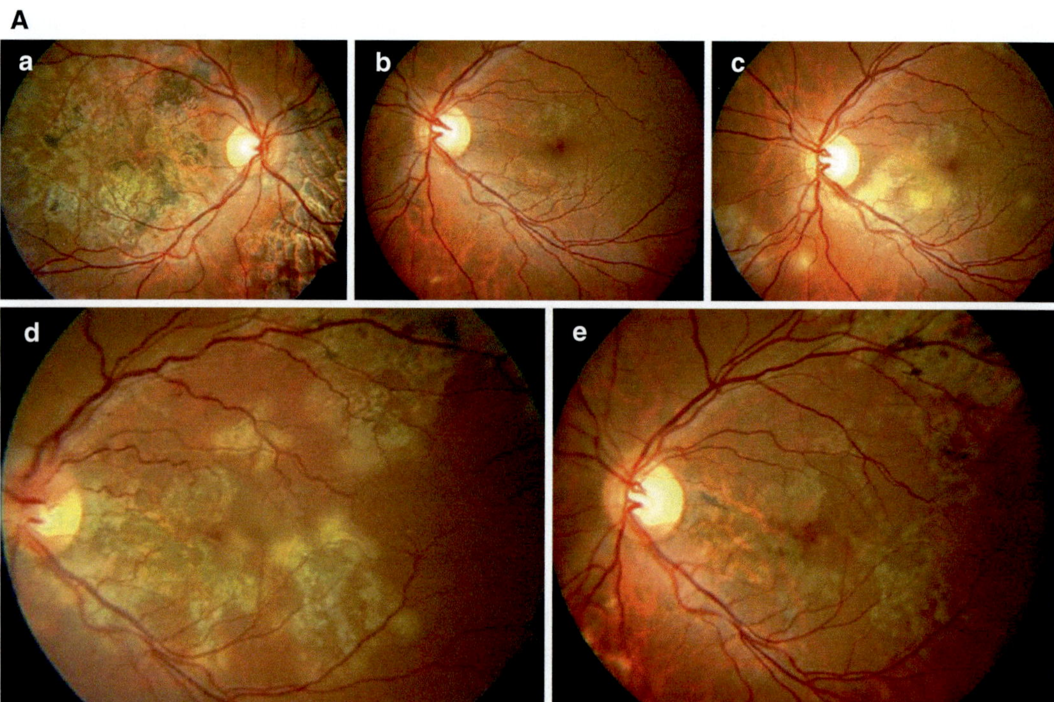

Fig. 10.10 (**A**) A 36-year-old man presented with extensive scarring of the right eye (**a**) and a healed choroiditis scar just above the fovea in the left eye (**b**). Within 8 weeks of presentation, he had blurring of vision in the left eye and showed plaque-like multifocal lesions in the left eye (**c**). The lesions showed a central healing and centrifugal spread at the margins (**d**). At 10 months following anti-TB treatment with oral corticosteroids, the lesions healed and did not recur (**e**). (**B**) The active choroiditis lesions (**f**) on FFA were hypofluorescent in the dye transit. Note speckled transmission hyperfluorescence in healed lesions (**g**). The hypolesions become hyperfluorescent in the late frames (h). (**C**) Left eye fundus photograph (a) and fundus autofluorescence (**b**) of a 45-year-old woman with a large placoid lesion in the macula and multifocal active lesions of serpiginous-like choroiditis. The active margins of the lesion are hypofluorescent in early (**c**) and hyperfluorescent in late phases (**d**). The centre of the lesion shows transmission hyperfluorescence, both in the early (**c**) and late phases (**d**). (Reproduced with the permission of the publishers from Bansal, R., Sharma, A., & Gupta, A. (2012). *Intraocular tuberculosis. Expert Review of Ophthalmology, 7(4), 341–349.* https://doi.org/10.1586/eop.12.42)

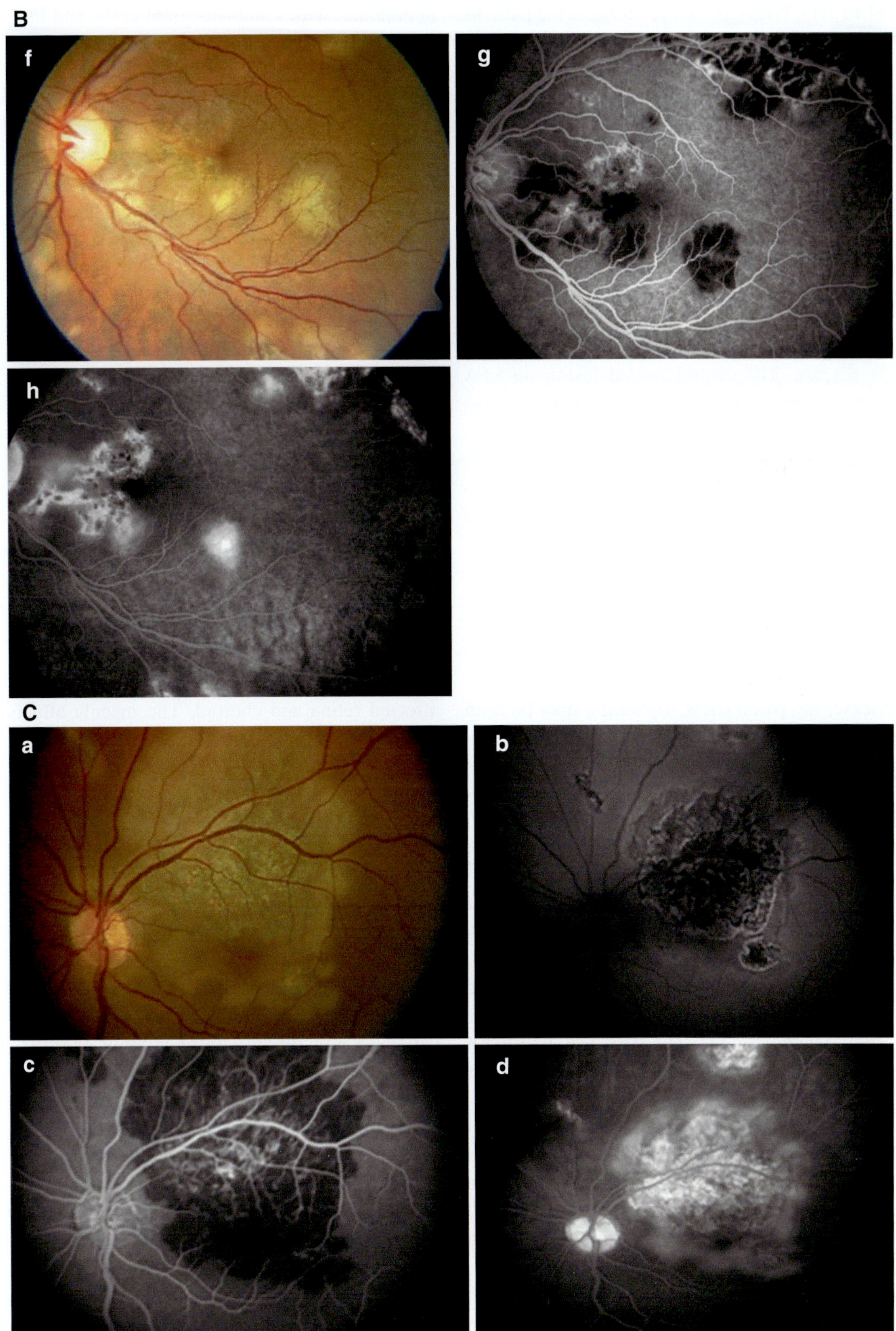

Fig. 10.10 (continued)

(M:F: 3:1). When first seen, >60% of the patients may have bilateral involvement, often one eye showing healed lesions that have gone unnoticed by the patient. In most patients, the lesions are non-contiguous to the optic disc. There is a variable amount of vitreous inflammation. Most lesions are located in the posterior pole, but in half of the patients, these lesions are also seen nasally to the optic disc. The lesions heal with retinal atrophy and a variable amount of pigmentation. Patients at presentation may have >6/12 visual acuity in the affected eye [128]. Notably, the foveal centre remains unaffected until late in the disease. The central healed lesion on FFA shows transmission mixed fluorescence, whereas the active advancing edge shows initial hypofluorescence with late staining. On ICG angiography, the lesions are hypofluorescent and remain hypofluorescent even in the late stages. The disease course is best followed on fundus autofluorescence, as the lesions become hypoautofluorescent from initial hyperfluorescence [129]. The TB-SLC lesions may progress after initiating anti-TB therapy [130]. If ultra-wide field fundus imaging is used to monitor the course of the disease, the paradoxical worsening may be seen in nearly 36% of the eyes [131]. On OCT angiography, the multifocal TB-SLC lesions show a flow deficit in the choriocapillaris layer corresponding to the hypofluorescent lesion on ICG angiography. As the lesions heal, the flow deficit areas are completely reversed, unlike in the placoid type of SLC, which shows the persistence of flow deficit consistent with atrophy of the choriocapillaris [132–134].

Anecdotal pathological reports indicate the presence of AFB in the RPE or choroid of the patients with TB-SLC. The AFB was first demonstrated from the homogenate of the choroid from an endo biopsy of a lesion initially diagnosed as a non-responsive viral retinitis but looked suspiciously like TB-SLC, an entity then unknown. Following anti-TB therapy, the lesion was completely healed [135]. In an enucleated eye, AFB was demonstrated from the necrotic RPE [136]. In a patient of SLC who showed paradoxical worsening following anti-TB therapy, a biopsy of the inner choroid revealed a caseous granuloma, with Langhans giant cells, and PCR for MTB DNA was positive from the subretinal fluid [137]. Using at least three different types of molecular techniques (rpo gene sequencing, GeneXpert and MTBDR plus assay), the MTB genome was detected from the undiluted vitreous samples obtained at pars plana vitreous surgery in patients with multifocal serpiginoid choroiditis (SLC) including drug-resistant MTB in three eyes [138].

The TB-SLC needs to be differentiated from the classic serpiginous choroiditis (CSC) seen in the TB-non-endemic regions of the world. It is a rare bilateral organ-specific recurrent autoimmune disorder seen in middle-aged persons that may show a relentless progression. Some patients respond to immunosuppressive therapy. The monofocal lesion typically starts in the peripapillary choroid, involves the overlying RPE and the outer retina, and shows a finger-like, serpentine, or jigsaw-like progression. There is no or minimal inflammatory reaction in the vitreous cavity. The advancing tip is greyish-white and hyperautofluorescent. The lesions heal with minimal pigmentation but leave a profound atrophy of the affected retina and choroid. The macula affects nearly 90% of patients with permanent vision loss [139].

Choroidal Granuloma

Choroidal granuloma is the most familiar phenotype of TBU to physicians as often these patients have systemic disseminated TB. The choroidal granuloma(s) are usually seen in the posterior pole near the arcades but could be present in the nasal retina. These are uncommon in the fundus periphery. Most patients will have a solitary large yellowish granuloma with or without exudative retinal detachment (Fig. 10.11). However, they are usually small if there is more than one granuloma. The most common cause of exudative retinal detachment in TBU is choroidal granuloma [140]. TB granulomas are usually associated with other signs of inflammation, including cells in the AC or the vitreous cavity, keratic precipitates, posterior synechiae, and retinal periphlebitis. Presenting visual acuity is usually less than 6/60 due to exudative retinal detachment involving the macula. One of the most characteristic features of the TB choroidal granuloma is the presence of small intraretinal haemorrhage(s) suggestive of increased vascularization of the granulomas. On FFA, the highly vascular nature of the TB choroidal granuloma is apparent and shows early hyperfluorescence with extensive staining and leakage of the dye in the late frames. On optical coherence tomography (OCT), the TB choroidal granulomas often show a dome-like elevation of the RPE and infiltration of the outer retina (Fig. 10.11c, d).

TB choroidal granulomas are amenable to 4-drug anti-TB therapy, with nearly 80% of the eyes responding to the treatment with the restoration of useful vision. Surgical interventions may be disastrous in such eyes [125]. A new paradigm of host-directed therapies is emerging in the treatment of tuberculosis. The TB granulomas are hypoxic and lead to overexpression of vascular endothelial growth factor (VEGF), resulting in increased granuloma vascularization. By restoring the endothelial barrier, anti-VEGF agents facilitate exchanges of small molecules, such as anti-TB drugs, to reach the core of the granuloma [141–143]. The first successful application of this strategy in clinical practice was achieved using anti-VEGF therapy as an adjunct in tubercular choroidal granulomas that showed paradoxical worsening on initiation of anti-TB therapy [144]. The granuloma vasculature may start exudation months or years later; hence, the patient needs to be kept under follow-up for any new symptoms [145]. Very high levels of VEGF have been found in the aqueous humour in these patients, and weekly anti-VEGF intravitreal injections combined with the conventional anti-TB therapy, corticosteroids, and intravitreal moxifloxacin led to prompt regression of these granulomas. Previously, the regressing TB granu-

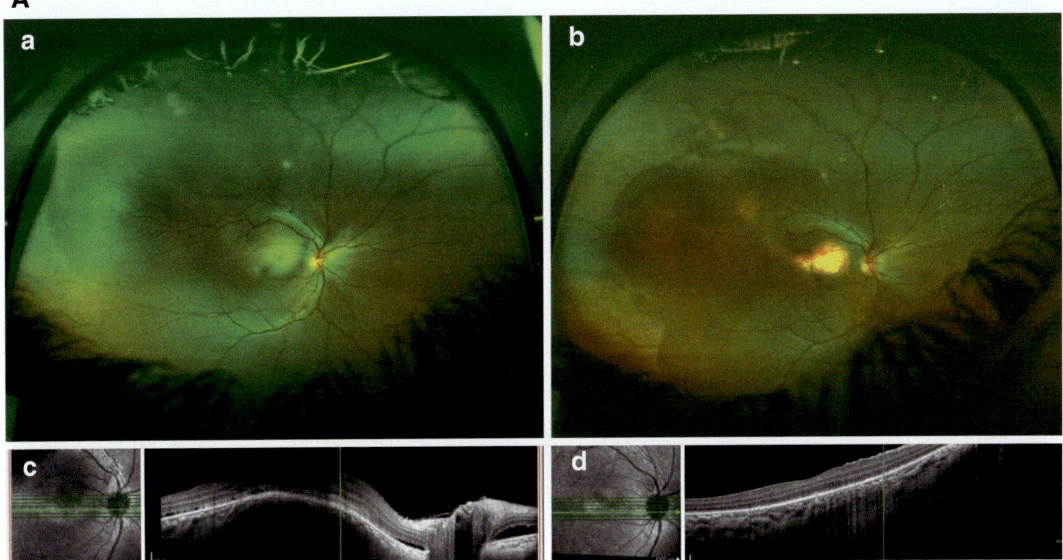

Fig. 10.11 (**A**) Tubercular choroidal granuloma seen as a solitary large yellowish granuloma in the posterior pole (**a**). Three weeks later, following initiation of systemic steroids and anti-tubercular therapy, the granuloma healed with scarring (**b**). OCT shows exudative retinal detachment (**c**) during active granuloma, and resolution of fluid (**d**) at 3 weeks during healing of granuloma. (**B**) Right eye fundus photograph of a 32-year-old man with choroidal granuloma and retinal vasculitis. The visual acuity was counting fingers and the QuantiFERON-TB Gold test was positive. After 9 months of anti-tubercular therapy and oral corticosteroids, the eye was quiescent with visual acuity 6/9. (Reproduced with permission from Bansal, R., Sharma, A., & Gupta, A. (2012). *Intraocular tuberculosis. Expert Review of Ophthalmology, 7(4), 341–349*. https://doi.org/10.1586/eop.12.42). (**C**) A case of TB choroidal granuloma with intraretinal haemorrhage (**a**). Fluorescein angiography shows the classical retinal angiomatous proliferation feeding the granuloma. (Images reproduced with permission of the publishers from Gupta, A., Gupta, V. (2016). Tuberculosis. In: Zierhut, M., Pavesio, C., Ohno, S., Orefice, F., Rao, N. (eds) Intraocular Inflammation. Springer, Berlin, Heidelberg. https://doi.org/10.1007/978-3-540-75387-2_105)

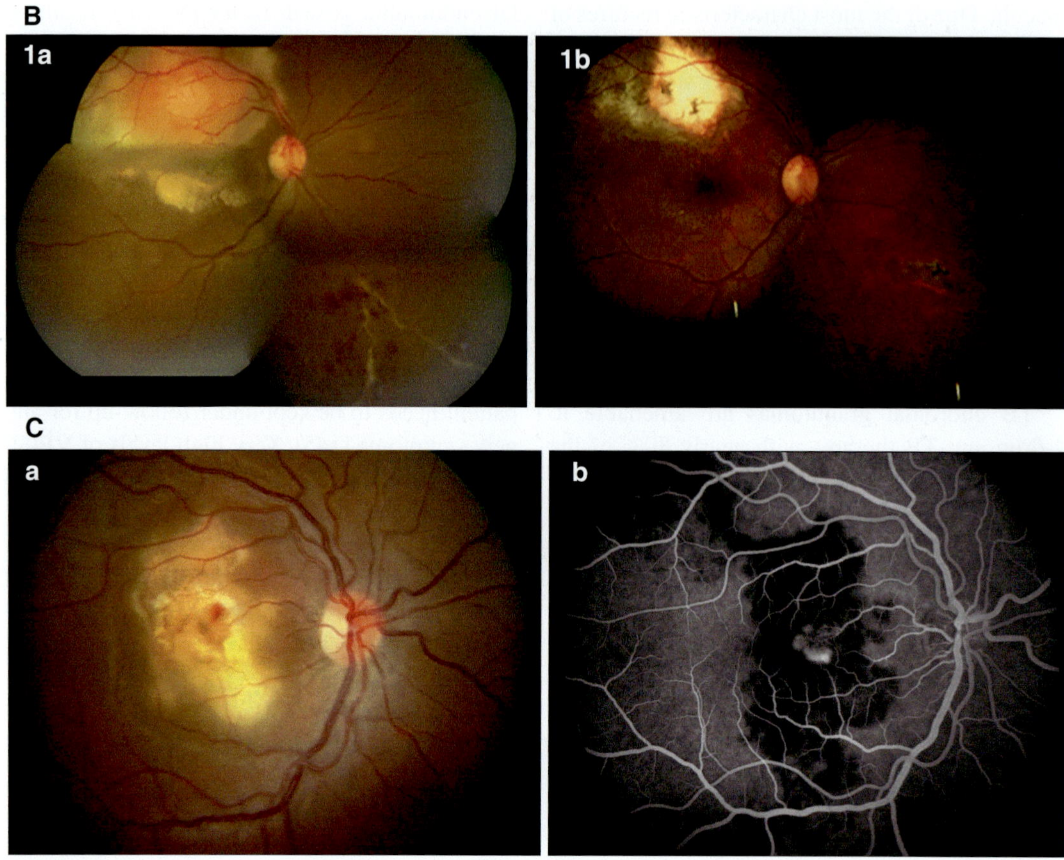

Fig. 10.11 (continued)

lomas showed a corresponding decrease in the aqueous humour VEGF levels [146]. Non-responding TB choroidal granuloma may harbour drug-resistant MTB, which can be detected using various PCR techniques, including semi-automated GeneXpert quantitative PCR, requiring multidrug-resistant treatment [147–149].

Retinal Periphlebitis

Henry Eales (1880) reported in Birmingham medical review four cases of recurrent vitreous haemorrhage and epistaxis in young, otherwise normal men who were habitually constipated. He noted dilated retinal veins and arteries in these patients. Except for one patient in whom he discovered 'thread-like retinal vessels' on the resolution of vitreous haemorrhage and who had sudden onset of glaucoma (most likely neovascular glaucoma), the other three had resolution of vitreous haemorrhage without leaving a trace (https://wellcomecollection.org/works/haupyuh9). Since then, idiopathic vitreous haemorrhage in young people has been labelled as Eales' disease. Except for his case # 1, none of the other patients he observed had any apparent cause of vitreous haemorrhage. A review of his description of the cases reveals that, except for case #1, none of them possibly resulted from retinal periphlebitis. Others likely represented examples of Valsalva retinopathy. For over 140 years,

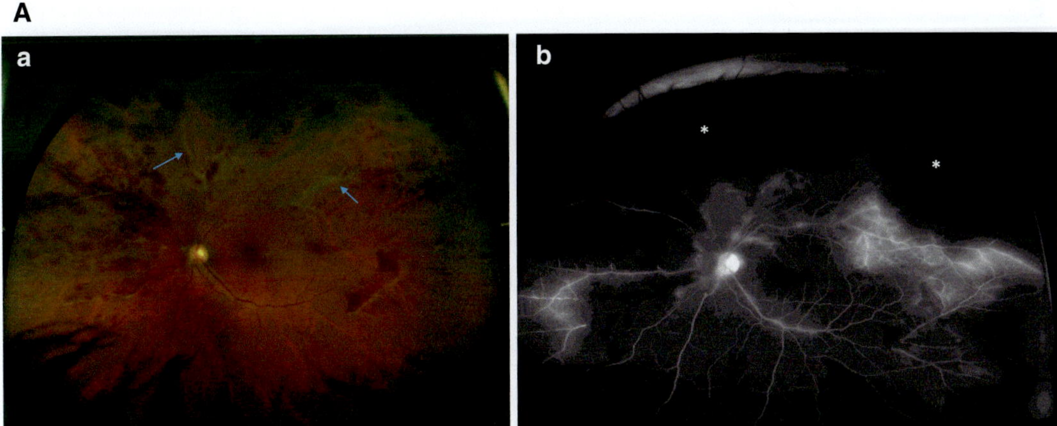

Fig. 10.12 (**A**) Tubercular retinal vasculitis (blue arrows) with periphlebitis, retinal haemorrhages, and perivascular cuffing (**a**). Fluorescein angiography shows extensive capillary non-perfusion (*) (**b**). (**B**) A 46-year-old man underwent successful pars plana vitreous surgery for the vitreous haemorrhage in the left eye (**a**) and recovered 20/20 visual acuity (**b**). Four years later, he returned with fresh symptoms. He showed multifocal choroiditis lesions along the retinal vessels (**c**). The FFA showed initial hypofluorescent (not shown) and intense fluorescein staining of the discrete chorioretinal lesions and retinal vessel wall staining nasal to the optic disc (**d**). His tuberculin skin test was positive at 13 × 15 mm. CT scan chest showed fibrotic opacities at the lung apices. Axillary glands were enlarged and were biopsied. On histopathology of the lymph node biopsy showed central areas of caseation necrosis, peripherally palisaded histiocytes along with epithelioid cell granulomas with Langhans giant cells. Stain for AFB was positive (**e**)

recurrent vitreous haemorrhage in young people has been erroneously labelled as Eales' disease, a misnomer for vitreous haemorrhage resulting from retinal periphlebitis, seen most commonly in TB-endemic countries like India. Biswas et al. [150], after an extensive review of the literature, suggested that this disease should be described as presumed tuberculous retinal periphlebitis.

Patients first present with vitreous haemorrhage and not earlier due to the mildly symptomatic or even asymptomatic nature of the peripheral retinal periphlebitis that may go unnoticed by young people. It is a bilateral but asymmetric disease. Examination of the contralateral eye in those presenting with vitreous haemorrhage will often reveal active periphlebitis or healed white thread-like occluded vessels in the peripheral retina. Acute-stage tubercular retinal vasculitis was characterized in patients who were PCR-positive for the MTB genome. These patients were treated with oral corticosteroids combined with anti-TB therapy and were followed up to monitor the course of the disease [122, 124]. In the acute stage, TB-periphlebitis is characterized by segmental exuberant perivenous infiltrates that involve one or more peripheral quadrants. Vitreous inflammatory cells, retinal haemorrhages, exudates, and macular oedema often accompany it. The most characteristic feature of this periphlebitis is the occlusion of the affected segments of the retinal veins resulting in extensive capillary non-perfusion (CNP) in the retinal periphery (Fig. 10.12). Nearly half of the patients may show perivascular discrete active or healed patches of chorioretinitis, which differentiates it from other causes of retinal vasculitis like Behcet's disease. Extensive CNP areas ultimately lead to the

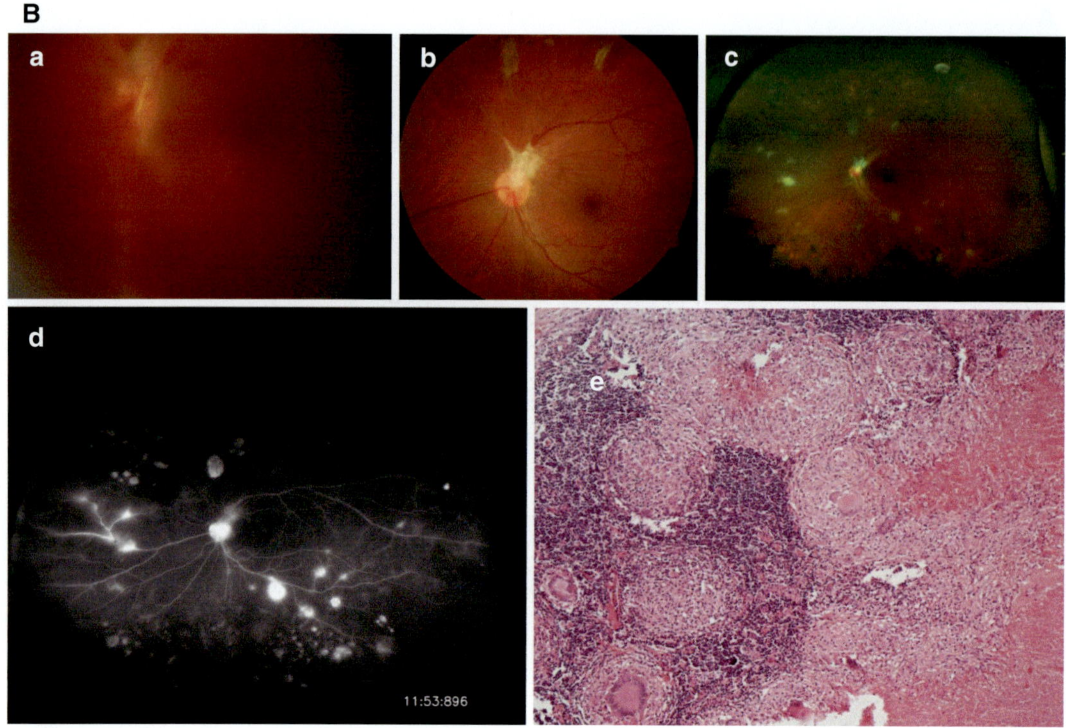

Fig. 10.12 (continued)

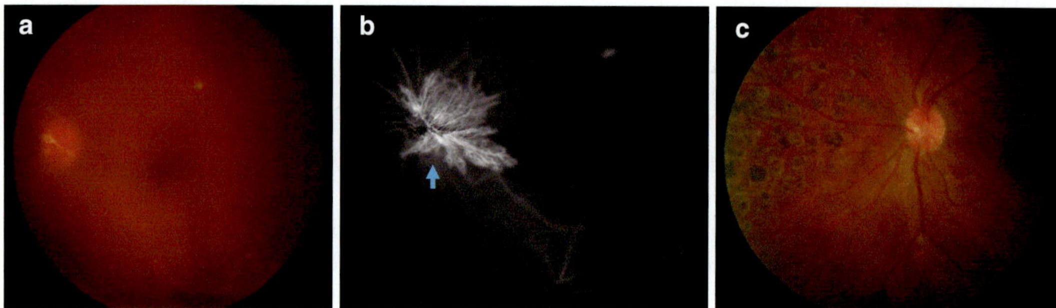

Fig. 10.13 Vitreous haemorrhage as the presentation of tubercular retinal vasculitis in a young man (**a**). Fluorescein angiography showed a large NVD (optic disc neovascularization, blue arrow) (**b**). Vitreous surgery with laser photocoagulation led to clearing of media and restoration of vision (**c**)

development of retinal neovessels elsewhere in the retina, which burst to cause sudden loss of vision from vitreous haemorrhage (Fig. 10.13). The new vessels are always accompanied by supporting connective tissue, which contracts and may lead to peripheral tractional retinal detachment. Undiluted vitreous samples from 57% of patients with the so-called Eales' disease were positive by quantitative PCR for the MTB genome, with copies varying from 1.52×10^4 to 1.01×10^6 [151]. Earlier, using the nested PCR technique, nearly 21% of the vitreous samples from patients with Eales' disease were positive for the MTB genome versus 4% from the control samples [152]. See Boxes 10.4 and 10.5 for clinical characteristics and the classification criteria of TB uveitis.

Box 10.4 Case Definitions for the Diagnosis of Tubercular Uveitis (TBU)

Proposed case definitions for diagnosing TBU
A. **Clinical signs consistent with TBU**
1. Broad posterior synechiae 2. Retinal periphlebitis with or without discrete chorioretinal lesions/scars 3. Multifocal serpiginoid choroiditis or SLC 4. Choroidal granuloma 5. Optic disc granuloma 6. Optic neuropathy
B. History of documented or undocumented exposure to TB within 48 months
C. Immunological tests—interferon gamma release assay or tuberculin skin test
D. Radiological evidence of active or past pulmonary TB
E. Histopathological evidence or AFB on smear or culture from extraocular sites
F. PCR or smear or culture + for MTB from ocular fluids
G. Response to treatment with anti-TB therapy assessed at 2 months after initiation

SLC serpiginous-like choroiditis, *TB* tuberculosis, *AFB* acid-fast bacilli, *PCR* polymerase chain reaction, *MTB* Mycobacterium tuberculosis

Ref. Adapted from Gupta et al. [99, 100] with permission of the publishers

Box 10.5 Classification Criteria for Tubercular Uveitis

Classification of TBU	
Clinical diagnostic group	Case definition criteria
Confirmed TBU (1 and 2)	1. At least one clinical sign suggestive of TBU 2. Microbiological confirmation of MTB from ocular fluids/tissues
Probable TBU (1, 2, and 3 together)	1. At least one clinical sign suggestive of TBU (other aetiologies excluded) 2. Radiological evidence consistent with TB infection or clinical evidence of extraocular TB or microbiological confirmation from sputum or extraocular sites 3. At least one of the following (a) Documented exposure to TB (b) Immunological evidence of TB
Possible TBU (1, 2, and 3) or (1 and 4)	1. At least one clinical sign suggestive of TBU (other aetiologies excluded) 2. Radiology not consistent with TB and no evidence of extraocular TB 3. A least one of the following (a) Documented exposure to TB (b) Immunological evidence of TB 4. Radiological evidence of TB but no documented exposure or immunological evidence of TB

TBU tubercular uveitis, *TB* tuberculosis, *MTB* Mycobacterium tuberculosis

Adapted from: Gupta A, Sharma A, Bansal R, Sharma K. Classification of intraocular tuberculosis. Ocul Immunol Inflamm. 2015 Feb;23(1):7–13. doi: 10.3109/09273948.2014.967358. Epub 2014 Oct 14. PMID: 25314361 with permission of the publishers

10.6.6.4 Laboratory Diagnosis of Infectious Uveitis Pathogen-Directed Polymerase Chain Reaction (PCR)

Necrotizing infections of the retina, especially in immunosuppressed individuals, are challenging to clinically differentiate, whether caused by herpes viruses, toxoplasmosis, or syphilis, as these often present with atypical features. Most organisms contain either DNA or RNA. Non-necrotizing infections by the herpes viruses in immunocompetent patients, although rare, may pose a diagnostic challenge [153]. Prespecified pathogen-directed polymerase chain reaction (PCR) from the ocular fluids has been a mainstay for more than three decades for detecting infections of the retina caused by HSV, VZV, and CMV with more than 95% sensitivity and nearly 100% specificity. [154–161]. The Ebola virus was found persisting in the aqueous humour of a patient who had recovered from the infection in the past [162]. More recently, a strip multiplex PCR to simultaneously test for 24 common eye infections produced comparable results to the conventional real-time PCR (RT-PCR) tests [163]. Suboptimal sensitivity of various PCR techniques in TBU, perhaps due to its paucibacillary pathology, has yet to find favour for these techniques for routine use in the clinics [151, 164, 165]. However, these have helped in characterizing the phenotypes of TBU. Moreover, the detection of a multidrug-resistant MTB genome by gene sequencing of the amplified DNA from the vitreous fluid helped successfully treat patients with non-responding TBU ([147, 149]; Sharma et al. 2019). Further, using mRNA multiplex PCR, viable MTB was reported from the vitreous fluid in over 40% of the suspected TBU cases [166], justifying the use of anti-tuberculosis drugs.

The yield of PCRs is higher from the vitreous fluid because of the proximity of the sampling site to the focus of infection. Micro-incisional pars plana vitreous surgery using either 23/25 or 27 gauge is a safe and effective procedure in patients with uveitis, especially infectious uveitis, where relatively larger volumes of fluid are required for carrying out many laboratory investigations [167, 168].

10.6.6.5 Next-Generation Sequencing (NGS)

Nearly 30 years after Sanger [169] introduced a technique, albeit slow and expensive, to identify the exact sequence of nucleotides in a genome, the introduction of NGS, a high-throughput technology capable of sequencing Gb size sequences of DNA by running millions of parallel sequences of 100–500 base pairs bits, it has begun to find its way into clinics to diagnose infections. Most of the sequenced DNA would be human, but an overabundance of microbial DNA indicates infection [170]. The major challenge is getting a sample not contaminated by bystander environmental organisms. It helps in detecting hitherto known or even unknown microbes. Deshmukh et al. [171] reported positivity rates of almost 88% from patients with endophthalmitis versus only 44% using conventional cultures.

10.6.6.6 Metagenomics Deep Sequencing (MDS)

An unbiased, comprehensive technique of NGS that can detect all species of microbes (viruses, bacteria, fungi and parasites) without any selection bias [172] led to the detection of organisms from 8 of the 36 (22%) archived vitreous samples that were negative by the conventional pathogen-directed PCR techniques. The technique has been validated by obtaining highly concordant results with the conventional pathogen-directed PCR [173]. The long-suspected rubella infection in patients of Fuchs' uveitis was confirmed by the MDS technique [172]. RNA-sequencing techniques have detected common and rare pathogens from the ocular fluids of patients with uveitis [173]. Using metagenomics sequencing, the same authors detected *Tropheryma whipplei* from the aqueous humour of a patient with Whipple's disease who presented with uveitis [174]. Arunasri et al. [175] found dysbiosis in the ocular microbiome in the vitreous fluid from patients with post-fever retinitis. Relapsing uveitis due to human T-lymphotropic virus type 1 in a patient living with HIV was diagnosed by metagenomic deep sequencing [176]. MDS has been one of the most exciting developments in microbial diagnostics. In the coming times, we expect to see a more extensive application of these techniques to detect offending microbes in the field of infectious uveitis and the yet-unknown microbes that drive non-infectious uveitis.

10.7 Non-infectious Choroiditis and Retinitis

Many rare non-infectious organ-specific immune-mediated disorders cause inflammation of the retina, choroid, or both. They include multiple evanescent white dot syndrome (MEWDS), punctate inner choroidopathy (PIC), multifocal choroiditis with panuveitis, acute posterior multifocal placoid pigment epitheliopathy (APMPPE), acute zonal occult outer retinopathy (AZOOR), and Birdshot chorioretinopathy. Commonly, Vogt-Koyanagi-Harada's (VKH) disease and sympathetic ophthalmia start first in the choroid and, during the disease, evolve into panuveitis involving both the anterior segment and the posterior segment. Retina and choroid often get involved in multisystem immune-mediated disorders such as systemic lupus erythematosus, Behcet's disease, and sarcoidosis.

10.7.1 Systemic Immune-Mediated Disorders

10.7.1.1 Systemic Lupus Erythematosus (SLE) Retinopathy

Rheumatological diseases are autoimmune multisystem inflammatory disorders, generally classified into arthritides, connective tissue disorders, and vasculitides. All three have significant, albeit variable, ocular involvement in different disorders. Of the major connective tissue disorders, namely SLE, scleroderma, polymyositis, dermatomyositis, and relapsing polychondritis, SLE is the most common affecting the eye. SLE predominantly affects young female patients in a ratio of 9:1. The incidence of SLE is ~5/100,000. It is 4–5 times higher in black and Asian ethnic groups than in the white races. The most characteristic feature of SLE is the development of autoantibodies years before the onset of clinical symptoms. The basic pathogenesis of SLE lies in the failure to handle the intracellular antigens (nucleosomes) from the apoptotic and necrotic cells. The macrophages take up these intracellular antigens and present them to the T and B lymphocytes to activate innate and adaptive immune responses to autoantigens [177]. Antinuclear antibodies are present in all patients with SLE, the highly specific anti-double stranded (ds) DNA antibodies are present in 70% of patients with SLE and only 0.5% of normal or even rheumatoid arthritis patients [178]. The level of the anti-ds DNA antibodies reflects the disease activity [179].

The anti-DS antibodies react with the released extracellular nucleosomes and activate complements that get deposited on the basement membrane and can involve any tissue, most commonly the kidneys, blood, and the brain. Any women presenting from 15 to 50 years of age with arthritis, skin rash, anaemia, thrombocytopenia, nephritis, seizures, or psychosis need to have SLE as a differential diagnosis [179]. The most common external feature of the disease is a skin malar rash. Nearly 33% of SLE patients have ocular involvement [180]. Before the availability of corticosteroids, nearly 50% of patients developed SLE retinopathy, but now the estimates vary from 3% in the well-controlled disease to 29% in the active disease [181]. SLE retinopathy is caused by immune complex deposition. Using immunofluorescent techniques, on the autopsy of a patient who had resolved SLE retinopathy, immune complexes were found deposited on the vascular walls of the entire choroidal vasculature, arterioles in the ciliary processes, and basement membrane of the bulbar conjunctiva [182]. SLE retinopathy is characterized by bilateral multiple cotton wool spots resulting from occlusion of the precapillary arterioles and manifests as SLE microangiopathy (see Chap. 3, Fig. 3.11).

SLE microangiopathy results from vascular endothelial injury from the deposition of immune complexes, leading to thrombosis. There may or may not be associated linear retinal haemorrhages. These changes are independent of hypertension, which is often present due to the involvement of kidneys by lupus. In addition, there may be infarcts in the visual pathways, ischaemic optic neuropathy, and internuclear ophthalmoplegia. There may be external eye involvement in keratoconjunctivitis sicca, episcleritis, or scleritis. There may also be small retinal arteriolar occlusion and venous thrombosis. Vision-threatening para macular acute middle maculopathy (PAMM) reflecting occlusion of deep retinal capillary plexus in the macula may be seen [183]. The retinal lesions in SLE indicate active disease and are a marker for poor survival. Nearly 75% of patients with SLE retinopathy have neuropsychiatric involvement [184]. On FFA, the retinal arterioles show stumping, indicating an obstruction to blood flow. Extensive occlusion of the vessels may rarely lead to the formation of new vessels on the optic disc and elsewhere, termed proliferative SLE retinopathy.

SLE may uncommonly present with choroidopathy, mostly bilateral, and presents with multifocal serous detachments of the retina that may mimic central serous chorioretinopathy [185, 186]. Usually, they are associated with active SLE disease. Choroidopathy may result from the deposition of immune complexes, antibodies against the RPE, or micro-thrombotic occlusion of choroidal vessels due to APLA. Most reported patients had associated systemic associations such as nephritis, CNS lupus, and hypertension. There is pinpoint leakage of fluorescein dye on FFA, and the ICG angiography shows non-filling of some of the choroidal vasculature. The OCT shows thickening of the choroid with loss of structural details and irregularities of the overlying of the RPE along with a collection of fluid under the retina and cystoid spaces in the outer plexiform layer [187].

Primary antiphospholipid syndrome (APS) is an autoimmune disorder caused by developing antiphospholipid antibodies (APLA), termed Lupus anticoagulant (LA), associated with arterial, venous thrombosis, and recurrent abortions. Secondary APLA is commonly associated with other autoimmune diseases like SLE and Sjogren's syndrome. Arterial and venous occlusions are significantly more common in primary or secondary APLA than SLE alone. While antinuclear antibodies (ANA) may be equally common in APS and SLE, LA is present in nearly two-thirds of the APS and very rare in SLE alone. Moreover, anti-cardiolipin antibodies are present in APS, not SLE [188]. It is essential to rule out APS if a retinal arterial or venous occlusion or any retinopathy is observed in a patient with SLE, as nearly 77% of patients of SLE who had retinopathy had associated APS [189]. See Box 10.6 for the classification criteria of SLE.

Box 10.6 Classification criteria for diagnosis of SLE

Entry criteria ANA + >1:80 on HEp-2 cells or equivalent	
If ANA is absent, do not classify it as SLE **If present, apply additive criteria** Do not apply additive criteria if there is a more likely explanation than SLE. Criteria occurrence on even one occasion is sufficient. They need not occur simultaneously. SLE classification requires at least one clinical criteria and >10 points. Within each domain, only the highest weighted criteria are counted	
Clinical domains and criteria Weight	**Immunological domain and criteria Weight**
Constitutional 2 Fever	**Antiphospholipid antibodies** Anti-cardiolipin antibodies **OR** Anti-β2GP1 antibodies **OR** Lupus anticoagulant 2
Haematologic Leukopenia 3 Thrombocytopenia 4 Autoimmune haemolysis 4	**Complement proteins** Low C3 or Low C4 3 Low C3 and C4 4
Neuropsychiatric Delirium 2 Psychosis 3 Seizure 5	**SLE-specific antibodies** Anti-dsDNA antibody Or Anti-Smith antibody 6

Mucocutaneous Non-scarring alopecia 2 Oral ulcers 2 Subacute cutaneous or discoid lupus 4 Acute cutaneous lupus 6	
Serosal Pleural or pericardial effusion 5 Acute pericarditis 6	
Musculoskeletal Joint involvement 6	
Renal Proteinuria >05 g/24 h 4 Renal biopsy class II **OR** 4 V lupus nephritis Renal biopsy class III **OR** IV lupus nephritis 8	
Classify as SLE with a score of 10 or more if entry criterion is fulfilled	

Adapted from Fig. 2 by Aringer et al. [190] with permission of the publishers

10.7.1.2 Sarcoidosis

Sarcoidosis is a systemic multiorgan granulomatous inflammatory disease that often involves the lungs, lymph nodes and skin. It affects people younger than 40 years of age. The pathogenesis of sarcoidosis is unknown, but as many as 2% of people of Afro-American ancestry have a lifetime risk of developing this disease. Compared to Caucasians, Blacks suffer more severe diseases. There are no definitive autoantibodies or markers for diagnosing or monitoring this disease. The granulomas are formed due to a Th1-type T-cell oligoclonal immune response to a poorly degradable antigen. Many triggers, including viruses (herpes, CMV, EBV, and retroviruses) or bacteria (MTB, Propionibacterium acnes, and Borrelia Burgdorferi), aluminium, zirconium, talc, pine tree pollens, or even soil, have been incriminated [191]. Sarcoidosis may mimic connective tissue disorders, vasculitis, or even a simultaneous autoimmune disease. Patients with sarcoidosis may have subtle constitutional symptoms, like low-grade fever, fatigue, cough, or breathlessness. Uncommonly, acute sarcoidosis may present as Lofgren syndrome characterized by fever, hilar lymphadenopathy, erythema nodosum, and ankle arthritis [192]. The lungs are involved in >90% of patients, lymph nodes in ~33%, the liver in 50–80%, eyes in 11–80%, CNS ~10%, skin ~25%, and less commonly may involve the heart and muscles [191]. In a series of 364 patients with sarcoid uveitis, more than 50% of patients had lung parenchymal disease, cutaneous involvement in 27% (lupus pernio, plaque-like, or nodular skin lesions), ~and arthritis and CNS in ~16%. Liver and cardiac involvement were seen involvement in 5–6%. Caucasian patients were older and had less granulomatous uveitis and less skin involvement [193].

Patients with sarcoidosis may present first to the ophthalmologist with visual symptoms. There are several, bilateral in nearly 90%, ocular signs that suggest a granulomatous inflammation of the eye, including mutton fat keratic precipitates, nodular iris granuloma in the inferior angle of the anterior chamber with a tent-like peripheral anterior synechiae (Berlin's nodule) [194, 195]. Koeppe's nodules at the pupillary border, broad posterior synechiae, vitritis with a string of pearls snowball opacities in the inferior vitreous gel, optic disc oedema, and focal nodular perivascular infiltrates like candle wax dripping, retinal arterial macroaneurysms, and choroidal granulomas (Fig. 10.14). In the external eye, they may also present with a dry eye due to lacrimal gland sarcoidosis. The age of presentation of sarcoidosis is shifting to a higher age in Western countries. Notably, patients above 65 present have fewer ocular signs than younger patients [196]. Taches de bougie lesions (candle wax spots) may be seen in nearly one-third of the ocular sarcoidosis as yellowish white streaks or discreet white spots in the inferior or inferonasal retina that may mimic birdshot chorioretinopathy or multifocal chorioretinitis [197]. Taches de bougie is present in the choroid in contrast to the perivascular candle wax drippings in the retina. In a large series of sarcoid uveitis, nearly two-thirds presented first to the

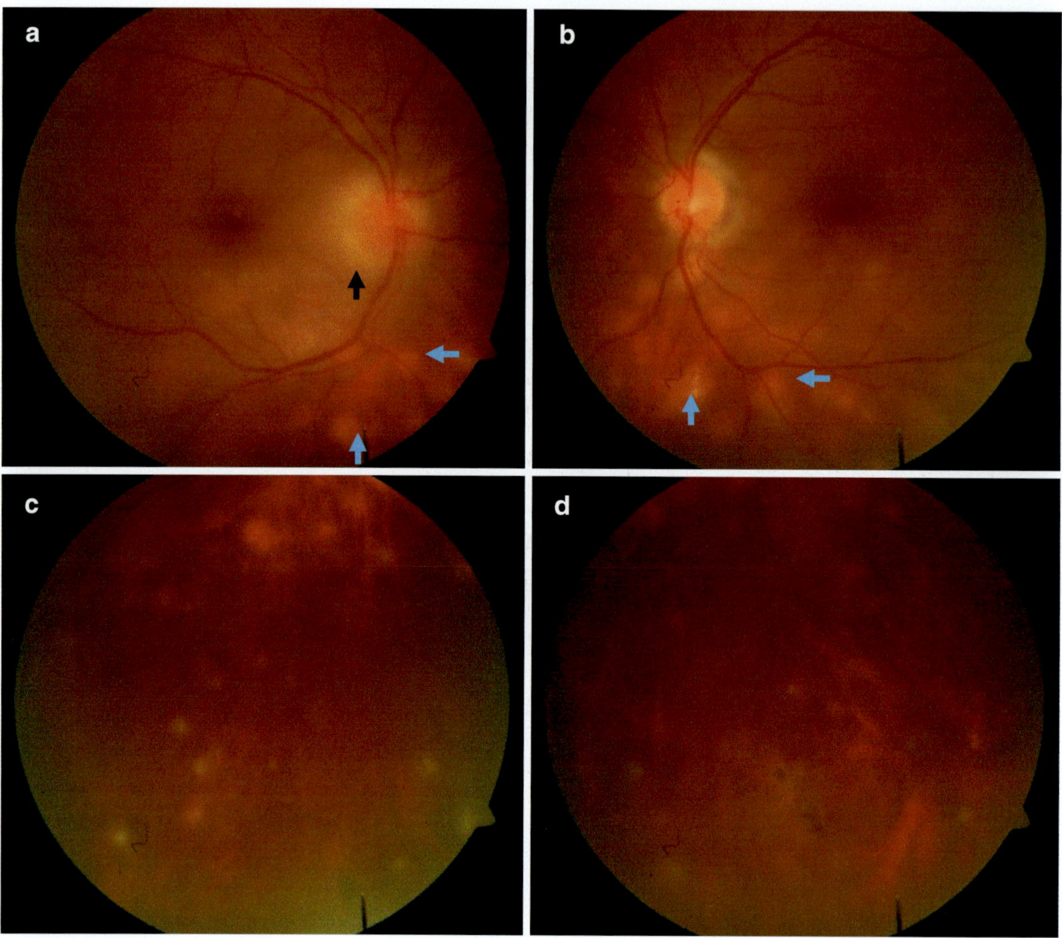

Fig. 10.14 Optic disc oedema (black arrow) and choroidal granulomas (blue arrows) in right (**a**) and left (**b**) eyes of a patient with sarcoidosis. Peripheral examination also revealed choroidal granulomas in right (**c**) and left (**d**) eyes

ophthalmologist. Granulomatous anterior uveitis was seen in ~48%, snowballs in vitreous ~46%, multifocal choroiditis in 43%, periphlebitis in 21%, and isolated optic nerve or choroidal granuloma in 11% [193]. In a study of 48 patients with multifocal choroiditis, 17% had retinal arteriolar macroaneurysms, and half had histopathologically proven sarcoidosis. Arterial macroaneurysms in sarcoidosis are associated with severe cardiovascular disease [198]. Most of these macroaneurysms are exudative [199].

Less commonly, sarcoid granuloma may be located on the optic disc and consists of epithelioid cells [200]. The choroid is thickened in sarcoidosis, and a disproportionate enlargement of the Sattler's layer (medium vessels layer of the choroid) in sarcoidosis can help differentiate it from TB choroiditis [201]. Choroidal granulomas on OCT are uniformly hyporeflective and may occupy the choroid's total or partial thickness (Fig. 10.15). Increased light transmission posterior to these hyporeflective spaces is a unique sign in sarcoid granulomas. The OCT also helps monitor the treatment response [202]. Sarcoidosis granulomas need to be differentiated from tubercular choroidal granulomas. The latter are often solitary, larger, lobulated, intense yellow in colour, perivascular in location, and vascularized (Fig. 10.11). Sarcoid granulomas are often multiple, oval in shape, dull yellow, and do not show retinal haemorrhages (Fig. 10.14). They remain under the RPE layer, unlike the TB granu-

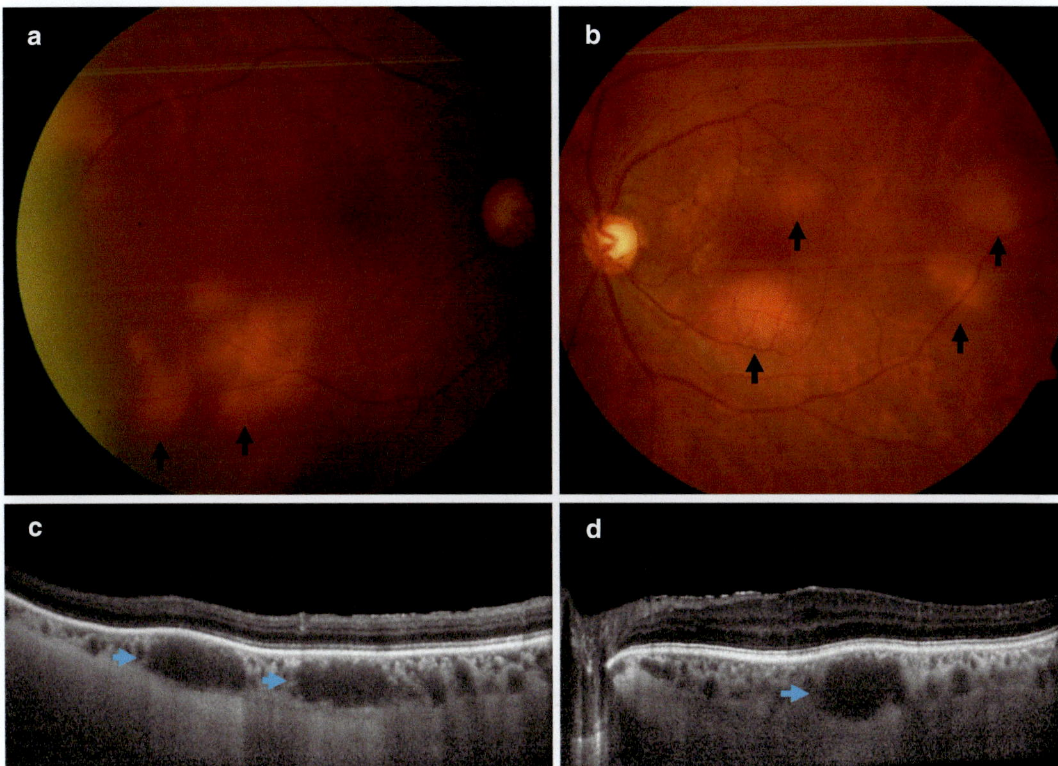

Fig. 10.15 A 59-year-old man, known case of skin sarcoidosis and calcified mediastinal lymph nodes, presented with bilateral choroidal granulomas (black arrows; **a**, **b**). On OCT, the sarcoid choroidal granulomas are uniformly hyporeflective (blue arrows) and occupy the choroid's total or partial thickness (**c**, **d**). Increased light transmission is seen posterior to these hyporeflective spaces

lomas that, on OCT, show hyperreflectivity in the outer retina indicative of the infiltrative nature of the TB granuloma [132–134].

Diagnostic Criteria for Ocular Sarcoidosis

An international workshop for ocular sarcoidosis (IWOS) suggested criteria for making a diagnosis of confirmed ocular sarcoidosis (biopsy proven); presumed—compatible uveitis with bilateral hilar lymphadenopathy (BHL) but biopsy not done; probable, no biopsy or BHL but three clinical signs and two laboratory tests positive; and possible, no biopsy, no BHL but four clinical signs and two laboratory tests [203]. However, in a large series of uveitis patients, 37% of those suspected to have sarcoidosis did not meet these IWOS criteria, and except for BHL, all clinical signs had low sensitivity [204]. The gold standard for diagnosing sarcoidosis remains a histopathological demonstration of non-caseating epithelioid cell granuloma from any available disease site. In recent years, a minimally invasive technique of endobronchial ultrasound-guided trans-bronchial needle aspiration (EBUS-TBNA) biopsy has been used with a diagnostic accuracy of almost 80%. It is recommended as a routine for diagnosing sarcoidosis wherever this facility is available [205]. The IWOS revised their criteria once again [206]. More recently, using machine learning algorithms, the Standardization of Uveitis Nomenclature (SUN) Working Group gave a new classification for sarcoidosis-associated uveitis with very high sensitivity and specificity for diagnosing sarcoidosis-associated uveitis. [60–63]. See Box 10.7 for investigations in a case of sarcoidosis and Box 10.8 for SUN classification criteria for diagnosis of sarcoidosis.

Box 10.7 Investigation in a Patient with a Suspected Diagnosis of Sarcoidosis or Autoimmune Disease

Laboratories	CBC; liver enzymes; creatinine; BUN; uric acid; creatine kinase; calcium; albumin; CRP Protein-electrophoresis ACE; sIL-2R Urine analysis for proteinuria, haematuria, and hypercalciuria RF; ACPA; ANA or ENA; IgG4 25(OH)D, 1,25(OH)D3
Imaging tests	X-ray chest; USG abdomen; CT chest Imaging studies of affected joints if required PET scan optional
Others	Pulmonary function tests
ECG	
Biopsy	Mediastinal lymph nodes, extrapulmonary nodes; skin lesion; liver; kidney

CBC complete blood counts, *BUN* blood urea nitrogen, *CRP* C-reactive proteins, *ACE* angiotensin-converting enzyme, *sIL-2R* soluble interleukin-2 receptor, *RF* rheumatoid factor, *ACPA* anti-citrullinated peptide antibodies, *ANA* antinuclear antibodies, *ENA* extractable nuclear antigen

Adapted from Korsten P, Tampe B, Konig MF, Nikiphorou E. Sarcoidosis and autoimmune diseases: differences, similarities and overlaps. Curr Opin Pulm Med. 2018 Sep;24(5):504–512. https://doi.org/10.1097/MCP.0000000000000500. PMID: 29985181 with permission of the publishers

Box 10.8 SUN Classification Criteria for Diagnosis of Ocular Sarcoidosis

Criteria	
Clinical	Compatible uveitis (a) Anterior (b) Intermediate or anterior-intermediate uveitis (c) Posterior uveitis either paucifocal or multifocal choroiditis (d) Panuveitis with choroiditis or retinal vascular sheathing or retinal vascular occlusion
Evidence	1. Tissue biopsy demonstrating non-caseating granuloma OR 2. BHL
Exclusion	1. Positive serology for syphilis 2. Evidence of infection with MTB (a) Histological or microbiological evidence of MTB OR (b) Positive IGRA OR (c) Positive tuberculin skin test (>10 mm induration)

SUN standardization of Uveitis Nomenclature, *BHL* bilateral hilar lymphadenopathy, *MTB* mycobacterium tuberculosis, *IGRA* interferon-γ release assay

Adapted from Standardization of Uveitis Nomenclature (SUN) Working Group. Classification Criteria for Sarcoidosis-Associated Uveitis, 2021. With permission of the publishers

10.7.1.3 Behçet's Syndrome

Epidemiology and Genetic Predisposition of Behçet's Syndrome

Behçet's syndrome (BS) is a multisystem autoinflammatory disorder seen worldwide, although its prevalence varies widely across regions. It is the most common cause of blinding panuveitis in regions along the old trading 'silk route' that extends from the countries around the Mediterranean Sea to the Middle East and the Far East. Its prevalence progressively decreases from a high of ~400 people per 100,000 population in North Turkey to 13.5 to 20/100,000 population in Saudi Arabia, Iran, China, and Japan and still lowers in the UK (0.64/100,000) and is least common in the USA (0.12–0.33/100,000). In Germany, its prevalence is estimated at 21/100,000 in people of Turkish origin versus 0.42–0.55/100,000 native Germans [207]. There is no single test to diagnose BS, but there is a strong association of BD with HLA-B*5101, and the prevalence of BS in the population runs parallel with the prevalence of this allele [208]. The highest prevalence of the HLA-B*51 allele is seen in Turkey and Saudi Arabia, where 24–26%

population has this allele versus 18–22% in Japan, 7.6–8.13% in India, 2.2–8.8 in different regions of China, and only 0.5% in Zimbabwe [209]. Notably, anecdotal cases have been reported from people of West African and Afro-Caribbean origin living for several years in the UK [209]. The exact aetiology remains unknown, but infectious antigen(s) (environmental factors) probably precipitate the disease in genetically predisposed people [210]. In the Japanese population, the frequency of HLA-B*51 varies according to the cluster of the symptom complex, with 50–52% in the dominant mucocutaneous, mucocutaneous arthritis, ocular, and CNS clusters compared to only 33% in the GI dominant BS [210]. Notably, with the rising number of women in their population, the HLA-B*51 frequency is decreasing.

Pathology of Behçet's Syndrome

The hallmark of Behcet's syndrome is the activation of neutrophils and expression of intercellular adhesion molecules on the endothelial cell lining of the blood vessels prompting the activated neutrophils and RBCs to extravasate from the vessels. Practically, all involved organs in BS show a significant infiltration with neutrophils. The other characteristic feature is the venous occlusions, likely related to the factor V Leiden mutation, which is seen more frequently in patients of BS with venous thrombosis [211].

There is a 14-fold rise in the risk of venous thrombosis in Behçet's syndrome compared to the normal controls [212]. All BS lesions in different organs show almost similar pathological changes. There is upregulation of cytokines like TNF-α, IL-Iβ, and Il-8 that are known to activate neutrophils. There are also increased levels of myeloperoxidase, which is generated by the neutrophils [208].

Systemic Signs of Behçet's Syndrome

The BS is characterized by recurrent panuveitis and oral and genital aphthous ulcers. Till 2018, Behçet's syndrome was known as Behçet's disease when the nomenclature was changed from a disease to a syndrome. The experts believe that Behçet's is not a single disease but a symptom complex with great variations in organ involvement in various regional and familial clusters [213]. There are fewer gastrointestinal symptoms in the Mediterranean basin, increased frequency of arthritis and skin ulcers in the familial cohorts in Japan, and less severe eye disease in the BS patients in the US and North European countries [214]. It is essentially a heterogeneous multisystem vasculitis affecting both the arteries (involvement of the vasa vasorum of large arteries leads to arterial aneurysms) and the veins (venous thrombosis) of all sizes. It runs a relapsing and remitting course and, besides the eye, involves skin (papulopustular or acne-like lesions, erythema nodosum and leg ulcers), joints (non-deforming acute mono- or poly-polyarthritis), gastrointestinal tract (inflammatory bowel disease), and central nervous system (parenchymal disease or venous thrombosis). It is predominantly seen in men in their early 20s to 30s who also carry a worse outcome than women. The involvement of the various organs may occur over several years. Besides, it runs a variable course and may sometimes show spontaneous remission. For these reasons, the treatment has to be organ-specific and individualized depending upon the severity of involvement. In general, the involvement of the skin, mucosa, and joints carries a much better prognosis than the involvement of the eyes, GI tract, and CNS [213]. It is now believed that the HLA-B*51 haplotype, which is closely associated with this syndrome, determines the clinical spectrum of the disease.

Recurrent, painful oral ulcers on the tongue, buccal, or labial mucosa, lasting for 7–10 days, are almost always present during the disease and may precede the onset of BS in other organs by years. Genial ulcers are seen on the scrotum and penis in men and the vulva in women, and anal ulcers may occur in both sexes. These are recurrent, painful, and larger than in the oral cavity. Genital ulcers usually heal with scarring, unlike oral ulcers, which do not leave behind any scarring. Other systemic involvement includes superficial venous thrombosis in the legs and arms, erythema nodosum, pseudofolliculitis, acneiform lesions, and ulceration [207]. Large joints may be involved as non-deforming mono- or polyarthri-

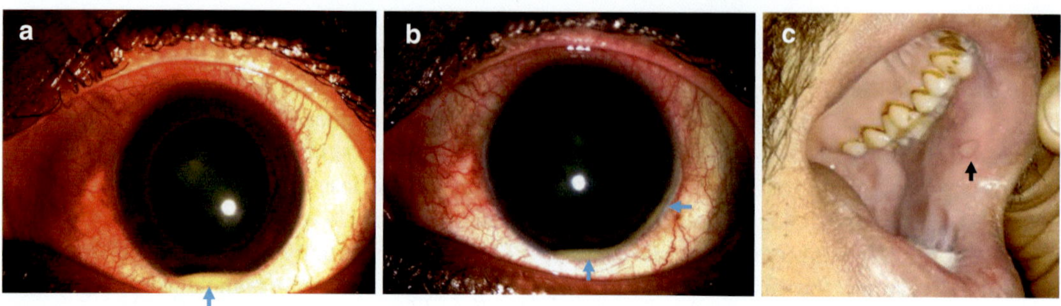

Fig. 10.16 Hypopyon (blue arrow) in a patient with Behcet's disease (**a**), which is shifting in nature (**b**), who had oral ulcers (black arrow; **c**)

tis. Patients may have inflammatory bowel disease (IBD) that mimics ulcerative colitis or Crohn's disease and present with diarrhoea or even GI perforation. HLA typing, the phenotype of uveitis and GI biopsy, may help distinguish the BS from other causes of IBD. A variety of nervous system symptoms, including meningitis, meningoencephalitis, venous thrombosis and brainstem involvement, may be seen in some patients. Neuropsychiatric symptoms ultimately lead to symptoms of dementia.

Ocular Signs of Behçet's Syndrome

In our single-centre experience in India from 1990 to 2006, BS was seen in 53 (1.25%) of the 4214 patients with uveitis [215]. It was seen as nearly three times more common in men than women at the mean age of 27 years (range 10–62 years). Ocular involvement was the most common in 92.4%, followed by oral ulcers in 88.7%, genital ulcers in 61.2%, skin lesions (erythema nodosum, acne, and folliculitis), and arthritis in 28.3% each. In our cohort, GI tract, CNS, and epididymis involvement was rare and seen only in two (3.7%) patients each.

In our experience, presenting ocular signs were panuveitis (57.1%), followed by posterior uveitis (26.5%) and anterior uveitis (16.3%) [215]. Although our cohort was much smaller than the Turkish report of 880 patients with BS, the ocular and systemic involvement was almost similar in the two cohorts [216]. The ocular involvement usually follows oral aphthous ulcers. However, it may be important to note that ocular involvement may be the first presentation or manifestation of the BS in about 20% of the cases. It is important to recognize this entity at the outset to prevent the long-term consequences of the disease (Tugal-Tutkun, 2022). BS uveitis may present as a painless, recurrent, and mobile hypopyon in one-third of the patients. In BS uveitis, the level of the hypopyon shifts with head tilting (Fig. 10.16). It is due to a lack of fibrin in the BS uveitis, unlike the painful acute anterior uveitis associated with HLA-B27 disease, in which the most dominant sign is a severe fibrinous reaction and a non-shifting streak hypopyon. The anterior uveitis in BS is non-granulomatous. Granulomatous reactions, such as mutton fat keratic precipitates, rule out the BS. The vitreous inflammatory reaction is variable. The most sight-threatening complication of BS uveitis is retinal vasculitis, which involves all retinal veins, capillaries, and retinal arterioles (Fig. 10.17). The complications include cystoid macular oedema (55.1%), occlusive vasculitis (44.8%), and optic atrophy (26.5%) [215]. There is a significant vitreous haze due to inflammatory cell infiltration of the vitreous gel, which may settle down as pearls. The retinal signs include transient greyish-white retinitis patches, which resolve without leaving any scarring. The vessels show perivascular infiltrates and a variable amount of haemorrhages. Retinal branch vein occlusions are more common than arterial occlusions. The retinal perivascular leakage and staining of the vessel walls of all types of small or large vessels characterize the fundus fluorescein angiography (FFA) in BS uveitis (Fig. 10.17). The 'fern-like' pattern of the retinal

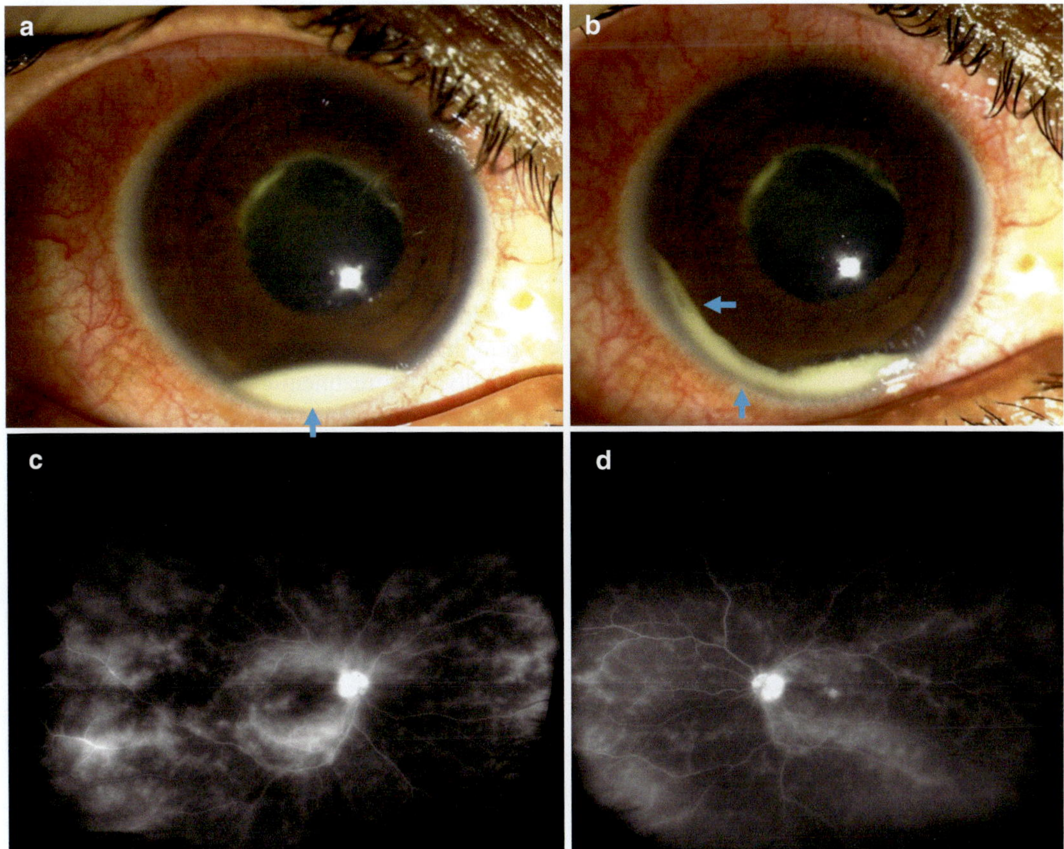

Fig. 10.17 A patient with Behcet's disease presented with hypopyon (blue arrows; **a**), which was shifting in nature (**b**). Fluorescein angiography showed leakage from vessels in fern pattern suggestive of active vasculitis in both eyes (**c**, **d**)

capillary leakage highly suggests subclinical inflammatory activity. Along with laser flare photometry, it is an important sign in apparently quiescent eyes, as these signs indicate an impending recurrence [217]. The FFA is also helpful in detecting and monitoring retinal vascular occlusions, capillary non-perfusion, and the development of new vessels. In recent years, ultra-wide-field FFA has been used to monitor the response to therapy [218]. Optical coherence tomography (OCT) helps detect cystoid macular oedema, frequently complicating Behçet's uveitis. It may also show defects in the ellipsoid zone, which may serve as a predictive sign for the final visual outcome. The OCT additionally may show defects in the external limiting membrane, RPE and epiretinal membrane disruption, and macular atrophy [219]. The role of OCT angiography is limited in BS uveitis as the most sensitive parameter of the disease activity; i.e., the retinal capillary leaks cannot be seen on OCTA. However, a recent meta-analysis showed that OCTA might be a valuable tool to monitor BS activity as it shows a decreased retinal capillary density in the superficial and deep capillary plexus in the macula, fovea, and parafovea [220]. The role of indocyanine green angiography (ICG) and fundus autofluorescence is limited as these do not provide any helpful information. Notably, Behçet's disease does not cause choroiditis, and if choroiditis is seen in BS suspects patients, we need to rule out syphilis and sarcoidosis as possible aetiology. See Box 10.9 for the classification criteria of Behcet's disease.

Box 10.9 Classification Criteria for Behçet's Uveitis

	Criteria
1	**Compatible uveitis syndrome** (a) Anterior uveitis (b) Anterior and intermediate uveitis (c) Posterior uveitis with retinal vasculitis and/or focal retinal infiltrates[a] (d) Panuveitis with retinal vasculitis and/or focal retinal infiltrates
2	**A diagnosis of Behçet's disease using ISG for Behçet's disease criteria** Recurrent oral ulcers observed by physician or patient at least three times in one 12-month period **Plus** any of the two criteria (a) Recurrent genital ulceration or scarring observed by physician or patient (b) Uveitis (anterior uveitis, posterior uveitis, or vitreous cells on slit-lamp examination or retinal vasculitis observed by physician) (c) Skin lesions (EN observed by patient or physician; pseudofolliculitis or papulopustular lesions or acneiform nodules observed by the physician in post-adolescent patients, not on corticosteroid treatment (d) Positive pathergy test read by physician at 24–48 h
Behçet's uveitis is diagnosed when criteria 1 and 2 are met	

ISG International study group for Behçet's disease, *EN* erythema nodosum

[a] Presence of choroiditis rules out Behçet's uveitis

Source:

1. Adapted from Standardization of Uveitis Nomenclature (SUN) Working Group. Classification Criteria for Behçet Disease Uveitis, 2021. With permission from the publishers
2. Adapted from Criteria for diagnosis of Behçet's disease. International Study Group for Behçet's Disease, 1990. With permission from the publishers [221]

Therapy of Behçet's Uveitis

The BS is a highly heterogeneous syndrome; hence, a multidisciplinary approach is required to diagnose, treat, and monitor response to therapy. Depending on the severity, as various systems may get affected over a considerable period, the therapy will usually be directed to the affected system. In the past, the treatment consisting of oral corticosteroids combined with immunomodulatory agents like cyclosporine or azathioprine has been used to control acute inflammation rapidly. The treatment goals in BS have been to achieve a temporary remission of inflammation, prevent recurrences and minimize complications. In recent years, increasingly biological agents like interferon-α and TNF-α blocking agents (infliximab or adalimumab) are being used to treat, especially the refractory cases of BS [222]. Tocilizumab has been used in patients who fail to respond to the anti-TNF-α antibodies. Although highly effective in uveitis, vascular and neurological disease is ineffective in many cases with oral or genital ulceration, arthritis, and skin and GI lesions. It worsened some of these patients' skin and oro-genital ulcers [223]. More recently, in a small pilot study of refractory Behçet's uveitis, cases have been successfully treated with tofacitinib, a JAK1/3 inhibitor, which targets both the innate and adaptive immune responses. It was suggested that being a small molecule, it can cross the blood-retinal barrier more efficiently than other biological agents. However, previously it failed to control the GI involvement in the BS [224]. These experiences strengthen the treatment philosophy of BS that being a highly heterogeneous disease, multiple inflammatory mechanisms may be involved in various systems, and therapeutic options should be chosen, keeping this fact in mind.

Visual Outcome of Behçet's Syndrome

BS is one of the most sight-threatening panuveitis. Thirty-eight per cent of the eyes in our own experience had less than 6/60 visual acuity at the final follow-up [215]. Likewise, most patients had panuveitis and bilateral involvement in a large international cohort with BS. At the final follow-up, 23–25% of these patients had less than 20/200 in the better eye. Men who were HLA-B 51 positive disease had more severe and blinding disease compared to women [225].

10.7.2 Organ-Specific (Ocular) Immune-Mediated Panuveitis with Multisystem Involvement

10.7.2.1 Vogt-Koyanagi-Harada (VKH) Disease

VKH disease is one of the most common causes of panuveitis and posterior uveitis in Asian and Hispanic populations and is distinctly uncommon in Caucasians. Although cases had been described independently in Japan by Vogt, Koyanagi, and Harada in the early decades of the twentieth century, it was only in the 1950s that a commonality was found in these cases, and the term VKH syndrome was coined. Its description as a 'syndrome' was replaced by 'disease' by the first international workshop on VKH disease held in 1999, which met to define its diagnostic criteria [226].

The VKH disease is characterized by an autoimmune T-cell response to tyrosinase family proteins contained in the melanocytes [227]. An experimental rat model of VKH disease has been successfully created by immunizing rats with tyrosinase family proteins [228]. Melanocytes are responsible for the colour of the skin and hair and also present in the meninges, choroid, and inner ear, and hence, the symptoms and signs in the VKH disease relate to these tissues. In the skin, the melanocytes are destroyed by an autoimmune response leading to the formation of vitiligo patches. Skin biopsy from skin vitiligo patches in patients with VKH disease revealed HLA-DR expressing T cells and CD4+ dominating over CD8+ T cells in a ratio of 3:1 [229]. In a rat model, electron microscopy showed an accumulation of lymphocytes and epithelioid cells around choroidal melanocytes [230]. In several populations, it has been associated with HLA-DRB1*0405, indicating a racial and genetic predilection. The exact trigger that causes loss of tolerance to the melanocytes is unknown. Exceptional cases of minor skin abrasions precipitating VKH have been reported [122, 124, 231]. VKH has followed vaccinations against BCG, hepatitis B and yellow fever, and viral infections such as the influenza A virus [232]. COVID-19 infection has led to the acute onset of VKH disease [233]. Even the administration of inactivated COVID-19 vaccine has not only led to the occurrence of the VKH disease [234] but an exacerbation of the existing VKH disease [235].

Interestingly, immune checkpoint inhibitors (ICIs) in patients with malignant melanoma have led to a picture mimicking VKH disease, including patients who developed alopecia, vitiligo, poliosis, exudative retinal detachment, and chronic uveitis [232]. The retinal detachment responded to the use of corticosteroids. The development of VKH-like disease following the use of CII was associated with regression of the melanomas and is considered an indicator of a good prognosis for the outcome of melanoma [236].

Clinical Presentations of VKH Disease

VKH disease has no specific diagnostic laboratory test; hence, clinical signs and symptoms are used to diagnose and classify VKH disease. Because of its spectrum of involving multiple systems has been classified as a complete, incomplete, or probable VKH disease [230]. See Box 10.10.

Box 10.10 Revised Diagnostic Criteria for Vogt-Koyanagi-Harada Disease

1.	No history of penetrating trauma or intraocular surgery before the onset of intraocular inflammation
2.	No clinical or laboratory evidence of any other disease
3.	Bilateral involvement (a) **OR** (b) must be met

	(a) **Early Manifestation**: I. Fundus examination: diffuse choroiditis, focal areas of SRF, bullous SRD **OR** If fundus exam is equivocal II. FFA signs of focal areas of delayed choroidal perfusion, pinpoint focal leakage, large placoid hyperfluorescence, and pooling of dye **AND** III. Diffuse choroidal thickening on USG. Rule out posterior scleritis
	(a) **Late manifestations:** History suggestive of prior disease as in (a). I. Sunset glow fundus; Sugiura's sign II. Nummular chorioretinal depigmented scars; recurrent or chronic anterior uveitis
4.	**Neurological sSymptoms:** meningismus, tinnitus or CSF pleocytosis (may have resolved)
5.	**Integumentary sSigns:** Must appear after the onset of ocular inflammation Vitiligo, poliosis, or alopecia
Complete VKH Disease: All the five criteria are present	
Incomplete VKH Disease: criteria 1, 2, and 3 with either 4 or 5	
Probable VKH Disease: criteria 1 to 3 are met	

Adapted from: O'Keefe GA, Rao NA. Vogt-Koyanagi-Harada disease. Surv Ophthalmol. 2017 Jan-Feb;62(1):1–25. https://doi.org/10.1016/j.survophthal.2016.05.002. Epub 2016 May 27. PMID: 27241814 with permission of the publishers

In a review of 120 patients with VKH disease seen in 10 years in our clinic from 2003–2012, it predominantly affected young women (W:M:2:1) at an average age of 35 years (range of 6–70 years) (unpublished data). We reached a diagnosis of probable VKH disease in 61% of the patients, incomplete VKH in 34%, and complete VKH disease only in 5% of the patients. The most differentiating features of VKH from other panuveitis are the nearly universal presence of bilateral exudative retinal detachment in the acute stage and sunset glow fundus in the chronic stage. The positive predictive value (PPV) of bilateral exudative retinal detachment in non-traumatic settings is 100% and the negative predictive value (NPV) of 88.4%. The PPV of sunset glow fundus was 94.5% and the NPV of 89.4% [237]. Irrespective of whether the VKH disease has been classified as complete, incomplete, or probable, it runs through a course of four stages [230]. These are (1) prodromal; (2) acute uveitic; (3) convalescent; and (4) chronic recurrent.

Prodromal Stage of VKH Disease

The prodromal stage of the VKH disease is characterized by symptoms suggestive of meningismus and includes headache, neck stiffness, nausea, and dysacusis (inability to perceive higher frequencies), which lasts for several days or weeks. The neck stiffness and headache symptoms may be so severe to land the patient in a neurology clinic. In a Japanese study, 84% of the patients in the prodromal stage showed lymphocytic pleocytosis in the cerebrospinal fluid (CSF), and 74% showed dysacusis [238]. However, being an invasive procedure, experts in many regions of the world do not currently insist on doing a CSF tap in patients suspected of the VKH disease. A simpler test is doing pure tone audiometry, which reveals loss of high-frequency sounds in nearly third-fourth of patients in the prodromal stage. The CSF changes and the audiometry changes persist well into the next stage, which brings the patients to the ophthalmologists.

Acute Uveitic Stage of VKH Disease

Some patients may not develop the prodromal stage and directly present with an acute uveitic stage characterized by multifocal exudative retinal detachments, which are always simultaneously bilateral. If unilateral, the contralateral eye may follow a few days later (Fig. 10.18a, b). There may be a presence of inflammatory cells in the anterior chamber and the vitreous cavity. This sign has 100% PPV for the diagnosis of VKH disease. The FFA shows the presence of initial patchy delayed filling of the choroid followed by numerous pinpoint leaks from the RPE and pooling of fluorescein dye in the subretinal space (Fig. 10.18c, d). A large majority of patients also

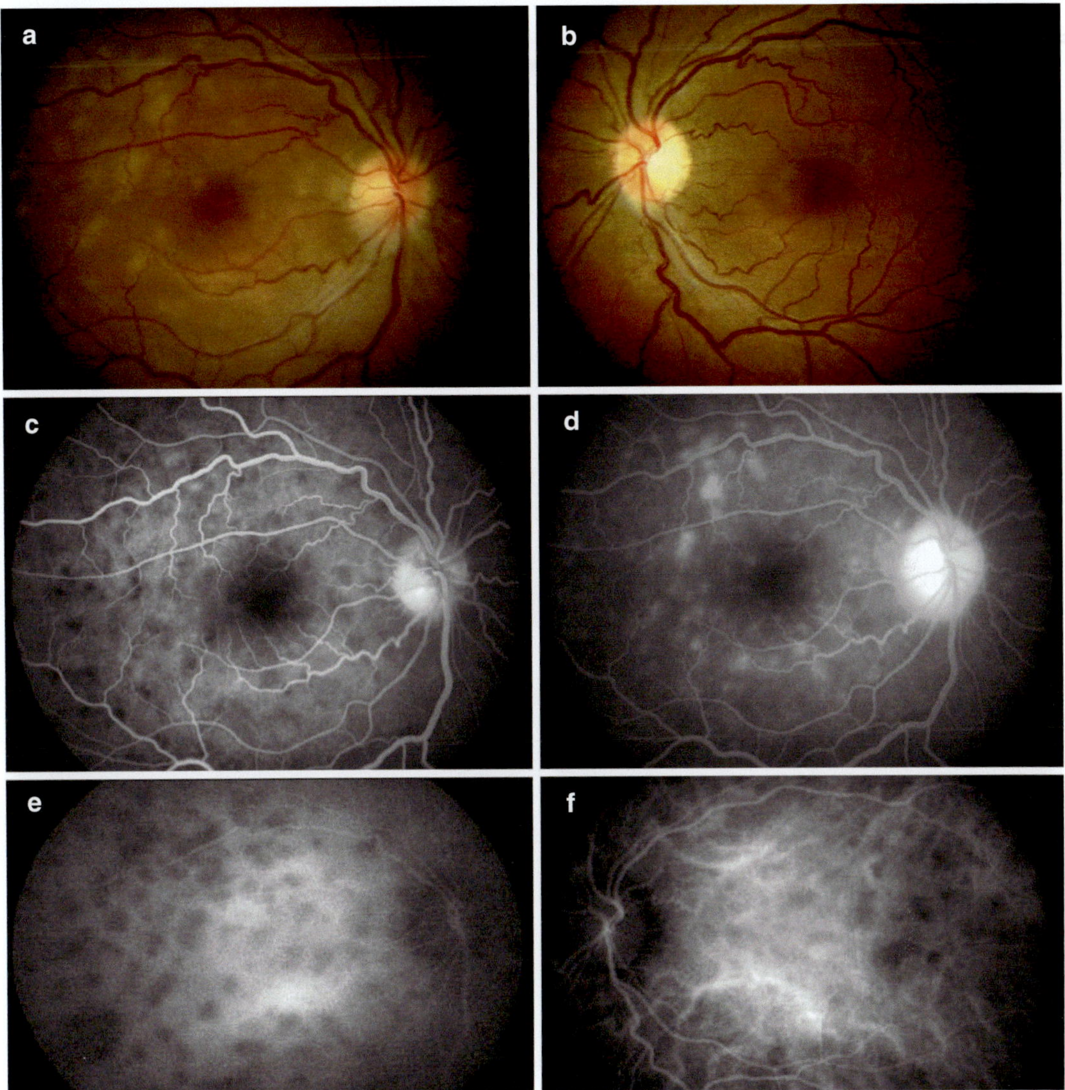

Fig. 10.18 Multifocal exudative retinal detachment in the acute uveitic stage of VKH disease in the right eye (**a**). The left eye looks clinically normal (**b**). Fluorescein angiography of the right eye shows hypofluorescent granulomas in the early phase (**c**), with pinpoint leaks in the late phase (**d**). ICG angiography shows hypocyanescent spots in the right (**e**) and left (**f**) eyes

show optic disc hyperfluorescence. The ICG angiography shows hypofluorescent spots in the early frames and remains hypofluorescent even in the late frames, suggestive of full-thickness stromal granulomas in the VKH disease (Fig. 10.18e, f) [239]. With aggressive therapy, these dark spots disappear only to appear later as the dose of corticosteroids is tapered, suggesting a subclinical recurrence of the disease [239]. Ultrasonography, if done at this stage, will show highly pathognomonic thickening of the choroid, which is maximum in the peripapillary choroid and shows progressive tapering towards the periphery [65, 66]. It corresponds to the distribution of the melanocytes in the choroid, which are found maximum in the peripapillary choroid and progressively decrease towards the periphery. The enhanced depth imaging in OCT (EDI-OCT) shows choroidal thickening along with pockets of serous subretinal fluid. The EDI-OCT can also be used to monitor the response to treatment and for regular follow-up [240]. Even before the patient becomes symptomatic with visual disturbance or return of inflammation, the EDI-OCT may indicate a disease recurrence by showing a thickening of the choroid. The swept-source OCT reveals bacillary layer detachment in more than 90% of the eyes, indicating a split in the myoid zone of the inner segments of the photoreceptors, a sign of inflammatory fluid collection [132–134]. Choroidal striations may be seen in the acute uveitic stage of the VKH disease due to choroidal thickening, which on FFA are seen as hypofluorescent lines. On OCT 3D mapping, undulations of the RPE are seen, which correspond to the choroidal striations [241]. Nearly 50% of older women may also develop a rise in intraocular pressure in the acute uveitic stage.

Convalescent Stage of VKH Disease

The eye enters a convalescent stage several weeks after the acute uveitis phase. During this time, the eye loses pigment in the choroid and appears orange-red, a highly sensitive and specific sign of the VKH disease termed the 'sunset' glow fundus (Fig. 10.19). Patients also develop integumentary changes during this stage, namely vitiligo (common site is the lower back) of the skin, poliosis (greying of the eyelashes), and patchy alopecia (Fig. 10.20a, b). The retinal periphery also shows nummular scars (Fig. 10.20c, d). Since most patients are treated with intensive corticosteroids and immunomodulatory therapy during the acute uveitis phase, the integumentary changes are not

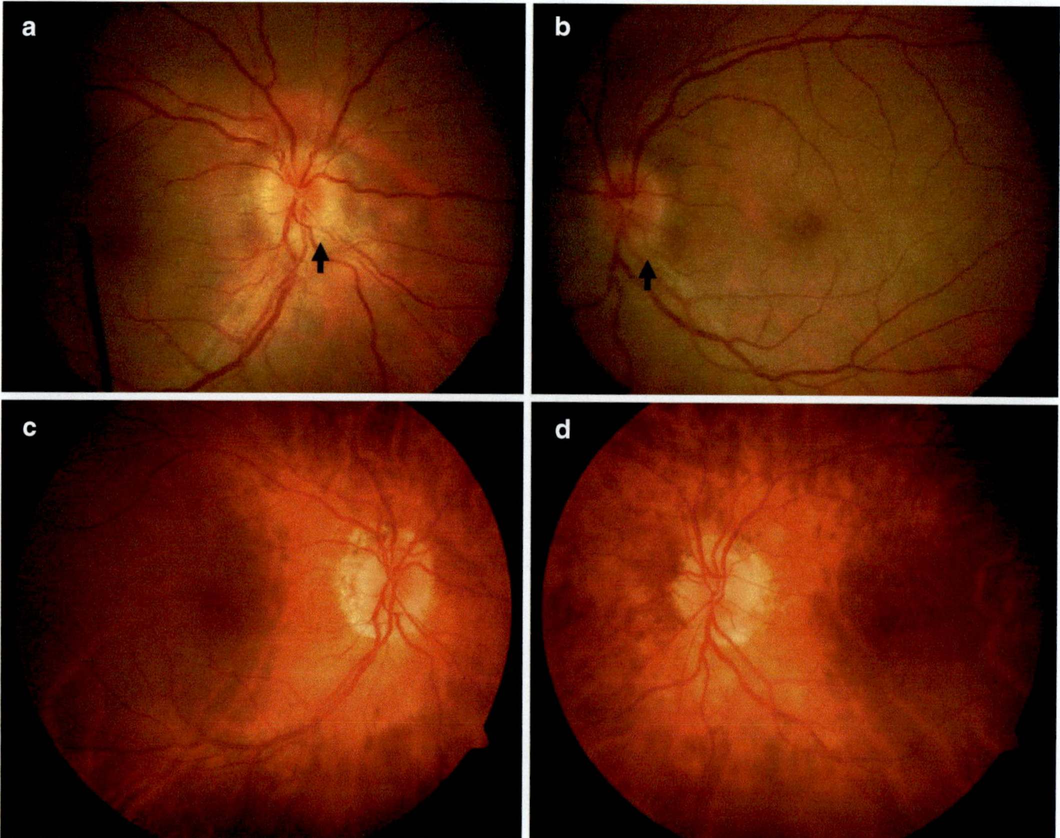

Fig. 10.19 Optic disc oedema (black arrows) with subclinical choroidal granulomas in acute presentation of VKH disease (**a** and **b**). Five years later, the patient developed sunset glow fundus and peripapillary atrophy (**c**, **d**)

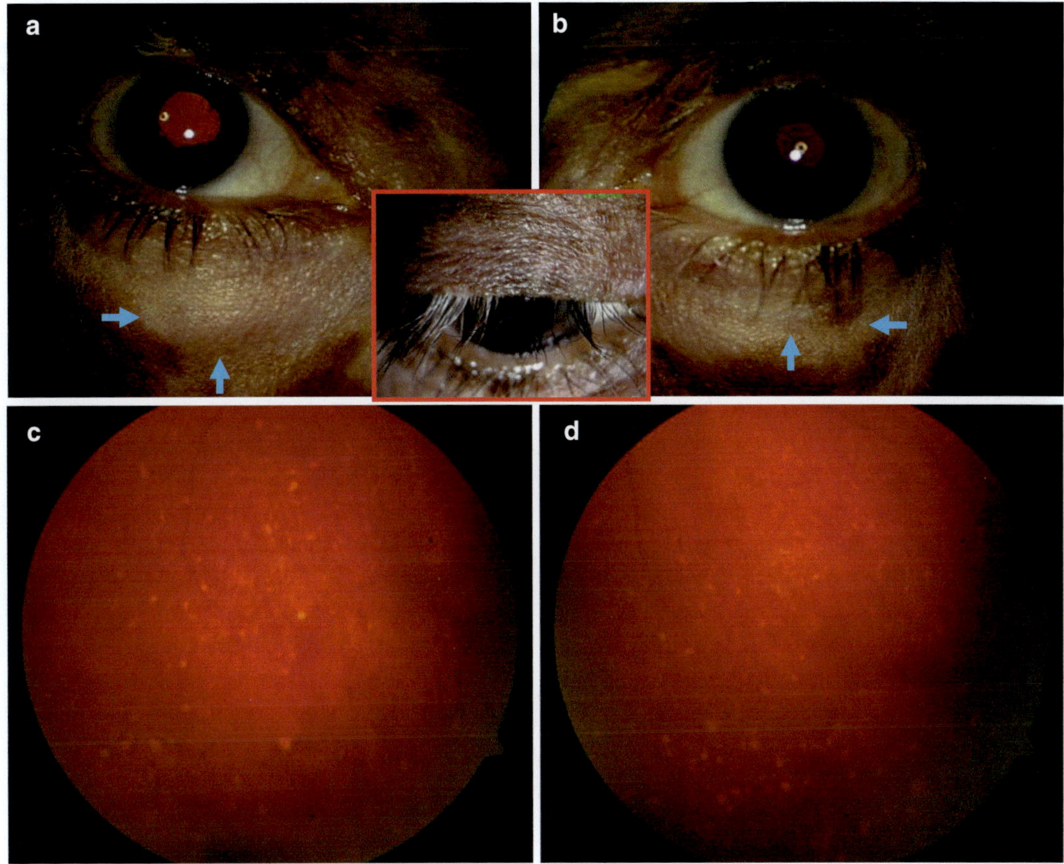

Fig. 10.20 Integumentary changes in chronic recurrent VKH, seen as vitiligo (blue arrows) and poliosis (inset), with sunset glow fundus (**a**, **b**). Nummular scars are seen in the periphery (**c**, **d**)

seen as frequently as recorded in the past. In our experience with the following 120 patients, only 5% developed integumentary changes. Nearly 31% of the patients who presented to us in the acute uveitic stage developed sunset glow fundus.

Chronic Recurrent Stage of VKH Disease

After several months, especially in those who have either early withdrawal or quick tapering of corticosteroids, patients enter into a chronic recurrent stage characterized by granulomatous anterior uveitis with keratic precipitates and development of posterior synechiae. During this stage, the patient may develop pigmentary changes and peripapillary atrophy, which may get complicated by the development of juxtapapillary CNV. Uncommonly, VKH eyes in the chronic recurrent phase may develop subretinal fibrosis within a median time of 6.5 months from the diagnosis in Hispanic population versus 6.5 years in the non-Hispanic population [242].

Complications of Acute Versus Late Presentation of VKH

Patients of VKH disease need early and highly aggressive therapy. Patients with aggressive therapy can be prevented from entering the chronic recurrent stage of VKH disease. Starting aggressive therapy when the patients have already reached the recurrent stage does not help in the further progression of various complications. Nearly one-third of the VKH disease patients presented to us in the chronic recurrent stage of VKH disease (unpublished data). The sunset glow fundus was already present in 67% of the eyes, and by the end of the follow-up, 79% of the eyes had developed this sign.

Further, 44% of eyes already had peripapillary atrophy, which increased to 62% of the eyes by the end of the follow-up. Nummular scars were present in 56% and increased to 76%. CNV had already complicated 5% of the eyes, and by the end of follow-up, 15% of these eyes had developed CNV. In contrast, in patients who reached us in the acute uveitic stage, no eye had sunset glow fundus, peripapillary atrophy or nummular scars at presentation. By the end of the follow-up, these patients who were intensively treated by us using induction therapy with intravenous methylprednisolone, followed by high-dose oral corticosteroids with slow tapering and institution of steroid-sparing immunomodulatory therapy, significantly less number of eyes developed sunset glow fundus (31%), peripapillary atrophy (27%), nummular scars (7%) and CNV (3%). With aggressive therapy, nearly 75% of the eyes attained 6/12 or better visual acuity.

10.7.2.2 Sympathetic Ophthalmia

Epidemiology of Sympathetic Ophthalmia (SO)

Sympathetic ophthalmia (SO) in the present times is extremely rare. A bilateral organ-specific autoimmune granulomatous pan uveitis follows penetrating ocular injuries or intraocular surgery. It is potentially a blinding disorder in one or both eyes if not detected, prevented, and treated appropriately. SO is a highly uncommon complication of penetrating ocular trauma and intraocular surgeries, especially glaucoma incisional and pars plana vitreous surgery. Intraocular surgery, especially vitreoretinal procedures, has become the dominant cause of SO in recent years. In a prospective surveillance study, the incidence of SO was 0.03/100,000 population [243]. Of the 18 patients for whom data were available, 11 followed surgery, and half followed retinal surgeries. Only seven patients of SO followed penetrating trauma. It is in sharp contrast to the earlier reports that suggested that 14–50% of all eye injuries sustained in the nineteenth-century wars developed SO [244]. In the pre-operating microscope era, Allen did not find a single case of SO among cataract surgeries done from 1933 to 1965 in his hospital. However, he did find 0.07% of all glaucoma surgeries, specifically 0.4% of the iris inclusion surgery (then a popular incisional glaucoma surgery) and 0.3 of all ocular injuries to develop SO [244]. Gass reported that over 5 years, every 2 of the 1000 enucleated eyeballs in the US pathology laboratories had evidence of SO [245]. Of the 53 eyes harbouring SO, 55% had sustained trauma, and 45% had undergone surgery [245]. In the National Eye Institute, Bethesda, USA, 32 cases of SO were seen over 10 years, of whom 23 followed trauma and nine followed surgery [246]. Prompt and meticulous repair of open globe injuries using modern microsurgical techniques has significantly reduced the risk of SO following trauma. However, it remains high at 0.24% in children who sustain open globe injuries [247]. Among all the ocular surgical procedures, the risk of repeat surgeries on the same eye is maximum with the vitreoretinal procedures with an attendant increasing risk of SO. Gass calculated that 0.06 of all vitreous surgeries were complicated by SO [245]. While only 0.008% of patients developed SO after a single vitreoretinal surgery, the risk of developing SO increased to 6.67% with seven procedures on the same eye [248].

Pathogenesis and Pathology of SO

The intraocular compartments lack lymphatics. Thus, the most critical step is the leakage of sequestrated soluble retinal antigens into the subconjunctival space following penetration of the ocular coats from where these are drained to the regional lymph nodes [249] followed by a T-cell-mediated immune response in both the exciting and sympathizing eyes. When injected in the subconjunctival space with a bacterial adjuvant, the soluble retinal antigen produced granulomatous uveitis but not when injected directly into the eye [249]. It also explains why the delay in repairing an open penetrating wound of the eye increases the risk of SO compared to those repaired within 24 h. Not only are the surfaces of the injured eye contaminated with bacteria, but the cell walls of the dead commensal bacteria may also act as adjuvants. Without adjuvants, injecting soluble retinal antigens fails to produce uveitis. The potential antigens include retinal-S antigen, interphotoreceptor-binding protein, recoverin, and melanin. Immunization with all these antigens has led to the development of autoimmune uveitis in animal models. Melanin proteins have been used to create a rat model of CD4+ T-cell-driven experimental autoimmune uveitis that mimics the pathology of SO [250].

The retinal-S antigen has been the most potential antigen studied of all the putative antigens, but its antibodies have not been detected in the sera of all SO patients [251].

Pathology of Sympathetic Ophthalmia

The pathology of SO was first described by Dalen and later by Fuchs as nodular aggregates beneath the RPE layer and essentially consist of macrophages. In the late stages, the macrophages may be accompanied by degenerated RPE cells and a few lymphocytes. However, these nodules are present only in one-third of the pathology samples of SO [251]. The choroid is thickened and infiltrated with lymphoid cells, epithelioid cells, and multinucleated giant cells. The iris likewise shows nodular infiltration with lymphoid cells, multinucleated giant cells, and epithelioid cells. The nodular collection of epithelioid cells under the RPE corresponds to the points of leakage on FFA from the RPE. On electron microscopy, the separation of tight junctions of RPE over the Dalen Fuchs nodules has also been seen [252]. In both sympathetic ophthalmia and VKH, despite heavy infiltration of the choroid with inflammatory cells, RPE and choriocapillaris are preserved. It was suggested that the RPE might modulate inflammation in these conditions and preserve the retina [253].

The mechanism of vision loss in SO remained unexplained as the retina is not primarily involved in SO. However, immune co-localization of TNF-α and its receptor inducible nitric synthase (iNOS) and the oxidative products nitrotyrosine have been localized to the photoreceptors of SO eyes explaining the apoptosis and photoreceptor cell death following oxidative stress in SO [254].

Clinical Picture of Sympathetic Ophthalmia

All patients who suffer from penetrating trauma should be counselled on reporting any symptoms in the contralateral eye for the early detection of SO. For several generations, SO has been described in the textbooks as a bilateral granulomatous pan uveitis that presents with mutton fat keratic precipitates, inflammatory cells in the anterior chamber, or the vitreous cavity has been misleading. Yellow-white lesions may be seen in the retinal periphery if ocular media permits. There may be papillitis, optic atrophy, retinal vasculitis, and retinal detachment. This description fits in with the stage of chronic recurrent uveitis. This description has led to ignoring the earliest presentation of the SO in the earliest stages, i.e. the acute uveitic stage.

Early Symptoms of Sympathetic Ophthalmia

The earliest symptoms in the sympathizing eye may be mild pain, blurred vision, and loss of accommodation. The signs include optic disc oedema, yellow-white discrete lesions deep to the retina, and multifocal serous retinal detachment (Fig. 10.21) [255].

In our tertiary care centre, we saw 40 patients with SO from 1989 to 2004, 75% of whom followed trauma and 25% followed surgery. Except for four cases, all presented in the acute stage of the disease. More than 50% of the sympathizing eyes presented only with posterior segment signs and had no anterior segment inflammation. There was mild vitreous inflammation in 75%, exudative retinal detachment in 73%, yellow-white peripheral lesions in 35%, optic disc oedema in 37%, and peripapillary CNV in 5% of the sympathizing eyes. All four patients who presented with a chronic stage of SO had sunset glow fundus and discrete white scars in the retina. FFA findings were similar to that seen in the VKH disease and were noted in 85% of the eyes. These consisted of delayed choroidal filling, pinpoint hyperfluorescence, and late pooling of the dye (Fig. 10.21). All 15 eyes that showed optic disc oedema showed optic disc staining on FFA. On ultrasonography,

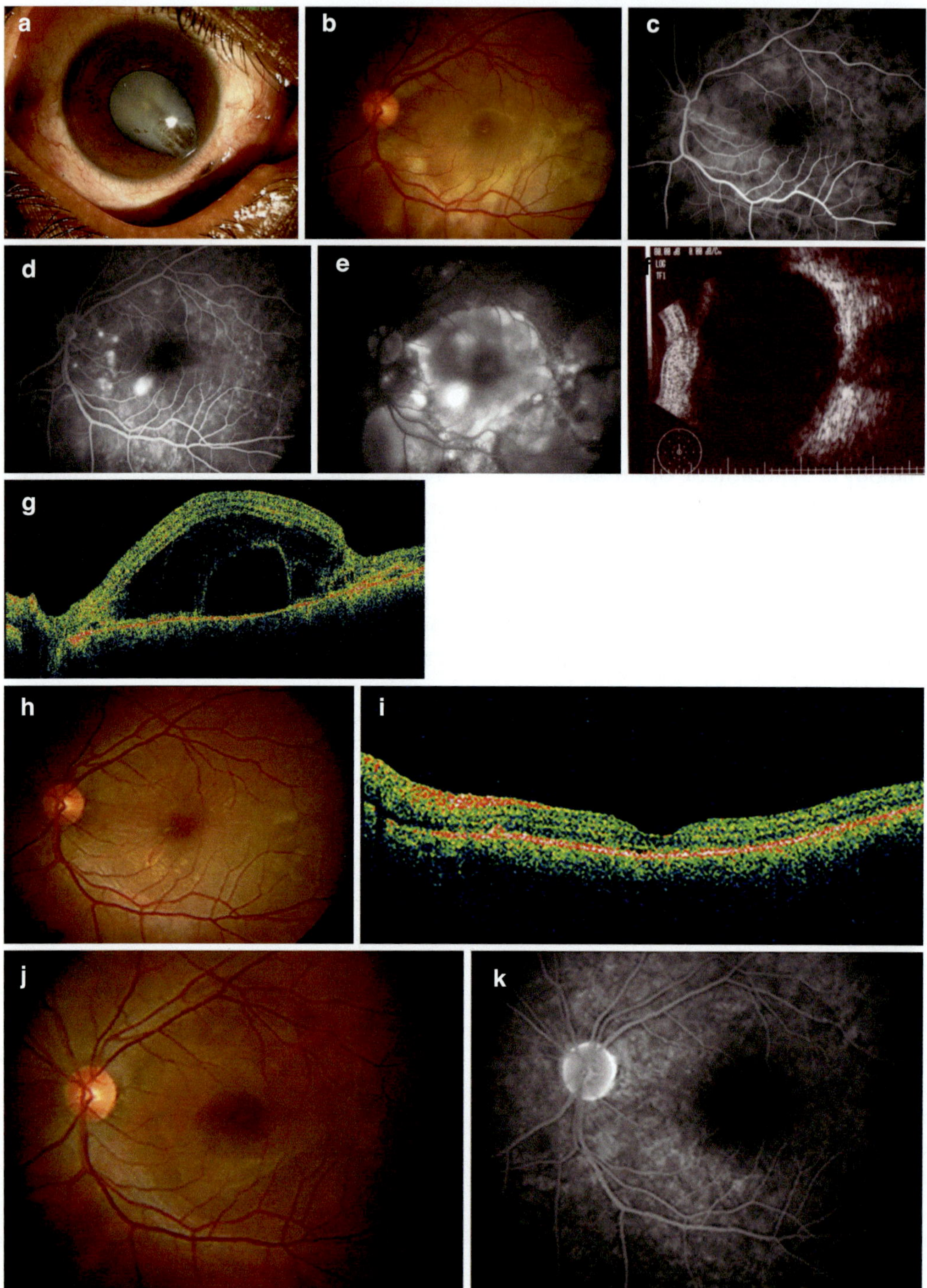

Fig. 10.21 (**a–g**): A 24-year-old man reported sustaining an open globe zone II injury in the right eye 2 days after hammering a chisel (**a**). Visual acuity was light perception in the right eye and 6/6 in the left eye. He underwent a primary repair. Twenty days later, he returned with multifocal retinal detachments in the left eye without any inflammatory reaction (**b**). FFA showed an initial hypofluorescent pinpoint lesions which became hyperfluorescent and pooled dye in late frames (**c–e**). USG showed choroidal thickening (**f**) and OCT showed subretinal fluid with septa (**g**). He was treated with intravenous methylprednisolone followed by oral corticosteroids. (**h–k**) A week later, his retinal detachment had resolved (**g**, **h**). Nine-month follow-up mild pigmentary changes (**i**, **j**)

63% of the eyes (12 of the 19 eyes) showed diffuse thickening of the choroid. The OCT was done in 10 eyes, and in all, it showed serous retinal detachment. Ten eyes were enucleated for histopathology, and all showed granulomatous infiltration of the choroid, with eosinophilic infiltration in four eyes and retinal perivascular infiltrates in one eye. The patients were treated with aggressive corticosteroid therapy and immunomodulatory therapy. Seventy-three percent of the eyes achieved final visual acuity of 6/12 or better in a median follow-up of 5 years. Thirty percent of the sympathizing eyes showed a severe granulomatous anterior uveitis recurrence on corticosteroid tapering. Notably, 5% of the eyes showed posterior segment recurrence in the form of exudative retinal detachment [256].

Similarity of Sympathetic Ophthalmia and the Acute Uveitic Stage of VKH Disease

The clinical picture of the acute stage of SO and the acute uveitic stage of the VKH disease are similar. The FFA in patients with SO is identical to those with VKH disease. The FFA is characterized by focal delayed choroidal filling and multifocal pinpoint dye leakage with late dye pooling in VKH disease and SO. Several cases of SO have been described in the past that showed similarity between the clinical features (vitiligo, poliosis, dysacusis, and meningitis-like symptoms) between the SO and the VKH disease [117, 118, 257]. The exciting eye was enucleated and subjected to histopathology in four SO patients who developed vitiligo, poliosis, dysacusis, and/or meningitis mimicking complete VKH disease. All the eyes revealed histopathological features of granulomatous choroiditis with chorioretinal adhesions and pigment migration into the retina and features also seen in the VKH eyes [258]. The only differentiating feature of SO from VKH is the history of penetrating trauma in the former.

Enucleation of the Injured Eye to Prevent Sympathetic Ophthalmia Is a Myth

The eye that undergoes trauma or surgery is termed the exciting eye, and the contralateral eye that develops granulomatous inflammation is termed the sympathizing eye. Both eyes show similar granulomatous pathology, except the injured eye also shows changes resulting from trauma. While nearly 50% of the eyes who have developed SO do so within 2 weeks to 3 months of injury, more than 90% of SO develop it in the first year. The rule of thumb is no longer valid, with little evidence that SO can be prevented in the contralateral eye if the traumatized eye is removed within 2 weeks. The SO may still happen despite the enucleation of the inciting eye [259]. The shortest interval between the traumatic event and the onset of SO has been 5 days [260]. Not only does the removal of the eye not exclude the risk of SO, but with the current surgical techniques, it is possible to put together even the badly injured eyes.

Moreover, even if the SO develops, powerful therapeutic drugs are now available to control and limit the damage in the sympathizing eye. If the injured eye is badly mutilated and the surgeon feels that anatomical integrity cannot be restored, then instead of enucleation with its psychological trauma and phantom pain, it should be eviscerated to allow for the implantation of a movable prosthesis [259]. Evisceration does not appear to increase the risk of SO. In one large series, not a single case of SO developed following evisceration of the 491 traumatized eyes [261].

10.7.3 Organ-Specific (Ocular) Immune-Mediated Disorders

Widely known as ‘white dot syndrome’, this is a group of disorders characterized by discreet white lesions deep in the retina, often bilateral, and often seen in young to middle-aged women. The salient clinical and imaging features of each of these disorders are given in Box 10.11. There is no anterior segment inflammation, although some have mild vitreous inflammation. Most of them cause photopsia or blurring of vision and scotomas. The availability of multimedia imaging tools has made it possible to differentiate them. The pathogenesis is unknown, but there is evidence of primary choriocapillaris involvement and loss of outer retinal microstructures. Differential diagnoses in the white dot syndromes include sarcoidosis, TB, syphilis, and primary vitreoretinal lymphoma, which may have clinical presentation indistinguishable from these syndromes and need to be

Box 10.11 Organ-Specific (Ocular) Immune-Mediated Inflammations

Disorder	Clinical characteristics	Imaging studies
MEWDS[a]	1. Young women > men 2. Photopsia, blurring of vision 3. Unilateral 4. Optic disc oedema 5. Macular granularity 6. Multifocal white lesions in paramacular and peripheral fundus 7. Spontaneous resolution in ~8 weeks	**FFA**: 1. Hyperfluorescent dots (<100 μ), in wreath configuration 2. OD staining 3. Minimum staining of white dots **ICG**: Hypofluorescent dots (>200 μ) in late frames **FAF**: Hyperautofluorescent **OCT**: Hyperreflective lesions cantered on the ellipsoid zone protruding from RPE into outer nuclear layer **OCTA**: Flow voids in CC All changes reversible on healing
APMPPE[b]	1. Young, preceding flu 2. Sudden loss of vision, photopsia, scotomas 3. Sequential bilateral creamy placoid lesions in outer retina 4. Lesions heal spontaneously with pigmentary changes	**FFA**: Initial hypofluorescent, late hyperfluorescence **ICG**: Hypofluorescent throughout **FAF**: Hypoautofluorescent with a ring of hyperautofluorescence **OCT**: Hyperreflective material in the outer retina, disruption of EZ and IZ; SRF+ **OCTA**: Flow void in CC All changes reversible on healing except transmission defects on FFA
PIC[c]	1. Young, myopic women 2. Blurring, photopsia, metamorphopsia 3. Discrete, 100-300μ multifocal outer retina and inner choroidal lesions in macula, heal with punched-out atrophic scars 4. Subfoveal haemorrhage 5. Serous macular RD	**FFA**: Hyperfluorescence in early and late frames; Type 2 CNV hyperfluorescence in macula **ICG**: Hypofluorescent lesion throughout **FAF**: Hyperautofluorescence **OCT**: Hyperreflective lesions in inner choroid with conical RPE elevation, with intact BM, photoreceptors not visible in active lesions **OCTA**: CNV between RPE and neurosensory retina
IMFC[d] (MFC with panuveitis)	1. Young myopic women 2. Photopsia, scotomas 3. Unilateral/bilateral/sequential 4. Multifocal choroiditis lesions or scars 5. Vitreous cells 6. Recurrent, progressive 7. CNV	**FFA**: Non-contributory in acute stage. Some hyperautofluorescence in late frames. Transmission defects in scars. Type 2 CNV **ICG**: Hypolesions from 50 to 400 μ, most remain hypofluorescent in late frames **FAF**: Hyperautofluorescence **OCT**: Hyperreflective material in the inner choroid elevating the RPE, with a rupture at the peak of BM/RPE and material extending into outer retina. Disruption of EZ, IZ, and ELM increased light transmission through the lesion **OCTA**: CC flow voids reversible in smaller lesions
AZOOR[d, e]	1. Young to middle-aged healthy women 2. Moving photopsia-lightening in a thunderstorm, photophobia, scotoma, blind spot in temp field, visual field loss, night vision problems 3. Bilateral asymmetric disease 4. Peripapillary normal or subtle lesion, white demarcation line between normal and affected retina may be prominent but transient; trizonal lesions are diagnostic 5. Bone specule pigment and atrophy	**FFA**: Non-contributory in acute, window defect in late stage **ICG:** Non-contributory in acute, trizonal pattern **FAF**: Patch hyperautofluorescence, progressive, later hypoautofluorescence, hyperautofluorescent demarcation line; normal outside the demarcation line **OCT**: Loss of EZ, thickening of outer plexiform layer and loss of outer nuclear layer; foveal centre may be spared for a long time loss of RPE in late stages

Disorder	Clinical characteristics	Imaging studies
BCR[f, g]	1. Middle-aged, F>M, Caucasians 2. HLA-A29*02 in >95% 3. Blurring of vision or floaters both eyes 4. Creamy oval/streak lesions choroidal 500–1500 μ radial to optic disc 5. Vitritis 6. CME 7. Retinal vasculitis 8. ODE 9. Cellophane maculopathy	**FFA**: delayed A-V transit; hypolesions in the early and mild hyperfluorescence in late frames; late OD staining; CME, retinal perivenous staining and leakage **ICG**: Most sensitive tool, hypofluorescent lesions corresponding to creamy lesions aligned with choroidal vessels. **FAF**: Linear hypoautofluorescence along retinal vessels **OCT**: Disruption of ellipsoid zone, focal to generalized; outer retinal atrophy **ERG**: Full field and mfERG shows delayed implicit time and decreased amplitude
AMN[h,i]	1. Young women 2. Unilateral or bilateral Paracentral scotomas after flu-like illness, transient or permanent 3. Fundus shows multiple reddish brown, sharp petaloid lesions deep in the retina centred around foveal centre 4. >100 μ outer retinal changes are often permanent	**NIR imaging**: Shows hyporeflective sharply defined lesions in the macula **FFA**: Normal **ICG**: Normal **FAF**: Normal **OCT**: Loss of ellipsoid zone/IZ and thinning of outer nuclear layer and OPL hyperreflectivity **OCTA:** Flow deficit in deep capillary plexiform layer. Flow may reverse but OCT changes may not revert **VF**: Paracentral scotoma

MEWDS multiple evanescent white dot syndrome, *FFA* fundus fluorescein angiography, *ICG* indocyanine angsiography, *FAF* fundus autofluorescence, *OCT* optical coherence tomography, *OCTA* optical coherence tomography angiography, *OD* optic disc, *CC* choriocapillaris, *PIC* punctate inner choroidopathy, *RD* retinal detachment, *CNV* choroidal neovascular membrane, *IMFC* idiopathic multifocal choroidopathy, *RPE* retinal pigment epithelium, *BM* Bruch's membrane, *EZ* ellipsoid zone, *IZ* interdigitating zone, *ELM* external limiting membrane, *AZOOR* acute zonal occult outer retinopathy, *BCR* birdshot chorioretinopathy, *ERG* electroretinography, *mfERG* multifocal ERG, *AMN* acute macular neuroretinitis, *NIR* near infrared, *OPL* outer plexiform layer

References

[a] Marsiglia et al. [262]; [b] Testi et al. [263]; [c] Ahnood et al. [264]; [d] Pichi et al. [202]; [e] Mrejen et al. [265]; [f] Minos et al. [266]; [g] Fogel-Levin et al. [267]; [h] Yzer et al. [268]; [i] Fawzi et al. [269]

excluded. Except for MFC and AZOOR, which require corticosteroids and immunosuppressive therapy, most white dot syndromes resolve spontaneously with or without residual changes.

10.8 Multiple Evanescent White Dot Syndrome (MEWDS)

Multiple evanescent white dot syndrome (MEWDS) is a rare disorder usually seen in young myopic women who present with photopsia and blurring vision (Fig. 10.22). The fundus examination reveals unilateral optic disc oedema and multiple white lesions in the paramacular and retinal periphery. The FAF imaging is highly diagnostic of MEWDS (Fig. 10.23). Most of these white dot syndromes have hyperautofluorescence due to exposure of the pigments in the RPE layer due to loss of the overlying photoreceptors and their pigments, which normally block the autofluorescence signals from the RPE [267]. Changes are reversible to a large extent in MEWDS (Fig. 10.23g).

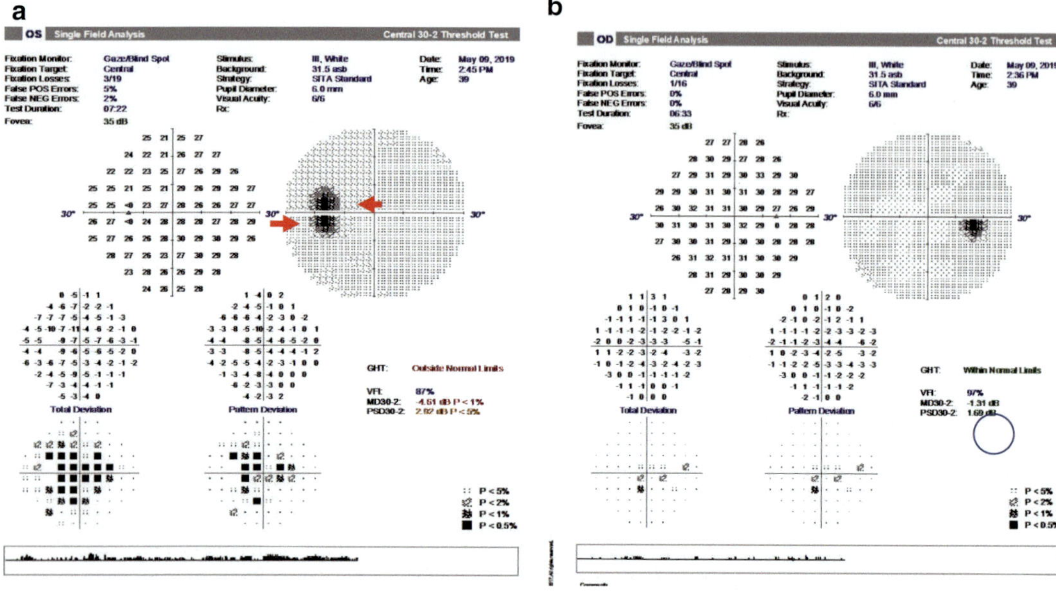

Fig. 10.22 A 39-year-old man presented with floaters in left eye for one week, with history of viral fever a few months ago. His visual acuity was 6/6/ in both eyes. Visual field testing revealed enlargement of blind spot (red arrow) in left eye (**a**). Right eye was normal (**b**). Imaging revealed a diagnosis of MEWDS. (Images courtesy of Dr. Padmamalini Mahendradas, Uveitis and Ocular Oncology, Narayana Nethralya, Bangalore, India)

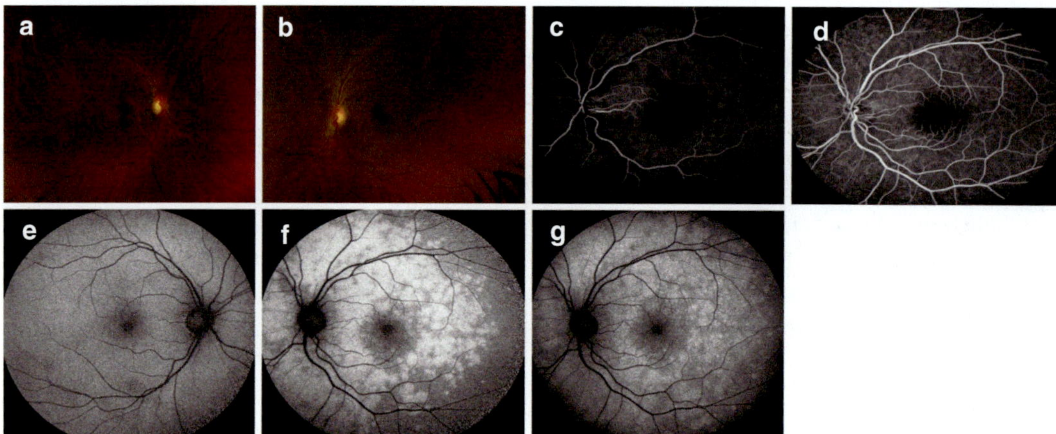

Fig. 10.23 Same patient with MEWDS as in Fig. 10.22, showing fundus photographs (**a**, **b**). Fluorescein angiography shows wreath-like pattern (blue arrows) (**c**, **d**). Fundus autofluorescence shows normal right eye (**e**) and characteristic hyperautofluorescent changes in left (**f**) eye. Follow-up at 6 months reveals near complete recovery of autofluorescence findings (**g**). (Images courtesy of Dr. Padmamalini Mahendradas, Uveitis and Ocular Oncology, Narayana Nethralya, Bangalore, India)

10.9 Acute Posterior Multifocal Placoid Pigment Epitheliopathy (APMPPE)

Acute posterior multifocal placoid pigment epitheliopathy (APMPPE) is characterized by the sudden onset of vision loss in young women preceded by a flu-like illness. It is usually bilateral, but the other eye may have sequential involvement within a few days of the onset. The fundus examination reveals multifocal creamy white placoid lesions in the outer retina (Fig. 10.24).

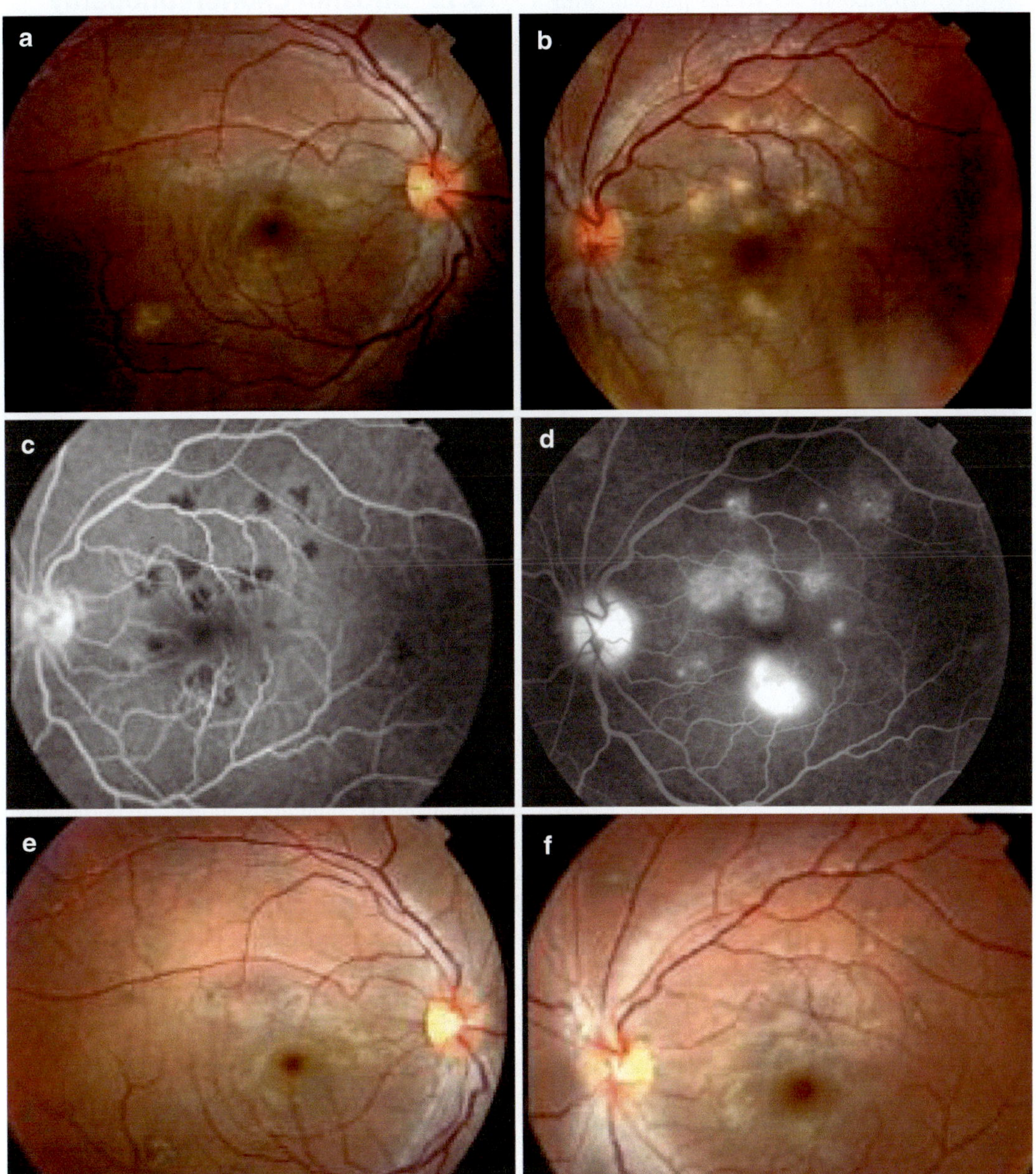

Fig. 10.24 Acute posterior multifocal placoid pigment epitheliopathy (APMPPE) in a 24-year-old man who had viral fever 8 days ago. There are asymmetric bilateral choroiditis lesions, with right eye (**a**) affected less than left eye (**b**). FFA shows hypofluorescent lesions in early phase (**c**), which become hyperfluorescent in late phase (**d**). A few weeks later, the choroiditis lesions resolved completely (**e**, **f**). (Images courtesy of Dr. Padmamalini Mahendradas, Uveitis and Ocular Oncology, Narayana Nethralya, Bangalore, India)

The lesions heal by restoring the photoreceptors' integrity and return of vision [262, 263, 270]. Many inflammatory diseases, autoimmune vasculitis, infections, and vaccines have been reported preceding the onset of APPMPPE [271]. A significantly higher frequency of HLA-B7, a class I antigen, and HLA-DR2, a class II antigen, has been reported in APMPPE patients with a relative risk of 3.38 and 3.34, respectively, lending support to a suggestion that this disorder may be caused by underlying immune mechanisms [272].

10.10 Punctate Inner Choroidopathy and Idiopathic Multifocal Choroidopathy (PIC and IMFC)

Most experts believe that punctate inner choroidopathy (PIC) and idiopathic multifocal choroiditis (IMFC) represent a spectrum of diseases. Idiopathic multifocal choroidopathy has been named in the past with various eponyms, including pseudo-presumed ocular histoplasmosis syndrome, multifocal choroiditis with panuveitis, and multifocal inner choroidopathy. Both of these disorders get complicated by the development of choroidal neovascular membranes (CNV) [202, 264]. The acute lesions of IMFC and PIC get picked up by the FAF imaging.

10.11 Acute Zonal Occult Outer Retinopathy (AZOOR)

The symptoms of moving photopsia, 'lightning strike in a thunderstorm', are highly suggestive of acute zonal occult outer retinopathy (AZOOR). They should prompt fundus autofluorescence studies as the fundus in the initial stages may look normal. A trizonal pattern of autofluorescence is highly characteristic of AZOOR [265]. Late stages of AZOOR result in retinal atrophy, bone-corpuscle pigmentation in the affected quadrants, and optic atrophy. These need to be differentiated from autoimmune retinopathies, retinal degenerations, and dystrophies like retinitis pigmentosa and optic neuropathies [265].

10.12 Birdshot Chorioretinopathy (BCR)

Birdshot chorioretinopathy (BCR) is strongly associated with HLA-A29*02 in Caucasians and rarely if ever, seen in Asians or Blacks. The diagnosis of BCR is often delayed due to very subtle clinical lesions that may be missed in a routine examination and need a high index of suspicion for making an early diagnosis. Patients are highly symptomatic even in the presence of normal or near-normal vision. It is a chronic recurrent inflammatory disease and needs immunosuppressive therapy to prevent retinal atrophy and optic atrophy [266, 267].

10.13 Acute Macular Neuroretinitis (AMN)

Acute macular neuroretinitis (AMN) is rare and often seen in young to middle-aged women. It often follows a flu-like illness or even a sudden hypotension attack may precipitate this disorder. While the fundus lesions may be very subtle, near-infrared imaging shows hyporeflective changes centred around the fovea. There are two types of AMN, type 1, also termed paracentral acute middle maculopathy (PAMM) due to occlusion of the deep capillary plexus and results in hyperreflectivity of the inner nuclear zone and the outer plexiform layer and type 2, which is characterized by the loss of outer nuclear layer and hyperreflectivity of the outer plexiform layer. Optical coherence tomography angiography shows flow voids in the deep retinal capillary plexus [273, 274]. The PAMM or AMN lesions may follow sickle cell disease [275].

References

1. Isaacs A, Lindenmann J, Valentine RC. Virus interference. II. Some properties of interferon. Proc R Soc Lond B Biol Sci. 1957, 147;(927):268–73. https://doi.org/10.1098/rspb.1957.0049. PMID: 13465721; Burke DC 2009. http://www.brainimmune.com/the--discovery-of-interferon-the-first-cytokine-by-alick-isaacs-and-jean-lindenmann-in-1957/.
2. di Giovine FS, Duff GW. Interleukin 1: the first interleukin. Immunol Today. 1990;11(1):13–20. https://doi.org/10.1016/0167-5699(90)90005-t. PMID: 2405873.
3. Ferreira VL, Borba HH, de F. Bonetti A, Leonart PL, Pontarolo R. Cytokines and interferons: types and functions. In: Khan WA, editor. Autoantibodies and cytokines [internet]. London: IntechOpen; 2018 [cited 2022 Oct 19]. https://doi.org/10.5772/intechopen.74550. https://www.intechopen.com/chapters/59914.
4. Gupta A. Bench to bedside research in ophthalmology in biomedical translational research: from disease diagnosis to treatment. In: Sobti RC, Ganju AK, editors. vol II. Springer Nature; 2022. p. 67–124.
5. Jawad S, Liu B, Agron E, Nussenblatt RB, Sen HN. Elevated serum levels of interleukin-17A in uveitis patients. Ocul Immunol Inflamm. 2013;21(6):434–9. https://doi.org/10.3109/09273948.2013.815786. Epub 2013 Aug 19. PMID: 23957503; PMCID: PMC5569243.
6. Kuiper JJ, Mutis T, de Jager W, de Groot-Mijnes JD, Rothova A. Intraocular interleukin-17 and proinflammatory cytokines in HLA-A29-associated birdshot chorioretinopathy. Am J Ophthalmol. 2011;152(2):177–182.e1. https://doi.org/10.1016/j.ajo.2011.01.031. Epub 2011 May 13. PMID: 21570674.
7. Ooi KG, Galatowicz G, Calder VL, Lightman SL. Cytokines and chemokines in uveitis: is there a correlation with clinical phenotype? Clin Med Res. 2006;4(4):294–309. https://doi.org/10.3121/cmr.4.4.294. PMID: 17210978; PMCID: PMC1764804.
8. Dinarello CA. Historical insights into cytokines. Eur J Immunol. 2007;37 Suppl 1(Suppl 1):S34–45. https://doi.org/10.1002/eji.200737772. PMID: 17972343; PMCID: PMC3140102.
9. Jabs DA, Nussenblatt RB, Rosenbaum JT, Standardization of Uveitis Nomenclature (SUN) Working Group. Standardization of uveitis nomenclature for reporting clinical data. Results of the first international workshop. Am J Ophthalmol. 2005;140(3):509–16. https://doi.org/10.1016/j.ajo.2005.03.057. PMID: 16196117; PMCID: PMC8935739.
10. Balasundaram MB, Andavar R, Palaniswamy M, Venkatapathy N. Outbreak of acquired ocular toxoplasmosis involving 248 patients. Arch Ophthalmol. 2010;128(1):28–32. https://doi.org/10.1001/archophthalmol.2009.354. Erratum in: Arch Ophthalmol 2010 Apr;128(4):508. PMID: 20065213.
11. Robert-Gangneux F, Dardé ML. Epidemiology of and diagnostic strategies for toxoplasmosis. Clin Microbiol Rev. 2012;25(2):264–96. https://doi.org/10.1128/CMR.05013-11. Erratum in: Clin Microbiol Rev. 2012 Jul;25(3):583. PMID: 22491772; PMCID: PMC3346298.
12. Acharya NR, Tham VM, Esterberg E, Borkar DS, Parker JV, Vinoya AC, Uchida A. Incidence and prevalence of uveitis: results from the Pacific Ocular Inflammation Study. JAMA Ophthalmol. 2013;131(11):1405–12. https://doi.org/10.1001/jamaophthalmol.2013.4237. PMID: 24008391.
13. Engelhard SB, Patel V, Reddy AK. Intermediate uveitis, posterior uveitis, and panuveitis in the mid-Atlantic USA. Clin Ophthalmol. 2015;9:1549–55. https://doi.org/10.2147/OPTH.S89428. PMID: 26345421; PMCID: PMC4556262.
14. Henderly DE, Genstler AJ, Smith RE, Rao NA. Changing patterns of uveitis. Am J Ophthalmol. 1987;103(2):131–6. https://doi.org/10.1016/s0002--9394(14)74217-5. PMID: 3812615.
15. Merrill PT, Kim J, Cox TA, Betor CC, McCallum RM, Jaffe GJ. Uveitis in the southeastern United States. Curr Eye Res. 1997;16(9):865–74. https://doi.org/10.1076/ceyr.16.9.865.5048. PMID: 9288447.
16. Rodriguez A, Calonge M, Pedroza-Seres M, Akova YA, Messmer EM, D'Amico DJ, Foster CS. Referral patterns of uveitis in a tertiary eye care center. Arch Ophthalmol. 1996;114(5):593–9. https://doi.org/10.1001/archopht.1996.01100130585016. PMID: 8619771.
17. Jones JL, Holland GN. Annual burden of ocular toxoplasmosis in the US. Am J Trop Med Hyg. 2010;82(3):464–5. https://doi.org/10.4269/ajtmh.2010.09-0664. PMID: 20207874; PMCID: PMC2829910.
18. Bodaghi B, Cassoux N, Wechsler B, Hannouche D, Fardeau C, Papo T, Huong DL, Piette JC, LeHoang P. Chronic severe uveitis: etiology and visual outcome in 927 patients from a single center. Medicine (Baltimore). 2001;80(4):263–70. https://doi.org/10.1097/00005792-200107000-00005. PMID: 11470987.
19. Sengün A, Karadağ R, Karakurt A, Saricaoğlu MS, Abdik O, Hasiripi H. Causes of uveitis in a referral hospital in Ankara, Turkey. Ocul Immunol Inflamm. 2005;13(1):45–50. https://doi.org/10.1080/09273940590909121. PMID: 15804769.
20. Al Dhahri H, Al Rubaie K, Hemachandran S, Mousa A, Gikandi PW, Al-Mezaine HS, Abu El-Asrar AM. Patterns of uveitis in a University-based Tertiary Referral Center in Riyadh, Saudi Arabia. Ocul Immunol Inflamm. 2015;23(4):311–9. https://doi.org/10.3109/09273948.2014.939197. Epub 2014 Jul 24. PMID: 25058456.

21. Al-Mezaine HS, Kangave D, Abu El-Asrar AM. Patterns of uveitis in patients admitted to a University Hospital in Riyadh, Saudi Arabia. Ocul Immunol Inflamm. 2010;18(6):424–31. https://doi.org/10.3109/09273948.2010.502284. Epub 2010 Aug 25. PMID: 20735294.
22. Çakar Özdal MP, Yazici A, Tüfek M, Öztürk F. Epidemiology of uveitis in a referral hospital in Turkey. Turk J Med Sci. 2014;44(2):337–42. https://doi.org/10.3906/sag-1302-132. PMID: 25536746.
23. Hamade IH, Elkum N, Tabbara KF. Causes of uveitis at a referral center in Saudi Arabia. Ocul Immunol Inflamm. 2009;17(1):11–6. https://doi.org/10.1080/09273940802491850. PMID: 19294567.
24. Jones JL, Bonetti V, Holland GN, Press C, Sanislo SR, Khurana RN, Montoya JG. Ocular toxoplasmosis in the United States: recent and remote infections. Clin Infect Dis. 2015;60(2):271–3. https://doi.org/10.1093/cid/ciu793. Epub 2014 Oct 9. PMID: 25301214.
25. Kazokoglu H, Onal S, Tugal-Tutkun I, Mirza E, Akova Y, Ozyazgan Y, Soylu M, Batioglu F, Apaydin C. Demographic and clinical features of uveitis in tertiary centers in Turkey. Ophthalmic Epidemiol. 2008;15(5):285–93. https://doi.org/10.1080/09286580802262821. PMID: 18850464.
26. Llorenç V, Mesquida M, Sainz de la Maza M, Keller J, Molins B, Espinosa G, Hernandez MV, Gonzalez-Martín J, Adán A. Epidemiology of uveitis in a Western urban multiethnic population. The challenge of globalization. Acta Ophthalmol. 2015;93(6):561–7. https://doi.org/10.1111/aos.12675. Epub 2015 Feb 15. PMID: 25683136.
27. Mercanti A, Parolini B, Bonora A, Lequaglie Q, Tomazzoli L. Epidemiology of endogenous uveitis in north-Eastern Italy. Analysis of 655 new cases. Acta Ophthalmol Scand. 2001;79(1):64–8. https://doi.org/10.1034/j.1600-0420.2001.079001064.x. PMID: 11167291.
28. Rothova A, Buitenhuis HJ, Meenken C, Brinkman CJ, Linssen A, Alberts C, Luyendijk L, Kijlstra A. Uveitis and systemic disease. Br J Ophthalmol. 1992;76(3):137–41. https://doi.org/10.1136/bjo.76.3.137. PMID: 1540555; PMCID: PMC504190.
29. Sittivarakul W, Bhurayanontachai P, Ratanasukon M. Pattern of uveitis in a university-based referral center in southern Thailand. Ocul Immunol Inflamm. 2013;21(1):53–60. https://doi.org/10.3109/09273948.2012.730651. PMID: 23323582.
30. Soheilian M, Heidari K, Yazdani S, Shahsavari M, Ahmadieh H, Dehghan M. Patterns of uveitis in a tertiary eye care center in Iran. Ocul Immunol Inflamm. 2004;12(4):297–310. https://doi.org/10.1080/092739490500174. PMID: 15621869.
31. Das D, Bhattacharjee H, Bhattacharyya PK, Jain L, Panicker MJ, Das K, Deka AC. Pattern of uveitis in North East India: a tertiary eye care center study. Indian J Ophthalmol. 2009;57(2):144–6. https://doi.org/10.4103/0301-4738.45506. PMID: 19237790; PMCID: PMC2684416
32. Biswas J, Narain S, Das D, Ganesh SK. Pattern of uveitis in a referral uveitis clinic in India. Int Ophthalmol. 1996;20(4):223–8. https://doi.org/10.1007/BF00175264. PMID: 9112191.
33. Rathinam SR, Namperumalsamy P. Global variation and pattern changes in epidemiology of uveitis. Indian J Ophthalmol. 2007;55(3):173–83. https://doi.org/10.4103/0301-4738.31936. PMID: 17456933.
34. Biswas J, Kharel Sitaula R, Multani P. Changing uveitis patterns in South India—comparison between two decades. Indian J Ophthalmol. 2018;66(4):524–7. https://doi.org/10.4103/ijo.IJO_851_17. PMID: 29582812; PMCID: PMC5892054.
35. Dogra M, Singh R, Agarwal A, Sharma A, Singh SR, Gautam N, Yangzes S, Samanta R, Sharma M, Aggarwal K, Sharma A, Sharma K, Bansal R, Gupta A, Gupta V. Epidemiology of uveitis in a Tertiary-Care Referral Institute in north India. Ocul Immunol Inflamm. 2017;25(sup1):S46–53. https://doi.org/10.1080/09273948.2016.1255761. Epub 2016 Dec 12. PMID: 27937033.
36. Singh R, Gupta V, Gupta A. Pattern of uveitis in a referral eye clinic in North India. Indian J Ophthalmol. 2004;52(2):121–5. PMID: 15283216.
37. Venkatesh P, Gogia V, Shah B, Gupta S, Sagar P, Garg S. Patterns of uveitis at the Apex Institute for Eye Care in India: results from a prospectively enrolled patient data base (2011-2013). Int Ophthalmol. 2016;36(3):365–72.https://doi.org/10.1007/s10792--015-0128-9. Epub 2015 Sep 25. PMID: 26408195.
38. Furtado JM, Smith JR, Belfort R Jr, Gattey D, Winthrop KL. Toxoplasmosis: a global threat. J Glob Infect Dis. 2011;3(3):281–4. https://doi.org/10.4103/0974-777X.83536. PMID: 21887062; PMCID: PMC3162817.
39. Smith JR, Ashander LM, Arruda SL, Cordeiro CA, Lie S, Rochet E, Belfort R Jr, Furtado JM. Pathogenesis of ocular toxoplasmosis. Prog Retin Eye Res. 2021;81:100882. https://doi.org/10.1016/j.preteyeres.2020.100882. Epub 2020 Jul 24. PMID: 32717377.
40. Harker KS, Ueno N, Lodoen MB. Toxoplasma gondii dissemination: a parasite's journey through the infected host. Parasite Immunol. 2015;37(3):141–9. https://doi.org/10.1111/pim.12163. PMID: 25408224.
41. Varikuti S, Jha BK, Holcomb EA, McDaniel JC, Karpurapu M, Srivastava N, McGwire BS, Satoskar AR, Parinandi NL. The role of vascular endothelium and exosomes in human protozoan parasitic diseases. Vessel Plus. 2020;4:28. https://doi.org/10.20517/2574-1209.2020.27. Epub 2020 Sep 27. PMID: 33089078; PMCID: PMC7575144.
42. Furtado JM, Bharadwaj AS, Chipps TJ, Pan Y, Ashander LM, et al. Toxoplasma gondii tachyzoites cross retinal endothelium assisted by intercellular

adhesion molecule-1 in vitro. Immunol Cell Biol. 2012;90:912–5.

43. Oliver GF, Ferreira LB, Vieira BR, Arruda S, Araújo M, Carr JM, Smith JR, Furtado JM. Posterior segment findings by spectral-domain optical coherence tomography and clinical associations in active toxoplasmic retinochoroiditis. Sci Rep. 2022;12(1):1156. https://doi.org/10.1038/s41598-022-05070-9. PMID: 35064148; PMCID: PMC8782858.
44. Babu K, Shah D, Bhagya M, Murthy KR. Near full thickness macular hole with an intact overlying internal limiting membrane following resolution of fulminant acquired toxoplasma retinitis—A unique finding. Indian J Ophthalmol. 2020;68(1):244–6. https://doi.org/10.4103/ijo.IJO_924_19. PMID: 31856540; PMCID: PMC6951158.
45. Dogra M, Singh SR. Commentary: internal limiting membrane sparing in necrotizing focal retinitis. Indian J Ophthalmol. 2020;68(1):246–7. https://doi.org/10.4103/ijo.IJO_2204_19. PMID: 31856541; PMCID: PMC6951161.
46. Bosch-Driessen LE, Berendschot TT, Ongkosuwito JV, Rothova A. Ocular toxoplasmosis: clinical features and prognosis of 154 patients. Ophthalmology. 2002;109(5):869–78.https://doi.org/10.1016/s0161--6420(02)00990-9. PMID: 11986090.
47. Elkins BS, Holland GN, Opremcak EM, Dunn JP Jr, Jabs DA, Johnston WH, Green WR. Ocular toxoplasmosis misdiagnosed as cytomegalovirus retinopathy in immunocompromised patients. Ophthalmology. 1994;101(3):499–507. https://doi.org/10.1016/s0161-6420(13)31267-6. PMID: 8127570.
48. Silveira C, Vallochi AL, da Silva UR, Muccioli C, Holland GN, Nussenblatt RB, Belfort R, Rizzo LV. Toxoplasma gondii in the peripheral blood of patients with acute and chronic toxoplasmosis. Br J Ophthalmol. 2011;95(3):396–400. https://doi.org/10.1136/bjo.2008.148205. Epub 2010 Jul 3. PMID: 20601663.
49. Bourdin C, Busse A, Kouamou E, Touafek F, Bodaghi B, Le Hoang P, Mazier D, Paris L, Fekkar A. PCR-based detection of Toxoplasma gondii DNA in blood and ocular samples for diagnosis of ocular toxoplasmosis. J Clin Microbiol. 2014;52(11):3987–91. https://doi.org/10.1128/JCM.01793-14. Epub 2014 Sep 10. PMID: 25210066; PMCID: PMC4313235.
50. Silva MD, Teixeira C, Gomes P, Borges M. Promising drug targets and compounds with anti-*Toxoplasma gondii* activity. Microorganisms. 2021;9(9):1960. https://doi.org/10.3390/microorganisms9091960. PMID: 34576854; PMCID: PMC8471693.
51. Doggett JS, Schultz T, Miller AJ, Bruzual I, Pou S, Winter R, Dodean R, Zakharov LN, Nilsen A, Riscoe MK, Carruthers VB. Orally bioavailable Endochin-like quinolone carbonate Ester prodrug reduces Toxoplasma gondii brain cysts. Antimicrob Agents Chemother. 2020;64(9):e00535–20. https://doi.org/10.1128/AAC.00535-20. PMID: 32540978; PMCID: PMC7449172.
52. Sangaré LO, Ólafsson EB, Wang Y, Yang N, Julien L, Camejo A, Pesavento P, Sidik SM, Lourido S, Barragan A, Saeij JPJ. In vivo CRISPR screen identifies TgWIP as a toxoplasma modulator of dendritic cell migration. Cell Host Microbe. 2019;26(4):478–492.e8. https://doi.org/10.1016/j.chom.2019.09.008. PMID: 31600500; PMCID: PMC7060943.
53. Seizova S, Ruparel U, Garnham AL, Bader SM, Uboldi AD, Coffey MJ, Whitehead LW, Rogers KL, Tonkin CJ. Transcriptional modification of host cells harboring Toxoplasma gondii bradyzoites prevents IFN gamma-mediated cell death. Cell Host Microbe. 2022;30(2):232–247.e6. https://doi.org/10.1016/j.chom.2021.11.012. Epub 2021 Dec 17. PMID: 34921775.
54. Caldas LA, de Souza W. A window to *Toxoplasma gondii* Egress. Pathogens. 2018;7(3):69. https://doi.org/10.3390/pathogens7030069. PMID: 30110938; PMCID: PMC6161258.
55. Young NJ, Bird AC. Bilateral acute retinal necrosis. Br J Ophthalmol. 1978;62(9):581–90. https://doi.org/10.1136/bjo.62.9.581. PMID: 708676; PMCID: PMC1043304.
56. Culbertson WW, Blumenkranz MS, Pepose JS, Stewart JA, Curtin VT. Varicella zoster virus is a cause of the acute retinal necrosis syndrome. Ophthalmology. 1986;93(5):559–69. https://doi.org/10.1016/s0161-6420(86)33701-1. PMID: 3014414.
57. Muthiah MN, Michaelides M, Child CS, Mitchell SM. Acute retinal necrosis: a national population-based study to assess the incidence, methods of diagnosis, treatment strategies and outcomes in the UK. Br J Ophthalmol. 2007;91(11):1452–5. https://doi.org/10.1136/bjo.2007.114884. Epub 2007 May 15. PMID: 17504853; PMCID: PMC2095441.
58. Lau CH, Missotten T, Salzmann J, Lightman SL. Acute retinal necrosis features, management, and outcomes. Ophthalmology. 2007;114(4):756–62. https://doi.org/10.1016/j.ophtha.2006.08.037. Epub 2006 Dec 20. PMID: 17184841.
59. Holland GN. Standard diagnostic criteria for the acute retinal necrosis syndrome. Executive Committee of the American Uveitis Society. Am J Ophthalmol. 1994;117(5):663–7. https://doi.org/10.1016/s0002--9394(14)70075-3. PMID: 8172275.
60. Standardization of Uveitis Nomenclature (SUN) Working Group. Classification criteria for acute retinal necrosis syndrome. Am J Ophthalmol. 2021;228:237–44. https://doi.org/10.1016/j.ajo.2021.03.057. Epub 2021 Apr 15. PMID: 33845012; PMCID: PMC8675365.
61. Standardization of Uveitis Nomenclature (SUN) Working Group. Classification criteria for sarcoidosis-associated uveitis. Am J Ophthalmol. 2021;228:220–30. https://doi.org/10.1016/j.ajo.2021.03.047. Epub 2021 May 11. PMID: 33845001; PMCID: PMC8594768.
62. Standardization of Uveitis Nomenclature (SUN) Working Group. Classification criteria for cytomeg-

alovirus retinitis. Am J Ophthalmol. 2021;228:245–54. https://doi.org/10.1016/j.ajo.2021.03.051. Epub 2021 May 11. PMID: 33845015; PMCID: PMC8594755.
63. Standardization of Uveitis Nomenclature (SUN) Working Group. Classification criteria for Behçet disease uveitis. Am J Ophthalmol. 2021;228:80–8. https://doi.org/10.1016/j.ajo.2021.03.058. Epub 2021 May 11. PMID: 33845008; PMCID: PMC8545705.
64. Duker JS, Shakin EP. Rapidly progressive outer retinal necrosis in the acquired immunodeficiency syndrome. Am J Ophthalmol. 1991;111(2):255–6. https://doi.org/10.1016/s0002-9394(14)72279-2. PMID: 1992756.
65. Forster DJ, Cano MR, Green RL, Rao NA. Echographic features of the Vogt-Koyanagi-Harada syndrome. Arch Ophthalmol. 1990;108(10):1421–6. https://doi.org/10.1001/archopht.1990.01070120069031. PMID: 2222275.
66. Forster DJ, Dugel PU, Frangieh GT, Liggett PE, Rao NA. Rapidly progressive outer retinal necrosis in the acquired immunodeficiency syndrome. Am J Ophthalmol. 1990;110(4):341–8. https://doi.org/10.1016/s0002-9394(14)77012-6. PMID: 2220967.
67. Jabs DA, Schachat AP, Liss R, Knox DL, Michels RG. Presumed varicella zoster retinitis in immunocompromised patients. Retina. 1987;7(1):9–13. PMID: 3602608.
68. Lei B, Zhou M, Wang Z, Chang Q, Xu G, Jiang R. Ultra-wide-field fundus imaging of acute retinal necrosis: clinical characteristics and visual significance. Eye (Lond). 2020;34(5):864–72. https://doi.org/10.1038/s41433-019-0587-8. Epub 2019 Sep 25. PMID: 31554945; PMCID: PMC7182555.
69. Zhao XY, Meng LH, Zhang WF, Wang DY, Chen YX. Retinal detachment after acute retinal necrosis and the efficacies of different interventions: a systematic review and metaanalysis. Retina. 2021;41(5):965–78. https://doi.org/10.1097/IAE.0000000000002971. PMID: 32932382.
70. Meghpara B, Sulkowski G, Kesen MR, Tessler HH, Goldstein DA. Long-term follow-up of acute retinal necrosis. Retina. 2010;30(5):795–800. https://doi.org/10.1097/IAE.0b013e3181c7013c. PMID: 20057342.
71. Fan S, Lin D, Wang Y. Role of prophylactic vitrectomy in acute retinal necrosis in preventing rhegmatogenous retinal detachment: systematic review and meta-analysis. Ocul Immunol Inflamm. 2022;30(2):515–9. https://doi.org/10.1080/09273948.2020.1800051. Epub 2020 Sep 23. PMID: 32966153.
72. Miserocchi E, Iuliano L, Fogliato G, Modorati G, Couto C, Schlaen A, Hurtado E, Llorenç V, Adan A, Bandello F. Bilateral acute retinal necrosis: clinical features and outcomes in a multicenter study. Ocul Immunol Inflamm. 2019;27(7):1090–8. https://doi.org/10.1080/09273948.2018.1501494. Epub 2018 Jul 30. PMID: 30059636.
73. Yawn BP, Wollan PC, Kurland MJ, St Sauver JL, Saddier P. Herpes zoster recurrences more frequent than previously reported. Mayo Clin Proc. 2011;86(2):88–93. https://doi.org/10.4065/mcp.2010.0618. Epub 2011 Jan 10. PMID: 21220354; PMCID: PMC3031432.
74. Kobayashi T, Sekar P, Meier J, Streit J. Acute retinal necrosis in a patient with remote severe herpes simplex encephalitis. BMJ Case Rep. 2019;12(5):e229137. https://doi.org/10.1136/bcr-2018-229137. PMID: 31138593; PMCID: PMC6557359.
75. Todokoro D, Kamei S, Goto H, Ikeda Y, Koyama H, Akiyama H. Acute retinal necrosis following herpes simplex encephalitis: a nationwide survey in Japan. Jpn J Ophthalmol. 2019;63(4):304–9. https://doi.org/10.1007/s10384-019-00668-5. Epub 2019 May 3. PMID: 31054049.
76. Klein A, Lefebvre P. Three consecutive episodes of acute retinal necrosis due to herpes simplex-1 over twelve years following herpetic encephalitis. Ocul Immunol Inflamm. 2007;15(5):411–3. https://doi.org/10.1080/09273940701662510. PMID: 17972228.
77. Kim SJ, Kang SW, Joo EY. An unusual case of herpes simplex viral encephalitis following acute retinal necrosis after administration of a systemic steroid. J Epilepsy Res. 2012;2(1):21–4. https://doi.org/10.14581/jer.12006. PMID: 24649457; PMCID: PMC3952316.
78. Matsuo T, Nakayama T, Baba T. Same eye recurrence of acute retinal necrosis syndrome. Am J Ophthalmol. 2001;131(5):659–61. https://doi.org/10.1016/s0002-9394(00)00847-3. PMID: 11336947.
79. Donovan CP, Levison AL, Lowder CY, Martin DF, Srivastava SK. Delayed recurrence of acute retinal necrosis (ARN): a case series. J Clin Virol. 2016;80:68–71. https://doi.org/10.1016/j.jcv.2016.04.021. Epub 2016 Apr 30. PMID: 27179886.
80. Okunuki Y, Usui Y, Kezuka T, Takeuchi M, Goto H. Four cases of bilateral acute retinal necrosis with a long interval after the initial onset. Br J Ophthalmol. 2011;95(9):1251–4. https://doi.org/10.1136/bjo.2010.191288. Epub 2011 Jan 17. PMID: 21242577.
81. Grinde B. Herpesviruses: latency and reactivation—viral strategies and host response. J Oral Microbiol. 2013;5. https://doi.org/10.3402/jom.v5i0.22766. PMID: 24167660; PMCID: PMC3809354.
82. Cohen JI. Herpesvirus latency. J Clin Invest. 2020;130(7):3361–9. https://doi.org/10.1172/JCI136225. PMID: 32364538; PMCID: PMC7324166.
83. Pirofski LA, Casadevall A. The state of latency in microbial pathogenesis. J Clin Invest. 2020;130(9):4525–31. https://doi.org/10.1172/

JCI136221. PMID: 32804154; PMCID: PMC7456213.

84. Wang K, Hoshino Y, Dowdell K, Bosch-Marce M, Myers TG, Sarmiento M, Pesnicak L, Krause PR, Cohen JI. Glutamine supplementation suppresses herpes simplex virus reactivation. J Clin Invest. 2017;127(7):2626–30. https://doi.org/10.1172/JCI88990. Epub 2017 Jun 5. PMID: 28581445; PMCID: PMC5490748.
85. Hoover DR, Peng Y, Saah A, Semba R, Detels RR, Rinaldo CR Jr, Phair JP. Occurrence of cytomegalovirus retinitis after human immunodeficiency virus immunosuppression. Arch Ophthalmol. 1996;114(7):821–7. https://doi.org/10.1001/archopht.1996.01100140035004. PMID: 8660165.
86. Downes KM, Tarasewicz D, Weisberg LJ, Cunningham ET Jr. Good syndrome and other causes of cytomegalovirus retinitis in HIV-negative patients—case report and comprehensive review of the literature. J Ophthalmic Inflamm Infect. 2016;6(1):3. https://doi.org/10.1186/s12348-016-0070-7. Epub 2016 Jan 25. PMID: 26809342; PMCID: PMC4726639.
87. Davis JL, Haft P, Hartley K. Retinal arteriolar occlusions due to cytomegalovirus retinitis in elderly patients without HIV. J Ophthalmic Inflamm Infect. 2013;3(1):17. https://doi.org/10.1186/1869-5760-3-17. PMID: 23514532; PMCID: PMC3605088.
88. Pathanapitoon K, Tesavibul N, Choopong P, Boonsopon S, Kongyai N, Ausayakhun S, Kunavisarut P, Rothova A. Clinical manifestations of cytomegalovirus-associated posterior uveitis and panuveitis in patients without human immunodeficiency virus infection. JAMA Ophthalmol. 2013;131(5):638–45. https://doi.org/10.1001/jamaophthalmol.2013.2860. PMID: 23494002.
89. Shapira Y, Mimouni M, Vishnevskia-Dai V. Cytomegalovirus retinitis in HIV-negative patients—associated conditions, clinical presentation, diagnostic methods and treatment strategy. Acta Ophthalmol. 2018;96(7):e761–7. https://doi.org/10.1111/aos.13553. Epub 2017 Oct 25. PMID: 29068151.
90. Gupta S, Vemulakonda GA, Suhler EB, Yeh S, Albini TA, Mandelcorn E, Flaxel CJ. Cytomegalovirus retinitis in the absence of AIDS. Can J Ophthalmol. 2013;48(2):126–9. https://doi.org/10.1016/j.jcjo.2012.12.002. PMID: 23561607.
91. Schneider EW, Elner SG, van Kuijk FJ, Goldberg N, Lieberman RM, Eliott D, Johnson MW. Chronic retinal necrosis: cytomegalovirus necrotizing retinitis associated with panretinal vasculopathy in non-HIV patients. Retina. 2013;33(9):1791–9. https://doi.org/10.1097/IAE.0b013e318285f486. PMID: 23584702.
92. Invernizzi A, Agarwal A, Ravera V, Oldani M, Staurenghi G, Viola F. Optical coherence tomography findings in cytomegalovirus retinitis: a longitudinal study. Retina. 2018;38(1):108–17. https://doi.org/10.1097/IAE.0000000000001503. PMID: 28145973.
93. Invernizzi A, Agarwal AK, Ravera V, Mapelli C, Riva A, Staurenghi G, McCluskey PJ, Viola F. Comparing optical coherence tomography findings in different aetiologies of infectious necrotising retinitis. Br J Ophthalmol. 2018;102(4):433–7. https://doi.org/10.1136/bjophthalmol-2017-310210. Epub 2017 Aug 1. PMID: 28765144.
94. Rao NA, Zhang J, Ishimoto S. Role of retinal vascular endothelial cells in development of CMV retinitis. Trans Am Ophthalmol Soc. 1998;96:111–23; discussion 124–6. PMID: 10360285; PMCID: PMC1298391.
95. Martin DF, Sierra-Madero J, Walmsley S, Wolitz RA, Macey K, Georgiou P, Robinson CA, Stempien MJ, Valganciclovir Study Group. A controlled trial of valganciclovir as induction therapy for cytomegalovirus retinitis. N Engl J Med. 2002;346(15):1119–26. https://doi.org/10.1056/NEJMoa011759. Erratum in: N Engl J Med 2002 Sep 12;347(11):862. PMID: 11948271.
96. Agarwal A, Kumari N, Trehan A, Khadwal A, Dogra MR, Gupta V, Sharma A, Gupta A, Singh R. Outcome of cytomegalovirus retinitis in immunocompromised patients without human immunodeficiency virus treated with intravitreal ganciclovir injection. Graefes Arch Clin Exp Ophthalmol. 2014;252(9):1393–401. https://doi.org/10.1007/s00417-014-2587-5. Epub 2014 Feb 21. PMID: 24557658.
97. Royston L, Royston E, Masouridi-Levrat S, Vernaz N, Chalandon Y, Van Delden C, Neofytos D. Letermovir primary prophylaxis in high-risk hematopoietic cell transplant recipients: a matched cohort study. Vaccines (Basel). 2021;9(4):372. https://doi.org/10.3390/vaccines9040372. PMID: 33921218; PMCID: PMC8069238.
98. Port AD, Orlin A, Kiss S, Patel S, D'Amico DJ, Gupta MP. Cytomegalovirus retinitis: a review. J Ocul Pharmacol Ther. 2017;33(4):224–34. https://doi.org/10.1089/jop.2016.0140. Epub 2017 Mar 29. PMID: 28355091.
99. Gupta A, Sharma A, Bansal R, Sharma K. Classification of intraocular tuberculosis. Ocul Immunol Inflamm. 2015;23(1):7–13. https://doi.org/10.3109/09273948.2014.967358. Epub 2014 Oct 14. PMID: 25314361.
100. Gupta MP, Coombs P, Prockop SE, Hasan AA, Doubrovina E, O'Reilly RJ, Cohen SH, Park SS, Kiss S. Treatment of cytomegalovirus retinitis with cytomegalovirus-specific T-lymphocyte infusion. Ophthalmic Surg Lasers Imaging Retina. 2015;46(1):80–2.https://doi.org/10.3928/23258160--20150101-14. PMID: 25559515; PMCID: PMC4373317.
101. Pepple KL, Van Gelder RN. T-cell therapy to the rescue. Ophthalmol Retina. 2021;5(9):835–7. https://doi.org/10.1016/j.oret.2021.07.001. PMID: 34503757.

102. Seo S, Smith C, Fraser C, Patheja R, Shah SP, Rehan S, Crooks P, Neller MA, Khanna R. Adoptive T-cell therapy for pediatric cytomegalovirus-associated retinitis. Blood Adv. 2019;3(11):1774–7. https://doi.org/10.1182/bloodadvances.2019000121. PMID: 31186253; PMCID: PMC6560354.
103. Kuthyar S, Anthony CL, Fashina T, Yeh S, Shantha JG. World Health Organization high priority pathogens: ophthalmic disease findings and vision health perspectives. Pathogens. 2021;10(4):442. https://doi.org/10.3390/pathogens10040442. PMID: 33917710; PMCID: PMC8068131.
104. Babu K, Kini R, Philips M, Subbakrishna DK. Clinical profile of isolated viral anterior uveitis in a south Indian patient population. Ocul Immunol Inflamm. 2014;22(5):356–9. https://doi.org/10.3109/09273948.2013.841482. Epub 2013 Oct 10. PMID: 24111839.
105. Mahendradas P, Shetty R, Malathi J, Madhavan HN. Chikungunya virus iridocyclitis in Fuchs' heterochromic iridocyclitis. Indian J Ophthalmol. 2010;58(6):545–7. https://doi.org/10.4103/0301-4738.71707. PMID: 20952847; PMCID: PMC2993993.
106. Ryan FJ, Carr JM, Furtado JM, Ma Y, Ashander LM, Simões M, Oliver GF, Granado GB, Dawson AC, Michael MZ, Appukuttan B, Lynn DJ, Smith JR. Zika virus infection of human iris pigment epithelial cells. Front Immunol. 2021;12:644153. https://doi.org/10.3389/fimmu.2021.644153. PMID: 33968035; PMCID: PMC8100333.
107. Furtado JM, Espósito DL, Klein TM, Teixeira-Pinto T, da Fonseca BA. Uveitis associated with Zika virus infection. N Engl J Med. 2016;375(4):394–6. https://doi.org/10.1056/NEJMc1603618. Epub 2016 Jun 22. PMID: 27332784.
108. Troumani Y, Touhami S, Jackson TL, Ventura CV, Stanescu-Segall DM, Errera MH, Rousset D, Bodaghi B, Cartry G, David T, Beral L. Association of anterior uveitis with acute Zika virus infection in adults. JAMA Ophthalmol. 2021;139(1):95–102. https://doi.org/10.1001/jamaophthalmol.2020.5131. PMID: 33237306; PMCID: PMC7689574.
109. Abroug N, Khairallah M, Zina S, Ksiaa I, Amor HB, Attia S, Jelliti B, Khochtali S, Khairallah M. Ocular manifestations of emerging arthropod-borne infectious diseases. J Curr Ophthalmol. 2021;33(3):227–35. https://doi.org/10.4103/joco.joco_134_21. PMID: 34765808; PMCID: PMC8579803.
110. Pattnaik A, Sahoo BR, Pattnaik AK. Current status of Zika virus vaccines: successes and challenges. Vaccines (Basel). 2020;8(2):266. https://doi.org/10.3390/vaccines8020266. PMID: 32486368; PMCID: PMC7349928.
111. Wolgemuth CW. Flagellar motility of the pathogenic spirochetes. Semin Cell Dev Biol. 2015;46:104–12. https://doi.org/10.1016/j.semcdb.2015.10.015. Epub 2015 Oct 17. PMID: 26481969; PMCID: PMC4994469.
112. Furtado JM, Simões M, Vasconcelos-Santos D, Oliver GF, Tyagi M, Nascimento H, Gordon DL, Smith JR. Ocular syphilis. Surv Ophthalmol. 2022;67(2):440–62. https://doi.org/10.1016/j.survophthal.2021.06.003. S0039-6257(21)00140–5. Epub ahead of print. PMID: 34147542.
113. Caplash S, Gangaputra S, Kesav N, Akanda M, Vitale S, Kodati S, Marques A, Sen HN. Usefulness of routine Lyme screening in patients with uveitis. Ophthalmology. 2019;126(12):1726–8. https://doi.org/10.1016/j.ophtha.2019.06.014. Epub 2019 Jun 27. PMID: 31358389; PMCID: PMC6875618.
114. Chu KM, Rathinam R, Namperumalsamy P, Dean D. Identification of Leptospira species in the pathogenesis of uveitis and determination of clinical ocular characteristics in South India. J Infect Dis. 1998;177(5):1314–21. https://doi.org/10.1086/515273. PMID: 9593018.
115. Rathinam SR. Leptospirosis. In: Chee SP, Khairallah M, editors. Emerging infectious uveitis. Cham: Springer; 2017. https://doi.org/10.1007/978-3-319-23416-8_8.
116. Oast SP. Concerning tuberculous lesions of the retina. Trans Am Ophthalmol Soc. 1932;30:503–27. PMID: 16692952; PMCID: PMC1316870.
117. Duke-Elder S, Perkins ES, editors. System of ophthalmology, diseases of the uvea, vol. IX. Henry Kimpton: London; 1966. p. 246–81.
118. Duke-Elder S, Perkins ES. System of ophthalmology, diseases of the uvea, vol. IX. London: Henry Kimpton; 1966. p. 574.
119. Wilder HC. Toxoplasma chorioretinitis in adults. AMA Arch Ophthalmol. 1952;48(2):127–36. https://doi.org/10.1001/archopht.1952.00920010132001. PMID: 14943320.
120. Zimmerman LE. Verhoeff's "terato-neuroma" a critical reappraisal in light of new observations and current concepts of embryonic tumors. Trans Am Ophthalmol Soc. 1971;69:210–36. PMID: 4116382; PMCID: PMC1310415.
121. Tsirouki T, Dastiridou A, Symeonidis C, Tounakaki O, Brazitikou I, Kalogeropoulos C, Androudi S. A focus on the epidemiology of uveitis. Ocul Immunol Inflamm. 2018;26(1):2–16. https://doi.org/10.1080/09273948.2016.1196713. Epub 2016 Jul 28. PMID: 27467180.
122. Gupta A, Gupta V, Arora S, Dogra MR, Bambery P. PCR-positive tubercular retinal vasculitis: clinical characteristics and management. Retina. 2001;21(5):435–44. https://doi.org/10.1097/00006982-200110000-00004. PMID: 11642371.
123. Gupta V, Arora S, Gupta A, Ram J, Bambery P, Sehgal S. Management of presumed intraocular tuberculosis: possible role of the polymerase chain reaction. Acta Ophthalmol Scand. 1998;76(6):679–82.https://doi.org/10.1034/j.1600--0420.1998.760609.x. PMID: 9881551.
124. Gupta V, Gupta A, Bambery P, Radotra BD, Pandav SS. Vogt-Koyanagi-Harada syndrome follow-

ing injury-induced progressive vitiligo. Indian J Ophthalmol. 2001;49:53–5.

125. Gupta V, Gupta A, Sachdeva N, Arora S, Bambery P. Successful management of tubercular subretinal granulomas. Ocul Immunol Inflamm. 2006;14(1):35–40. https://doi.org/10.1080/09273940500269939. PMID: 16507489.
126. Alli HD, Ally N, Mayet I, Dangor Z, Madhi SA. Global prevalence and clinical outcomes of tubercular uveitis: a systematic review and meta-analysis. Surv Ophthalmol. 2022;67(3):770–92. https://doi.org/10.1016/j.survophthal.2021.10.001. Epub 2021 Oct 7. PMID: 34626620.
127. Gupta V, Gupta A, Arora S, Bambery P, Dogra MR, Agarwal A. Presumed tubercular serpiginous-like choroiditis: clinical presentations and management. Ophthalmology. 2003;110(9):1744–9. https://doi.org/10.1016/S0161-6420(03)00619-5. PMID: 13129872.
128. Bansal R, Gupta A, Gupta V, Dogra MR, Sharma A, Bambery P. Tubercular serpiginous-like choroiditis presenting as multifocal serpiginoid choroiditis. Ophthalmology. 2012;119(11):2334–42. https://doi.org/10.1016/j.ophtha.2012.05.034. Epub 2012 Aug 11. PMID: 22892153.
129. Gupta A, Bansal R, Gupta V, Sharma A. Fundus autofluorescence in serpiginouslike choroiditis. Retina. 2012;32(4):814–25. https://doi.org/10.1097/IAE.0b013e3182278c41. PMID: 22080913.
130. Gupta V, Bansal R, Gupta A. Continuous progression of tubercular serpiginous-like choroiditis after initiating antituberculosis treatment. Am J Ophthalmol. 2011;152(5):857–63.e2. https://doi.org/10.1016/j.ajo.2011.05.004. Epub 2011 Jul 26. PMID: 21794847.
131. Aggarwal K, Agarwal A, Deokar A, Singh R, Bansal R, Sharma A, Sharma K, Dogra MR, Gupta V. Ultra-wide field imaging in paradoxical worsening of tubercular multifocal Serpiginoid choroiditis after the initiation of anti-tubercular therapy. Ocul Immunol Inflamm. 2019;27(3):365–70. https://doi.org/10.1080/09273948.2017.1373829. Epub 2017 Oct 11. PMID: 29020501.
132. Agarwal A, Aggarwal K, Mandadi SKR, Kumar A, Grewal D, Invernizzi A, Bansal R, Sharma A, Sharma K, Gupta V, for OCTA Study Group. Longitudinal follow-up of tubercular serpiginous-like choroiditis using optical coherence tomography angiography. Retina. 2021;41(4):793–803. https://doi.org/10.1097/IAE.0000000000002915. PMID: 32833411.
133. Agarwal A, Aggarwal K, Pichi F, Meng T, Munk MR, Bazgain K, Bansal R, Agrawal R, Gupta V. Clinical and multimodal imaging clues in differentiating between tuberculomas and sarcoid choroidal granulomas. Am J Ophthalmol. 2021;226:42–55. https://doi.org/10.1016/j.ajo.2021.01.025. Epub 2021 Jan 30. PMID: 33529591.
134. Agarwal A, Freund KB, Kumar A, Aggarwal K, Sharma D, Katoch D, Bansal R, Gupta V, OCTA Study Group. Bacillary layer detachment in acute Vogt-Koyanagi-Harada disease: a novel swept-source optical coherence tomography analysis. Retina. 2021;41(4):774–83. https://doi.org/10.1097/IAE.0000000000002914. PMID: 32833410.
135. Barondes MJ, Sponsel WE, Stevens TS, Plotnik RD. Tuberculous choroiditis diagnosed by chorioretinal endobiopsy. Am J Ophthalmol. 1991;112(4):460–1. https://doi.org/10.1016/s0002--9394(14)76260-9. PMID: 1928253.
136. Rao NA, Saraswathy S, Smith RE. Tuberculous uveitis: distribution of Mycobacterium tuberculosis in the retinal pigment epithelium. Arch Ophthalmol. 2006;124(12):1777–9. https://doi.org/10.1001/archopht.124.12.1777. PMID: 17159041.
137. Kawali A, Emerson GG, Naik NK, Sharma K, Mahendradas P, Rao NA. Clinicopathologic features of Tuberculous serpiginous-like choroiditis. JAMA Ophthalmol. 2018;136(2):219–21. https://doi.org/10.1001/jamaophthalmol.2017.5791. PMID: 29270629.
138. Bansal R, Sharma K, Gupta A, Sharma A, Singh MP, Gupta V, Mulkutkar S, Dogra M, Dogra MR, Kamal S, Sharma SP, Fiorella PD. Detection of Mycobacterium tuberculosis genome in vitreous fluid of eyes with multifocal serpiginoid choroiditis. Ophthalmology. 2015;122(4):840–50. https://doi.org/10.1016/j.ophtha.2014.11.021. Epub 2015 Jan 9. PMID: 25578256.
139. Nazari Khanamiri H, Rao NA. Serpiginous choroiditis and infectious multifocal serpiginoid choroiditis. Surv Ophthalmol. 2013;58(3):203–32. https://doi.org/10.1016/j.survophthal.2012.08.008. Epub 2013 Mar 27. PMID: 23541041; PMCID: PMC3631461.
140. Song JH, Koreishi AF, Goldstein DA. Tuberculous uveitis presenting with a bullous exudative retinal detachment: a case report and systematic literature review. Ocul Immunol Inflamm. 2019;27(6):998–1009. https://doi.org/10.1080/09273948.2018.1485958. Epub 2018 Jul 3. PMID: 29969330.
141. Datta M, Via LE, Kamoun WS, Liu C, Chen W, Seano G, Weiner DM, Schimel D, England K, Martin JD, Gao X, Xu L, Barry CE 3rd, Jain RK. Anti-vascular endothelial growth factor treatment normalizes tuberculosis granuloma vasculature and improves small molecule delivery. Proc Natl Acad Sci U S A. 2015;112(6):1827–32. https://doi.org/10.1073/pnas.1424563112. Epub 2015 Jan 26. PMID: 25624495; PMCID: PMC4330784.
142. Hortle E, Oehlers SH. Host-directed therapies targeting the tuberculosis granuloma stroma. Pathog Dis. 2020;78(2):ftaa015. https://doi.org/10.1093/femspd/ftaa015. PMID: 32149337.
143. Oehlers SH. Revisiting hypoxia therapies for tuberculosis. Clin Sci (Lond). 2019;133(12):1271–80. https://doi.org/10.1042/CS20190415. PMID: 31209098.
144. Babu K, Murthy PR, Murthy KR. Intravitreal bevacizumab as an adjunct in a patient with presumed vascularised choroidal tubercular granuloma. Eye

(Lond). 2010;24(2):397–9. https://doi.org/10.1038/eye.2009.83. Epub 2009 Apr 17. PMID: 19373263.
145. Bansal R, Beke N, Sharma A, Gupta A. Intravitreal bevacizumab as an adjunct in the management of a vascular choroidal granuloma. BMJ Case Rep. 2013;2013:bcr2013200255. https://doi.org/10.1136/bcr-2013-200255. PMID: 24014333; PMCID: PMC3794147.
146. Agarwal M, Gupta C, Mohan KV, Upadhyay PK, Jha V. Correlation of vascular endothelial growth factor with the clinical regression of tubercular granuloma. Indian J Ophthalmol. 2020;68(9):2037–40. https://doi.org/10.4103/ijo.IJO_1261_20. PMID: 32823472; PMCID: PMC7690512.
147. Sharma K, Bansal R, Sharma A, Gupta A, Fiorella PD. Successful treatment of rifampicin-resistant intraocular tuberculosis. Ocul Immunol Inflamm. 2015;23(1):93–6. https://doi.org/10.3109/09273948.2014.888084. Epub 2014 Mar 21. PMID: 24654625.
148. Sharma K, Gupta A, Sharma M, Sharma A, Bansal R, Sharma SP, Singh RD, Gupta V. The emerging challenge of diagnosing drug-resistant tubercular uveitis: experience of 110 eyes from North India. Ocul Immunol Inflamm. 2021;29(1):107–14. https://doi.org/10.1080/09273948.2019.1655581. Epub ahead of print. PMID: 31580170.
149. Sharma K, Sharma A, Bansal R, Fiorella PD, Gupta A. Drug-resistant tubercular uveitis. J Clin Microbiol. 2014;52(11):4113–4. https://doi.org/10.1128/JCM.01918-14. Epub 2014 Sep 3. PMID: 25187635; PMCID: PMC4313252.
150. Biswas J, Ravi RK, Naryanasamy A, Kulandai LT, Madhavan HN. Eales' disease—current concepts in diagnosis and management. J Ophthalmic Inflamm Infect. 2013;3(1):11. https://doi.org/10.1186/1869--5760-3-11. PMID: 23514227; PMCID: PMC3605068.
151. Singh R, Toor P, Parchand S, Sharma K, Gupta V, Gupta A. Quantitative polymerase chain reaction for Mycobacterium tuberculosis in so-called Eales' disease. Ocul Immunol Inflamm. 2012;20(3):153–7. https://doi.org/10.3109/09273948.2012.658134. Epub 2012 Apr 9. PMID: 22486260.
152. Madhavan HN, Therese KL, Kavitha D. Further investigations on the association of Mycobacterium tuberculosis with Eales' disease. Indian J Ophthalmol. 2002;50:35–9.
153. Bodaghi B, Rozenberg F, Cassoux N, Fardeau C, LeHoang P. Nonnecrotizing herpetic retinopathies masquerading as severe posterior uveitis. Ophthalmology. 2003;110(9):1737–43. https://doi.org/10.1016/S0161-6420(03)00580-3. PMID: 13129871.
154. Biswas J, Mayr AJ, Martin WJ, Rao NA. Detection of human cytomegalovirus in ocular tissue by polymerase chain reaction and in situ hybridization. Graefes Arch Clin Exp Ophthalmol. 1993;231:66–70.
155. Fenner TE, Garweg J, Hufert FT, Boehnke M, Schmitz H. Diagnosis of human cytomegalovirus-induced retinitis in human immunodeficiency virus type 1-infected subjects by using the polymerase chain reaction. J Clin Microbiol. 1991;29(11):2621–2. https://doi.org/10.1128/JCM.29.11.2621-2622.1991. PMID: 1663513; PMCID: PMC270387.
156. Fox GM, Crouse CA, Chuang EL, Pflugfelder SC, Cleary TJ, Nelson SJ, Atherton SS. Detection of herpesvirus DNA in vitreous and aqueous specimens by the polymerase chain reaction. Arch Ophthalmol. 1991;109(2):266–71. https://doi.org/10.1001/archopht.1991.01080020112054. PMID: 1847043.
157. Knox CM, Chandler D, Short GA, Margolis TP. Polymerase chain reaction-based assays of vitreous samples for the diagnosis of viral retinitis. Use in diagnostic dilemmas. Ophthalmology. 1998;105(1):37–44; discussion 44–5. PMID: 9442777. https://doi.org/10.1016/s0161-6420(98)71127-2.
158. McCann JD, Margolis TP, Wong MG, Kuppermann BD, Luckie AP, Schwartz DM, Irvine AR, Ai E. A sensitive and specific polymerase chain reaction-based assay for the diagnosis of cytomegalovirus retinitis. Am J Ophthalmol. 1995;120(2):219–26. https://doi.org/10.1016/s0002-9394(14)72610-8. PMID: 7639306.
159. Montoya JG, Parmley S, Liesenfeld O, Jaffe GJ, Remington JS. Use of the polymerase chain reaction for diagnosis of ocular toxoplasmosis. Ophthalmology. 1999;106(8):1554–63. https://doi.org/10.1016/S0161-6420(99)90453-0. PMID: 10442904.
160. Nishi M, Hanashiro R, Mori S, Masuda K, Mochizuki M, Hondo R. Polymerase chain reaction for the detection of the varicella-zoster genome in ocular samples from patients with acute retinal necrosis. Am J Ophthalmol. 1992;114(5):603–9. https://doi.org/10.1016/s0002-9394(14)74491-5. PMID: 1332482.
161. Short GA, Margolis TP, Kuppermann BD, Irvine AR, Martin DF, Chandler D. A polymerase chain reaction-based assay for diagnosing varicella-zoster virus retinitis in patients with acquired immunodeficiency syndrome. Am J Ophthalmol. 1997;123(2):157–64.https://doi.org/10.1016/s0002--9394(14)71031-1. PMID: 9186120.
162. Varkey JB, Shantha JG, Crozier I, Kraft CS, Lyon GM, Mehta AK, Kumar G, Smith JR, Kainulainen MH, Whitmer S, Ströher U, Uyeki TM, Ribner BS, Yeh S. Persistence of Ebola virus in ocular fluid during convalescence. N Engl J Med. 2015;372(25):2423–7. https://doi.org/10.1056/NEJMoa1500306. Epub 2015 May 7. Erratum in: N Engl J Med 2015 Jun 18;372(25):2469. PMID: 25950269; PMCID: PMC4547451.
163. Nakano S, Tomaru Y, Kubota T, Takase H, Mochizuki M, Shimizu N, Sugita S, Strip PCR Project Group. Evaluation of a multiplex strip PCR test for infectious uveitis: a prospective multicenter study. Am J Ophthalmol. 2020;213:252–9. https://

doi.org/10.1016/j.ajo.2019.10.031. Epub 2019 Nov 28. PMID: 31785234.

164. Sharma K, Gupta V, Bansal R, Sharma A, Sharma M, Gupta A. Novel multi-targeted polymerase chain reaction for diagnosis of presumed tubercular uveitis. J Ophthalmic Inflamm Infect. 2013;3(1):25. https://doi.org/10.1186/1869-5760-3-25. PMID: 23514226; PMCID: PMC3605072.

165. Therese KL, Jayanthi U, Madhavan HN. Application of nested polymerase chain reaction (nPCR) using MPB 64 gene primers to detect Mycobacterium tuberculosis DNA in clinical specimens from extrapulmonary tuberculosis patients. Indian J Med Res. 2005;122(2):165–70. PMID: 16177475.

166. Sharma K, Gupta A, Sharma M, Singh S, Sharma A, Singh R, Gupta V. Detection of viable Mycobacterium tuberculosis in ocular fluids using mRNA-based multiplex polymerase chain reaction. Indian J Med Microbiol. 2022;40(2):254–7. https://doi.org/10.1016/j.ijmmb.2021.12.019. Epub 2022 Jan 17. PMID: 35058073.

167. Bansal R, Gupta A, Gupta V, Mulkutkar S, Dogra M, Katoch D, Dogra MR, Sharma K, Singh MP, Sharma A, Kamal S, Sharma SP. Safety and outcome of microincision vitreous surgery in uveitis. Ocul Immunol Inflamm. 2017;25(6):775–84. https://doi.org/10.3109/09273948.2016.1165259. Epub 2016 May 18. PMID: 27191861.

168. Zhao XY, Xia S, Chen YX. Role of diagnostic pars plana vitrectomy in determining the etiology of uveitis initially unknown. Retina. 2020;40(2):359–69. https://doi.org/10.1097/IAE.0000000000002372. PMID: 31972807.

169. Sanger F, Nicklen S, Coulson AR. DNA sequencing with chain-terminating inhibitors. Proc Natl Acad Sci U S A. 1977;74(12):5463–7. https://doi.org/10.1073/pnas.74.12.5463. PMID: 271968; PMCID: PMC431765.

170. Gu W, Miller S, Chiu CY. Clinical metagenomic next-generation sequencing for pathogen detection. Annu Rev Pathol. 2019;14:319–38. https://doi.org/10.1146/annurev-pathmechdis-012418-012751. Epub 2018 Oct 24. PMID: 30355154; PMCID: PMC6345613.

171. Deshmukh D, Joseph J, Chakrabarti M, Sharma S, Jayasudha R, Sama KC, Sontam B, Tyagi M, Narayanan R, Shivaji S. New insights into culture negative endophthalmitis by unbiased next generation sequencing. Sci Rep. 2019;9(1):844. https://doi.org/10.1038/s41598-018-37502-w. PMID: 30696908; PMCID: PMC6351655.2416-4. PMID: 29515160; PMCID: PMC5841358.

172. Valdes L, Bispo P, Sobrin L. Application of metagenomic sequencing in the diagnosis of infectious uveitis. Semin Ophthalmol. 2020;35(5–6):276–9. https://doi.org/10.1080/08820538.2020.1818795. Epub 2020 Oct 18. PMID: 33073643.

173. Doan T, Sahoo MK, Ruder K, Huang C, Zhong L, Chen C, Hinterwirth A, Lin C, Gonzales JA, Pinsky BA, Acharya NR. Comprehensive pathogen detection for ocular infections. J Clin Virol. 2021;136:104759. https://doi.org/10.1016/j.jcv.2021.104759. Epub 2021 Feb 11. PMID: 33609933; PMCID: PMC7954984.

174. Gonzales JA, Doan T, VanZante A, Stewart JM, Sura A, Reddy A, Rasool N. Detection of *Tropheryma whipplei* genome from the aqueous humor by metagenomic sequencing. Ann Intern Med. 2021;174(9):1329–30. https://doi.org/10.7326/L20--1470. Epub 2021 Jun 15. PMID: 34125575.

175. Arunasri K, Mahesh M, Sai Prashanthi G, Jayasudha R, Kalyana Chakravarthy S, Tyagi M, Pappuru RR, Shivaji S. Comparison of the vitreous fluid bacterial microbiomes between individuals with post fever retinitis and healthy controls. Microorganisms. 2020;8(5):751. https://doi.org/10.3390/microorganisms8050751. PMID: 32429503; PMCID: PMC7285296.

176. Phadke VK, Shantha JG, O'Keefe G. Relapsing uveitis due to human T-lymphotropic virus type 1 in a patient living with HIV diagnosed by metagenomic deep sequencing. Open Forum Infect Dis. 2020;7(3):ofaa078. https://doi.org/10.1093/ofid/ofaa078. PMID: 32206676; PMCID: PMC7081385.

177. D'Cruz DP, Khamashta MA, Hughes GR. Systemic lupus erythematosus. Lancet. 2007;369(9561):587–96. https://doi.org/10.1016/S0140-6736(07)60279-7. PMID: 17307106.

178. Isenberg DA, Manson JJ, Ehrenstein MR, Rahman A. Fifty years of anti-ds DNA antibodies: are we approaching journey's end? Rheumatology (Oxford). 2007;46(7):1052–6. https://doi.org/10.1093/rheumatology/kem112. Epub 2007 May 11. PMID: 17500073.

179. Rahman A, Isenberg DA. Systemic lupus erythematosus. N Engl J Med. 2008;358(9):929–39. https://doi.org/10.1056/NEJMra071297. PMID: 18305268.

180. Dammacco R. Systemic lupus erythematosus and ocular involvement: an overview. Clin Exp Med. 2018;18(2):135–49.https://doi.org/10.1007/s10238--017-0479-9. Epub 2017 Dec 14. PMID: 29243035.

181. Lee I, Zickuhr L, Hassman L. Update on ophthalmic manifestations of systemic lupus erythematosus: pathogenesis and precision medicine. Curr Opin Ophthalmol. 2021;32(6):583–9. https://doi.org/10.1097/ICU.0000000000000810. PMID: 34545846.

182. Aronson AJ, Ordoñez NG, Diddie KR, Ernest JT. Immune-complex deposition in the eye in systemic lupus erythematosus. Arch Intern Med. 1979;139(11):1312–3. PMID: 159674.

183. Chin D, Gan NY, Holder GE, Tien M, Agrawal R, Manghani M. Severe retinal vasculitis in systemic lupus erythematosus leading to vision threatening paracentral acute middle maculopathy. Mod Rheumatol Case Rep. 2021;5(2):265–71. https://doi.org/10.1080/24725625.2021.1893961. Epub 2021 Mar 15. PMID: 33627049.

184. Stafford-Brady FJ, Urowitz MB, Gladman DD, Easterbrook M. Lupus retinopathy. Patterns,

associations, and prognosis. Arthritis Rheum. 1988;31(9):1105–10. https://doi.org/10.1002/art.1780310904. PMID: 3422014.

185. Edouard S, Douat J, Sailler L, Arlet P, Astudillo L. Bilateral choroidopathy in systemic lupus erythematosus. Lupus. 2011;20(11):1209–10. https://doi.org/10.1177/0961203311398510. Epub 2011 Apr 21. PMID: 21511760.
186. Nguyen QD, Uy HS, Akpek EK, Harper SL, Zacks DN, Foster CS. Choroidopathy of systemic lupus erythematosus. Lupus. 2000;9(4):288–98. https://doi.org/10.1191/096120300680199024. PMID: 10866100.
187. Hasanreisoglu M, Gulpinar Ikiz GD, Kucuk H, Varan O, Ozdek S. Acute lupus choroidopathy: multimodal imaging and differential diagnosis from central serous chorioretinopathy. Int Ophthalmol. 2018;38(1):369–74.https://doi.org/10.1007/s10792--016-0433-y. Epub 2017 Jan 3. PMID: 28050729.
188. Kucukkomurcu E, Unal AU, Esen F, Ozen G, Direskeneli H, Kazokoglu H. Ocular posterior segment involvement in patients with antiphospholipid syndrome and systemic lupus erythematosus. Ocul Immunol Inflamm. 2020;28(1):86–91. https://doi.org/10.1080/09273948.2018.1552759. Epub 2018 Dec 17. PMID: 30556792.
189. Montehermoso A, Cervera R, Font J, Ramos-Casals M, García-carrasco M, Formiga F, Callejas JL, Jorfán M, Griñó MC, Ingelmo M. Association of antiphospholipid antibodies with retinal vascular disease in systemic lupus erythematosus. Semin Arthritis Rheum. 1999;28(5):326–32. https://doi.org/10.1016/s0049-0172(99)80017-1. PMID: 10342390.
190. Aringer M, Costenbader K, Daikh D, Brinks R, Mosca M, Ramsey-Goldman R, Smolen JS, Wofsy D, Boumpas DT, Kamen DL, Jayne D, Cervera R, Costedoat-Chalumeau N, Diamond B, Gladman DD, Hahn B, Hiepe F, Jacobsen S, Khanna D, Lerstrøm K, Massarotti E, McCune J, Ruiz-Irastorza G, Sanchez-Guerrero J, Schneider M, Urowitz M, Bertsias G, Hoyer BF, Leuchten N, Tani C, Tedeschi SK, Touma Z, Schmajuk G, Anic B, Assan F, Chan TM, Clarke AE, Crow MK, Czirják L, Doria A, Graninger W, Halda-Kiss B, Hasni S, Izmirly PM, Jung M, Kumánovics G, Mariette X, Padjen I, Pego-Reigosa JM, Romero-Diaz J, Rúa-Figueroa Fernández Í, Seror R, Stummvoll GH, Tanaka Y, Tektonidou MG, Vasconcelos C, Vital EM, Wallace DJ, Yavuz S, Meroni PL, Fritzler MJ, Naden R, Dörner T, Johnson SR. 2019 European League Against Rheumatism/American College of Rheumatology classification criteria for systemic lupus erythematosus. Arthritis Rheumatol. 2019;71(9):1400–12. https://doi.org/10.1002/art.40930. Epub 2019 Aug 6. PMID: 31385462; PMCID: PMC6827566.
191. Costabel U, Hunninghake GW. ATS/ERS/WASOG statement on sarcoidosis. Sarcoidosis Statement Committee. American Thoracic Society. European Respiratory Society. World Association for Sarcoidosis and Other Granulomatous Disorders. Eur Respir J. 1999;14(4):735–7. https://doi.org/10.1034/j.1399-3003.1999.14d02.x. PMID: 10573213.
192. Korsten P, Tampe B, Konig MF, Nikiphorou E. Sarcoidosis and autoimmune diseases: differences, similarities and overlaps. Curr Opin Pulm Med. 2018;24(5):504–12. https://doi.org/10.1097/MCP.0000000000000500. PMID: 29985181.
193. Niederer RL, Ma SP, Wilsher ML, Ali NQ, Sims JL, Tomkins-Netzer O, Lightman SL, Lim LL. Systemic associations of sarcoid uveitis: correlation with uveitis phenotype and ethnicity. Am J Ophthalmol. 2021;229:169–75. https://doi.org/10.1016/j.ajo.2021.03.003. Epub 2021 Mar 15. PMID: 33737030.
194. Kassa E, Elner VM, Moroi SE, Sun Y. Diffuse Berlin nodules: unusual presentation of ocular sarcoidosis. Br J Ophthalmol. 2013;97(9):1214, 1223–4. Epub 2013 May 31. PMID: 23728905. https://doi.org/10.1136/bjophthalmol-2013-303112.
195. Mahendradas P, Thomas R, Kawali A, Shetty BK. Berlin nodule in sarcoidosis. Indian J Ophthalmol. 2019;67(7):1180. https://doi.org/10.4103/ijo.IJO_1756_18. PMID: 31238450; PMCID: PMC6611251.
196. Takayama K, Harimoto K, Sato T, Sakurai Y, Taguchi M, Kanda T, Takeuchi M. Age-related differences in the clinical features of ocular sarcoidosis. PLoS One. 2018;13(8):e0202585. https://doi.org/10.1371/journal.pone.0202585. PMID: 30138345; PMCID: PMC6107189.
197. Vrabec TR, Augsburger JJ, Fischer DH, Belmont JB, Tashayyod D, Israel HL. Taches de bougie. Ophthalmology. 1995;102(11):1712–21. https://doi.org/10.1016/s0161-6420(95)30804-4. PMID: 9098267.
198. Rothova A, Lardenoye C. Arterial macroaneurysms in peripheral multifocal chorioretinitis associated with sarcoidosis. Ophthalmology. 1998;105(8):1393–7. https://doi.org/10.1016/S0161-6420(98)98018-6. PMID: 9709748.
199. Yamanaka E, Ohguro N, Kubota A, Yamamoto S, Nakagawa Y, Tano Y. Features of retinal arterial macroaneurysms in patients with uveitis. Br J Ophthalmol. 2004;88(7):884–6. https://doi.org/10.1136/bjo.2003.035923. PMID: 15205230; PMCID: PMC1772231.
200. Gass JD, Olson CL. Sarcoidosis with optic nerve and retinal involvement. A clinicopathologic case report. Trans Am Acad Ophthalmol Otolaryngol. 1973;77(6):OP739–50. PMID: 4772534.
201. Mehta H, Sim DA, Keane PA, Zarranz-Ventura J, Gallagher K, Egan CA, Westcott M, Lee RW, Tufail A, Pavesio CE. Structural changes of the choroid in sarcoid- and tuberculosis-related granulomatous uveitis. Eye (Lond). 2015;29(8):1060–8. https://doi.org/10.1038/eye.2015.65. Epub 2015 May 29. PMID: 26021867; PMCID: PMC4541349.

202. Pichi F, Invernizzi A, Tucker WR, Munk MR. Optical coherence tomography diagnostic signs in posterior uveitis. Prog Retin Eye Res. 2020;75:100797. https://doi.org/10.1016/j.preteyeres.2019.100797. Epub 2019 Sep 9. PMID: 31513851.
203. Herbort CP, Rao NA, Mochizuki M, Members of Scientific Committee of First International Workshop on ocular sarcoidosis. International criteria for the diagnosis of ocular sarcoidosis: results of the first international workshop on ocular sarcoidosis (IWOS). Ocul Immunol Inflamm. 2009;17(3):160–9. https://doi.org/10.1080/09273940902818861. PMID: 19585358.
204. Acharya NR, Browne EN, Rao N, Mochizuki M, International Ocular Sarcoidosis Working Group. Distinguishing features of ocular sarcoidosis in an international cohort of uveitis patients. Ophthalmology. 2018;125(1):119–26. https://doi.org/10.1016/j.ophtha.2017.07.006. Epub 2017 Aug 16. PMID: 28823384.
205. Agarwal R, Srinivasan A, Aggarwal AN, Gupta D. Efficacy and safety of convex probe EBUS-TBNA in sarcoidosis: a systematic review and meta-analysis. Respir Med. 2012;106(6):883–92. https://doi.org/10.1016/j.rmed.2012.02.014. Epub 2012 Mar 13. PMID: 22417738.
206. Mochizuki M, Smith JR, Takase H, Kaburaki T, Acharya NR, Rao NA, International Workshop on Ocular Sarcoidosis Study Group. Revised criteria of international workshop on ocular sarcoidosis (IWOS) for the diagnosis of ocular sarcoidosis. Br J Ophthalmol. 2019;103(10):1418–22. https://doi.org/10.1136/bjophthalmol-2018-313356. Epub 2019 Feb 23. PMID: 30798264.
207. Sakane T, Takeno M, Suzuki N, Inaba G. Behçet's disease. N Engl J Med. 1999;341(17):1284–91. https://doi.org/10.1056/NEJM199910213411707. PMID: 10528040.
208. Verity DH, Wallace GR, Vaughan RW, Stanford MR. Behçet's disease: from Hippocrates to the third millennium. Br J Ophthalmol. 2003;87(9):1175–83. https://doi.org/10.1136/bjo.87.9.1175. PMID: 12928293; PMCID: PMC1771837.
209. Poon W, Verity DH, Larkin GL, Graham EM, Stanford MR. Behçet's disease in patients of west African and Afro-Caribbean origin. Br J Ophthalmol. 2003;87(7):876–8. https://doi.org/10.1136/bjo.87.7.876. PMID: 12812890; PMCID: PMC1771753.
210. Takeno M. The association of Behçet's syndrome with HLA-B51 as understood in 2021. Curr Opin Rheumatol. 2022;34(1):4–9. https://doi.org/10.1097/BOR.0000000000000846. PMID: 34690278; PMCID: PMC8635258.
211. Gül A, Ozbek U, Oztürk C, Inanç M, Koniçe M, Ozçelik T. Coagulation factor V gene mutation increases the risk of venous thrombosis in Behçet's disease. Br J Rheumatol. 1996;35(11):1178–80. https://doi.org/10.1093/rheumatology/35.11.1178. PMID: 8948311.
212. Ames PR, Steuer A, Pap A, Denman AM. Thrombosis in Behçet's disease: a retrospective survey from a single UK centre. Rheumatology (Oxford). 2001;40(6):652–5. https://doi.org/10.1093/rheumatology/40.6.652. PMID: 11426022.
213. Hatemi G, Christensen R, Bang D, Bodaghi B, Celik AF, Fortune F, Gaudric J, Gul A, Kötter I, Leccese P, Mahr A, Moots R, Ozguler Y, Richter J, Saadoun D, Salvarani C, Scuderi F, Sfikakis PP, Siva A, Stanford M, Tugal-Tutkun I, West R, Yurdakul S, Olivieri I, Yazici H. 2018 update of the EULAR recommendations for the management of Behçet's syndrome. Ann Rheum Dis. 2018;77(6):808–18. https://doi.org/10.1136/annrheumdis-2018-213225. Epub 2018 Apr 6. PMID: 29625968.
214. Yazici H, Ugurlu S, Seyahi E. Behçet syndrome: is it one condition? Clin Rev Allergy Immunol. 2012;43(3):275–80.https://doi.org/10.1007/s12016--012-8319-x. PMID: 22674015.
215. Sachdev N, Kapali N, Singh R, Gupta V, Gupta A. Spectrum of Behçet's disease in the Indian population. Int Ophthalmol. 2009;29(6):495–501. https://doi.org/10.1007/s10792-008-9273-8. Epub 2008 Oct 21. PMID: 18936879.
216. Tugal-Tutkun I, Onal S, Altan-Yaycioglu R, Huseyin Altunbas H, Urgancioglu M. Uveitis in Behçet disease: an analysis of 880 patients. Am J Ophthalmol. 2004;138(3):373–80. https://doi.org/10.1016/j.ajo.2004.03.022. PMID: 15364218.
217. Tugal-Tutkun I. Imaging in the diagnosis and management of Behçet disease. Int Ophthalmol Clin. 2012;52(4):183–90. https://doi.org/10.1097/IIO.0b013e318265d56a. PMID: 22954940.
218. Kim BH, Park UC, Park SW, Yu HG. Ultra-Widefield fluorescein angiography to monitor therapeutic response to adalimumab in Behcet's uveitis. Ocul Immunol Inflamm. 2022;30:1347–53. https://doi.org/10.1080/09273948.2021.1872652. Epub ahead of print. PMID: 33793368.
219. Yalçındağ FN, Temel E, Şekkeli MZ, Kar İ. Macular structural changes and factors affecting final visual acuity in patients with Behçet uveitis. Graefes Arch Clin Exp Ophthalmol. 2021;259(3):715–21. https://doi.org/10.1007/s00417-020-04958-4. Epub 2020 Oct 10. PMID: 33037921.
220. Ji KB, Hu Z, Zhang QL, Mei HF, Xing YQ. Retinal microvasculature features in patients with Behcet's disease: a systematic review and meta-analysis. Sci Rep. 2022;12(1):752. https://doi.org/10.1038/s41598-021-04730-6. PMID: 35031636; PMCID: PMC8760269.
221. International Study Group for Behçet's Disease. Criteria for diagnosis of Behçet's disease. Lancet. 1990;335(8697):1078–80. PMID: 1970380.
222. Tugal-Tutkun I. Uveitis in Behçet disease—an update. Curr Opin Rheumatol. 2023;35:17. https://doi.org/10.1097/BOR.0000000000000911. Epub ahead of print. PMID: 36255985.
223. Akiyama M, Kaneko Y, Takeuchi T. Effectiveness of tocilizumab in Behcet's disease: a system-

atic literature review. Semin Arthritis Rheum. 2020;50(4):797–804. https://doi.org/10.1016/j.semarthrit.2020.05.017. Epub 2020 Jun 5. PMID: 32544751.
224. Zou J, Lin CH, Wang Y, Shen Y, Guan JL. Correspondence on 'A pilot study of tofacitinib for refractory Behçet's syndrome'. Ann Rheum Dis. 2023;82:e100. https://doi.org/10.1136/annrheumdis-2020-219810. Epub ahead of print. PMID: 33495153.
225. Kitaichi N, Miyazaki A, Iwata D, Ohno S, Stanford MR, Chams H. Ocular features of Behcet's disease: an international collaborative study. Br J Ophthalmol. 2007;91(12):1579–82. https://doi.org/10.1136/bjo.2007.123554. PMID: 18024808; PMCID: PMC2095523.
226. Read RW, Holland GN, Rao NA, Tabbara KF, Ohno S, Arellanes-Garcia L, Pivetti-Pezzi P, Tessler HH, Usui M. Revised diagnostic criteria for Vogt-Koyanagi-Harada disease: report of an international committee on nomenclature. Am J Ophthalmol. 2001;131(5):647–52.https://doi.org/10.1016/s0002--9394(01)00925-4. PMID: 11336942.
227. Yamaki K, Gocho K, Hayakawa K, Kondo I, Sakuragi S. Tyrosinase family proteins are antigens specific to Vogt-Koyanagi-Harada disease. J Immunol. 2000;165(12):7323–9. https://doi.org/10.4049/jimmunol.165.12.7323. PMID: 11120868.
228. Yamaki K, Kondo I, Nakamura H, Miyano M, Konno S, Sakuragi S. Ocular and extraocular inflammation induced by immunization of tyrosinase related protein 1 and 2 in Lewis rats. Exp Eye Res. 2000;71(4):361–9. https://doi.org/10.1006/exer.2000.0893. PMID: 10995557.
229. Okada T, Sakamoto T, Ishibashi T, Inomata H. Vitiligo in Vogt-Koyanagi-Harada disease: immunohistological analysis of inflammatory site. Graefes Arch Clin Exp Ophthalmol. 1996;234(6):359–63. https://doi.org/10.1007/BF00190711. PMID: 8738701.
230. O'Keefe GA, Rao NA. Vogt-Koyanagi-Harada disease. Surv Ophthalmol. 2017;62(1):1–25. https://doi.org/10.1016/j.survophthal.2016.05.002. Epub 2016 May 27. PMID: 27241814.
231. Rathinam SR, Namperumalsamy P, Nozik RA, Cunningham ET Jr. Vogt-Koyanagi-Harada syndrome after cutaneous injury. Ophthalmology. 1999;106(3):635–8. https://doi.org/10.1016/S0161--6420(99)90129-X. PMID: 10080227.
232. Lim JA, Tan WC, Nor NM. Hints from the skin beneath: Vitiligo in Vogt–Koyanagi–Harada disease. Dermatol Sin [serial online]. 2022 [cited 2022 Oct 31];40:78–84. https://www.dermsinica.org/text.asp?2022/40/2/78/347097.
233. Anthony E, Rajamani A, Baskaran P, Rajendran A. Vogt Koyanagi Harada disease following a recent COVID-19 infection. Indian J Ophthalmol. 2022;70(2):670–2. https://doi.org/10.4103/ijo.IJO_2550_21. PMID: 35086262; PMCID: PMC9023905.
234. Chen X, Wang B, Li X. Acute-onset Vogt-Koyanagi-Harada like uveitis following Covid-19 inactivated virus vaccination. Am J Ophthalmol Case Rep. 2022;26:101404. https://doi.org/10.1016/j.ajoc.2022.101404. Epub 2022 Feb 9. PMID: 35165663; PMCID: PMC8826601.
235. De Domingo B, López M, Lopez-Valladares M, Ortegon-Aguilar E, Sopeña-Perez-Argüelles B, Gonzalez F. Vogt-Koyanagi-Harada disease exacerbation associated with COVID-19 vaccine. Cells. 2022;11(6):1012. https://doi.org/10.3390/cells11061012. PMID: 35326462; PMCID: PMC8947156.
236. Gambichler T, Seifert C, Lehmann M, Lukas C, Scheel C, Susok L. Concurrent Vogt-Koyanagi-Harada disease and impressive response to immune checkpoint blockade in metastatic melanoma. Immunotherapy. 2020;12(7):439–44. https://doi.org/10.2217/imt-2019-0206. Epub 2020 Apr 19. PMID: 32308086.
237. Rao NA, Gupta A, Dustin L, Chee SP, Okada AA, Khairallah M, Bodaghi B, Lehoang P, Accorinti M, Mochizuki M, Prabriputaloong T, Read RW. Frequency of distinguishing clinical features in Vogt-Koyanagi-Harada disease. Ophthalmology. 2010;117(3):591–9, 599.e1. Epub 2009 Dec 24. PMID: 20036008; PMCID: PMC2830365. https://doi.org/10.1016/j.ophtha.2009.08.030.
238. Ohno S, Minakawa R, Matsuda H. Clinical studies of Vogt-Koyanagi-Harada's disease. Jpn J Ophthalmol. 1988;32(3):334–43. PMID: 3230720.
239. Herbort CP, Mantovani A, Bouchenaki N. Indocyanine green angiography in Vogt-Koyanagi-Harada disease: angiographic signs and utility in patient follow-up. Int Ophthalmol. 2007;27(2–3):173–82. https://doi.org/10.1007/s10792-007-9060-y. Epub 2007 Apr 25. PMID: 17457515.
240. Silpa-Archa S, Ittharat W, Chotcomwongse P, Preble JM, Foster CS. Analysis of three-dimensional choroidal volume with enhanced depth imaging findings in patients with recurrent Vogt-Koyanagi-Harada disease. Curr Eye Res. 2021;46(7):1010–7. https://doi.org/10.1080/02713683.2020.1849732. Epub 2020 Nov 20. PMID: 33215546.
241. Gupta V, Gupta A, Gupta P, Sharma A. Spectral-domain cirrus optical coherence tomography of choroidal striations seen in the acute stage of Vogt-Koyanagi-Harada disease. Am J Ophthalmol. 2009;147(1):148–153.e2. https://doi.org/10.1016/j.ajo.2008.07.028. Epub 2008 Oct 2. PMID: 18834577.
242. Kuo IC, Rechdouni A, Rao NA, Johnston RH, Margolis TP, Cunningham ET Jr. Subretinal fibrosis in patients with Vogt-Koyanagi-Harada disease. Ophthalmology. 2000;107(9):1721–8. https://doi.org/10.1016/s0161-6420(00)00244-x. PMID: 10964836.
243. Kilmartin DJ, Dick AD, Forrester JV. Prospective surveillance of sympathetic ophthalmia in the

UK and Republic of Ireland. Br J Ophthalmol. 2000;84(3):259–63. https://doi.org/10.1136/bjo.84.3.259. PMID: 10684834; PMCID: PMC1723405.
244. Allen JC. Sympathetic ophthalmia, a disappearing disease. JAMA. 1969;209(7):1090. PMID: 5819666.
245. Gass JD. Sympathetic ophthalmia following vitrectomy. Am J Ophthalmol. 1982;93(5):552–8. https://doi.org/10.1016/s0002-9394(14)77368-4. PMID: 7081353.
246. Chan CC, Roberge RG, Whitcup SM, Nussenblatt RB. 32 cases of sympathetic ophthalmia. A retrospective study at the National Eye Institute, Bethesda, MD, from 1982 to 1992. Arch Ophthalmol. 1995;113(5):597–600. https://doi.org/10.1001/archopht.1995.01100050065032. Erratum in: Arch Ophthalmol 1995 Dec;113(12):1507. PMID: 7748129.
247. Kumar K, Mathai A, Murthy SI, Jalali S, Sangwan V, Reddy Pappuru R, Pathangay A. Sympathetic ophthalmia in pediatric age group: clinical features and challenges in management in a tertiary center in southern India. Ocul Immunol Inflamm. 2014;22(5):367–72. https://doi.org/10.3109/09273948.2013.841958. Epub 2013 Oct 16. PMID: 24131076.
248. Anikina E, Wagner SK, Liyanage S, Sullivan P, Pavesio C, Okhravi N. The risk of sympathetic ophthalmia after vitreoretinal surgery. Ophthalmol Retina. 2022;6(5):347–60. https://doi.org/10.1016/j.oret.2022.01.012. Epub 2022 Jan 31. PMID: 35093583.
249. Rao NA, Robin J, Hartmann D, Sweeney JA, Marak GE Jr. The role of the penetrating wound in the development of sympathetic ophthalmia experimental observations. Arch Ophthalmol. 1983;101(1):102–4. https://doi.org/10.1001/archopht.1983.01040010104019. PMID: 6849641.
250. Chan CC, Hikita N, Dastgheib K, Whitcup SM, Gery I, Nussenblatt RB. Experimental melanin-protein-induced uveitis in the Lewis rat. Immunopathologic processes. Ophthalmology. 1994;101(7):1275–80. https://doi.org/10.1016/s0161-6420(94)31199-7. PMID: 7913541.
251. Chu XK, Chan CC. Sympathetic ophthalmia: to the twenty-first century and beyond. J Ophthalmic Inflamm Infect. 2013;3(1):49. https://doi.org/10.1186/1869-5760-3-49. PMID: 23724856; PMCID: PMC3679835.
252. Goto H, Rao NA. Sympathetic ophthalmia and Vogt-Koyanagi-Harada syndrome. Int Ophthalmol Clin. 1990;30(4):279–85. https://doi.org/10.1097/00004397-199030040-00014. PMID: 2228475.
253. Rao NA. Mechanisms of inflammatory response in sympathetic ophthalmia and VKH syndrome. Eye (Lond). 1997;11(Pt 2):213–6. https://doi.org/10.1038/eye.1997.54. PMID: 9349415.
254. Parikh JG, Saraswathy S, Rao NA. Photoreceptor oxidative damage in sympathetic ophthalmia. Am J Ophthalmol. 2008;146(6):866–75.e2. https://doi.org/10.1016/j.ajo.2008.03.026. Epub 2008 Jun 2. PMID: 18514610.
255. Kumaradas M, Rao NA. Chapter 81. Sympathetic ophthalmia. In: Levin LA, Albert DM, editors. Ocular disease. Edinburgh: W.B. Saunders; 2010. p. 635–41. https://doi.org/10.1016/B978-0-7020--2983-7.00081-4. https://www.sciencedirect.com/science/article/pii/B9780702029837000814.
256. Gupta V, Gupta A, Dogra MR. Posterior sympathetic ophthalmia: a single centre long-term study of 40 patients from North India. Eye (Lond). 2008;22(12):1459–64. https://doi.org/10.1038/sj.eye.6702927. Epub 2007 Jul 6. PMID: 17618240.
257. Freedman J. A clinical approach to the aetiology of uveitis in Bantu adults. Br J Ophthalmol. 1976;60(1):64–9. https://doi.org/10.1136/bjo.60.1.64. PMID: 1268163; PMCID: PMC1017469.
258. Rao NA, Marak GE. Sympathetic ophthalmia simulating vogt-Koyanagi-Harada's disease: a clinicopathologic study of four cases. Jpn J Ophthalmol. 1983;27(3):506–11. PMID: 6656012.
259. Jordan DR, Dutton J. The ruptured globe, sympathetic ophthalmia, and the 14-day rule. Ophthalmic Plast Reconstr Surg. 2022;38(4):315–24. https://doi.org/10.1097/IOP.0000000000002068. Epub 2022 Sep 28. PMID: 34593714.
260. Williams AM, Shepler AM, Chu CT, Nischal KK. Sympathetic ophthalmia presenting 5 days after penetrating injury. Am J Ophthalmol Case Rep. 2020;19:100816. https://doi.org/10.1016/j.ajoc.2020.100816. PMID: 32695926; PMCID: PMC7363657.
261. du Toit N, Motala MI, Richards J, Murray AD, Maitra S. The risk of sympathetic ophthalmia following evisceration for penetrating eye injuries at Groote Schuur hospital. Br J Ophthalmol. 2008;92(1):61–3. https://doi.org/10.1136/bjo.2007.120600. Epub 2007 Jun 25. PMID: 17591674.
262. Marsiglia M, Gallego-Pinazo R, Cunha de Souza E, Munk MR, Yu S, Mrejen S, Cunningham ET Jr, Lujan BJ, Goldberg NR, Albini TA, Gaudric A, Francais C, Rosen RB, Freund KB, Jampol LM, Yannuzzi LA. Expanded clinical spectrum of multiple evanescent white dot syndrome with multimodal imaging. Retina. 2016;36(1):64–74. https://doi.org/10.1097/IAE.0000000000000685. PMID: 26166804.
263. Testi I, Vermeirsch S, Pavesio C. Acute posterior multifocal placoid pigment epitheliopathy (APMPPE). J Ophthalmic Inflamm Infect. 2021;11(1):31. https://doi.org/10.1186/s12348-021-00263-1. PMID: 34524577; PMCID: PMC8443720.
264. Ahnood D, Madhusudhan S, Tsaloumas MD, Waheed NK, Keane PA, Denniston AK. Punctate inner choroidopathy: a review. Surv Ophthalmol. 2017;62(2):113–26. https://doi.org/10.1016/j.survophthal.2016.10.003. Epub 2016 Oct 15. PMID: 27751823.

265. Mrejen S, Khan S, Gallego-Pinazo R, Jampol LM, Yannuzzi LA. Acute zonal occult outer retinopathy: a classification based on multimodal imaging. JAMA Ophthalmol. 2014;132(9):1089–98. https://doi.org/10.1001/jamaophthalmol.2014.1683. PMID: 24945598.
266. Minos E, Barry RJ, Southworth S, Folkard A, Murray PI, Duker JS, Keane PA, Denniston AK. Birdshot chorioretinopathy: current knowledge and new concepts in pathophysiology, diagnosis, monitoring and treatment. Orphanet J Rare Dis. 2016;11(1):61. https://doi.org/10.1186/s13023-016-0429-8. PMID: 27175923; PMCID: PMC4866419.
267. Fogel-Levin M, Sadda SR, Rosenfeld PJ, Waheed N, Querques G, Freund BK, Sarraf D. Advanced retinal imaging and applications for clinical practice: a consensus review. Surv Ophthalmol. 2022;67(5):1373–90. https://doi.org/10.1016/j.survophthal.2022.02.004. Epub 2022 Feb 17. PMID: 35183611.
268. Yzer S, Freund KB, Engelbert M. Imaging in the diagnosis and management of acute macular neuroretinopathy. Int Ophthalmol Clin. 2012;52(4):269–73. https://doi.org/10.1097/IIO.0b013e31826704a4. PMID: 22954950.
269. Fawzi AA, Pappuru RR, Sarraf D, Le PP, McCannel CA, Sobrin L, Goldstein DA, Honowitz S, Walsh AC, Sadda SR, Jampol LM, Eliott D. Acute macular neuroretinopathy: long-term insights revealed by multimodal imaging. Retina. 2012;32(8):1500–13. https://doi.org/10.1097/IAE.0b013e318263d0c3. PMID: 22846801.
270. Klufas MA, Phasukkijwatana N, Iafe NA, Prasad PS, Agarwal A, Gupta V, Ansari W, Pichi F, Srivastava S, Freund KB, Sadda SR, Sarraf D. Optical coherence tomography angiography reveals choriocapillaris flow reduction in placoid chorioretinitis. Ophthalmol Retina. 2017;1(1):77–91. https://doi.org/10.1016/j.oret.2016.08.008. Epub 2016 Oct 17. PMID: 31047399.
271. Steiner S, Goldstein DA. Imaging in the diagnosis and management of APMPPE. Int Ophthalmol Clin. 2012;52(4):211–9. https://doi.org/10.1097/IIO.0b013e318265d45a. PMID: 22954943.
272. Wolf MD, Folk JC, Panknen CA, Goeken NE. HLA-B7 and HLA-DR2 antigens and acute posterior multifocal placoid pigment epitheliopathy. Arch Ophthalmol. 1990;108(5):698–700. https://doi.org/10.1001/archopht.1990.01070070084040. PMID: 2334328.
273. Nemiroff J, Sarraf D, Davila JP, Rodger D. Optical coherence tomography angiography of acute macular neuroretinopathy reveals deep capillary ischemia. Retin Cases Brief Rep. 2018;12 Suppl 1:S12–5. https://doi.org/10.1097/ICB.0000000000000706. PMID: 29561336.
274. Ramtohul P, Comet A, Denis DL. Optical coherence tomography angiography recovery pattern of acute macular neuroretinopathy. JAMA Ophthalmol. 2020;138(2):221–3. https://doi.org/10.1001/jamaophthalmol.2019.5066. PMID: 31855236.
275. Ong SS, Ahmed I, Scott AW. Association of acute macular neuroretinopathy or paracentral acute middle maculopathy with sickle cell disease. Ophthalmol Retina. 2021;5(11):1146–55. https://doi.org/10.1016/j.oret.2021.01.003. Epub 2021 Jan 19. PMID: 33476854.

11 Macular Oedema

11.1 Anatomical Considerations

The retina is a highly organized, multi-layered innermost lining of the eyeball. It converts photons into electrical signals to transmit to the visual cortex located in the occipital lobes of the brain for ultimately transforming reflected light from the objects around into their 3D visual perception. Maintaining the light path transparency is critical to achieving sharp and high-resolution images. Several anatomical and physiological factors must work in perfect harmony to project a sharp image of the object on the photoreceptors. These factors include a powerful fixed concavo-convex lens-transparent cornea, variability of the pupillary aperture to control the quantum of light entering the eye, the transparent double convex crystalline lens with its capacity to change power, a clear vitreous gel, and the size of the eyeball. The retina consists of two layers, the transparent neurosensory retina anteriorly and a dark retinal pigment epithelial (RPE) layer posteriorly, separated by a potential space. The neurosensory retina is a multi-layered structure consisting of several highly organized cells of neural and glial origin and their processes. The light has to pass through from front to back, the internal limiting membrane (footplates of the macroglia, the Muller cells), the retinal nerve fibre layer (RNFL, the axons of the ganglion cells), ganglion cells, the inner plexiform layer (the synaptic junction of the dendrites of the ganglion cells, amacrine cells and axons of the bipolar cells), the bipolar cell layer (it also has the cell bodies of the Muller cells, amacrine, and horizontal cells), the outer plexiform layer (the synaptic junctions of the dendrites of the bipolar cells, and the axons of the photoreceptor rods and cones; with horizontal cell processes controlling transmission), the external limiting membrane (Muller cell apical processes joining each other and the inner segments of the photoreceptors), the outer nuclear layer (ONL), and the cell bodies of the rods and cones. The neurosensory retina is further divided into an inner retina up to the outer border of the inner nuclear layer and the outer retina, from the outer plexiform layer (OPL) to the photoreceptor layer. The neural cells and fibres are tightly packed in all the layers and are oriented vertically in the outer retina but become near parallel in the anterior retina. The blood supply is also layered. The anterior neurosensory retina gets its blood supply from the central retinal vessels that run their course in the RNFL and supply the inner retina through four capillary plexuses. The superficial plexus (SCP) in the ganglion cells layer, the intermediate plexus (ICP) at the inner border of the inner nuclear layer (INL), and the deep plexus (DCP) at the outer border of the INL and the radial capillaries from the optic disc vessels for peripapillary RNFL provide the blood supply. If the cilioretinal artery is present, it supplies nutrients and oxygen to all the layers of the macula. The retinal capillaries do not cross beyond the

A. Gupta et al., *Ophthalmic Signs in Practice of Medicine*,
https://doi.org/10.1007/978-981-99-7923-3_11

inner one-third of the OPL, also known as the middle limiting membrane.

The OPL in the fovea is known as the Henle fibre layer. The cones and the Muller cell fibres have a radial orientation in this zone. The retinal vessels have tight endothelial junctions (inner blood-retinal barrier) and do not allow macromolecules, cellular elements, and fluid movement into the extravascular space. The central 400–500 μm of the anterior neurosensory retina is called the foveal avascular zone and is a vessel-free zone. The outer retina is avascular and receives nutrition and oxygen requirement from the choroid. The OPL is avascular and falls in the watershed zone of the two vascular supply systems. The dark RPE at the back of the neurosensory retina has tight junctions and maintains the outer blood-retinal barrier. The vertebrate outer limiting membrane (OLM) also has adherent and tight junction proteins. It provides a partial semi-permeable barrier function that allows diffusion of only small protein molecules (<35 radius Angstrom units) that are present in the extracellular space around the photoreceptors [1].

11.2 Homeostasis in the Retinal Microenvironment

Microenvironmental homeostasis keeps the retina in a balanced hydrous state. The Muller cells processes extend throughout the thickness of the neurosensory retina and maintain very intimate contact with the capillary endothelial cells, retinal ganglion cells, bipolar cells, horizontal cells, the amacrine cells, and the photoreceptors to form a neuro-glia-vascular unit or commonly called as a neurovascular unit [2]. The primary function of this unit is to maintain metabolic homeostasis in the retina by controlling glucose metabolism. The Muller cells remove the toxic glutamate, prevent oxidative damage, and recycle neurotrophic factors critical for cell survival [3]. The inactivated resident microglia are generally present in the IPL and the OPL. However, once activated, they assume the functions of macrophages and move around freely throughout the thickness of the retina. Normal homeostasis may get disturbed by several metabolic, inflammatory, post-surgical, vascular occlusions, and pharmacological or degenerative conditions that lead to a collection of the intraretinal and the subretinal fluid. The collection of fluid in the extracellular space and some swelling of the cellular elements in the neurosensory retina is called macular oedema (ME). It causes significant visual disturbances [2]. The OPL in the watershed zone is the most favoured site for collecting fluid, the following common site being the INL.

11.3 Examination of Retina and Documentation of Macular Oedema

The retina is amenable to examination and documentation by various techniques, from ophthalmoscopic examination and ultra-wide fundus photography to fundus fluorescein angiography, optical coherence tomography (OCT), and OCT angiography. These techniques are now routinely used to detect and monitor ME.

11.3.1 Clinical Examination of the Macula

Even now, the standard clinical technique to detect macular thickening in ophthalmology clinics is a biomicroscopy stereoscopic fundus examination either using a −64D Goldmann contact lens or a macula lens that provides a high resolution, virtual and erect, 3-D view of the macula, albeit with a limited field of view. Fundus examination on the slit lamp requires a minimal angle between the microscope and the illuminating arm. The illuminating and the reflected beam path overlap can be removed using the short mirror and tilting the illuminating arm in the Haag Streit 900 slit lamp. Unlike the long mirror, the short deviating mirror does not block the observation path and provides a stereoscopic view. In the Zeiss slit lamps, the path of the illuminating beam is changed by rotating down the illuminating column. A minus-contact lens neutralizes the cornea's power and provides the highest-resolution image of the macula. The magnification can be changed using the magnification changer of the slit lamp (Galilean systems).

A non-contact movable preset −58.6D planoconcave Hruby lens can be attached to the slit lamp to provide a virtual erect image of the vitreous and the macula. Now, the use of this lens has become very rare in practice. Preset or hand-held high plus lenses were first introduced by El-Bayadi [4], Schmidt [5], and at present, a wide variety of these lenses is available as +60D, +78D, or +90D lenses. High + lenses currently remain the most prevalent clinical technique for the stereoscopic fundus examination. It is convenient but provides a lower resolution than a contact lens. The high plus objective lens provides a real, inverted, and laterally reversed image of the macula in front of this lens and needs the experience to master the technique. A +90D lens provides a field of view of ~90°, a working distance of 7 mm from the cornea, and a magnification factor of 0.76×. Because of the lens's small diameter and metallic ring, it is convenient to hold it for a long time and can be used even in an undilated pupil. A wider area of the retina can be screened by asking the patient to move his eye in different directions. The +78D lens is bigger and can have a field of view of 81/97° and a magnification factor of 0.93× at 8 mm from the cornea. However, it requires a dilated pupil and may be tiring if required to hold it for a long time.

Apart from being highly subjective, the major limitation of assessing macular thickness on clinical examination is the inability to be sure of the presence of macular oedema till the retina is thickened at least 1.5 times its average thickness. However, there are indirect clinical clues to macular oedema, such as loss of the foveal reflex, loss of transparency of the retina in the area of thickening, presence of hard exudates, retinal haemorrhages, and a cluster of MAS. Cystic macular oedema (CME) may appear as tiny cystic lesions arranged around a larger foveal cyst in a petaloid pattern. Physicians and many comprehensive ophthalmologists use a monocular direct ophthalmoscope. It is a handy tool for bedside fundus examination of critically ill patients. Alternatively, trained ophthalmologists can use a portable binocular indirect ophthalmoscope. The direct ophthalmoscope offers a magnification of 15× but only a 5° field of view. In the hands of an experienced physician, it can detect the retinal MAS and tiny dot haemorrhages besides detecting fine new vessels on the optic disc. If any abnormality is detected on direct ophthalmoscopy, it calls for a referral to a retina specialist for a detailed retinal examination.

11.3.2 Documentation of Macular Oedema-Fundus Photography

In the past, 30° standard 7-field, colour film-based fundus photography was done to document retinal diseases and objectively document the effect of the therapeutic interventions on retinal pathology. The seven fields included the one centred on the optic disc, macula, and temporal to the macula. Four images were taken tangentially to lines forming a cross passing at the upper and lower pole of the optic disc. Non-simultaneous stereoscopic pictures were taken of all the fields. The colour transparencies were developed, mounted, and kept in plastic slide holders and sent to the fundus photograph reading centres to be evaluated by trained readers [6]. Many trials used stereoscopic fundus imaging, including the diabetic retinopathy study, ETDRS, Diabetes Control and Complications Trial (DCCT), and Macular Photocoagulation Study. In recent years, there have been revolutionary changes in the multiple ways the retina is imaged, termed multimedia imaging. These include using blue, green, or red reflectance images of the retina. Using a near-infrared light source, autofluorescence imaging can be obtained. It exploits the fluorescent properties of various natural pigments and the degraded lipofuscin that results from processing the retinal photoreceptor outer segments. Incorporating various laser wavelengths in the scanning laser ophthalmoscope in the digital cameras can obtain blue reflectance (for superficial structures like epiretinal membranes), green reflectance (for blood vessels, RNFL, and exudates), and near-infrared reflectance (for deeper retina and choroidal structures) images to highlight retinal structures located in different layers of the retina. Besides, these systems now obtain a wide angle (retinal field of view including vortex vein ampulla) or ultra-wide (includes retina field of view anterior to the entry of vertex veins) image of the entire retina (~200°) in a single exposure.

Availability and rapid developments in optical coherence tomography (OCT) in the last 20 years have revolutionized how macular pathology is documented. A systematic review of studies comparing the stereoscopic examination of the fundus with OCT to detect diabetic macular oedema (DME) found that the positive likelihood ratio of 6.5 and the negative likelihood ratio of 0.24 strongly favoured the use of OCT to diagnose DME [7]. From the time domain to the spectral domain, now, the swept-source technology has supplanted stereo retinal photography with OCT for recording the thickness of the macula and the ultrastructural changes in the macula and rest of the retina in an objective and reproducible manner.

11.3.3 Fundus Fluorescein Angiography

Photographic documentation of the retinal vasculature by injecting a bolus of fluorescein dye into the antecubital vein called the fundus fluorescein angiography (FFA) was the first disruptive technological breakthrough since the discovery of the direct ophthalmoscope more than 100 years before that. The technique gave a significant fillip to the in vivo study of the retinal vascular involvement in many systemic and ophthalmological disorders [8, 9]. The FFA involves injecting a 3 mL bolus of a water-soluble fluorescent dye (fluorescein sodium 20%) intravenously and taking fundus photographs through a special camera equipped with matched narrow-band excitation and barrier filters. As the dye flows in the retinal vessels, it is excited by blue light, which in turn emits light at a higher wavelength (the green spectrum) which was earlier captured on a photographic B&W film and at present captured on a digital camera. Availability of the FFA made it possible to visualize in vivo the retinal microaneurysms, retinal capillaries, and the areas of retinal ischaemia, which till then had been seen and documented only on trypsin digestion studies of the retina. Most importantly, FFA can demonstrate any breakdown in the tight blood-retinal barrier (BRB) and fluid leakage into the extravascular space. To date, the FFA remains the most sensitive technique to demonstrate the competence of the BRB. Moreover, the fluorescein dye stains the site of the fluid leakage and the leaked fluid, whether in the interstitial retinal tissue or its pooling in the potential spaces. The FFA is used even today to diagnose and document cystoid macular oedema and its response to therapy. The limitations of the degree of retinal field captured in film-based systems have been overcome with the development of digital ultra-wide field FFA, which can show vascular changes in the extreme peripheral retina. However, the FFA is an invasive technique. Though rare, it has its share of minor and major adverse events, including nausea, vomiting, allergic hives, or hypotension in 5–9% of the patients [10]. Even fatal anaphylactic reactions have been recorded in 0.04% of the patients undergoing the FFA [11]. For nearly 40 years, the FFA remained the most favoured technique till it got supplanted with non-invasive optical coherence tomography.

11.3.4 Optical Coherence Tomography

Optical coherence tomography (OCT) was the second most disruptive technology after the FFA that has revolutionized the practice of ophthalmology. The introduction of OCT was akin to the profound changes in the practice of medicine brought about by the development of imaging technologies like ultrasonography, computerized tomography (CT scan), and magnetic resonance imaging (MRI). Before the introduction of OCT, the retina was seen as a two-dimensional structure. Now, it has become possible to look into the microstructure of the retina. Huang et al. [12]

developed OCT technology to examine the cross-sectional details of biological tissues non-invasively. The basic principle of the use of OCT was similar to the use of ultrasonography. Like the sound waves, the reflected light signals are detected as a low-coherence light beam passes through the retina, which either gets reflected or transmitted. The initial time-domain technology used a time-of-flight delay between the reflected light from a standard mirror and the time the light took to reflect from the various structural interfaces in the retina. It gave an axial resolution of ~10μ. Rapid technological developments have taken place in this field. The spectral domain technology replaced the time-domain technology. It used a broad-band near-infrared superluminescent diode as a light source and a spectrometer to detect the Fourier transformation of the reflected light from the tissue interfaces. The axial resolution improved to 1–3μ. At the same time, there was a tremendous change in the acquisition time to obtain information from each point of the retinal structures enabling a 3D construct of the retina. Apart from the cross-sectional image of the various microstructures, a layer-by-retinal layer information is obtained as en face imaging. On the other hand, the swept-source OCT (SS-OCT) uses a narrow band of a tunable laser source. The higher acquisition speed with SS-OCT to 100,000 scans/second compared to 50,000 scans/s with the SD-OCT has allowed a 12 × 12 mm wider scan line compared to a 6 × 6 mm line scan with SD-OCT. Using a higher wavelength of 1050 nm than the SD-OCT (840 nm), SS-OCT gives higher resolution images (1μ) of the deeper retinal structures and choroid and can delineate even the choroido-scleral interface [13, 14].

11.3.5 Measuring the Central Subfield Thickness (CST) with OCT

Presently, the OCT has wholly replaced stereographic photography, which, at best, gave a rough estimate of the macular thickness. Because of the relatively consistent and reproducible measurements, it has become standard practice to use OCT to study thickness and microstructure in all retinal studies. The ETDRS grid is used to define the various sectors of the macula. The area within the innermost central 1-mm-diameter circle is the central subfield (CSF), the inner subfield is the area between the innermost circle, and a circle of 3-mm-diameter centred on the fovea and the outer subfield is the area between the 3-mm circle and the outer circle of 6-mm diameter. Each of these circles is further subdivided into sectors. The measurements of macular thickness with OCT come with an important caveat that different OCT machines come with different resolutions and different algorithms to identify reflective interfaces; hence, the results obtained from one machine cannot be transposed to the other machine. Likewise, racial, gender, and age factors may vary the CST measurements [15]. The TD-OCT (Stratus; Carl Zeiss Meditec, Inc.) machine used an algorithm that measured the distance between the ILM and the IS/OS junction. This junction is now named the ellipsoid zone. This zone of the outer segments has the maximum density of mitochondria. This OCT gave a CST of 176.4μ in a North China population [16]. The SD-OCT machine (Cirrus; Carl Zeiss Meditec, Inc., Dublin, CA) measures the retinal thickness between the ILM and the mean reflectance of the outer segment/RPE junction. It thus gives a higher value of CST by ~60μ than the Stratus [17].

In a follow-up of the Handan population-based study, using an SD-OCT machine (RTVue 100–2, Optovue, Fremont, California; V.4.0) the mean CSF thickness was 237μ [18]. These results were consistent with the Japanese population study [17] cited above, which also used a Cirrus machine. The mean CST thickness has varied from 240 to 265 μm using the Cirrus SD-OCT machine in various normal populations. Using a Spectralis OCT (Heidelberg Engineering, Heidelberg, Germany), the mean CST has varied from 260 μm in a Chinese population [19] to 280 μm in an all-White Italian population [20].

11.4 Causes of Macular Oedema

Macular oedema is broadly divided into two types, those associated with fluid leakage from the retinal capillaries (vasogenic) and those that do not show any leakage from the retinal capillaries (non-vasogenic). The leakage of fluid is demonstrated on the FFA. The leaked fluid accumulates in the extravascular space. Furthermore, the ME results from intracellular swelling for those who do not show fluid leakage from the retinal vessels.

A. Associated with leakage from retinal vessels
   1. Diabetic retinopathy
   2. Branch or central retinal vein occlusion
   3. Uveitis
   4. Post-intraocular surgery
   5. Drug-induced
   6. Neovascular age-related macular degeneration
   7. Laser photocoagulation and cryopexy
   8. Vitreoretinal traction, epiretinal membrane, impending macular hole
   9. Trauma
   10. Choroidal melanoma, von Hippel-Lindau's disease, Coats' disease
B. Without leakage from retinal vessels [21, 22]
   1. Retinitis pigmentosa
   2. Bestrophinopathies
   3. X-linked retinoschisis
   4. Enhanced S-cone dystrophy
   5. Choroideremia
   6. Gyrate atrophy
   7. Biettí crystalline dystrophy
   8. Drug-induced ME

11.4.1 Diabetic Macular Oedema

Diabetic macular oedema (DME) is the leading cause of moderate visual loss in patients with diabetes. According to the International Diabetes Federation, in 2021, 537 million people worldwide were living with diabetes, estimated to go up to 783 million by 2045. Moreover, 541 million people were estimated to have impaired glucose tests in 2021 [23]. A pooled analysis of 35 studies (22,896 individuals with DM) from across the world showed a prevalence of any diabetic retinopathy (DR) in 34.6% and DME in 6.8% [24].

11.4.1.1 Development of Diabetic Macular Oedema-Breakdown in Retinal Homeostasis

As discussed above, the normal retina maintains a stable hydrous state of the retina and transparency, allowing the light to reach the photoreceptors unhindered. However, a persistent hyperglycaemic state in diabetes mellitus (DM) over several years brings about systemic and local changes in the metabolic, biochemical, haemorheological, immunological, and inflammatory pathways that have a profound impact on the normal haemostasis and subject the retinal microstructure to oxidative stress and create a state of relative hypoxia leading to the development of diabetic retinopathy.

11.4.1.2 Thickening of Basement Membrane in Diabetes Mellitus

One of the earliest pathological changes of DM is the thickening of the basement membrane (BM) surrounding the endothelial cells. The thickening of BM is seen in the capillaries across the organs but is most pronounced in the retinal capillaries. The BM plays a significant role in maintaining homeostasis, provides an additional blood-retinal permeability barrier, controls pericyte contraction, promotes cell-to-cell communication, plays a role in apoptosis, and is a repository of growth factors that promote new vessel growth [25]. The non-enzymatic glycation of proteins in long-term hyperglycaemia results in the deposition of the extracellular matrix (ECM) proteins and the advanced glycation end products (AGE) in the BM of the capillaries and causes thickening of the BM. These proteins are found more abundant in the area of the retinal microaneurysms. Two components of the complement family, C4 and C9, are also exclusively detected in the diabetic BM, suggesting a role for complement-mediated chronic inflammation in diabetic retinopathy.

11.4.1.3 Consequences of the Basement Membrane Thickening

One of the consequences of the thickened BM is the loss of pericytes due to poor cell-matrix adhesions. It is one of the earliest pathological lesions in diabetic retinopathy [26, 27].

A thickened BM also disrupts the cell-to-cell communication between the Muller cells, the pericytes, and the endothelial cells, leading to a loss of the autoregulatory control by this neurovascular unit resulting in a state of hypoxia which also leads to activation of the microglia, and Muller cells throughout the retina [28]. Once activated, the microglia assume phagocytic activity and release pro-inflammatory cytokines. The hypoxic milieu in the retina in diabetic retinopathy leads to overexpression of hypoxia-inducible factor 1-α (HIF-1α) in the endothelial and Muller cells. HIF-1α is a regulator of vascular endothelial growth factor (VEGF). Hypoxic Muller cells also produce VEGF, which promotes endothelial cell proliferation and breakdown of the tight endothelial junctions [29].

11.4.1.4 Loss of Pericytes and Endothelial Cells and Microaneurysm Formation

Pericytes are intimately connected with endothelial cells and, by their contractile properties, play a significant role in the control of microcirculation [30]. Pericytes are buried in the basement of the endothelial cells and cover more than 85% of the retinal endothelial cells [31]. Pericytes play a significant role in checking endothelial cell proliferation. Besides, the pericytes regulate the expression of tight junction proteins that maintain the inner blood-retinal barrier. Pores (gap junctions) in the extracellular matrix (ECM) of the basement membrane (BM) allow for the cell-to-cell crosstalk between the pericytes and the endothelial cells [28]. A thickened BM results in the loss of pericyte matrix adhesion, facilitating the loss of pericytes.

Unlike endothelial cells, pericytes do not have the potential to regenerate. The vascular endothelial cells and pericytes share similar insulin receptors. One of the significant characteristics of diabetic microvascular disease is insulin resistance by the endothelial cells and impaired endothelial repair by the endothelial progenitor cells [32]. Persistent hyperglycaemia leads to the accumulation of AGE products first in the BM and then intracellularly in the pericytes and the endothelial cells. The AGE activates the PKC pathway and induces the enzyme inducible nitric oxide synthase (iNOS), leading to the overproduction of the highly cytotoxic nitric oxide (NO) and release of the reactive oxygen species that ultimately cause loss of both pericytes and endothelial cells [33]. Additional factors include the expression of inflammatory cytokines, released by the activated microglia, on the endothelial cells, leading to the adhesion of leukocytes and leukostasis in the capillaries. Thus, capillaries may become either acellular hollow tubes from loss of pericytes and endothelial cells or get occluded by leukostasis. Microaneurysms (MAs) are usually formed around the area of acellular capillaries by a fusiform or saccular dilatation of the capillaries, which may be cellular or acellular. The endothelial cells lining the MAs lack junctional proteins and leak fluid and macromolecules like lipoproteins.

11.4.1.5 Focal Versus Diffuse Diabetic Macular Oedema and Clinically Significant Macular Oedema

Diabetic macular oedema (DME) is seen in 5% of patients within 5 years of the diagnosis of type 2 DM and up to 15% by 15 years of the diagnosis [34]. The hallmark of non-proliferative diabetic retinopathy is the formation of retinal microaneurysms. In diabetes, the retinal capillaries are not affected uniformly across the retina but do so in patches. Starling's law governs the movement of fluids across capillaries based on the hydrostatic and the oncotic pressure in the intra- and extravascular spaces. The fluid and macromolecules in the diabetic retina leak into the extravascular space from the MAs and the affected capillary segments. While the extravasated fluid returns to the intravascular space at the venous end of the unaffected capillaries, the macromolecules—the

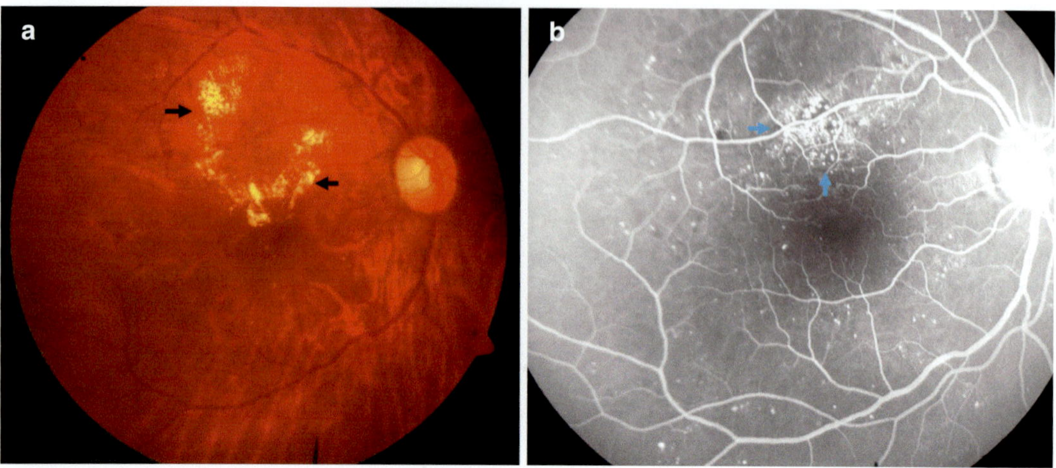

Fig. 11.1 Circinate ring of hard exudates (black arrows) with retinal thickening (**a**). Fluorescein angiography confirms focal (blue arrows) diabetic macular oedema (**b**)

lipoproteins, once leaked into the extravascular space—cannot return to vessels again. These are carted away by the usual phagocytic mechanisms. Since the leakage and absorption are a continuous process, an equilibrium is reached soon, and the lipoproteins get deposited around the leakage site in a circinate fashion, which may be incomplete or complete. The retina is thickened in the centre of the circinate ring and is labelled focal oedema (Fig. 11.1).

On the other hand, if several segments of the retinal capillaries lose their tight endothelial junctions, there is widespread leakage of fluid, called diffuse macular oedema (Fig. 11.2). There has never been a precise and reproducible definition of focal and diffuse macular oedema. The researchers have used clinical examination parameters such as the circinate rings, the macular thickness on stereoscopic examination, the pattern and extent of leakage on FFA, or a combination of these [35]. Moreover, a variable component of focal and diffuse leakage often contributes to macular oedema. Several systemic associations of DM, such as hypertension and nephropathy, favour excessive fluid extravasation into the extravascular space. Drugs like pioglitazone and rosiglitazone, currently banned, were highly effective in controlling type 2 DM but led to excessive fluid retention in the body when given in combination with insulin, especially in patients with nephropathy and worsened the DME, among other adverse effects [36, 37]. Irrespective of the renal status measured by the urinary albumin creatinine ratio and the estimated glomerular filtration rates, patients with DM tend to have higher extracellular water to total body water ratio that may contribute to the DME [38].

The early treatment of diabetic retinopathy study (ETDRS) defined clinically significant macular oedema (CSME) nearly 40 years ago as (1) thickening of the macula at or within 500μ of the centre or (2) hard exudates at or within 500 if associated with retinal thickening or (3) a zone or zones of macular thickening 1DD or larger if within 1 DD of the foveal centre. This definition of DME was based on stereoscopic fundus pictures [39]. The definition of DME was based on subjective evaluation of the stereoscopic fundus photographs by the trained graders and was not reproducible.

11.4.1.6 The New Classification of Diabetic Macular Oedema

Diabetic retinopathy clinical research network participants discovered during several multicentric controlled trials conducted by it that the thickness of the central subfield of the macula impacted the visual outcome of therapeutic interventions. Hence, the group proposed that the

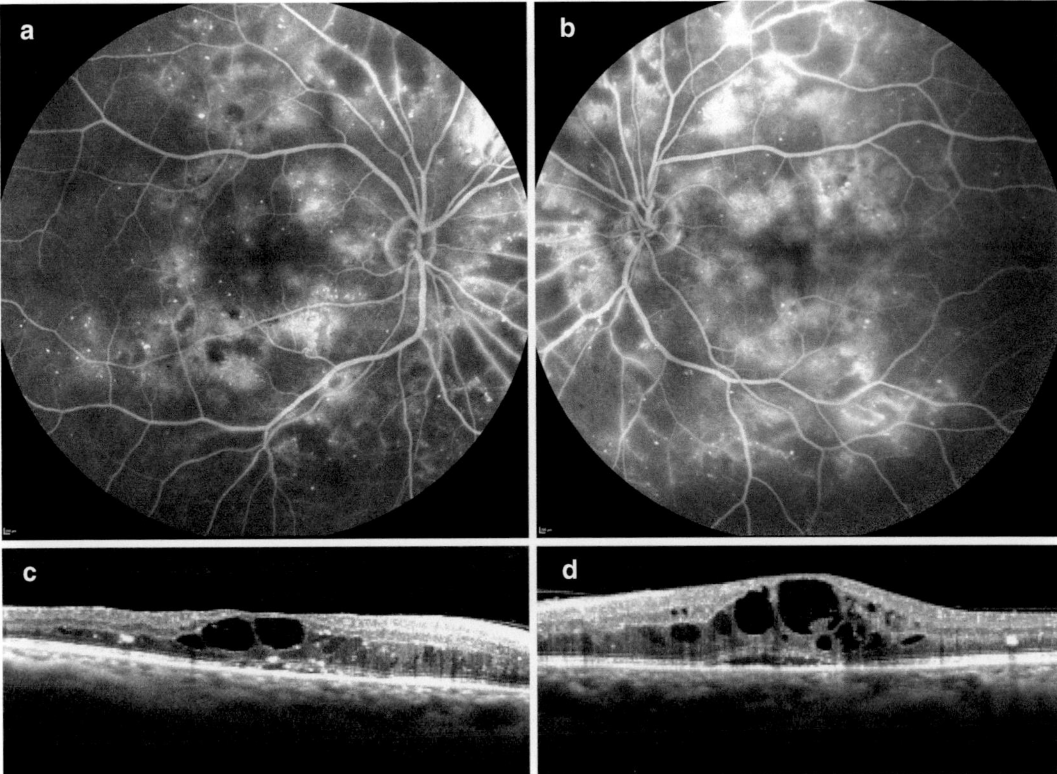

Fig. 11.2 Fluorescein angiography showing diffuse macular oedema in both eyes (**a**, **b**). OCT shows corresponding cystoid spaces in both eyes (**c**, **d**)

DME should be classified based on whether there was significant involvement of the central 1 mm (central subfield). In patients with no or minimal diabetic retinopathy and who did not have clinically detectable DME, the mean central subfield thickness (CST) was 270 μm on SD-OCT, which was 70 μm higher than the Stratus OCT [40]. It was proposed that any thickness above two standard deviations of the mean thickness taken as 320 μm for men and 305 μm on SD-OCT (Spectralis, Heidelberg Engineering, Heidelberg, Germany) be classified as centre-involving DME (CI-DME). Values less than these are considered non-centre-involving DME (nci-DME). Notably, the errors in automated measurements of DME were minor even with the Stratus OCT, compared to the manual technique used earlier, and were not likely to affect the results of trials. Thus, there was no need to send the OCT images to the centralized reading centres [41].

11.4.1.7 The OCT Biomarkers in DME

Till the availability of the OCT, patients with DME who did not respond to the then standard of care focal/grid laser photocoagulation were labelled as recalcitrant macular oedema. One of the primary reasons for the recalcitrance was the presence of a thick glistening membrane in the macula labelled as a taut posterior hyaloid membrane (PHM), which caused significant traction on the macula. These taut membranes often accompany the regressed proliferative diabetic retinopathy. No amount of laser photocoagulation was effective in such patients. It required pars plana vitreous surgery to release the traction on the macula (Fig. 11.3a–d). These taut hyaloid membranes were only sometimes discernible on clinical biomicroscopic examination. Even the first-generation TD-OCT could easily detect all the vitreoretinal interface abnormalities, including thickening of the PHM, posterior vitreoschi-

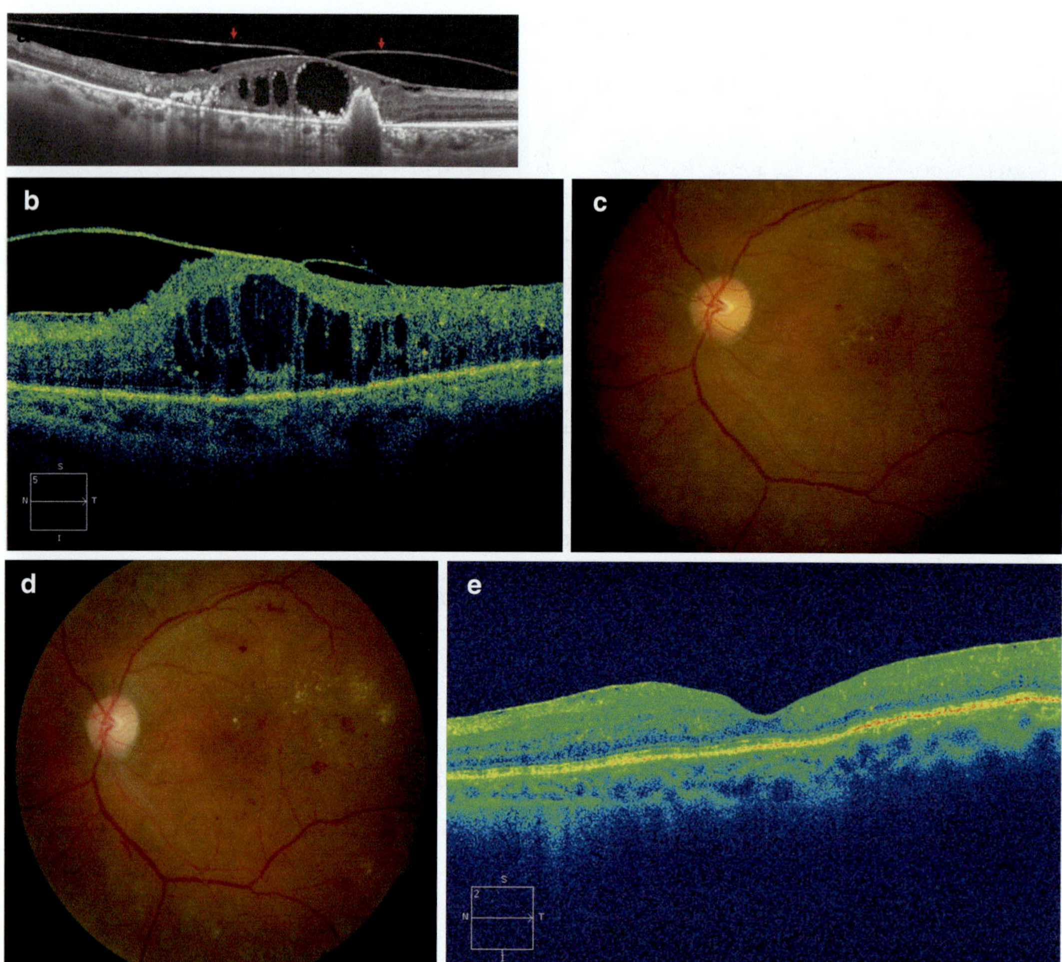

Fig. 11.3 A taut posterior hyaloid membrane (TPHM) is a thick membrane (red arrows) in the macula that causes significant traction on the macula and is often responsible for recalcitrant diabetic macular oedema (**a**). A 62-year-old woman with type 2 diabetes for 15 years had undergone pan-retinal photocoagulation in both eyes for proliferative diabetic retinopathy. She was pseudophakic in both eyes and had DM for 15 years. Her visual acuity in the left eye was 6/60. She had a clinically unapparent taut post-hyaloid membrane (**b**), which on OCT showed traction on the macula. Macular thickness was increased to 726 μm (**c**). She underwent pars plan vitreous surgery to remove the taut posterior hyaloid membrane. At 18 months, her visual acuity had improved to 6/18, there was no CME (**d**), and OCT showed a normal foveal contour, and macular thickness had reduced to 226 μm (**e**). Another patient with an apparent taut posterior hyaloid membrane (TPHM) was already treated for proliferative diabetic retinopathy with PRP in the right eye. Visual acuity was reduced to counting fingers at one metre. The OCT showed tractional macular detachment with complete disturbance of the macular architecture (**f**, **h**). She underwent pars plana vitreous surgery for removal of the tractional elements and at 3 weeks improved to 6/24 visual acuity with restoration of the foveal contour (**g**, **i**)

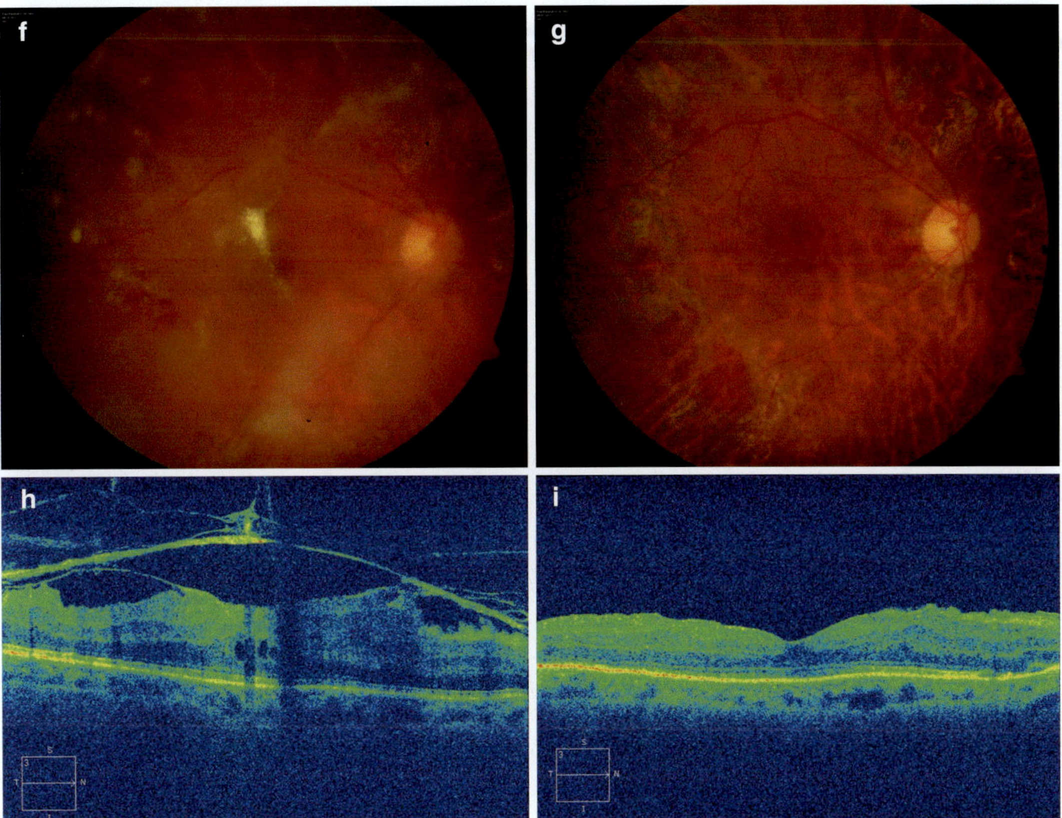

Fig. 11.3 (continued)

sis, and tractional detachment of the macula. It is, thus, essential first to rule out these tractional elements in DME because no pharmacotherapy is effective in such cases, and they require surgery. The SD-OCT and the SS-OCT give highly accurate and reproducible measurements of the CST, which is a measurable critical parameter to study the therapy outcome.

Leakage from MAs in the deep capillary plexus (DCP) leaks into the outer plexiform layer and in the ONL, which on OCT is seen as hyporeflective comparatively large cystic cavities. Intraretinal fluid in the inner nuclear layer appears as smaller hyporeflective cystic spaces due to a breakdown of BRB in the superficial capillary plexus (SCP) and DCP. Later, cysts appear in the OPL as well. Fluid may also accumulate in the potential space between the outer nuclear layer and the RPE layer, termed the subretinal fluid [42]. The SRF may be present in 25–30% of the eyes with DME. The significance of SRF is still not clearly understood. It may result from either a failure of the RPE pump or the breakdown of tight junctions of the RPE. Larger intraretinal cysts are associated with chronic DME [42].

In patients with long-standing DME, there are often disruptions of the inner retinal layers (DRIL), a significant biomarker for predicting the visual outcome following any therapeutic intervention. It is proposed that DRIL develop when the thickening of the retina stretches the bipolar cells beyond their limit of elasticity. DRIL of ≥50% of the central 1-mm area (CSF) carries an inferior visual outcome. DRIL is present if the boundaries between the various retinal layer interfaces in the inner retina cannot be identified, for example, between ganglion cell layer (GCL), IPL, and INL or INL and OPL or OPL and ONL. These are present irrespective of the cystic cavities in the retina [43]. Any improvement or worsening in the DRIL >300 μm in the CFS was associated with long-term improvement or worsening, respectively. DRIL may represent the retinal cells' disorganization that hinders the photoreceptors' signal transmission to the ganglion cells [43]. After the resolution of DME in patients with DRIL, increased FAZ in both superficial and deep capillaries is seen, suggesting that DRIL is possibly caused by ischaemia [44]. The other OCT parameters associated with DRIL are disruption of the ELM and EZ.

Small, round, or oval hyperreflective foci (HRF) in the retinal layers and choroid also predict visual outcomes in DME. These are believed to be activated microglia and are also present in inflammatory diseases and age-related macular degeneration. These could also represent migrating RPE cells, lipid-laden macrophages, extracellular proteinaceous, or lipid material. However, HRFs are usually less than 30 μm in size without any shadowing and are more likely to be of inflammatory origin [45]. These HRFs are not visible on biomicroscopy or the fundus photographs till they become confluent. They are seen on the outer border of the ONL and OPL and detected within the walls of the retinal MAs and may thus be the microglia filled with lipids [46]. The higher number of HRF in the outer retinal layers is also a predictor of poor visual outcomes [45]. These must be differentiated from the hard exudates, which are larger and generally show a shadow. Baseline higher numbers of HRF in the choroid and a low choroidal vascularity index, both indicating inflammatory activity, predict a good response to the treatment of DME with fluocinolone acetonide (FA) inserts [47]. If associated with DME, the hard exudates respond better to intravitreal (IVT) injection of corticosteroids than the anti-VEGF agents [48].

11.4.1.8 OCT Angiography in Diabetic Macular Oedema

OCT angiography (OCTA) is a non-invasive technique of visualizing the depth-resolved flow of RBCs in the regular or abnormal retinal/choroidal vessels without injecting any dye. The OCTA seeks to replace the FFA in day-to-day clinical practice. It has several advantages over the conventional FFA as the segmented en face view can show layer by layer the retinal capillaries and larger vessels that were not seen in FFA because of the obscuration of the deeper vessels by the dye. It has been shown that MAs in the deep capillary plexus are majorly responsible for DME. Wide-angle OCTA can quantify the extent of ischaemia in DR (Fig. 11.4). It can show the extent of the ischaemic macula at the SCP and DCP layers, which carries significant prognostic implications for the visual outcome.

Several OCTA parameters are larger in DME, such as FAZ area and irregularity of its contour, average vessel calibre, higher vessel tortuosity, and a low vessel density (VD) in the SCP. Higher VD in SCP carries a better visual outcome following anti-VEGF therapy [49]. Large cystic spaces in DME introduce artefacts and pose a significant challenge in interpreting the OCTA images in ~25% of the DME eyes [50]. The VD in DCP may artifactually show a higher VD in eyes with DME [51]. Patients with DME, nonresponders to anti-VEGF treatment, have capillary non-perfusion in the DCP layer and more MAs in this layer [52]. The OCTA does not show any significant reperfusion of the ischaemic areas of the retina following the use of the anti-VEGF agents for DME [53]. On the other hand, it has been claimed that IVT corticosteroids (Iluvien) may reopen capillaries blocked by leukostasis and improve perfusion in DME [54]. Although anti-VEGF therapy has become the gold standard treatment for DR, there is some evidence that using anti-VEGF agents may affect retinal perfusion in the DCP [55].

11.4.1.9 Role of Vascular Endothelial Growth Factor in DME

The discovery of VEGF in 1989 [56] and its humanized antibody in 1997 [57] brought about a paradigm shift in managing several eye disorders, including ARMD, DME, retinal vascular occlusion, and proliferative diabetic retinopathy. The VEGF mRNA levels were nearly 3.2 times higher in the retina of a diabetic rat model, and the retinal vascular permeability was 1.8 times higher in the diabetic rats versus the control animals. Highly specific antibodies against the VEGF

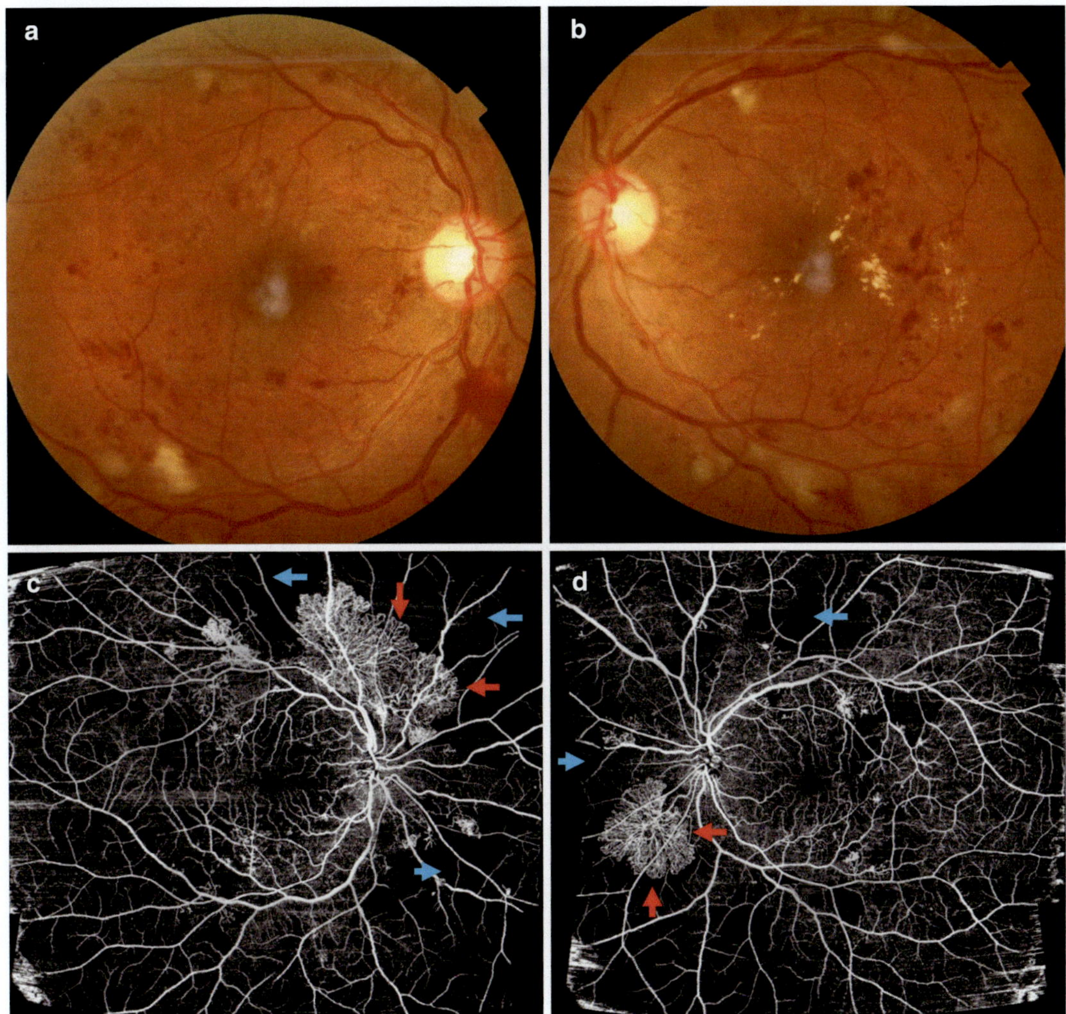

Fig. 11.4 Fundus photographs of right (**a**) and left (**b**) eyes of a patient with proliferative diabetic retinopathy. Montage of OCT angiography, a dyeless angiography, quantifying the extent of ischaemia (blue arrows), and retinal neovascularization (red arrows) in both eyes (**c**, **d**)

blocked the increased permeability. The authors concluded that anti-VEGF antibodies could become a potent tool for treating patients with a blood-retinal barrier breakdown [58]. Earlier, it had been shown that intravitreal injection of VEGF led to overexpression of intercellular adhesion molecules (ICAM) on the retinal vascular endothelium promoting leukostasis in retinal capillaries [59]. Moreover, vitreous levels of VEGF, ICAM-1, IL-6, and monocyte chemotactic protein-1(MCP-1) were significantly higher in patients with DME than in non-diabetic controls. Of these, the VEGF and the ICAM-1 level were also significantly associated with the severity of DME [60, 61].

11.4.1.10 Anti-VEGF Therapy in Diabetic Macular Oedema

Many patients who have CI-DME still maintain a visual acuity of 20/20. Such patients should be followed every 2–3 months, and treatment should be instituted if the VA drops to 20/30 or worse [62]. In a prospective, controlled trial, patients with CI-DME but visual acuity ≥20/25 randomized to receive either aflibercept every 4 weeks or laser photocoagulation or observation had visual acuity of 20/20 in 77%, 71%, and 66%, respectively, at the end of 2 years. By this time, the probability of receiving aflibercept as a rescue treatment in the laser and observation group was 26% and 36%, respectively [63]. Interestingly, nearly two-third of the patients in the observation group maintained their visual acuity and giving them injections would have been unnecessary. Thus, patients with CI-DME and good visual acuity should be observed [64]. Besides the cost factor, IVT interventions carry a definitive, minimal risk of endophthalmitis. Thus, these patients must be counselled to maintain control of their HbA1c and other comorbid conditions to delay injections and maintain good vision as long as possible [65].

A sham-controlled, masked, double-blind controlled trial in DME (VA 20/32–20/160) showed that IVT injection of 0.5 mg ranibizumab administered every month led to ≥15 ETDRS letter improvement in 22.6% of the eyes and 53% achieved ≥20/40 at the end of 1 year compared to 8.2% and 23.6% eyes, respectively, by the laser photocoagulation alone. There was no advantage to combining laser therapy with ranibizumab [66]. Two parallel multicentric phase 3 RISE (NCT00473330) and RIDE (NCT00473382) pivotal trials established the role of IVT injections of ranibizumab 0.3 or 0.5 mg every month for treating DME. Seventy percent of the patients who were followed up to 4 years showed a sustained effect of 0.5 mg ranibizumab given on a PRN basis after the initial 1-monthly dosage schedule [67]. The US FDA approved IVT Lucentis 0.3 mg (ranibizumab) prefilled syringe to treat DME in August 2012.

A novel anti-VEGF molecule was created by fusing VEGFR1 and VEGFR2 receptors to the Fc region of the human IgG. In addition to binding all isoforms of VEGF, it also bound the placenta-derived growth factor and was called VEGF-Trap. Not only it prevented the activity of VEGF on its receptors in the endothelial cells, but it also reversed the leukostasis [68]. This novel anti-VEGF agent, named aflibercept (Eylea), was US FDA approved in 2019 for the treatment of DME following two phase 3 parallel randomized controlled trials, VIVID and VISTA, in which more than 40% of patients showed ≥15 letters of improvement in visual acuity score compared to the laser photocoagulation. Intravitreal injections of Eylea 2.0 mg/0.05 mL given every 8/16 weeks for moderately severe or severe DR without DME have also resulted in consistent improvement in DR severity scores (DRSS) and prevented the development of DME (Fig. 11.5). Eighty percent of the eyes which received IVT Eylea injection every 8 weeks and 65% of eyes every 16 weeks had improvement in DRSS by ≥2 steps. Moreover, only 16% of patients developed DME at the end of 1 year versus 50% in the untreated control group [69].

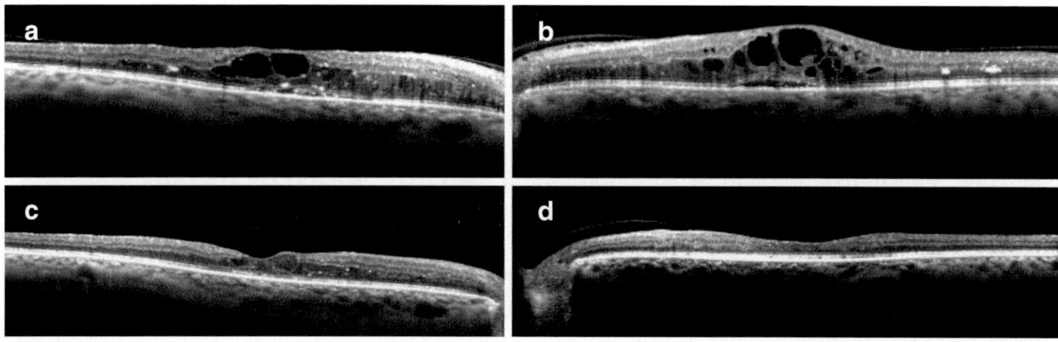

Fig. 11.5 OCT showing bilateral diabetic macular oedema (DME) at presentation (**a**, **b**) and resolution of DME 2 years following anti-VEGF therapy with aflibercept (**c**, **d**)

Bevacizumab (Avastin) is the first anti-VEGF agent developed for oncology use. It is available as 40 mg/mL vial. Fractionated from this vial, a 1.25 mg/0.1 mL dose has improved or stabilized the visual acuity of patients with DME [70]. It has to be sourced from compounding pharmacies. Although not approved by the FDA for IVT injections, being the most cost-effective anti-VEGF, it remains the most commonly used IVT anti-VEGF agent worldwide. A head-to-head comparison of bevacizumab (Avastin), ranibizumab (Lucentis), and aflibercept (Eylea) in a randomized control trial (DRCR-protocol T) did not show any difference in the visual outcome or safety in patients with DME at the end of 2 years if the initial VA was 20/40 or better. However, in patients with 20/50 or worse, Eylea was superior to Avastin. However, 64%, 52%, and 41% of eyes required focal laser photocoagulation for persistent DME beyond 6 months in the eyes that received Avastin, Lucentis, and Eylea, respectively [71].

Moreover, a post hoc analysis of this study revealed that the CST contributed only a small part to the improvement in visual acuity and cannot be a surrogate marker for evaluating the visual acuity change following IVT anti-VEGF therapy in DME [72]. Nearly two-third of the patients in protocol T were followed up for 2 years and received treatment at the investigator's discretion for the next 3 years. While the reduced macular thickness obtained at 2 years was maintained at 5 years, there was a mean loss of 4.6 letters of visual acuity between the 2 and 5 years. The results emphasized the need for better strategies for the long-term management of DME [73].

The DRCR Retina network protocol W looked at whether aflibercept could prevent the development of PDR and CI-DME in patients who had only NPDR and NCI-DME. At the end of 2 years, there was a three-fold decrease in the risk of developing CI-DME or PDR compared to the sham group, which received aflibercept only as rescue therapy. However, after 4 years, although a significant risk reduction in sight-threatening DR was evident, there was no meaningful visual gain from using aflibercept as a preventive strategy [74].

11.4.1.11 Newer Therapeutic Paradigms for the Treatment of DME

The major challenge of using anti-VEGF agents in treating DME is the treatment burden for the patients and the healthcare systems as the disease they treat is chronic, and the effect of the anti-VEGF agents is short-lived and does not last beyond 4 weeks. Thus, there has been a continuous search for new treatment paradigms and drugs. In recent years, the angiopoietin-Tie signalling pathway has emerged as an effective mechanism for controlling endothelial barrier function [75]. Angiopoietin-Tie (tunica interna endothelial kinase) signalling pathway controls vascular endothelial permeability and stability. Ang-1 is a natural ligand for Tie-2 (a transmembrane receptor on vascular endothelial cells). By binding Tie-2, it activates it by phosphorylation and promotes the endothelial cells' viability, junctions, and barrier functions. Vascular endothelium protein tyrosine phosphatase (VE-PTP) and Ang-2 are upregulated in hypoxia and inflammation.

While VE-PTP inactivates Tie-2 by dephosphorylation, Ang-2 blocks its action by binding with it, both preventing the action of Tie-2 in keeping the vascular endothelium stable and thus causing its instability and loss of barrier function [76, 77]. Newer agents that target the Ang-2/Tie pathway have been developed to regulate and stabilize the endothelial barrier [77]. In a phase II clinical trial, monthly IVT injections of a bispecific antibody that targets angiopoietin-2 and VEGF-A (Faricimab, 0.6 mg) were found superior to ranibizumab (0.3 mg) in the treatment of DME [78]. In a phase III trial, IVT injections of Faricimab given every 8 weeks or at personalized intervals up to every 16 weeks were found non-inferior to aflibercept given every 8 weeks, thus demonstrating the possibility of extending the treatment interval up to 16 weeks. Sixty percent of the patients in these trials could achieve a dosing interval of 16 weeks while maintaining a durable improvement of vision and reduction in DME at 2 years [79].

In an in vitro study, a Tie-2 agonist, a Tie2.1-hexamer, was effective in normalizing and stabilizing the intercellular junctions of a stressed endothelial cells monolayer. Preclinical studies found it effectively restored barrier function in a mouse and a non-human primate model. Moreover, it was found effective when anti-VEGF agents were ineffective in restoring endothelial barrier function. It has an extended presence in the vitreous humour and is a new potential therapeutic agent for treating DME [80]. Several trials evaluating newer molecules and drug delivery systems have been recently reviewed [81].

11.4.1.12 Is There a Role for Laser Photocoagulation for DME?

Until 2010, the standard of care for DME was focal/grid laser photocoagulation. The ETDRS recommended focal laser photocoagulation of MAs in focal DME and grid laser photocoagulation in diffuse DME as it prevented moderate visual loss by 50% at the end of the 3-year follow-up. Twelve percent of the DME patients who were treated had a significant loss of vision (≥15 letters on ETDRS) compared to 24% who were not treated [39]. However, laser photocoagulation led to only stabilization of vision, and by the end of 3 years, only 44% of eyes gained ≥10 ETDRS letters and 16% lost vision. A modified grid with greater spacing, less intense treatment, and direct laser photocoagulation of MAs and not treating anywhere closer than 500 μm from the foveal centre is recommended. Although no controlled trials have been done, laser photocoagulation is recommended for NCI-DME [62]. A recent Cochrane analysis concluded that modified laser protocol for focal/grid laser photocoagulation prevented further loss of vision and led to partial or complete resolution of DME compared to no intervention at 1–3 years [82]. A mild macular grid without directly treating the MAs is not recommended as it is not an effective strategy [83]. Following focal laser photocoagulation, nearly 90% of the MAs close by 3 months (Fig. 11.6). The reduction of CST on OCT rather than the MAs leakage on FFA at 2 weeks predicts the final CST at 3 months [84]. One of the significant complications of laser photocoagulation is an expansion of the scars, and if treatment is done too close to the foveal centre, it may compromise the vision. Inadvertent photocoagulation of the fovea centre is a distinct possibility, especially in an eye with severe macula oedema where the landmarks of the fovea may not be clearly defined.

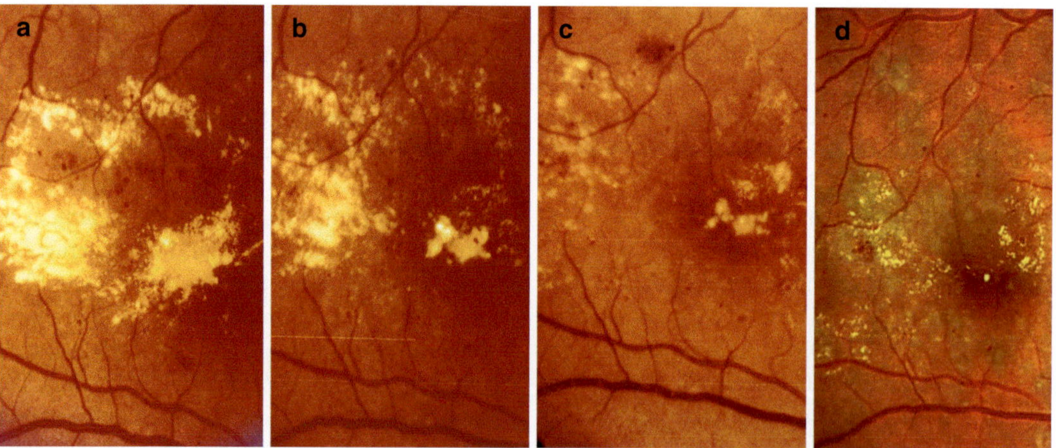

Fig. 11.6 A 46-year-old man with type 2 diabetes and dyslipidaemia presented with macular oedema with massive hard exudates in the macula (**a**). His visual acuity was reduced to counting fingers close to his face. He was treated with statins, which significantly reduced hard exudates at 6 weeks with an improvement in visual acuity to 6/60 (**b**). At this stage, he was treated with focal laser photocoagulation. His visual acuity had improved to 6/36 with further reduced hard exudates (**c**). At 18 months, his visual acuity had improved to 6/12 with the resolution of macular oedema and minimal hard exudates (**d**)

11.4.1.13 Role of Corticosteroids in Diabetic Macular Oedema

To reduce the frequency of IVT injections, long-acting corticosteroids such as triamcinolone acetonide (TA) or sustained-release biodegradable dexamethasone implants or non-biodegradable fluocinolone acetonide (FA) inserts have been evaluated in randomized clinical trials. In one such trial, focal laser photocoagulation yielded better visual outcomes at the end of 2 years than the TA (IVT inj of 1 mg or 4 mg). Nearly 51% of the phakic eyes receiving IVT injections of 4 mg of TA (23% in the 1 mg group) had to undergo cataract surgery, and 33% and 16%, respectively, in the 4 mg vs 1 mg, developed a 10 mm of Hg rise of intraocular pressure [85]. The outcome was not changed at 3 years of follow-up [86]. However, in a subset of the pseudophakic eyes, TA combined with prompt focal/grid laser yielded results similar to IVT Lucentis [87].

Despite one macular photocoagulation treatment, patients with persistent DME were randomized to a slow-release low-dose (0.2 μg/day) or high-dose (0.5 μg/day) FA insert versus a sham IVT injection. At the end of 2 years, 26% of patients with FA receiving either insert compared to 13% of the sham had >15 ETDRS letters improving visual acuity. The low-dose group had a better risk-benefit profile. Of those phakic at baseline, cataract surgery was required in 41–51% of patients in the low and high doses, respectively. Glaucoma incisional surgery was required in the low and high doses in 3.7% and 8.1%, respectively [88]. By the end of 3 years, the incidence of high pressure did not change much, but practically all phakic patients had to undergo cataract surgery. Improvement by ETDRS ≥15 letters in 34% of treated eyes versus 13% of sham-treated eyes [89]. In a subgroup analysis, in patients who had chronic DME (diagnosis ≥3 years), the low-dose inserts improved VA by ≥15 ETDRS letters in 34% vs 13% in the sham group and 22% vs 28%, respectively, in the non-chronic DME [90]. In September 2014, the Iluvien implant (0.2 μg/day) was US FDA-approved for patients with DME who had not previously shown a corticosteroid-induced rise in intraocular pressure.

A slow-release dexamethasone implant (0.7 or 0.35 mg) was tested in two randomized sham-controlled, parallel phase 3 clinical trials. It showed that 22% of the study eyes vs 12% of the sham-treated eyes showed improvement in VA by ≥15 ETDRS letters at the end of 3 years. On average, four implants were required by the end of 3 years. The rates of cataract development were 68%, 64%, and 20% in the high, low, and sham groups, respectively. A significant rise in intraocular pressure was seen in 0.6% and 0.3% of the high and low doses, respectively [91] (Fig. 11.7a, b). However, when Dexa implant (0.7 mg) was added to the continued Lucentis treatment in patients who showed persistent macular oedema even after three injections of Lucentis, although macular oedema improved, there was no change in the visual acuity [92]. In a single-centre study of recalcitrant DME, a single IVT of Ozurdex (0.7 mg) implant led to significant improvement in the CST over 6 months. The VA improved from a mean of 0.82 ± 0.46 log MAR before the implant to 0.68 ± 0.49 log MAR at 6 months of follow-up. Maximum improvement in VA was seen at 4 weeks, and the maximum reduction in CST was at 6 weeks [93]. Corticosteroids are no longer recommended as primary therapy in DME but are favoured as second-line therapy in non-responders to the conventional anti-VEGF treatment [62]. Patients with DME who are planned for cataract surgery may be benefitted from an IVT Ozurdex implant at the time of surgery [94].

11.4.1.14 Control of Diabetes and Other Comorbid Conditions

Multifactorial interventions to control blood sugar levels, blood pressure, lipids, and proteinuria lead to a decrease in DME. If done before treatment with laser photocoagulation, decreased retinal thickness facilitates the application of low energy laser beam [95] (Fig. 11.6). In a prospective study, patients with DME were encouraged to reach the target values of HbA1c, lipids, blood pressure, Hb, and proteinuria through extensive

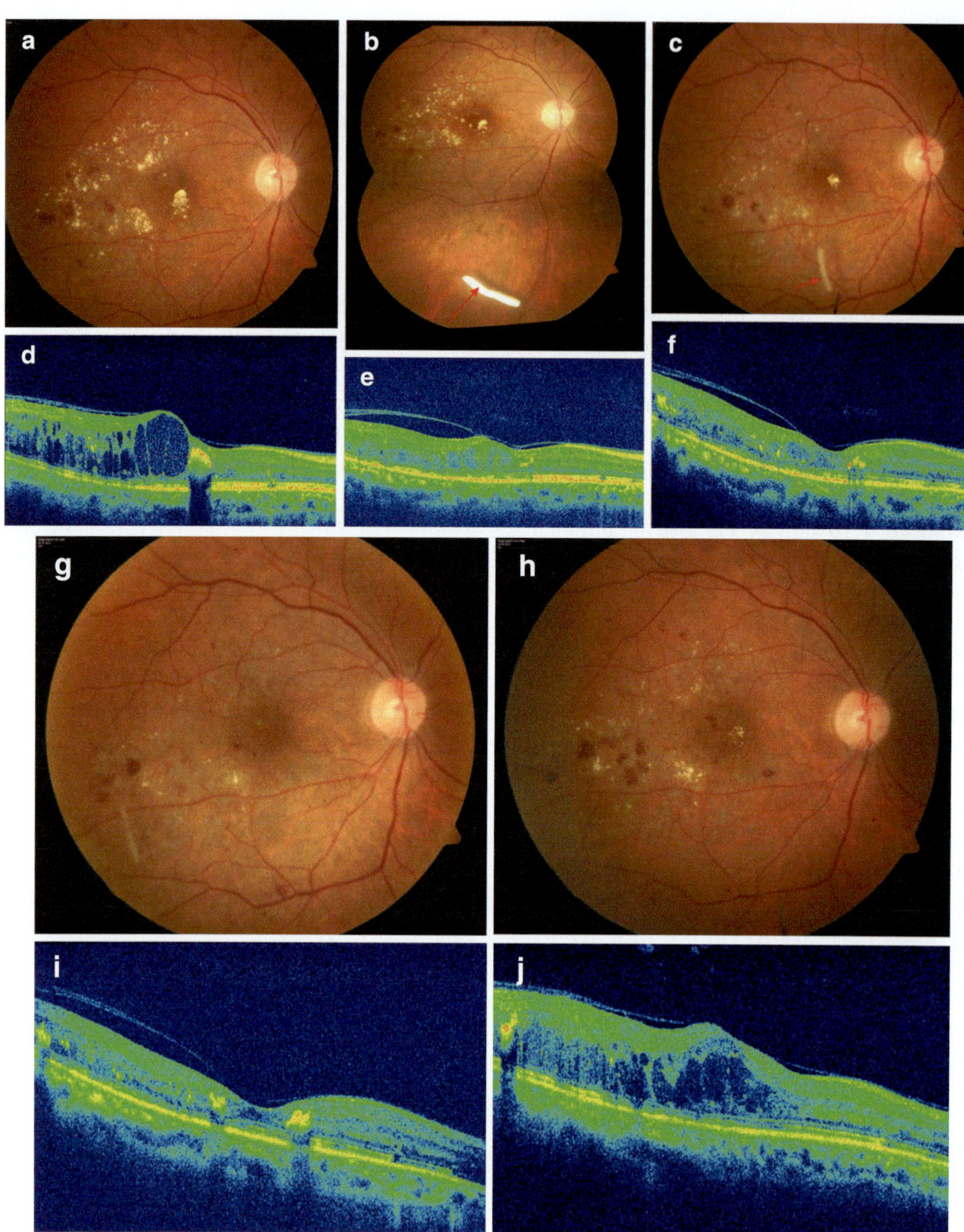

Fig. 11.7 (**A**) A 56-year-old man with type 2 DM for 20 years had received focal laser thrice, and multiple anti-VEGF injections and yet continued to have macular oedema in the right eye. Visual acuity was 6/24 and the central foveal thickness was 512 μm (**a**, **d**). He received an intravitreal implant of Ozurdex (red arrow, **b**). A month later, visual acuity improved to 6/18. Note a reduction in the hard exudates and macular thickness (**b**, **e**). At 3 months, hard exudates had resolved except at the foveal centre (**f**). Visual acuity improved to 6/12. Note the residual implant inferiorly (red arrow) (**b**, **c**). Four months after the Ozurdex implant, there were no hard exudates, and visual acuity improved to 6/12. Macular thickness had decreased to 218 μm (**g**, **i**). However, at 6 months post-Ozurdex implant, the macular oedema returned, visual acuity decreased to 6/18, and the CST measured 498 μm (**h**, **j**)

multifactorial interventions over 4–6 weeks before subjecting them to focal/grid laser photocoagulation. Of those who achieved complete control of the target values, 29% of the eyes had improvement in VA by three lines or more versus 21% of those with incomplete control [96].

Elevated HbA1C is known to increase the risk of DME. Often the focal DME is accompanied by massive hard exudates (HEX). There is a risk of subfoveal migration of hard exudates following laser therapy. The HEX under the fovea can damage photoreceptors and promote subfoveal fibrosis. The use of statins before focal laser photocoagulation is known to reduce the severity of HEX even before the laser and prevent subfoveal migration [97]. Statins reduce the risk of progression of diabetic retinopathy and DME. They also reduce the need for laser photocoagulation, any treatment for diabetic retinopathy, and vitreous surgery in these patients [98, 99]. Diabetes is a systemic disease, and its comorbid systemic associations profoundly affect the progression of diabetic retinopathy. It needs a multidisciplinary team approach for preventing, progressing, and controlling diabetic retinopathy. Control of blood sugar levels and hypertension significantly impacts the course of diabetic retinopathy and the need for therapeutic interventions [100].

11.4.2 Macular Oedema in Retinal Vein Occlusions

Retinal vein occlusions, the branch as well as the central retinal vein, and the hemispheric retinal vein occlusion are the second most common cause of macular oedema. Macular oedema is the commonest cause of visual disturbance in these patients (Fig. 11.8). By 3 months of the onset, most of the retinal haemorrhages get absorbed by the usual phagocytic mechanisms and depending upon the net balance of fluid leakage from the broken/decompensated endothelial cell barrier and the capacity of the collateral vessels that form in deep capillary plexus to drain it; macular oedema may resolve or continue to persist. There are no collateral channels identified on OCTA in the superficial venous plexus. The fluid moves in the interstitial tissue from the SCP to the DCP. The fluid first collects in the INL and then moves to the OPL. A pioneering study showed that compared to 0.3 mg, the effect of IVT injection of 0.5 mg Lucentis in reducing ME was quicker and lasted longer. Moreover, there is a direct correlation between the severity of ME and the baseline aqueous humour VEGF levels, suggesting that VEGF was a major driver of ME and laid grounds for establishing the role of anti-VEGF therapy for the resolution of macular oedema, albeit for a short duration (~1 month) in both the BRVO and the CRVOs [101].

11.4.2.1 Macular Oedema in Branch Retinal Vein Occlusions

The visual acuity improves spontaneously in many BRVO eyes without intervention. Still, improvement beyond 20/40 visual acuity is uncommon [102].

In the natural course, the median time to resolve macular oedema was 18 months in the macular vein occlusion and 21 months for the major BRVO [103]. Major BRVO eyes show a

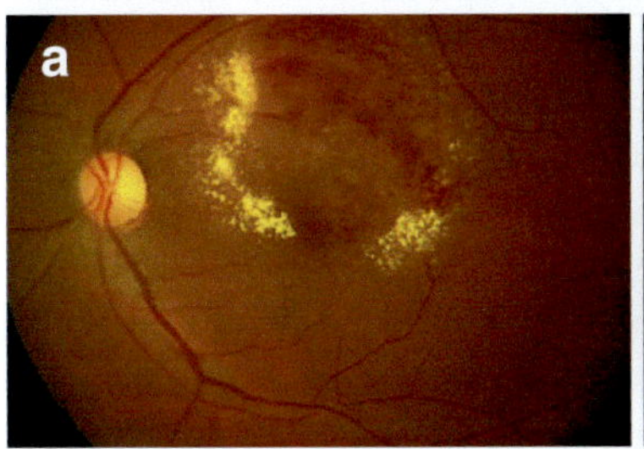

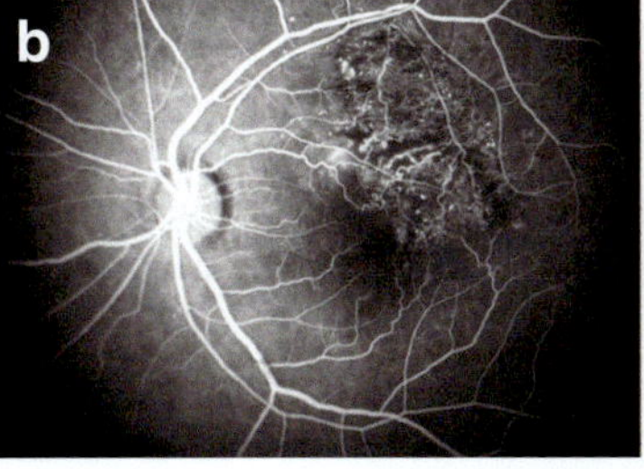

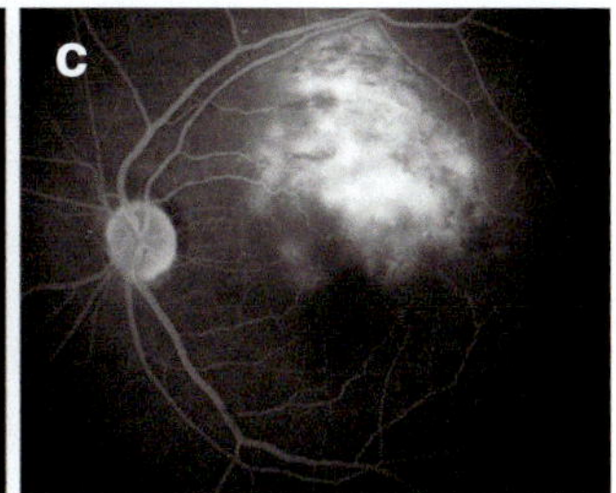

Fig. 11.8 A 54-year-old man presented 4 months after a left eye upper temporal branch vein occlusion. He showed residual linear haemorrhages and an incomplete ring of hard exudates around an area of macular oedema (**a**). FFA showed telangiectatic vessels and multiple microaneurysms (**b**) and diffuse staining of the macula in the affected quadrant in the late frames of FFA (**c**). Such macular oedema in branch retinal vein occlusion will only rarely if at all show a spontaneous resolution

higher aqueous VEGF and inflammatory cytokine level than the macular BRVO. The major BRVO eyes also show a higher chance of DRIL, EZ disruption, and SRF and require several anti-VEGF injections [104]. In terms of visual improvement, in the branch vein occlusion study, a multicentric controlled trial, there was spontaneous improvement ≥20/40 in 34% of the untreated eyes versus 60% who had undergone a grid laser photocoagulation in the area of macular oedema [105]. The persisting macular oedema does not follow a zonal distribution and collects in the centre of the macula. Spontaneous resolution in up to 40% of the affected eyes may restore near-normal visual acuity [103]. However, with the anti-VEGF treatment, ME may resolve completely, persist, or recur after initial resolution. Persistent or recurrent ME is associated with collateral formation in the intermediate capillary plexus and the DCP, where these capillary networks show increased density and thickening of the retinal layer [106, 107]. Moreover, the BRVO eyes that show recurrence of ME also show a greater loss of the perifoveal capillary network, especially in the DCP [108]. Eyes that show more gap vessels (capillaries present in the SCP but corresponding capillaries absent in the DCP) also tend to show a persistent ME [109, 110].

Clinical diagnosis of macular vein occlusion, especially if the patient presents late, may pose a challenge to differentiate it from diabetic retinopathy. Notably, the retinal veins follow a strict quadrantic pattern. The haemorrhages and the microaneurysms, unlike macular oedema, are strictly limited to the affected quadrant above or below the horizontal raphe, as the case may be. In diabetic retinopathy, the microaneurysms and haemorrhages do not follow this rule and are seen across the horizontal raphe. One notable exception is the formation of hard exudates in the BRVO. If oedema persists, hard exudates may be seen deposited in a circinate pattern around the site of persisting retinal oedema from the decompensated capillary bed and/or microaneurysms and cross the horizontal raphe. The formation of microaneurysms is a risk factor for the development of refractory macula oedema [111]. In the BRVO eyes with macular oedema and increased subfoveal choroidal thickness, elevated levels of VEGF and IL-8 were seen as predictors of good outcomes following anti-VEGF therapy [112].

The BRVO eyes that show non-perfusion areas on ultra-wide FFA show a good correlation with the CNP in the SCP and the DCP. Thus, OCTA alone can provide a fair idea of the ischaemic status of the eye in patients with BRVO [113].

Optical coherence tomography (OCT) is often used to diagnose and monitor the presence of macular oedema (central subfield thickness, CST). Notably, the smoothness of the interface between INL and OPL on SD-OCT may indicate fewer chances of ME or its recurrence [114]. Additionally, the OCT may show some structural alterations, including disorganization of the internal retinal layers (DRIL) and disruptive changes in the photoreceptors and the external limiting membrane that may limit visual improvement, including contrast sensitivity following therapeutic interventions [115, 116].

There is level 1 evidence for using pharmacotherapy to treat ME in BRVO [117]. In the last 15 years, intravitreal injections of anti-VEGF agents have supplanted gird laser photocoagulation for treating macular oedema due to BRVO. Many such agents have been tested in several controlled trials. They have found almost equivalent results using ranibizumab, bevacizumab, or aflibercept that need to be given initially every month for three injections and followed by a PRN (pro re nata) basis protocol. Visual improvement and reduction in CST, the usual parameters to monitor the response, have shown more significant results with the use of pharmacotherapy compared to laser gird therapy [118, 119].

A more recent Cochrane review of randomized controlled trials has endorsed the recommendations of the earlier studies that, compared to no treatment or treatment with grid laser photocoagulation, treatment with any of the anti-VEGF agents or depot corticosteroids was more effective in improving visual acuity, the CST, and quality of life up to 12 months. Because of the spontaneous improvement of ME in many eyes, investigators in the past usually waited for

3–4 months before starting anti-VEGF therapy. It has been seen that an early start of intervention gives a superior visual outcome with a lesser number of injections than delaying the treatment [120]. Compared to corticosteroids, anti-VEGF agents are more effective. Moreover, there is evidence that steroids lead to high intraocular pressure and cataract formation [121]. Although highly effective, these injections have increased the burden on patients and care providers. Additional macular laser photocoagulation can reduce the number of intravitreal injections [122] (Fig. 11.9a, b).

11.4.2.2 Macular Oedema in Central Retinal Vein Occlusion

Raised intravascular pressure in the CRVO leads to a breakdown of the blood-retinal barrier and increased fluid leakage into the retina's interstitial tissues. Eyes with CRVO, which maintain a foveal depression on structural OCT, have a better outcome as these require fewer injections of IVT anti-VEGF than those without preserved foveal depression. In CRVO, extensive RNFL haemorrhages compared to deep retinal haemorrhages provide an easy clinical clue to the eventual worse visual outcome, severe ME, and ischaemic complications [123].

The increased pressure interferes with the perfusion in the retinal tissues, especially in the DCP. It leads to hypoxia and the release of hypoxia-inducible factor 1-alpha, causing overexpression of the vascular endothelial growth factor (VEGF). Discovered in 1989, the VEGF is expressed in response to hypoxia and is a potent endothelial cell-specific stimulant that causes increased vascular permeability, endothelial cell proliferation, formation of new vessels, and recruitment of leukocytes [124].

Vascular endothelial growth factor (VEGF) was found elevated in the ocular fluids in the patients with proliferative diabetic retinopathy and CRVO [125, 126] and related with the severity of the retinal vein occlusion [127]. Although initial reports had found elevated VEGF levels in the RVOs, it was unknown how much of the fluid in the interstitial fluid is contributed by the increased hydrostatic pressure or the cytokines in the retina. The discovery of VEGF led to the development of an antigen-binding protein against VEGF (bevacizumab) and later a special antigen-binding fragment (ranibizumab), especially for intraocular use [57, 128]. Initial small, controlled trials with 3-monthly IVT injections of ranibizumab, an anti-VEGF agent, led to remarkable improvement in the vision and the reduction in central retinal thickness irrespective of the duration of the RVO.

One of the earliest studies found vitreous levels of IL-6 and VEGF elevated in eyes with CRVO [129]. Subsequently, aqueous humour levels of sVEGFR-1 and sVEGFR-2, placental growth factor (PlGF), and platelet-derived growth factor (PDGF) and inflammatory cytokines were also found elevated in the CRVO eyes and related to ME [130]. The inflammatory cytokines keep increasing in the CRVO and account for persistent and refractory ME. Moreover, the blood flow velocity of leukocytes slows, converting many non-ischaemic CRVO into the ischaemic variety [131]. There is level 1 evidence that early treatment with anti-VEGF agents is a safe and effective therapy in CRVO. It needs to be initiated early rather than late. It has also been shown that anti-VEGF therapy leads to decreased retinal venous pressure in eyes with CRVO [132].

Several controlled clinical trials have been done both with anti-VEGF agents that last about 1 month and intravitreal injections of depot steroids (triamcinolone acetonide, 1 mg Kenalog) or sustained-release dexamethasone implants (Ozurdex) to overcome the increased burden of the monthly injections [133].

There is a significant risk of cataract formation and raised intraocular pressure with intravitreal depot steroids. The anti-VEGF agents to date remain the first line of therapy for persistent macular oedema in RVOs, depot steroids being reserved only for patients who are resistant to the anti-VEGF agents [134]. A post hoc analysis comparing the efficacy of Avastin, Eylea, and Lucentis in CRVO ME showed that ~61% of eyes still showed recurrent ME, 28% were completely dry, and 11% had persistent ME at the end of 2 years. Of the three agents, persistent ME was seen in ~18% of eyes treated with Avastin, compared to 8% with Lucentis and 5% with Eylea [135]. There is strong evidence for a treat and extend strategy as only ~8 injections were required in the first year and 13 by the end of second year of therapy [136].

However, most patients continue to receive injections even after 5 years [137] and still require at least four injections per year at the end of 8 years [138]. The search for innovative drug delivery systems continues in an attempt to reduce the treatment burden (Fig. 11.9a, b).

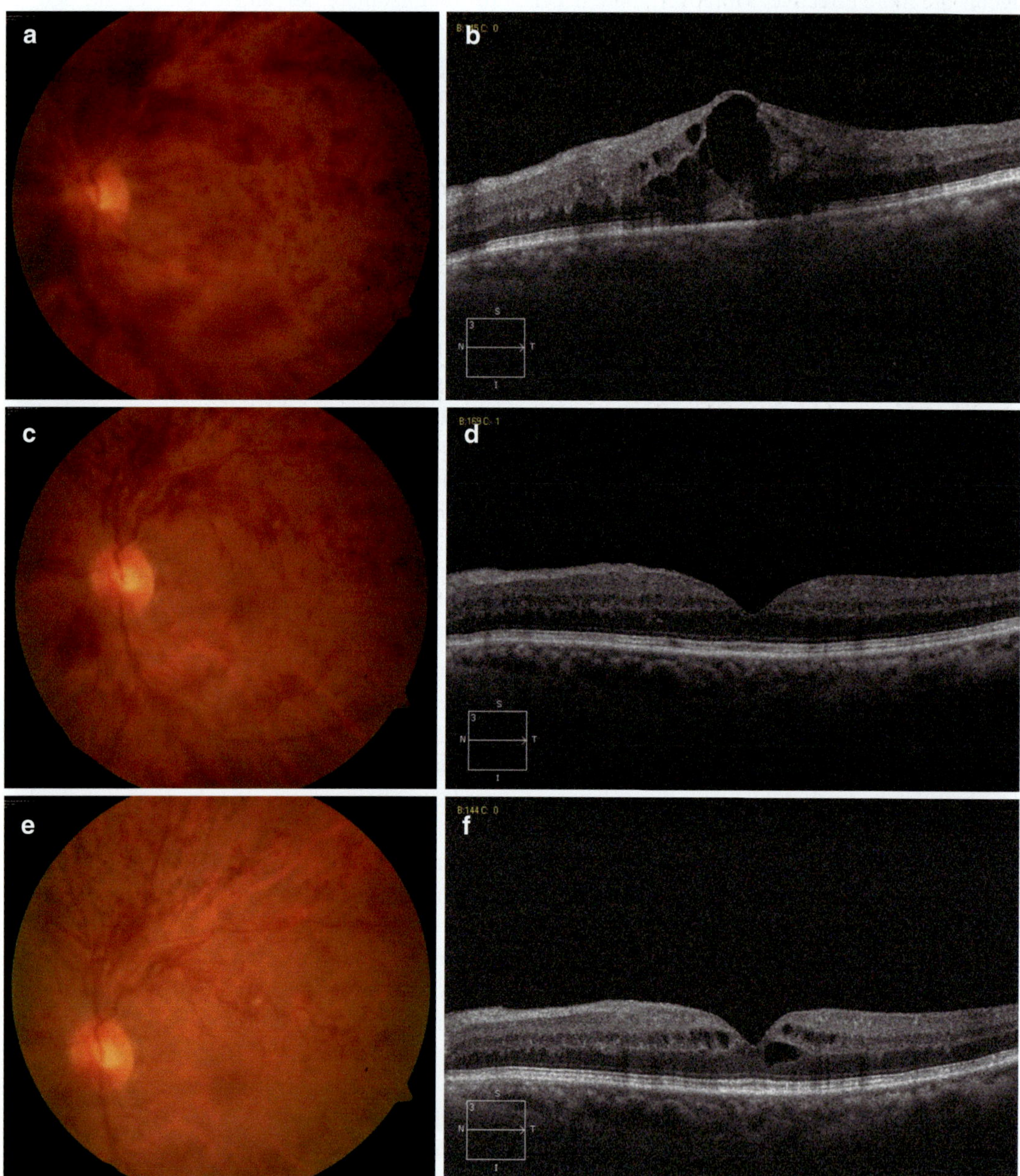

Fig. 11.9 A 65-year-old man presented with left eye non-ischaemic central retinal vein occlusion with CME and visual acuity of 6/24 (**a**, **b**). He received intravitreal inj bevacizumab and showed incomplete resolution of haemorrhages and a normal foveal contour on OCT at 4 weeks (**c**, **d**). Six weeks later, the CME returned, and he received another IVT bevacizumab (**e**, **f**). He received seven injections in the first year of CRVO on a pro re nata basis. Course during the second year shown (**g**–**j**) and the third year (**k**–**m**). In 34 months of follow-up, he required bevacizumab injections in decreasing frequency, totalling ten injections. He maintained a visual acuity of 6/6 and a dry macula

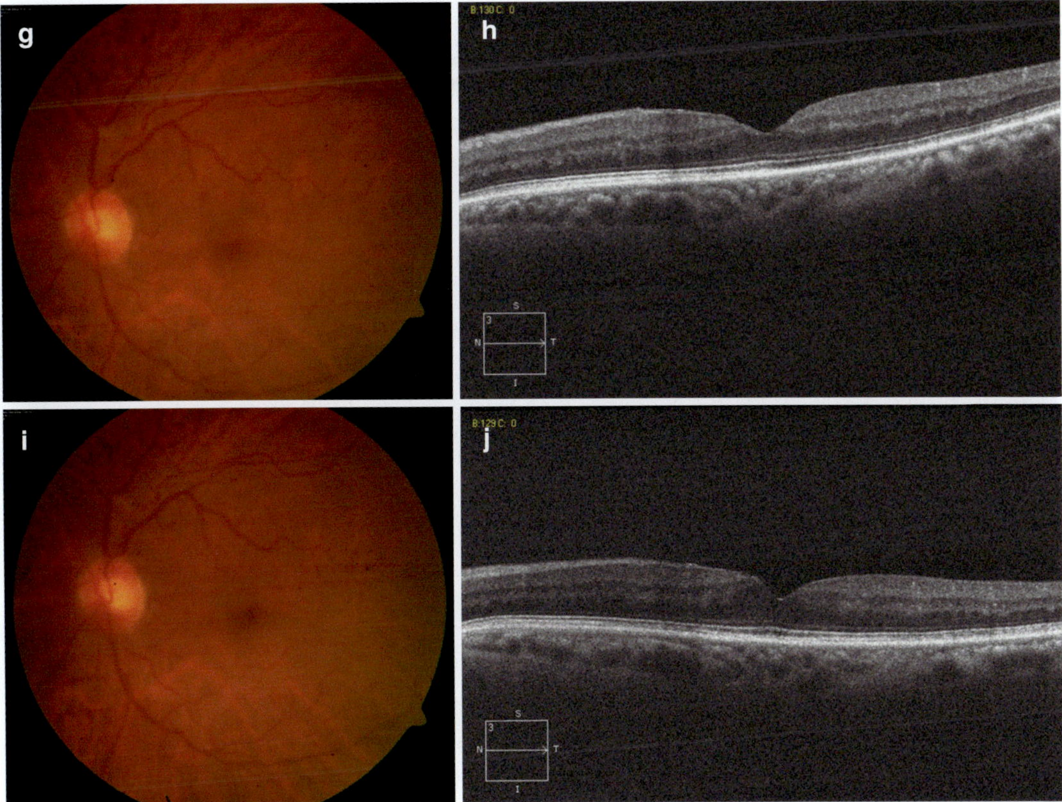

Fig. 11.9 (continued)

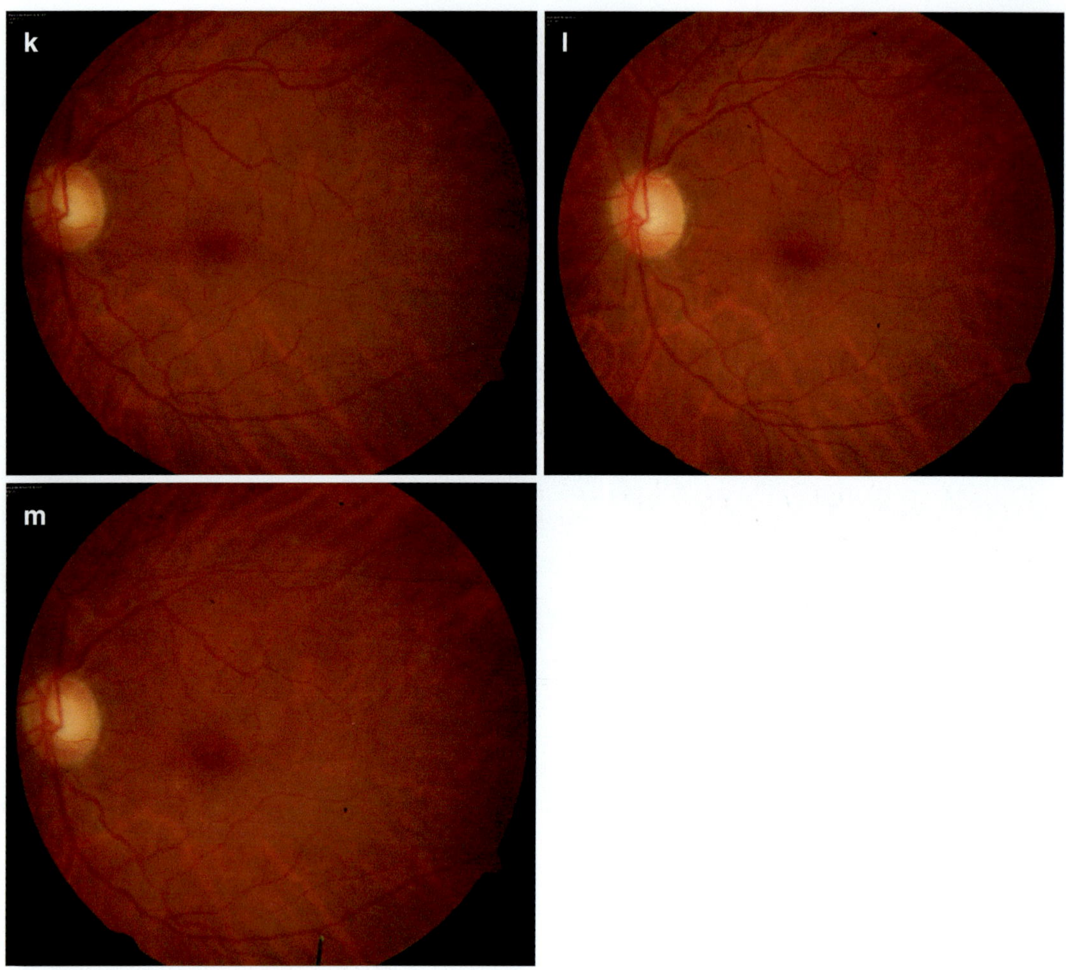

Fig. 11.9 (continued)

11.5 Macular Oedema in Uveitis

Macular oedema in uveitis is a leading cause of blindness in the industrialized world and may account for 10–15% of blindness [139, 140]. One of the most frequent causes of impaired vision in uveitis is the development of cystoid macular oedema (CME), which may occur in >40% of the eyes [140, 141]. The CME is often seen in older patients with long-duration chronic uveitis, uncommon in acute cases (Figs. 11.10 and 11.11). Smoking is a significant risk factor for the development of uveitis CME [142]. The most frequent anatomical location of uveitis complicated by the development of CME is intermediate uveitis, posterior and pan uveitis, the least common being anterior uveitis. The estimates of the prevalence of CME for each anatomical location have varied widely. The prevalence of CME in uveitis has varied from 9% to 28% in the anterior, 25% to 70% in intermediate uveitis, 19% to 34% in the posterior, and 18% to 66% in the posterior [140, 143–145]. There are many reasons for these variations. Unlike macular oedema with a clear media in DM, vascular occlusions, or cataract surgery, uveitis CME (UME) is difficult to diagnose clinically as the media is often hazy due to vitritis, posterior synechiae, complicated cataract, hypotony, or band-shaped keratopathy. The latter is a frequent complication of juvenile idiopathic arthritis-associated uveitis in young children.

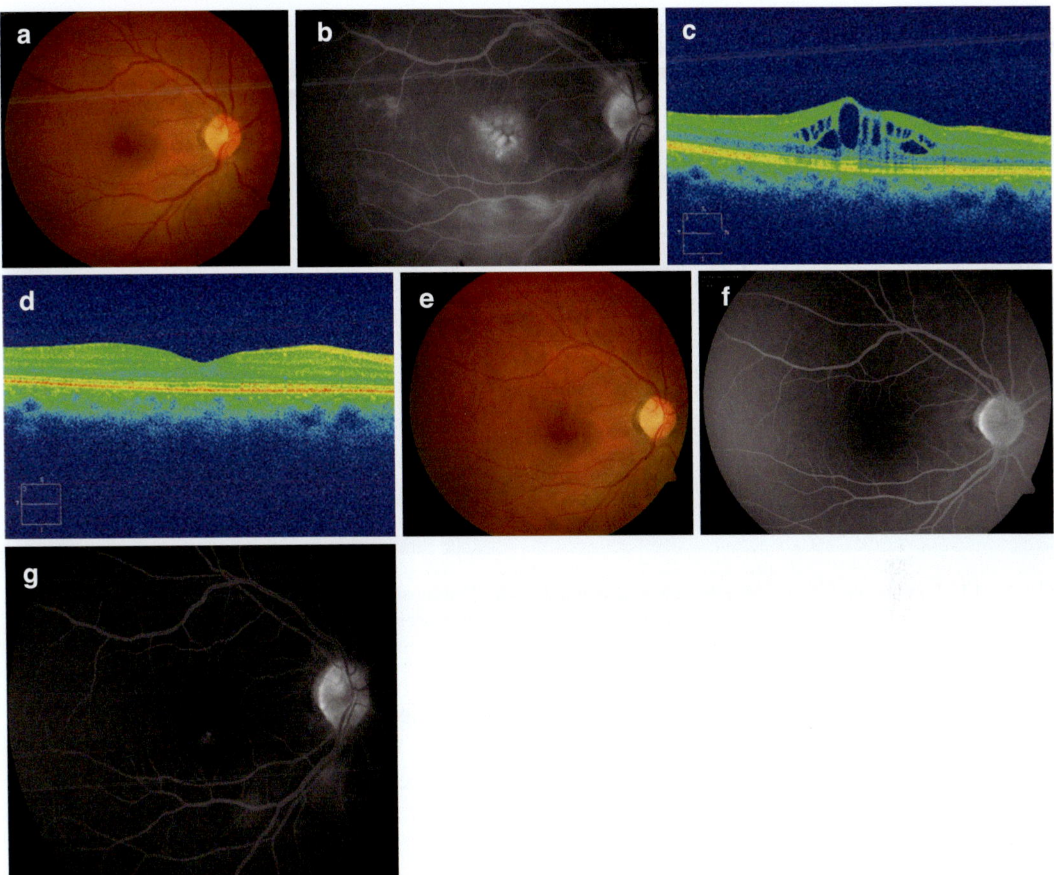

Fig. 11.10 A 56-year-old woman presented with a diminution of visual acuity in BE for 6 days. She had been treated for uveitis 18 years ago with oral steroids. Visual acuity was 6/18, and vitreous cells and CME in the right eye (**a**). FFA showed a petaloid pattern of dye collection and perivascular leak from retinal vessels (**b**). The OCT showed CME (**c**). Her tuberculin skin test was positive at +20 × 23 mm. Since she showed no response to oral corticosteroids and anti-TB therapy, she was given an Ozurdex implant. CME resolved at 1 week (**d**) and remained CME-free till 12 weeks (**e**, **f**) with Ozurdex, but CME recurrence started at 16 weeks (**g**)

11.5.1 Diagnosis of Macular Oedema in Uveitis

Apart from the biomicroscopic examination, the FFA and OCT are employed frequently to diagnose UME. However, in uveitis, the dye leakage from retinal vessels on FFA does not always increase macular thickness on the OCT, especially if the macula is already atrophic or if the leakage is only mild. Concordance between the FFA and OCT may be seen only in half of the patients. In birdshot chorioretinopathy, an autoimmune panuveitis, FFA shows mild leakage from the retinal vessels, but the OCT may not show increased central subfield thickness (CST). On the other hand, in intermediate uveitis, the OCT shows the presence of CME, but the FFA may not show any leakage [146]. If the media is clear, over 80% of uveitis eyes may show concordance between FFA and OCT observations [147] (Figs. 11.10 and 11.11). Generally, uveitis eyes with diffuse macular oedema have a poorer outcome than those with CME. Since ~10% of eyes may also show SRF, it creates a challenge in estimating the exact CST [147]. Of the three modalities, helpful information for CME diagnosis was obtained in 90% with Stratus-3 OCT, 77% with FFA, and 76% with the biomicroscopic examination. Nearly one-third of

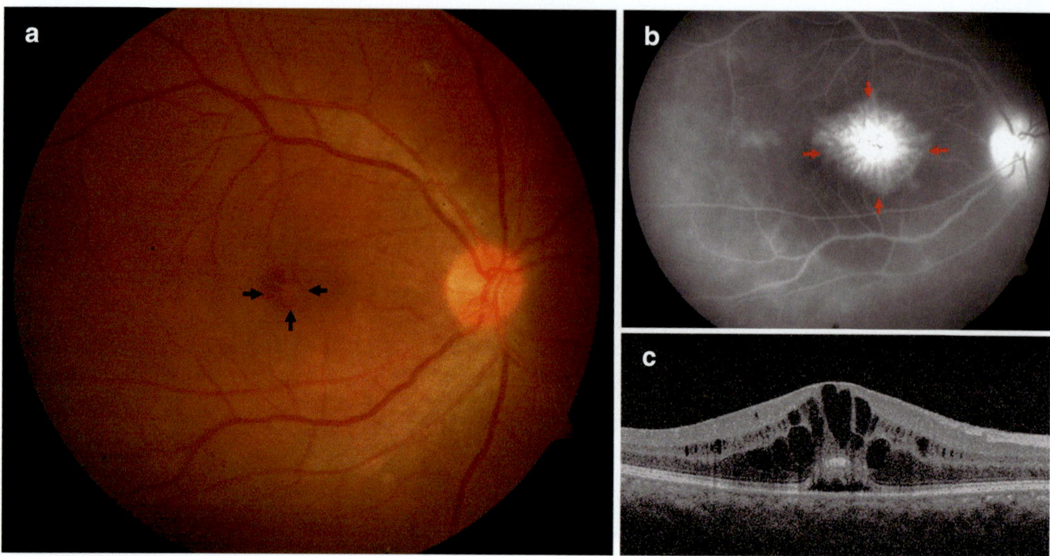

Fig. 11.11 Fundus photograph of a 46-year-old woman with decreased vision of 6/24 in right eye showing media haze due to vitritis and a dull foveal reflex (black arrows) (**a**). Diagnosis of cystoid macular oedema was confirmed by fluorescein angiography (red arrows) that also showed leakage from retinal vessels (**b**), and OCT (**c**)

the patients with fluorescein leak did not show macular thickness on OCT, and one-third of those with macular thickness did not show fluorescein leakage. Therapeutic decisions should ideally be made after obtaining information from FFA and OCT [148].

11.5.2 OCT Biomarkers in Uveitis Macular Oedema

In non-infectious uveitis, the most critical OCT biomarkers to predict VA improvement are the intact ellipsoid zone and cystic spaces in the macula's central subfield (CSF) and the subretinal fluid (SRF). OCT biomarkers, including disruption of the retinal inner layers in both horizontal and vertical extent, CST, presence of intraretinal cysts, disruptions of the ellipsoid zone and ELM, and presence of hyperreflective foci, are significant surrogate markers for VA improvement in UME [149].

11.5.3 Treatment of Uveitis Macular Oedema

Topical treatment with difluprednate 0.05% is a reasonably good first line of therapy for treating UME. It led to a reduction of ≥20% in UME or resolution (≤320 μm without cysts) in 69% and 43%, respectively, by 3 months. The rise of IOP in 11% of the eyes above 24 mm Hg was a significant concern, and these eyes need to be watched [150].

Resolution of UME is a reasonable goal of treatment efficacy in non-infectious uveitis. Patients who participated in the multicentric uveitis steroids treatment trial (MUST) received either an intravitreal Retisert implant (Fluocinolone acetonide 0.59 mg) or oral corticosteroids (Fig. 11.12). The cumulative UME resolution rate was seen in 94% of the eyes with initial UME (defined on TD-OCT as ≥240 μm), followed by annual OCT measurements up to 7 years. However, >40% of eyes had recurrences. The VA improved if the CST improved, but not otherwise. An epiretinal membrane had a lower likelihood of improving the CST [151].

Steroid-sparing antimetabolite treatment improved macular thickness at 6 and 12 months of initiation, but 50% of the eyes still had persistent UME [152].

Triamcinolone acetonide suspension (TA) delivered as a periocular or intravitreal injection has been used for a long time in treating

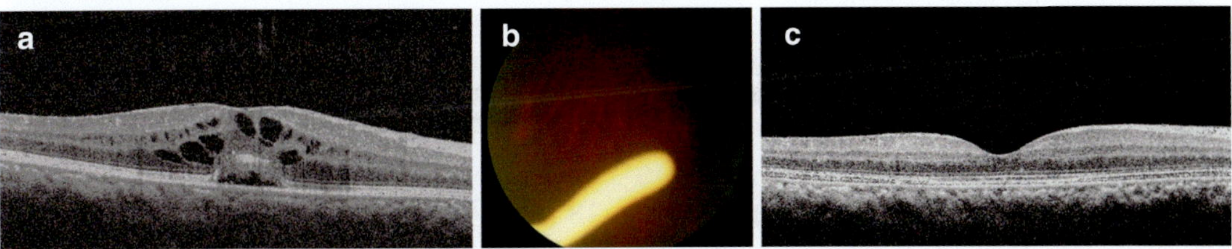

Fig. 11.12 A case of uveitic cystoid macular oedema (**a**). Following an injection of intravitreal dexamethasone implant (**b**), and the macular oedema remains resolved at 3 months (**c**)

UME. Development of ptosis in the former and a rise in intraocular pressure in both techniques have been significant challenges. By 24 months with one or more IVT-TA, the incidence of raised IOP >21 mmHg had increased to ~45% [153]. Fifty-three percent of the eyes had resolution of UME following a single injection of 1 mL of periocular TA (40 mg/mL) at 1 month. More than 40% required repeat injections. Of those which had shown a good initial response, more than 50% of eyes had a recurrence of UME in a median time of 20 weeks. Nearly 16% of eyes developed ptosis, and 59% had IOP rise beyond 22 mm of Hg, half above 30 mm of Hg [154]. While the IVT-TA (4 mg/0.1 mL) was a reasonably safe option to treat UME, half the eyes had persistent UME at the mean follow-up of 18 months. Nearly 20% of eyes had shown cataract progression [155].

In the POINT trial, the head-to-head efficacy of three common strategies to treat UME, namely the posterior subtenon TA, IVT-TA, or IVT Dexa implant, was tested. All eyes showed a reduction in CST. At 8 weeks, the CST reduced from the baseline by 23%, 39%, and 46%, respectively. PST treatment strategy was inferior to both IVT treatment strategies but showed a lower rise in intraocular pressure compared to the IVT groups [156].

11.5.4 Sustained-Release Corticosteroid Implants

Presently, three sustained-release corticosteroid implants are available.

11.5.4.1 Biodegradable Dexamethasone Implant

These include a slow-release biodegradable dexamethasone implant (DEX implant, Ozurdex, Allergan, Inc., Irvine, California) injected into the vitreous cavity through a preloaded 22-gauge syringe. In patients with non-infectious uveitis, it led to a significant reduction in the vitreous haze score. There was a mean reduction of the CST by >90 μm at 8 weeks, but by the end of the study at 26 weeks, the mean reduction was only 50 μm. This study had no significant incidence of cataract formation or rise in IOP [157]. US FDA approved Ozurdex in September 2010 for the treatment of non-infectious uveitis. The Ozurdex was designed to release dexamethasone over 6 months. Still, in practice, the effect did not last that long and required repeated IVT implantation at 3–4 months for sustained effect on control of inflammation. It reportedly controlled inflammation in 72% of the eyes and was considered a valuable adjunct to systemic therapy [158]. 85% of the eyes sustained improvement in VA and decreased CST over the 5-year follow-up. However, 30% of eyes had raised IOP [159].

In refractory UME in both adults and children, the IVT Ozurdex was a safe and effective adjunctive therapy [160].

In a preliminary study, the IVT Ozurdex implant at the time of cataract surgery in uveitis eyes was as effective as oral corticosteroids in preventing any exacerbation of inflammation following surgery [161]. In a prospective controlled study, IVT Ozurdex showed a significant reduction of postoperative flare in uveitis cataract surgery. Nearly 37% of the eyes in the standard of care group developed UME, vs none in the Dexa group [162]. In a meta-analysis of cataract surgery in uveitis, intravitreal therapy (TA or Ozurdex) controlled postoperative inflammation more effectively than systemic anti-inflammatory therapy [163].

11.5.4.2 Non-biodegradable Implants

The two US FDA-approved non-degradable inserts are similar in construct, with the core containing fluocinolone acetonide (FA) 0.18 mg (Yutiq) and 0.19 mg (Iluvien). Both are inserted into the vitreous cavity with a 25-gauge preloaded applicator. The Yutiq implant initially releases FA at 0.25 μg/day and later at 0.2 μg/day for 3 years. The Iluvien insert releases 0.2 μg/day, and the effect also lasts for 3 years. Randomized controlled study data is available only for the Yutiq implant. By the end of 3 years, mean recurrences of uveitis were 1.7 per implant eye vs 5.3 per sham-treated eye. The time to the first recurrence was 657 vs 70.5 days. Nearly 65.5% of the implanted eyes had a recurrence of uveitis versus 97.5% of the sham-treated eyes. The implant effectively resolved UME in 75% of the eyes with UME at the baseline vs 54% in the sham-controlled group. Only 13% of the implanted eyes had persistent UME at the end of 3 years versus 27.3% of the control eyes. However, by 3 years, nearly three-fourth of patients required cataract surgery and 26% required IOP-lowering medications. VA had no loss or gain [164, 165].

11.5.5 Suprachoroidal Injection of Triamcinolone Acetonide Suspension

Suprachoroidal space is a potential space between the sclera and the choroid, a non-immune-privileged site. In recent years, this site has been a favourite route for drug delivery, including gene therapies. Suprachoroidal injection of triamcinolone acetonide (TA) 4 mg/0.1 mL in suspension form is a novel treatment modality and is FDA approved for the treatment of ME (Xipeer®, Clearside Biomedical, Alpharetta, GA, USA). It involves injecting the TA in the superotemporal quadrant 4 mm from the limbus of 0.1 mL of the TA suspension using a micro-needle length varying from 0.9 to 1.1 mm. Suprachoroidal injections of CLS-TA, a suprachoroidal suspension of triamcinolone acetonide, decreased CST by 154 μm compared to 18 μm in the control group. The VA improved ≥15 ETDRS letters in 47% of the patients in the treatment group vs 16% in the sham-treated control group. The treatment-related rise in intraocular pressure or cataract formation was not significantly different in the treatment and the control arms [166]. CLS-TA led to improvement in the CST preceding improvement in VA. Interestingly, the >50 μm improvement in CST at 4 weeks could predict the outcome at 24 weeks [167].

11.5.6 Alternative Strategies to Treat UME

Repeated IVT injections of bevacizumab (1.25 mg/0.1 mL) or TA (4 mg/0.1 mL) were equally effective for persistent UME [168]. In patients with refractory UME, anti-IL-6 receptor, tocilizumab (8 mg/kg body weight), was given as an intravenous infusion over 1 h every 4 weeks for 9 months. This therapy was effective either alone or in addition to the current immunosuppressive therapy. This therapy led to a reduction in CST from a mean of 415 to 259 μm. Sixty percent of the eyes had remission of CME [169]. Other therapies that have been found helpful in refractory uveitis and UME include IVT methotrexate (400 μg/0.1 mL) [170].

11.6 Post-surgical Macular Oedema

Although first suspected on slit-lamp biomicroscopy by Irvine [171], the advent of FFA and later the OCT in clinical practice helped define pathogenesis mechanisms of macular oedema following surgical procedures. Cataract surgery is the most common cause of post-surgery ME (Fig. 11.13). Patients who undergo pars plana vit-

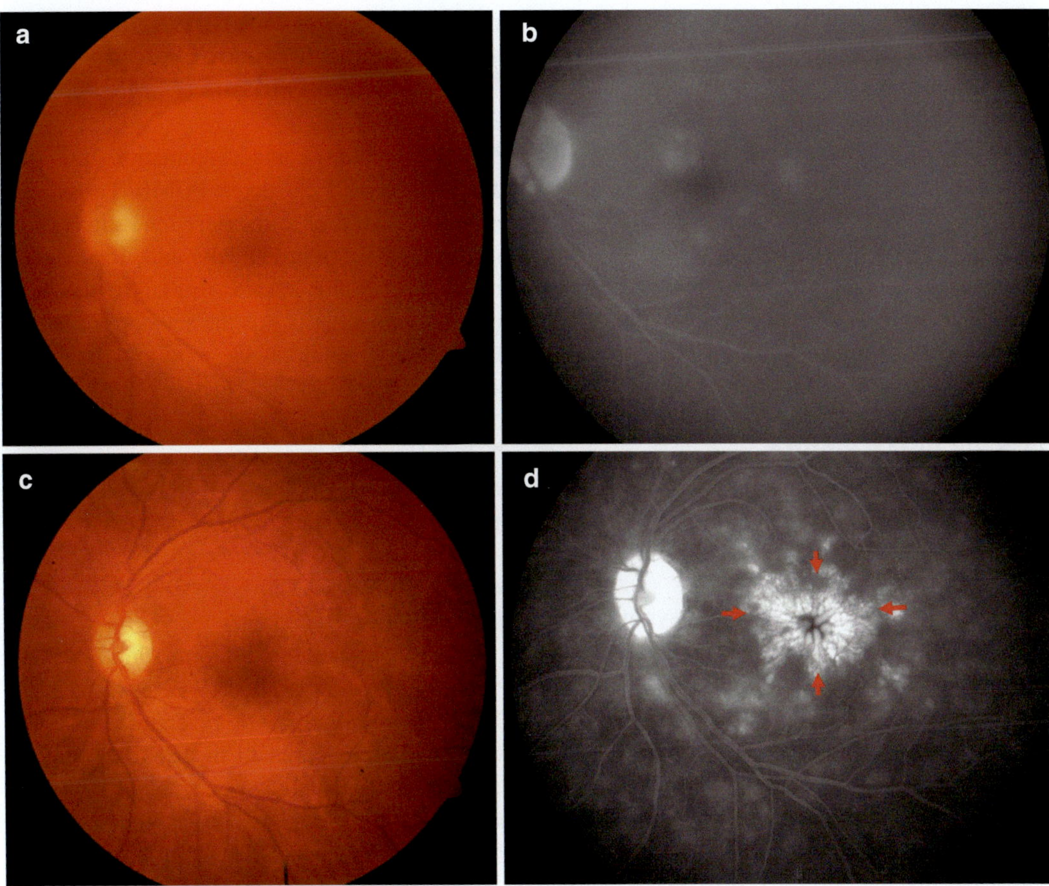

Fig. 11.13 Fundus photograph (**a**) and fluorescein angiography (**b**) showing media haze due to senile cataract. Six weeks following cataract surgery, the media clarity was restored (**c**), but fluorescein angiography showed petaloid pattern (red arrows) of CME (**d**)

reous surgery with or without phacoemulsification have a significantly higher risk of ME than the scleral buckle alone. In more than two-third of the patients, the CME resolved within 12 months of the surgery [172, 173].

11.6.1 Historical Perspective: Role of Vitreous Traction

It was believed that post-surgical vitreoretinal traction on the macula due to vitreous incarceration in the cataract surgery wound resulted in ME. Irvine [171] noted a rupture of the anterior hyaloid face and late adhesions of the cortical vitreous fibres to the cataract wound following uneventful intracapsular cataract surgery. He noted ‘macular degeneration’ in 19% of eyes that did not show any rupture of the anterior vitreous face vs 45% of those with a rupture of the vitreous face. He showed late adhesions of the vitreous strands to the corneal wound [171]. Tolentino and Schepens [174] described the incidence of ME in 1.7% of all cataract surgeries. They found that the area of macular oedema was often larger than the size of the adhesion of vitreous strands to the macula and that spontaneous release of the traction often led to the resolution of the ME. The posterior vitreous face is firmly adherent to the macula and margins of the optic disc. Cataract surgery precipitates a posterior vitreous detachment. However, the vitreous may remain attached to the macula via a thin strand or a broader adhesion [174].

Traction on the macula and the optic disc may cause fluid leakage from the perifoveal capillaries [175]. Based on extensive anatomical and clinical studies of the vitreous anatomy, it was hypothesized that cortical vitreous fibres directly transmit traction on the Muller cells. They also speculated that inflammation or noxious anterior uveal agents might also play an essential role in the pathogenesis of ME [176].

11.6.2 Clinical Picture and Fluorescein Angiography in CME Following Cataract Surgery

The patients typically become symptomatic 4–12 weeks after uneventful cataract surgery. The patients complain of blurring of vision. The visual acuity (VA) may vary from 20/30 to 20/70. Macular oedema associated with VA better than 20/40 is not clinically significant. On biomicroscopic examination, the ME is characterized by an absent foveal reflex, forward bulging of the macula, with a yellowish spot in the fovea. It is surrounded by a few intraretinal cystoid spaces [177]. During FFA, there is leakage of dye from the perifoveal capillaries. The dye accumulates in the cystic spaces in a petaloid pattern. It may take 5–15 min and sometimes up to 30 min in some cases to show the full extent of the CME. The fine retinal vessels stand out as dark lines against the accumulated dye (Fig. 11.13). Using FFA, Gass, and Norton, for the first time, showed that the ME resulted from fluid leakage from the perifoveal retinal capillaries. In the late phases of FFA, dye accumulates in the cystic spaces [177]. The eosinophilic material-filled cystic spaces were found on pathology in Henle's outer plexiform layer and the INL. Contrary to the observation of Tolentino and Schepens [174], Gass did not find any significant vitreous traction on pathological examination of the eyes [177].

11.6.3 Objective Measurement of Pseudophakic Cystoid Macular Oedema (PCME)

Clinical biomicroscopic examination, the FFA and now the OCT can detect PCME. The OCT is a non-invasive tool to measure the retinal thickness accurately, reproducibly, and, importantly, the CST. It yields results similar to the FFA, which, until recently, was the standard of care in diagnosing pseudophakic cystoid macular oedema (PCME) [178]. However, the VA does not always correlate with the measurement of CST. It is fairly common to see a minor increase in the perifoveal thickness [179], which resolves spontaneously. Generally, a 30% increase in CST over the baseline is significant. PCME in the presence of VA >20/40 is generally considered non-significant.

OCTA could help in differentiating DME and PCME. Both show a larger FAZ at the level of DCP, which is significantly reversible in patients with PCME compared to the DME. There are capillary abnormalities and capillary non-perfusion in DME, which is not seen in PCME. Disruptions of the parafoveal capillary network and cystoid spaces in the DCP are seen more frequently in eyes with DME compared to PCME [180]. The OCTA studies have shown decreased vessel density in both the SCP and the DCP in PCME [181].

11.6.4 Incidence and Risk Factor for Post-surgery Macular Oedema

Defining a significant CME (Irvine-Gass) syndrome as a 30% increase in the CST on SD-OCT, the incidence of significant CME was 2.3% following phacoemulsification and non-significant in 6.8%. The major risk factors were diabetes, capsular dehiscence, and the epiretinal membrane [182]. A preexisting epiretinal membrane (ERM) is a risk factor for pseudophakic CME [183]. The ERM should be removed before the cataract surgery rather than afterwards. The former technique improves visual outcomes [184]. Following uneventful phacoemulsification, the development of PCME is not an uncommon cause of visual disturbance. The incidence has varied depending on the technique of cataract surgery, the post-surgery interval, the type of intraocular lens implant, and the technique used to diagnose [185]. The visual acuity may or may not be significantly affected. Preexisting uveitis, ERM, retinal vascular occlusion, post-retinal detachment surgery eyes, or posterior capsular dehiscence with or without vitreous loss during surgery increases the risk of CME [186].

Patients with DM, especially those with NPDR, are at a higher risk of developing PCME. In one of the largest real-world series of nearly 82,000 consecutive cataract surgeries, the incidence of PCME in uneventful cataract surgery without any other predisposing factor was 1.17% and was significantly higher at 1.56% in eyes with at least one risk factor other than DM. Nearly 4% of patients with DM developed PCME, irrespective of the presence or absence of diabetic retinopathy [187].

The risk and severity of oedema increased with the increasing severity of diabetic retinopathy [187]. These patients should receive non-steroidal anti-inflammatory agents (NSAIDs) starting before cataract surgery and continuing for several weeks. Those with DME should also receive preoperative IVT anti-VEGF or corticosteroid treatment before cataract surgery.

11.6.5 Role of Inflammatory Mediators and Prostaglandins in Surgical Trauma

Any traumatic event, including surgical trauma, is followed hours later by the initiation of the process of wound healing. Inflammation is an integral part of this process. It involves releasing and recruiting many inflammatory cells, namely platelets, neutrophils, and monocytes, and their activation into macrophages and fibroblasts. Several inflammatory mediators, such as chemokines, cytokines, and growth factors, are generated. Arachidonic acid, a fatty acid, is released from the cell plasma membrane by phospholipase. The arachidonic acid is metabolized by the cyclooxygenase (COX) to generate prostaglandins. The prostaglandins are generated even before the recruitment of the inflammatory cells into the wound. The level of prostaglandins is low in healthy tissues but increases immediately following trauma, even before the recruitment of the leukocytes. PGE_2 is the primary prostaglandin involved in inflammation. In cataract surgery, the prostaglandins are released from the iris and the lens epithelium [188]. The primary function of prostaglandins is to increase blood flow and vascular endothelial permeability through their action on histamine. Applying topical prostaglandins was shown to cause the breakdown of the blood-aqueous barrier and cause miosis of the pupil [189]. The prostaglandins are much smaller molecules, quickly diffuse into tissues, and find receptors on practically all tissues in the eye.

Once they diffuse into the vitreous cavity and reach the retina, prostaglandins cause the breakdown of the blood-retinal barrier, resulting in fluid leakage in the OPL and the INL [188]. Non-steroidal anti-inflammatory agents block the action of COX-1 and COX-2 and thus prevent the generation of prostaglandins [190, 191]. Apart from the prostaglandins, other mediators of inflammation may also play a significant role in the formation of CME. In a mouse model of extracapsular lens extraction, IL-1β and chemokine CCL2 were upregulated in the retina, and the complement pathway was activated within 30 min of the surgery. The IL-1β is known to cause the breakdown of the blood-retinal barrier. Both are acute innate immune responses to injury and may play a role in the PCME [192].

11.6.6 Pathogenesis and Prevention of PCME

A better understanding of the pathogenesis of inflammation and the mechanism of wound healing has led to a constant evolution of the surgical techniques in cataract surgery from intracapsular surgery with almost 15 mm scleral incision to extracapsular surgery (ECCE) to progressively smaller self-sealing clear corneal incision, phacoemulsification, and placement of the intraocular lens implants within the capsular bag. The degree of inflammation leading to a breakdown of the blood-retinal barrier and the release of proteinaceous fluid into the anterior chamber can be objectively measured using the laser flare metre. Compared to the ECCE, the flare levels in phacoemulsification were low and lasted for a significantly shorter time [193]. Likewise, clear corneal incisions in phacoemulsification produced much lower flare levels than the conventional corneoscleral incisions [194]. Even in patients with DM, phacoemulsification led to lower inflammation than ECCE in the opposite eye [195]. In a prospective controlled trial, patients preoperatively received three instillations of eye drops of either ketorolac 0.45%, fluorometholone 0.1% (FML), or a combination of ketorolac and FML or no eye drops. In the aqueous samples obtained during surgery, the IL-6 and the TNF-α values were similar in all four groups. The IL-8 levels were low in eyes receiving FML alone or in combination with ketorolac. Likewise, the PGE_2 levels were low in eyes receiving ketorolac alone or in combination with FML but not in eyes receiving FML or the control group establishing the role of topical NSAID in blocking PGE_2. Notably, immediately after the Femto laser application in Femto laser-assisted cataract surgery, there was a significant rise in the PGE_2 levels in the aqueous humour [196]. A systematic review and meta-analysis of randomized controlled trials have shown that in both diabetic and non-diabetic populations, compared to topical steroids, topical NSAIDs are more effective in preventing the onset of PCME after cataract surgery. Adding either the TA or anti-VEGF agents to the topical NSAIDs was no additional benefit, which remains the standard of care in preventing PCME [197]. Another topical NSAID agent, bromfenac, decreased postoperative inflammation and CME [198]. Topical use of nepafenac, another NSAID, in the perioperative period was highly effective in preventing PCME in patients with DR [199]. In two large parallel, randomized vehicle-controlled trials of cataract surgery in patients with diabetic retinopathy, a significant increase in CST (>30% increase over baseline) was seen in 4% with the use of nepafenac vs 16% in the control group [200].

11.6.7 Treatment of PCME

Most PCMEs resolve with the continuation of the topical NSAID within 3 months of the surgery. However, PCME that persists beyond 6 months is unlikely to resolve spontaneously. These patients need intervention beyond a topical NSAID. Posterior subtenon placement of a single injection of TA 40 mg/mL through a conjunctival peritomy is an effective treatment modality for PCME. It led to the resolution of PCME in 90% of the eyes [201]. As discussed above, patients with DM have a higher risk of developing PCME, which usually does not resolve spontaneously and needs definitive interventions in the form of corticosteroids, which can be prophylactically administered at the time of surgery to thwart the development of PCME. In the postoperative period, the PCME and the progression of diabetic retinopathy may overlap, emanating from an exaggeration of downstream inflammatory pathways. The IVT injection of TA 4 mg at the time of cataract surgery in patients with DM resulted in a significant reduction in CST and improved visual outcomes [202, 203]. Similar results were obtained with the DEXA implant used during surgery [94, 204]. The Dexa implant's effect lasts at least 3 months [205]. Since the PCME majorly results from an inflammatory pathway, the IVT inj of Lucentis, an anti-VEGF agent, given simultaneously with cataract surgery in DME eyes, showed no appreciable difference [206]. However, IVT injections of 1.25 mg of bevacizumab and 2 mg of TA effectively reduced the CST and improved VA 3 months after surgery [207].

11.7 Macular Oedema in Vitreoretinal Traction

The FFA, in a majority of such cases, fails to demonstrate any fluid leakage. However, the thickened retina can be easily diagnosed on OCT. Mechanical traction on the macula in vitreomacular traction disorders such as epiretinal membranes, impending macular holes, diabetic traction maculopathy, and

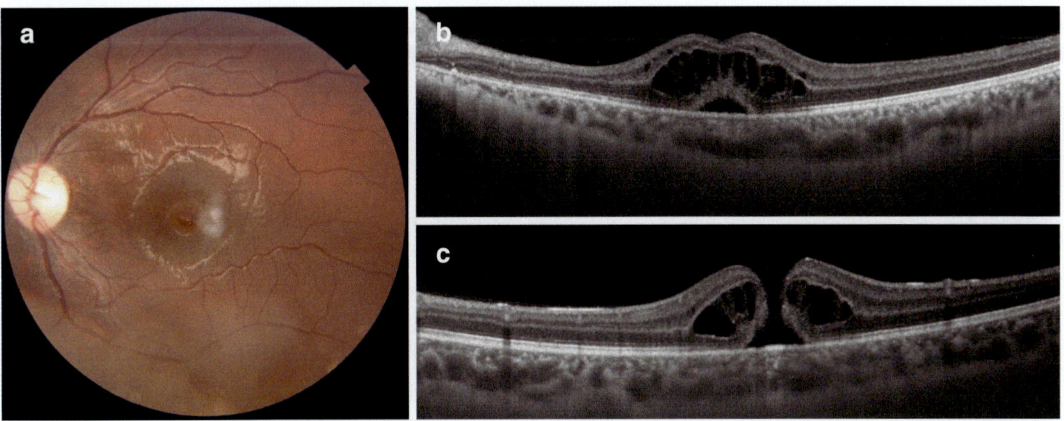

Fig. 11.14 Optic disc pallor and macular oedema in a 16-year-old man who had trauma to left eye by a ball 3 months ago (**a**). OCT showed cystoid macular oedema (**b**) with a macular hole (**c**)

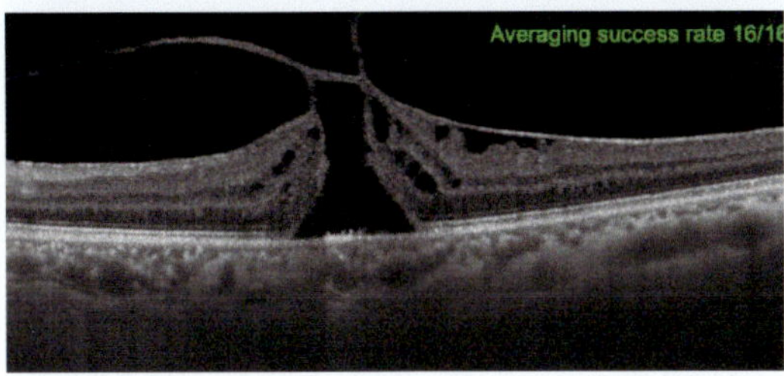

Fig. 11.15 Macular oedema caused by vitreomacular traction

myopic foveoschisis also leads to cystic changes in the macula [21] (Figs. 11.14 and 11.15). The foveal cysts may disappear on the spontaneous release of the vitreoretinal traction or require surgical intervention. In some cases, leakage from the retinal capillaries may also occur.

11.8 Macular Cystic Changes in Inherited Macular Dystrophies

Intracellular fluid accumulation may also be seen in many inherited retinal diseases, especially retinitis pigmentosa (RP). Nearly 20–50% of autosomal dominant or recessive RP patients may show cystic cavities in the inner nuclear layer. Some of these patients may show retinal capillary leakage. Topical dorzolamide or oral acetazolamide reverses macular oedema with improvement in central vision. Interestingly, cystic cavities are not seen in the X-linked RP. In autosomal recessive bestrophinopathies, there is a collection of hyperautofluorescent vitelliform material and subretinal fluid. In X-linked foveoschisis, schisis cavities are seen in the inner nuclear layer. Patients with enhanced S-cone syndrome, a rare autosomal recessive disorder, present with night blindness due to loss of rod photoreceptors, foveomacular schisis (Fig. 11.16), yellow-white dots, and torpedo-like lesions [208]. More than 50% of patients with X-linked choroideremia show topical dorzolamide-responsive cystoid macular oedema in the outer plexiform and inner nuclear layers [209]. For more detailed information on the rare inherited macular disorders that present with cystic changes in the macula, the readers may refer to recent reviews [21, 22].

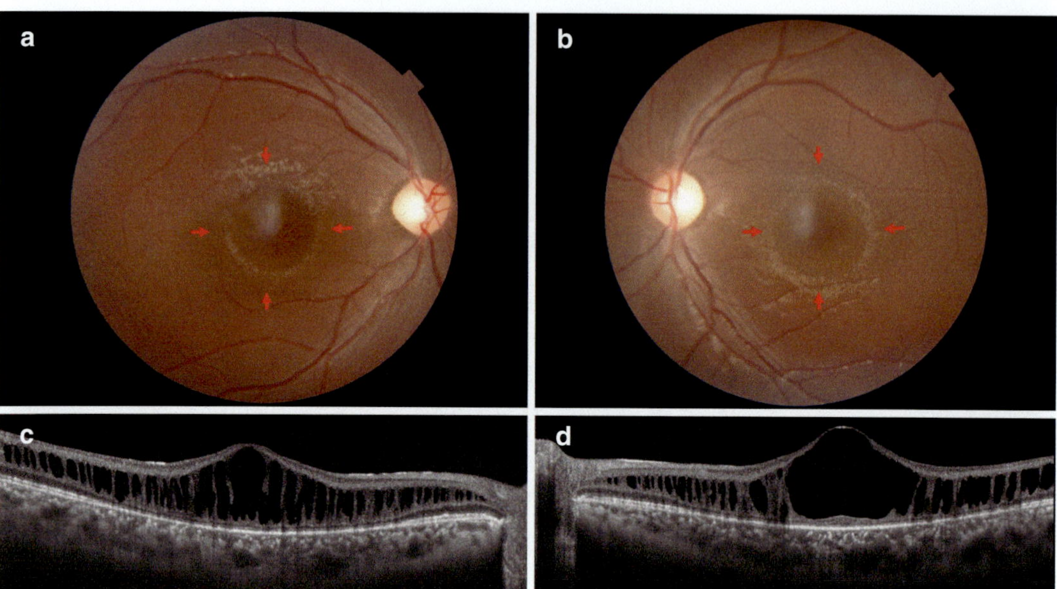

Fig. 11.16 Spoke-wheel pattern (red arrows) of macular oedema in a 12-year-old boy with X-linked retinoschisis, which is bilaterally symmetrical (**a**, **b**). OCT shows schisis cavities in the inner nuclear layer in both eyes (**c**, **d**)

11.9 Drug-Induced Macular Oedema

The retinal thickness increases most commonly because of the breakdown of the retinal barriers with the extravasation of fluid from the retinal vessels. This fluid accumulates in the extracellular spaces, and the macular thickening represents the outcome of total ingress and egress of the fluid. The fluid is mainly removed from the inner retinal layer through the retinal Muller glial (RMG) cells and from the outer retinal layers by an active metabolic pump in the RPE. High oncotic pressure in the choroid facilitates fluid movement from the vitreous across the retina and RPE. Fluid leakage from the vessels can be seen on FFA. The RMG end feet and microglia processes in the inner retina form intimate contact with the neuronal cells, the capillary endothelial cells, and the pericytes. This neuro-vascular glial unit is responsible for maintaining normal homeostasis in the retina. It allows transcellular transportation of nutrients and oxygen to the retinal cells without going through the interstitial or extracellular space [21]. The fluid generated from the retina's normal cellular metabolism exits via the RMG. Insult to the K^+ channels in the RMG cell's end feet may cause a reversal of fluid flow from the blood into the RMG, bringing about swelling of the RMG and formation of cystic spaces [210]. The toxic effects of several drugs may lead to intracellular accumulation of fluid, causing the thickness of the retina, especially the macula, which creates cystic spaces [21, 211].

In hormone receptor-positive breast carcinoma, which accounts for nearly third-fourth of all such patients, the foveal cystic changes on OCT are estimated to occur in 12% of all who received tamoxifen. This incidence is much higher than earlier believed [212]. The changes in the fovea are similar to the Mac Tel type 2, suggesting tamoxifen toxicity to RMG cells [213]. Several other drugs, including Niacin (used for dyslipidaemia), Paclitaxel, and Docetaxel (anticancer drugs), are also toxic to the retinal Muller cells. The fluorescein angiogram in these patients shows no capillary leak, thus labelled as nonvasogenic maculopathy. The macular oedema in these patients can only be seen on

OCT. Discontinuation of the drug or using acetazolamide may reverse the CME in some patients.

Hydroxychloroquine (HCQ) is often prescribed to patients with autoimmune disorders, rheumatoid arthritis, and systemic lupus erythematosus as an immunomodulatory drug. HCQ toxicity has varied from 1.5% to 10% [214]. Patients with HCQ toxicity may have ethnic differences, the white Caucasians showing more perifoveal and Asians showing a more peripheral pericentral distribution of changes in the loss of the photoreceptors. A wide-angle volume OCT scan was recommended not to miss more peripheral lesions of HCQ toxicity [215]. Cystic changes may occur in HCQ toxicity even after drug withdrawal [216, 217]. Occasionally, late stages of HCQ toxicity may present as macular oedema and show vessel leakage. Such patients may respond to oral acetazolamide [216].

Fingolimod used in remitting-relapsing multiple sclerosis may cause cystoid macular oedema within months. It is an immunomodulatory drug. It significantly reduces the relapse rates of multiple sclerosis. It is US FDA-approved for MS. In the controlled trials, 1.6% of those receiving 1.25 mg/day developed macular oedema, but none developed ME at a lower dose of 0.5 mg/day. It appears to have dose-dependent toxicity. It is recommended that patients undergo a baseline ophthalmological examination and again after 3–4 months, at 6 months, and 1 yearly after that [211, 218]. The oedema is reversible once the drug is stopped [219].

After many years of use for interstitial cystitis, pentosan polysulphate sodium used may cause cystoid macular oedema, areas of complete RPE, and outer retinal atrophy and needs to be differentiated from geographic atrophy seen in AMD. The area of atrophy may progress even after stopping the drug [220].

There are many anecdotal reports of the development of ME following the use of imatinib for chronic myeloid leukaemia, leflunomide for rheumatoid arthritis, rifabutin for Mycobacterium avium complex lung disease, and rituximab for polyangiitis with granulomatous [211].

References

1. Omri S, Omri B, Savoldelli M, Jonet L, Thillaye-Goldenberg B, Thuret G, Gain P, Jeanny JC, Crisanti P, Behar-Cohen F. The outer limiting membrane (OLM) revisited: clinical implications. Clin Ophthalmol. 2010;4:183–95. https://doi.org/10.2147/opth.s5901.
2. Daruich A, Matet A, Moulin A, Kowalczuk L, Nicolas M, Sellam A, Rothschild PR, Omri S, Gélizé E, Jonet L, Delaunay K, De Kozak Y, Berdugo M, Zhao M, Crisanti P, Behar-Cohen F. Mechanisms of macular edema: beyond the surface. Prog Retin Eye Res. 2018;63:20–68. https://doi.org/10.1016/j.preteyeres.2017.10.006. Epub 2017 Nov 7.
3. Jayaram H, Jones MF, Eastlake K, Cottrill PB, Becker S, Wiseman J, Khaw PT, Limb GA. Transplantation of photoreceptors derived from human Muller glia restore rod function in the P23H rat. Stem Cells Transl Med. 2014;3(3):323–33. https://doi.org/10.5966/sctm.2013-0112. Epub 2014 Jan 29.
4. El-Bayadi G. New method of slit-lamp micro-ophthalmoscopy. Br J Ophthalmol. 1953;37(10):625–8. https://doi.org/10.1136/bjo.37.10.625.
5. Schmidt TA. On slit-lamp microscopy. Doc Ophthalmol. 1975;39(1):117–53. https://doi.org/10.1007/BF00578760.
6. Early Treatment Diabetic Retinopathy Study Research Group. Grading diabetic retinopathy from stereoscopic color fundus photographs—an extension of the modified Airlie House classification. ETDRS report number 10. Early Treatment Diabetic Retinopathy Study Research Group. Ophthalmology. 1991;98(5 Suppl):786–806.
7. Virgili G, Menchini F, Dimastrogiovanni AF, Rapizzi E, Menchini U, Bandello F, Chiodini RG. Optical coherence tomography versus stereoscopic fundus photography or biomicroscopy for diagnosing diabetic macular edema: a systematic review. Invest Ophthalmol Vis Sci. 2007;48(11):4963–73. https://doi.org/10.1167/iovs.06-1472.
8. Dollery CT, Hodge JV, Engel M. Studies of the retinal circulation with fluorescein. Br Med J. 1962;2(5314):1210–5. https://doi.org/10.1136/bmj.2.5314.1210.
9. Novotny HR, Alvis DL. A method of photographing fluorescence in circulating blood in the human retina. Circulation. 1961;24:82–6. https://doi.org/10.1161/01.cir.24.1.82.
10. Marcus DF, Bovino JA, Williams D. Adverse reactions during intravenous fluorescein angiography. Arch Ophthalmol. 1984;102(6):825. https://doi.org/10.1001/archopht.1984.01040030651010.
11. Kwiterovich KA, Maguire MG, Murphy RP, Schachat AP, Bressler NM, Bressler SB, Fine SL. Frequency of adverse systemic reactions after fluorescein angiography. Results of a prospective

study. Ophthalmology. 1991;98(7):1139–42. https://doi.org/10.1016/s0161-6420(91)32165-1.
12. Huang D, Swanson EA, Lin CP, Schuman JS, Stinson WG, Chang W, Hee MR, Flotte T, Gregory K, Puliafito CA, et al. Optical coherence tomography. Science. 1991;254(5035):1178–81. https://doi.org/10.1126/science.1957169.
13. Tan CS, Ngo WK, Cheong KX. Comparison of choroidal thicknesses using swept source and spectral domain optical coherence tomography in diseased and normal eyes. Br J Ophthalmol. 2015;99(3):354–8. https://doi.org/10.1136/bjophthalmol--2014-305331. Epub 2014 Oct 1.
14. Tan CS, Sadda SVR. Swept-source optical coherence tomography. In: Meyer CH, Saxena S, Sadda SR, editors. Spectral domain optical coherence tomography in macular diseases. New Delhi: Springer; 2017. p. 59–77.
15. Wong KH, Tham YC, Nguyen DQ, Dai W, Tan NYQ, Mathijia S, Neelam K, Cheung CY, Sabanayagam C, Schmetterer L, Wong TY, Cheng CY. Racial differences and determinants of macular thickness profiles in multiethnic Asian population: the Singapore Epidemiology of Eye Diseases Study. Br J Ophthalmol. 2019;103(7):894–9. https://doi.org/10.1136/bjophthalmol-2018-312447. Epub 2018 Aug 10.
16. Duan XR, Liang YB, Friedman DS, Sun LP, Wong TY, Tao QS, Bao L, Wang NL, Wang JJ. Normal macular thickness measurements using optical coherence tomography in healthy eyes of adult Chinese persons: the Handan Eye Study. Ophthalmology. 2010;117(8):1585–94. https://doi.org/10.1016/j.ophtha.2009.12.036. Epub 2010 May 15.
17. Kakinoki M, Sawada O, Sawada T, Kawamura H, Ohji M. Comparison of macular thickness between cirrus HD-OCT and stratus OCT. Ophthalmic Surg Lasers Imaging. 2009;40(2):135–40. https://doi.org/10.3928/15428877-20090301-09.
18. Wu J, Lin C, Du Y, Fan SJ, Pan L, Pan Q, Cao K, Wang N. Macular thickness and its associated factors in a Chinese rural adult population: the Handan Eye Study. Br J Ophthalmol. 2022; https://doi.org/10.1136/bjo-2022-321766. Epub ahead of print.
19. Wang Q, Wei WB, Wang YX, Yan YN, Yang JY, Zhou WJ, Chan SY, Xu L, Jonas JB. Thickness of individual layers at the macula and associated factors: the Beijing Eye Study 2011. BMC Ophthalmol. 2020;20(1):49. https://doi.org/10.1186/s12886-019-1296-6.
20. Invernizzi A, Pellegrini M, Acquistapace A, Benatti E, Erba S, Cozzi M, Cigada M, Viola F, Gillies M, Staurenghi G. Normative data for retinal-layer thickness maps generated by spectral-domain OCT in a white population. Ophthalmol Retina. 2018;2(8):808–815.e1. https://doi.org/10.1016/j.oret.2017.12.012. Epub 2018 Feb 6.
21. Gaudric A, Audo I, Vignal C, Couturier A, Boulanger-Scemama É, Tadayoni R, Cohen SY. Non-vasogenic cystoid maculopathies. Prog Retin Eye Res. 2022;91:101092. https://doi.org/10.1016/j.preteyeres.2022.101092. Epub 2022 Aug 1.
22. Naseripour M, Hemmati S, Chaibakhsh S, Gordiz A, Miri L, Abdi F. Cystoid macular oedema without leakage in fluorescein angiography: a literature review. Eye (Lond). 2022;37:1519. https://doi.org/10.1038/s41433-022-02230-z. Epub ahead of print.
23. International Diabetes Federation. IDF diabetes atlas. 10th ed. Brussels: International Diabetes Federation; 2021.
24. Yau JW, Rogers SL, Kawasaki R, Lamoureux EL, Kowalski JW, Bek T, Chen SJ, Dekker JM, Fletcher A, Grauslund J, Haffner S, Hamman RF, Ikram MK, Kayama T, Klein BE, Klein R, Krishnaiah S, Mayurasakorn K, O'Hare JP, Orchard TJ, Porta M, Rema M, Roy MS, Sharma T, Shaw J, Taylor H, Tielsch JM, Varma R, Wang JJ, Wang N, West S, Xu L, Yasuda M, Zhang X, Mitchell P, Wong TY, Meta-Analysis for Eye Disease (META-EYE) Study Group. Global prevalence and major risk factors of diabetic retinopathy. Diabetes Care. 2012;35(3):556–64. https://doi.org/10.2337/dc11--1909. Epub 2012 Feb 1.
25. Roy S, Kim D. Retinal capillary basement membrane thickening: role in the pathogenesis of diabetic retinopathy. Prog Retin Eye Res. 2021;82:100903. https://doi.org/10.1016/j.preteyeres.2020.100903. Epub 2020 Sep 18.
26. Beltramo E, Buttiglieri S, Pomero F, Allione A, D'Alù F, Ponte E, Porta M. A study of capillary pericyte viability on extracellular matrix produced by endothelial cells in high glucose. Diabetologia. 2003;46(3):409–15.https://doi.org/10.1007/s00125--003-1043-6. Epub 2003 Feb 26.
27. Beltramo E, Pomero F, Allione A, D'Alù F, Ponte E, Porta M. Pericyte adhesion is impaired on extracellular matrix produced by endothelial cells in high hexose concentrations. Diabetologia. 2002;45(3):416–9. https://doi.org/10.1007/s00125-001-0761-x.
28. Lechner J, O'Leary OE, Stitt AW. The pathology associated with diabetic retinopathy. Vis Res. 2017;139:7–14. https://doi.org/10.1016/j.visres.2017.04.003. Epub 2017 Apr 29.
29. Rodrigues M, Xin X, Jee K, Babapoor-Farrokhran S, Kashiwabuchi F, Ma T, Bhutto I, Hassan SJ, Daoud Y, Baranano D, Solomon S, Lutty G, Semenza GL, Montaner S, Sodhi A. VEGF secreted by hypoxic Müller cells induces MMP-2 expression and activity in endothelial cells to promote retinal neovascularization in proliferative diabetic retinopathy. Diabetes. 2013;62(11):3863–73. https://doi.org/10.2337/db13-0014. Epub 2013 Jul 24.
30. Trost A, Lange S, Schroedl F, Bruckner D, Motloch KA, Bogner B, Kaser-Eichberger A, Strohmaier C, Runge C, Aigner L, Rivera FJ, Reitsamer HA. Brain and retinal Pericytes: origin, function and role. Front Cell Neurosci. 2016;10:20. https://doi.org/10.3389/fncel.2016.00020.

31. Frank RN, Turczyn TJ, Das A. Pericyte coverage of retinal and cerebral capillaries. Invest Ophthalmol Vis Sci. 1990;31(6):999–1007.
32. Cubbon RM, Ali N, Sengupta A, Kearney MT. Insulin- and growth factor-resistance impairs vascular regeneration in diabetes mellitus. Curr Vasc Pharmacol. 2012;10(3):271–84. https://doi.org/10.2174/157016112799959305.
33. Stitt AW, Curtis TM, Chen M, Medina RJ, McKay GJ, Jenkins A, Gardiner TA, Lyons TJ, Hammes HP, Simó R, Lois N. The progress in understanding and treatment of diabetic retinopathy. Prog Retin Eye Res. 2016;51:156–86. https://doi.org/10.1016/j.preteyeres.2015.08.001. Epub 2015 Aug 18.
34. Aiello LP, Gardner TW, King GL, Blankenship G, Cavallerano JD, Ferris FL 3rd, Klein R. Diabetic retinopathy. Diabetes Care. 1998;21(1):143–56. https://doi.org/10.2337/diacare.21.1.143.
35. Browning DJ, Altaweel MM, Bressler NM, Bressler SB, Scott IU, Diabetic Retinopathy Clinical Research Network. Diabetic macular edema: what is focal and what is diffuse? Am J Ophthalmol. 2008;146(5):649–55, 655.e1–6. https://doi.org/10.1016/j.ajo.2008.07.013. Epub 2008 Sep 5.
36. Colucciello M. Vision loss due to macular edema induced by rosiglitazone treatment of diabetes mellitus. Arch Ophthalmol. 2005;123(9):1273–5. https://doi.org/10.1001/archopht.123.9.1273.
37. Fong DS, Contreras R. Glitazone use associated with diabetic macular edema. Am J Ophthalmol. 2009;147(4):583–586.e1. https://doi.org/10.1016/j.ajo.2008.10.016. Epub 2009 Feb 1.
38. Yao J, Peng Q, Li Y, Liang A, Xie J, Zhuang X, Chen R, Chen Y, Wang Z, Zhang L, Cao D. Clinical relevance of body fluid volume status in diabetic patients with macular edema. Front Med (Lausanne). 2022;9:857532. https://doi.org/10.3389/fmed.2022.857532.
39. Early Treatment Diabetic Retinopathy Study Research Group. Photocoagulation for diabetic macular edema. Early Treatment Diabetic Retinopathy Study report number 1. Arch Ophthalmol. 1985;103(12):1796–806.
40. Chalam KV, Bressler SB, Edwards AR, Berger BB, Bressler NM, Glassman AR, Grover S, Gupta SK, Nielsen JS, Diabetic Retinopathy Clinical Research Network. Retinal thickness in people with diabetes and minimal or no diabetic retinopathy: Heidelberg Spectralis optical coherence tomography. Invest Ophthalmol Vis Sci. 2012;53(13):8154–61. https://doi.org/10.1167/iovs.12-10290.
41. Glassman AR, Beck RW, Browning DJ, Danis RP, Kollman C, Diabetic Retinopathy Clinical Research Network Study Group. Comparison of optical coherence tomography in diabetic macular edema, with and without reading center manual grading from a clinical trials perspective. Invest Ophthalmol Vis Sci. 2009;50(2):560–6. https://doi.org/10.1167/iovs.08-1881. Epub 2008 Jun 19.
42. Munk MR, Somfai GM, de Smet MD, Donati G, Menke MN, Garweg JG, Ceklic L. The role of intravitreal corticosteroids in the treatment of DME: predictive OCT biomarkers. Int J Mol Sci. 2022;23(14):7585. https://doi.org/10.3390/ijms23147585.
43. Sun JK, Lin MM, Lammer J, Prager S, Sarangi R, Silva PS, Aiello LP. Disorganization of the retinal inner layers as a predictor of visual acuity in eyes with center-involved diabetic macular edema. JAMA Ophthalmol. 2014;132(11):1309–16. https://doi.org/10.1001/jamaophthalmol.2014.2350.
44. Moein HR, Novais EA, Rebhun CB, Cole ED, Louzada RN, Witkin AJ, Baumal CR, Duker JS, Waheed NK. Optical coherence tomography angiography to detect macular capillary ischemia in patients with inner retinal changes after resolved diabetic macular edema. Retina. 2018;38(12):2277–84. https://doi.org/10.1097/IAE.0000000000001902.
45. Fragiotta S, Abdolrahimzadeh S, Dolz-Marco R, Sakurada Y, Gal-Or O, Scuderi G. Significance of hyperreflective foci as an optical coherence tomography biomarker in retinal diseases: characterization and clinical implications. J Ophthalmol. 2021;2021:6096017. https://doi.org/10.1155/2021/6096017.
46. Bolz M, Schmidt-Erfurth U, Deak G, Mylonas G, Kriechbaum K, Scholda C, Diabetic Retinopathy Research Group Vienna. Optical coherence tomographic hyperreflective foci: a morphologic sign of lipid extravasation in diabetic macular edema. Ophthalmology. 2009;116(5):914–20. https://doi.org/10.1016/j.ophtha.2008.12.039.
47. Arrigo A, Capone L, Lattanzio R, Aragona E, Zollet P, Bandello F. Optical coherence tomography biomarkers of inflammation in diabetic macular edema treated by fluocinolone acetonide intravitreal drug-delivery system implant. Ophthalmol Ther. 2020;9(4):971–80. https://doi.org/10.1007/s40123--020-00297-z. Epub 2020 Sep 10.
48. Shin YU, Hong EH, Lim HW, Kang MH, Seong M, Cho H. Quantitative evaluation of hard exudates in diabetic macular edema after short-term intravitreal triamcinolone, dexamethasone implant or bevacizumab injections. BMC Ophthalmol. 2017;17(1):182. https://doi.org/10.1186/s12886-017-0578-0.
49. Hsieh YT, Alam MN, Le D, Hsiao CC, Yang CH, Chao DL, Yao X. OCT angiography biomarkers for predicting visual outcomes after ranibizumab treatment for diabetic macular edema. Ophthalmol Retina. 2019;3(10):826–34. https://doi.org/10.1016/j.oret.2019.04.027. Epub 2019 May 7.
50. Podkowinski D, Beka S, Mursch-Edlmayr AS, Strauss RW, Fischer L, Bolz M. A swept source optical coherence tomography angiography study: imaging artifacts and comparison of non-perfusion areas with fluorescein angiography in diabetic macular edema. PLoS One. 2021;16(4):e0249918. https://doi.org/10.1371/journal.pone.0249918.

51. Maltsev DS, Kulikov AN, Kazak AA, Freund KB. Suspended scattering particles in motion may influence optical coherence tomography angiography vessel density metrics in eyes with diabetic macular edema. Retina. 2021;41(6):1259–64. https://doi.org/10.1097/IAE.0000000000003016.
52. Lee J, Moon BG, Cho AR, Yoon YH. Optical coherence tomography angiography of DME and its association with anti-VEGF treatment response. Ophthalmology. 2016;123(11):2368–75. https://doi.org/10.1016/j.ophtha.2016.07.010. Epub 2016 Sep 6.
53. Couturier A, Rey PA, Erginay A, Lavia C, Bonnin S, Dupas B, Gaudric A, Tadayoni R. Widefield OCT-angiography and fluorescein angiography assessments of nonperfusion in diabetic retinopathy and edema treated with anti-vascular endothelial growth factor. Ophthalmology. 2019;126(12):1685–94. https://doi.org/10.1016/j.ophtha.2019.06.022. Epub 2019 Jun 26.
54. Brambati M, Borrelli E, Capone L, Querques L, Sacconi R, Battista M, Bandello F, Querques G. Changes in macular perfusion after ILUVIEN® intravitreal implant for diabetic macular edema: An OCTA study. Ophthalmol Ther. 2022;11(2):653–60. https://doi.org/10.1007/s40123-022-00455-5. Epub 2022 Jan 28.
55. Song J, Huang BB, Ong JX, Konopek N, Fawzi AA. Hemodynamic effects of anti-vascular endothelial growth factor injections on optical coherence tomography angiography in diabetic macular edema eyes. Transl Vis Sci Technol. 2022;11(10):5. https://doi.org/10.1167/tvst.11.10.5.
56. Ferrara N, Henzel WJ. Pituitary follicular cells secrete a novel heparin-binding growth factor specific for vascular endothelial cells. Biochem Biophys Res Commun. 1989;161(2):851–8. https://doi.org/10.1016/0006-291x(89)92678-8.
57. Ferrara N. From the discovery of vascular endothelial growth factor to the introduction of avastin in clinical trials—an interview with Napoleone Ferrara by Domenico Ribatti. Int J Dev Biol. 2011;55(4–5):383–8. https://doi.org/10.1387/ijdb.103216dr.
58. Qaum T, Xu Q, Joussen AM, Clemens MW, Qin W, Miyamoto K, Hassessian H, Wiegand SJ, Rudge J, Yancopoulos GD, Adamis AP. VEGF-initiated blood-retinal barrier breakdown in early diabetes. Invest Ophthalmol Vis Sci. 2001;42(10):2408–13.
59. Lu M, Perez VL, Ma N, Miyamoto K, Peng HB, Liao JK, Adamis AP. VEGF increases retinal vascular ICAM-1 expression in vivo. Invest Ophthalmol Vis Sci. 1999;40(8):1808–12.
60. Funatsu H, Noma H, Mimura T, Eguchi S, Hori S. Association of vitreous inflammatory factors with diabetic macular edema. Ophthalmology. 2009;116(1):73–9. https://doi.org/10.1016/j.ophtha.2008.09.037.
61. Funatsu H, Yamashita H, Ikeda T, Mimura T, Eguchi S, Hori S. Vitreous levels of interleukin-6 and vascular endothelial growth factor are related to diabetic macular edema. Ophthalmology. 2003;110(9):1690–6. https://doi.org/10.1016/S0161-6420(03)00568-2.
62. Flaxel CJ, Adelman RA, Bailey ST, Fawzi A, Lim JI, Vemulakonda GA, Ying GS. Diabetic retinopathy preferred practice pattern®. Ophthalmology. 2020;127(1):P66–P145. https://doi.org/10.1016/j.ophtha.2019.09.025. Epub 2019 Sep 25. Erratum in: Ophthalmology. 2020;127(9):1279.
63. Baker CW, Glassman AR, Beaulieu WT, Antoszyk AN, Browning DJ, Chalam KV, Grover S, Jampol LM, Jhaveri CD, Melia M, Stockdale CR, Martin DF, Sun JK, DRCR Retina Network. Effect of initial management with aflibercept vs laser photocoagulation vs observation on vision loss among patients with diabetic macular edema involving the center of the macula and good visual acuity: a randomized clinical trial. JAMA. 2019;321(19):1880–94. https://doi.org/10.1001/jama.2019.5790.
64. Peto T, Chakravarthy U. New findings from diabetic retinopathy clinical research retina network protocol V confirm a role for focal laser photocoagulation or observation for eyes with center-involved diabetic macular edema and good visual acuity: new is not always best. JAMA Ophthalmol. 2019;137(7):838–9. https://doi.org/10.1001/jamaophthalmol.2019.1876.
65. Chew EY. Patients with good vision and diabetic macular edema involving the center of the macula: to treat or not to treat? JAMA. 2019;321(19):1873–5. https://doi.org/10.1001/jama.2019.5793.
66. Mitchell P, Bandello F, Schmidt-Erfurth U, Lang GE, Massin P, Schlingemann RO, Sutter F, Simader C, Burian G, Gerstner O, Weichselberger A, RESTORE Study Group. The RESTORE study: ranibizumab monotherapy or combined with laser versus laser monotherapy for diabetic macular edema. Ophthalmology. 2011;118(4):615–25. https://doi.org/10.1016/j.ophtha.2011.01.031.
67. Sun JK, Wang PW, Taylor S, Haskova Z. Durability of diabetic retinopathy improvement with as-needed ranibizumab: open-label extension of RIDE and RISE studies. Ophthalmology. 2019;126(5):712–20. https://doi.org/10.1016/j.ophtha.2018.10.041. Epub 2018 Nov 9.
68. Holash J, Davis S, Papadopoulos N, Croll SD, Ho L, Russell M, Boland P, Leidich R, Hylton D, Burova E, Ioffe E, Huang T, Radziejewski C, Bailey K, Fandl JP, Daly T, Wiegand SJ, Yancopoulos GD, Rudge JS. VEGF-Trap: a VEGF blocker with potent antitumor effects. Proc Natl Acad Sci U S A. 2002;99(17):11393–8. https://doi.org/10.1073/pnas.172398299. Epub 2002 Aug 12.
69. Brown DM, Wykoff CC, Boyer D, Heier JS, Clark WL, Emanuelli A, Higgins PM, Singer M, Weinreich DM, Yancopoulos GD, Berliner AJ, Chu K, Reed K, Cheng Y, Vitti R. Evaluation of intravitreal aflibercept for the treatment of severe nonproliferative diabetic retinopathy: results from the PANORAMA randomized clinical trial. JAMA Ophthalmol. 2021;139(9):946–55. https://doi.org/10.1001/jamaophthalmol.2021.2809.

70. Arevalo JF, Fromow-Guerra J, Quiroz-Mercado H, Sanchez JG, Wu L, Maia M, Berrocal MH, Solis-Vivanco A, Farah ME, Pan-American Collaborative Retina Study Group. Primary intravitreal bevacizumab (Avastin) for diabetic macular edema: results from the Pan-American Collaborative Retina Study Group at 6-month follow-up. Ophthalmology. 2007;114(4):743–50. https://doi.org/10.1016/j.ophtha.2006.12.028.
71. Wells JA, Glassman AR, Ayala AR, Jampol LM, Bressler NM, Bressler SB, Brucker AJ, Ferris FL, Hampton GR, Jhaveri C, Melia M, Beck RW, Diabetic Retinopathy Clinical Research Network. Aflibercept, bevacizumab, or Ranibizumab for diabetic macular edema: two-year results from a comparative effectiveness randomized clinical trial. Ophthalmology. 2016;123(6):1351–9. https://doi.org/10.1016/j.ophtha.2016.02.022. Epub 2016 Feb 27.
72. Bressler NM, Odia I, Maguire M, Glassman AR, Jampol LM, MacCumber MW, Shah C, Rosberger D, Sun JK, Retina DRCR, Network. Association between change in visual acuity and change in central subfield thickness during treatment of diabetic macular edema in participants randomized to aflibercept, bevacizumab, or ranibizumab: a post hoc analysis of the protocol T randomized clinical trial. JAMA Ophthalmol. 2019;137(9):977–85. https://doi.org/10.1001/jamaophthalmol.2019.1963.
73. Glassman AR, Wells JA 3rd, Josic K, Maguire MG, Antoszyk AN, Baker C, Beaulieu WT, Elman MJ, Jampol LM, Sun JK. Five-year outcomes after initial aflibercept, bevacizumab, or ranibizumab treatment for diabetic macular edema (Protocol T Extension Study). Ophthalmology. 2020;127(9):1201–10. https://doi.org/10.1016/j.ophtha.2020.03.021. Epub 2020 Mar 29.
74. Tan TE, Sivaprasad S, Wong TY. Anti-vascular endothelial growth factor therapy for complications of diabetic retinopathy-from treatment to prevention? JAMA Ophthalmol. 2023;141:223. https://doi.org/10.1001/jamaophthalmol.2023.0496. Epub ahead of print.
75. Zhang Y, Kontos CD, Annex BH, Popel AS. Angiopoietin-Tie signaling pathway in endothelial cells: a computational model. iScience. 2019;20:497–511. https://doi.org/10.1016/j.isci.2019.10.006. Epub 2019 Oct 3.
76. Campochiaro PA, Peters KG. Targeting Tie2 for treatment of diabetic retinopathy and diabetic macular edema. Curr Diab Rep. 2016;16(12):126. https://doi.org/10.1007/s11892-016-0816-5.
77. Khan M, Aziz AA, Shafi NA, Abbas T, Khanani AM. Targeting angiopoietin in retinal vascular diseases: a literature review and summary of clinical trials involving faricimab. Cell. 2020;9(8):1869. https://doi.org/10.3390/cells9081869.
78. Sahni J, Patel SS, Dugel PU, Khanani AM, Jhaveri CD, Wykoff CC, Hershberger VS, Pauly-Evers M, Sadikhov S, Szczesny P, Schwab D, Nogoceke E, Osborne A, Weikert R, Fauser S. Simultaneous inhibition of angiopoietin-2 and vascular endothelial growth factor-A with faricimab in diabetic macular edema: Boulevard phase 2 randomized trial. Ophthalmology. 2019;126(8):1155–70. https://doi.org/10.1016/j.ophtha.2019.03.023. Epub 2019 Mar 21.
79. Wykoff CC, Abreu F, Adamis AP, Basu K, Eichenbaum DA, Haskova Z, Lin H, Loewenstein A, Mohan S, Pearce IA, Sakamoto T, Schlottmann PG, Silverman D, Sun JK, Wells JA, Willis JR, Tadayoni R, YOSEMITE and RHINE Investigators. Efficacy, durability, and safety of intravitreal faricimab with extended dosing up to every 16 weeks in patients with diabetic macular oedema (YOSEMITE and RHINE): two randomised, double-masked, phase 3 trials. Lancet. 2022;399(10326):741–55. https://doi.org/10.1016/S0140-6736(22)00018-6. Epub 2022 Jan 24.
80. Agard NJ, Zhang G, Ridgeway J, Dicara DM, Chu PY, Ohri R, Sanowar S, Vernes JM, Chi H, Zhang J, Holz E, Paluch M, He G, Benson Y, Zhang J, Chan P, Tang N, Javale P, Wilson B, Barrett K, Rowntree RK, Hang J, Meng YG, Hass P, Fuh G, Piskol R, Bantseev V, Loyet KM, Tran JC, Wu C, Indjeian VB, Shivva V, Yan M. Direct Tie2 agonists stabilize vasculature for the treatment of diabetic macular edema. Transl Vis Sci Technol. 2022;11(10):27. https://doi.org/10.1167/tvst.11.10.27.
81. Iglicki M, González DP, Loewenstein A, Zur D. Next-generation anti-VEGF agents for diabetic macular oedema. Eye (Lond). 2022;36(2):273–7. https://doi.org/10.1038/s41433-021-01722-8. Epub 2021 Aug 9.
82. Jorge EC, Jorge EN, Botelho M, Farat JG, Virgili G, El Dib R. Monotherapy laser photocoagulation for diabetic macular oedema. Cochrane Database Syst Rev. 2018;10(10):CD010859. https://doi.org/10.1002/14651858.CD010859.pub2.
83. Writing Committee for the Diabetic Retinopathy Clinical Research Network, Fong DS, Strauber SF, Aiello LP, Beck RW, Callanan DG, Danis RP, Davis MD, Feman SS, Ferris F, Friedman SM, Garcia CA, Glassman AR, Han DP, Le D, Kollman C, Lauer AK, Recchia FM, Solomon SD. Comparison of the modified early treatment diabetic retinopathy study and mild macular grid laser photocoagulation strategies for diabetic macular edema. Arch Ophthalmol. 2007;125(4):469–80. https://doi.org/10.1001/archopht.125.4.469.
84. Sachdev N, Gupta V, Abhiramamurthy V, Singh R, Gupta A. Correlation between microaneurysm closure rate and reduction in macular thickness following laser photocoagulation of diabetic macular edema. Eye (Lond). 2008;22(7):975–7. https://doi.org/10.1038/sj.eye.6702801. Epub 2007 Apr 6.
85. Diabetic Retinopathy Clinical Research Network. A randomized trial comparing intravitreal triamcinolone acetonide and focal/grid photocoagulation for diabetic macular edema. Ophthalmology.

2008;115(9):1447–9, 1449.e1–10. https://doi.org/10.1016/j.ophtha.2008.06.015. Epub 2008 Jul 26.

86. Diabetic Retinopathy Clinical Research Network (DRCR.net), Beck RW, Edwards AR, Aiello LP, Bressler NM, Ferris F, Glassman AR, Hartnett E, Ip MS, Kim JE, Kollman C. Three-year follow-up of a randomized trial comparing focal/grid photocoagulation and intravitreal triamcinolone for diabetic macular edema. Arch Ophthalmol. 2009;127(3):245–51. https://doi.org/10.1001/archophthalmol.2008.610.
87. Diabetic Retinopathy Clinical Research Network, Elman MJ, Aiello LP, Beck RW, Bressler NM, Bressler SB, Edwards AR, Ferris FL 3rd, Friedman SM, Glassman AR, Miller KM, Scott IU, Stockdale CR, Sun JK. Randomized trial evaluating ranibizumab plus prompt or deferred laser or triamcinolone plus prompt laser for diabetic macular edema. Ophthalmology. 2010;117(6):1064–1077.e35. https://doi.org/10.1016/j.ophtha.2010.02.031. Epub 2010 Apr 28.
88. Campochiaro PA, Brown DM, Pearson A, Ciulla T, Boyer D, Holz FG, Tolentino M, Gupta A, Duarte L, Madreperla S, Gonder J, Kapik B, Billman K, Kane FE, FAME Study Group. Long-term benefit of sustained-delivery fluocinolone acetonide vitreous inserts for diabetic macular edema. Ophthalmology. 2011;118(4):626–635.e2. https://doi.org/10.1016/j.ophtha.2010.12.028.
89. Campochiaro PA, Brown DM, Pearson A, Chen S, Boyer D, Ruiz-Moreno J, Garretson B, Gupta A, Hariprasad SM, Bailey C, Reichel E, Soubrane G, Kapik B, Billman K, Kane FE, Green K, FAME Study Group. Sustained delivery of fluocinolone acetonide vitreous inserts provide benefit for at least 3 years in patients with diabetic macular edema. Ophthalmology. 2012;119(10):2125–32. https://doi.org/10.1016/j.ophtha.2012.04.030. Epub 2012 Jun 21.
90. Cunha-Vaz J, Ashton P, Iezzi R, Campochiaro P, Dugel PU, Holz FG, Weber M, Danis RP, Kuppermann BD, Bailey C, Billman K, Kapik B, Kane F, Green K, FAME Study Group. Sustained delivery fluocinolone acetonide vitreous implants: long-term benefit in patients with chronic diabetic macular edema. Ophthalmology. 2014;121(10):1892–903. https://doi.org/10.1016/j.ophtha.2014.04.019. Epub 2014 Jun 14.
91. Boyer DS, Yoon YH, Belfort R Jr, Bandello F, Maturi RK, Augustin AJ, Li XY, Cui H, Hashad Y, Whitcup SM, Ozurdex MEAD Study Group. Three-year, randomized, sham-controlled trial of dexamethasone intravitreal implant in patients with diabetic macular edema. Ophthalmology. 2014;121(10):1904–14. https://doi.org/10.1016/j.ophtha.2014.04.024. Epub 2014 Jun 4.
92. Maturi RK, Glassman AR, Liu D, Beck RW, Bhavsar AR, Bressler NM, Jampol LM, Melia M, Punjabi OS, Salehi-Had H, Sun JK, Diabetic Retinopathy Clinical Research Network. Effect of adding dexamethasone to continued ranibizumab treatment in patients with persistent diabetic macular edema: a DRCR network phase 2 randomized clinical trial. JAMA Ophthalmol. 2018;136(1):29–38. https://doi.org/10.1001/jamaophthalmol.2017.4914.
93. Bansal P, Gupta V, Gupta A, Dogra MR, Ram J. Efficacy of Ozurdex implant in recalcitrant diabetic macular edema—a single-center experience. Int Ophthalmol. 2016;36(2):207–16. https://doi.org/10.1007/s10792-015-0103-5. Epub 2015 Aug 2.
94. Agarwal A, Gupta V, Ram J, Gupta A. Dexamethasone intravitreal implant during phacoemulsification. Ophthalmology. 2013;120(1):211, 211.e1–5. https://doi.org/10.1016/j.ophtha.2012.08.002.
95. Singh R, Abhiramamurthy V, Gupta V, Gupta A, Bhansali A. Effect of multifactorial intervention on diabetic macular edema. Diabetes Care. 2006;29(2):463–4. https://doi.org/10.2337/diacare.29.02.06.dc05-1931.
96. Singh R, Gupta V, Gupta A, Sachdev N, Dogra MR, Bhansali A. Multifactorial interventions before laser photocoagulation improve outcome of diabetic macular edema. Diabetes Care. 2006;29(12):2758–9. https://doi.org/10.2337/dc06-1302.
97. Gupta A, Gupta V, Thapar S, Bhansali A. Lipid-lowering drug atorvastatin as an adjunct in the management of diabetic macular edema. Am J Ophthalmol. 2004;137(4):675–82. https://doi.org/10.1016/j.ajo.2003.11.017.
98. Kawasaki R, Konta T, Nishida K. Lipid-lowering medication is associated with decreased risk of diabetic retinopathy and the need for treatment in patients with type 2 diabetes: a real-world observational analysis of a health claims database. Diabetes Obes Metab. 2018;20(10):2351–60. https://doi.org/10.1111/dom.13372. Epub 2018 Jun 21.
99. Vail D, Callaway NF, Ludwig CA, Saroj N, Moshfeghi DM. Lipid-lowering medications are associated with lower risk of retinopathy and ophthalmic interventions among United States patients with diabetes. Am J Ophthalmol. 2019;207:378–84. https://doi.org/10.1016/j.ajo.2019.05.029. Epub 2019 Jun 10.
100. Aiello LP, Cahill MT, Wong JS. Systemic considerations in the management of diabetic retinopathy. Am J Ophthalmol. 2001;132(5):760–76. https://doi.org/10.1016/s0002-9394(01)01124-2.
101. Campochiaro PA, Hafiz G, Shah SM, Nguyen QD, Ying H, Do DV, Quinlan E, Zimmer-Galler I, Haller JA, Solomon SD, Sung JU, Hadi Y, Janjua KA, Jawed N, Choy DF, Arron JR. Ranibizumab for macular edema due to retinal vein occlusions: implication of VEGF as a critical stimulator. Mol Ther. 2008;16(4):791–9. https://doi.org/10.1038/mt.2008.10. Epub 2008 Feb 5.
102. Rogers SL, McIntosh RL, Lim L, Mitchell P, Cheung N, Kowalski JW, Nguyen HP, Wang JJ, Wong TY. Natural history of branch retinal vein occlusion: an evidence-based systematic review.

Ophthalmology. 2010;117(6):1094–1101.e5. https://doi.org/10.1016/j.ophtha.2010.01.058.
103. Hayreh SS, Zimmerman MB. Branch retinal vein occlusion: natural history of visual outcome. JAMA Ophthalmol. 2014;132(1):13–22. https://doi.org/10.1001/jamaophthalmol.2013.5515.
104. Choi YJ, Jee D, Kwon JW. Characteristics of major and macular branch retinal vein occlusion. Sci Rep. 2022;12(1):14103. https://doi.org/10.1038/s41598-022-18414-2.
105. The Branch Vein Occlusion Study Group. Argon laser photocoagulation for macular edema in branch vein occlusion. Am J Ophthalmol. 1984;98(3):271–82. https://doi.org/10.1016/0002-9394(84)90316-7.
106. Freund KB, Sarraf D, Leong BCS, Garrity ST, Vupparaboina KK, Dansingani KK. Association of optical coherence tomography angiography of collaterals in retinal vein occlusion with major venous outflow through the deep vascular complex. JAMA Ophthalmol. 2018;136(11):1262–70. https://doi.org/10.1001/jamaophthalmol.2018.3586.
107. Tsuboi K, Sasajima H, Kamei M. Collateral vessels in branch retinal vein occlusion: anatomic and functional analyses by OCT angiography. Ophthalmol Retina. 2019;3(9):767–76. https://doi.org/10.1016/j.oret.2019.04.015. Epub 2019 Apr 18.
108. Jang JH, Kim YC, Shin JP. Correlation between macular edema recurrence and macular capillary network destruction in branch retinal vein occlusion. BMC Ophthalmol. 2020;20(1):341. https://doi.org/10.1186/s12886-020-01611-w.
109. Tsuboi K, Ishida Y, Kamei M. Gap in capillary perfusion on optical coherence tomography angiography associated with persistent macular edema in branch retinal vein occlusion. Invest Ophthalmol Vis Sci. 2017;58(4):2038–43. https://doi.org/10.1167/iovs.17-21447.
110. Yeung L, Wu WC, Chuang LH, Wang NK, Lai CC. Novel optical coherence tomography angiography biomarker in branch retinal vein occlusion macular edema. Retina. 2019;39(10):1906–16. https://doi.org/10.1097/IAE.0000000000002264.
111. Tomiyasu T, Hirano Y, Yoshida M, Suzuki N, Nishiyama T, Uemura A, Yasukawa T, Ogura Y. Microaneurysms cause refractory macular edema in branch retinal vein occlusion. Sci Rep. 2016;6:29445. https://doi.org/10.1038/srep29445.
112. An Y, Park SP, Kim YK. Aqueous humor inflammatory cytokine levels and choroidal thickness in patients with macular edema associated with branch retinal vein occlusion. Int Ophthalmol. 2021;41(7):2433–44. https://doi.org/10.1007/s10792-021-01798-x. Epub 2021 Mar 19.
113. Ryu G, Park D, Lim J, van Hemert J, Sagong M. Macular microvascular changes and their correlation with peripheral nonperfusion in branch retinal vein occlusion. Am J Ophthalmol. 2021;225:57–68. https://doi.org/10.1016/j.ajo.2020.12.026. Epub 2021 Jan 4.
114. Sasajima H, Tsuboi K, Kiyosawa R, Fukutomi A, Murotani K, Kamei M. Smooth borders between inner nuclear layer and outer plexiform layer predict fewer macular edema recurrences in branch retinal vein occlusion. Sci Rep. 2021;11(1):15987. https://doi.org/10.1038/s41598-021-95501-w.
115. Moussa M, Leila M, Bessa AS, Lolah M, Abou Shousha M, El Hennawi HM, Hafez TA. Grading of macular perfusion in retinal vein occlusion using en-face swept-source optical coherence tomography angiography: a retrospective observational case series. BMC Ophthalmol. 2019;19(1):127. https://doi.org/10.1186/s12886-019-1134-x.
116. Wang J, Cui Y, Vingopoulos F, Kasetty M, Silverman RF, Katz R, Kim L, Miller JB. Disorganisation of retinal inner layers is associated with reduced contrast sensitivity in retinal vein occlusion. Br J Ophthalmol. 2022;106(2):241–5. https://doi.org/10.1136/bjophthalmol-2020-317615. Epub 2020 Nov 10.
117. Yeh S, Kim SJ, Ho AC, Schoenberger SD, Bakri SJ, Ehlers JP, Thorne JE. Therapies for macular edema associated with central retinal vein occlusion: a report by the American Academy of Ophthalmology. Ophthalmology. 2015;122(4):769–78. https://doi.org/10.1016/j.ophtha.2014.10.013. Epub 2015 Jan 8.
118. Schmidt-Erfurth U, Garcia-Arumi J, Gerendas BS, Midena E, Sivaprasad S, Tadayoni R, Wolf S, Loewenstein A. Guidelines for the management of retinal vein occlusion by the European Society of Retina Specialists (EURETINA). Ophthalmologica. 2019;242(3):123–62. https://doi.org/10.1159/000502041. Epub 2019 Aug 14.
119. Tan MH, McAllister IL, Gillies ME, Verma N, Banerjee G, Smithies LA, Wong WL, Wong TY. Randomized controlled trial of intravitreal ranibizumab versus standard grid laser for macular edema following branch retinal vein occlusion. Am J Ophthalmol. 2014;157(1):237–247.e1. https://doi.org/10.1016/j.ajo.2013.08.013. Epub 2013 Oct 7.
120. Khan MA, Mallika V, Joshi D. Comparison of immediate versus deferred intravitreal bevacizumab in macular oedema due to branch retinal vein occlusion: a pilot study. Int Ophthalmol. 2018;38(3):943–9. https://doi.org/10.1007/s10792-017-0538-y. Epub 2017 Apr 21.
121. Shalchi Z, Mahroo O, Bunce C, Mitry D. Anti-vascular endothelial growth factor for macular oedema secondary to branch retinal vein occlusion. Cochrane Database Syst Rev. 2020;7(7):CD009510. https://doi.org/10.1002/14651858.CD009510.pub3.
122. Zou W, Du Y, Ji X, Zhang J, Ding H, Chen J, Wang T, Ji F, Huang J. Comparison of the efficiency of anti-VEGF drugs intravitreal injections treatment with or without retinal laser photocoagulation for macular edema secondary to retinal vein occlusion: A systematic review and meta-analysis. Front Pharmacol. 2022;13:948852. https://doi.org/10.3389/fphar.2022.948852.

123. Au A, Hilely A, Scharf J, Gunnemann F, Wang D, Chehaibou I, Iovino C, Grondin C, Farecki ML, Falavarjani KG, Phasukkijwatana N, Battista M, Borrelli E, Sacconi R, Powell B, Hom G, Greenlee TE, Conti TF, Ledesma-Gil G, Teke MY, Choudhry N, Fung AT, Krivosic V, Baek J, Lee MY, Sugiura Y, Querques G, Peiretti E, Rosen R, Lee WK, Yannuzzi LA, Zur D, Loewenstein A, Pauleikhoff D, Singh R, Modi Y, Hubschman JP, Ip M, Sadda S, Freund KB, Sarraf D. Relationship between nerve fiber layer hemorrhages and outcomes in central retinal vein occlusion. Invest Ophthalmol Vis Sci. 2020;61(5):54. https://doi.org/10.1167/iovs.61.5.54.
124. Ferrara N. Vascular endothelial growth factor: basic science and clinical progress. Endocr Rev. 2004;25(4):581–611. https://doi.org/10.1210/er.2003-0027.
125. Aiello LP, Avery RL, Arrigg PG, Keyt BA, Jampel HD, Shah ST, Pasquale LR, Thieme H, Iwamoto MA, Park JE, et al. Vascular endothelial growth factor in ocular fluid of patients with diabetic retinopathy and other retinal disorders. N Engl J Med. 1994;331(22):1480–7. https://doi.org/10.1056/NEJM199412013312203.
126. Funk M, Kriechbaum K, Prager F, Benesch T, Georgopoulos M, Zlabinger GJ, Schmidt-Erfurth U. Intraocular concentrations of growth factors and cytokines in retinal vein occlusion and the effect of therapy with bevacizumab. Invest Ophthalmol Vis Sci. 2009;50(3):1025–32. https://doi.org/10.1167/iovs.08-2510. Epub 2008 Dec 5.
127. Ehlken C, Rennel ES, Michels D, Grundel B, Pielen A, Junker B, Stahl A, Hansen LL, Feltgen N, Agostini HT, Martin G. Levels of VEGF but not VEGF(165b) are increased in the vitreous of patients with retinal vein occlusion. Am J Ophthalmol. 2011;152(2):298–303.e1. https://doi.org/10.1016/j.ajo.2011.01.040. Epub 2011 May 28.
128. Ferrara N, Damico L, Shams N, Lowman H, Kim R. Development of ranibizumab, an anti-vascular endothelial growth factor antigen binding fragment, as therapy for neovascular age-related macular degeneration. Retina. 2006;26(8):859–70. https://doi.org/10.1097/01.iae.0000242842.14624.e7.
129. Noma H, Funatsu H, Mimura T, Harino S, Hori S. Vitreous levels of interleukin-6 and vascular endothelial growth factor in macular edema with central retinal vein occlusion. Ophthalmology. 2009;116(1):87–93. https://doi.org/10.1016/j.ophtha.2008.09.034.
130. Noma H, Mimura T, Yasuda K, Shimura M. Role of soluble vascular endothelial growth factor receptor signaling and other factors or cytokines in central retinal vein occlusion with macular edema. Invest Ophthalmol Vis Sci. 2015;56(2):1122–8. https://doi.org/10.1167/iovs.14-15789.
131. Noma H, Yasuda K, Shimura M. Cytokines and pathogenesis of central retinal vein occlusion. J Clin Med. 2020;9(11):3457. https://doi.org/10.3390/jcm9113457.
132. Kida T, Flammer J, Konieczka K, Ikeda T. Retinal venous pressure is decreased after anti-VEGF therapy in patients with retinal vein occlusion-related macular edema. Graefes Arch Clin Exp Ophthalmol. 2021;259(7):1853–8. https://doi.org/10.1007/s00417-020-05068-x. Epub 2021 Jan 15.
133. Gale R, Gill C, Pikoula M, Lee AY, Hanson RLW, Denaxas S, Egan C, Tufail A, Taylor P, UK EMR Database Users Group. Multicentre study of 4626 patients assesses the effectiveness, safety and burden of two categories of treatments for central retinal vein occlusion: intravitreal anti-vascular endothelial growth factor injections and intravitreal Ozurdex injections. Br J Ophthalmol. 2021;105(11):1571–6. https://doi.org/10.1136/bjophthalmol-2020-317306. Epub 2020 Sep 22.
134. Qian T, Zhao M, Xu X. Comparison between anti-VEGF therapy and corticosteroid or laser therapy for macular oedema secondary to retinal vein occlusion: a meta-analysis. J Clin Pharm Ther. 2017;42(5):519–29. https://doi.org/10.1111/jcpt.12551. Epub 2017 Jun 22.
135. Gurudas S, Patrao N, Nicholson L, Sen P, Ramu J, Sivaprasad S, Hykin P. Visual outcomes associated with patterns of macular edema resolution in central retinal vein occlusion treated with anti-vascular endothelial growth factor therapy: a post hoc analysis of the lucentis, eylea, avastin in vein occlusion (LEAVO) trial. JAMA Ophthalmol. 2022;140(2):143–50. https://doi.org/10.1001/jamaophthalmol.2021.5619.
136. Nanji K, Khan M, Khalid MF, Xie JS, Sarohia GS, Phillips M, Thabane L, Garg SJ, Kaiser P, Sivaprasad S, Wykoff CC, Chaudhary V. Treat-and-extend regimens of anti-vascular endothelial growth factor therapy for retinal vein occlusions: a systematic review and meta-analysis. Acta Ophthalmol. 2022;100(6):e1199–208. https://doi.org/10.1111/aos.15068. Epub 2021 Nov 29.
137. Scott IU, VanVeldhuisen PC, Oden NL, Ip MS, Blodi BA, SCORE2 Investigator Group. Month 60 outcomes after treatment initiation with anti-vascular endothelial growth factor therapy for macular edema due to central retinal or hemiretinal vein occlusion. Am J Ophthalmol. 2022;240:330–41. https://doi.org/10.1016/j.ajo.2022.04.001. Epub 2022 Apr 21.
138. Spooner KL, Fraser-Bell S, Hong T, Wong JG, Chang AA. Long-term outcomes of anti-VEGF treatment of retinal vein occlusion. Eye (Lond). 2022;36(6):1194–201. https://doi.org/10.1038/s41433-021-01620-z. Epub 2021 Jun 11.
139. Nussenblatt RB. The natural history of uveitis. Int Ophthalmol. 1990;14(5–6):303–8. https://doi.org/10.1007/BF00163549.
140. Rothova A, Suttorp-van Schulten MS, Frits Treffers W, Kijlstra A. Causes and frequency of blindness in patients with intraocular inflammatory disease. Br J Ophthalmol. 1996;80(4):332–6. https://doi.org/10.1136/bjo.80.4.332.

141. Tomkins-Netzer O, Lightman S, Drye L, Kempen J, Holland GN, Rao NA, Stawell RJ, Vitale A, Jabs DA, Multicenter Uveitis Steroid Treatment Trial Research Group. Outcome of treatment of uveitic macular edema: the multicenter uveitis steroid treatment trial 2-year results. Ophthalmology. 2015;122(11):2351–9. https://doi.org/10.1016/j.ophtha.2015.07.036. Epub 2015 Sep 7.
142. Thorne JE, Daniel E, Jabs DA, Kedhar SR, Peters GB, Dunn JP. Smoking as a risk factor for cystoid macular edema complicating intermediate uveitis. Am J Ophthalmol. 2008;145(5):841–6. https://doi.org/10.1016/j.ajo.2007.12.032. Epub 2008 Mar 5.
143. Lardenoye CW, van Kooij B, Rothova A. Impact of macular edema on visual acuity in uveitis. Ophthalmology. 2006;113(8):1446–9. https://doi.org/10.1016/j.ophtha.2006.03.027.
144. Levin MH, Pistilli M, Daniel E, Gangaputra SS, Nussenblatt RB, Rosenbaum JT, Suhler EB, Thorne JE, Foster CS, Jabs DA, Levy-Clarke GA, Kempen JH, Systemic Immunosuppressive Therapy for Eye Diseases Cohort Study. Incidence of visual improvement in uveitis cases with visual impairment caused by macular edema. Ophthalmology. 2014;121(2):588–95.e1. https://doi.org/10.1016/j.ophtha.2013.09.023. Epub 2013 Dec 12.
145. Pivetti-Pezzi P, Accorinti M, La Cava M, Colabelli Gisoldi RA, Abdulaziz MA. Endogenous uveitis: an analysis of 1,417 cases. Ophthalmologica. 1996;210(4):234–8. https://doi.org/10.1159/000310715.
146. Ossewaarde-van Norel J, Camfferman LP, Rothova A. Discrepancies between fluorescein angiography and optical coherence tomography in macular edema in uveitis. Am J Ophthalmol. 2012;154(2):233–9. https://doi.org/10.1016/j.ajo.2012.02.003. Epub 2012 Apr 27.
147. Tran TH, de Smet MD, Bodaghi B, Fardeau C, Cassoux N, Lehoang P. Uveitic macular oedema: correlation between optical coherence tomography patterns with visual acuity and fluorescein angiography. Br J Ophthalmol. 2008;92(7):922–7. https://doi.org/10.1136/bjo.2007.136846.
148. Kempen JH, Sugar EA, Jaffe GJ, Acharya NR, Dunn JP, Elner SG, Lightman SL, Thorne JE, Vitale AT, Altaweel MM, Multicenter Uveitis Steroid Treatment (MUST) Trial Research Group. Fluorescein angiography versus optical coherence tomography for diagnosis of uveitic macular edema. Ophthalmology. 2013;120(9):1852–9. https://doi.org/10.1016/j.ophtha.2013.01.069. Epub 2013 May 21.
149. Grewal DS, O'Sullivan ML, Kron M, Jaffe GJ. Association of disorganization of retinal inner layers with visual acuity in eyes with uveitic cystoid macular edema. Am J Ophthalmol. 2017;177:116–25. https://doi.org/10.1016/j.ajo.2017.02.017. Epub 2017 Feb 22.
150. Schallhorn JM, Niemeyer KM, Browne EN, Chhetri P, Acharya NR. Difluprednate for the treatment of uveitic cystoid macular edema. Am J Ophthalmol. 2018;191:14–22. https://doi.org/10.1016/j.ajo.2018.03.027. Epub 2018 Mar 24.
151. Tomkins-Netzer O, Lightman SL, Burke AE, Sugar EA, Lim LL, Jaffe GJ, Altaweel MM, Kempen JH, Holbrook JT, Jabs DA, Multicenter Steroid Treatment Trial and Follow-up Study Research Group. Seven-year outcomes of uveitic macular edema: the multicenter uveitis steroid treatment trial and follow-up study results. Ophthalmology. 2021;128(5):719–28. https://doi.org/10.1016/j.ophtha.2020.08.035. Epub 2020 Sep 10.
152. Tsui E, Rathinam SR, Gonzales JA, Thundikandy R, Kanakath A, Balamurugan S, Vedhanayaki R, Lim LL, Suhler EB, Al-Dhibi HA, Doan T, Keenan J, Ebert CD, Kim E, Madow B, Porco TC, Acharya NR, FAST Research Group. Outcomes of uveitic macular edema in the first-line antimetabolites as steroid-sparing treatment uveitis trial. Ophthalmology. 2022;129(6):661–7. https://doi.org/10.1016/j.ophtha.2022.02.002. Epub 2022 Feb 8.
153. Roth DB, Verma V, Realini T, Prenner JL, Feuer WJ, Fechtner RD. Long-term incidence and timing of intraocular hypertension after intravitreal triamcinolone acetonide injection. Ophthalmology. 2009;116(3):455–60. https://doi.org/10.1016/j.ophtha.2008.10.002. Epub 2009 Jan 20.
154. Leder HA, Jabs DA, Galor A, Dunn JP, Thorne JE. Periocular triamcinolone acetonide injections for cystoid macular edema complicating noninfectious uveitis. Am J Ophthalmol. 2011;152(3):441–448.e2. https://doi.org/10.1016/j.ajo.2011.02.009. Epub 2011 Jun 8.
155. Androudi S, Letko E, Meniconi M, Papadaki T, Ahmed M, Foster CS. Safety and efficacy of intravitreal triamcinolone acetonide for uveitic macular edema. Ocul Immunol Inflamm. 2005;13(2–3):205–12. https://doi.org/10.1080/09273940590933511.
156. Thorne JE, Sugar EA, Holbrook JT, Burke AE, Altaweel MM, Vitale AT, Acharya NR, Kempen JH, Jabs DA, Multicenter Uveitis Steroid Treatment Trial Research Group. Periocular triamcinolone vs. intravitreal triamcinolone vs. intravitreal dexamethasone implant for the treatment of uveitic macular edema: the PeriOcular vs. INTravitreal corticosteroids for uveitic macular edema (POINT) trial. Ophthalmology. 2019;126(2):283–95. https://doi.org/10.1016/j.ophtha.2018.08.021. Epub 2018 Sep 27.
157. Lowder C, Belfort R Jr, Lightman S, Foster CS, Robinson MR, Schiffman RM, Li XY, Cui H, Whitcup SM, Ozurdex HURON Study Group. Dexamethasone intravitreal implant for noninfectious intermediate or posterior uveitis. Arch Ophthalmol. 2011;129(5):545–53. https://doi.org/10.1001/archophthalmol.2010.339. Epub 2011 Jan 10.
158. Tsang AC, Virgili G, Abtahi M, Gottlieb CC. Intravitreal dexamethasone implant for the treatment of macular edema in chronic non-infectious uveitis. Ocul Immunol Inflamm. 2017;25(5):685–

92. https://doi.org/10.3109/09273948.2016.1160130. Epub 2016 May 18.
159. Alba-Linero C, Sala-Puigdollers A, Romero B, Llorenç V, Adan A, Zarranz-Ventura J. Long-term intravitreal dexamethasone implant outcomes in uveitis. Ocul Immunol Inflamm. 2020;28(2):228–37. https://doi.org/10.1080/09273948.2019.1578380. Epub 2019 Apr 17.
160. Ratra D, Barh A, Banerjee M, Ratra V, Biswas J. Safety and efficacy of intravitreal dexamethasone implant for refractory uveitic macular edema in adults and children. Ocul Immunol Inflamm. 2018;26(7):1034–40. https://doi.org/10.1080/09273948.2018.1424342. Epub 2018 Feb 2.
161. Gupta A, Ram J, Gupta A, Gupta V. Intraoperative dexamethasone implant in uveitis patients with cataract undergoing phacoemulsification. Ocul Immunol Inflamm. 2013;21(6):462–7. https://doi.org/10.3109/09273948.2013.822087. Epub 2013 Aug 13.
162. Gupta G, Ram J, Gupta V, Singh R, Bansal R, Gupta PC, Gupta A. Efficacy of intravitreal dexamethasone implant in patients of uveitis undergoing cataract surgery. Ocul Immunol Inflamm. 2019;27(8):1330–8. https://doi.org/10.1080/09273948.2018.1524498. Epub 2018 Sep 21.
163. Hsieh YH, Jhou HJ, Chen PH, Hwang YS. Intravitreal injection versus systematic treatment in patients with uveitis undergoing cataract surgery: a systematic review and meta-analysis. Graefes Arch Clin Exp Ophthalmol. 2022;261:809. https://doi.org/10.1007/s00417-022-05852-x. Epub ahead of print.
164. Jaffe GJ, Pavesio CE, Study Investigators. Effect of a fluocinolone acetonide insert on recurrence rates in noninfectious intermediate, posterior, or panuveitis: three-year results. Ophthalmology. 2020;127(10):1395–404. https://doi.org/10.1016/j.ophtha.2020.04.001. Epub 2020 Apr 17.
165. Steeples LR, Pockar S, Jones NP, Leal I. Evaluating the safety, efficacy and patient acceptability of intravitreal fluocinolone acetonide (0.2mcg/day) implant in the treatment of non-infectious uveitis affecting the posterior segment. Clin Ophthalmol. 2021;15:1433–42. https://doi.org/10.2147/OPTH.S216912.
166. Yeh S, Khurana RN, Shah M, Henry CR, Wang RC, Kissner JM, Ciulla TA, Noronha G, PEACHTREE Study Investigators. Efficacy and safety of suprachoroidal CLS-TA for macular edema secondary to noninfectious uveitis: phase 3 randomized trial. Ophthalmology. 2020;127(7):948–55. https://doi.org/10.1016/j.ophtha.2020.01.006. Epub 2020 Jan 10.
167. Ciulla TA, Kapik B, Barakat MR, Khurana RN, Nguyen QD, Grewal DS, Albini T, Cunningham ET Jr, Goldstein DA. Optical coherence tomography anatomic and temporal biomarkers in uveitic macular edema. Am J Ophthalmol. 2022;237:310–24. https://doi.org/10.1016/j.ajo.2021.10.024. Epub 2021 Nov 3.
168. Lasave AF, Schlaen A, Zeballos DG, Díaz-Llopis M, Couto C, El-Haig WM, Arevalo JF. Twenty-four months follow-up of intravitreal bevacizumab injection versus intravitreal triamcinolone acetonide injection for the management of persistent non-infectious uveitic cystoid macular edema. Ocul Immunol Inflamm. 2019;27(2):294–302. https://doi.org/10.1080/09273948.2017.1400073. Epub 2017 Nov 20.
169. Vegas-Revenga N, Calvo-Río V, Mesquida M, Adán A, Hernández MV, Beltrán E, Valls Pascual E, Díaz-Valle D, Díaz-Cordovés G, Hernandez-Garfella M, Martínez-Costa L, Calvo I, Atanes A, Linares LF, Modesto C, González-Vela C, Demetrio-Pablo R, Aurrecoechea E, Cordero M, Domínguez-Casas LC, Atienza-Mateo B, Martín-Varillas JL, Loricera J, Palmou-Fontana N, Hernández JL, González-Gay MA, Blanco R. Anti-IL6-receptor tocilizumab in refractory and noninfectious uveitic cystoid macular edema: multicenter study of 25 patients. Am J Ophthalmol. 2019;200:85–94. https://doi.org/10.1016/j.ajo.2018.12.019. Epub 2019 Jan 17.
170. Taylor SR, Habot-Wilner Z, Pacheco P, Lightman SL. Intraocular methotrexate in the treatment of uveitis and uveitic cystoid macular edema. Ophthalmology. 2009;116(4):797–801. https://doi.org/10.1016/j.ophtha.2008.10.033.
171. Irvine SR. A newly defined vitreous syndrome following cataract surgery. Am J Ophthalmol. 1953;36(5):599–619. https://doi.org/10.1016/0002-9394(53)90302-x.
172. Gharbiya M, Visioli G, Iannetti L, Iannaccone A, Tamburrelli AC, Marenco M, Albanese GM. Comparison between scleral buckling and vitrectomy in the onset of cystoid macular edema and epiretinal membrane after rhegmatogenous retinal detachment repair. Retina. 2022;42(7):1268–76. https://doi.org/10.1097/IAE.0000000000003475. Epub 2022 Mar 11.
173. Merad M, Vérité F, Baudin F, Ghezala IB, Meillon C, Bron AM, Arnould L, Eid P, Creuzot-Garcher C, Gabrielle PH. Cystoid macular edema after rhegmatogenous retinal detachment repair with pars plana vitrectomy: rate, risk factors, and outcomes. J Clin Med. 2022;11(16):4914. https://doi.org/10.3390/jcm11164914.
174. Tolentino FI, Schepens CL. Edema of posterior pole after cataract extraction. A biomicroscopic study. Arch Ophthalmol. 1965;74(6):781–6. https://doi.org/10.1001/archopht.1965.00970040783008.
175. Schepens CL, Avila MP, Jalkh AE, Trempe CL. Role of the vitreous in cystoid macular edema. Surv Ophthalmol. 1984;28(Suppl):499–504. https://doi.org/10.1016/0039-6257(84)90232-7.
176. Sebag J, Balazs EA. Pathogenesis of cystoid macular edema: an anatomic consideration of vitreoretinal adhesions. Surv Ophthalmol. 1984;28(Suppl):493–8. https://doi.org/10.1016/0039-6257(84)90231-5.
177. Gass JD, Norton EW. Cystoid macular edema and papilledema following cataract extraction. A

fluorescein fundoscopic and angiographic study. Arch Ophthalmol. 1966;76(5):646–61. https://doi.org/10.1001/archopht.1966.03850010648005.

178. Antcliff RJ, Stanford MR, Chauhan DS, Graham EM, Spalton DJ, Shilling JS, Ffytche TJ, Marshall J. Comparison between optical coherence tomography and fundus fluorescein angiography for the detection of cystoid macular edema in patients with uveitis. Ophthalmology. 2000;107(3):593–9. https://doi.org/10.1016/s0161-6420(99)00087-1.

179. Biro Z, Balla Z, Kovacs B. Change of foveal and perifoveal thickness measured by OCT after phacoemulsification and IOL implantation. Eye (Lond). 2008;22(1):8–12. https://doi.org/10.1038/sj.eye.6702460. Epub 2006 Jun 2.

180. Sacconi R, Corbelli E, Carnevali A, Mercuri S, Rabiolo A, Querques L, Marchini G, Bandello F, Querques G. Optical coherence tomography angiography in pseudophakic cystoid macular oedema compared to diabetic macular oedema: qualitative and quantitative evaluation of retinal vasculature. Br J Ophthalmol. 2018;102(12):1684–90. https://doi.org/10.1136/bjophthalmol-2017-311240. Epub 2018 Feb 20.

181. Serra R, Sellam A, Coscas F, Bruyère E, Sieiro A, Coscas GJ, Souied EH. Evaluation of pseudophakic cystoid macular edema using optical coherence tomography angiography. Eur J Ophthalmol. 2018;28(2):234–40. https://doi.org/10.5301/ejo.5001068. Epub 2017 Jan 11.

182. Bellocq D, Mathis T, Voirin N, Bentaleb ZM, Sallit R, Denis P, Kodjikian L. Incidence of Irvine Gass syndrome after phacoemulsification with spectral-domain optical coherence tomography. Ocul Immunol Inflamm. 2019;27(8):1224–31. https://doi.org/10.1080/09273948.2019.1634215. Epub 2019 Aug 15.

183. Copete S, Martí-Rodrigo P, Muñiz-Vidal R, Pastor-Idoate S, Rigo J, Figueroa MS, García-Arumí J, Zapata MA. Preoperative vitreoretinal interface abnormalities on spectral domain optical coherence tomography as risk factor for pseudophakic cystoid macular edema after phacoemulsification. Retina. 2019;39(11):2225–32. https://doi.org/10.1097/IAE.0000000000002298.

184. Chen YC, Chen SJ, Li AF, Huang YM. Visual outcomes and incidence of pseudophakic cystoid macular oedema in eyes with cataract and idiopathic epiretinal membrane after two-step sequential surgery. Eye (Lond). 2022;36(8):1597–603. https://doi.org/10.1038/s41433-021-01673-0. Epub 2021 Jul 21.

185. Flach AJ. The incidence, pathogenesis and treatment of cystoid macular edema following cataract surgery. Trans Am Ophthalmol Soc. 1998;96:557–634.

186. Henderson BA, Kim JY, Ament CS, Ferrufino-Ponce ZK, Grabowska A, Cremers SL. Clinical pseudophakic cystoid macular edema. Risk factors for development and duration after treatment. J Cataract Refract Surg. 2007;33(9):1550–8. https://doi.org/10.1016/j.jcrs.2007.05.013.

187. Chu CJ, Johnston RL, Buscombe C, Sallam AB, Mohamed Q, Yang YC, United Kingdom Pseudophakic Macular Edema Study Group. Risk factors and incidence of macular edema after cataract surgery: a database study of 81984 eyes. Ophthalmology. 2016;123(2):316–23. https://doi.org/10.1016/j.ophtha.2015.10.001. Epub 2015 Dec 8.

188. Miyake K, Ibaraki N. Prostaglandins and cystoid macular edema. Surv Ophthalmol. 2002;47(Suppl 1):S203–18. https://doi.org/10.1016/s0039-6257(02)00294-1.

189. Hall DW, Bonta IL. Prostaglandins and ocular inflammation. Doc Ophthalmol. 1977;44(2):421–34. https://doi.org/10.1007/BF00230091.

190. Ricciotti E, FitzGerald GA. Prostaglandins and inflammation. Arterioscler Thromb Vasc Biol. 2011;31(5):986–1000. https://doi.org/10.1161/ATVBAHA.110.207449.

191. Sun BK, Siprashvili Z, Khavari PA. Advances in skin grafting and treatment of cutaneous wounds. Science. 2014;346(6212):941–5. https://doi.org/10.1126/science.1253836.

192. Xu H, Chen M, Forrester JV, Lois N. Cataract surgery induces retinal pro-inflammatory gene expression and protein secretion. Invest Ophthalmol Vis Sci. 2011;52(1):249–55. https://doi.org/10.1167/iovs.10-6001.

193. Chee SP, Ti SE, Sivakumar M, Tan DT. Postoperative inflammation: extracapsular cataract extraction versus phacoemulsification. J Cataract Refract Surg. 1999;25(9):1280–5. https://doi.org/10.1016/s0886-3350(99)00161-3.

194. Dick HB, Schwenn O, Krummenauer F, Krist R, Pfeiffer N. Inflammation after sclerocorneal versus clear corneal tunnel phacoemulsification. Ophthalmology. 2000;107(2):241–7. https://doi.org/10.1016/s0161-6420(99)00082-2.

195. Dowler JG, Hykin PG, Hamilton AM. Phacoemulsification versus extracapsular cataract extraction in patients with diabetes. Ophthalmology. 2000;107(3):457–62. https://doi.org/10.1016/s0161-6420(99)00136-0.

196. Schultz T, Joachim SC, Kuehn M, Dick HB. Changes in prostaglandin levels in patients undergoing femtosecond laser-assisted cataract surgery. J Refract Surg. 2013;29(11):742–7. https://doi.org/10.3928/1081597X-20131021-03.

197. Wielders LH, Lambermont VA, Schouten JS, van den Biggelaar FJ, Worthy G, Simons RW, Winkens B, Nuijts RM. Prevention of cystoid macular edema after cataract surgery in nondiabetic and diabetic patients: a systematic review and meta-analysis. Am J Ophthalmol. 2015;160(5):968–981.e33. https://doi.org/10.1016/j.ajo.2015.07.032. Epub 2015 Jul 29.

198. Endo N, Kato S, Haruyama K, Shoji M, Kitano S. Efficacy of bromfenac sodium ophthalmic solu-

tion in preventing cystoid macular oedema after cataract surgery in patients with diabetes. Acta Ophthalmol. 2010;88(8):896–900. https://doi.org/10.1111/j.1755-3768.2009.01582.x.

199. Singh R, Alpern L, Jaffe GJ, Lehmann RP, Lim J, Reiser HJ, Sall K, Walters T, Sager D. Evaluation of nepafenac in prevention of macular edema following cataract surgery in patients with diabetic retinopathy. Clin Ophthalmol. 2012;6:1259–69. https://doi.org/10.2147/OPTH.S31902. Epub 2012 Aug 3.
200. Singh RP, Lehmann R, Martel J, Jong K, Pollack A, Tsorbatzoglou A, Staurenghi G, Cervantes-Coste Cervantes G, Alpern L, Modi S, Svoboda L, Adewale A, Jaffe GJ. Nepafenac 0.3% after cataract surgery in patients with diabetic retinopathy: results of 2 randomized phase 3 studies. Ophthalmology. 2017;124(6):776–85. https://doi.org/10.1016/j.ophtha.2017.01.036. Epub 2017 Mar 6.
201. Erden B, Çakır A, Aslan AC, Bölükbaşı S, Elçioğlu MN. The efficacy of posterior Subtenon triamcinolone acetonide injection in treatment of Irvine-Gass syndrome. Ocul Immunol Inflamm. 2019;27(8):1235–41. https://doi.org/10.1080/09273948.2019.1620786. Epub 2019 Aug 14.
202. Lam DS, Chan CK, Mohamed S, Lai TY, Lee VY, Lai WW, Fan DS, Chan WM. Phacoemulsification with intravitreal triamcinolone in patients with cataract and coexisting diabetic macular oedema: a 6-month prospective pilot study. Eye (Lond). 2005;19(8):885–90. https://doi.org/10.1038/sj.eye.6701686.
203. Nunome T, Sugimoto M, Kondo M, Suto C. Short-term results of intravitreal triamcinolone acetonide combined with cataract surgery for diabetic macular edema in Japan: in the era of anti-vascular endothelial growth factor therapy. Ophthalmologica. 2018;240(2):73–80. https://doi.org/10.1159/000487548. Epub 2018 Apr 5.
204. Sze AM, Luk FO, Yip TP, Lee GK, Chan CK. Use of intravitreal dexamethasone implant in patients with cataract and macular edema undergoing phacoemulsification. Eur J Ophthalmol. 2015;25(2):168–72. https://doi.org/10.5301/ejo.5000523. Epub 2014 Oct 21.
205. Panozzo GA, Gusson E, Panozzo G, Dalla MG. Dexamethasone intravitreal implant at the time of cataract surgery in eyes with diabetic macular edema. Eur J Ophthalmol. 2017;27(4):433–7. https://doi.org/10.5301/ejo.5000920. Epub 2016 Dec 16.
206. Rauen PI, Ribeiro JA, Almeida FP, Scott IU, Messias A, Jorge R. Intravitreal injection of ranibizumab during cataract surgery in patients with diabetic macular edema. Retina. 2012;32(9):1799–803. https://doi.org/10.1097/IAE.0b013e31824bebb8.
207. Akinci A, Muftuoglu O, Altınsoy A, Ozkılıc E. Phacoemulsification with intravitreal bevacizumab and triamcinolone acetonide injection in diabetic patients with clinically significant macular edema and cataract. Retina. 2011;31(4):755–8. https://doi.org/10.1097/IAE.0b013e3182006da1.
208. de Carvalho ER, Robson AG, Arno G, Boon CJF, Webster AA, Michaelides M. Enhanced S-cone syndrome: spectrum of clinical, imaging, electrophysiologic, and genetic findings in a retrospective case series of 56 patients. Ophthalmol Retina. 2021;5(2):195–214. https://doi.org/10.1016/j.oret.2020.07.008. Epub 2020 Jul 15.
209. Genead MA, Fishman GA. Cystic macular oedema on spectral-domain optical coherence tomography in choroideremia patients without cystic changes on fundus examination. Eye (Lond). 2011;25(1):84–90. https://doi.org/10.1038/eye.2010.157. Epub 2010 Oct 22.
210. Bringmann A, Reichenbach A, Wiedemann P. Pathomechanisms of cystoid macular edema. Ophthalmic Res. 2004;36(5):241–9. https://doi.org/10.1159/000081203.
211. Makri OE, Georgalas I, Georgakopoulos CD. Drug-induced macular edema. Drugs. 2013;73(8):789–802. https://doi.org/10.1007/s40265-013-0055-x.
212. Kim HA, Lee S, Eah KS, Yoon YH. Prevalence and risk factors of tamoxifen retinopathy. Ophthalmology. 2020;127(4):555–7. https://doi.org/10.1016/j.ophtha.2019.10.038. Epub 2019 Nov 7.
213. Doshi RR, Fortun JA, Kim BT, Dubovy SR, Rosenfeld PJ. Pseudocystic foveal cavitation in tamoxifen retinopathy. Am J Ophthalmol. 2014;157(6):1291–1298.e3. https://doi.org/10.1016/j.ajo.2014.02.046. Epub 2014 Feb 26.
214. Alieldin RA, Boonarpha N, Saedon H. Outcomes of screening for hydroxychloroquine retinopathy at the Manchester Royal Eye Hospital: 2 years' audit. Eye (Lond). 2022; https://doi.org/10.1038/s41433-022-02159-3. Epub ahead of print.
215. Ahn SJ, Joung J, Lim HW, Lee BR. Optical coherence tomography protocols for screening of hydroxychloroquine retinopathy in Asian patients. Am J Ophthalmol. 2017;184:11–8. https://doi.org/10.1016/j.ajo.2017.09.025. Epub 2017 Sep 28.
216. Hong EH, Ahn SJ, Lim HW, Lee BR. The effect of oral acetazolamide on cystoid macular edema in hydroxychloroquine retinopathy: a case report. BMC Ophthalmol. 2017;17(1):124. https://doi.org/10.1186/s12886-017-0517-0.
217. Kellner S, Weinitz S, Farmand G, Kellner U. Cystoid macular oedema and epiretinal membrane formation during progression of chloroquine retinopathy after drug cessation. Br J Ophthalmol. 2014;98(2):200–6. https://doi.org/10.1136/bjophthalmol-2013-303897. Epub 2013 Nov 1.
218. Jain N, Bhatti MT. Fingolimod-associated macular edema: incidence, detection, and management. Neurology. 2012;78(9):672–80. https://doi.org/10.1212/WNL.0b013e318248deea.
219. Wang C, Deng Z, Song L, Sun W, Zhao S. Diagnosis and management of fingolimod-associated macular

edema. Front Neurol. 2022;13:918086. https://doi.org/10.3389/fneur.2022.918086.

220. Jung EH, Lindeke-Myers A, Jain N. Two-year outcomes after variable duration of drug cessation in patients with maculopathy associated with pentosan polysulfate use. JAMA Ophthalmol. 2023;141:260. https://doi.org/10.1001/jamaophthalmol.2022.6093. Epub ahead of print.

12 Subretinal Fluid and Retinal Detachment

12.1 Developmental, Anatomical, and Physiological Aspects in Brief

Subretinal fluid is a collection of fluid in the potential space between the neurosensory (NS) retina and the retinal pigment epithelium (RPE), leading to the separation of the neurosensory retina from the RPE cell layer. Embryologically, the vertebrate eyes develop from the neural crest as an evagination from the ventral aspect of the forebrain to first form the optic vesicle. The lens placode, arising from the surface ectoderm, invaginates into the distal aspect of the optic vesicle to form a double-layered optic cup with a space between the two layers. The distal aspect of the optic cup develops into the NS retina, and the proximal layer of the cup forms the RPE, the only pigmented tissue in the body to develop from the neural crest. The eye is fully formed by integrating the surrounding mesenchyme [1]. The subretinal space is thus a creation of the embryological development of the retina. While the NSR is a transparent multi-layered tissue, the RPE is a mono-layered pigmented membrane. The two have intimate contact in the normal physiological state, with each RPE cell in contact with ~30 photoreceptors. The retina is a transparent structure tightly packed with cellular elements and neuronal fibres, allowing unhindered light access to the photoreceptors.

Among its diverse functions, the most critical function of the RPE is participation in the visual cycle. The apical villi of the RPE phagocytose the outer segments of the photoreceptors. When the light falls on the photoreceptors, it bleaches a visual pigment, rhodopsin, to split into all-trans-retinal and opsin. It triggers a nerve impulse carried onto the brain to be perceived as vision (phototransduction). The all-trans-retinal is converted to all-trans-retinol and is transported to the RPE, where it isomerized to the 11-cis retinal, stored in the RPE cells, and transported across the subretinal space to get back into outer photoreceptor segments to form rhodopsin, and the cycle continues. On the other hand, in the day vision photoreceptors, the cone chromophore is recycled in the Muller glial cells, where it is stored and converted to all-trans-retinal and esterified to the 11-cis-retinal and transported back to the cones to combine with the opsin to form the cone pigment [2].

12.2 The Flow of Aqueous Fluid in the Eye

The ciliary processes secrete aqueous humour into the eye's posterior chamber to meet the micronutrient and metabolic requirements of the various intraocular structures besides keeping the eyeball inflated at an intraocular pressure (~15 mmHg) within a narrow range of diurnal

A. Gupta et al., *Ophthalmic Signs in Practice of Medicine*,
https://doi.org/10.1007/978-981-99-7923-3_12

variations. The formation rate of aqueous humour varies from 3 μL/min in the morning to 1.5 μL/min at night [3]. The non-pigmented ciliary epithelium forms most of the aqueous humour by secretion, which is actively transported by the aquaporin water channels. The aqueous humour is responsible for maintaining homeostasis in the anterior segment. The bulk of the aqueous humour follows a pressure gradient. It flows through the anterior route via the trabecular meshwork at the anterior chamber's angle and ~40% through the uveoscleral outflow through an osmotic gradient through the anterior face of the ciliary muscles into the suprachoroidal space [4]. Contrary to popular belief held till recently that there is no posterior aqueous flow, current evidence suggests that almost the same amount of aqueous flows out (2.5 μL/min) through the vitreous cavity as the anterior route. The posteriorly directed fluid moves through the neurosensory retina (NSR), is pumped out by the RPE, and finally exits the eye through vortex veins [5].

12.3 Factors That Keep the Retina Attached to RPE and the Accumulation of Subretinal Fluid (SRF)

The photoreceptors contact the microvilli of the RPE through interdigitation. On the OCT, it is seen as the zone of interdigitation. An interphotoreceptor protein matrix consisting of glycoproteins and proteoglycans with high concentrations of glycosaminoglycans acts as a glue between the photoreceptor outer segments and the RPE microvilli [6, 7]. The NSR and the RPE remain adherent throughout life despite the absence of anatomic adhesions. However, within no time of the eye removal or death, the NSR can be easily peeled off from the RPE at 37 °C. Metabolic activity and oxygen are crucial in maintaining the adhesion of the NSR and the RPE [8]. Lowering the temperature to 4 °C makes it difficult to peel off the NSR, possibly because of the shutting down of the Na+ pump, which causes cellular swelling and thus tightens the grip of microvilli on the outer segments of the photoreceptors [9]. Several factors play a role in keeping the subretinal space dry. The most important is an active pump located at the apical aspect of the RPE cells capable of pumping balanced salt solution fluid from the subretinal space at a rate of 0.12 μL/mm^2/h. The RPE pump removes 70% of the SRF. The rest of the fluid moves into the choroid because of the high oncotic pressure in the choroid [10]. A posteriorly directed pressure gradient is created by maintaining a posteriorly directed fluid flow. In addition to these factors, the retina offers resistance to fluid flow, and the intraocular pressure pushes the retina posteriorly against the eye wall [7].

The fact that the retina offers resistance to the fluid flow across the retina has become a matter of debate. The outflow rate from the RPE is almost the same as the anterior route outflow. In patients with retinal detachment subjected to pars plana vitreous surgery, the vitreous cavity is often filled with silicone oil as a vitreous substitute. Many of these eyes show a rise in IOP. The IOP rises because the normal posterior outflow channel through the retina is no longer available. Apart from the anterior outflow, the flow of aqueous humour through the retina also plays a crucial role in maintaining IOP. The pressure gradient across the NSR and RPE cannot be easily measured [5]; thus, there is no way of knowing whether fluid is transported across the NSR. Some fluid, albeit small in quantity, generated in the NSR from the very high cellular metabolic activity is undoubtedly transported across NSR through the retinal Muller glial cell processes. The Muller cell processes link with the photoreceptors to form the outer retina's external limiting membrane (ELM).

It has been estimated that in non-drainage retinal detachment surgery, 261 μL/mm^2/day can be transported by the RPE and absorbed by the choroid, which is half the volume of the vitreous cavity suggesting a very active RPE pump for removal of SRF [11].

IFN-γ is a significant regulator on the posterolateral aspect of the RPE cells that keeps the subretinal space dry. IFN-γ is activated by nitric oxide, continuously produced in the retina and the choriocapillaris [12].

Acetazolamide, when systemically administered, also enhances the apical to basal fluid flow in the RPE by blocking the cell membrane carbonic anhydrase and lowering the pH in the subretinal space [13, 14]. However, it is more effective in drying SRF due to RPE dysfunction than the macular detachment due to retinal vessel leakage.

12.4 Causes of Subretinal Fluid

The major causes of the accumulation of fluid in the subretinal space (SRF) are (A) exudative, (B) tractional, and (C) rhegmatogenous retinal detachment. Besides, several systemic diseases present with subretinal fluid accumulation. See Box 12.1.

A. **Exudative (serous) retinal detachment**
   1. Central serous chorioretinopathy; pachychoroid spectrum disorder in young
   2. Neovascular age-related macular degeneration in old
   3. Retinal disorders—diabetic macular oedema; retinal venous occlusions; retinal angiomas; Coats' disease; and retinal inflammations
   4. Malignant hypertension and pregnancy-induced hypertension
   5. Uveal inflammations (anterior uveitis; choroiditis; choroidal granulomas; inflammatory choroidal neovascular membrane)
   6. Choroidal metastatic lesions; choroidal tumours
B. **Tractional causes of retinal detachment**
   1. Proliferative diabetic retinopathy
   2. Branch retinal vein occlusion
   3. Retinopathy of prematurity; familial exudative vitreoretinopathy (FEVR)
   4. Retinal vasculitis; sickle cell retinopathy
   5. Myopic tractional detachment
C. **Rhegmatogenous retinal detachment**

Box 12.1 Systemic Disorders Associated with Serous Macular Detachment

1	Malignant hypertension[a]
2	Diabetes mellitus[a]
3	Pregnancy-induced hypertension[b]
4	Systemic lupus erythematosus[c]
5	Chronic renal disease/end-stage renal disease[d]
6	Drug-induced: phosphodiesterase type 5 inhibitors; anticancer drugs[e,f]
7	Hypercortisolism: endogenous or exogenous (corticosteroids)[a]
8	Disseminated intravascular coagulopathy[a]
9	Thrombocytopenic purpura[a]
10	Systemic vasculitis[a]
11	Paraproteinemias/hyperviscosity syndromes[a]
12	Glomerulonephritis; IgA nephropathy[a]
13	Metastatic disease; leukaemias[a]

[a] Wolfensberger and Tufail [170]
[b] Roos et al. [171]
[c] Jabs et al. [172]
[d] Chang et al. [111]
[e] da Cruz et al. [173]
[f] Fortes et al. [174]

12.4.1 Central Serous Chorioretinopathy

Central serous chorioretinopathy is a common idiopathic condition seen at least six times more common in men <50 years of age who present with acute onset of metamorphopsia and blurring of vision. In a nationwide study of the Japanese population over 8 years, 76% were men, and 24% were women. The incidence rate of CSC was 54.2 and 15.7 per 100,000 population in men and women, respectively. The mean age at onset was higher in women at 54.7 ± 13.5 vs 50.5 ± 12.5 years in men, the peak incidence being in 40–44 years in men and 50–54 in women [15]. Forty percent of patients with CSC have bilateral disease [16]. A 3D single-layer RPE scan on SD-OCT has shown RPE bumps in 94% of the asymptomatic eyes [17].

Fundus examination reveals a serous detachment of the macula from the subretinal fluid

(SRF) collection (Fig. 12.1). Most patients show spontaneous resolution within 6 months without any intervention. On fundus fluorescein angiography, following an initial delay in the choroidal filling, there is either a single or multiple points of fluorescein leakage, which increases in size as an ink blot or has a classical smoke stack appearance as the dye is seen rising as a plume of smoke under the retina and fills a sharply defined PED and late pooling of the dye in the subretinal space. The ICG shows increased hyperpermeability of the choroidal vessels. In most acute cases of CSC, there is an associated single or multiple leaks in pigment epithelial detachments (PEDs) overlying the area of choroidal hyperpermeability [18, 19]. The yellow dot-like precipitates seen in the SRF of CSC correspond to hyperautofluorescent dots seen in CSC and represent the outer segments of photoreceptors [20]. On resolution, the NSR quickly establishes contact with the microvilli of the RPE. The hyperautofluorescent shed photoreceptor outer segments in the SRF may remain visible for a long time under the NSR. Exposure to corticosteroids leads to massive exudation in CSC [21]. Subretinal fibrinous exudation with or without corticosteroid exposure, especially in the young, is often associated with RPE rips, which may be giant at times [22–26].

12.4.1.1 Risk Factors for CSC

The risk factors for CSC include male gender, hyperopia, short axial length [27], thick sclera, type A personality [28], corticosteroid use and pregnancy [29], and stress [30] (Fig. 12.1b, c). Frequent and vigorous physical activity increases the risk of CSC. Increased blood pressure and sympathetic activity due to vigorous exercise might contribute to decompensating the choroidal vessels [31]. Exercise is known to activate the renin-angiotensin-aldosterone pathway and induce hypertension. The choroid may be the target organ for frequent attacks of exercise-induced hypertension variability. The sclera is significantly thinner in the steroid-associated CSC than in the non-steroid-associated CSC, suggesting that steroid-associated CSC is unrelated to

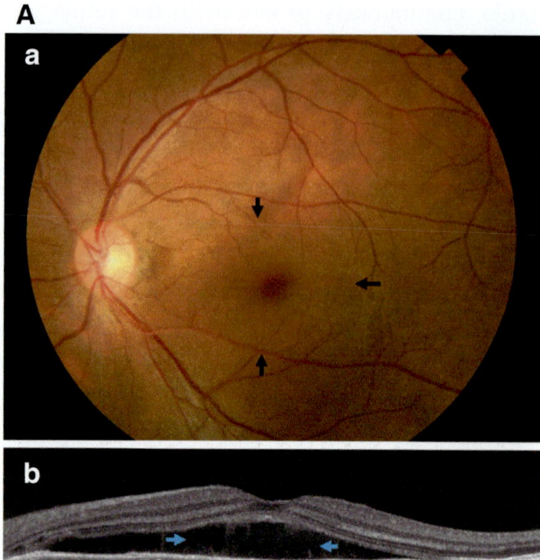

Fig. 12.1 (**A**) Serous retinal detachment in the macula (black arrows) in a 32-year-old man suggestive of acute central serous chorioretinopathy (CSC) in the left eye (**a**). OCT shows subretinal fluid (blue arrows) (**b**). (**B**) A 44-year-old man presented with a diminution of vision in the right eye and had received corticosteroids elsewhere with a mistaken diagnosis of choroiditis. The right eye at presentations showed subretinal fluid with massive yellow-coloured subretinal fibrin (**a**). FFA shows an area of hyperfluorescence (red arrow) and outlining of the pigment epithelial detachments (PEDS), white arrows in (**b**). Late frames of FFA show filling of the PEDs and a reverse smokestack hyperfluorescence from the site of leakage shown in 'b' with a red arrow (**c**). He was asked to stop oral corticosteroids which led to spontaneous resolution of the SRF and left behind only a streak of fibrin (blue arrow) (**d**). (**C**) A 42-year-old woman had a diminution of vision in both eyes for 3 months. She had been diagnosed with bilateral choroiditis elsewhere and treated with oral corticosteroids, leading to further vision deterioration in both eyes. The right eye posterior pole shows subretinal fluid, folds of the internal limiting membrane and subretinal fibrin. Note clear dot-like spaces in the fibrin (a, red arrows). Similar subretinal fibrin and exudative detachment are seen in the left eye (**b**). On FFA, the right eye shows expanding dots of fluid leakage (**c**, **d**). Note that the red arrows in 'c' correspond to the clear dots in the fibrin seen in 'a'. FFA in the left eye also shows similar expanding dots and pooling fluorescein dye under the retina (**e**–**h**). (**i**, **j**) The patient was advised to stop oral corticosteroids which led to resolution of the subretinal fluid in both eyes. The right eye shows a subretinal residual contracted fibrinous membrane (red arrows)

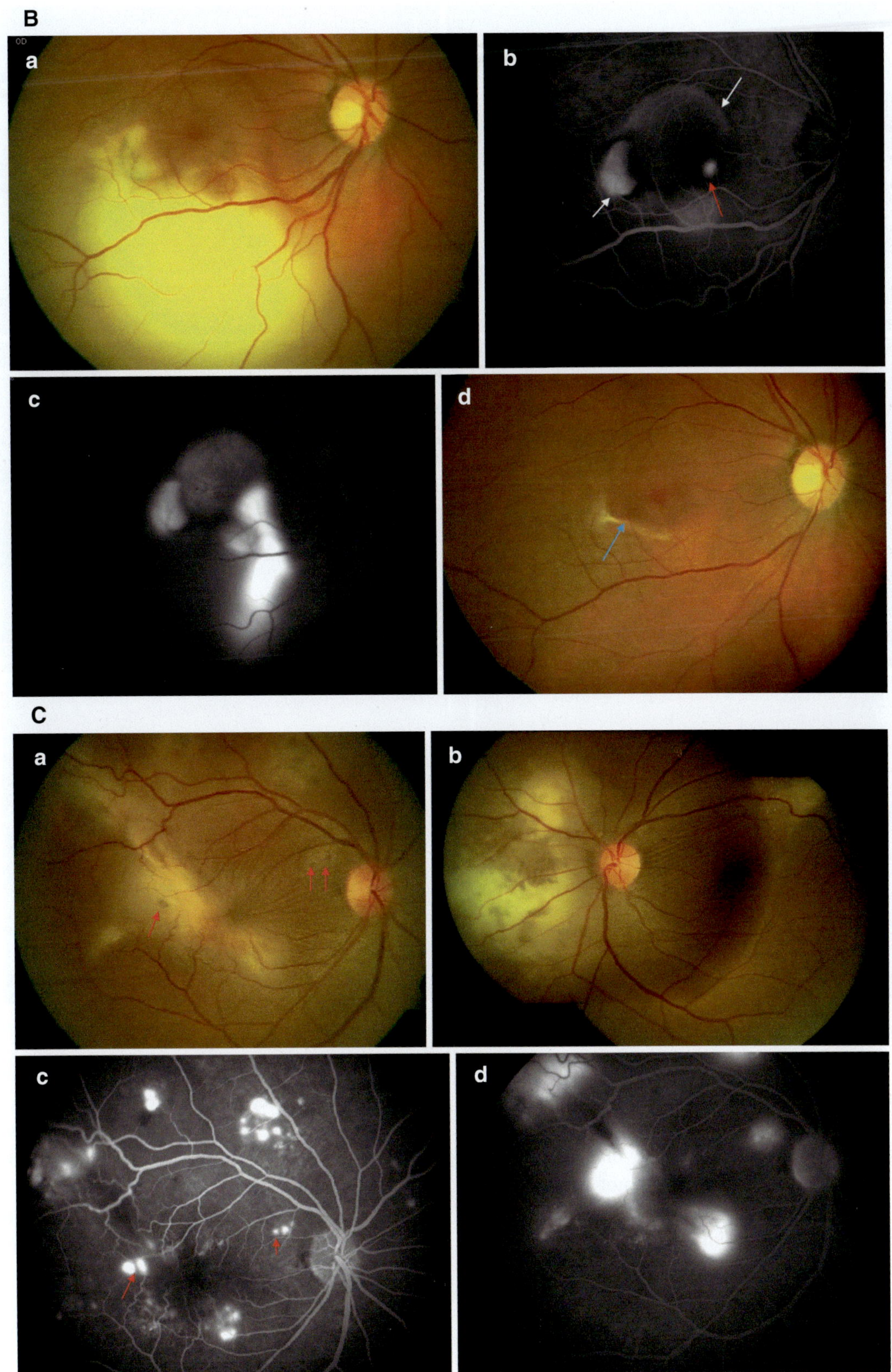

Fig. 12.1 (continued)

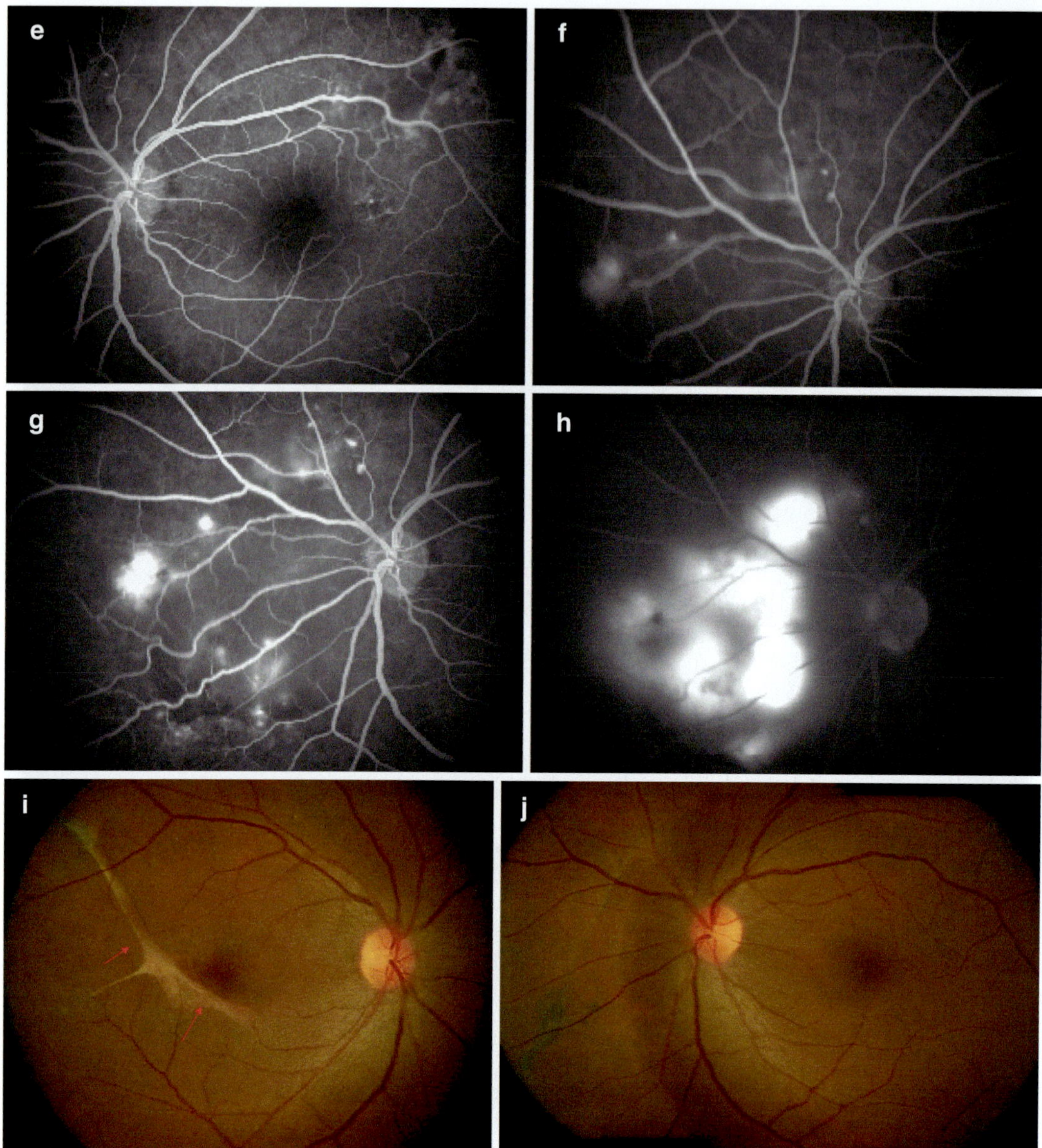

Fig. 12.1 (continued)

increased scleral thickness [32]. Proportionately, more women than men are affected in steroid-associated CSC. The precise mechanisms that cause CSC with steroid use are not known. It may be due to sympathetic overactivity. Stress and type A persons are long-recognized risk factors for CSC. The choroidal blood supply is autonomic and responds to parasympathetic and sympathetic control. Applying topical 2% homatropine increased subfoveal thickness within 30–60 min [33]. In anecdotal reports, recurrent PED has followed the application of topical phenylephrine 2.5% [34, 35].

On the contrary, a controlled study has shown that topical tropicamide 1% and phenylephrine 2.5% decreased the subfoveal choroidal thickness [36]. Epinephrine has been used to create an animal model that mimics CSC [37]. In vitro experiments have shown that epinephrine causes apoptosis of RPE cells by elevating the cyclic adenosine monophosphate in the RPE [38]. Dexamethasone, when applied directly to the RPE cells, did not cause apoptosis, but cortisols work by upregulating the β-adrenergic receptors on a variety of cells. It has long been known that endogenous blood and urine cortisol levels are higher in patients with CSC [39].

12.4.1.2 OCT in CSC

Nearly 50% of the CSC eyes may show a micro-rip in the RPE corresponding to the FFA leak. Spontaneous closure of the micro-rip leads to the resolution of the SRF [40]. Others have noted a lower incidence of micro-rips and seen them more often in chronic CSC (6%) than in acute CSC (2%) [41, 42]. One of the earliest studies using enhanced depth imaging on SD-OCT revealed increased subfoveal choroidal thickness and decreased innermost choroidal layer. A double-layer sign consisting of undulating RPE and intact Bruch's membrane was seen in 75% of the eyes with chronic CSC [42], which shall now be interpreted as representing a polypoidal choroidal vasculopathy (PCV). PCV is considered a stage in pachychoroid syndrome. PCV has been mimicking the CSC in the past [43].

12.4.1.3 Pathogenesis of SRF in CSC

The source of the SRF can be either the NSR or the choroid. The increased hydrostatic pressure under the RPE because of a choroidal pathology may overcome the adherence forces that keep the NSR and the RPE in contact. The serous retinal detachment develops when the RPE barrier breaks, and the fluid leaks through the RPE into the subretinal space. It is usually seen in all those conditions with increased hydrostatic pressure in the choroid, such as venous outflow choroidopathy, pachychoroid spectrum disorders, or choroidal inflammations. A normal functioning RPE will dry out this leakage of SRF in no time. However, it is not the case in patients with CSC. The persistent SRF indicates a more widespread metabolic dysfunction of the RPE that fails to pump out the SRF. An equilibrium may reach when the inflow into the subretinal space matches the outflow. It is hypothesized that increased choroidal pressure and choriocapillaris ischaemia, coupled with an RPE metabolic dysfunction around the leak's site, allow the fluid accumulation in the subretinal space. It may accumulate far away from the site of leakage [44].

It is believed that acute CSC is the first stage of a pachychoroid spectrum disease. Notably, the sclera in CSC eyes is significantly thickened compared to non-CSC eyes [45]. Recently, ~20% of the eyes with CSC were shown to have cilio-choroidal effusion. Ciliochoroidal effusion and exudative retinal detachment are features of uveal effusion syndrome (UES) [46]. Hyperopia, short axial length and increased scleral thickness are risk factors for both UES and CSC. Increased scleral thickness suggests that CSC, like UES, may be the outcome of venous outflow choroidopathy [47].

Moreover, thick sclera and increased subfoveal choroidal thickness are associated with pockets of fluid in the outer choroid, indicating that CSC is a stage in the pachychoroid spectrum [48, 49]. Plasma leakage into the choroidal interstitial tissue likely leads to decreased blood flow, raising the pressure in the Haller vessels and consequent dilatation of these vessels (pachyvessels), a thick choroid and compression of the choriocapillaris [50]. The loculation of fluid in the posterior choroid may be due to a decrease in the trans-scleral outflow of fluid due to a thick sclera.

In the choroid, the venous drainage is segmental. It drains into the vortex veins, each segment drained by 1–2 vortex veins. The availability of wide-angle ICG has made it possible to study the vortex veins. An outflow obstruction in the vortex veins leads to congestion of the choroidal veins. Intervortex veins form anastomotic channels across the horizontal watershed to compensate for the congested veins. These vessels are dilated (pachyvessels) and show hyperpermeability on ICG. Given the similarity of imaging features in CSC and obstruction in the vortex vein blood flow outside the eye as in carotid-cavernous fistula (CCF), a view is emerging that CSC is likely an outcome of venous overload choroidopathy [51, 52].

12.4.1.4 Formation of Choroidal New Vessels in CSC

One of the consequences of pachyvessels is the compression of the choriocapillaris, causing ischaemia [53]. It is evident on ICG angiography; all eyes with pachyvessels show patchy delayed filling of the choriocapillaris, and new vessels (pachychoroid neovasculopathy) were seen in all areas that showed delayed filling [54]. In patients who present with a clinical picture consistent with type I CNV without drusen, the characteristics of their CNV are more like polypoidal choroidal neovasculopathy (PCN). Patients with chronic CSC may either present with PCN or develop this complication after an interval varying from 7 to 365 months [55].

The development of CNV is a sight-threatening complication in the so-called benign spontaneously resolving disease. The anti-VEGF therapy treats CNV successfully. It needs a high suspicion index, especially in older patients and those with a chronic course of CSC. In the past, using ICG angiography, the formation of choroidal new vessels (CNVs) was seen in ~9% of patients. Patients older than 50, chronic CSC patients, and patients who showed thickened RPE, pigmentary changes, and subretinal lipid deposits developed CNV [56]. The diagnosis of CNV in chronic CSC is difficult as the clinical picture of the two overlaps. On FFA, there is no specific leakage pattern of the CNV to differentiate it from the CSC leaks. The FFA, therefore, has poor sensitivity and only moderate specificity to detect CNV [57]. On OCT angiography, the incidence of CNV has varied from 21% to 23% [57, 58]. However, in CSC lasting more than 6 months, as many as 30% of eyes had CNV [59]. Ill-defined leakage on FFA and irregular flat PED on structural OCT and OCTA findings can help detect CNV in CSC [58]. Non-homogeneous hyperreflectivity either in the choriocapillaris layer or under a shallow irregular pigment epithelial detachment of any length and height may be used as a marker of CNV and treated with ant-VEGF therapy [60–63]. While two-thirds of the chronic CSC fellow eyes may show irregular shallow PED, internal hyperreflectivity in these lesions suggests CNV. Nearly one-fourth of the fellow eyes of chronic CSC may also show an asymptomatic CNV network on the OCTA. Hence, OCTA should always be done in both eyes, even if only one is symptomatic. Notably, these networks are difficult to be picked up on conventional angiography [64].

12.4.1.5 Treatment of CSC

Most patients show spontaneous resolution and are usually watched without intervention (Fig. 12.2). Lifestyle changes are suggested to reduce stress. Previously, mild focal laser photocoagulation was applied to non-resolving CSC patients. Various cells in the retina and choroid express mineralocorticoid (MR) and glucocorticoid receptors (GR). While aldosterone is a natural ligand for the MR, cortisol also binds the MR. Because cortisol levels are often raised in CSC and get aggravated by corticosteroids, blocking the MR is a logical approach to treating patients with CSC. However, there are no biomarkers to know either the MR pathway's activation or their antagonists' bioavailability in various eye compartments [65].

The possibility for the role of MR in the pathophysiology of CSC has led to using eplerenone to block the mineralocorticoid receptors. Eplerenone is better tolerated than another aldosterone-blocking drug, Spironolactone. The other drugs used to treat CSC include ketoconazole (inhibitor of steroid synthesis) and mifepristone—a glucocorticoid receptor-blocking drug [66]. Anti-VEGF therapy has now supplanted photodynamic therapy for the treatment of CSC neovasculopathy. Both pulse laser and eplerenone treatment were equally effective short-term strategies in chronic CSC in resolving SRF [67]. However, compared to half-dose PDT, eplerenone therapy was not well tolerated and resolved SRF only in 17% vs 78% in the PDT group [68]. Previously, in a randomized placebo-controlled trial, eplerenone was no better than the placebo in improving the best corrected visual acuity [69]. Intact EZ and outer retina may predict a good response to eplerenone [70]. Case

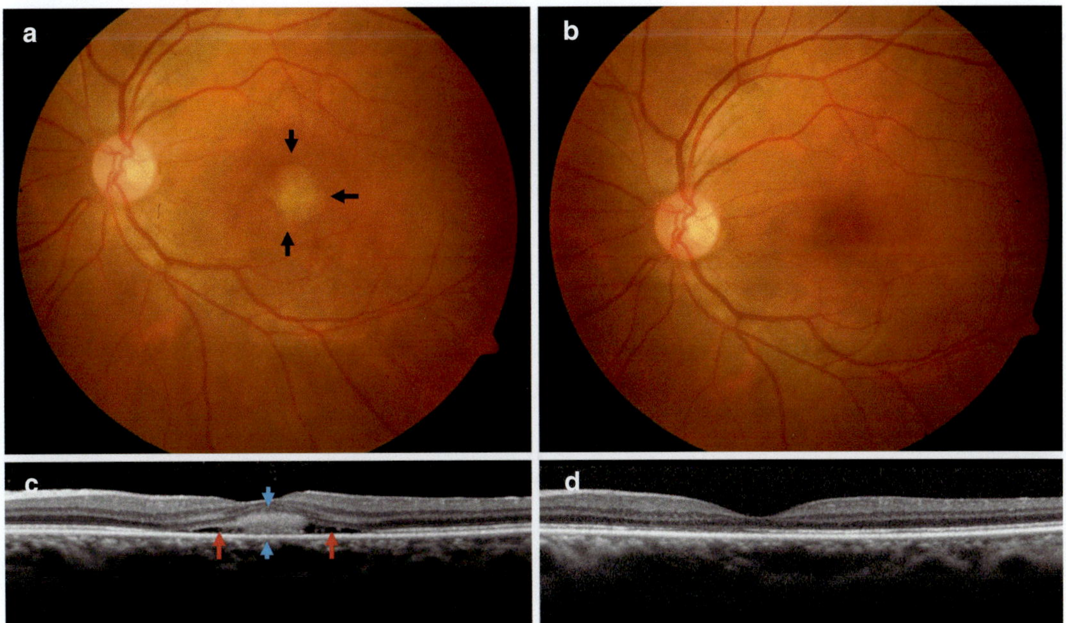

Fig. 12.2 Fibrinous deposits (black arrows) in the fovea in a steroid-exposed (using steroid cream for a skin disease) patient with central serous chorioretinopathy (**a**). Following cessation of steroid therapy, the fibrinous deposits resolved spontaneously and completely at 3 months (**b**). OCT shows subretinal fibrin (blue arrows) and subretinal fluid (red arrows) at presentation (**c**). At 3 months, there was complete resolution of fibrin and SRF in the macula (**d**)

selection is a major challenge in testing any drug therapy in chronic CSC. Most of the studies in the past rule out neovasculopathy OCT angiography, which is a frequent complication of chronic CSC and is unlikely to respond to MR blocker drugs.

12.4.2 Subretinal Fluid in Choroidal Neovascular Membranes

In choroidal neovascular membranes, the endothelial cells activate, migrate through Bruch's membrane (BM), and establish contact with the RPE cells. Capillary endothelial cells in contact with the RPE cells express soluble VEGF, which compromises RPE barrier function, thus causing SRF accumulation, reversible with anti-VEGF agents (Fig. 12.3) [71]. Thickening of the Bruch's membrane due to the deposition of lipids (esterified > unesterified) is an age-related phenomenon. It offers resistance to the fluid passage from the subretinal space to the choroid and leads to fluid formation under the RPE, termed pigment epithelial detachment (PED) [72]. This phenomenon is akin to atherosclerosis, where the deposits of esterified cholesterol are several times higher than the blood levels. A free exchange of serum lipids from the blood to the RPE cells and the cell membrane lipids from the digested photoreceptor segments occurs. However, the lipid in the BM is more like LDL than the membrane lipids [73]. One of the other primary functions of the RPE is keeping the NS and the subretinal space dry with the help of an active pump for optimal retina functioning. Up to 150 μm of the SRF on OCT in patients with wet age-related macular degeneration has minimal impact on vision [74]. However, beyond 200 μm, the SRF affects vision only if there is no associated outer retinal atrophy or subretinal hyperreflective material (SHRM). However, if there is atrophy of NSR or SHRM, the presence of SRF has no additional detrimental effect [75]. It is crucial since giving additional injections of anti-VEGF agents in the ARMD to completely dry out the subretinal space only adds

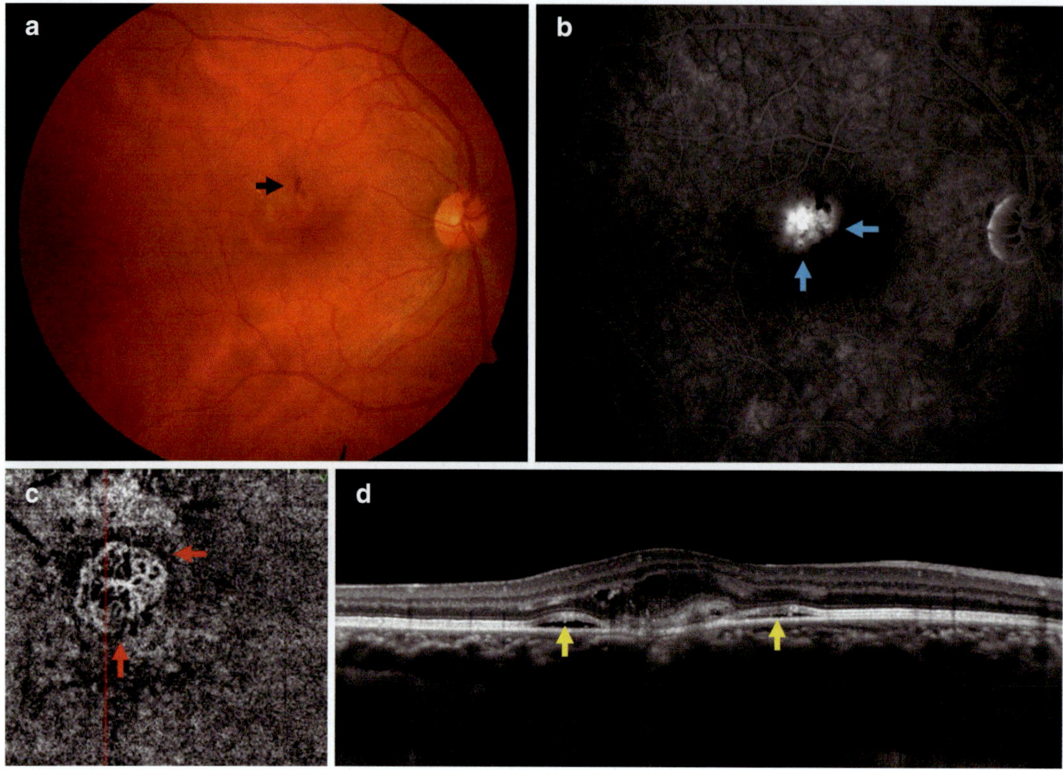

Fig. 12.3 A tiny retinal haemorrhage (black arrow) above the fovea in an eye with choroidal neovascular membrane (CNVM) (**a**). Fluorescein angiography showing leak (blue arrow) from the CNVM (**b**). OCT angiography shows the neovascular complex (red arrow) (**c**). OCT shows subretinal fluid (yellow arrows) along with cystic spaces in the macula (**d**)

to the treatment burden without gaining any vision. On the other hand, treatment-resistant SRF is protective against macular atrophy [76]. The SRF carries a better visual outcome than intraretinal fluid (IRF) which impacts the vision unfavourably [77]. The IRF results from damage to the retinal Muller glial cells affecting the photoreceptor functioning and neural transmission [78]. A breach in the external limiting membrane (ELM) contributes to the IRF. At the same time, an SRF indicates an intact ELM, integrity of the ellipsoid zone, and better visual outcome [79].

12.4.3 Subretinal Fluid in Diabetic Macular Oedema

One-third to two-thirds of patients with diabetic macular oedema (DME) may be accompanied by serous retinal detachment (SRD) (Fig. 12.4). The source of the SRF in these patients has remained a matter of debate. The disruptions in the ellipsoid zone (EZ), ELM, the number of hyperreflective foci (HRF), and increased subfoveal choroidal thickness are significantly associated with the presence of SRF in DME. The increased fovea avascular zone, either in the SCP or DCP, has no influence. However, whenever there was SRF, disruptions of the retinal inner layers were less commonly seen [80]. Significantly patients of DME with SRF show high vitreous levels of IL-6, suggesting an inflammatory origin of this fluid [81]. High systolic and diastolic blood pressure may be an independent and significant risk factor for developing SRF in DME [82].

The FFA in patients of DME with SRF shows diffuse leakage from retinal vessels compared to an ischaemic pattern in DR eyes which do not show SRF. When treated with intravitreal (IVT) Lucentis, the visual gains in DME + SRF eyes are poorer than the DME − no SRF [83]. DME eyes that are resistant to Lucentis show resolution of

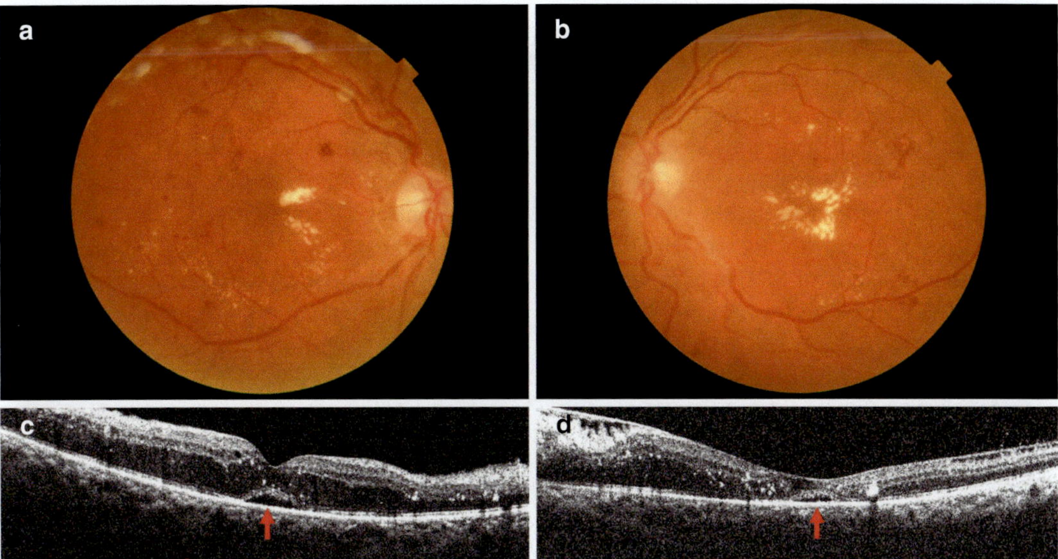

Fig. 12.4 Bilateral moderate non-proliferative diabetic retinopathy with diabetic macular oedema (**a**, **b**). OCT shows a cone-shaped pocket of subretinal fluid (red arrow) beneath the fovea, along with intraretinal cystoid spaces and hard exudates (**c**, **d**)

SRF with IVT DEX implant [84]. The SRF and the hyperreflective foci (HRF) are markers of inflammation. In eyes treated with anti-VEGF injections, those with SRF and HRF at the baseline have significantly more recurrences [85]. However, in treating naïve DME with inflammatory markers (SRF and HRF), anatomical results are better with IVT DEX implant, although the visual improvement is more significant with Eylea injections [86]. The DME eyes with SRF, intact EZ, and no HRF respond much better to the IVT DEX implant compared to those who do not have these features [87].

12.4.4 Subretinal Fluid in Retinal Vein Occlusions

Macular oedema often complicates eyes with retinal vein occlusions (RVO). In the past, exudative retinal detachments were only occasionally reported in eyes with central retinal vein occlusion (CRVO) [88]. The availability of OCT revealed that many more patients with branch retinal vein occlusion (BRVO) or central retinal vein occlusion (CRVO) develop SRF [89]. Most RVO eyes develop SRF under the fovea as a cone-shaped detachment that later becomes dome-shaped (Fig. 12.5). It is hypothesized that this SRF may result from fluid leakage through the retinal Muller glial cells [90]. A thicker sub-

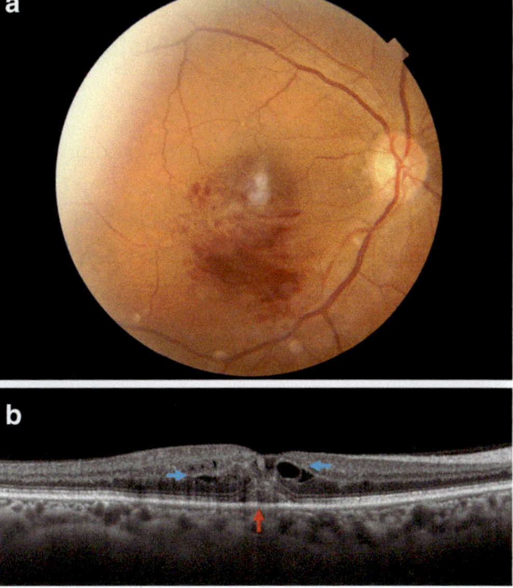

Fig. 12.5 Retinal haemorrhages due to macular BRVO (**a**), with cystoid macular oedema (blue arrows) and a cone-shaped pocket of subretinal fluid (red arrow) on OCT (**b**)

foveal choroidal thickness is a good prognostic indicator for response to treatment with anti-VEGF agents in eyes with retinal vein occlusion (RVO) that shows SRF [91]. Increased vascular permeability due to high vitreous levels of VEGF, soluble intercellular adhesion molecules (sICAM), and downregulation of pigment epithelial-derived growth factor (PEDF) may result in the formation of SRF in eyes with RVO [92, 93]. The visual acuity is mainly affected by macular oedema (ME) in RVO than by the presence of SRF, which often accompanies the ME [94]. Both IVT Eylea and IVT DEX implants lead to the resolution of the SRF in CRVO, but the visual results are superior with Eylea [95]. Eylea is also more effective in BRVO with SRF than Lucentis [96]. Triamcinolone acetonide (TA) is also effective in resolving SRF in eyes with RVO [97]. While TA led to a better morphological outcome in BRVO eyes with ME and SRF, the visual outcome was good irrespective of the presence of SRF [98].

12.4.5 Subretinal Fluid in Malignant Hypertension

Recognizing exudative retinal detachment as a manifestation of malignant hypertension (MH) is vital. An undiagnosed patient may first present with sudden onset of bilateral loss of vision due to exudative retinal detachment. For more than 125 years since Liebreich's first description of 'albuminuric retinitis' in MH, retinal arteriolar changes in hypertension had remained the focus of physicians' attention until Hayreh first described choroidopathy as a manifestation of accelerated hypertension in a monkey model of renal hypertension [99]. Exudative retinal detachment and RPE infarction were the most characteristic feature of hypertensive choroidopathy. The changes were first detected after a median interval of 36 days after clamping the renal artery when the systolic blood pressure (BP) reached a median of 180–190 mmHg. There was widespread occlusion of the choroidal arteries, infarction of the choriocapillaris and RPE, and exudative retinal detachment. On FFA, there was delayed filling of the choroid, mainly in the post-pole. Multifocal, small, round pale or white RPE changes were seen in the macula or temporal to the macula, which leaked fluorescein in the late phase and showed dye pooling in the subretinal space. The choroidal vasculature is under autonomic control. The renin-angiotensin-aldosterone system is the primary regulator of blood pressure control. Hayreh, in his experiments, produced acute ischaemic injury of the kidney by clamping one or both renal arteries, which led to the release of renin. This proteolytic enzyme cleaves angiotensin I from angiotensinogen, further converted by the angiotensin-converting enzyme to angiotensin II. Angiotensin II has widespread activity in the sympathetic system and promotes the release and potentiation of norepinephrine-induced vasoconstrictor activity. It ultimately leads to the occlusion of arterioles.

Papilloedema and exudative retinal detachment besides the cotton wool spots and the retinal haemorrhages characterize the fundus changes in malignant hypertension (see Chap. 8, Fig. 8.7a–d). If the fundus examination is unavailable, high blood pressure (usually systolic BP >200 mmHg and diastolic BP >120 mmHg) with at least three end-organ damage, including kidneys, heart, and brain and thrombotic microangiopathy. Despite the availability of potent antihypertensive therapy for more than four decades, the incidence of MH has not decreased, especially in underserved regions and communities. Three-fourths of the MH is caused by essential hypertension. The less common causes include oestrogen contraception, renal artery stenosis, primary hyperaldosteronism, IgA nephropathy, and pheochromocytoma [100]. The end-organ damage due to MH in the eyes, kidneys, and brain shows a high degree of concurrency. It is believed to be due to hyperperfusion-induced capillary leakage, which causes posterior reversible encephalopathy syndrome, proteinuria, and exudative retinal detachment. These changes are reversible with the control of BP (see Chap. 8, Fig. 8.7e–h). The reversible damage is due to an elevated BP beyond the autoregulatory control of the arterioles leading to capillary hyperperfusion. The choroid already has the highest blood flow tissue in the eye. A laser speckle flowgraphy has shown increased choroidal blood flow when the untreated blood pressure is very high [101, 102]. On the other hand, many believe that lesions of hypertensive choroidopathy are due to ischaemic insult [103, 104]. Multimodal imaging shows SRF and the presence of hyperreflective deposits on Bruch's membrane, which persist after the resolution of the SRF. The OCT angiography also shows the hyperreflective deposits in the choriocapillaris layer. These are seen as autofluorescent spots on FAF and are likely due to fibrin deposits [105, 106]. The electron microscopy in the monkey model of hypertensive choroidopathy also showed fibrin deposits [107]. On OCT angiography, the retinal circulation showed extensive flow voids in the choriocapillaris of a patient with MH who showed massive SRF. Concurrent with the normalization of BP, the perfusion in the choriocapillaris improved, SRF resolved, and the visual acuity improved but flow deficit persisted in the retina [108]. Reperfusion of choriocapillaris was also seen in a patient with pregnancy-induced hypertension [109]. Hypertensive choroidopathy frequently complicates pregnancy-induced hypertension (preeclampsia). These patients develop choroidopathy at a BP lower than in age-matched non-pregnant hypertensive patients who present more often with hypertensive retinopathy. On OCT angiography, these patients may not have complete reperfusion of choriocapillaris. Both ischaemic and hyperperfusion mechanisms may likely be responsible for hypertensive choroidopathy [110]. Patients with end-stage renal disease who are on dialysis have a higher risk of developing serous retinal detachment, perhaps because of hyperperfusion in the choroid [111].

12.4.6 Subretinal Fluid in Uveitis

The most common cause of SRF/exudative retinal detachment (ERD) is VKH disease which accounts for nearly 40% of the cases of ERD in uveitis. The other less common causes are panuveitis (15%), posterior scleritis (4%), necrotizing scleritis (2%), retinochoroiditis (2%), and sympathetic ophthalmia (1%) [112].

The SRF develops in around 40–65% of eyes with uveitis CME [113]. Unlike other causes of ME (RVO; Irvine-Gass syndrome) that show the presence of hyperreflective deposits in the SRF, only a minority of uveitis ME (UME) does so [114]. In patients with uveitis who develop cystoid macular oedema (CME), SRF appears first before they develop CME [115]. It is an early sign of UME and generally carries a favourable prognosis. Patients with worse vision and thicker retinas on presentation respond well to treatment with improved visual acuity [113]. They respond well to periocular or IVT corticosteroids. Macular oedema affects vision more than SRF. The SRF does not appear to have a direct effect on visual acuity. However, eyes with ME with SRF respond better to treatment than eyes with intraretinal thickening without SRF [116]. However, increasing central subfield thickness (CST) had a greater chance of disruptions of EZ and the interdigitating zone (IZ), leading to irreversible visual loss [117].

The OCT has shown that more than 80% of the eyes with juvenile idiopathic arthritis-associated chronic uveitis (JIA uveitis) may be associated with macular oedema and show SRF in 18% [118]. SRF may be the only manifestation, or it may be associated with perifoveolar macular thickening or CME. Patients respond well to increased immunomodulatory therapy [119].

Even Bartonella henselae neuroretinitis rarely may present as a monofocal choroiditis lesion with overlying serous detachment in the macula appearing as a helioid lesion (SUN-like) [120, 121].

The patients with VKH disease show thickening of the choroid due to infiltration by granulomatous inflammatory cells (Fig. 12.6). FFA and the ICG angiography show initial delayed filling of the choroid and pinpoint leakage from the RPE in mid-phase with pooling of the dye in multifocal SRF pockets.

A similar phenomenon is seen in the tubercular (TB) choroidal granulomas, which are hypoxic and highly vascularized. TB granulomas

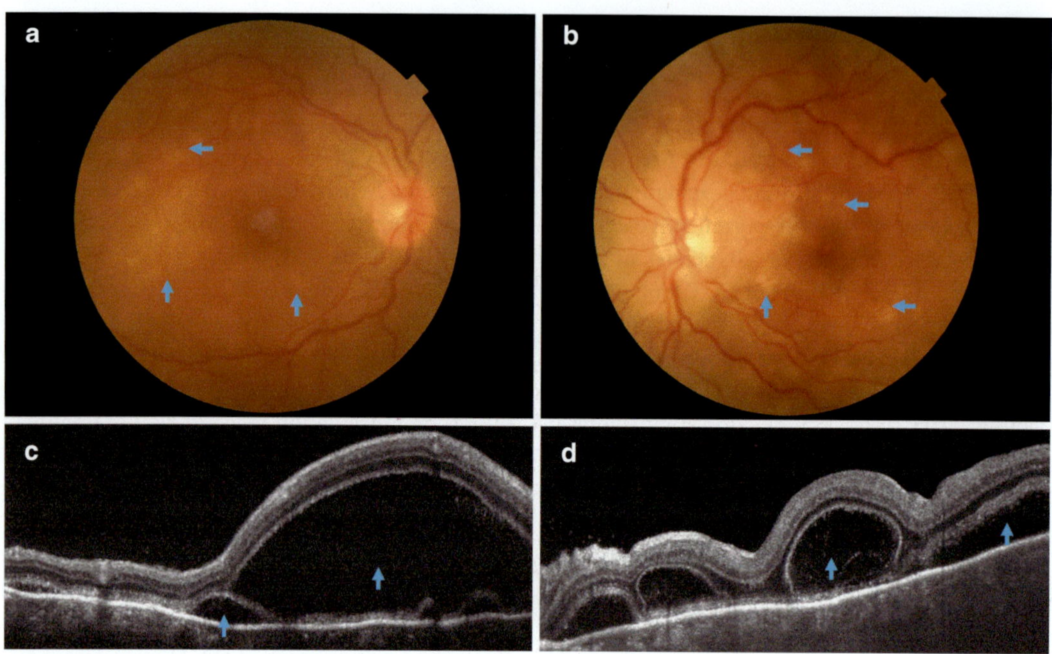

Fig. 12.6 Multifocal pockets of subretinal fluid (blue arrows) are seen in both eyes in acute VKH disease on fundus photography (**a**, **b**) and OCT (**c**, **d**)

are often associated with the accumulation of SRF, leading to a variable extent of exudative retinal detachment (see Chap. 10, Figs. 10.1b and 10.2b) [122–124]. In experimental models of TB granulomas, the VEGF was overexpressed by the overlying RPE of TB granulomatous choroidal inflammation [125]. On FFA, these granulomas show initial hypofluorescence followed by intense hyperfluorescence and pooling of dye in the subretinal space. On the IC angiography, these granulomas remain hypofluorescent throughout the study.

12.4.7 Subretinal Fluid in Metastatic Cancer

Choroid is a common and preferred site for breast and lung cancer metastasis. Renal cell carcinoma may metastasize to choroid years before the first presentation or several years after the patient's nephrectomy for cancer. These metastases have a characteristic orange-red colour [126]. Nearly 8–10% of all cancers metastasize to the choroid because of its rich blood supply. Nearly 28–73% present with SRF [127]. The unrestricted proliferation of the cancer cells increases the metabolic requirements, expresses VEGF, and forms new vessels. The RPE barrier breaks, and the patient presents with vision loss due to exudative retinal detachment [128]. The FFA shows early hypofluorescence, multifocal pinpointing points in the mid-phase, and hyperfluorescence in the late phase (Fig. 12.7). On ICG angiography, the metastatic lesions remain hypofluorescent throughout the study [127]. On OCT angiography, the choroidal metastasis lesions show no flow in the mass lesion, which may be due to the masking effect of the RPE. However, on colour flow mapping, 100% of the metastatic lesions in the choroid show high vascularity [129]. Several successful cases of choroidal metastasis treatment have been reported when anti-VEGF therapy was combined with systemic chemotherapy [127]. Subretinal fluid may be the presenting sign of lung cancer and renal cell carcinoma metastasis to the choroid (Fig. 12.7b, c).

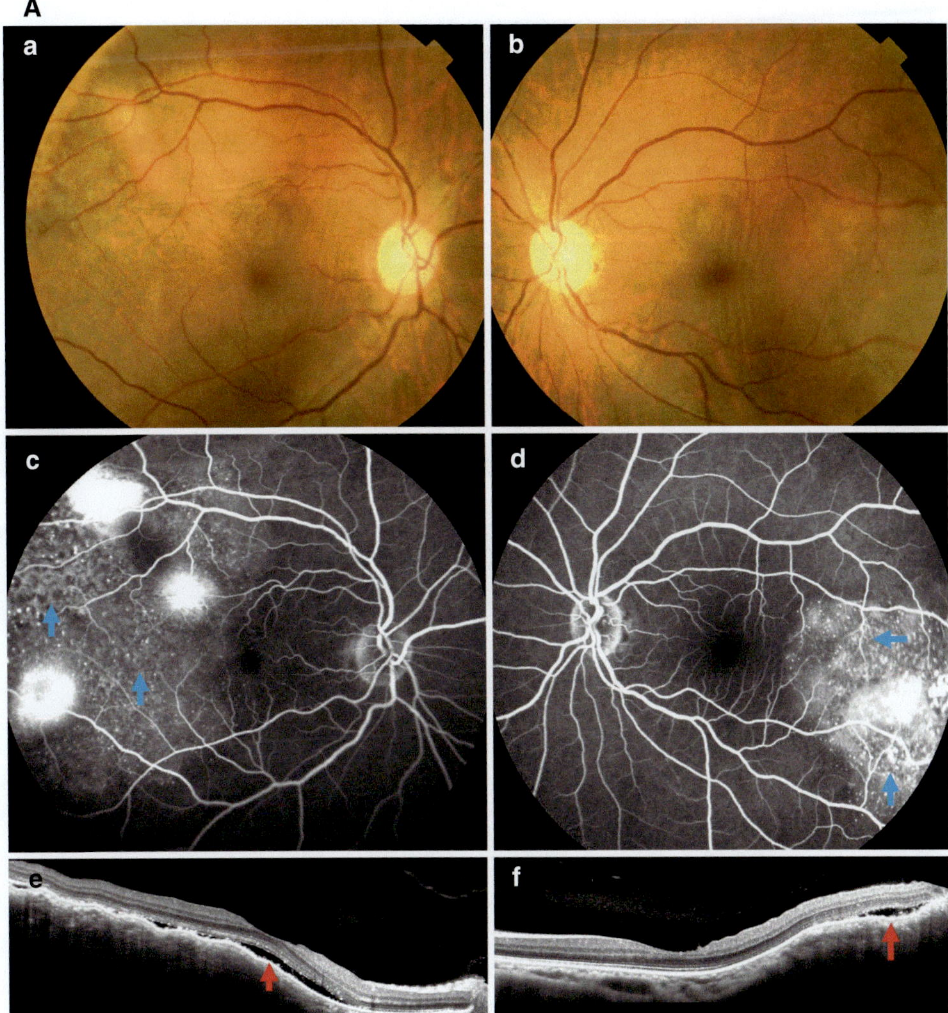

Fig. 12.7 (**A**) A 52-year-old female, who completed chemotherapy for breast carcinoma, presented with bilateral exudative retinal detachment (**a**, **b**), suggestive of metastatic cancer. FFA showed multifocal pinpoint leaking points (blue arrows) and hyperfluorescence in the late phase (**c**, **d**). OCT showed subretinal fluid (red arrows) (**e**, **f**). (**B**) A 48-year-old man presented three months following a total nephrectomy for renal clear cell carcinoma. In the past, he had received laser photocoagulation in the right eye for a diagnosis of central serous choroidopathy (**a**, arrow). His visual acuity was 6/18 and 6/9 in the right and left eyes, respectively. On fluorescein angiography, there was punctate hyperfluorescence between the optic disc and the fovea with leakage of dye above the optic disc (**b**). The OCT scan shows minimum subretinal fluid and increased choroidal thickness (**c**). The left eye showed similar changes (**d**–**f**). There is increased choroidal thickness and intra- and subretinal fluid (**g**). (**C**) A 60-year-old non-smoker presented with 15 days of diminution of vision in his left eye. Fundus examination of the left eye showed a flat subretinal lesion (arrow), approximately one-disc diameter in size, located upper and temporal to the optic disc (**a**, black arrow). The FFA showed initial punctate hyperfluorescence and faint staining in late frames (**b**, arrow). Optical coherence tomography (OCT) showed subretinal fluid involving the fovea (**c**). CT scan of the thorax showed a spiculated mass in the right lower lobe extending up to the visceral pleura (**d**). Fine-needle biopsy of the lung mass revealed a loosely cohesive cluster of tumour cells with moderate-to-abundant vacuolated cytoplasm (arrow) (May Grünwald-Giemsa stain; 40×). Inset shows a papillary cluster of tumour cells with coarse chromatin and conspicuous nucleoli (haematoxylin and eosin stain; 40×) consistent with adenocarcinoma (**e**). Complete lesion regression was observed on repeat fundus examination after four cycles of chemotherapy (**f**). (Reproduced with permission of the publishers from Singh N, Kulkarni P, Aggarwal AN, Mittal BR, Gupta N, Behera D, Gupta A. Choroidal metastasis as a presenting manifestation of lung cancer: a report of 3 cases and systematic review of the literature. Medicine (Baltimore). 2012;91(4):179–194. https://doi.org/10.1097/MD.0b013e3182574a0b. PMID: 22732948)

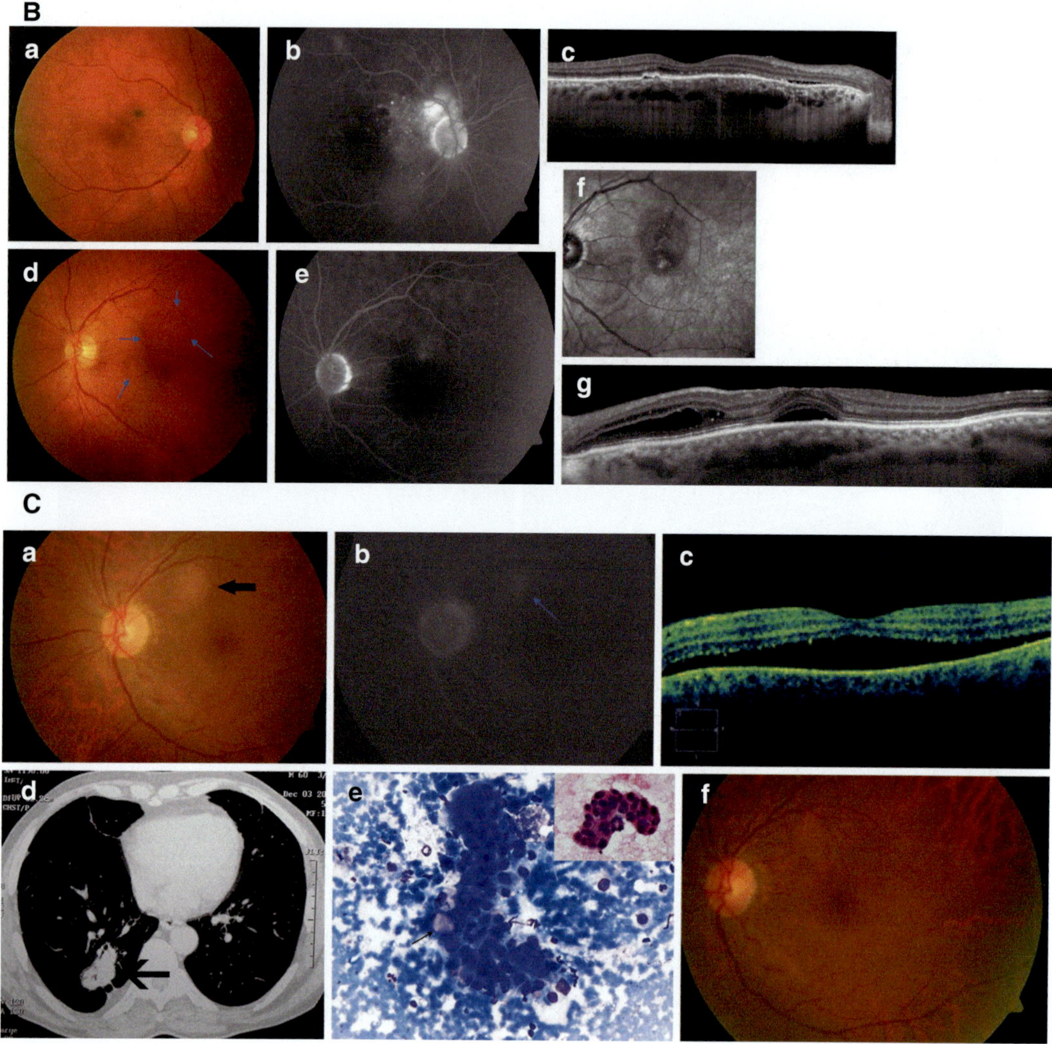

Fig. 12.7 (continued)

12.5 Consequence of Subretinal Fluid

In rhegmatogenous retinal detachment, within 24 h of separating the photoreceptor from the RPE, the photoreceptors' outer nuclear layer is lost due to apoptosis [130]. In acute cases of central serous chorioretinopathy (CSC), if the outer border of the photoreceptor layer is smooth, with minimum thinning of the foveal ONL compared to the normal contralateral eye, they usually have good vision. On the other hand, patients with thickening of the outer border or granular appearance (shaggy border) have thinning of the foveal ONL and have loss of vision. The worst outcome is seen in those who show granular deposits on the ELM and have a maximum thinning of the foveal ONL [131].

12.5.1 Tractional Retinal Detachment

The simultaneous upregulation of the fibroblastic growth factor and the vascular endothelial growth factor (VEGF) in response to the ischaemic retina leads to the development of new retinal vessels accompanied by fibrous proliferation. The most common causes of retinal neovascularization

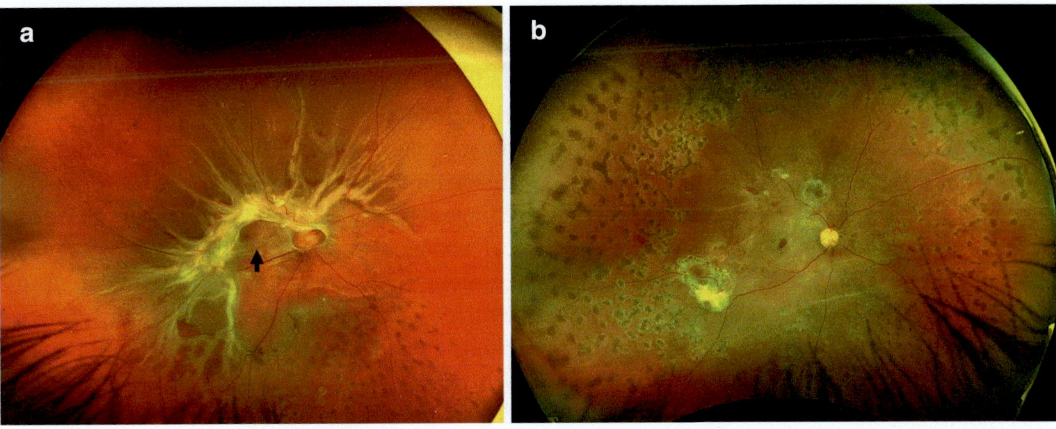

Fig. 12.8 Tractional retinal detachment (TRD) in the right eye of a patient with proliferative diabetic retinopathy along the major vascular arcades (**a**). The macula is lifted (black arrow) into a table-top TRD. Following pars plana vitrectomy, the retina was attached with laser scars in periphery (**b**)

include proliferative diabetic retinopathy (PDR), branch retinal vein occlusion, retinopathy of prematurity (ROP), familial exudative vitreoretinopathy (FEVR), sickle cell anaemia, and ischaemic retinal periphlebitis. Effective treatment strategies to regress the new vessels include ablation of the ischaemic retina with laser photocoagulation or intravitreal injections of anti-VEGF agents. However, the accompanying fibrous tissue does not regress. TRD develops along the major vascular arcades in PDR and lifts the macula into a table-top TRD (Fig. 12.8a). Fibrous proliferation on the posterior hyaloid surface of the vitreous leads to the formation of a taut posterior hyaloid membrane which causes macular oedema with a shallow macular detachment. Post-treatment with either PRP or anti-VEGF therapy, there is often a visible regression of the new vessels. Still, the fibrous membranes lying flat on the posterior pole are only sometimes evident on clinical examination. In such cases, the OCT can show the presence of fibrous membranes, their adherence to the underlying retina, and the extent of the retina elevation.

There is as yet no medical treatment available not only to prevent the formation but also the contraction of these fibrous membranes. The fibrous membranes are firmly anchored to the new vessels' growth sites and grow along the posterior hyaloid surface, which provides a scaffold for these proliferating fibrocytes. The growth of the new vessels along the posterior hyaloid face leads to partial vitreous detachment and contraction of the posterior hyaloid face. The contracting fibrous membranes exert antero-posteriorly or tangentially oriented forces that overcome the adhesion forces between the NSR and the RPE and form tractional retinal detachment (TRD). Clinically, the TRD appear taut and concave anteriorly due to the forward pulling traction of the fibrosis and the posterior pulling forces of the RPE pump. At times, the contraction of these membranes may be so severe to create a break (hole) in the retina and develop a combined rhegmatogenous and tractional retinal detachment.

The formation of a hole in the retina allows the aqueous fluid to go behind the retina, with a consequent change in the configuration of the RD. This phenomenon is seen in diabetic retinopathy more commonly than other causes of TRD.

Patients of DR who reach a stage of TRD generally have poor systemic health. The 5-year mortality in these patients after surgery varies from 25.3% [132] to 57% [133].

Patients with BRVO, sickle cell retinopathy, and FEVR often develop peripheral TRDs. The ischaemic peripheral vasculitis produces highly complex peripheral TRD. In contrast to the diabetic TRDs that form in the posterior pole or the post-equatorial retina, the post-vasculitic TRDs are often pre-equatorial. If not treated in time, preterm babies with ROP develop peripheral tractional retinal detachment that involves the macula. Eventually, the contracting fibrous tissue may detach the entire retina, causing total retinal detachment to lie just behind the crystalline lens.

In juvenile idiopathic arthritis-associated uveitis, fibrous membranes are often formed on the peripheral retina and the ciliary body. These form fibrous cyclitic membranes that cause tractional detachment of the pars plicata and peripheral tractional retinal detachment. Inferior traction retinal detachment may develop in the retina's inferior periphery, complicating longstanding pars plana exudates in intermediate uveitis.

The larva migrans of Toxocara canis often present as a peripheral TRD or a juxtapapillary TRD.

12.5.2 Myopic Tractional Maculopathy

For the clear perception of objects, the parallel rays of reflected light from the objects located at infinity (the far point of the normal eye, generally taken as 6 m) must be sharply focused on the NSR. The light rays from objects closer than 6 m are divergent, but the accommodative power of the crystalline lens focuses the image on the NSR (the eye's focal point). Many factors contribute to the focus of the image on NSR. The axial length of the eyeball is the most important of all. If the eyeball's size is longer than average, the eye's focal point moves anterior to the NSR, the light rays from the far point are focused in front of the retina, and the image is perceived as a blur. This error of refraction is called myopia. Myopia is corrected by placing a minus-powered (diverging) lens to move the far point to infinity. The average axial length of the emmetropic eye is 23 mm (22–24 mm). An increase in the eyeball's axial length by 0.35 mm leads to an error of refraction −1D [134]. The newborns are born with a short eye which continues to grow in size till it achieves most of the emmetropic size by 3 years and, after that, slowly continues to grow till adolescence. Myopia is fast emerging as a public health challenge in Asian countries where 80–90% of school-leaving children have myopia, and 10–20% have pathological myopia [135]. High myopia is defined when a ≥6D minus lens must be placed in front of the cornea to focus the image on the NSR. In many patients, axial length elongation leads to sight-threatening pathological changes in the retina, namely the myopic crescent, chorioretinal atrophy, cracks in the Bruch's membrane (Lacquer cracks), subfoveal choroidal neovessels, macular hole, macular schisis or macular traction retinal detachment, and outpouching of the posterior sclera (posterior staphyloma). If any of these changes are present, it is called 'pathological myopia' [135]. More than the axial length, the eyeball's abnormal shape is responsible for pathological changes [134].

One-third of the patients with high myopia may show tractional maculopathy. In myopic tractional maculopathy (MTM), the posterior hyaloid membrane is thickened and firmly adherent to the NSR. Due to the abnormal shape, two opposing forces are generated in the vulnerable eyes, laterally directed tangential and anterior-posterior traction by the post-hyaloid face of the vitreous. The relatively rigid ILM and anterior retina stretch across the posterior staphyloma while the more compliant outer retina lines the staphyloma leading to tractional detachment of the anterior retinal layers. Vertical stretching of Henle's fibres gives the appearance of a schisis-like appearance. The inner retina may show cystic changes. The macular hole may develop in some patients. The MTM was only recognized after the availability of OCT.

The treatment of MTM involves 3-port PPV with posterior hyaloid removal. It has excellent outcomes following pars plana vitreous surgery to relieve macular traction with complete resolution of the MTM and improve visual acuity [136, 137]. The ILM is not peeled over the foveal centre for fear of creating an iatrogenic macular hole. Fovea-sparing ILM peeling leads to significant visual improvement compared to when the ILM over the fovea is also peeled [138, 139].

12.5.3 Treatment of Tractional Retinal Detachment

Treating TRD, epiretinal fibrous membranes, or the taut hyaloid membranes requires surgical intervention. The complexity of the surgery varies from case to case, and the surgical plan is individualized. The basic steps of surgery involve a three-port pars plana vitreous (PPV) surgery to remove the entire vitreous gel, release all the fibrous tractional membranes and bands, remove the posterior hyaloid face, obtain haemostasis, and close all the preexisting or iatrogenic retinal holes with the application of laser photocoagulation. If there are no retinal breaks, often releasing the tractional forces will lead to reattachment of the NSR to the RPE (Fig. 12.8b). However, it may take several months to completely absorb the SRF [140].

Surgery of TRD is highly variable in complexity; iatrogenic breaks are not uncommon and may be seen in nearly 25% of the eyes. The surgery requires careful removal of the posterior hyaloid face and the scar tissue. To ensure complete reattachment of the retina on the table, some surgeons prefer to create retinal breaks to drain all the SRF during the fluid gas exchange and replace the vitreous cavity with a long-acting gas or silicone oil. Some surgeons may place a 360° scleral buckle to counteract unseen residual traction. Any residual traction on the retina will not allow the entire retina to reattach. If the residual TRD is in the periphery or in the nasal retina, many surgeons prefer to leave it as such if it is not compromising the vision.

The single surgery success rate in diabetic TRD has improved over the years and is ~85% [141, 142]. The PPV with suture less 25G+ technique also was effective and safe in reaching success in 91% [143] to 99% [144].

Despite excellent surgical outcomes, visual acuity better than 20/50 was achievable only in 23% [142]. Postoperative vitreous haemorrhage is a significant complication of PPV in diabetic TRD. To reduce the risk of postoperative haemorrhage, many surgeons favour preoperative or intraoperative use of intravitreal injection anti-VEGF agents [145]. The current surgical techniques show a significant decrease in postoperative haemorrhage at 13%. However, visual acuity better than 20/50 was achieved in only 19.5% of eyes, although it stabilized in 96%. Only 1.2% lost light perception [146]. Instead of leaving the eye filled with a balanced salt solution at the end of the surgery, replacing it with 20–30% SF6 gas reduced the postoperative haemorrhage from 33% to 11% [147].

In a series of 74 eyes with post-retinal vasculitis RD, one-third were combined tractional and rhegmatogenous RD. Although 90% of the eyes achieved anatomical success following pars plana vitreous surgery, significant visual acuity improvement was seen only in 70% of the eyes [148].

Confluent laser photocoagulation of the ischaemic retina with or without concurrent use of intravitreal anti-VEGF therapy is highly effective in preventing the progression of ROP to stage 4, i.e. peripheral TRD without (4A) or with macular involvement (4B). Bilateral sequential lens sparing 25/27G PPV in the same surgical session is a highly effective strategy in stage 4 ROP. In one such series, the macula was still attached in 90% of eyes, and complete resolution of TRD was achieved in 63% of eyes at the end of 45 weeks of surgery [149]. A Turkish group obtained similar results and achieved anatomical success in 96% of 4A and 85% in 4B ROP [150]. This strategy was found highly effective in the paediatric age group PPV to achieve anatomical success in 90% of cases [151].

12.5.4 Rhegmatogenous Retinal Detachment

Rhegmatogenous retinal detachment (RRD) is a collection of fluid between the neurosensory retina and the RPE caused by a retinal tear or a hole (Fig. 12.9). RRD is a common cause of sudden loss of vision in older people. The main symptom of acute RD is a dark curtain rising in front of the eye.

The mere presence of a retinal hole is not enough to create an RRD, as the hole remains plugged by a healthy vitreous. Typically, the corti-

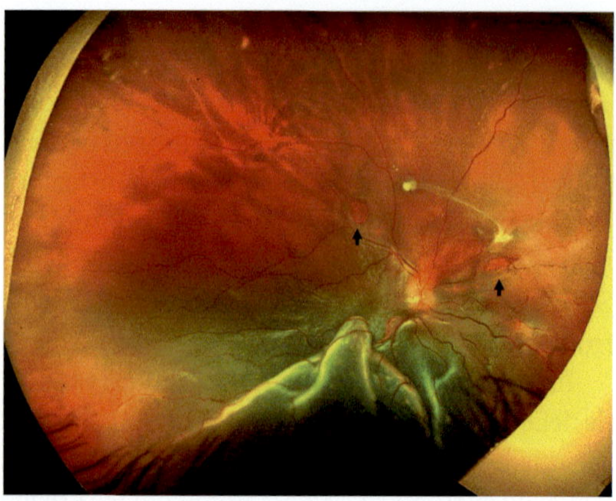

Fig. 12.9 Subretinal fluid in an eye with rhegmatogenous retinal detachment, caused by a retinal tear or a hole (black arrows)

cal vitreous is firmly adherent at the optic disc margins and the vitreous base where it straddles the ora serrata (transition from the NSR to the non-pigmented ciliary epithelium). The vitreous is also lightly attached to the retinal surface over the macula and the retinal vessels. The cortical vitreous adheres firmly to areas of retinal degeneration, especially at the borders of the lattice degeneration. It is also adherent at sites of chorioretinal scars. Nearly one-third of the patients with myopia of ≥6D–8D and 6–10% of the normal population have circumferentially or occasionally radially oriented patches of lattice degeneration. These areas of retinal atrophy, crisscross white lines, and variable pigmentation may have atrophic holes. Nearly 54% have lesions in both eyes, equally distributed among men and women [152].

The vitreous gel undergoes syneresis (liquefaction) with old age. In eyes with high myopia, vitreous liquefaction occurs at a much younger age. There is also a thinning out of the posterior cortical vitreous in front of the macula where an opening may form, allowing the misdirected aqueous to move behind the posterior hyaloid membrane, peeling it off from the ILM. The age-related liquefaction of the anterior vitreous may weaken Wiegert's ligament attachment on the posterior surface of the crystalline lens. The misdirected aqueous then gets access to flow through the Cloquet's canal to the Martegiani space in front of the optic disc to communicate with the pocket of liquefied vitreous in front of the macula [153]. Movement of the partially detached PHM due to saccadic eye movements of the eye exerts a constant force on its posterior attachment to the optic disc margin. Separation of the vitreous attachment to the optic disc margin is an acute event termed posterior vitreous detachment (PVD) and is a common phenomenon between the ages of 45 and 65.

The PVD happens earlier in myopic eyes and post-trauma [154]. Following uneventful cataract surgery, nearly 75% of eyes without preexisting PVD developed PVD within 5 years and, more often, if they had preexisting asymptomatic lattice degeneration [155].

The patients often become aware of the PVD by the sudden appearance of a floating partial or complete ring shadow (Weiss ring) and dark spots (floaters) in their field of vision. A sudden movement of the head may bring on a lightning streak. The lightning streak appears due to the pull on the retinal elements by the still adherent vitreous strands. The light flashes in themselves are not significant except when floaters accompany these. Opacities cause floaters in the vitreous due to leakage of blood from the rupture of retinal capillaries, especially in areas where the vitreous is firmly attached to the retina. The leaked blood is seen as a thin horizontal layer inferiorly on the retina's surface. The PVD needs urgent consultation with a retina specialist for binocular indirect ophthalmoscopy with scleral depression to rule out the presence of a retinal tear, especially if there are pigmented cells or blood in the vitreous cavity or retina. These symptomatic tears lead to retinal detachment in the next few days. However, if it is detected and sealed with laser photocoagulation, the development of RRD can be prevented.

12.5.5 Pathogenesis of Rhegmatogenous Retinal Detachment

The formation of a round atrophic hole does not always lead to retinal detachment. Acute flap tears develop during acute PVD, and adherent vitreous pulls on the degenerated/atrophic retina. The vitreous strands can be seen attached to the apex of the arrowhead-shaped flap, with its apex directed posteriorly. These tears tend to extend anteriorly towards the ora serrata; hence, if detected before they result in RRD, they should be sealed using laser photocoagulation that must extend anteriorly up to the ora serrata. The raised flap sets up eddy currents during the saccades and facilitates entry of the misdirected aqueous into the subretinal space. In the past, only the liquefied vitreous was believed to have entered the subretinal space. However, it needs a more accurate explanation as the RPE constantly absorbs the SRF, and the fresh one moves in, a phenomenon impossible with a limited quantity of the vitreous [153].

12.5.6 Risk Factors for Rhegmatogenous Retinal Detachment

Myopia with lattice degeneration is the most significant risk factor; nearly 20–30% with RRD show this sign. Familial cases of RRD are seen in Stickler's syndrome, a genetic disorder with defective collagen production, and Wagner's syndrome, an autosomal dominant disorder. Clear lens extraction as treatment of very high myopia also raises the risk of RRB fourfold [156]. Nearly 1% of the patients undergoing cataract surgery, especially those with axial myopia or intraoperative complications like capsular dehiscence or vitreous loss, may also develop RRD [154]. Nd:Yag laser capsulotomy led to a fourfold increase in the risk for RRD, especially in young people [157], and led to RRD in 2% of eyes [158]. RRD may follow trauma to the eye from tears in the vitreous base. Lateral eyeball expansion following blunt trauma may cause disinsertion of the vitreous base and retinal dialysis or giant retinal tears [159].

12.5.7 Clinical Diagnosis of Rhegmatogenous Retinal Detachment

Unlike the exudative retinal detachment with a smooth elevation, fresh RRD appears as an undulating semitransparent membrane with folds of the outer retina, giving it a corrugated appearance [160, 161]. These have a highly characteristic appearance on the OCT and are likely due to the hydration of the interphotoreceptor matrix proteins [162]. The SRF arising from the retinal tears above the horizontal meridian (superior retinal breaks/tears) first appears around the retina break, extends up to the ora serrata, and then gravitates inferiorly to give a bullous appearance to the RRD. These RRDs rapidly expand to involve the macula. In contrast, those arising from the inferior breaks are generally shallow, expand slowly, and do not show a corrugated appearance. These are called inferior RRDs and may show high water marks at the upper border. The most critical step in managing RRD is locating all the retinal breaks. The contours of the RRD are drawn on an Amsler chart using a binocular indirect ophthalmoscope with a +20D condensing lens [163].

The key to locating a retinal break is first to determine if it is a bullous RRD or a shallow RD, i.e. whether it is arising from a superior break or an inferior break, respectively, and draw the contours of the subretinal fluid. Next is to find out whether the RRD is total or subtotal and, if subtotal, the number of quadrants involved, and whether the macula is 'On' or 'Off'. Most of the retinal breaks are located in the upper temporal quadrant. There may be more than one retinal break, and all-out efforts are made to locate all the breaks.

The superior RRD in the early stage may be localized to only one quadrant. The most superior break dictates the configuration of the RRD and generally follows Lincoff's rule [164]. In brief, if the bullous RRD is located in the superior half, determine which side has the lower SRF level. In the superior breaks, generally, the fluid will not cross the midline, gravitate inferiorly, rise on the opposite inferior quadrant, and then move up. The retinal break is located on the side with a higher fluid level. However, if the retinal break is located at the 12 O'clock meridian, the fluid level crosses the midline, and the inferior fluid levels are the same on either side. In the inferior bullous RRD, the retinal break is located on the side, which shows a higher fluid level and shall always be above the horizontal meridian. In shallow inferior RRD, the retinal break is located on the side of the higher upper fluid level, but if the retinal break is at 6 O'clock, the fluid levels are equal on either side.

12.5.8 Development of Proliferative Vitreoretinopathy in RRD

The development of fibrous membranes on the anterior and posterior surfaces of the detached retina often complicates the RRDs. It is termed proliferative vitreoretinopathy (PVR). In the RRD, the RPE cells migrate into the vitreous cavity through the retinal tear, undergo fibrous metaplasia, and form layers on the anterior and posterior retinal surfaces. The RPE cells produce many inflammatory cytokines that promote fibrous proliferation. Because of the gravitation, these fibroblasts most often settle on the inferior retina and form tractional membranes in the inferior retina more than the superior retina. The retina is dragged into the contracted epicentre of the scar tissue to create a highly characteristic appearance of the detached retina termed 'star fold'. These contracting membranes are circumferentially oriented in the pre-equatorial retina and labelled 'anterior PVR'.

Depending upon the number of quadrants involved and the resultant configuration of the RRD, these changes are classified into various grades. The significant risk factors for the development of PVR include young age, myopia, larger and more posterior breaks, giant retinal tears, choroidal detachment, long duration of RRD, hypotony, vitreous haemorrhage, inflammation, failed surgery and repeated PPV, and RRDs resulting from penetrating trauma and retained intraocular foreign bodies [165].

12.5.9 Treatment of RRD

Gonin laid down the principles of surgery for RRD more than 100 years ago and demonstrated that retinal tears were primarily responsible for RRD. Sealing of retinal breaks led to retina reattachment [166]. The primary goal of the surgery is to locate all the retinal breaks during surgery and seal them by retinopexy, either using cryopexy, laser photocoagulation, or even diathermy in the past. Traction on the retinal tear is relaxed by external support using either a local or a 360° scleral buckle (SB). Depending upon the surgeon's preference, external transscleral drainage of the SRF ensures that the SB supports the retinal breaks during the surgery. Scleral buckling procedures combined with cryopexy lead to ~90% anatomical success rates in fresh localized RRDs, which are not complicated by PVR or the PVR changes are limited up to two quadrants. More extensive PVR changes, inadequately supported or missed breaks may not allow retina reattachment. Progression of PVR following surgery may open the retinal break and lead to redetachment. More advanced stages of PVR, including the open or closed funnel configuration of RD, large giant tears, posterior tears, and a macular hole or choroidal coloboma-associated retinal detachments, require more complex surgical procedures such as PPV with or without an SB. The principles of PPV include complete removal of the vitreous gel, separation of the PHM, dissection and excision of the fibrous membranes from both surfaces of the retina, reattaching the retina preoperatively by doing a fluid gas exchange and using laser photocoagulation to seal the retinal breaks. At the end of the surgery, the air is exchanged with a mixture of non-expansile concentrations of long-acting gas SF6 (20–30%) or C3F8 (14%) or silicone oil. With the current techniques, including small gauge PPV (23, 25, or 27G), wide-angle viewing systems, disposable microinstruments, and highly controlled microfluidics of the vitrectomy machines, anatomical success can be achieved in more than 90% of eyes with a single surgery and nearly 98% with repeat surgeries [167]. A recent meta-analysis found single surgery success rates to be higher with PPV combined with a scleral buckle than the PPV alone. Ultimately, however, there was no difference between the success rates or complications [168]. Of the two techniques used to reattach the retina, the scleral buckle alone or PPV alone, the eyes with scleral buckles have a better visual outcome, and both achieve ~85%

reattachment rates with a single surgery and ~98% following repeat surgeries.

Complications like choroidal detachment, subretinal haemorrhage, and persistent SRF are more common with SB, but iatrogenic breaks are more common with PPV [169].

References

1. Fuhrmann S. Eye morphogenesis and patterning of the optic vesicle. Curr Top Dev Biol. 2010;93:61–84. https://doi.org/10.1016/B978-0-12-385044-7.00003-5.
2. Tsin A, Betts-Obregon B, Grigsby J. Visual cycle proteins: Structure, function, and roles in human retinal disease. J Biol Chem. 2018;13016–21. https://doi.org/10.1074/jbc.AW118.003228. Epub2018 Jul 12. PMID:30002120; PMCID: PMC6109927.
3. Brubaker RF. Flow of aqueous humor in humans [The Friedenwald Lecture]. Invest Ophthalmol Vis Sci. 1991;32(13):3145–66.
4. Goel M, Picciani RG, Lee RK, Bhattacharya SK. Aqueous humor dynamics: a review. Open Ophthalmol J. 2010;4:52–9. https://doi.org/10.2174/1874364101004010052.
5. Smith DW, Lee CJ, Gardiner BS. No flow through the vitreous humor: how strong is the evidence? Prog Retin Eye Res. 2020:100845. https://doi.org/10.1016/j.preteyeres.2020.100845. Epub ahead of print.
6. Adler AJ, Klucznik KM. Proteins and glycoproteins of the bovine interphotoreceptor matrix: composition and fractionation. Exp Eye Res. 1982;34:423–34.
7. Marmor MF. Chapter 19: Mechanisms of normal retinal adhesion. In: Ryan SJ, Sadda SVR, Hinton DR, Schachat AP, Wilkinson CP, Wiedemann P, editors. Retina. 5th ed. W.B. Saunders; 2013. p. 447–64. ISBN: 9781455707379. https://www.sciencedirect.com/science/article/pii/B9781455707379000199. https://doi.org/10.1016/B978-1-4557-0737-9.00019-9.
8. Marmor MF, Abdul-Rahim AS, Cohen DS. The effect of metabolic inhibitors on retinal adhesion and subretinal fluid resorption. Invest Ophthalmol Vis Sci. 1980;19(8):893–903.
9. Marmor MF, Yao XY. The enhancement of retinal adhesiveness by ouabain appears to involve cellular edema. Invest Ophthalmol Vis Sci. 1989;30(7):1511–4.
10. Negi A, Marmor MF. Quantitative estimation of metabolic transport of subretinal fluid. Invest Ophthalmol Vis Sci. 1986;27(11):1564–8.
11. Chihara E, Nao-i N. Resorption of subretinal fluid by transepithelial flow of the retinal pigment epithelium. Graefes Arch Clin Exp Ophthalmol. 1985;223(4):202–4. https://doi.org/10.1007/BF02174060.
12. Soubrane G, Coscas G. Chapter 30: Pathogenesis of serous detachment of the retina and pigment epithelium. In: Ryan SJ, Sadda SVR, Hinton DR, Schachat AP, Wilkinson CP, Wiedemann P, editors. Retina. 5th ed. W.B. Saunders; 2013. p. 618–23. ISBN: 9781455707379. https://www.sciencedirect.com/science/article/pii/B9781455707379000308. https://doi.org/10.1016/B978-1-4557-0737-9.00030-8.
13. Marmor MF, Maack T. Enhancement of retinal adhesion and subretinal fluid resorption by acetazolamide. Invest Ophthalmol Vis Sci. 1982;23(1):121–4.
14. Wolfensberger TJ, Chiang RK, Takeuchi A, Marmor MF. Inhibition of membrane-bound carbonic anhydrase enhances subretinal fluid absorption and retinal adhesiveness. Graefes Arch Clin Exp Ophthalmol. 2000;238(1):76–80. https://doi.org/10.1007/s004170050013.
15. Kido A, Miyake M, Tamura H, Hiragi S, Kimura T, Ohtera S, Takahashi A, Ooto S, Kawakami K, Kuroda T, Tsujikawa A. Incidence of central serous chorioretinopathy (2011-2018): a nationwide population-based cohort study of Japan. Br J Ophthalmol. 2022;106(12):1748–53. https://doi.org/10.1136/bjophthalmol-2021-319403. Epub 2021 Jul 14.
16. Gäckle HC, Lang GE, Freissler KA, Lang GK. Chorioretinopathia centralis serosa. Klinische, fluoreszeinangiographische und demographische Aspekte [Central serous chorioretinopathy. Clinical, fluorescein angiography and demographic aspects]. Ophthalmologe. 1998;95(8):529–33. German. https://doi.org/10.1007/s003470050310.
17. Gupta P, Gupta V, Dogra MR, Singh R, Gupta A. Morphological changes in the retinal pigment epithelium on spectral-domain OCT in the unaffected eyes with idiopathic central serous chorioretinopathy. Int Ophthalmol. 2010;30(2):175–81. https://doi.org/10.1007/s10792-009-9302-2. Epub 2009 Jan 30.
18. Guyer DR, Yannuzzi LA, Slakter JS, Sorenson JA, Ho A, Orlock D. Digital indocyanine green videoangiography of central serous chorioretinopathy. Arch Ophthalmol. 1994;112(8):1057–62. https://doi.org/10.1001/archopht.1994.01090200063023.
19. Piccolino FC, Borgia L. Central serous chorioretinopathy and indocyanine green angiography. Retina. 1994;14(3):231–42. https://doi.org/10.1097/00006982-199414030-00008.
20. Matsumoto H, Kishi S, Sato T, Mukai R. Fundus autofluorescence of elongated photoreceptor outer segments in central serous chorioretinopathy. Am J Ophthalmol. 2011;151(4):617–623.e1. https://doi.org/10.1016/j.ajo.2010.09.031. Epub 2011 Jan 22.
21. Gass JD, Little H. Bilateral bullous exudative retinal detachment complicating idiopathic central serous chorioretinopathy during systemic corticosteroid therapy. Ophthalmology. 1995;102(5):737–47. https://doi.org/10.1016/s0161-6420(95)30960-8.

22. Gupta P, Gupta A, Gupta V, Singh R. Successful outcome of giant retinal pigment epithelium rip in idiopathic central serous chorioretinopathy. Retina. 2008;28(2):364–5. https://doi.org/10.1097/IAE.0b013e31815960d5.
23. Ishida Y, Kato T, Minamoto A, Yokoyama T, Jian K, Mishima HK. Retinal pigment epithelial tear in a patient with central serous chorioretinopathy treated with corticosteroids. Retina. 2004;24(4):633–6. https://doi.org/10.1097/00006982-200408000-00028.
24. Lim Z, Wong D. Retinal pigment epithelial rip associated with idiopathic central serous chorioretinopathy. Eye (Lond). 2008;22(3):471–3. https://doi.org/10.1038/sj.eye.6703020. Epub 2007 Nov 9.
25. Parchand S, Gupta V, Gupta A, Dogra MR. Bilateral giant retinal pigment epithelial rip in idiopathic central serous chorioretinopathy. Retina. 2011;31(9):1977–8. https://doi.org/10.1097/IAE.0b013e31822352b9.
26. Shanmugam MP, Bhende M. Retinal pigment epithelial tears associated with idiopathic central serous chorioretinopathy. Indian J Ophthalmol. 2000;48(4):315–7.
27. Terao N, Koizumi H, Kojima K, Kusada N, Nagata K, Yamagishi T, Yoneda K, Yoshii K, Kinoshita S, Sotozono C. Short axial length and hyperopic refractive error are risk factors of central serous chorioretinopathy. Br J Ophthalmol. 2020;104(9):1260–5. https://doi.org/10.1136/bjophthalmol-2019-315236. Epub 2019 Nov 28.
28. Yannuzzi LA. Type-A behavior and central serous chorioretinopathy. Retina. 1987;7(2):111–31. https://doi.org/10.1097/00006982-198700720-00009.
29. Haimovici R, Koh S, Gagnon DR, Lehrfeld T, Wellik S, Central Serous Chorioretinopathy Case-Control Study Group. Risk factors for central serous chorioretinopathy: a case-control study. Ophthalmology. 2004;111(2):244–9. https://doi.org/10.1016/j.ophtha.2003.09.024.
30. Spahn C, Wiek J, Burger T, Hansen L. Psychosomatic aspects in patients with central serous chorioretinopathy. Br J Ophthalmol. 2003;87(6):704–8. https://doi.org/10.1136/bjo.87.6.704.
31. Piccolino FC, Fruttini D, Eandi C, Nicolò M, Mariotti C, Tito S, Lupidi M. Vigorous physical activity as a risk factor for central serous chorioretinopathy. Am J Ophthalmol. 2022;244:30–7. https://doi.org/10.1016/j.ajo.2022.08.002. Epub ahead of print.
32. Sawaguchi S, Terao N, Imanaga N, Wakugawa S, Tamashiro T, Yamauchi Y, Koizumi H. Scleral thickness in steroid-induced central serous chorioretinopathy. Ophthalmol Sci. 2022;2(2):100124. https://doi.org/10.1016/j.xops.2022.100124.
33. Sander BP, Collins MJ, Read SA. The effect of topical adrenergic and anticholinergic agents on the choroidal thickness of young healthy adults. Exp Eye Res. 2014;128:181–9. https://doi.org/10.1016/j.exer.2014.10.003. Epub 2014 Oct 7.
34. German O, Jampol LM. Relapsing pigment epithelial detachment in central serous chorioretinopathy after dilated eye examination. JAMA Ophthalmol. 2020;138(10):1106–7. https://doi.org/10.1001/jamaophthalmol.2020.3024.
35. Watson MJG, Yellachich D. Relapsing pigment epithelial detachment in central serous chorioretinopathy after dilated eye examination. JAMA Ophthalmol. 2020;138(3):318–9. https://doi.org/10.1001/jamaophthalmol.2019.5946.
36. Kara N, Demircan A, Karatas G, Ozgurhan EB, Tatar G, Karakucuk Y, Basci A, Demirok A. Effects of two commonly used mydriatics on choroidal thickness: direct and crossover effects. J Ocul Pharmacol Ther. 2014;30(4):366–70. https://doi.org/10.1089/jop.2013.0093. Epub 2014 Jan 29.
37. Yoshioka H, Katsume Y, Akune H. Experimental central serous chorioretinopathy in monkey eyes: fluorescein angiographic findings. Ophthalmologica. 1982;185(3):168–78. https://doi.org/10.1159/000309239.
38. Sibayan SA, Kobuch K, Spiegel D, Eckert E, Leser R, Monzer J, Gabel VP. Epinephrine, but not dexamethasone, induces apoptosis in retinal pigment epithelium cells in vitro: possible implications on the pathogenesis of central serous chorioretinopathy. Graefes Arch Clin Exp Ophthalmol. 2000;238(6):515–9. https://doi.org/10.1007/pl00007893.
39. Garg SP, Dada T, Talwar D, Biswas NR. Endogenous cortisol profile in patients with central serous chorioretinopathy. Br J Ophthalmol. 1997;81(11):962–4. https://doi.org/10.1136/bjo.81.11.962.
40. Gupta V, Gupta P, Dogra MR, Gupta A. Spontaneous closure of retinal pigment epithelium microrip in the natural course of central serous chorioretinopathy. Eye (Lond). 2010;24(4):595–9. https://doi.org/10.1038/eye.2009.193. Epub 2009 Jul 31.
41. Ranjan R, Agarwal M, Verma N. Microrip of retinal pigment epithelium in central serous chorioretinopathy. JAMA Ophthalmol. 2020;138(6):e193120. https://doi.org/10.1001/jamaophthalmol.2019.3120. Epub 2020 Jun 11.
42. Yang L, Jonas JB, Wei W. Optical coherence tomography-assisted enhanced depth imaging of central serous chorioretinopathy. Invest Ophthalmol Vis Sci. 2013;54(7):4659–65. https://doi.org/10.1167/iovs.12-10991.
43. Yannuzzi LA, Freund KB, Goldbaum M, Scassellati-Sforzolini B, Guyer DR, Spaide RF, Maberley D, Wong DW, Slakter JS, Sorenson JA, Fisher YL, Orlock DA. Polypoidal choroidal vasculopathy masquerading as central serous chorioretinopathy. Ophthalmology. 2000;107(4):767–77. https://doi.org/10.1016/s0161-6420(99)00173-6.
44. Marmor MF. On the cause of serous detachments and acute central serous chorioretinopathy. Br J Ophthalmol. 1997;81(10):812–3. https://doi.org/10.1136/bjo.81.10.812.

45. Imanaga N, Terao N, Nakamine S, Tamashiro T, Wakugawa S, Sawaguchi K, Koizumi H. Scleral thickness in central serous chorioretinopathy. Ophthalmol Retina. 2021;5(3):285–91. https://doi.org/10.1016/j.oret.2020.07.011. Epub 2020 Jul 16.
46. Bansal R, Menia NK, Gupta A. Familial nanophthalmos presenting with spontaneous uveal effusion syndrome. Ocul Immunol Inflamm. 2020;28(2):191–3. https://doi.org/10.1080/09273948.2018.1552761. Epub 2018 Dec 17.
47. Terao N, Imanaga N, Wakugawa S, Sawaguchi S, Tamashiro T, Yamauchi Y, Koizumi H. Ciliochoroidal effusion in central serous chorioretinopathy. Retina. 2022;42(4):730–7. https://doi.org/10.1097/IAE.0000000000003376.
48. Imanaga N, Terao N, Sawaguchi S, Tamashiro T, Wakugawa S, Yamauchi Y, Koizumi H. Clinical factors related to loculation of fluid in central serous chorioretinopathy. Am J Ophthalmol. 2022;235:197–203. https://doi.org/10.1016/j.ajo.2021.09.009. Epub 2021 Sep 20.
49. Spaide RF, Ryan EH Jr. Loculation of fluid in the posterior choroid in eyes with central serous chorioretinopathy. Am J Ophthalmol. 2015;160(6):1211–6. https://doi.org/10.1016/j.ajo.2015.08.018. Epub 2015 Aug 20.
50. Nishi O, Yasukawa T. Comment on: Clinical factors related to loculation of fluid in central serous chorioretinopathy. Am J Ophthalmol. 2022;241:293–4. https://doi.org/10.1016/j.ajo.2022.04.028. Epub 2022 Jun 21.
51. Imanaga N, Koizumi H. Reply to "Comment on clinical factors related to loculation of fluid in central serous chorioretinopathy". Am J Ophthalmol. 2022;241:295. https://doi.org/10.1016/j.ajo.2022.06.012. Epub 2022 Jun 22.
52. Spaide RF, Gemmy Cheung CM, Matsumoto H, Kishi S, Boon CJF, van Dijk EHC, Mauget-Faysse M, Behar-Cohen F, Hartnett ME, Sivaprasad S, Iida T, Brown DM, Chhablani J, Maloca PM. Venous overload choroidopathy: a hypothetical framework for central serous chorioretinopathy and allied disorders. Prog Retin Eye Res. 2022;86:100973. https://doi.org/10.1016/j.preteyeres.2021.100973. Epub 2021 May 21.
53. Kishi S, Matsumoto H. A new insight into pachychoroid diseases: remodeling of choroidal vasculature. Graefes Arch Clin Exp Ophthalmol. 2022;260(11):3405–17. https://doi.org/10.1007/s00417-022-05687-6. Epub 2022 May 16.
54. Matsumoto H, Hoshino J, Mukai R, Nakamura K, Kishi S, Akiyama H. Chronic choriocapillaris ischemia in dilated vortex vein region in pachychoroid neovasculopathy. Sci Rep. 2021;11(1):16274. https://doi.org/10.1038/s41598-021-95904-9.
55. Fung AT, Yannuzzi LA, Freund KB. Type 1 (sub-retinal pigment epithelial) neovascularization in central serous chorioretinopathy masquerading as neovascular age-related macular degeneration. Retina. 2012;32(9):1829–37. https://doi.org/10.1097/IAE.0b013e3182680a66.
56. Spaide RF, Campeas L, Haas A, Yannuzzi LA, Fisher YL, Guyer DR, Slakter JS, Sorenson JA, Orlock DA. Central serous chorioretinopathy in younger and older adults. Ophthalmology. 1996;103(12):2070–9; discussion 2079–80. https://doi.org/10.1016/s0161-6420(96)30386-2.
57. Bansal R, Dogra M, Mulkutkar S, Katoch D, Singh R, Gupta V, Dogra MR, Gupta A. Optical coherence tomography angiography versus fluorescein angiography in diagnosing choroidal neovascularization in chronic central serous chorioretinopathy. Indian J Ophthalmol. 2019;67(7):1095–100. https://doi.org/10.4103/ijo.IJO_1238_18.
58. Ng DS, Ho M, Chen LJ, Yip FL, Teh WM, Zhou L, Mohamed S, Tsang CW, Brelén ME, Chen H, Pang CP, Lai TYY. Optical coherence tomography angiography compared with multimodal imaging for diagnosing neovascular central serous chorioretinopathy. Am J Ophthalmol. 2021;232:70–82. https://doi.org/10.1016/j.ajo.2021.05.029. Epub 2021 Jun 9.
59. Bonini Filho MA, de Carlo TE, Ferrara D, Adhi M, Baumal CR, Witkin AJ, Reichel E, Duker JS, Waheed NK. Association of choroidal neovascularization and central serous chorioretinopathy with optical coherence tomography angiography. JAMA Ophthalmol. 2015;133(8):899–906. https://doi.org/10.1001/jamaophthalmol.2015.1320.
60. Dansingani KK, Balaratnasingam C, Klufas MA, Sarraf D, Freund KB. Optical coherence tomography angiography of shallow irregular pigment epithelial detachments in pachychoroid spectrum disease. Am J Ophthalmol. 2015;160(6):1243–1254.e2. https://doi.org/10.1016/j.ajo.2015.08.028. Epub 2015 Aug 28.
61. Hagag AM, Rasheed R, Chandra S, Jeffery G, Sivaprasad S. The diagnostic accuracy of double-layer sign in detection of macular neovascularization secondary to central serous chorioretinopathy. Am J Ophthalmol. 2022;236:271–80. https://doi.org/10.1016/j.ajo.2021.10.021. Epub 2021 Oct 23.
62. Zhang Y, Zhang J, Sun X. The efficacy of anti-VEGF therapy for putative or visible CNV in central serous chorioretinopathy by optical coherence tomography angiography. J Ophthalmol. 2022;2022:1272524. https://doi.org/10.1155/2022/1272524.
63. Zhao Z, Zhang J. Nonhomogenous hyperreflectivity in the choriocapillaris layer on optical coherence tomography angiography implies early treatment with anti-VEGF for central serous chorioretinopathy. Ophthalmic Res. 2022;65(5):506–15. https://doi.org/10.1159/000524488. Epub 2022 Apr 11.
64. Mandadi SKR, Singh SR, Sahoo NK, Mishra SB, Sacconi R, Iovino C, Berger L, Munk MR, Querques G, Peiretti E, Chhablani J. Optical coherence tomography angiography findings in fellow eyes of choroidal neovascularisation associated with central serous chorioretinopathy. Br J Ophthalmol.

2021;105(9):1280–5. https://doi.org/10.1136/bjophthalmol-2018-313576. Epub 2019 Feb 23.
65. Behar-Cohen F, Zhao M. Mineralocorticoid pathway in retinal health and diseases. Br J Pharmacol. 2022;179(13):3190–204. https://doi.org/10.1111/bph.15770. Epub 2022 Jan 28.
66. Bousquet E, Beydoun T, Zhao M, Hassan L, Offret O, Behar-Cohen F. Mineralocorticoid receptor antagonism in the treatment of chronic central serous chorioretinopathy: a pilot study. Retina. 2013;33(10):2096–102. https://doi.org/10.1097/IAE.0b013e318297a07a.
67. Toto L, D'Aloisio R, De Nicola C, Evangelista F, Ruggeri ML, Cerino L, Simonelli MB, Aharrh-Gnama A, Di Nicola M, Porreca A, Mastropasqua R. Short-term comparison between navigated subthreshold microsecond pulse laser and oral eplerenone for chronic central serous chorioretinopathy. Sci Rep. 2022;12(1):4727. https://doi.org/10.1038/s41598-022-08764-2.
68. van Rijssen TJ, van Dijk EHC, Tsonaka R, Feenstra HMA, Dijkman G, Peters PJH, Diederen RMH, Hoyng CB, Schlingemann RO, Boon CJF. Half-dose photodynamic therapy versus eplerenone in chronic central serous chorioretinopathy (SPECTRA): a randomized controlled trial. Am J Ophthalmol. 2022;233:101–10. https://doi.org/10.1016/j.ajo.2021.06.020. Epub 2021 Jun 29.
69. Lotery A, Sivaprasad S, O'Connell A, Harris RA, Culliford L, Ellis L, Cree A, Madhusudhan S, Behar-Cohen F, Chakravarthy U, Peto T, Rogers CA, Reeves BC, VICI Trial Investigators. Eplerenone for chronic central serous chorioretinopathy in patients with active, previously untreated disease for more than 4 months (VICI): a randomised, double-blind, placebo-controlled trial. Lancet. 2020;395(10220):294–303. https://doi.org/10.1016/S0140-6736(19)32981-2.
70. Gergely R, Kovács I, Récsán Z, Sándor GL, Czakó C, Nagy ZZ, Ecsedy M. Predictive factors of selective mineralocorticoid receptor antagonist treatment in chronic central serous chorioretinopathy. Sci Rep. 2020;10(1):16621. https://doi.org/10.1038/s41598-020-73959-4.
71. Hartnett ME, Lappas A, Darland D, McColm JR, Lovejoy S, D'Amore PA. Retinal pigment epithelium and endothelial cell interaction causes retinal pigment epithelial barrier dysfunction via a soluble VEGF-dependent mechanism. Exp Eye Res. 2003;77(5):593–9. https://doi.org/10.1016/s0014-4835(03)00189-1.
72. Curcio CA, Millican CL, Bailey T, Kruth HS. Accumulation of cholesterol with age in human Bruch's membrane. Invest Ophthalmol Vis Sci. 2001;42(1):265–74.
73. Meng LH, Chen YX. Lipid accumulation and protein modifications of Bruch's membrane in age-related macular degeneration. Int J Ophthalmol. 2021;14(5):766–73. https://doi.org/10.18240/ijo.2021.05.19.
74. Guymer RH, Markey CM, McAllister IL, Gillies MC, Hunyor AP, Arnold JJ, Investigators FLUID. Tolerating subretinal fluid in neovascular age-related macular degeneration treated with ranibizumab using a treat-and-extend regimen: FLUID study 24-month results. Ophthalmology. 2019;126(5):723–34. https://doi.org/10.1016/j.ophtha.2018.11.025. Epub 2018 Nov 29.
75. Aslam TM, Mahmood S, Balaskas K, Hoyle DC. Statistical modelling of the visual impact of subretinal fluid and associated features. Ophthalmol Ther. 2021;10(1):127–35. https://doi.org/10.1007/s40123-020-00327-w. Epub 2021 Jan 9.
76. Zarbin MA, Hill L, Maunz A, Gliem M, Stoilov I. Anti-VEGF-resistant subretinal fluid is associated with better vision and reduced risk of macular atrophy. Br J Ophthalmol. 2022;106(11):1561–6. https://doi.org/10.1136/bjophthalmol-2020-318688. Epub 2021 May 26.
77. Chaudhary V, Matonti F, Zarranz-Ventura J, Stewart MW. Impact of fluid compartments on functional outcomes for patients with neovascular age-related macular degeneration: a systematic literature review. Retina. 2022;42(4):589–606. https://doi.org/10.1097/IAE.0000000000003283.
78. Bringmann A, Wiedemann P. Müller glial cells in retinal disease. Ophthalmologica. 2012;227(1):1–19. https://doi.org/10.1159/000328979. Epub 2011 Sep 15.
79. Riedl S, Cooney L, Grechenig C, Sadeghipour A, Pablik E, Seaman JW 3rd, Waldstein SM, Schmidt-Erfurth U. Topographic analysis of photoreceptor loss correlated with disease morphology in neovascular age-related macular degeneration. Retina. 2020;40(11):2148–57. https://doi.org/10.1097/IAE.0000000000002717.
80. Xu M, Xu H, Li X, Chen F. Characteristics of macular morphology and microcirculation in diabetic macular edema patients with serous retinal detachment. BMC Ophthalmol. 2022;22(1):299. https://doi.org/10.1186/s12886-022-02523-7.
81. Sonoda S, Sakamoto T, Yamashita T, Shirasawa M, Otsuka H, Sonoda Y. Retinal morphologic changes and concentrations of cytokines in eyes with diabetic macular edema. Retina. 2014;34(4):741–8. https://doi.org/10.1097/IAE.0b013e3182a48917.
82. Gupta A, Raman R, Kulothungan V, Sharma T. Association of systemic and ocular risk factors with neurosensory retinal detachment in diabetic macular edema: a case-control study. BMC Ophthalmol. 2014;14:47. https://doi.org/10.1186/1471-2415-14-47.
83. Gündoğdu KÖ, Doğan E, Çelik E, Alagöz G. Effect of intravitreal ranibizumab on serous retinal detachment in diabetic macular edema. J Diabetes Complicat. 2022;36(7):108228. https://doi.

org/10.1016/j.jdiacomp.2022.108228. Epub 2022 Jun 7.

84. Bayat AH, Elçioğlu MN. Effects of dexamethasone treatment on serous retinal detachment in ranibizumab-resistant diabetic macular edema. Ther Adv Ophthalmol. 2020;12:2515841420971936. https://doi.org/10.1177/2515841420971936.
85. Maggio E, Mete M, Sartore M, Bauci F, Guerriero M, Polito A, Pertile G. Temporal variation of optical coherence tomography biomarkers as predictors of anti-VEGF treatment outcomes in diabetic macular edema. Graefes Arch Clin Exp Ophthalmol. 2022;260(3):807–15. https://doi.org/10.1007/s00417-021-05387-7. Epub 2021 Oct 18.
86. Ozsaygili C, Duru N. Comparison of intravitreal dexamethasone implant and aflibercept in patients with treatment-naive diabetic macular edema with serous retinal detachment. Retina. 2020;40(6):1044–52. https://doi.org/10.1097/IAE.0000000000002537.
87. Zur D, Iglicki M, Busch C, Invernizzi A, Mariussi M, Loewenstein A, International Retina Group. OCT biomarkers as functional outcome predictors in diabetic macular edema treated with dexamethasone implant. Ophthalmology. 2018;125(2):267–75. https://doi.org/10.1016/j.ophtha.2017.08.031. Epub 2017 Sep 19
88. Weinberg D, Jampol LM, Schatz H, Brady KD. Exudative retinal detachment following central and hemicentral retinal vein occlusions. Arch Ophthalmol. 1990;108(2):271–5. https://doi.org/10.1001/archopht.1990.01070040123045. Erratum in: Arch Ophthalmol 1990;108(4):563.
89. Spaide RF, Lee JK, Klancnik JK Jr, Gross NE. Optical coherence tomography of branch retinal vein occlusion. Retina. 2003;23(3):343–7. https://doi.org/10.1097/00006982-200306000-00009.
90. Tsujikawa A, Sakamoto A, Ota M, Kotera Y, Oh H, Miyamoto K, Kita M, Yoshimura N. Serous retinal detachment associated with retinal vein occlusion. Am J Ophthalmol. 2010;149(2):291–301.e5. https://doi.org/10.1016/j.ajo.2009.09.007.
91. Chen L, Yuan M, Sun L, Chen Y. Choroidal thickening in retinal vein occlusion patients with serous retinal detachment. Graefes Arch Clin Exp Ophthalmol. 2021;259(4):883–9.https://doi.org/10.1007/s00417--020-04983-3. Epub 2020 Nov 18.
92. Noma H, Funatsu H, Mimura T, Eguchi S. Vitreous inflammatory factors and serous retinal detachment in central retinal vein occlusion: a case control series. J Inflamm (Lond). 2011;8:38. https://doi.org/10.1186/1476-9255-8-38.
93. Noma H, Funatsu H, Mimura T, Tatsugawa M, Shimada K, Eguchi S. Vitreous inflammatory factors and serous macular detachment in branch retinal vein occlusion. Retina. 2012;32(1):86–91. https://doi.org/10.1097/IAE.0b013e31821801de.
94. Noma H, Funatsu H, Mimura T, Shimada K. Visual function and serous retinal detachment in patients with branch retinal vein occlusion and macular edema: a case series. BMC Ophthalmol. 2011;11:29. https://doi.org/10.1186/1471-2415-11-29.
95. Bayat AH, Akpolat Ç, Livan H, Bölükbaşı S, Elçioğlu MN. Comparison of the effects of aflibercept and dexamethasone in central retinal vein occlusion with serous retinal detachment. Clin Exp Optom. 2022;105(4):404–9. https://doi.org/10.1080/08164622.2021.1927676. Epub 2021 Jun 17.
96. Küçük B, Sirakaya E, Karaca C. Comparison of ranibizumab versus aflibercept in treating macular edema among patients with serous retinal detachment secondary to branch retinal vein occlusion. Ocul Immunol Inflamm. 2021;29(2):403–10. https://doi.org/10.1080/09273948.2019.1681474. Epub 2019 Nov 13.
97. Karacorlu M, Karacorlu SA, Ozdemir H, Senturk F. Intravitreal triamcinolone acetonide for treatment of serous macular detachment in central retinal vein occlusion. Retina. 2007;27(8):1026–30. https://doi.org/10.1097/IAE.0b013e3180645905.
98. Noma H, Funatsu H, Mimura T, Shimada K. Comparison of the efficacy of intravitreal triamcinolone acetonide for cystoid macular edema with versus without serous retinal detachment in branch retinal vein occlusion: influence on macular sensitivity and morphology. BMC Ophthalmol. 2012;12:39. https://doi.org/10.1186/1471-2415-12-39.
99. Hayreh SS, Servais GE, Virdi PS. Fundus lesions in malignant hypertension. VI. Hypertensive choroidopathy. Ophthalmology. 1986;93(11):1383–400. https://doi.org/10.1016/s0161-6420(86)33554-1.
100. Rubin S, Cremer A, Boulestreau R, Rigothier C, Kuntz S, Gosse P. Malignant hypertension: diagnosis, treatment and prognosis with experience from the Bordeaux cohort. J Hypertens. 2019;37(2):316–24. https://doi.org/10.1097/HJH.0000000000001913.
101. Mishima E, Funayama Y, Suzuki T, Mishima F, Nitta F, Toyohara T, Kikuchi K, Kunikata H, Hashimoto J, Miyazaki M, Harigae H, Nakazawa T, Ito S, Abe T. Concurrent analogous organ damage in the brain, eyes, and kidneys in malignant hypertension: reversible encephalopathy, serous retinal detachment, and proteinuria. Hypertens Res. 2021;44(1):88–97. https://doi.org/10.1038/s41440-020-0521-2. Epub 2020 Jul 27.
102. Saito M, Noda K, Saito W, Hirooka K, Hashimoto Y, Ishida S. Increased choroidal blood flow and choroidal thickness in patients with hypertensive chorioretinopathy. Graefes Arch Clin Exp Ophthalmol. 2020;258(2):233–40. https://doi.org/10.1007/s00417-019-04511-y. Epub 2019 Nov 14.
103. Bourke K, Patel MR, Prisant LM, Marcus DM. Hypertensive choroidopathy. J Clin Hypertens (Greenwich). 2004;6(8):471–2. https://doi.org/10.1111/j.1524-6175.2004.3749.x.
104. Dewilde E, Huygens M, Cools G, Van Calster J. Hypertensive choroidopathy in pre-eclampsia: two consecutive cases. Ophthalmic Surg Lasers Imaging Retina. 2014;45(4):343–6. https://doi.

org/10.3928/23258160-20140617-02. Epub 2014 Jun 30.

105. Rotsos T, Andreanos K, Blounas S, Brouzas D, Ladas DS, Ladas ID. Multimodal imaging of hypertensive chorioretinopathy by swept-source optical coherence tomography and optical coherence tomography angiography: case report. Medicine (Baltimore). 2017;96(39):e8110. https://doi.org/10.1097/MD.0000000000008110.
106. Velazquez-Villoria D, Marti Rodrigo P, DeNicola ML, Zapata Vitori MA, Segura García A, García-Arumí J. Swept source optical coherence tomography evaluation of chorioretinal changes in hypertensive choroidopathy related to Hellp syndrome. Retin Cases Brief Rep. 2019;13(1):30–3. https://doi.org/10.1097/ICB.0000000000000524.
107. Kishi S, Tso MO, Hayreh SS. Fundus lesions in malignant hypertension. I. A pathologic study of experimental hypertensive choroidopathy. Arch Ophthalmol. 1985;103(8):1189–97. https://doi.org/10.1001/archopht.1985.01050080101029.
108. Viruni N, Ong SS, Wu JH, Liu TYA. Longitudinal optical coherence tomography angiography findings in malignant hypertension choroidopathy: a case report. Case Rep Ophthalmol. 2022;13(1):276–81. https://doi.org/10.1159/000524115.
109. Saito M, Ishibazawa A, Kinouchi R, Yoshida A. Reperfusion of the choriocapillaris observed using optical coherence tomography angiography in hypertensive choroidopathy. Int Ophthalmol. 2018;38(5):2205–10. https://doi.org/10.1007/s10792-017-0705-1. Epub 2017 Sep 11.
110. Lee CS, Choi EY, Lee M, Kim H, Chung H. Serous retinal detachment in preeclampsia and malignant hypertension. Eye (Lond). 2019;33(11):1707–14. https://doi.org/10.1038/s41433-019-0461-8. Epub 2019 May 14.
111. Chang YS, Weng SF, Chang C, Wang JJ, Chen HI, Ko SY, Tu IT, Chien CC, Wang JJ, Wang CM, Jan RL. Risk of serous retinal detachment in patients with end-stage renal disease on dialysis. PLoS One. 2017;12(6):e0180133. https://doi.org/10.1371/journal.pone.0180133.
112. Shah DN, Al-Moujahed A, Newcomb CW, Kaçmaz RO, Daniel E, Thorne JE, Foster CS, Jabs DA, Levy-Clarke GA, Nussenblatt RB, Rosenbaum JT, Sen HN, Suhler EB, Bhatt NP, Kempen JH. Systemic immunosuppressive therapy for eye diseases research group exudative retinal detachment in ocular inflammatory diseases: risk and predictive factors. Am J Ophthalmol. 2020;218:279–87. https://doi.org/10.1016/j.ajo.2020.06.019. Epub 2020 Jul 2.
113. Lehpamer B, Moshier E, Goldberg N, Ackert J, Godbold J, Jabs DA. Subretinal fluid in uveitic macular edema: effect on vision and response to therapy. Am J Ophthalmol. 2013;155(1):143–9. https://doi.org/10.1016/j.ajo.2012.06.028. Epub 2012 Sep 27.
114. Munk MR, Sacu S, Huf W, Sulzbacher F, Mittermüller TJ, Eibenberger K, Rezar S, Bolz M, Kiss CG, Simader C, Schmidt-Erfurth U. Differential diagnosis of macular edema of different pathophysiologic origins by spectral domain optical coherence tomography. Retina. 2014;34(11):2218–32. https://doi.org/10.1097/IAE.0000000000000228.
115. Ossewaarde-van Norel J, Berg EM, Sijssens KM, Rothova A. Subfoveal serous retinal detachment in patients with uveitic macular edema. Arch Ophthalmol. 2011;129(2):158–62. https://doi.org/10.1001/archophthalmol.2010.337.
116. Weldy EW, Patnaik JL, Pecen PE, Palestine AG. Quantitative effect of subretinal fluid and intraretinal edema on visual acuity in uveitic cystoid macular edema. J Ophthalmic Inflamm Infect. 2021;11(1):38. https://doi.org/10.1186/s12348-021-00266-y.
117. Alvarez-Guzman C, Bustamante-Arias A, Colorado-Zavala MF, Rodriguez-Garcia A. The impact of central foveal thickness and integrity of the outer retinal layers in the visual outcome of uveitic macular edema. Int J Retina Vitreous. 2021;7(1):36. https://doi.org/10.1186/s40942-021-00306-8.
118. Ducos de Lahitte G, Terrada C, Tran TH, Cassoux N, LeHoang P, Kodjikian L, Bodaghi B. Maculopathy in uveitis of juvenile idiopathic arthritis: an optical coherence tomography study. Br J Ophthalmol. 2008;92(1):64–9. https://doi.org/10.1136/bjo.2007.120675. Epub 2007 Jun 21. Erratum in: Br J Ophthalmol. 2008;92(8):1159.
119. Liang F, Terrada C, Ducos de Lahitte G, Quartier P, Lehoang P, Thorne JE, Bodaghi B. Foveal serous retinal detachment in juvenile idiopathic arthritis-associated uveitis. Ocul Immunol Inflamm. 2016;24(4):386–91. https://doi.org/10.3109/09273948.2015.1012297. Epub 2015 Jul 14.
120. Kalogeropoulos C, Koumpoulis I, Mentis A, Pappa C, Zafeiropoulos P, Aspiotis M. Bartonella and intraocular inflammation: a series of cases and review of literature. Clin Ophthalmol. 2011;5:817–29. https://doi.org/10.2147/OPTH.S20157. Epub 2011 Jun 16.
121. Pollock SC, Kristinsson J. Cat-scratch disease manifesting as unifocal helioid choroiditis. Arch Ophthalmol. 1998;116(9):1249–51.
122. Gupta V, Gupta A, Arora S, Sachdeva N, Bambery P. Simultaneous choroidal tuberculoma and epididymo-orchitis caused by Mycobacterium tuberculosis. Am J Ophthalmol. 2005;140(2):310–2. https://doi.org/10.1016/j.ajo.2005.01.023.
123. Gupta V, Gupta A, Sachdeva N, Arora S, Bambery P. Successful management of tubercular subretinal granulomas. Ocul Immunol Inflamm. 2006;14(1):35–40. https://doi.org/10.1080/09273940500269939.
124. Song JH, Koreishi AF, Goldstein DA. Tuberculous uveitis presenting with a bullous exudative retinal detachment: a case report and systematic literature review. Ocul Immunol Inflamm. 2019;27(6):998–1009. https://doi.org/10.1080/09273948.2018.1485958. Epub 2018 Jul 3.
125. Thayil SM, Albini TA, Nazari H, Moshfeghi AA, Parel JM, Rao NA, Karakousis PC. Local ischemia and increased expression of vascular

endothelial growth factor following ocular dissemination of Mycobacterium tuberculosis. PLoS One. 2011;6(12):e28383. https://doi.org/10.1371/journal.pone.0028383. Epub 2011 Dec 5.

126. Haimovici R, Gragoudas ES, Gregor Z, Pesavento RD, Mieler WF, Duker JS. Choroidal metastases from renal cell carcinoma. Ophthalmology. 1997;104(7):1152–8. https://doi.org/10.1016/s0161-6420(97)30169-9.

127. Mathis T, Jardel P, Loria O, Delaunay B, Nguyen AM, Lanza F, Mosci C, Caujolle JP, Kodjikian L, Thariat J. New concepts in the diagnosis and management of choroidal metastases. Prog Retin Eye Res. 2019;68:144–76. https://doi.org/10.1016/j.preteyeres.2018.09.003. Epub 2018 Sep 19.

128. Vicini G, Nicolosi C, Pieretti G, Mazzini C. Large choroidal metastasis with exudative retinal detachment as presenting manifestation of small cell lung cancer: a case report. Respir Med Case Rep. 2020;30:101074. https://doi.org/10.1016/j.rmcr.2020.101074.

129. Neudorfer M, Waisbourd M, Anteby I, Liran A, Goldenberg D, Barak A, Kessler A. Color flow mapping: a non-invasive tool for characterizing and differentiating between uveal melanomas and choroidal metastases. Oncol Rep. 2011;25(1):91–6.

130. Arroyo JG, Yang L, Bula D, Chen DF. Photoreceptor apoptosis in human retinal detachment. Am J Ophthalmol. 2005;139(4):605–10. https://doi.org/10.1016/j.ajo.2004.11.046.

131. Yu J, Jiang C, Xu G. Correlations between changes in photoreceptor layer and other clinical characteristics in central serous chorioretinopathy. Retina. 2019;39(6):1110–6. https://doi.org/10.1097/IAE.0000000000002092.

132. Gollamudi SR, Smiddy WE, Schachat AP, Michels RG, Vitale S. Long-term survival rate after vitreous surgery for complications of diabetic retinopathy. Ophthalmology. 1991;98(1):18–22. https://doi.org/10.1016/s0161-6420(91)32349-2.

133. Vote BJ, Gamble GD, Polkinghorne PJ. Auckland proliferative diabetic vitrectomy fellow eye study. Clin Exp Ophthalmol. 2004;32(4):397–403. https://doi.org/10.1111/j.1442-9071.2004.00845.x.

134. Atchison DA, Jones CE, Schmid KL, Pritchard N, Pope JM, Strugnell WE, Riley RA. Eye shape in emmetropia and myopia. Invest Ophthalmol Vis Sci. 2004;45(10):3380–6. https://doi.org/10.1167/iovs.04-0292.

135. Morgan IG, Ohno-Matsui K, Saw SM. Myopia. Lancet. 2012;379(9827):1739–48. https://doi.org/10.1016/S0140-6736(12)60272-4.

136. Johnson MW. Myopic traction maculopathy: pathogenic mechanisms and surgical treatment. Retina. 2012;32(Suppl 2):S205–10. https://doi.org/10.1097/IAE.0b013e31825bc0de.

137. Panozzo G, Mercanti A. Vitrectomy for myopic traction maculopathy. Arch Ophthalmol. 2007;125(6):767–72. https://doi.org/10.1001/archopht.125.6.767.

138. Chen G, Mao S, Tong Y, Jiang F, Yang J, Li W. Fovea sparing versus complete internal limiting membrane peeling for myopic traction maculopathy: a meta-analysis. Int Ophthalmol. 2022;42(3):765–73. https://doi.org/10.1007/s10792-021-02042-2. Epub 2021 Oct 8.

139. Iwasaki M, Miyamoto H, Okushiba U, Imaizumi H. Fovea-sparing internal limiting membrane peeling versus complete internal limiting membrane peeling for myopic traction maculopathy. Jpn J Ophthalmol. 2020;64(1):13–21. https://doi.org/10.1007/s10384--019-00696-1. Epub 2019 Nov 4.

140. Barzideh N, Johnson TM. Subfoveal fluid resolves slowly after pars plana vitrectomy for tractional retinal detachment secondary to proliferative diabetic retinopathy. Retina. 2007;27(6):740–3. https://doi.org/10.1097/IAE.0b013e318030c663.

141. Meleth AD, Carvounis PE. Outcomes of vitrectomy for tractional retinal detachment in diabetic retinopathy. Int Ophthalmol Clin. 2014;54(2):127–39. https://doi.org/10.1097/IIO.0000000000000021.

142. Sokol JT, Schechet SA, Rosen DT, Ferenchak K, Dawood S, Skondra D. Outcomes of vitrectomy for diabetic tractional retinal detachment in Chicago's county health system. PLoS One. 2019;14(8):e0220726. https://doi.org/10.1371/journal.pone.0220726.

143. Mikhail M, Ali-Ridha A, Chorfi S, Kapusta MA. Long-term outcomes of sutureless 25-G+ pars-plana vitrectomy for the management of diabetic tractional retinal detachment. Graefes Arch Clin Exp Ophthalmol. 2017;255(2):255–61. https://doi.org/10.1007/s00417-016-3442-7. Epub 2016 Aug 2.

144. Dikopf MS, Patel KH, Setlur VJ, Lim JI. Surgical outcomes of 25-gauge pars plana vitrectomy for diabetic tractional retinal detachment. Eye (Lond). 2015;29(9):1213–9. https://doi.org/10.1038/eye.2015.126. Epub 2015 Jul 17.

145. Gupta A, Bansal R, Gupta V, Dogra MR. Six-month visual outcome after pars plana vitrectomy in proliferative diabetic retinopathy with or without a single preoperative injection of intravitreal bevacizumab. Int Ophthalmol. 2012;32(2):135–44. https://doi.org/10.1007/s10792-012-9541-5. Epub 2012 Mar 27.

146. Rush RB, Rush SW, Reinauer RM, Bastar PG, Browning DJ. Vitrectomy for diabetic complications: a pooled analysis of randomized controlled trials using modern techniques and equipment. Retina. 2022;42(7):1292–301. https://doi.org/10.1097/IAE.0000000000003471.

147. Rush RB, Velazquez JC, Rosales CR, Rush SW. Gas tamponade for the prevention of postoperative vitreous hemorrhaging after diabetic vitrectomy: a randomized clinical trial. Am J Ophthalmol. 2022;242:173–80. https://doi.org/10.1016/j.ajo.2022.06.015. Epub 2022 Jun 25.

148. Bansal R, Moharana B, Katoch D, Gupta V, Dogra MR, Gupta A. Outcome of pars plana vitrectomy in patients with retinal detachments secondary to retinal vasculitis. Indian J Ophthalmol. 2020;68(9):1905–11. https://doi.org/10.4103/ijo.IJO_551_20.
149. Chandra P, Kumawat D, Tewari R, Sinha R. Surgical outcomes of immediate sequential bilateral vitreoretinal surgery for advancing retinopathy of prematurity. Indian J Ophthalmol. 2019;67(6):903–7. https://doi.org/10.4103/ijo.IJO_741_18.
150. Özdek Ş, Özmen MC, Yalınbaş D, Atalay HT, Coşkun D. Immediate sequential bilateral vitrectomy surgery for retinopathy of prematurity: a single surgeon experience. Turk J Ophthalmol. 2021;51(4):225–30. https://doi.org/10.4274/tjo.galenos.2020.07377.
151. Yonekawa Y, Wu WC, Kusaka S, Robinson J, Tsujioka D, Kang KB, Shapiro MJ, Padhi TR, Jain L, Sears JE, Kuriyan AE, Berrocal AM, Quiram PA, Gerber AE, Paul Chan RV, Jonas KE, Wong SC, Patel CK, Abbey AM, Spencer R, Blair MP, Chang EY, Papakostas TD, Vavvas DG, Sisk RA, Ferrone PJ, Henderson RH, Olsen KR, Hartnett ME, Chau FY, Mukai S, Murray TG, Thomas BJ, Meza PA, Drenser KA, Trese MT, Capone A Jr. Immediate sequential bilateral pediatric vitreoretinal surgery: an international multicenter study. Ophthalmology. 2016;123(8):1802–8. https://doi.org/10.1016/j.ophtha.2016.04.033. Epub 2016 May 22.
152. Celorio JM, Pruett RC. Prevalence of lattice degeneration and its relation to axial length in severe myopia. Am J Ophthalmol. 1991;111(1):20–3. https://doi.org/10.1016/s0002-9394(14)76891-6.
153. Tabibian D, Hoogewoud F, Mavrakanas N, Schutz JS. Misdirected aqueous flow in rhegmatogenous retinal detachment: a pathophysiology update. Surv Ophthalmol. 2015;60(1):51–9. https://doi.org/10.1016/j.survophthal.2014.07.002. Epub 2014 Aug 10.
154. Flaxel CJ, Adelman RA, Bailey ST, Fawzi A, Lim JI, Vemulakonda GA, Ying GS. Posterior vitreous detachment, retinal breaks, and lattice degeneration preferred practice pattern®. Ophthalmology. 2020;127(1):P146–81. https://doi.org/10.1016/j.ophtha.2019.09.027. Epub 2019 Sep 25. Erratum in: Ophthalmology. 2020;127(9):1279.
155. Ripandelli G, Coppé AM, Parisi V, Olzi D, Scassa C, Chiaravalloti A, Stirpe M. Posterior vitreous detachment and retinal detachment after cataract surgery. Ophthalmology. 2007;114(4):692–7. https://doi.org/10.1016/j.ophtha.2006.08.045. Epub 2007 Jan 17.
156. Colin J, Robinet A, Cochener B. Retinal detachment after clear lens extraction for high myopia: seven-year follow-up. Ophthalmology. 1999;106(12):2281–4; discussion 2285. https://doi.org/10.1016/S0161-6420(99)90526-2.
157. Javitt JC, Tielsch JM, Canner JK, Kolb MM, Sommer A, Steinberg EP. National outcomes of cataract extraction. Increased risk of retinal complications associated with Nd:YAG laser capsulotomy. The Cataract Patient Outcomes Research Team. Ophthalmology. 1992;99(10):1487–97; discussion 1497–8. https://doi.org/10.1016/s0161-6420(92)31775-0.
158. Ficker LA, Vickers S, Capon MR, Mellerio J, Cooling RJ. Retinal detachment following Nd:YAG posterior capsulotomy. Eye (Lond). 1987;1(Pt 1):86–9. https://doi.org/10.1038/eye.1987.13.
159. Cooling RJ. Traumatic retinal detachment—mechanisms and management. Trans Ophthalmol Soc U K (1962). 1986;105(Pt 5):575–9.
160. Barbosa GC, Gomes da Silva A, Rocha de Sousa J, Machado CG, Gomes AV. Enlightening new underpinnings in hydration retinal folds. Eur J Ophthalmol. 2022;32(6):3510–3. https://doi.org/10.1177/11206721221086239. Epub 2022 Mar 4.
161. Muni RH, Darabad MN, Oquendo PL, Hamli H, Lee WW, Nagel F, Bansal A, Melo IM, Ramachandran A. Outer retinal corrugations in rhegmatogenous retinal detachment: the retinal pigment epithelium-photoreceptor dysregulation theory. Am J Ophthalmol. 2022;245:14–24. https://doi.org/10.1016/j.ajo.2022.08.019. Epub ahead of print.
162. Dalvin LA, Spaide RF, Yannuzzi LA, Freund KB, Pulido JS. Hydration folds in rhegmatogenous retinal detachment. Retin Cases Brief Rep. 2020;14(4):355–9. https://doi.org/10.1097/ICB.0000000000000711.
163. Majumder PD. https://www.eophtha.com/posts/documentation-drawing-in-ophthalmology. Accessed 5 Dec 2022.
164. Lincoff H, Gieser R. Finding the retinal hole. Arch Ophthalmol. 1971;85(5):565–9. https://doi.org/10.1001/archopht.1971.00990050567007.
165. Nagasaki H, Shinagawa K, Mochizuki M. Risk factors for proliferative vitreoretinopathy. Prog Retin Eye Res. 1998;17(1):77–98. https://doi.org/10.1016/s1350-9462(97)00007-4.
166. Amsler M. The heritage of Gonin. Proc R Soc Med. 1960;53(12):1043–6.
167. Lumi X, Lužnik Z, Petrovski G, Petrovski BÉ, Hawlina M. Anatomical success rate of pars plana vitrectomy for treatment of complex rhegmatogenous retinal detachment. BMC Ophthalmol. 2016;16(1):216. https://doi.org/10.1186/s12886-016-0390-2.
168. Eshtiaghi A, Dhoot AS, Mihalache A, Popovic MM, Nichani PAH, Sayal AP, Yu HJ, Wykoff CC, Kertes PJ, Muni RH. Pars plana vitrectomy with and without supplemental scleral buckle for the repair of rhegmatogenous retinal detachment: a meta-analysis. Ophthalmol Retina. 2022;6(10):871–85. https://doi.org/10.1016/j.oret.2022.02.009. Epub 2022 Feb 26.
169. Dhoot AS, Popovic MM, Nichani PAH, Eshtiaghi A, Mihalache A, Sayal AP, Yu H, Wykoff CC, Kertes PJ, Muni RH. Pars plana vitrectomy versus scleral buckle: A comprehensive meta-analysis of 15,947 eyes. Surv Ophthalmol. 2022;67(4):932–49. https://doi.org/10.1016/j.survophthal.2021.12.005. Epub 2021 Dec 9.

170. Wolfensberger TJ, Tufail A. Systemic disorders associated with detachment of the neurosensory retina and retinal pigment epithelium. Curr Opin Ophthalmol. 2000;11(6):455–61. https://doi.org/10.1097/00055735-200012000-00012.
171. Roos NM, Wiegman MJ, Jansonius NM, Zeeman GG. Visual disturbances in (pre)eclampsia. Obstet Gynecol Surv. 2012;67(4):242–50. https://doi.org/10.1097/OGX.0b013e318250a457.
172. Jabs DA, Hanneken AM, Schachat AP, Fine SL. Choroidopathy in systemic lupus erythematosus. Arch Ophthalmol. 1988;106(2):230–4. https://doi.org/10.1001/archopht.1988.01060130240036.
173. da Cruz NFS, Polizelli MU, Cezar LM, Cardoso EB, Penha F, Farah ME, Rodrigues EB, Novais EA. Effects of phosphodiesterase type 5 inhibitors on choroid and ocular vasculature: a literature review. Int J Retina Vitreous. 2020;6:38. https://doi.org/10.1186/s40942-020-00241-0.
174. Fortes BH, Tailor PD, Dalvin LA. Ocular toxicity of targeted anticancer agents. Drugs. 2021;81(7):771–823. https://doi.org/10.1007/s40265-021-01507-z. Epub 2021 Mar 31. Erratum in: Drugs. 2022;82(3):355.

13 Macular Degeneration, Geographic Atrophy, and Inherited Retinal Disorders

13.1 Introduction

Many disorders that lead to primary retinal atrophy affect the retina bilaterally and involve either the macula, the peripheral retina, or both the macula and the peripheral retina. The most common of these is dry age-related macular degeneration (AMD) which leads to irreversible loss of central vision and is a significant public health concern in the fast-growing ageing populations in the developed and developing regions of the world. The incident late AMD significantly impacts the vision-related quality of life regarding reading, mobility, and emotional well-being [1]. Several inherited retinal disorders (IRD) affect the macula or the peripheral retina. These have a variable age of onset and lead to irreversible loss of either central or peripheral vision. The most typical example of IRD is retinitis pigmentosa (RP) which affects millions of children worldwide and makes them blind in their youth.

Till recently, none of these could have been treated. Rapid strides in cell biology, biotechnology, and genetics in the past few decades have led to remarkable progress in understanding the pathophysiology of these disorders. Often labelled orphan diseases, many IRDs have remained neglected because of their rarity. However, innovative therapeutic interventions are being developed to treat these hitherto blinding disorders and should be available in the foreseeable future. Among the first FDA-approved gene therapies is Luxturna for RP, and its beneficial results have been sustained through almost 5 years of follow-up. For those patients who have lost photoreceptors, a new field of optogenetics has made it possible to express the opsin gene (the protein involved in phototransduction) in inner retinal cells, and the first human trials have already started. Cell-based therapies have been initiated to replace the retinal pigment epithelium (RPE). This chapter will not discuss secondary retinal atrophies and degenerations secondary to the involvement of the retina, choroid or optic nerve by diabetes mellitus, vascular occlusions, inflammation, infections, drug toxicities, cancer-associated retinopathies, and trauma.

13.2 Anatomical Considerations

The neurosensory retina (NSR) is a highly organized multilayered tissue consisting of highly organized neural cells and their fibres, namely the photoreceptors rods and cones (first neuron), bipolar cells (second neuron), horizontal cells, amacrine cells, and the retinal ganglion cells (third neuron). The glial cells include the Muller glial cells spanning the entire NSR, microglia, and astrocytes. The retinal cells are post-mitotic and do not regenerate once they undergo degeneration. The processes of the Muller cells and the microglia (up to the inner nuclear layer) and astrocytes only in the superficial capillary

A. Gupta et al., *Ophthalmic Signs in Practice of Medicine*,
https://doi.org/10.1007/978-981-99-7923-3_13

plexus form very intimate contact with pericytes, capillary endothelial cell, and neural cells (the neuro-glia-vascular unit) that maintains the metabolic and immune homeostasis of the retina. The photoreceptor outer segments are in intimate contact with the microvilli of the RPE cells. Each RPE cell receives the photoreceptor outer segments from 20 to 30 rods and cones. The RPE phagocytose the rod and cone outer segment membranes. The rod visual pigment is recycled in the RPE cells, whereas the Muller cell bodies recycle the cone visual pigment. The RPE cell layer is a single layer of post-mitotic cells that do not regenerate once they degenerate. The RPE layer is vital for the survival of the photoreceptors.

The visual impulse is generated when the light falls on the photoreceptors, where the visual pigment is split into opsin and all-trans-retinal, the process known as phototransduction. The visual signal is transmitted from the photoreceptors to the visual cortex via the visual pathways, involving the first three neurons in the retina and their synapses. The axons of the ganglion cells exit the eye to form the optic nerve, which conducts the signals up to the lateral geniculate nucleus, where the fourth neuron is located. The optic radiation from the geniculate body further transmits signals to the visual cortex located in the occipital lobe, where the signals are perceived as the image of the objects.

The NSR, up to the inner third of the outer plexiform layer, receives its oxygen and micronutritional requirements from the capillary plexus derived from the retinal vessels. The RPE and the outer retina are avascular and get their oxygen and micro-nutritional requirements from the choroidal blood supply through a single layer of closed-fenestrated wide lumen capillaries 10–30 μm in thickness. Compared to the retinal capillaries, the choriocapillaris (ChC) offers less resistance to blood flow and ensures oxygen and metabolic substrate supply to the outer retina [2]. The ChC's closed-fenestrations (which are covered with a diaphragm) are larger than the capillaries elsewhere in the body and face the Bruch's membrane (BM), which separates them from the RPE cells. Unlike the sinusoidal capillaries in the liver, these closed fenestrations do not allow blood plasma to pass into the interstitial tissue. The ChC allows diffusion of small-sized macromolecules but does not allow larger macromolecules to enter interstitial space. The scleral side of the endothelial cells has gap junctions and discontinuous tight junctions [2].

The choroid has the highest blood flow in the body and very high oxygen saturation, which is only 2–3% less than the arterial blood. A high gradient of oxygen saturation ensures efficient diffusion of oxygen into the outer retina [3]. The blood flow in ChC is vital for sustaining the RPE and the photoreceptors. The innermost layer of the five-layered BM is constituted by the basement membrane of the RPE cells, followed by the inner collagenous layer, the middle elastic layer, an outer collagenous layer, and the outermost layer by the basement membrane of the endothelial cells of the ChC. The BM allows only the passive transport of molecules between the ChC and the RPE by diffusion, concentration gradient, and hydrostatic pressure. It does not allow the movement of cells across it.

13.3 Complement Pathway-Basics

Complement pathways are essential in the pathogenesis of AMD. Complements are small proteins manufactured in the liver by hepatocytes and circulate in the blood as precursors. Complement pathways are an integral component of the innate immune defence system. In the past, their role was limited to the opsonization of the invading bacteria for their elimination by phagocytosis. Later it was realized that complement pathways also play a significant role in eliminating the stressed tissue cells in the body. Regulatory failure of complement factor H can amplify the inflammatory reaction.

The complement (C) pathways involve the action of the proteolytic enzymes on substrates generated by the degradation of cells. There are mainly three mechanisms which activate the complement pathways. The classical pathway

(CP) is through the binding of C1q, a fragment of C1, with an antigen-antibody complex or substrates. The microglia and macrophages express the C1q in RPE and outer photoreceptors [4]. Additionally, there may be leakage and deposition of systemic complements in the ocular tissues.

In the retina, various substrates like C-reactive proteins, phosphatidyl serine and other phospholipids, clustered IgG, amyloid, and hydroxyapatite are generated from the phagocytosis of the photoreceptor outer segments, and the lysosomal degradation of their cell membranes. These are opsonized by C1q to initiate the CP [4].

In the Lectin pathway (LP), instead of the C1q, mannose-binding lectin (MBL) binds to the carbohydrate residues on the organism's surface and activates serine proteases like the CP. The alternate pathway (AP) involves spontaneous hydrolysis of C3, which maintains a low-level activity at all times and does not require binding to specific receptors.

All three pathways of complement activation lead to the formation of complement convertase C3bBb, which cleaves C3 to C3a and C3b. Factor B binds with C3b to form C3bB. Factor B is cleaved by factor D to form Bb, which binds to C3b to form C3 convertase C3bBb. C3b enters into an amplification loop with increasing amounts of the C3 convertase formation, which cleaves C5 to C5a and C5b. Fragments C3a and C5a are anaphylatoxins chemoattractants for the microglia and the macrophages. Factor C5b combines with C6–C9 to form a membrane attack complex (MAC) which disrupts the cell walls' bilipid layer, resulting in the cell death of RPE cells, photoreceptors, and the endothelial cells of the ChC [5].

Increased complement activity also leads to the release of anaphylatoxins C3a and C5a, which also recruit inflammatory cells, microglial, and macrophages in the subretinal space. The phagocytes recognize the opsonization of the stressed target cells (photoreceptors, RPE cells, and ChC endothelial cells) by the complement fragments such as C3b, iC3b, and C4b [5]. There is some evidence that the C1q fragment, the initiating molecule in the classic pathway, maybe a significant pathway in AMD pathogenesis. C1q activating ligands are present at the photoreceptor synapses, outer segments of photoreceptors, RPE, and drusen. The microglia and macrophages also express C1q in these locations [4].

In normal circumstances, the complement activity should cease once the substrate has been completely removed. However, in GA, waste products are produced continuously in the drusen and the stressed cell membranes, resulting in continuous complement activation and inflammasome activation within the RPE cells. These lead to the recruitment of microglia and macrophages, cell wall lysis, and phagocytic activity [4].

The protein Properdin increases the survival time of C3 convertase and plays a role in promoting inflammation. On the contrary, Factor H is a regulatory protein for blocking the C3b fragment cleaved from C3 and thus plays a significant role in containing innate inflammatory activity [5]. Patients with the Factor H variant gene and who did not develop the disease were found to lack Factor B, another critical component required for generating C3 convertase [6].

There needed to be more information on the exact transcriptome-wide associations or the gene expressions directly responsible for the causation of AMD pathology [7]. Only recently have transcriptome studies been done on RPE cells derived from the induced pluripotent stem cells (iPSC) developed from the geographic atrophy patients' fibroblasts. These derived RPE cells have all five significant protein quantitative loci that regulate protein expression in mitochondrial biology and neurodegeneration, suggesting a role for mitochondrial dysfunction in GA [8].

13.4 Age-Related Changes in the Retina

Significant changes occur in the retina with ageing. More significant changes occur in the outer retina compared to the inner retina. The density of cones in the macular area is reduced closer to the foveal centre, although their thickness increases [9]. There is thinning of the ChC, which is compensated by increased passive transfers between the outer retina and the Choroid [2]. Histological studies of eyes from 6 to 100 years old have shown an increase in the thickness of BM from 2 to 4.7 μm and a decrease in the ChC density by 47%. The thickening of BM is related only to age and not to AMD [10]. The decrease in the ChC density with ageing corresponds to a similar loss of the rod photoreceptors. There is a loss of hydraulic conductivity due to the deposition of lipids in the BM. With ageing, there is a significant reduction in the size of the macromolecules that can pass through the BM [2].

13.5 Age-Related Macular Degeneration (AMD)

13.5.1 Epidemiology

Age-related macular degeneration (AMD) is a major public health challenge with significant ethnic and racial differences. Globally, 196 million people are estimated to have AMD, likely reaching 288 million by 2040 [11]. Nearly 8.7% of persons above 30 had any documented AMD, with 8% having an early and 0.37% having a late AMD. Any stage AMD is more common in Europeans (11.2%) compared to Asians (6.8%) and Africans (7.2%). Geographic atrophy (GA) was noted in 1.11% of Europeans versus 0.21% of Asians, 0.16% of Hispanics, and 0.14% of Africans [11].

13.5.2 Role of Complement Pathways in AMD

In a significant breakthrough, a single-point mutation in the genes coding for complement factor H was first reported in 2005. This discovery first pointed out the role of genetics in the causation of AMD [12–14]. The discovery of many components of the alternative complement pathway in drusen, a precursor of AMD, has strongly suggested a role for innate inflammation in AMD [15].

In addition to the mutations in the complement factor H, single nucleotide polymorphisms (SNPs) in rs10490924, in the ARMS2 gene located on Chromosome 10, is highly associated with AMD. This gene mediates the opsonization of necrotic and apoptotic cells [16, 17]. A deficiency of the normal ARMS2 protein may be responsible for drusen formation [17].

A two-level model hypothesis recently suggested that the primary insult in the AMD is due to local oxidative stress in the outer retina modulated by an unbridled inflammatory response due to SNPs in the complement factor H. Hence the treatment strategies to control AMD target the involved complement pathways [18].

13.5.3 Risk Factors for AMD and Its Pathogenesis

The retina is a tissue with the highest metabolic rate in the body and is highly vulnerable to oxidative stress. Ageing results in a decrease in the choroidal blood flow and thinning of the choroid, thickening of the BM with a consequent slowdown of the exchange of oxygen, metabolic substrates, and waste products between the choroid and the photoreceptors. Rozing et al. [18] have reviewed the subject extensively.

AMD is a complex multifactorial disease with significant genetic and environmental risk factors. Besides ageing, several preventable risk factors such as family history, hypertension, smoking, obesity, and a sedentary lifestyle are common between AMD and cardiovascular diseases. These cause systemic low-grade chronic inflammation and increased oxidative stress [19]. The Mediterranean diet recommended for preventing CVD, consisting of leafy vegetables, fruits, fish, and legumes, has also been shown to reduce the incidence of late AMD by almost 40% [20]. Additionally, prospective population-based cohorts have shown beneficial effects of high levels of physical activity in preventing the occurrence of early AMD [21]. Obesity and smoking in people who show SNPs in CFH Y402H and ARMS 2 (LOC387715 A69S) genes raise the risk of progressive AMD by 19-fold [22].

In a large European cohort, nearly two-third of the patients with late AMD had risk allele rs3750486 at the ARMS2/HTRA1 locus. Homozygous carriers had an odds ratio of 8.6 for geographic atrophy and 11.2 for neovascular AMD (nAMD). The lifetime risk of developing advanced AMD was 4.4 for non-genotype, 9.4 for heterozygous, and 26.8 for homozygous carriers. The homozygotes also had the onset of late AMD almost 10 years earlier. This gene variant plays the role of a strong catalyst in patients with early changes of AMD [23].

In ageing RPE, there is an accumulation of lipid peroxidation products which are deposited between the basement membrane of RPE and BM. It has been proposed that environmental factors with defective innate and adaptive immune mechanisms in aged people due to their genetic predisposition lead to low-grade systemic inflammation, which in the eye leads to AMD. The same factors also lead to systemic atherosclerosis, which explains the high risk of CVD in patients with AMD.

The cellular debris is deposited under the retina in the BM as well-defined hard drusen, ill-defined soft drusen, or densely packed small reticular drusen. On the other hand, subretinal drusenoid deposits (SDD), earlier known as pseudo reticular drusen, are deposited under the NSR and above the RPE. The latter differs from the classical drusen in their location and lipid composition. The SDD may breach the ellipsoid zone (EZ) and extend into the NSR. The SDD is associated with type 3 new vessels and geographic atrophy [24]. The site where the drusen will appear does not appear to be a random phenomenon but relates to the areas of choroidal ischaemia. Although histopathological studies in the past had shown thinning of ChC in the AMD eyes, more recently, imaging studies using OCT angiography have shown significant flow deficits in ChC underlying the existing drusen, expanding drusen or even those that will appear in future, suggesting that choroidal ischaemia is a critical event in the development of AMD [25]. Age-related thickening of BM, deposition of advanced glycosylated end products (AGE) and extracellular debris as basal laminar deposits, and increased expression of VEGF from the RPE and microglia in an ischaemic microenvironment lead to the formation of pathological new vessels that grow most commonly under the RPE (type1), less commonly under the NSR (type 2) or even from the retina (type 3). These vessels do not have tight endothelial junctions and leak fluid and blood under the macula.

13.5.4 Epigenetic Factors in Dry AMD

The allele variants associated with AMD are regulatory proteins and not structural proteins. Smoking, nutritional, and other environmental factors are strong epigenetic factors for the expression of regulatory proteins and increase the risk for the development of AMD in carriers of these alleles.

In the first 10 years since the original studies in 2005, large genome-wide association studies discovered 52 independent common and rare gene variants distributed across 34 loci [26]; at present, the number has gone up to 90 allele variants spread over 55 independent loci [8]. Most of the loci discovered in AMD are involved in either complement-mediated inflammation or lipid metabolism.

13.5.5 Clinical Diagnosis of AMD

The non-exudative AMD is asymptomatic in the early and intermediate stages. It gets diagnosed in patients who may visit an ophthalmology/optometry clinic for a routine examination/screening for cataracts and glaucoma. The non-exudative AMD is a symmetric bilateral disease, and 90% of patients do not progress to an exudative stage. Drusen are the hallmark of AMD and vary in size from <63μ to nearly 1000μm. Small drusen, <63μ, are seen in the macula as yellow-white discrete dot lesions and are commonly seen in older people (Fig. 13.1). These are called drupelets and usually are not seen on fundus fluorescein angiography (FFA). These stay unaltered for several years and may show mineralization. On structural

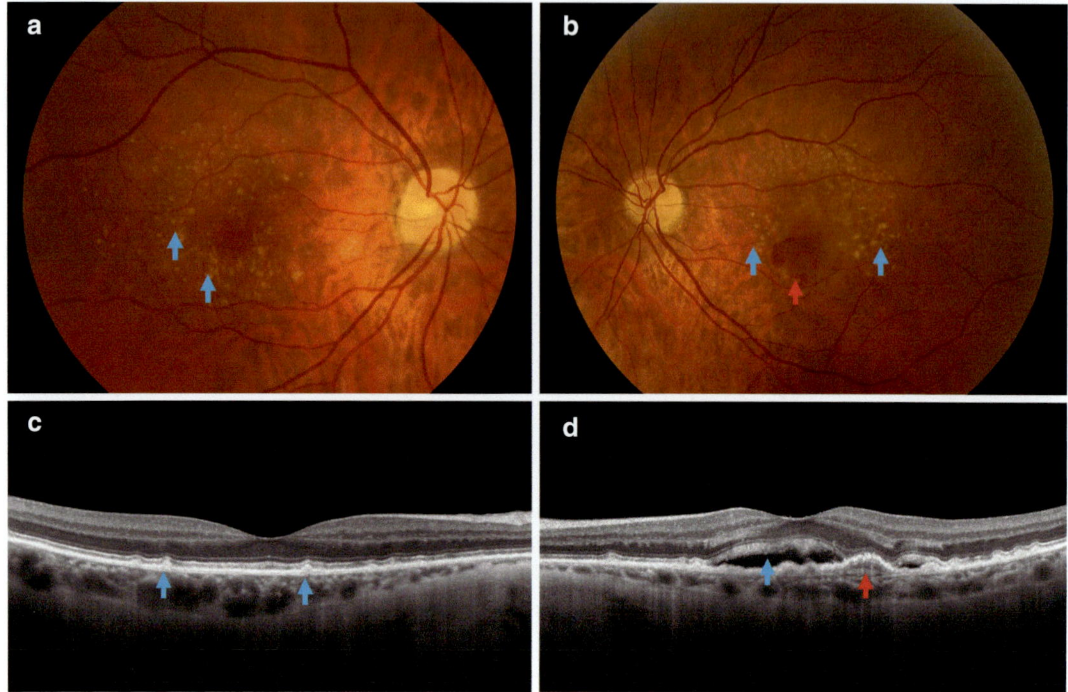

Fig. 13.1 Right eye shows (**a**) hard drusen (blue arrows), and the left eye (**b**) shows hard drusen (blue arrows) along with a subretinal haemorrhage (red arrow) suggestive of a CNVM. OCT shows sub-RPE drusenoid deposits (blue arrows) in the right eye (**c**), and a CNVM complex (red arrow) with subretinal fluid (blue arrow) in the left eye (**d**). (Images courtesy of Dr Anita Agarwal, West Coast Retina Medical Group, San Francisco, CA)

OCT, these appear as tiny nodular elevations over the BM. These do not progress further to the GA or predispose to choroidal neovascular membrane (CNVM) formation. Soft drusen are made of a similar lipoproteins debris but are larger than 63μ, are pale yellow and have indistinct borders. The presence of soft drusen <125μ is labelled as early AMD (Fig. 13.2). These may become confluent over time and increase in numbers. More than 20 soft drusen >63–124μ or multiple small with a single large soft druse >125μ is classified as an intermediate stage of AMD (Fig. 13.3). Pigmentary changes may accompany the soft drusen. Both hyper and hypopigmentation may be seen. The soft drusen are mound-like deposits over the BM on structural OCT. On autofluorescence, some of these may show a central hypoautofluorescencewitharingofhyperautofluorescence. A thin layer of basilar linear deposits connects the soft drusen. The most significant type of drusen is the SDD under the NSR and overlie the RPE. These were characterized only after the availability of the structural OCT. These may be best seen on blue light reflectance images rather than colour fundus photographs or IR reflectance images [24].

Gass [27] first showed the development of nAMD in 18% of eyes with drusen at an average age of 75 years and an average follow-up of nearly 5 years. These eyes were characterized by the development of sub-RPE and subretinal exudation through either an intact BM or the growth of new vessels through breaks in the BM causing exudative and haemorrhagic detachment of the RPE and the NSR [27].

13.5.6 Classification of AMD

AMD is mainly of two types. More than 90% of the cases have a gradually progressive non-exudative or dry type of AMD, and 10% have an

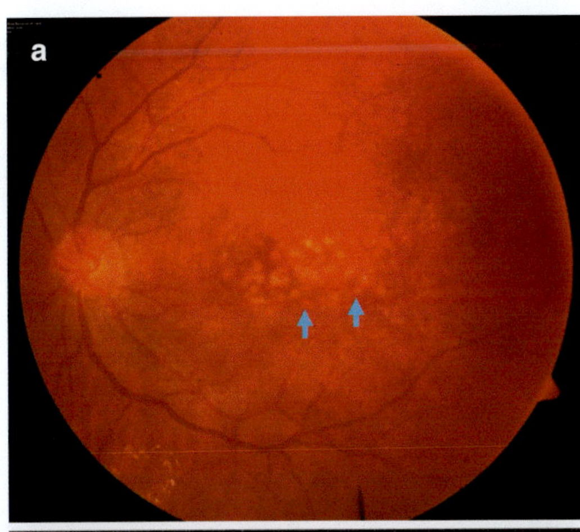

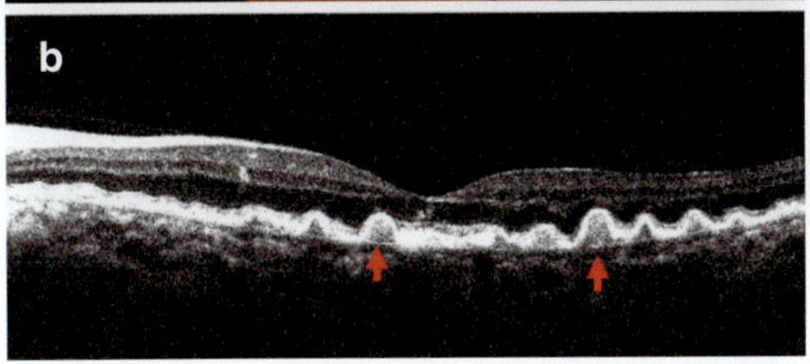

Fig. 13.2 Early AMD: a 59-year-old female presented with 6/24 vision and distortion of images in left eye. Fundus examination (**a**) revealed soft drusens (blue arrows) in the macula, seen as pale yellow lesions with indistinct borders. Optical coherence tomography (**b**) showed mound-like deposits over the Bruch's membrane (red arrows)

immediate vision-threatening wet type of neovascular AMD (nAMD). The hallmark of the AMD is the development of drusen, which are extracellular deposits of metabolic waste products between the basement membrane of the RPE and the BM. These also get deposited between the RPE and the NSR as SDD and have been termed reticular pseudodrusen. A macular research committee reached the following consensus classification to bring uniformity in investigators' usage of various AMD stages [28].

No apparent ageing changes: If there are no drusen or pigmentary changes. Pigmentary changes are considered significant only if associated with medium or large drusen.

Normal ageing changes: Drusen <63 μm in size without any pigmentary changes. These are called drupelets.

Early AMD: Medium drusen >63 μm but ≤125 μm and no pigmentary changes.

Intermediate AMD: Large drusen >125 μm or any pigmentary changes associated with medium or large drusen.

Late AMD: Geographic atrophy and/or neovascular AMD.

13.5.6.1 Geographic Atrophy (GA)

Geographic atrophy (GA) is a late stage of non-exudative AMD and causes irreversible loss of central vision. It manifests as complete loss of the choriocapillaris (ChC), RPE, and the overlying photoreceptors. It is defined as sharply demarcated area/s of atrophy of RPE, minimum one-eighth optic disc size, with baring of the large choroidal vessels without any new choroidal vessels [29]. There is a sharp demarcation of the normal and atrophic retina (Fig. 13.4). For this reason, it can be accurately measured on both colour fundus pictures (CFP), fundus autofluorescence (FAF), and OCT. On SD-OCT, the border of the GA is marked by a sharp descent of the external limiting membrane (ELM) and piling up of the RPE cells and the SDDs (Fig. 13.5). The gap between the hypoautofluorescent region on FAF and the OCT marks the junctional zone, the next area to degenerate [30]. Recently, based on OCT characteristics, GA has been classified into two stages, an incomplete RPE and outer retinal atrophy (iRORA) and a complete RPE and outer retinal atrophy (cRORA). For diagnosing, iRORA, three OCT signs include vertically aligned increased light signal transmission into the choroid, RPE attenuation or disruption, with overlying photoreceptor degeneration and subsidence of the INL, OPL, and ONL. If these changes are at least 250 μm in size, these will qualify for the diagnosis of cRORA [31].

AMD is a progressive disease, and irrespective of the successful use of intravitreal injection of anti-VEGF to regress the new vessels, there is no proven therapy to arrest the progression of the GA. Notably, the macular atrophy progression in eyes with macular new vessels (MNV) is significantly slower than the GA in eyes without MNV, highly suggestive of a protective role for MNV in preventing macular atrophy [32].

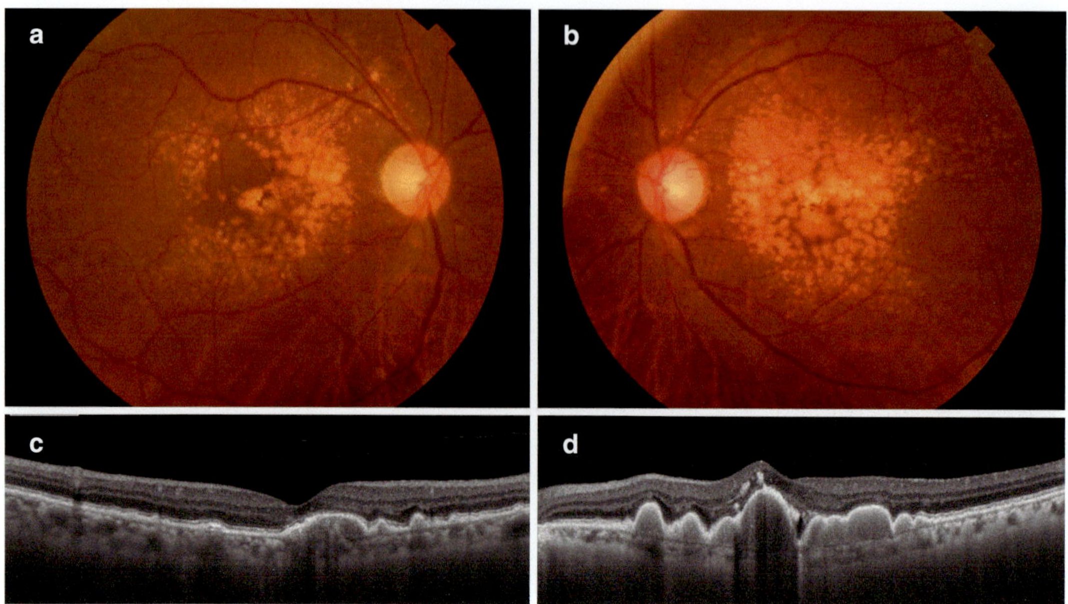

Fig. 13.3 Intermediate AMD: a 75-year-old male presented with large, confluent, soft drusen in the macula, seen as pale-yellow lesions in both eyes (**a**, **b**). Optical coherence tomography showed large, mound-like deposits over Bruch's membrane in both eyes (**c**, **d**)

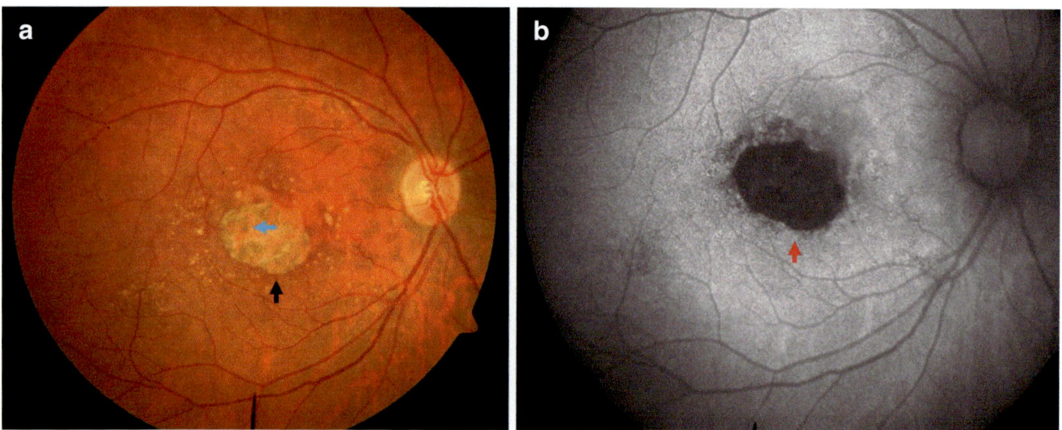

Fig. 13.4 Geographic atrophy: a sharply demarcated area (black arrow) of RPE atrophy with baring (blue arrow) of the large choroidal vessels (**a**), seen as a dark hypoautofluorescent area (red arrow) on fundus autofluorescence (**b**)

Macular atrophy is distinct from GA. The macular atrophy develops in about one-fourth of the patients receiving anti-VEGF therapy over 12–24 months. By 7–8 years of follow-up, in MNV patients, who continue to receive anti-VEGF therapy, 100% of eyes may show macular atrophy. The persistence of a shallow subretinal fluid >25 μm appears protective against macular atrophy development [33, 34].

Among the patients with GA, a new clinical phenotype has been identified, which occurs in relatively younger patients. They do not have drusen and show features of pachychoroid and hyperpermeability of choroidal vessels. The risk

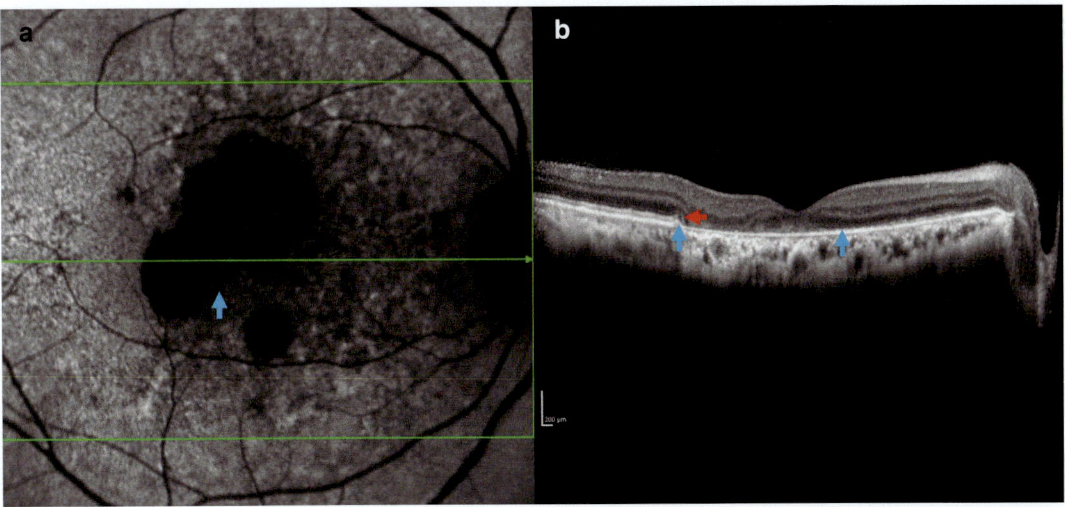

Fig. 13.5 OCT of geographic atrophy: through the dark hypoautofluorescent area (blue arrow) of geographic atrophy (**a**), the OCT shows complete loss (blue arrows) of outer retinal layers and RPE (**b**). The border of GA is marked by a sharp descent of ELM (red arrow)

allele ARMS2A69S was less frequent in these patients than in conventional GA. These patients have associated pachychoroid pigment epitheliopathy and may even have pachychoroid neovasculopathy. Unlike inherited retinal dystrophies, these are asymmetric [35].

13.5.6.2 Progression of Dry AMD to GA

The risk factors for progression from intermediate AMD to GA at 2 years include drusen volume, SDD, intraretinal hyperreflective dots, hyporeflective core of drusen, and a thin double layer sign observed on volume scans on OCT [36].

For any interventional studies, the outcome measure in GA is the rate of progression of GA. In the age-related eye disease study (AREDS2), 6.2% of eyes had pre-existing GA, which was either central (33%) or non-central (67%). The configuration was small (36%), unifocal (26%), multifocal (24%), horseshoe (9%), or indeterminate (6%). Of those who did not have GA at the onset, the 5-year incident rate of GA was 19%. The 4-year risk of central involvement was 57% for those eyes that started with non-central GA. The rate of progression of GA, irrespective of pre-existing or incident GA, was ~0.28 mm^2/year. The significant risk factors for progression were non-central lesions, bilaterality, and multifocality of the lesions. The progression was faster in the ARMS2 risk genotype and C3 non-risk and APOE non-risk genotypes [29]. The ARMS2 allele and the reticular pseudodrusen are strong yet independent risk factors for progression. The subretinal drusenoid deposits (reticular pseudodrusen) are a significant risk factor for the fast progression of non-central GA [37]. Patients with no reticular pseudodrusen and no ARMS2 risk allele have the lowest risk of GA progression [37].

In a large multicentric cohort, 4.5–16.5% of patients with AMD showed progression over a minimum follow-up of 2 years. Patients with early or intermediate AMD in both eyes at presentation progressed to GA at 2/100 person-years and nAMD 3.2/100 person-years. However, if they already had GA in one eye, they progressed at 11.2/100 person-years. In the presence of the nAMD eye and early/intermediate AMD in the other eye, they progressed at 4.1/100 person-years. If they had mixed GA + nAMD in one eye and early/intermediate AMD in the fellow eye, they progressed at 7.8/100 person-years. The major risk factor for progression to GA was the presence of GA in the fellow eye [38]. A prospective natural history study of patients with at least >125 μm^2 area of GA measured progression by FAF, CFP, or both. The GA progressed by 0.88 mm^2 at 6 months, 1.85 mm^2 at 12 months, and 3.14 mm^2 at 18 months. When measured by the CFP, the corresponding rates were 0.78, 1.57, and 3.17 mm^2, respectively. The main risk factor for progression was the presence of multifocal areas of GA [39]. A similar progression (3.85 mm^2) was noted at 2 years in a prospective multicentric global observation study if both eyes had GA at the onset. The progression rate was 3.55 mm^2 if the fellow eye had nAMD and 2.96 mm^2 if the fellow eye had intermediate AMD [40].

Even before the RPE atrophy, there is a loss of the EZ beyond the borders of RPE atrophy and thinning of the outer segments, which can be quantified on SD-OCT and predict future progression [41].

13.5.6.3 Treatment of GA

Nutritional Supplement

Consumption of the Mediterranean diet, whole fruits, a greater proportion of monounsaturated fats, and alcohol intake within defined intervals of g/day led to a significant decrease in the progression of the GA. On the other hand, red meat consumption was associated with a faster progression of GA [42]. Increasing consumption of lutein and zeaxanthin-containing green leafy vegetables and fish oil reduces the risk of AMD, whereas supplementary calcium may increase the risk of AMD [43].

Role of AMD Genotyping

Genotyping is not recommended in patients with AMD for several reasons, including the non-availability of any genotyping-based treatment. Patients with no AMD with genetic variants and AMD clinical phenotypes with strong correlations for progression have little value added by genotyping [43]. Genotyping remains as yet a research tool. A genetic risk score can be calculated by adding up the weighted value (depending upon the strength of association) of the presence of the gene variants [43].

Complement Inhibition in AMD

Many complement factors have been targeted to halt the progression of GA. The most common complement fragments targeted in clinical phase 1/2 trials are C3 and C5. Although successful in a phase 2 trial, the factor D blocking agent, Lampalizumab, in two parallel phase 3 trials failed to halt the progression of GA over 48 weeks of follow-up [44].

Pegcetacoplan is a C3 inhibitor and blocks all complement pathways. In a phase 2b study, the use of intravitreal (IVT) injection of 15 mg Pegcetacoplan every month or every other month led to a significant decrease (29%) in the progression of geographic atrophy. Every month treatment was more effective than every other month. However, nearly 20% of the monthly treated eyes developed new-onset exudative AMD at 12 months versus 1.2% of the sham-treated eyes. The safety and efficacy of this therapy need further evaluation in phase 3 studies [45].

A C5 inhibitor drug Avacincaptad pegol (Zimura, Iveric bio), was tested in a phase 2/3 trial among 286 patients of GA. It showed a 27–28% reduction in progression rates of GA at 12 months compared to the sham group [46]. However, at the 18-month follow-up, 8–16% in the treatment group developed exudative AMD compared to 2% in the sham group. A post hoc analysis revealed the presence of pre-existing macular new vessels in the fellow eyes and the double layer sign in the study eye as significant risk factors for developing exudative AMD in the Pegcetacoplan-treated eyes [47]. In any case, anti-VEGF treatment was highly effective in controlling the exudative AMD in these eyes.

Earlier, Eculizumab, a systemic inhibitor of complement C5 although well tolerated for 6 months, was ineffective in preventing geographic atrophy's expansion [48].

Monoclonal antibodies to block Properdin failed in the phase 2 clinical trial, and the trial was stopped. Several trials are underway or have been completed to study the efficacy of blocking various complement pathways in AMD [49].

Deep learning algorithms have been developed for automated quantification of the segmented RPE and photoreceptor layers on SD-OCT volume modelling to monitor the therapeutic efficacy of various treatment strategies [50].

RPE Cell Implantation in Dry AMD

Another approach was successfully tested in preclinical studies, and limited human studies have shown that implanted RPE cells retain their functionality. The RPE cells can be derived from various sources, including human embryonic stem cells, iPSC from adipose fibroblasts or bone marrow CD34+ cells. These can be injected in intravitreal, subretinal or suprachoroidal space as a cellular suspension or transplanted on a bioengineered monolayer under the retina to rescue the degenerating photoreceptors. Meta-analysis for early trials for dry AMD patients has shown these to be a safe and effective strategy with modest improvement in visual acuity [51]. Many human phase 1/2 studies are underway to study the role of RPE transplant in restoring vision in patients with advanced macular degeneration [52].

In one such study, human embryonic cells-derived RPE cells on an ultrathin parylene substrate were implanted under the retina as an outdoor procedure in patients with advanced dry AMD. The follow-up was available for 1 year. The implant successfully improved visual acuity in 27% of eyes. Loss of vision >5 letters was seen in 47% of untreated eyes versus 33% of treated eyes. Four of the 16 eyes had severe ocular adverse events, including RPE detachment, haemorrhage, and oedema [53]. However, long-term outcomes have yet to be discovered. One of the significant concerns of cellular transplants remains the risk of tumorigeneses.

13.6 Inherited Retinal Disorders

13.6.1 Introduction

Inherited retinal disorders (IRD) affect millions of people worldwide. Most of them suffer from retinitis pigmentosa (RP), a disease characterized by progressive degeneration of predominantly the rod or cone photoreceptors (Fig. 13.6). Most patients have night blindness in the early stages, but eventually, many go blind. RP has been recognized ever since the invention of the ophthalmoscope in 1851. Although it is not an inflammatory disease, the term retinitis pigmentosa, suggested more than 165 years ago, has stayed [54]. The familial nature of the disease has been known for more than 100 years, and the focus was on Mendelian inheritance patterns. The most common RP is an autosomal recessive disorder with early onset and is the most severe. The autosomal dominant pattern is comparatively less common and milder. X-linked RP is rarely seen but has the most severe phenotype. In the early 1980s, the database of RP (all ages) in Philadelphia (US) and childhood RP in Toronto (Canada) was created. The turning point was the discovery of a point mutation in the rhodopsin gene in patients with an autosomal dominant form of RP [55] that focused attention on clinical genotype-phenotype correlation.

It became apparent that IRDs predominantly involving the macula, or the peripheral retina, is a group of heterogeneous genetic disorders with varying ages of onset, severity, and progression. These may affect vision early in life, or the vision may be preserved until late. There is often discordance between genotypes and phenotypes; many genetic mutations may give rise to a similar phenotype, or several mutant genes may cause a single phenotype. Even in the same family, phenotypical discordance may be seen. The pathogenic variants in the same gene may cause different phenotypes. For instance, pathogenic variants in the PRPH2 gene may cause many pattern dystrophies and peripheral retinitis pigmentosa [56]. With the increasing sophistication of gene sequencing technology, the phenotype-genotype correlation has become more crucial. There are variations in genes that are of no consequence (non-pathogenic); there are pathogenic and likely pathogenic variants. Thus, an extensive database of the various phenotypes and genotypes of IRDs is necessary.

In the past, most patients with IRD were dismissed with a remark that ‘nothing can be done’.

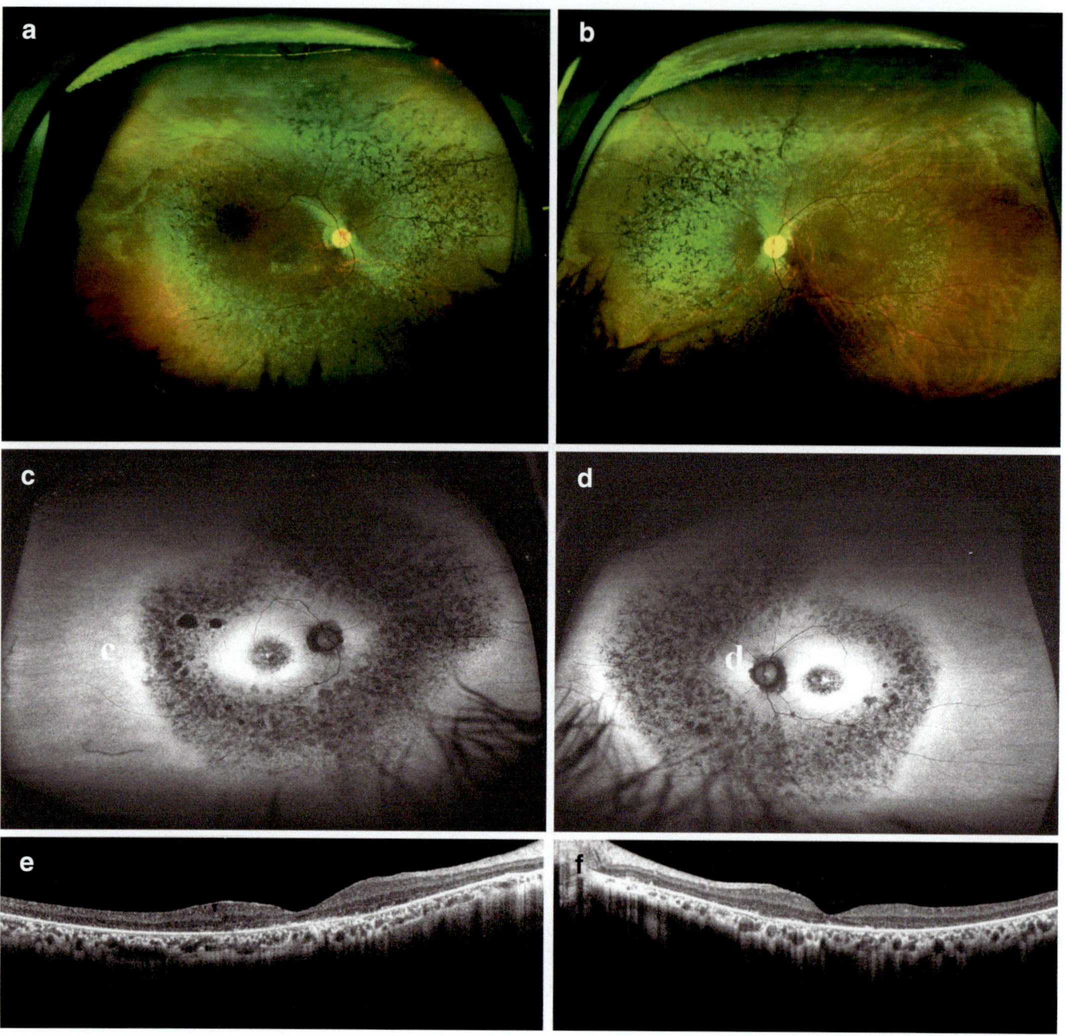

Fig. 13.6 A 30-year-old male had an insidious progressive diminution of vision in both eyes since childhood. Visual acuity was reduced to HM in the right and CF in the left eye. He had temporal disc pallor, attenuation of retinal vessels and bony spicule pigmentation in both eyes (**a**, **b**), with corresponding changes on fundus autofluorescence (**c**, **d**). OCT shows loss of the photoreceptors in both eyes (**e**, **f**)

Recent advances in genetics, molecular biology, and gene therapy have rekindled interest in IRDs. Ultra-widefield (UWF) fundus imaging, FAF studies, SD-OCT, perimetry, and electrophysiology provide tools to document clinical phenotypes accurately. Close collaboration is required for systemic evaluation by paediatricians and physicians to detect systemic involvement. Geneticists and bioinformatics experts analyze and interpret the humongous data which is generated. Rapid advances have taken place in molecular gene testing, such as 'Sanger sequencing' to confirm the gene variation with almost 100% accuracy, 'next-generation sequencing' (NGS), and 'whole exome sequencing' (WES) to now more comprehensive 'whole genome sequencing' (WGS).

Even with all the advances, the genetic defect remains unknown in many patients with IRD. Until 2006, only 100 mutant genes were known for inherited ocular disorders. In 2006, the National Institutes of Health (NIH) created an 'eyeGENE' network to create a database of clinical manifestations and a repository of molecular genetic data from patients with inherited ocular disorders and their families from the USA and Canada [57].

In a multigene panel testing of 85 unrelated paediatric-age patients with syndromic or non-syndromic IRD, the molecular test was positive in nearly 80% of the patients, which included 67% with the autosomal recessive, 25% with X-linked and 7.5% of autosomal dominant IRD. Often it was successful in differentiating stationary from progressive disease. Since molecular genetic testing is likely to be more positive in early-onset disease (paediatric age group), it was recommended that if IRD is clinically suspected based on the phenotype or electroretinography, multipanel gene testing should be done early in the course of the disease [58].

Performing a WGS will likely improve the diagnostic yield of single-nucleotide variants in IRD over and above the targeted panel NGS technique [59]. In a cohort of 1000 families with IRD, clinically focused molecular testing found that 76% harbour a pathogenic variant. Of the 104 genes detected in this cohort, 75% were small enough to be packed in an attenuated adenovirus (AAV) vector with implications for future gene therapy. Nearly 23% of the families had mutations in the ABCA4 gene. Eighty genes caused phenotype in less than five families each [60].

At present, >250 defective genes are known to cause retinal degeneration. Large NGS panels can determine the genetic basis in up to 76% of IRD cases [56]. Among more than 6000 patients from 5385 families with 30 different inherited eye disorders, the most common IRD was retinitis pigmentosa (Fig. 13.6), Stargardt's disease (Fig. 13.7), cone-rod dystrophy, Best disease (Fig. 13.8), pattern macular dystrophies (Fig. 13.9), and choroideremia (Fig. 13.10). Among >5000 patients tested for defective genes, pathogenic or likely pathogenic genes were seen in 62%, and 30% had gene variants of uncertain significance. Notably, ten pathogenic genes account for 68% of all the pathogenic or likely pathogenic variants in the database. Based on the current gene therapy trials, nearly one-fifth of the patients would be eligible for clinical trials [57].

13.6.2 Ancillary Lab Testing in Inherited Retinal Disorders

The three most useful ancillary tests for evaluating IRD in the office of the ophthalmologist include electroretinography, fundus imaging, and optical coherence tomography (OCT).

13.6.2.1 Electroretinography [61]

Electroretinography (ERG) is the most critical investigation in patients with IRD. Briefly, full-field ERG (ffERG) involves the recording of electrical signals from the retina on exposure of almost the entire retina to a uniform light stimulus in the dark-adapted (20 min to eliminate cone function) and light-adapted (10 min to eliminate rod function) states of the retina. The pupil is maximally dilated. After anaesthetizing the cornea, the recording electrode is placed on the conjunctiva. Alternatively, the electrode embedded in a corneal contact lens can be used. A negative electrode is placed on the skin on the lower orbit margin. In the dark-adapted eye, three recordings of DA 0.01, DA 7.5, and DA 10 are done by increasing the flash intensity from 0.025, 7.5, and 25 cd/m^2, respectively. The duration of each flash should not exceed 5 ms, and intervals between flashes ≥2, ≥10, and ≥20 s, respectively, with increasing intensity. The response is recorded as implicit time (ms) from the flash's onset to the response's generation. The amplitude is measured in μV. Essentially, the ERG response consists of a negative 'a' wave and a positive 'b' wave. In the dark-adapted eye, ERG records responses mainly from rod photoreceptors. A weak light intensity (DA 0.01) elicits no 'a' wave, and the first positive response is a 'b' wave generated by the ON bipolar cells. Increasing the light intensity generates a negative 'a' wave response from rods and cones, but predominantly from the rods. It is followed by a positive 'b' wave from ON/OFF bipolar cells. The amplitude of 'a' is measured from the baseline (0 μV) to the trough of the maximum response. The implicit time for the 'b' wave is from the flash's onset to the wave's peak. The 'b' wave amplitude is measured from the trough of the negative 'a' wave to the peak

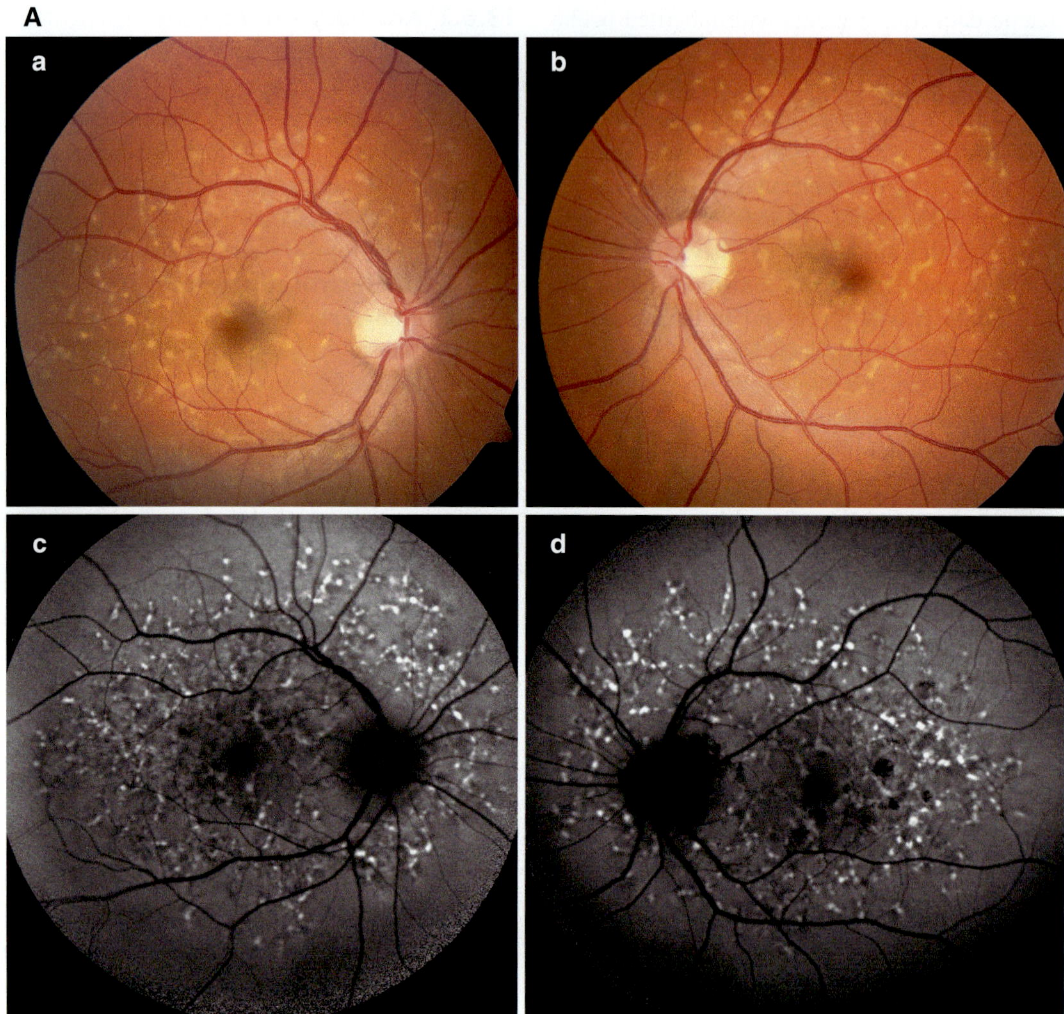

Fig. 13.7 (**A**) Right and left fundus photos demonstrating pisciform flecks typical of Stargardt's disease (**a**, **b**). Some flecks have lost the vitelliform material. FAF shows the hyper autofluorescent flecks and a few areas of hypo autofluorescent non-central atrophy (**c**, **d**). Dark choroid of the background fundus seen on fluorescein angiogram (**e**, **f**). OCT shows a thick RPE layer with patchy ellipsoid line loss and some thinning of the overlying outer nuclear layer (**g**, **h**). (**B**) ABCA4 dystrophy with atrophy. Both eyes' macula shows islands of atrophy with a few flecks around them (**a**, **d**). The FAF image shows hypo autofluorescence corresponding to the atrophy and a few hyper autofluorescent flecks (**b**, **e**). OCT shows atrophy of the RPE, the overlying photoreceptors, some inner nuclear loss, and the choriocapillaris thinning (**c**, **f**). (Images courtesy of Dr Anita Agarwal, West Coast Retina Medical Group, San Francisco, CA)

of the positive 'b' wave. Similar recordings are done for the light-adapted eye using the light intensity of 3 cd/m^2 and 31 Hz flicker frequency, eliminating the rod response. In the flicker ERG in light-adapted eyes, the amplitude is measured from the trough to the peak of each wave. The light-adapted ERG's implicit time and amplitude are also measured as described above for the dark-adapted eye. In the light-adapted eye, the negative 'a' wave is mainly from cones and the 'b' wave from the On/Off bipolar cells.

In retinitis pigmentosa, the scotopic ERG responses are abnormal and may be undetectable. The light-adapted responses are also generally abnormal. In the advanced stage of RP, there are no ERG responses in dark or light-adapted eyes. Leber's congenital amaurosis has no ERG responses early in infancy.

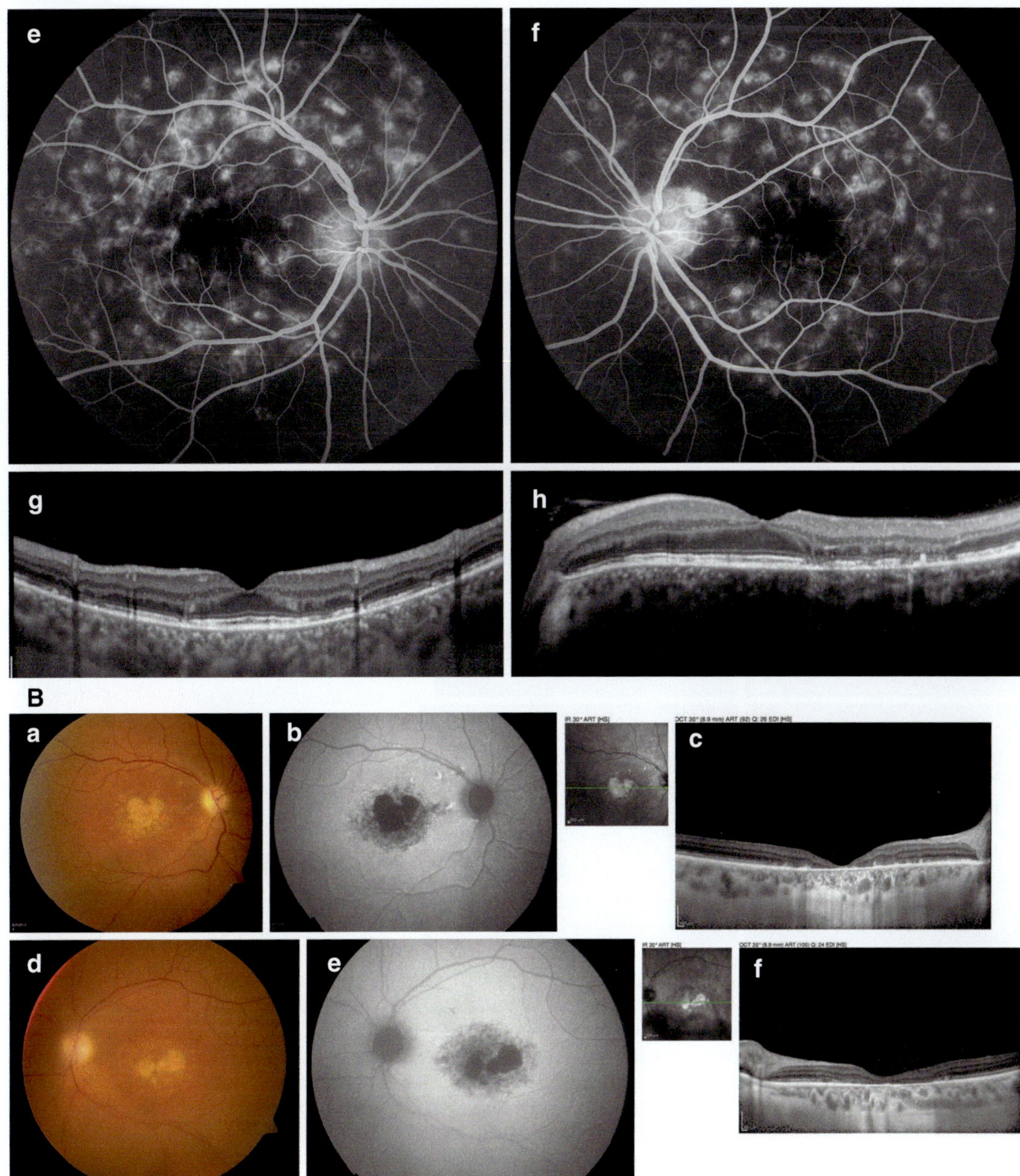

Fig. 13.7 (continued)

In cone-rod RP, the light-adapted responses are more affected than the dark-adapted eyes. In cone dystrophy, on the other hand, only the light-adapted responses are affected with nearly normal dark-adapted responses. https://eyewiki.aao.org/Electroretinogram, accessed on Dec 17, 2022.

13.6.2.2 Fundus Imaging and Fundus Autofluorescence

Fundus imaging is essential in documenting the clinical picture of IRDs, and the course of the disease in follow-up. The traditional fundus cameras capture only 30–55° colour fundus pictures of the post pole and required the preparation of

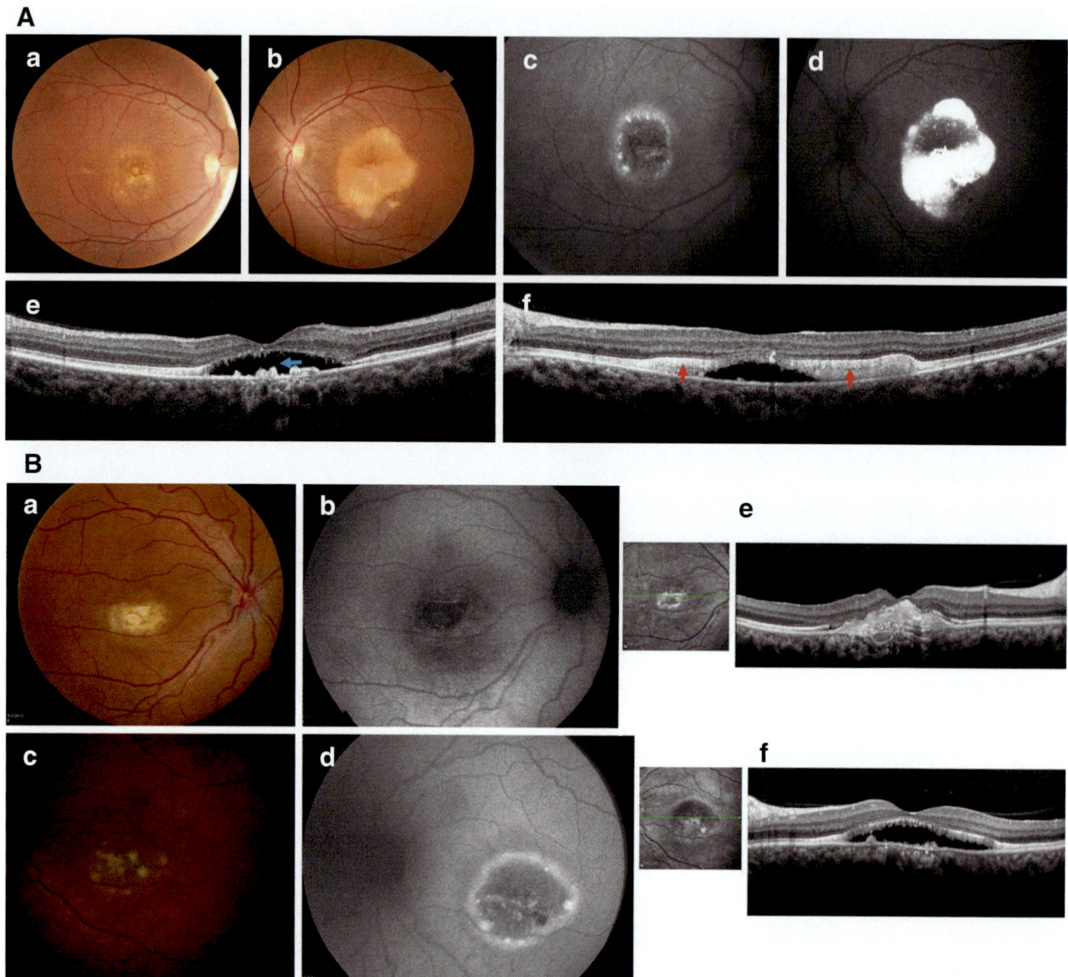

Fig. 13.8 (**A**) Best vitelliform macular dystrophy seen as subretinal yellow deposits in the right eye (**a**) and egg-yolk appearance in the macula in the left eye (**b**). The vitelliform material appears brightly hyperautofluorescent (**c**, **d**). The OCT shows subretinal fluid (blue arrow) in the right eye (**e**) and deposition of vitelliform material (red arrows) in subretinal space in the left eye (**f**). (**B**) Right eye with subretinal fibrosis from a prior choroidal neovascular membrane and scrambled egg stage of Best disease (**a**, **b**). Left eye with scrambled egg stage of the Best disease (**c**). Fundus autofluorescence of the left eye with a ring of hyper autofluorescence corresponding to the residual vitelliform material (**d**). OCT of the right eye with subretinal fibrosis (**e**) and OCT of the left eye with persistent vitelliform space seen in Best disease (**f**). (Images 13.8 B courtesy of Dr Anita Agarwal, West Coast Retina Medical Group, San Francisco, CA)

manual or automated montages to capture the retinal periphery from multiple images. Widefield cameras capture images of the retina up to 100, marked by the posterior edge of the vortex vein ampulla. Ultra-widefield fundus (UWF) imaging with Optomap (Optos Inc., Marlborough, MA 01752, USA) uses a low-power laser (Blue, 488 nm; green, 532 nm; and red, 633) to capture the macula and the retinal periphery up to 200° in one frame. In one capture, it covers 80% of the retina and makes an automated 220° montage. In addition, it can capture red-free images, choroidal images, FFA, ICG, and fundus autofluorescence (FAF), and recently an integrated 23 mm swept-source OCT line scan can also be done. The confocal scanning laser ophthalmoscope (Spectralis, Heidelberg Engineering Inc. Franklin, MA 02038, USA) uses infrared, green

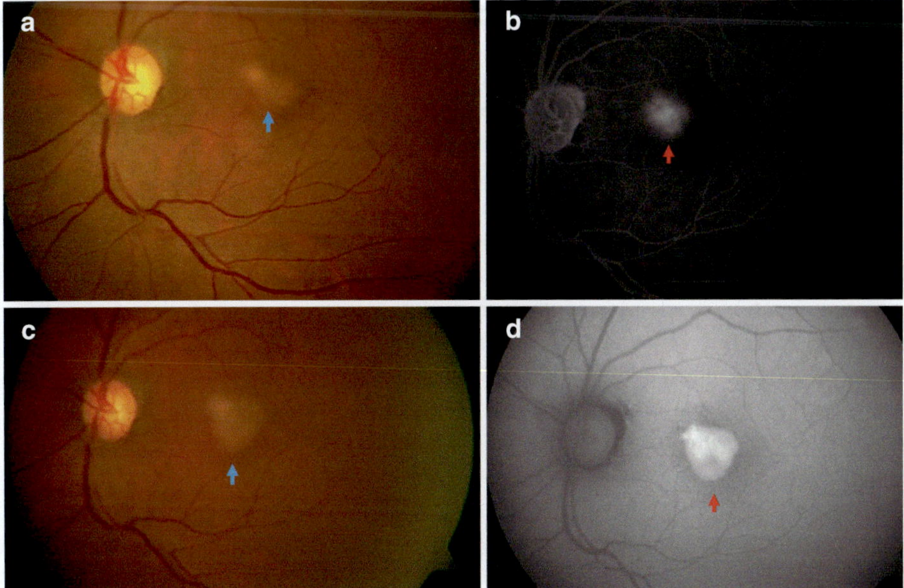

Fig. 13.9 A 75-year-old woman with metamorphopsia presented with a vitelliform lesion (blue arrow) in the macula of left eye suggestive of adult-onset foveomacular vitelliform degeneration (**a**). Fundus fluorescein angiography showed hyperfluorescence (red arrow) of the lesion (**b**). Three years later, there was an increase in the size (blue arrow) of the lesion (**c**) which was intensely hyper autofluorescent (red arrow) on fundus autofluorescence (**d**)

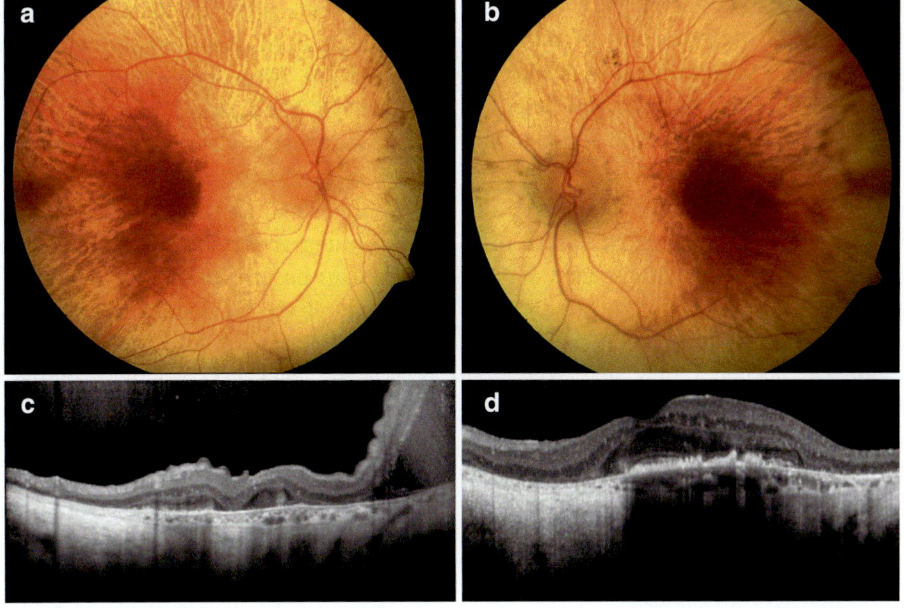

Fig. 13.10 A patient with choroideremia (**a**, **b**), showing diffuse chorioretinal atrophy sparing an island of foveal and parafoveal centre on OCT (**c**, **d**). (Images courtesy of Dr Anita Agarwal, West Coast Retina Medical Group, San Francisco, CA)

and blue wavelengths to capture images of the different retinal layers and generates a high-quality and contrast multicolour image. It captures a wide-field view (105°) which can be automatically montaged to generate ultra-widefield images. It is convenient for small children and uncooperative patients. The UWF FFA and ICG angiography can also be done. For IRDs, FAF imaging is crucial for clinically differentiating the functioning from dead areas of photoreceptors and RPE (Fig.e 13.6). A2E is an autofluorescent component of lipofuscin, an end product of the phagocytosed outer segments of photoreceptors which accumulate in the RPE throughout a person's life. RPE cells under stress produce more A2E than usual, and these areas appear hyperautofluorescent on SW FAF imaging. The areas that have dead RPE cells appear dark. In patients with IRD, the FAF pattern can provide a map of the A2E deposits in the RPE and provide a more accurate phenotype assessment than the colour fundus picture. It is advantageous in delineating subclinical lesions in Stargardt's disease and the progression of the Best disease. In patients with Rod-cone dystrophy, a ring of hyperautofluorescence (Robson-Holder ring) marks the boundary of the dead peripheral RPE and the central area where the RPE is still viable [62]. Outside the ring, the ELM lies next to the RPE layer as the photoreceptors are lost.

Notably, in the light-adapted normal retina, the pigments in the photoreceptors absorb blue light and obscure the autofluorescence signals from the RPE layer; thus, the posterior pole appears dark. The photopigments are bleached in the dark-adapted normal retina, and excitation with SW-FAF image reveals the autofluorescence from the RPE. In patients with RP, wide-field hypoautofluorescence areas correspond to the visual field scotoma [63]. The FAF images are used to monitor the progression of lesions.

13.6.2.3 Optical Coherence Tomography

Optical coherence tomography (OCT) is a non-invasive imaging tool to obtain cross-sectional microstructural details of the different layers of the retina and choroid. Currently, two technologies are being used to obtain OCT images. The spectral domain technology uses a broad-band near-infrared super luminescent diode as a light source and a spectrometer to detect the Fourier transformation of the reflected light from the tissue interfaces. The axial resolution with SD-OCT is 1–3μ. Fast acquisition time has enabled obtaining information from each point of the retinal structures to construct a 3-D retina model. Apart from the cross-sectional image of the various microstructures, layer-by-retinal-layer information can be obtained as en face imaging. The swept-source OCT uses a narrow band of a tunable laser source. The higher acquisition speed with SS-OCT to 100,000 scans/s compared to 50,000 scans/s with the SD-OCT has allowed a 12 × 12 mm wider scan line compared to a 6 × 6 mm line scan with SD-OCT. Using a higher wavelength of 1050 nm than the SD-OCT (840 nm), SS-OCT gives higher resolution images (1μ) of the deeper retinal structures and choroid and can delineate even the choroido-scleral interface [64, 65].

In patients with RP, the OCT delineates the absence of an EZ that correlates with visual acuity centrally. More importantly, the absence of ELM on OCT indicates a more severe phenotype. Besides, it detects CME as a complication, especially in syndromic RP. Most patients with RP show abnormalities of the vitreoretinal interface [66]. Further, in RP, the interdigitation zone (IZ), the first to be affected, is the shortest line, the next to go is the EZ and the longest is the ELM, indicating that in RP, the first structural change is seen at the level of IZ, followed by the EZ, and finally the ELM. Histopathological changes in RP also show that the outer segments of the retina are affected first. The SD-OCT also shows findings consistent with this observation [67]. The next change in the order of a progressive disease is thinning of the outer nuclear layer (ONL). The thinning of ONL is accompanied by normal or even thicker inner retinal layers, possibly due to glia-neuronal remodelling. Moreover, hyperreflective foci in the ONL correspond to the RPE changes [67].

13.6.2.4 Genetics of Non-syndromic Retinitis Pigmentosa

In non-syndromic RP, the most common pathologic variants are USH2A, BBS8, and RP1 genes. The other affected genes are ARL6, BBS1, BBS9, C2orf71, C8orf7, CLRN1, FAM161A, MAK, OFD1, RP2, RPGR, TOPORS, TULP1. Pathogenic variants have been found in the RPGR gene localized to the connecting cilium, which can lead to both the cone RP and rod-cone RP. Variants have also been found in genes RPGRIP1, C8orf37, RAB28, and TTLL5 localized to the cilium base in patients with cone-rod RP. Pathologic variants in Leber's congenital amaurosis involve CEP290 [68].

Patients with macular dystrophy (MD) need to be differentiated from RP. In MD, gene variants have been found in RPGR and RP1L1. MD patients have colour vision defects and loss of central vision ([68].).

The IRDs may be isolated or associated with systemic disorders involving multiple organs, the former termed non-syndromic IRDs and the latter syndromic IRDs. Nearly 23% of working-age persons in Australia with low vision had IRD. Of these, non-syndromic RP accounted for 54%, and Stargardt's Disease for 12% [69].

13.6.3 Non-syndromic Retinitis Pigmentosa: Clinical Signs

Retinitis pigmentosa (RP) is one of the commonest IRDs, with a prevalence of nearly 1:3000–1:4000 population in the USA and Europe. It is estimated that nearly 2 million people worldwide may be suffering from RP. The disease usually manifests in the second decade when the patients complain of night blindness. The onset is insidious, and the initial symptoms of difficulty navigating in the dark may be ignored. In the early stages of RP, the retina may appear normal without any pigmentary changes. Without a family history, the diagnosis of RP is often ignored. It most commonly affects rod photoreceptors followed by cones and is termed Rod-Cone degeneration. Day vision is normal in patients with rod-cone degeneration (Fig. 13.11).

In some cases, it may primarily affect the cones first when it is termed cone-rod degeneration. These patients are detected earlier as they have daylight photophobia and reading vision challenges. It is a progressive disease, although the rate of progression may vary from one patient to the other. In the later stages, fundus examination reveals pigmentary changes in the mid-retinal periphery, which may involve all four quadrants or be limited to even one quadrant.

The pigmentary changes are typically described as bone-spicule. In the late stages, there is attenuation of retinal arterioles, retinal atrophy, and optic disc pallor [70]. The perimetry in the early stages reveals a ring scotoma; eventually, as the disease progresses, patients may be left with tunnel vision. The development of a complicated cataract or cystoid macular oedema may affect central vision. Over several decades, RP eventually leads to blindness.

Autosomal dominant forms are the mildest and start late in life. Autosomal recessive ones start early so does the X-linked RP. The most common gene involved in AD RP is RHO, responsible for 25% of the cases; USH2A, for 20% of the AR cases; and RPGR, responsible for most of the X-linked RP cases [71].

Autosomal recessive RP (arRP) with RP1 mutations and X-linked RP (xLRP) with RPGR or RP2 mutations have significant myopia compared to the arRP with other genetic mutations [72].

13.6.4 Leber Congenital Amaurosis

Leber congenital amaurosis (LCA) is one of the severest non-syndromic RP with an early onset and is characterized by very poor vision, nystagmus, and an oculodigital sign. The affected children rub their eyes with their fingers to generate a sensation of light (phosphene). The wave formation on ffERG is either absent or grossly subnormal. Over 25 genes have been identified, accounting for 70–80% of all LCA cases. The

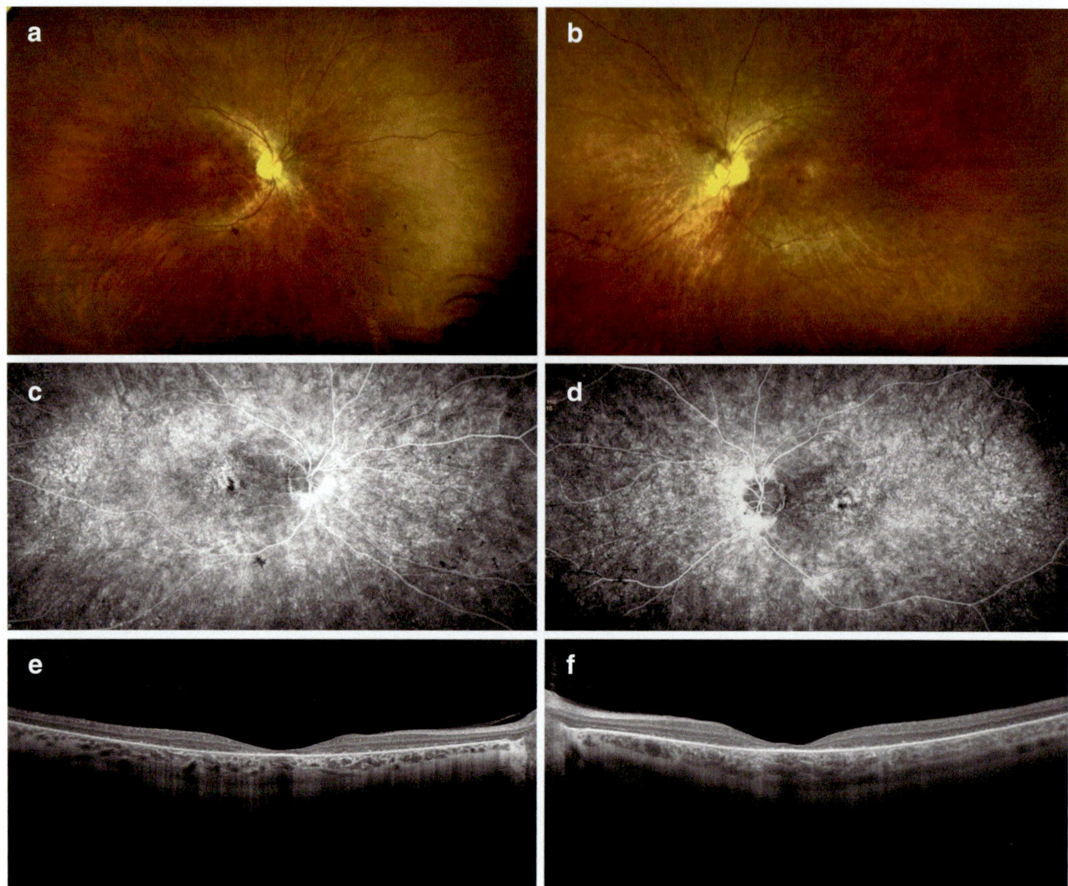

Fig. 13.11 Fundus photographs (**a**, **b**) and fluorescein angiography (**c**, **d**) of cone-rod dystrophy, with OCT (**e**, **f**) showing foveal atrophy and diffuse loss of photoreceptors. (Images courtesy of Dr Anita Agarwal, West Coast Retina Medical Group, San Francisco, CA)

severest form of LCA leads to visual disability that does not allow daily activities before 3 years. If the child has limited vision but is not disabled for up to 10 years, it is termed severe early childhood onset retinal dystrophy (SECORD). If the affected child does not become blind by ten, it has been termed early childhood onset retinal dystrophy (ECORD) [60]. Given the heterogeneity in phenotypes and genotypes, the LCA is best described as a phenotype-genotype (Kumaran et al.2017).

The most frequent genes associated with LCA include GUCY2D, followed by CRB1, AIPL1, and NMNAT1. Frequent genes associated with SECORD include RPE65, RDH12, and LRAT [73]. GUCY2D and AIPL1 are involved in phototransduction, the former in the cones and the latter in the rods. The genes RPE65, RDH12, and LRAT are involved in the retinoid cycle in the RPE cells.

GUCY2D is the most frequent LCA genotype and encodes for a retina-specific membrane protein, guanylate cyclase, which is expressed in the outer segments of cone/rod photoreceptors. A deficiency of the protein leads to phototoxicity. Heterozygous mutations of this gene are associated with autosomal dominant cone dystrophy and autosomal dominant cone-rod degeneration [74]. The patients present with relatively preserved rod function but lose central and colour vision. In a comparative study of the OCT in GUCY2D, RPE65, CEP290 or AIPL1-related

LCA, all three patients with GUCY2D mutations showed preserved retinal layers and the ellipsoid zone, although the vision was poor. The other three genotypes had disorganized lamellar structures of the retina. Patients with CEP290 mutations had preserved the outer nuclear layer in the fovea with macular thickening. The macular thickness was markedly reduced in patients with RPE65 and AIPL1 mutations [75].

13.6.5 RPE 65-Associated LCA

RPE 65-associated LCA accounts for ~5% of all RP patients and is seen in 1:80,000 normal population. RPE 65 gene participates in the RPE's visual cycle and encodes for a protein retinoid isomerohydrolase. This protein binds retinal esters to isomerase and generates11-cis-retinal. Mutations in RPE65 lead to a deficiency of 11-cis-retinal. RPE65 has been targeted for gene supplementation and is in clinical use for several years. These children have preserved cone function but have night blindness. Mild pendular nystagmus is noted. They have variable visual acuity defects, varying from 20/200 to 20/100. Colour vision is affected to a variable extent. In very early cases, the fundus may appear normal, but later, the pigmentary changes, retinal atrophy, and waxy pallor of the optic disc become apparent (Fig. 13.12). Parafoveal areas of retinal atrophy may be seen. On perimetry, the peripheral visual field is lost. Even with a large object size, it is restricted to the central 20–40°. On OCT, the ONL may be preserved in the macular area in the ECORD phenotype, with significant thinning in the paramacular area. In other patients, the outer nuclear layer may become thinner with an approximation of the EZ with the RPE. There is a lack of hyperautofluorescence on short-wave FAF, signifying a lack of lipofuscin in the RPE in these patients [76].

Compared to the RPE 65-associated LCA, the LRAT-associated RP is generally milder and may show preservation of the parafoveal outer retinal layers. LRAT encodes for the lecithin-retinol acyltransferase, a key enzyme in vitamin A metabolism and production of the retinyl esters. The fundus appearance is variable. Nearly half of them may show white dots. They reach blindness levels late in life. The ffERG is undetectable in all. The OCT shows thinning of retinal layers with preservation of parafoveal outer retinal layers [77].

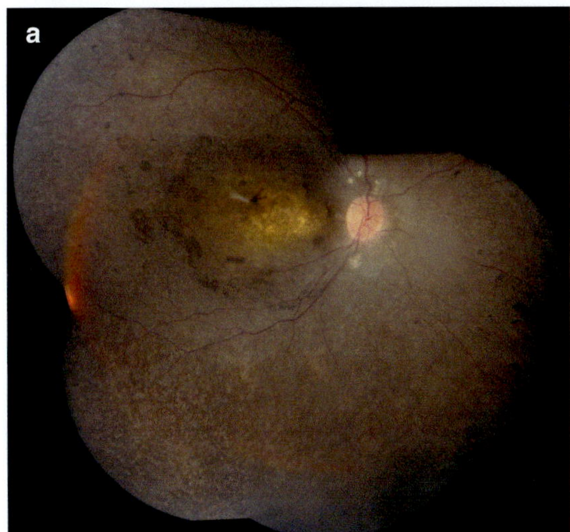

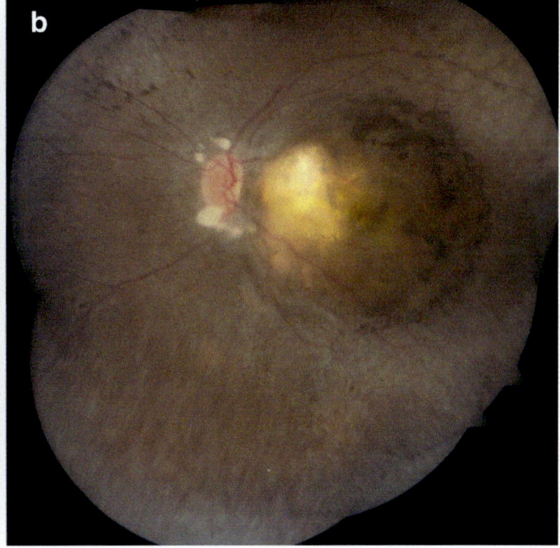

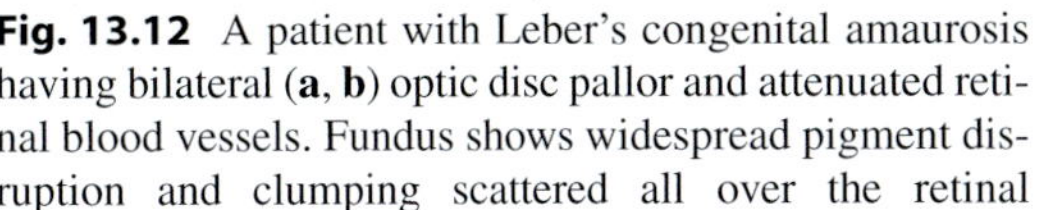

Fig. 13.12 A patient with Leber's congenital amaurosis having bilateral (**a**, **b**) optic disc pallor and attenuated retinal blood vessels. Fundus shows widespread pigment disruption and clumping scattered all over the retinal periphery. Macula in both eyes shows extensive atrophic changes. (Images courtesy of Dr Anita Agarwal, West Coast Retina Medical Group, San Francisco, CA)

13.6.6 CEP290-Associated Retinal Dystrophy

CEP290 encodes for a centrosomal protein found in the connecting cilia of photoreceptors and regulates the transport of proteins between the inner and outer segments of photoreceptors. Abnormal gene expression of CEP290 in other organs can result in syndromic RP, such as Bardet-Biedl Syndrome, Meckel-Gruber Syndrome, and Senior-Loken syndromes (discussed in the syndromic RP). Biallelic loss of CEP290 can result in a severe form of early-onset RP termed LCA10. It may be responsible for up to 30% of all LCA cases. The clinical picture is heterogeneous [78].

13.6.7 Primary Ciliopathies and RP

Visual transduction occurs in the outer segment, with hundreds of discs carrying a vast amount of visual pigment. The RPE cells phagocytose nearly 10% of the outer segment discs daily. The mRNA transcription synthesizes proteins in the inner segments transported through the connecting cilium to the outer segments. There are several proteins in photoreceptors such as rhodopsin, subunits α and β of rod phosphodiesterase, subunits α and β of cGMP, cytoskeleton proteins, trafficking RPGR, RP1, RP2, and many others involved in the differentiation of photoreceptors, extracellular matrices, lipid, and other metabolic pathways. All these must function in a much-regulated fashion to transduce visual signals [70].

In contrast to non-vertebrates, non-motile cilia are present in all vertebrate cells. Long considered redundant, only in the last two decades the role of these sensors in maintaining homeostasis and health has emerged [79]. These cilia act as sensors to provide information from the extracellular to the intracellular or within the intracellular compartment. The cilia cannot produce proteins but transport them along the axoneme (Intraflagellar transport). They also act as signal transducers. The highly metabolic photoreceptor inner segments have cell bodies packed with mitochondria. There is a high turnover of protein transcription in the inner segments. The photoreceptors' outer segments in the retina are specialized cilia forming a photoreceptor sensory cilium complex. Genetic mutations or pathological variants in the cilia genes are called primary ciliopathies and lead to syndromic and non-syndromic disorders involving multiple organs, including the eye, brain, heart, kidneys, liver, and other structures. It is estimated that genes involved in the structure or function of primary cilia account for nearly one-third of IRD [80].

13.6.8 Systemic Diseases Associated with Inherited Retinal Degeneration

Patients at the time of IRD diagnosis may already have systemic organ involvement. A team approach involving an ophthalmologist, geneticist, and primary care physician is required for early diagnosis, genetic testing, counselling, and early and appropriate management [81]. The major syndromic RP are discussed below. See Boxes 13.1, 13.2, 13.3, and 13.4.

Box 13.1 Syndromic Inherited Retinal Degenerations and the Genes in Primary Ciliopathies

Syndrome	Inheritance	Gene/locus
Bardet-Biedl syndrome (BBS)	AR	CCDC28B; SDCCAG8; IFT172; WDPCP; BBS5; LZTFL1; ARL6; BBS7; BBS12; PTHB1; TMEM67; CFAP418; IFT74; TRIM32; BBIP1; **BBS1**; BBS10; CEP290; TTC8; BBS4; BBS2; MKS1; MKKS; IFT27
Alström syndrome (ALMS)	AR	**ALMS1**
Senior-Loken syndrome (SLS)	AR	**NPHP1**; NPHP4; SDCCAG8; TRAF3IPI; IQCB1; SLSN3; WDR19; CEP290; RPRGRIP1L/NPHP8; SDCCAG8/NPHP10; BBS14; BBS16
Joubert syndrome (JBS)	AR	**INPP5E**; CEP104; NPHP1; TMEM237; ARMC9; PDE6D; ARL13B; CC2D2A; CPLANE1; CEP120; AHI1; CEP41; CSPP1; TMEM67; IFI74; FAM149B1; TCTN3; SUFU; ARL3; TMEM138; TMEM216; TMEM218; CEP290; TECT1; TECT2; PIBF1; TOGARAMI; KIAA0586; KIF7; KATNIP; ZNF423; RPGRIP1L; TMEM231; KIAA0753; TMEM231; TMEM107; B9D1; MKS1; B9D2; OFD1
Jeune syndrome or asphyxiating thoracic dystrophy (JATD)	AR	TTC21B; NPHP12; **WDR19**; NPHP13; **IFT80**; DYNC2H1; IFT140; TTC21B
Meckel-Gruber syndrome (MKS)	AR	CC2D2A; CEP290/BBS14/NPHP6; **CSPP1**; MKS1/BBS13; NPHP3; RPGRIP1L/NPHP8; TMEM216/MKS2; PHP11; TMEM 67/MKS3 as modifier; WDPCP/BBS15

Reference: Werdich et al. [81]

Box 13.2 Bardet-Biedl Syndrome: Salient Clinical Features

Organ	Abnormality	Frequency
Eye	Rod-cone dystrophy	>90%
Gonads	Hypogenitalism; delayed puberty	~90%
Obesity	Overweight/obesity	>75%
Limbs	Polydactyly Brachydactyly	~70% ~46%
CNS	Ataxia; abnormal gait	30–40%
Kidney	Calyceal clubbing, parenchymal cysts, etc.	24–46%
Dental	High arched palate	>80%
Speech	High pitched	~50%
Behaviour	Immaturity	~30%
Development	Delayed	50%
Learning	Mild to moderate difficulty	~60%

Adapted from Beales et al. [82]

Box 13.3 Alström Syndrome-Salient Systemic Involvement

Organ	Abnormality	Frequency
Eye[a]	Cone-rod dystrophy; nystagmus; photophobia	Early 100%
Hearing[a]	Deafness by 7 years	88%
Heart[a]	Infantile cardiomyopathy, adolescent/adult	42% 18%

Organ	Abnormality	Frequency
Diabetes[a]	Second to third decade; insulin resistance; hyperinsulinemia	~82% 92%[a]
Gonads	Hypogonadism Reduced fertility[b] Gynecomastia[a]	77%[a] 100%
Obesity[b]	Infantile obesity	~90%
Limbs[b]	Short stature	~32%
CNS[a]	Clonic tics Muscle weakness	20% 29%
Kidney/liver	Chronic nephropathy; rapid decline in eGFR; ESRD Hepatitis	49[a]–63%[c]
Dental		
Speech[a]	Motor delays	46%
Behaviour	Delays	
Development	Delays	46%
Learning	Language and cognitive	11–16%

[a] Adapted from Marshall et al. [83]
[b] Adapted from Russell-Eggitt et al. [84]
[c] Adapted from Baig et al. [88]

Box 13.4 Differential Diagnosis of Dual Sensory Impairment Syndromes

Ocular phenotype	Hearing impairment	Associated systemic features
Usher syndrome (USH1B-H and K; USH2A,C,D: USH 3A; USH 4) RP in the first decade in USH1 and second decade in USH2; post-pubertal in USH3 and at 40 years in USH 4	Congenital deafness in USH1 Deafness in second decade in USH2 Late-onset deafness in USH3	Vestibular dysfunction in first decade in USH1. No or variable vestibular dysfunction in USH2. Congenital vestibular dysfunction in USH 3 and no vestibular dysfunction in USH4.
Bardet Biedl syndrome Age at diagnosis of RP ~10 years and blindness by ~15 years.	Hearing loss in 21%; mostly conductive due to otitis media; rarely sensory-neural deafness	Renal dysfunction, obesity, hypogonadism, polydactyly, brachydactyly, and cognitive impairment.
Alström syndrome Cone-rod dystrophy early onset; nystagmus	Progressive sensory-neural deafness in 90% beginning in the first decade; conductive loss due to otitis media	Obesity; hypogonadism; brachydactyly; type2 DM; cardiomyopathy
Stickler syndrome High myopia; vitreoretinal degeneration; membranous or beaded vitreous; RD	Sensorineural or conductive hearing loss	Underdeveloped jaw; backward displacement of the tongue that frequently blocks the airway (Pierre-Robin face); cardiac and skeletal abnormalities
Waaredenburg syndrome Heterochromia; choroidal hypopigmentation	Sensorineural deafness increased from 69% in WS type 1 to 87% in WS type 2	White forelock; partial albinism; flat root of nose; telecanthus; synophrys eyebrows; musculoskeletal abnormalities
MIDD syndrome Pattern dystrophy; punctate hyper and hypofluorescent dots; continuous or discontinuous areas of pericentral chorioretinal atrophy	Deafness in 75% develops at a young age	Type 2 diabetes
Alport syndrome Flecked retina; lenticonus; foveal hypoplasia; giant macular holes	Variable hearing loss	Haematuria; progressive fibrosis of kidneys with renal failure

Reference: Guimaraes et al. [90]

13.6.8.1 Bardet-Biedl Syndrome

Bardet-Biedl syndrome (BBS) is a highly heterogeneous, autosomal recessive syndrome which may have variations in clinical manifestations in the same family. BBS1 is the most frequently affected gene on the long arm of chromosome 11 (11q13.2), modified by genes CCDC28B (1p35.2) and ARL6 (3.q11.2). There are more than 20 known phenotypes of BBS. (https://omim.org/phenotypicSeries/PS209900). At times, clinical diagnosis of BBS may be difficult. They present with night blindness and a fundus picture of RP. The major clinical features include retinitis pigmentosa, polydactyly (hands/feet), obesity, hypogonadism, renal anomalies, and learning disability. Minor/rare features include high arched palate, dental crowding, hepatic fibrosis, speech delay, and mental disorders. Four major or three major and two minor clinical features make the diagnosis of BBS. The salient clinical features and systemic associations include rod-cone dystrophy, hypogonadism, and delayed puberty in more than 90% of the affected patients. Others include obesity, polydactyly, and mild to moderate learning disability [82].

13.6.8.2 Alström Syndrome

Alström syndrome (ALS) is a rare autosomal recessive disorder caused by biallelic mutations or compound heterogeneous mutation in a single-gene ALMS1 located on the short arm of chromosome 2 (2p13.1). Unlike BBS, RP in Alström syndrome has an early onset and is characterized by the predominant involvement of cones. They present with photophobia and nystagmus in early childhood because of early involvement of the macula. The diagnosis of Alström syndrome is difficult due to the slow unfolding of the complete phenotypes [83]. Unlike BBS, these children do not have polydactyly but may have gynecomastia and infertility. They have type 2 diabetes, increasing insulin resistance, obesity, and deafness. Most of these children have early-onset cardiomyopathy and die of heart failure [84]. Nearly 50% of non-obese Alström patients have a deficiency of growth hormone, leading to short stature [85]. As the ALMS1 gene regulates insulin transport, these patients have extreme insulin resistance [86]. There is a gradual progression from obesity to diabetes because of the progressive decline in insulin from pancreatic β-cells [87]. Salient features of ALS syndrome include cone-rod dystrophy, nystagmus, deafness by 7 years of life, cardiomyopathy, and type 2 diabetes mellitus in their 20s due to insulin resistance and hyperinsulinemia [83]. Chronic nephropathy may vary from 49% to 66% [83, 88]. The other common feature is infantile obesity. Nearly one-third may have short stature [84].

13.6.8.3 Differentiating BBS from Alström Syndrome

Differentiating the two syndromes, Bardet-Biedl from the rarer Alström Syndrome, is important because children need early care for systemic complications. Both have retinal dystrophy, are obese, and suffer from hypogonadism. Alström Syndrome has an onset earlier than BBS, and they present with nystagmus due to cone-rod dystrophy, unlike BBS, which causes rod-cone dystrophy. Developmental delays are more frequent in BBS than in Alström Syndrome. BBS has both polydactyly and brachydactyly, whereas Alström Syndrome has only brachydactyly. The Alström Syndrome is characterized by type 2 diabetes mellitus in most patients and has cardiomyopathy more frequently than BBS. Hearing loss is more common in Alström Syndrome than in BBS [89].

13.6.8.4 Usher Syndrome

It is an autosomal recessive disorder characterized by RP and sensorineural deafness and occasional disturbance in vestibular functions. This is also called dual sensory impairment syndrome. It is caused by mutations in USH protein network located in the periciliary region of the photoreceptors. Several syndromes have dual sensory impairments with variable frequency. Apart from Usher syndrome, most patients with Alström syndrome also have progressive sensorineural deafness starting in the first decade, and nearly three-fourth of those with maternally inherited diabetes and deafness (MIDD) and type 2 Waardenburg syndromes have impaired hearing. Hearing loss is less frequent in Bardet-Biedl,

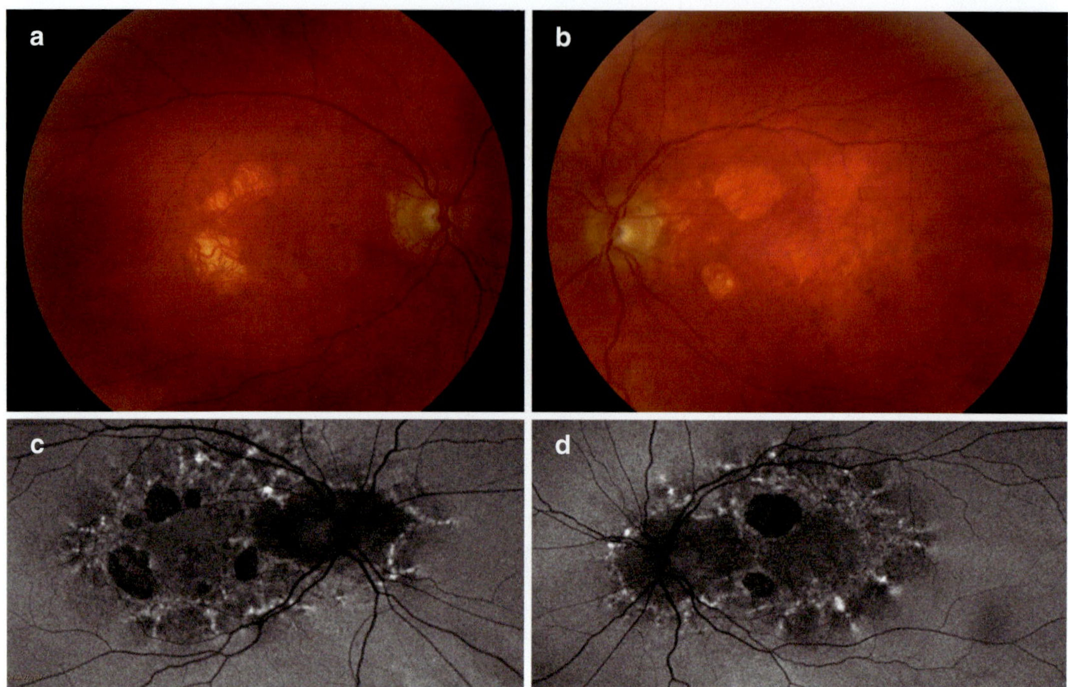

Fig. 13.13 An individual with macular dystrophy due to MIDD having macular and peripapillary depigmented lesions in both eyes (**a**, **b**). Fundus autofluorescence shows mixed areas of increased (subretinal deposits) and decreased (atrophy) autofluorescence (**c**, **d**). (Images courtesy of Dr Anita Agarwal, West Coast Retina Medical Group, San Francisco, CA)

Alport's, and Stickler's syndromes. Apart from hearing loss, each has highly characteristic signs (Fig. 13.13) [90].

At least four USH ocular phenotypes have been identified. USH2 is the commonest phenotype and accounts for most of the non-syndromic RP (Fig. 13.14). While deafness starts in the first decade, the RP starts in the second decade. USH1 is the severest and has congenital neurosensory deafness. As a consequence, these children do not learn to speak. The RP in USH1 starts in the first decade. They also have vestibular dysfunction. USH3 and USH4 are rare. The USH3 is associated with the late onset of progressive RP but has congenital vestibular dysfunction. The RP in USH4 starts in the fourth decade. Vestibular dysfunctions lead to problems with posture, balance, hand-eye coordination, and even reading or eye tracking [90]. Nearly 32% of patients with early-onset IRD are complicated by the development of cystoid macular oedema and more so in Usher's syndrome [91] (Fig. 13.15).

13.6.8.5 Senior-Loken Syndrome (SLS)

Senior-Loken syndrome (SLS) is a rare ciliopathy wherein LCA type RP is associated with inflammation and scarring of the kidneys (nephronophthisis). It is also called hereditary renal–retinal dysplasia. It was initially described as 'familial juvenile nephronophthisis' [92], characterized by progressive renal function deterioration with minimal or no haematuria and albuminuria. The autopsy reveals marked thinning of the cortex and peri glomerular fibrosis, and interstitial fibrosis. The association of tapetoretinal degeneration was described in six of the 13 children in a family with nephronophthisis by Senior et al. [93]. In the same year, two siblings died of renal dysplasia at 8 and 9 years, one of

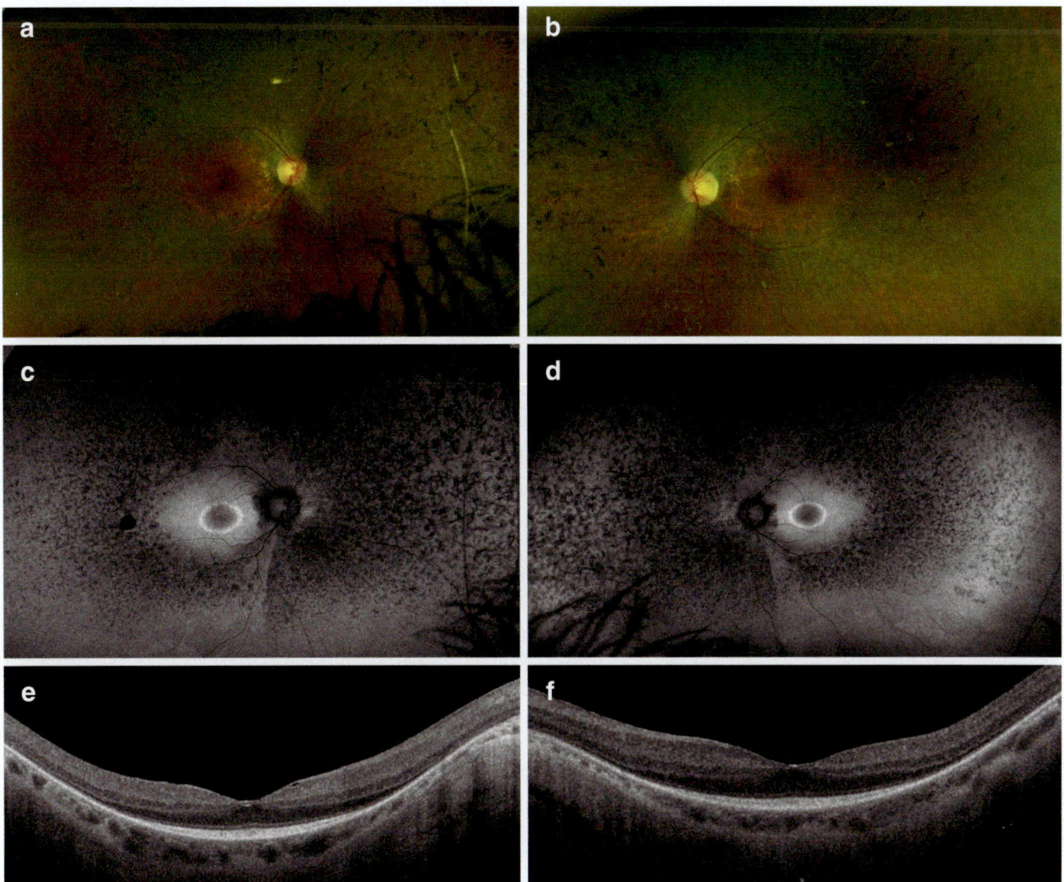

Fig. 13.14 Retinitis pigmentosa in a patient with Usher's syndrome as seen on fundus photograph (**a**, **b**), fundus autofluorescence (**c**, **d**) and OCT (**e**, **f**). (Images courtesy of Dr Anita Agarwal, West Coast Retina Medical Group, San Francisco, CA)

whom showed retinal dysplasia and, on autopsy, showed loss of the outer nuclear layer of the retina and rod photoreceptors [94]. The Senior-Loken patients present with night blindness, bone-spicule pigmentation of the peripheral retina, arterial attenuation, and optic disc pallor. The median age of the patients is 13 years when they present with polydipsia, polyuria, and thirst.

The gene NPH1 encodes for the nephrocystin1 protein located on 2q13.

SLS is the commonest cause of inherited end-stage renal disease in childhood and adolescence. On ultrasonography of the kidneys, it is difficult to differentiate the renal cortex from the medulla and may show the presence of cysts. Eight of the 13 known nephrocystins genes are located in the cilium of photoreceptors and cilia and the centrosomes of the renal epithelium cells. Mutations in the nephrocystins affect protein transport in the cilia. In the eye, it accumulates rhodopsin and transducin in the inner segment, which is not transported to the outer segments. Outer segments of the photoreceptors are not formed, leading to photoreceptor retinal degeneration [95]. Although SLS accounts for only 1% of retinal dystrophies, these children are not routinely screened for renal involvement. In one of the reported families, whole exome sequencing in a sibling affected with RP led to the discovery of two deletions in the IQCB1 gene, one of the

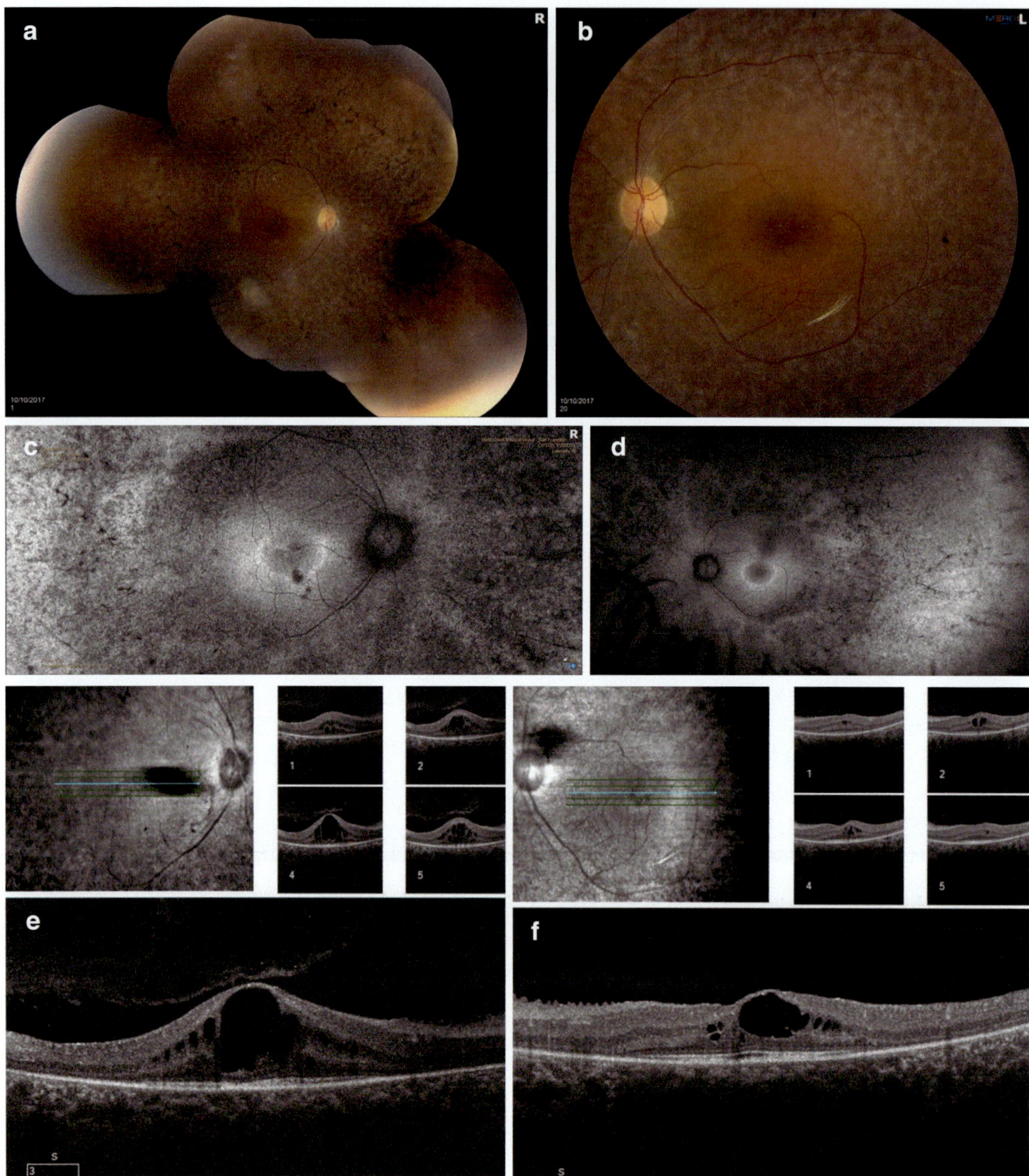

Fig. 13.15 A case of retinitis pigmentosa showing pigmentary changes in both eyes (**a**, **b**). Note hyperautofluorescent ring around the fovea in both eyes (**c**, **d**). OCT shows cystoid macular edema in both eyes (**e**, **f**). (Images courtesy of Dr Anita Agarwal, West Coast Retina Medical Group, San Francisco, CA)

nephrocystins associated with SLS. His younger sibling presented with nocturnal enuresis, fatigue, and slow growth. The timely discovery of the genetic mutation led to the early detection of nephronophthisis. An early renal transplant saved the dialysis dependency of the child [59].

13.6.8.6 Joubert Syndrome (JBTS)

Joubert et al. [96] first described four children in a family with remote consanguinity, characterized by abnormal breathing (episodic hyperpnoea with spells of apnoea), mental retardation, ataxia, and nystagmus associated with the absence of vermis on autopsy in one sibling and on imaging of the brain in others. Children with this rare autosomal recessive syndrome present with ataxia, abnormal breathing (episodic hyperpnoea), hypotonia, and nystagmus due to maldevelopment or absence of cerebellar vermis and malformations of the brain stem. There are remarkable developmental delays in both motor skills and cognition. The axial MRI gives a characteristic 'molar tooth' sign because of the lack of normal decussating cerebellar peduncles and a missing vermis. The most significant ocular features include the inability to move eyes voluntarily (ocular motor apraxia, periodic alternating nystagmus) in 80%, followed by strabismus in 74%, ptosis in 43%, chorioretinal coloboma in 33%, RP in 38%, and optic atrophy in 22% [97].

A homozygous mutation in the INPP5E gene on chromosome 9q34 causes Joubert Syndrome (JBTS). JBTS is a highly heterogeneous syndrome with at least 40 subtypes of JBTS known due to pathological variants in different genes/loci [81]. Of the many subtypes, including JS-Ret, the predominant eye involvement is retinitis pigmentosa or JS-Ren with nephronophthisis or JS-OR with both oculorenal involvements. There are other subtypes as well. More than 40 genes have been described in JBTS, concerned with the cilia's structural proteins (https://omim.org/entry/213300?search=Joubert%20Syndrome&highlight=joubert%20syndrome%20syndromic, accessed Dec 16, 2022, https://rarediseases.org/rare-diseases/joubert-syndrome/, accessed Dec 15, 2022). In a family with developmental delay, hypotonia, oculomotor abnormality, and cerebellar dysplasia, whole exome sequencing led to the detection of new pathogenic disease variants in four genes, confirming the diagnosis of JBTS in four siblings. This helped in genetic counselling and guidance for future pregnancy [98].

13.6.8.7 Jeune Syndrome or the Asphyxiating Thoracic Dystrophy (JATD) and Meckel-Gruber Syndrome (MGS)

Jeune syndrome, asphyxiating thoracic dystrophy (JATD), and Meckel-Gruber syndrome (MGS) are rare primary ciliopathies with severe systemic manifestations. However, RP is only rarely a part of these syndromes. The JATD is diagnosed before or shortly after birth and is characterized by skeletal abnormalities that primarily affect the rib cage forming a bell-shaped chest, short limbs, abnormal pelvis, and brachydactyly. Retinal pigmentary dystrophy is seen only occasionally. They have serious breathing difficulties. The gene variants causing the JATD include IFT80, DYNC2H1, WDR19, IFT140, and TTC21B. https://rarediseases.info.nih.gov/diseases/3049/jeune-syndrome.

The MGS is the severest ciliopathy and often results in stillbirth, or the babies die soon after birth. It has highly heterogeneous manifestations and displays allelism with other ciliopathies like BBS and JBTS. It is characterized by posterior encephalocele, polydactyly (hands and feet), and other craniofacial abnormalities. Other salient manifestations include renal cystic dysplasia that causes massive enlargement of the kidneys and hepatic abnormalities/fibrosis. In the eye, it causes choroidal coloboma. Variants in the genes C5orf42, CSPP1, and CEP55 are responsible for most MGS cases [99].

13.7 Inherited Macular Dystrophies

Several well-characterized and poorly characterized macular dystrophies present with loss of central vision in the young or even later in life. These may have autosomal dominant, autosomal recessive or X-linked inheritance. The variants in the affected genes have been identified for many of them. Phenotypic expression of the disease may vary among the family members. In general, macular dystrophies with autosomal dominant transmission have milder symptoms. Salient features of macular dystrophies are given in Boxes 13.5 and 13.6.

13.7.1 Stargardt's Disease and Fundus Flavimaculatus (ABCA4 Disorders)

Of all the macular dystrophies, Stargardt's disease (STGD) is one of the most common macular dystrophies seen in young people, with an esti-

Box 13.5 Salient Features of Inherited Macular Dystrophies-1

Ocular phenotype	Salient clinical signs	Inheritance	Gene/locus
Stargardt's disease/fundus flavimaculatus if no central atrophy	Commonest macular dystrophy; progressive decline in VA; yellow flecks; bronze-beaten foveal atrophy; HAF flecks	AR; rare AD	ABCA4 1p21–22
Best vitelliform macular dystrophy (Best disease)	Childhood-onset; egg-yellow vitelliform lesion, progresses to pseudohypopyon, vitelliruptive, atrophic stages; VA decline in stages 3–5; HAF vitelline material EOG: light/dark ratio <1.5	AD	Bestrophin1 (BEST1) 11q12.3
AD-vitreoretinal-choroidopathy	VA not affected 360° peripheral pigmentary changes; demarcation line at the equator; vitreous cells; no night blindness Normal ERG; ±ERG	AD	BEST1
Adult vitelliform macular dystrophy	Asymptomatic >50% Mild VA symptoms in the third to fifth decade Heterogeneous phenotypes; variable shapes of yellow-white lesions with pigmentation; HAF; ERG/EOG normal	AR	RDS/PRPH2 6p21
Autosomal recessive bestrophinopathy	Onset first decade or later; serous macular detachment; HAF dot lesions EOG: light rise absent or grossly reduced ERG: pattern-ERG mild to severely reduced amplitude; ffERG: delayed and low amplitude	AR	BEST 1 11q12
Occult macular dystrophy[a] (Miyake disease) East Asia	The median age of onset 25 years (range 2–73) Median VA: Log MAR 0.65 (range: 0.08–1.22); Snellen 20/24–20/330 (median 20/90) Fundus: normal; FFA: normal; VF: central scotoma; OCT: blurred EZ and absent IZ ffERG: normal; mfERG: central decrease in amplitude	AD	RP1L1 8p23
Late-onset macular dystrophy[b] Late-onset dominant RP; or AD-LCA	Age of onset 20–60 years; photophobia; loss of central vision, rapid in old age Bull's eye maculopathy; central hypoautofluorescence and ring of HAF OCT: loss of outer retinal layers in the fovea; subretinal hyperreflective material. ffERG and mfERG low amplitude; pERG, non-recordable	AD	CRX

Source: Johnson et al. [110]

VA visual acuity, *HAF* hyperautofluorescent, *AR* autosomal recessive, *AD* autosomal dominant, *ABCA4* ATP-binding cassette subfamily A member 4, *EOG* electrooculography, *ERG* electroretinography, *RDS* retinal degeneration slow, *PRPH2* peripherin 2, *HAF* hyperautofluorescence, *ffERG* full-field ERG, *OCT* optical coherence tomography, *EZ* ellipsoid zone, *IZ* interdigitating zone, *mfERG* multifocal ERG, *RP1L1* retinitis pigmentosa-1-like-1, *CRX* cone-rod homeobox, *LCA* leber congenital amaurosis, *pERG* pattern ERG

[a] Fujinami et al. [136]

[b] Yahya et al. [137], Sohocki et al. [138]

Box 13.6 Salient Features of Inherited Macular Dystrophies-2

Ocular phenotype	Salient clinical signs	Inheritance	Gene/locus
Malattia leventinese/ autosomal dominant drusen/Doyne honeycomb retinal dystrophy	Early adulthood onset; radial-oriented small drusen in temporal macula and around optic disc; FFA drusen show early discrete hyperfluorescence; subretinal fibrous dysplasia; late-onset macular atrophy; CNVM; visual loss	AD	EFEMP1 2p R345W
North Carolina macular dystrophy (MCDR1)	Variable: small drusen-like deposits to large confluent, coloboma; CNVM ERG/EOG: normal	AD	Duplication of PRDM13 in MCDR1 locus 6q16
Sorsby fundus dystrophy[a]	Late-onset; fourth-decade; phenotypic variations; night blindness reversed by Vit A; inability to discriminate shades of blue and yellow early sign; macular oedema; atrophy; haemorrhage, progressive chorioretinal atrophy; pigment proliferation; reticular pseudodrusen in retinal periphery; hypoautofluorescent; OCT: subretinal deposits which are hyporeflective on NIR;disease reversal with adalimumab	AD	TIMP3 22q12.3
Central areolar choroidal atrophy[b]	Three phenotypes; pigment mottling in macula; photoreceptors degeneration followed by well-defined RPE and ChC atrophy by 30–60 years	AD	GUCY2D (17p13.1) PRPH2 (6p21.1)
Dominant cystoid macular oedema[c]	CME in the second to fourth decade with good VA; perifoveal leakage on FFA; high hyperopia; squint; later stages decrease in CME; progressive atrophy 'beaten bronze' macula; normal ERG	AD	7p15–p21
X-linked juvenile retinoschisis[d]	Infancy or early childhood; only males; spoke wheel-like foveal schisis; peripheral retinoschisis and pigmentary changes in 50%; vascular occlusion; hyperopia; Mizuo phenomenon ERG: 'a' wave larger than 'b' wave	XLR	RS1 (cell adhesion protein expressed on photoreceptors and bipolar cells) Xp22.13

Adapted from Michaelides et al. [68]

AD autosomal dominant, *EFEMP1* EGF containing fibrulin extracellular matrix protein1, *MCDR1* macular dystrophy retinal 1 (North Carolina), *PRDM13* PR domain-containing protein 13, *TIMP3* tissue inhibitor of matrix metalloproteinase 3, *RS1* retinoschisin 1, *ERG* electroretinography

[a] https://www.omim.org/entry/136900. Spaide [139]

[b] https://www.omim.org/entry/215500, https://www.omim.org/entry/613105, https://www.omim.org/entry/613144

[c] https://www.omim.org/entry/153880

[d] https://www.omim.org/entry/312700

mated prevalence of 1:4,000–1:10,000 people. However, a recent prospective population-based study in the UK found a low incidence ranging from 0.110 to 0.128 per 100,000 people at a median age of 27. Patients were evaluated with FAF and ERG [100]. It is an autosomal recessive disorder caused by variants in the ATP-binding cassette subfamily A type 4 gene (ABCA4) locatewd on the short arm of chromosome 1 (1p21–p22). In the autosomal dominant phenotype, a milder STGD is seen in older adults; the gene variants are ELOVL4 (6q14) and PROML1 (4p) [100]. ABCA4 is a transport gene involved in transporting/flipping the product of 11-trans-retinal (*N*-retinal phosphatidylethanolamine) from the luminal side of the outer segments to the cytoplasmic surface, where it is reduced to 11-trans retinol before reaching the RPE during phagocytosis. The protein has a similar role in the RPE. In the absence of the protein encoded by ABCA4 protein, there is an excessive collection of 11-cis-retinal and N-retinal phosphatidylethanolamine in the outer segments of the photoreceptors and RPE where these get oxidized, resulting in A2E accumulation (lipofuscin) [101].

This phenomenon starts in the retinal periphery and proceeds centrally, eventually involving the macula. Yellow flecks in the posterior pole characterize the fundus picture (Fig. 13.7). The flecks are hyperautofluorescent on FAF imaging. On FFA, the most significant sign is 'dark choroid' due to the obscuration of choroidal circulation by the lipofuscin deposits in the RPE. Over time, the yellow flecks caused by lipofuscin accumulation in the RPE cells undergo atrophy and appear as transmission defects on FFA and areas of decreased autofluorescence on FAF imaging. Histopathological studies have also shown somewhat similar findings. So long as the disease is confined to the retinal mid-periphery without atrophy, it is termed fundus flavimaculatus. Eventually, central macular atrophy develops when it is termed STGD. In a retrospective analysis of 217 patients of STGD drawn from the US, the UK, and Europe, questionably decreased autofluorescence (DAF) areas developed over a mean of 6 years. However, those without definitive areas of DAF developed definitive areas of DAF in 4.9 years. Nearly 50% of the eyes will progress in less than 5 years. Areas of decreased autofluorescence can be used to monitor the progression of the disease [102]. STGD has been classified based on the colour fundus pictures, ERG changes, and FAF imaging with either Heidelberg or Optos. More recently, it has been graded as type I, limited to central atrophy with or without flecks confined to the posterior pole (within 55°); type II, central atrophy with flecks outside the posterior pole; and type III, central atrophy extending outside the posterior pole and significant extramacular flecks [103].

13.7.1.1 Treatment of STGD

STGD patients' significant challenge is a progressive decline in central vision, making physical activities like driving and reading difficult, which causes great mental stress [104]. Patients need counselling to accept the disease and encouragement to use magnifiers and electronic devices for reading. There is, as yet no approved treatment available for SGTD.

One of the significant steps in the visual cycle is the isomerization of all-trans retinyl esters to 11-cis-retinol by RPE65, an isomerohydrolase. Blocking the RPE65 is expected to interrupt the visual cycle, stop the regeneration of rhodopsin, and thereby reduce the accumulation of toxic lipofuscin fluorophore, A2E. Emixustat is a small molecule which blocks the activity of RPE65. Successful interruption of the visual cycle can be seen on ERG as the recovery of the suppressed rod b wave. In a multicentric controlled study, Emixustat 10 mg oral was found to be biologically active and has paved the way for a phase 3 clinical trial [105].

Delayed dark adaptation is a known side effect of isotretinoin, a commonly used drug for acne. This prompted its use in a mouse model of STGD to successfully block A2E accumulation in the RPE [106]. However, there are no clinical reports to suggest its efficacy in humans.

A novel RPE65-61, a non-retinoid compound, led to slower chromophore regeneration after light bleach in a mouse model of STGD [107].

It is yet early days in cell replacement therapies. Human embryonic stem cell-derived RPE cells were implanted under the macula in 12 patients with STGD and were followed for 12 months but failed to show a benefit [108]. Although successful in salvaging the photoreceptors in the animal models, in small human studies, the autologous or allogeneic RPE cells suspension or layered on biocompatible scaffolds, although found safe, had no proven efficacy [109].

13.7.2 Bestrophinopathies

Mutations in the Best1 gene are associated with five distinct clinical phenotypes, namely (1) Best vitelliform macular dystrophy (BVMD); (2) Adult onset vitelliform macular dystrophy (AVMD); (3) Autosomal recessive bestrophinopathy (ARB); (4) Autosomal dominant vitreoretinochoroidopathy (ADVIRC); and (5) Autosomal dominant micro cornea rod-cone dystrophy staphyloma syndrome (ADMRCS). There is no treatment available for any of the bestrophinopathies as yet. We give here a brief outline of the three relatively common bestrophinopathies. For more detailed information, the readers may refer to a review on this subject by Johnson et al. [110].

13.7.2.1 Best Vitelliform Macular Dystrophy

Best vitelliform macular dystrophy (BVMD) is not an uncommon autosomal dominantly inherited macular dystrophy seen in early childhood. At least five phenotypes are known to be caused by a heterozygous mutation in the Bestrophin gene (BEST1, VMD2) located on the long arm of chromosome 11 (11q12.3). https://www.omim.org/entry/153700?search=Best%20vitelliform%20macualr%20dystrophy&highlight=best%20dystrophy%20macualr%20vitelliform.

The typical presentation is of an egg-yolk appearance of a lesion located in the macula of both eyes (Fig. 13.8). A rarer phenotype which is a more multifocal variety is seen as autosomal recessive dystrophy. At the egg-yolk stage, the disease is largely asymptomatic. Later in the years, the egg-yolk appearance changes to a pseudohypopyon-like, followed by a scrambled egg appearance and is later replaced by an atrophic pigmented scar. At this stage, the central vision is significantly affected. The ERG studies are normal, but EOG studies show a reduced Arden ratio (light rise/dark trough ratio) usually less than 1.5. The normal Arden ratio is 1.85–2.5 or more. The deposition of vitelliform material under the RPE causes the egg-yolk appearance. During the scrambled egg appearance, there is a disruption of the photoreceptors responsible for the visual symptoms [111]. Histopathological studies have shown a widespread accumulation of vitelliform material in the RPE cells and between Bruch's membrane and RPE cells. A rupture of the RPE cells possibly allows this material to move into the subretinal space and damage the photoreceptors [112]. Five stages of BVMD are recognized. Stage 1, pre-vitelliform; stage 2, vitelliform; stage 3, pseudohypopyon; stage 4, vitelliruptive; stage 5, atrophic. Visual acuity is maintained up to stage 2 [113], with progressive decline. In stages 1–2, only a few eyes may show disruption in EZ and RPE, but practically all eyes in stages 3–5 show disruption of the outer retinal layers and RPE. Most stage 5 eyes show the absence of outer retinal layers. The vitelliform material is seen in stages 2–3 and is reduced after that [113]. A vitelliform space called the Best space is present under the NSR in all stages except after fibrosis from a secondary CNVM.

The subfoveal RPE-BM thickness is significantly reduced from the pre-vitelliform to the vitelliform stage. In the pre-vitelliform stage, the zone between the RPE and the EZ is thickened, which corresponds to the interdigitating zone (IZ). The EZ overlying the vitelliform lesion shows disruption. Over time, during the pseudohypopyon stage, the RPE is separated from BM with a hyporeflective space. During the vitelliruptive stage, it is difficult to distinguish the RPE, vitelliform material, and the photoreceptors [114]. The vitelliform material is hyperautofluorescent on short wavelength FAF.

13.7.2.2 Autosomal Recessive Bestrophinopathy

Autosomal recessive bestrophinopathy (ARB), first described by Burgess et al. [115], is an autosomal recessive disorder due to a homozygous or compound heterozygous mutation in the BEST1 gene located on chromosome 11(11q12). BEST1 gene is located on the basolateral aspect of the RPE cells and controls Cl (−) channel responsible for maintaining the cell volume. ARB is a null phenotype, i.e. there is a total loss of formation of the functional protein. Patients with ARB present in the first decade of life with visual symptoms. One of the characteristic lesions in ARB is a collection of serous fluid in the macula accompanied by a cluster of hyperautofluorescent dots around the faint yellowish central lesion. On fundus examination, there are areas of atrophy of RPE and subretinal yellow-white dot lesions in the macula and periphery. On FAF, the areas of RPE atrophy appear dark, while the yellow-white lesions correspond to the hyperautofluorescent dots. None of these patients shows vitelliform lesions, highly characteristic of the Best disease. The FFA shows increased transmission hyperfluorescence suggestive of RPE atrophy. The SRF in the macula also shows hyperfluorescence. There may be a central scar due to the development of the CNVM. On EOG, the light rise is absent or grossly reduced. Pattern ERG shows mild to severe reduction in amplitude. The ffERG show delayed implicit times and reduced amplitude. Many patients with ARB are hyperopes, have a shallow anterior chamber, and may develop angle closure glaucoma.

The severity of lesions on ultrahigh SD-OCT reflects the severity of the clinical picture. In the perifoveal area EZ, cone IZ and rod IZ are preserved. However, in the area of serous fluid, the cone IZ are missing, and the cone outer segments are elongated. Hyperreflective dots appear in the cone's outer segments. The more severe changes include the cone outer segments' disappearance and the EZ's disruption into fragments. The fragmented EZ is replaced by hyperreflective dots that hang like icicles initially from the EZ. With the disappearance of the EZ, these dots appear to hang from the ELM [116].

13.7.2.3 Adult Onset Vitelliform Dystrophy

Adult vitelliform macular dystrophy (AVMD), also termed vitelliform macular dystrophy-3 or Adult foveomacular vitelliform dystrophy is an autosomal dominant dystrophy caused by a mutation in the RDS gene (PRPH2) located on the short arm of chromosome 6 (6p21). Patients become mildly symptomatic in the third to the fifth decade. https://www.omim.org/entry/608161?search=Adult%20onset%20vitelliform%20macular%20dystrophy&highlight=adult%20dystrophy%20macular%20onset%20vitelliform.

These have also been grouped as pattern dystrophies and named depending on the pattern of pigment distribution. Pattern dystrophies can present with variable phenotypic heterogeneity. The pattern in the two eyes of the same patient or different members of the same family may be different. The most common pattern is a small one-third to one disc diameter, a variable-shaped egg-yolk-like lesion, which may have pigmentation in its centre (Fig. 13.9). There may be smaller paramacular fleck lesions in addition. On FAF, the lesions are intensely hyperautofluorescent. On FFA, the lesions show central hypofluorescence and hyperfluorescence at the margins. In more than one-half of the patients, the lesions may be asymptomatic or have only mild visual symptoms [117]. Unlike the significantly reduced Arden ratio (light rise to the dark trough of electric potential) in EOG in Best disease, it is nearly normal in AVMD. The ERG is also normal. Patients have normal colour vision. Progression has been demonstrated on SD-OCT in AVMD, similar to the BVMD. The OCT shows subretinal hyperreflective material, which is highly hyperautofluorescent. With the development of the pseudohypopyon stage, the vitelliform material is sedimented inferiorly. The upper part of the lesion becomes hypoautofluorescent and hypo reflective on the OCT. There is variable hypo-reflective space between the NSR and the RPE. Disruption of the EZ is seen early in the course of AVMD. Additionally, focal hyperreflective nodules between BM and RPE are also seen [118].

On histopathology, loss of photoreceptors and pigment migration into the NSR is seen. Besides, a chorioretinal adhesion in the centre of the lesion accounts for the hyperpigmented spot seen clinically in the centre of the lesion. A focal drusen-like lesion may be seen. There is no change in the ChC layer [119]. Histopathology also confirmed the presence of lipofuscin-laden RPE cells, a zone of RPE atrophy ringed by a zone of RPE hypertrophy and photoreceptor degeneration overlying the atrophic RPE. Ultraviolet fluorescent microscopy has confirmed the presence of autofluorescent material in the hypertrophic RPE and the overlying atrophic photoreceptor layer [120].

It has been proposed that the patients who present with AVMD and have a mutation in the BEST1 gene should be considered milder versions of the BVMD [110]. RPE aperture has been noted to complicate AVMD [121]. For detailed information on inherited macular dystrophies, readers may refer to a review by Michaelides et al. [68].

13.8 Mitochondrial Retinal Dystrophies

Somatic mutations in mitochondrial DNA (mtDNA) are fairly common in normal people. The paternal mtDNA is lost during fertilization and plays no role. Mutations in the maternal mtDNA lead to a state wherein the normal mtDNA is mixed with the mutated DNA in all the cells of the body tissues. This is called heteroplasmy. Various clinical phenotypes manifest depending upon the proportion of the normal and mutated mtDNA. It is a dynamic process, and clinical phenotypes will appear when the mutated mtDNA becomes more abundant than normal. In the eye, these manifest as macular dystrophies and are associated with systemic features. Diagnosing these dystrophies may pose a challenge especially if the systemic features are mildly manifested. Fundus examination may provide the first clue to the existence of mitochondrial dystrophy. In type 1 macular dystrophy, the patients are asymptomatic and have discrete fleck-like lesions that show hyperautofluorescence surrounded by hypoautofluorescence. There are disturbances at the level of the interdigitating zone (IZ) and the RPE on OCT. The ERG is normal at this stage.

In type 2, in addition to the flecks, sharp areas of chorioretinal atrophy (GA) appear in the paracentral macula which may be discontinuous or continuous and spare the foveal centre, along with peripapillary hypofluorescence. The changes are limited to the posterior pole. The patients may or may not be symptomatic. The ERG is normal. In type 3, the changes are more widespread with granular lesions that extend beyond the arcades. The atrophic areas extend into the fovea. The photopic and scotopic ERG are subnormal [122]. Many of these syndromes have overlapping macular and systemic signs. The salient features of the mitochondrial dystrophies and others associated with systemic features are given in Box 13.7.

Box 13.7 Systemic Associations of Mitochondrial and Other Macular Dystrophies

Phenotype	Salient features Ocular[a]	Salient features Systemic	Inheritance/gene/ locus
MIDD[b]	Pattern macular dystrophy: progressive lesions Butterfly/reticular Punctate/pigmented dots/ continuous or discontinuous perifoveal circular areas of GA FAF shows HFA dots, OCT hyperreflective deposits in RPE	Diabetes; deafness; men and women are equally affected	A point mutation in mtDNA TL1, A3243G MT-TK; MT-TE
MELAS[b]	Pigmentary dystrophy as in MIDD; optic atrophy progressive external ophthalmoplegia	Onset before 20 years; recurrent stroke-like episodes; lactic acidosis-muscle fatigue; and pain, vomiting; breathing issues; confusion; slow dementia	Point mutation mtDNA[a] MT-TL-1 A3243G
MERRF[b]	Pattern dystrophy Chronic progressive external ophthalmoplegia	Onset young to adults; myoclonic jerks legs/arms/body; epilepsy; ataxia; myopathy; cardiomyopathy; hearing loss; muscle biopsy shows red-ragged fibres	A point mutation in mtDNA MT-TK
Kearns-Sayre syndrome[c]	Onset before 20 years Pigmentary retinal degeneration in the macula On pathology, pigment hypertrophy and loss of pigment in RPE, FFA transmission hyperfluorescence Ptosis; progressive external ophthalmoplegia ERG: subnormal	Cardiomyopathy; microcephaly; short stature; hearing loss; cerebellar ataxia; seizures; sensory and motor neuropathy; muscle weakness; muscle biopsy shows red-ragged fibres; lactic acidosis; increased CSF proteins	Most cases are sporadic multiple deletions in mtDNA MTTL1 in AD cases
Alport's syndrome	Lenticonus, PSC; post polymorphous corneal dystrophy; small yellow-white flecks in the superficial perifoveal macula and deeper flecks in the peripheral retina; giant macular holes	85% are male; haematuria; progressive renal failure; and hearing loss	Deletion of COL4A5/COL4A6 on Xq22, gene for collagen IV
Aicardi's syndrome	Circular 1/10–2 DD, white chorioretinal lacunae; symmetrical; bilateral, no pigmentation	Only in females; infantile flexion spasms, agenesis of the corpus callosum; seizures; microcephaly; postural defects due to costovertebral defects	XLD inheritance; lethal in males Xp22
Sjögren-Larsson syndrome	Early childhood-hyperautofluorescent glistening white dots and yellow pigmentary changes in the macula Photophobia; ERG/EOG normal	Ichthyosis of skin; low-grade mental disability; spastic paresis of legs; speech difficulty; dental and osseous dysplasia	ALDH3A2 gene 17p11.2 • Fatty aldehyde dehydrogenase deficiency

Source: https://rarediseases.org/rare-diseases/

Bryan et al. [140], Ambonville et al. [141], Agarwal [142]

MIDD maternally inherited deafness and diabetes, *MELAS* mitochondrial encephalomyopathy lactic acidosis and stroke-like episodes, *MERRF* myoclonic epilepsy with red-ragged fibres, *MT-TL* mitochondrially encoded transfer RNA leucine 1, *MT-TK* mitochondrially encoded transfer RNA lysine, *COL* collagen, *DD* disc diameter, *XLD* X-linked autosomal dominant, *ALDH* aldehyde dehydrogenase

[a] Heteroplasmy exists. Mutated and normal mtDNA co-exists in the same cell. Symptoms appear when mutated mtDNA is significantly more than the normal mtDNA

[b] All three syndromes frequently show overlap and may have similar pigmentary dystrophy

[c] https://www.omim.org/entry/530000

13.9 Treatment of Inherited Retinal Disorders

In the last nearly 30 years, rapid advances in gene sequencing technologies have facilitated the identification of the genes responsible for many retinal and macular dystrophies. Animal models for several genetic disorders have been created to test the efficacy of various therapeutic interventions. More are still required for estimating optimal dosage. Many approaches are being tested in preclinical studies, including gene supplements, an antisense oligonucleotide (AON), gene editing (gene repair), cell therapy, neurotrophic factors, and optogenetics.

More recently, inducible pluripotent stem cells (iPSC) from patients and normal people have been used to create a 2-D cell culture of RPE and 3-D retina organoids to study the IRDs [123]. The iPSC and organoids that contain multilayered retinal structures can be used as a source of cells for cell replacement therapy. The iPSC derived from fibroblasts or the patient's blood with IRD can be reprogrammed (repaired) using CRISPR-Cas9 editing technology. It has successfully corrected a pathological variant in CEP 290, a mutation responsible for a type of LCA and a gain of function mutation Pro23His rhodopsin (RHO) mutation responsible for autosomal dominant RP. The gene editing restored the mRNA transcription [124]. This approach prevents overexpression of the supplemented gene. Moreover, this approach can overcome limitations imposed by the size of genes the AAV vector can package. These cells can be used for autologous transplantation of cells [124].

13.9.1 Gene Supplement Therapy

Monogenic defects (caused by a mutation in a specific gene) cause nearly 80% of genetic disorders. These are the first being targeted for gene therapy. The initial clinical studies in such patients involved gene supplemental therapy. Among all genetic disorders, the treatment of Leber congenital amaurosis (LCA) caused by mutations in RPE65 was the first to complete successful clinical trials leading to the FDA approval of the first gene supplement therapy in December 2017. It involved an injection of an adeno-associated vector to package an RPE 65 gene, Luxturna (voretigene neparvovec-rzyl, Spark Therapeutics), into the subretinal space. Recently, the three decade-journey of the genetics of IRD, gene therapy, selection and safety of vectors, and preclinical studies finally leading to the clinical trials were reviewed [125]. The subretinal injection of Luxturna has been found safe, and the maximum improvement was reached in 30 days.

No adverse effects were noted, and the effect was maintained in 4 years of follow-up [126]. The success of this therapy has prompted a change in terminology that involves specifying the gene in the diagnosis of IRD so that specific information can be shared with all the stakeholders [127]. The term LCA2 has been changed to RPE65 retinopathy. The term gene therapy is no longer used. It is preferred to use 'Gene augmentation' or 'Gene replacement'. More recently, microstructural and visual improvements were reported at day 30/45 and 6 months following the subretinal injection of Voretigene-neparvovek in six children in biallelic RPE65 retinopathy. There was an increase in the central foveal ring macular thickness and the outer nuclear layer [128].

In a cohort of 18 eyes of 10 patients, progressive subretinal atrophy developed, although all eyes showed a consistent increase in the full-field stimulus threshold. Scotomas were reported in three eyes related to the chorioretinal trophy [129]. In a real-world study of 27 eyes of 14 patients, there was an improvement in full-field stimulus threshold, visual acuity, and the Goldmann visual fields in each eye. The main adverse effects were the rise in intraocular pressure in 59% of eyes, inflammation in 15%, and vitreous opacities in 26%, which resolved over several months [130]. The 3-year follow-up of subretinal gene supplement therapy for ABCA4 mutant Stargardt's disease found the treatment safe in the first 22 cases of a five-family cohort. However, six of the treated eyes showed progression of chorioretinal atrophy more than the control eyes. None of the patients had changes in visual acuity, perimetry or ERG attributable to treatment. Subretinal injection involves raising a serous retinal bleb into which the vector carrying the gene is injected. In some patients, it may lead to RPE atrophy [131].

A phase1/2 trial of intravitreal rAAV2tYF-CB-hRS1, a recombinant adeno-associated virus vector expressing retinoschisin (RS1) was tested in 22 adults and five children suffering from X-linked retinoschisis. The adverse event noted was mild to moderate ocular inflammation requiring immunosuppressive therapy; however, at 1-year follow-up, no measurable improvement was in any of the parameters [132].

13.9.2 Antisense Oligonucleotide Treatment

Mutations in USH2-exon13 often cause Usher syndrome and non-syndromic RP. ProQR reported positive results in a phase 1/2 trial. QR-421a, an RNA therapy that skips the mutated exon13 and restores the usherin protein, was well tolerated and showed improved visual acuity, perimetry, and OCT parameters. https://www.proqr.com/press-releases/proqr-announces-positive-results-from-clinical-trial-of-qr-421a-in-usher-syndrome-and-plans-to-start-pivotal-trials.

13.9.3 Optogenetics

The current technologies can target only a specific gene through gene supplementation, antisense oligonucleotides or gene repair using CRISPR cas9 technology. However, the number of defective genes in IRD exceed 250 and targeting these specific genes in individual patients, although possible, is not a practical solution. One of the unique characteristics of IRD is the survival of the inner retinal cells and their circuits for a long time despite the complete loss of the outer retina. Nearly 30% of the ganglion cells and 78–88% of the inner nuclear cells are present even in moderate to severe RP [133]. Optogenetics involves programming the ganglion cells to express opsin, the photosensitive protein, by injecting a gene carried by an AAV vector into either the intravitreal or the subretinal space [134]. It has the potential to restore partial vision in patients who are blind. The first successfully treated case of advanced RP with optogenetic technology was reported in 2021. This person, a 58-year-old blind, had been diagnosed with RP 40 years previously and had only light perception vision. He was administered intravitreal injection of an optogenetic AAV vector (serotype 2.7m8) that encoded ChrimsonR (channelrhodopsin protein fused to the red fluorescent protein tdTomat). Seven months after the treatment, he was given visual training using light stimulation goggles. The partial vision was restored in the treated eye [135].

In 2021, Nanoscope announced the successful optogenetic treatment of 11 RP patients, restoring clinically meaningful results at 52 weeks of follow-up. https://nanostherapeutics.com/2021/06/03/nanoscopes-optogenetic-gene-therapy-restores-clinically-meaningful-vision/.

Another phase 2 trial has enrolled 14 advanced RP patients who were administered a single intravitreal injection of RST001, a therapeutic optogenetic gene and the results are awaited. https://clinicaltrials.gov/ct2/show/NCT02556736. Bionic sight also reported successfully treating four patients. First Four Patients In Bionic Sight's Optogenetic Gene (https://globenewswire.com).

References

1. Man REK, Gan ATL, Fenwick EK, Teo KYC, Tan ACS, Cheung GCM, Teo ZL, Kumari N, Wong TY, Cheng CY, Lamoureux EL. Impact of incident age-related macular degeneration and associated vision loss on vision-related quality of life. Br J Ophthalmol. 2022;106(8):1063–8. https://doi.org/10.1136/bjophthalmol-2020-318269. Epub 2021 Feb 26.
2. Zouache MA. Variability in retinal neuron populations and associated variations in mass transport systems of the retina in health and aging. Front Aging

Neurosci. 2022;14:778404. https://doi.org/10.3389/fnagi.2022.778404.
3. Bill A, Sperber G, Ujiie K. Physiology of the choroidal vascular bed. Int Ophthalmol. 1983;6(2):101–7. https://doi.org/10.1007/BF00127638.
4. Yednock T, Fong DS, Lad EM. C1q and the classical complement cascade in geographic atrophy secondary to age-related macular degeneration. Int J Retina Vitreous. 2022;8(1):79. https://doi.org/10.1186/s40942-022-00431-y.
5. Kim BJ, Mastellos DC, Li Y, Dunaief JL, Lambris JD. Targeting complement components C3 and C5 for the retina: key concepts and lingering questions. Prog Retin Eye Res. 2021;83:100936. https://doi.org/10.1016/j.preteyeres.2020.100936. Epub 2020 Dec 13.
6. Gold B, Merriam JE, Zernant J, Hancox LS, Taiber AJ, Gehrs K, Cramer K, Neel J, Bergeron J, Barile GR, Smith RT, AMD Genetics Clinical Study Group, Hageman GS, Dean M, Allikmets R. Variation in factor B (BF) and complement component 2 (C2) genes is associated with age-related macular degeneration. Nat Genet. 2006;38(4):458–62. https://doi.org/10.1038/ng1750. Epub 2006 Mar 5.
7. Strunz T, Kiel C, Sauerbeck BL, Weber BHF. Learning from fifteen years of genome-wide association studies in age-related macular degeneration. Cell. 2020;9(10):2267. https://doi.org/10.3390/cells9102267.
8. Senabouth A, Daniszewski M, Lidgerwood GE, Liang HH, Hernández D, Mirzaei M, Keenan SN, Zhang R, Han X, Neavin D, Rooney L, Lopez Sanchez MIG, Gulluyan L, Paulo JA, Clarke L, Kearns LS, Gnanasambandapillai V, Chan CL, Nguyen U, Steinmann AM, McCloy RA, Farbehi N, Gupta VK, Mackey DA, Bylsma G, Verma N, MacGregor S, Watt MJ, Guymer RH, Powell JE, Hewitt AW, Pébay A. Transcriptomic and proteomic retinal pigment epithelium signatures of age-related macular degeneration. Nat Commun. 2022;13(1):4233. https://doi.org/10.1038/s41467-022-31707-4.
9. Chui TY, Song H, Clark CA, Papay JA, Burns SA, Elsner AE. Cone photoreceptor packing density and the outer nuclear layer thickness in healthy subjects. Invest Ophthalmol Vis Sci. 2012;53(7):3545–53. https://doi.org/10.1167/iovs.11-8694.
10. Ramrattan RS, van der Schaft TL, Mooy CM, de Bruijn WC, Mulder PG, de Jong PT. Morphometric analysis of Bruch's membrane, the choriocapillaris, and the choroid in aging. Invest Ophthalmol Vis Sci. 1994;35(6):2857–64.
11. Wong WL, Su X, Li X, Cheung CM, Klein R, Cheng CY, Wong TY. Global prevalence of age-related macular degeneration and disease burden projection for 2020 and 2040: a systematic review and meta-analysis. Lancet Glob Health. 2014;2(2):e106–16. https://doi.org/10.1016/S2214-109X(13)70145-1. Epub 2014 Jan 3.
12. Edwards AO, Ritter R 3rd, Abel KJ, Manning A, Panhuysen C, Farrer LA. Complement factor H polymorphism and age-related macular degeneration. Science. 2005;308(5720):421–4. https://doi.org/10.1126/science.1110189. Epub 2005 Mar 10.
13. Haines JL, Hauser MA, Schmidt S, Scott WK, Olson LM, Gallins P, Spencer KL, Kwan SY, Noureddine M, Gilbert JR, Schnetz-Boutaud N, Agarwal A, Postel EA, Pericak-Vance MA. Complement factor H variant increases the risk of age-related macular degeneration. Science. 2005;308(5720):419–21. https://doi.org/10.1126/science.1110359. Epub 2005 Mar 10.
14. Klein RJ, Zeiss C, Chew EY, Tsai JY, Sackler RS, Haynes C, Henning AK, SanGiovanni JP, Mane SM, Mayne ST, Bracken MB, Ferris FL, Ott J, Barnstable C, Hoh J. Complement factor H polymorphism in age-related macular degeneration. Science. 2005;308(5720):385–9. https://doi.org/10.1126/science.1109557. Epub 2005 Mar 10.
15. Anderson DH, Radeke MJ, Gallo NB, Chapin EA, Johnson PT, Curletti CR, Hancox LS, Hu J, Ebright JN, Malek G, Hauser MA, Rickman CB, Bok D, Hageman GS, Johnson LV. The pivotal role of the complement system in aging and age-related macular degeneration: hypothesis re-visited. Prog Retin Eye Res. 2010;29(2):95–112. https://doi.org/10.1016/j.preteyeres.2009.11.003. Epub 2009 Dec 2.
16. Fritsche LG, Loenhardt T, Janssen A, Fisher SA, Rivera A, Keilhauer CN, Weber BH. Age-related macular degeneration is associated with an unstable ARMS2 (LOC387715) mRNA. Nat Genet. 2008;40(7):892–6. https://doi.org/10.1038/ng.170. Epub 2008 May 30.
17. Micklisch S, Lin Y, Jacob S, et al. Age-related macular degeneration associated polymorphism rs10490924 in ARMS2 results in deficiency of a complement activator. J Neuroinflammation. 2017;14:4. https://doi.org/10.1186/s12974-016-0776-3.
18. Rozing MP, Durhuus JA, Krogh Nielsen M, Subhi Y, Kirkwood TB, Westendorp RG, Sørensen TL. Age-related macular degeneration: a two-level model hypothesis. Prog Retin Eye Res. 2020;76:100825. https://doi.org/10.1016/j.preteyeres.2019.100825. Epub 2019 Dec 30.
19. Mauschitz MM, Finger RP. Age-related macular degeneration and cardiovascular diseases: revisiting the common soil theory. Asia Pac J Ophthalmol (Phila). 2022;11(2):94–9. https://doi.org/10.1097/APO.0000000000000496. Epub 2022 Feb 23.
20. Merle BMJ, Colijn JM, Cougnard-Grégoire A, de Koning-Backus APM, Delyfer MN, Kiefte-de Jong JC, Meester-Smoor M, Féart C, Verzijden T, Samieri C, Franco OH, Korobelnik JF, Klaver CCW, Delcourt C, EYE-RISK Consortium. Mediterranean diet and incidence of advanced age-related macular degeneration: the EYE-RISK Consortium. Ophthalmology. 2019;126(3):381–90. https://doi.org/10.1016/j.ophtha.2018.08.006. Epub 2018 Aug 13.
21. Mauschitz MM, Schmitz MT, Verzijden T, Schmid M, Thee EF, Colijn JM, Delcourt C, Cougnard-

Grégoire A, Merle BMJ, Korobelnik JF, Gopinath B, Mitchell P, Elbaz H, Schuster AK, Wild PS, Brandl C, Stark KJ, Heid IM, Günther F, Peters A, Klaver CCW, Finger RP, European Eye Epidemiology (E3) Consortium. Physical activity, incidence, and progression of age-related macular degeneration: a multicohort study. Am J Ophthalmol. 2022;236:99–106. https://doi.org/10.1016/j.ajo.2021.10.008. Epub 2021 Oct 22.

22. Seddon JM, Francis PJ, George S, Schultz DW, Rosner B, Klein ML. Association of CFH Y402H and LOC387715 A69S with progression of age-related macular degeneration. JAMA. 2007;297(16):1793–800. https://doi.org/10.1001/jama.297.16.1793. Erratum in: JAMA (2007) 297(23):2585.
23. Thee EF, Colijn JM, Cougnard-Grégoire A, Meester-Smoor MA, Verzijden T, Hoyng CB, Fauser S, Hense HW, Silva R, Creuzot-Garcher C, Ueffing M, Delcourt C, den Hollander AI, Klaver CCW, European Eye Epidemiology Consortium and EYE-RISK Project. The phenotypic course of age-related macular degeneration for ARMS2/HTRA1: the EYE-RISK Consortium. Ophthalmology. 2022;129(7):752–64. https://doi.org/10.1016/j.ophtha.2022.02.026. Epub 2022 Mar 1.
24. Spaide RF, Ooto S, Curcio CA. Subretinal drusenoid deposits AKA pseudodrusen. Surv Ophthalmol. 2018;63(6):782–815. https://doi.org/10.1016/j.survophthal.2018.05.005. Epub 2018 May 31.
25. Nassisi M, Tepelus T, Nittala MG, Sadda SR. Choriocapillaris flow impairment predicts the development and enlargement of drusen. Graefes Arch Clin Exp Ophthalmol. 2019;257(10):2079–85. https://doi.org/10.1007/s00417-019-04403-1. Epub 2019 Jul 1.
26. Fritsche LG, Igl W, Bailey JN, Grassmann F, Sengupta S, Bragg-Gresham JL, Burdon KP, Hebbring SJ, Wen C, Gorski M, Kim IK, Cho D, Zack D, Souied E, Scholl HP, Bala E, Lee KE, Hunter DJ, Sardell RJ, Mitchell P, Merriam JE, Cipriani V, Hoffman JD, Schick T, Lechanteur YT, Guymer RH, Johnson MP, Jiang Y, Stanton CM, Buitendijk GH, Zhan X, Kwong AM, Boleda A, Brooks M, Gieser L, Ratnapriya R, Branham KE, Foerster JR, Heckenlively JR, Othman MI, Vote BJ, Liang HH, Souzeau E, McAllister IL, Isaacs T, Hall J, Lake S, Mackey DA, Constable IJ, Craig JE, Kitchner TE, Yang Z, Su Z, Luo H, Chen D, Ouyang H, Flagg K, Lin D, Mao G, Ferreyra H, Stark K, von Strachwitz CN, Wolf A, Brandl C, Rudolph G, Olden M, Morrison MA, Morgan DJ, Schu M, Ahn J, Silvestri G, Tsironi EE, Park KH, Farrer LA, Orlin A, Brucker A, Li M, Curcio CA, Mohand-Saïd S, Sahel JA, Audo I, Benchaboune M, Cree AJ, Rennie CA, Goverdhan SV, Grunin M, Hagbi-Levi S, Campochiaro P, Katsanis N, Holz FG, Blond F, Blanché H, Deleuze JF, Igo RP Jr, Truitt B, Peachey NS, Meuer SM, Myers CE, Moore EL, Klein R, Hauser MA, Postel EA, Courtenay MD, Schwartz SG, Kovach JL, Scott WK, Liew G, Tan AG, Gopinath B, Merriam JC, Smith RT, Khan JC, Shahid H, Moore AT, McGrath JA, Laux R, Brantley MA Jr, Agarwal A, Ersoy L, Caramoy A, Langmann T, Saksens NT, de Jong EK, Hoyng CB, Cain MS, Richardson AJ, Martin TM, Blangero J, Weeks DE, Dhillon B, van Duijn CM, Doheny KF, Romm J, Klaver CC, Hayward C, Gorin MB, Klein ML, Baird PN, den Hollander AI, Fauser S, Yates JR, Allikmets R, Wang JJ, Schaumberg DA, Klein BE, Hagstrom SA, Chowers I, Lotery AJ, Léveillard T, Zhang K, Brilliant MH, Hewitt AW, Swaroop A, Chew EY, Pericak-Vance MA, DeAngelis M, Stambolian D, Haines JL, Iyengar SK, Weber BH, Abecasis GR, Heid IM. A large genome-wide association study of age-related macular degeneration highlights contributions of rare and common variants. Nat Genet. 2016;48(2):134–43. https://doi.org/10.1038/ng.3448. Epub 2015 Dec 21.
27. Gass JD. Drusen and disciform macular detachment and degeneration. Trans Am Ophthal Soc 1972;70:409–36.
28. Ferris FL 3rd, Wilkinson CP, Bird A, Chakravarthy U, Chew E, Csaky K, Sadda SR, Beckman Initiative for Macular Research Classification Committee. Clinical classification of age-related macular degeneration. Ophthalmology. 2013;120(4):844–51. https://doi.org/10.1016/j.ophtha.2012.10.036. Epub 2013 Jan 16.
29. Keenan TD, Agrón E, Domalpally A, Clemons TE, van Asten F, Wong WT, Danis RG, Sadda S, Rosenfeld PJ, Klein ML, Ratnapriya R, Swaroop A, Ferris FL 3rd, Chew EY, AREDS2 Research Group. Progression of geographic atrophy in age-related macular degeneration: AREDS2 report number 16. Ophthalmology. 2018;125(12):1913–28. https://doi.org/10.1016/j.ophtha.2018.05.028. Epub 2018 Jul 27.
30. Reiter GS, Told R, Schranz M, Baumann L, Mylonas G, Sacu S, Pollreisz A, Schmidt-Erfurth U. Subretinal drusenoid deposits and photoreceptor loss detecting global and local progression of geographic atrophy by SD-OCT imaging. Invest Ophthalmol Vis Sci. 2020;61(6):11. https://doi.org/10.1167/iovs.61.6.11.
31. Guymer RH, Rosenfeld PJ, Curcio CA, Holz FG, Staurenghi G, Freund KB, Schmitz-Valckenberg S, Sparrow J, Spaide RF, Tufail A, Chakravarthy U, Jaffe GJ, Csaky K, Sarraf D, Monés JM, Tadayoni R, Grunwald J, Bottoni F, Liakopoulos S, Pauleikhoff D, Pagliarini S, Chew EY, Viola F, Fleckenstein M, Blodi BA, Lim TH, Chong V, Lutty J, Bird AC, Sadda SR. Incomplete retinal pigment epithelial and outer retinal atrophy in age-related macular degeneration: classification of atrophy meeting report 4. Ophthalmology. 2020;127(3):394–409. https://doi.org/10.1016/j.ophtha.2019.09.035. Epub 2019 Sep 30.
32. Airaldi M, Corvi F, Cozzi M, Nittala MG, Staurenghi G, Sadda SR. Differences in long-term progression of atrophy between neovascular and nonneovascular age-related macular degeneration.

Ophthalmol Retina. 2022;6(10):914–21. https://doi.org/10.1016/j.oret.2022.04.012. Epub 2022 Apr 20.
33. Foss A, Rotsos T, Empeslidis T, Chong V. Development of macular atrophy in patients with wet age-related macular degeneration receiving anti-VEGF treatment. Ophthalmologica. 2022;245(3):204–17. https://doi.org/10.1159/000520171. Epub 2021 Oct 25.
34. Rofagha S, Bhisitkul RB, Boyer DS, Sadda SR, Zhang K, SEVEN-UP Study Group. Seven-year outcomes in ranibizumab-treated patients in ANCHOR, MARINA, and HORIZON: a multicenter cohort study (SEVEN-UP). Ophthalmology. 2013;120(11):2292–9. https://doi.org/10.1016/j.ophtha.2013.03.046. Epub 2013 May 3.
35. Takahashi A, Ooto S, Yamashiro K, Tamura H, Oishi A, Miyata M, Hata M, Yoshikawa M, Yoshimura N, Tsujikawa A. Pachychoroid geographic atrophy: clinical and genetic characteristics. Ophthalmol Retina. 2018;2(4):295–305. https://doi.org/10.1016/j.oret.2017.08.016. Epub 2017 Nov 22.
36. Hirabayashi K, Yu HJ, Wakatsuki Y, Marion KM, Wykoff CC, Sadda SR. OCT risk factors for development of atrophy in eyes with intermediate age-related macular degeneration Ophthalmol Retina 2022. pii: S2468-6530(22)00486-9. https://doi.org/10.1016/j.oret.2022.09.007. Epub ahead of print.
37. Agrón E, Domalpally A, Cukras CA, Clemons TE, Chen Q, Swaroop A, Lu Z, Chew EY, Keenan TDL, AREDS and AREDS2 Research Groups. Reticular Pseudodrusen status, ARMS2/HTRA1 genotype, and geographic atrophy enlargement: age-related eye disease study 2 report 32. Ophthalmology. 2022. pii: S0161-6420(22)00932-0. doi: https://doi.org/10.1016/j.ophtha.2022.11.026. Epub ahead of print.
38. Chakravarthy U, Bailey CC, Scanlon PH, McKibbin M, Khan RS, Mahmood S, Downey L, Dhingra N, Brand C, Brittain CJ, Willis JR, Venerus A, Muthutantri A, Cantrell RA. Progression from early/intermediate to advanced forms of age-related macular degeneration in a large UK cohort: rates and risk factors. Ophthalmol Retina. 2020;4(7):662–72. https://doi.org/10.1016/j.oret.2020.01.012. Epub 2020 Jan 25.
39. Schmitz-Valckenberg S, Sahel JA, Danis R, Fleckenstein M, Jaffe GJ, Wolf S, Pruente C, Holz FG. Natural history of geographic atrophy progression secondary to age-related macular degeneration (geographic atrophy progression study). Ophthalmology. 2016;123(2):361–8. https://doi.org/10.1016/j.ophtha.2015.09.036. Epub 2015 Nov 3.
40. Holekamp N, Wykoff CC, Schmitz-Valckenberg S, Monés J, Souied EH, Lin H, Rabena MD, Cantrell RA, Henry EC, Tang F, Swaminathan B, Martin J, Ferrara D, Staurenghi G. Natural history of geographic atrophy secondary to age-related macular degeneration: results from the prospective proxima A and B clinical trials. Ophthalmology. 2020;127(6):769–83. https://doi.org/10.1016/j.ophtha.2019.12.009. Epub 2019 Dec 14.
41. Pfau M, von der Emde L, de Sisternes L, Hallak JA, Leng T, Schmitz-Valckenberg S, Holz FG, Fleckenstein M, Rubin DL. Progression of photoreceptor degeneration in geographic atrophy secondary to age-related macular degeneration. JAMA Ophthalmol. 2020;138(10):1026–34. https://doi.org/10.1001/jamaophthalmol.2020.2914.
42. Agrón E, Mares J, Chew EY, Keenan TDL, AREDS2 Research Group. Adherence to a Mediterranean diet and geographic atrophy enlargement rate: age-related eye disease study 2 report 29. Ophthalmol Retina. 2022;6(9):762–70. https://doi.org/10.1016/j.oret.2022.03.022. Epub 2022 Apr 4.
43. Fleckenstein M, Keenan TDL, Guymer RH, Chakravarthy U, Schmitz-Valckenberg S, Klaver CC, Wong WT, Chew EY. Age-related macular degeneration. Nat Rev Dis Primers. 2021;7(1):31. https://doi.org/10.1038/s41572-021-00265-2.
44. Holz FG, Sadda SR, Busbee B, Chew EY, Mitchell P, Tufail A, Brittain C, Ferrara D, Gray S, Honigberg L, Martin J, Tong B, Ehrlich JS, Bressler NM, Chroma and Spectri Study Investigators. Efficacy and safety of lampalizumab for geographic atrophy due to age-related macular degeneration: chroma and spectri phase 3 randomized clinical trials. JAMA Ophthalmol. 2018;136(6):666–77. https://doi.org/10.1001/jamaophthalmol.2018.1544.
45. Liao DS, Grossi FV, El Mehdi D, Gerber MR, Brown DM, Heier JS, Wykoff CC, Singerman LJ, Abraham P, Grassmann F, Nuernberg P, Weber BHF, Deschatelets P, Kim RY, Chung CY, Ribeiro RM, Hamdani M, Rosenfeld PJ, Boyer DS, Slakter JS, Francois CG. Complement C3 inhibitor pegcetacoplan for geographic atrophy secondary to age-related macular degeneration: a randomized phase 2 trial. Ophthalmology. 2020;127(2):186–95. https://doi.org/10.1016/j.ophtha.2019.07.011. Epub 2019 Jul 16.
46. Jaffe GJ, Westby K, Csaky KG, Monés J, Pearlman JA, Patel SS, Joondeph BC, Randolph J, Masonson H, Rezaei KA. C5 inhibitor avacincaptad pegol for geographic atrophy due to age-related macular degeneration: a randomized pivotal phase 2/3 trial. Ophthalmology. 2021;128(4):576–86. https://doi.org/10.1016/j.ophtha.2020.08.027. Epub 2020 Sep 1.
47. Wykoff CC, Rosenfeld PJ, Waheed NK, Singh RP, Ronca N, Slakter JS, Staurenghi G, Monés J, Baumal CR, Saroj N, Metlapally R, Ribeiro R. Characterizing new-onset exudation in the randomized phase 2 FILLY trial of complement inhibitor pegcetacoplan for geographic atrophy. Ophthalmology. 2021;128(9):1325–36. https://doi.org/10.1016/j.ophtha.2021.02.025. Epub 2021 Mar 10.
48. Yehoshua Z, de Amorim Garcia Filho CA, Nunes RP, Gregori G, Penha FM, Moshfeghi AA, Zhang

K, Sadda S, Feuer W, Rosenfeld PJ. Systemic complement inhibition with eculizumab for geographic atrophy in age-related macular degeneration: the COMPLETE study. Ophthalmology. 2014;121(3):693–701. https://doi.org/10.1016/j.ophtha.2013.09.044. Epub 2013 Nov 26.

49. Halawa OA, Lin JB, Miller JW, Vavvas DG. A review of completed and ongoing complement inhibitor trials for geographic atrophy secondary to age-related macular degeneration. J Clin Med. 2021;10(12):2580. https://doi.org/10.3390/jcm10122580.
50. Riedl S, Vogl WD, Mai J, Reiter GS, Lachinov D, Grechenig C, McKeown A, Scheibler L, Bogunović H, Schmidt-Erfurth U. The effect of pegcetacoplan treatment on photoreceptor maintenance in geographic atrophy monitored by artificial intelligence-based OCT analysis. Ophthalmol Retina. 2022;6(11):1009–18. https://doi.org/10.1016/j.oret.2022.05.030. Epub 2022 Jun 3.
51. Li L, Yu Y, Lin S, Hu J. Changes in best-corrected visual acuity in patients with dry age-related macular degeneration after stem cell transplantation: systematic review and meta-analysis. Stem Cell Res Ther. 2022;13(1):237. https://doi.org/10.1186/s13287-022-02931-y.
52. Van Gelder RN, Chiang MF, Dyer MA, Greenwell TN, Levin LA, Wong RO, Svendsen CN. Regenerative and restorative medicine for eye disease. Nat Med. 2022;28(6):1149–56. https://doi.org/10.1038/s41591-022-01862-8. Epub 2022 Jun 17. Erratum in: Nat Med. 2022;28(10):2218.
53. Kashani AH, Lebkowski JS, Rahhal FM, Avery RL, Salehi-Had H, Chen S, Chan C, Palejwala N, Ingram A, Dang W, Lin CM, Mitra D, Pennington BO, Hinman C, Faynus MA, Bailey JK, Mohan S, Rao N, Johnson LV, Clegg DO, Hinton DR, Humayun MS. One-year follow-up in a phase 1/2a clinical trial of an allogeneic RPE cell bioengineered implant for advanced dry age-related macular degeneration. Transl Vis Sci Technol. 2021;10(10):13. https://doi.org/10.1167/tvst.10.10.13.
54. Duke-Elder S, Dobree JH. Diseases of the retina. In: Duke-Elder, Ed., System of Ophthalmology. Henry Kimpton, London. 1967;10:126–7.
55. Dryja TP, McGee TL, Reichel E, Hahn LB, Cowley GS, Yandell DW, Sandberg MA, Berson EL. A point mutation of the rhodopsin gene in one form of retinitis pigmentosa. Nature. 1990;343(6256):364–6. https://doi.org/10.1038/343364a0.
56. Branham K, Schlegel D, Fahim AT, Jayasundera KT. Genetic testing for inherited retinal degenerations: triumphs and tribulations. Am J Med Genet C Semin Med Genet. 2020;184(3):571–7. https://doi.org/10.1002/ajmg.c.31835. Epub 2020 Aug 31.
57. Goetz KE, Reeves MJ, Gagadam S, Blain D, Bender C, Lwin C, Naik A, Tumminia SJ, Hufnagel RB. Genetic testing for inherited eye conditions in over 6,000 individuals through the eyeGENE network. Am J Med Genet C Semin Med Genet. 2020;184(3):828–37. https://doi.org/10.1002/ajmg.c.31843. Epub 2020 Sep 7.
58. Taylor RL, Parry NRA, Barton SJ, Campbell C, Delaney CM, Ellingford JM, Hall G, Hardcastle C, Morarji J, Nichol EJ, Williams LC, Douzgou S, Clayton-Smith J, Ramsden SC, Sharma V, Biswas S, Lloyd IC, Ashworth JL, Black GC, Sergouniotis PI. Panel-based clinical genetic testing in 85 children with inherited retinal disease. Ophthalmology. 2017;124(7):985–91. https://doi.org/10.1016/j.ophtha.2017.02.005. Epub 2017 Mar 22.
59. Ellingford JM, Sergouniotis PI, Lennon R, Bhaskar S, Williams SG, Hillman KA, O'Sullivan J, Hall G, Ramsden SC, Lloyd IC, Woolf AS, Black GC. Pinpointing clinical diagnosis through whole exome sequencing to direct patient care: a case of Senior-Loken syndrome. Lancet. 2015;385(9980):1916. https://doi.org/10.1016/S0140-6736(15)60496-2.
60. Stone EM, Andorf JL, Whitmore SS, DeLuca AP, Giacalone JC, Streb LM, Braun TA, Mullins RF, Scheetz TE, Sheffield VC, Tucker BA. Clinically focused molecular investigation of 1000 consecutive families with inherited retinal disease. Ophthalmology. 2017;124(9):1314–31. https://doi.org/10.1016/j.ophtha.2017.04.008. Epub 2017 May 27.
61. Robson AG, Frishman LJ, Grigg J, Hamilton R, Jeffrey BG, Kondo M, Li S, McCulloch DL. ISCEV standard for full-field clinical electroretinography (2022 update). Doc Ophthalmol. 2022;144(3):165–77. https://doi.org/10.1007/s10633-022-09872-0. Epub 2022 May 5.
62. Yung M, Klufas MA, Sarraf D. Clinical applications of fundus autofluorescence in retinal disease. Int J Retina Vitreous. 2016;2:12. https://doi.org/10.1186/s40942-016-0035-x.
63. Ogura S, Yasukawa T, Kato A, Usui H, Hirano Y, Yoshida M, Ogura Y. Wide-field fundus autofluorescence imaging to evaluate retinal function in patients with retinitis pigmentosa. Am J Ophthalmol. 2014;158(5):1093–8. https://doi.org/10.1016/j.ajo.2014.07.021. Epub 2014 Jul 22.
64. Tan CS, Ngo WK, Cheong KX. Comparison of choroidal thicknesses using swept source and spectral domain optical coherence tomography in diseased and normal eyes. Br J Ophthalmol. 2015;99(3):354–8. https://doi.org/10.1136/bjophthalmol--2014-305331. Epub 2014 Oct 1.
65. Tan CS, Sadda SR. Swept source optical coherence tomography. In: Meyer CH, Saxena S, Sadda SVR, editors. Spectral domain optical coherence tomography in macular diseases. New Delhi: Springer; 2017. p. 59–77.
66. Triolo G, Pierro L, Parodi MB, De Benedetto U, Gagliardi M, Manitto MP, Bandello F. Spectral-domain optical coherence tomography findings in patients with retinitis pigmentosa.

Ophthalmic Res. 2013;50(3):160–4. https://doi.org/10.1159/000351681. Epub 2013 Aug 28.
67. Liu G, Liu X, Li H, Du Q, Wang F. Optical coherence tomographic analysis of retina in retinitis pigmentosa patients. Ophthalmic Res. 2016;56(3):111–22. https://doi.org/10.1159/000445063. Epub 2016 Jun 29.
68. Michaelides M, Hunt DM, Moore AT. The genetics of inherited macular dystrophies. J Med Genet. 2003;40(9):641–50. https://doi.org/10.1136/jmg.40.9.641.
69. Heath Jeffery RC, Mukhtar SA, McAllister IL, Morgan WH, Mackey DA, Chen FK. Inherited retinal diseases are the most common cause of blindness in the working-age population in Australia. Ophthalmic Genet. 2021;42(4):431–9. https://doi.org/10.1080/13816810.2021.1913610. Epub 2021 May 3. Erratum in: Ophthalmic Genet. 2021:1.
70. Hamel C. Retinitis pigmentosa. Orphanet J Rare Dis. 2006;1:40. https://doi.org/10.1186/1750-1172-1-40.
71. Hartong DT, Berson EL, Dryja TP. Retinitis pigmentosa. Lancet. 2006;368(9549):1795–809. https://doi.org/10.1016/S0140-6736(06)69740-7.
72. Chassine T, Bocquet B, Daien V, Avila-Fernandez A, Ayuso C, Collin RW, Corton M, Hejtmancik JF, van den Born LI, Klevering BJ, Riazuddin SA, Sendon N, Lacroux A, Meunier I, Hamel CP. Autosomal recessive retinitis pigmentosa with RP1 mutations is associated with myopia. Br J Ophthalmol. 2015;99(10):1360–5. https://doi.org/10.1136/bjophthalmol-2014-306224. Epub 2015 Apr 16.
73. Kumaran N, Moore AT, Weleber RG, Michaelides M. Leber congenital amaurosis/early-onset severe retinal dystrophy: clinical features, molecular genetics and therapeutic interventions. Br J Ophthalmol. 2017;101(9):1147–54. https://doi.org/10.1136/bjophthalmol-2016-309975. Epub 2017 Jul 8. Erratum in: Br J Ophthalmol. 2019;103(6):862.
74. Kitiratschky VB, Wilke R, Renner AB, Kellner U, Vadalà M, Birch DG, Wissinger B, Zrenner E, Kohl S. Mutation analysis identifies GUCY2D as the major gene responsible for autosomal dominant progressive cone degeneration. Invest Ophthalmol Vis Sci. 2008;49(11):5015–23. https://doi.org/10.1167/iovs.08-1901. Epub 2008 May 16.
75. Pasadhika S, Fishman GA, Stone EM, Lindeman M, Zelkha R, Lopez I, Koenekoop RK, Shahidi M. Differential macular morphology in patients with RPE65-, CEP290-, GUCY2D-, and AIPL1-related Leber congenital amaurosis. Invest Ophthalmol Vis Sci. 2010;51(5):2608–14. https://doi.org/10.1167/iovs.09-3734. Epub 2009 Dec 3.
76. Maguire AM, Bennett J, Aleman EM, Leroy BP, Aleman TS. Clinical perspective: treating RPE65-associated retinal dystrophy. Mol Ther. 2021;29(2):442–63. https://doi.org/10.1016/j.ymthe.2020.11.029. Epub 2020 Dec 3.
77. Talib M, van Schooneveld MJ, van Duuren RJG, Van Cauwenbergh C, Ten Brink JB, De Baere E, Florijn RJ, Schalij-Delfos NE, Leroy BP, Bergen AA, Boon CJF. Long-term follow-up of retinal degenerations associated with *LRAT* mutations and their comparability to phenotypes associated with *RPE65* mutations. Transl Vis Sci Technol. 2019;8(4):24. https://doi.org/10.1167/tvst.8.4.24.
78. Leroy BP, Birch DG, Duncan JL, Lam BL, Koenekoop RK, Porto FBO, Russell SR, Girach A. Leber congenital amaurosis due to CEP290 mutations-severe vision impairment with a high unmet medical need: a review. Retina. 2021;41(5):898–907. https://doi.org/10.1097/IAE.0000000000003133.
79. May-Simera H, Nagel-Wolfrum K, Wolfrum U. Cilia—the sensory antennae in the eye. Prog Retin Eye Res. 2017;60:144–80. https://doi.org/10.1016/j.preteyeres.2017.05.001. Epub 2017 May 11.
80. Estrada-Cuzcano A, Roepman R, Cremers FP, den Hollander AI, Mans DA. Non-syndromic retinal ciliopathies: translating gene discovery into therapy. Hum Mol Genet. 2012;21(R1):R111–24. https://doi.org/10.1093/hmg/dds298. Epub 2012 Jul 26.
81. Werdich XQ, Place EM, Pierce EA. Systemic diseases associated with retinal dystrophies. Semin Ophthalmol. 2014;29(5–6):319–28. https://doi.org/10.3109/08820538.2014.959202.
82. Beales PL, Elcioglu N, Woolf AS, Parker D, Flinter FA. New criteria for improved diagnosis of Bardet-Biedl syndrome: results of a population survey. J Med Genet. 1999;36(6):437–46.
83. Marshall JD, Bronson RT, Collin GB, Nordstrom AD, Maffei P, Paisey RB, Carey C, Macdermott S, Russell-Eggitt I, Shea SE, Davis J, Beck S, Shatirishvili G, Mihai CM, Hoeltzenbein M, Pozzan GB, Hopkinson I, Sicolo N, Naggert JK, Nishina PM. New Alström syndrome phenotypes based on the evaluation of 182 cases. Arch Intern Med. 2005;165(6):675–83. https://doi.org/10.1001/archinte.165.6.675.
84. Russell-Eggitt IM, Clayton PT, Coffey R, Kriss A, Taylor DS, Taylor JF. Alström syndrome. Report of 22 cases and literature review. Ophthalmology. 1998;105(7):1274–80. https://doi.org/10.1016/S0161-6420(98)97033-6.
85. Romano S, Maffei P, Bettini V, Milan G, Favaretto F, Gardiman M, Marshall JD, Greggio NA, Pozzan GB, Collin GB, Naggert JK, Bronson R, Vettor R. Alström syndrome is associated with short stature and reduced GH reserve. Clin Endocrinol (Oxf). 2013;79(4):529–36. https://doi.org/10.1111/cen.12180. Epub 2013 Mar 26.
86. Dassie F, Favaretto F, Bettini S, Parolin M, Valenti M, Reschke F, Danne T, Vettor R, Milan G, Maffei P. Alström syndrome: an ultra-rare monogenic disorder as a model for insulin resistance, type 2 diabetes mellitus and obesity. Endocrine. 2021;71(3):618–25. https://doi.org/10.1007/s12020-021-02643-y. Epub 2021 Feb 10.
87. Bettini V, Maffei P, Pagano C, Romano S, Milan G, Favaretto F, Marshall JD, Paisey R, Scolari F, Greggio NA, Tosetto I, Naggert JK, Sicolo N,

Vettor R. The progression from obesity to type 2 diabetes in Alström syndrome. Pediatr Diabetes. 2012;13(1):59–67. https://doi.org/10.1111/j.1399--5448.2011.00789.x. Epub 2011 Jul 3.

88. Baig S, Paisey R, Dawson C, Barrett T, Maffei P, Hodson J, Rambhatla SB, Chauhan P, Bolton S, Dassie F, Francomano C, Marshall RP, Belal M, Skordilis K, Hayer M, Price AM, Cramb R, Edwards N, Steeds RP, Geberhiwot T. Defining renal phenotype in Alström syndrome. Nephrol Dial Transplant. 2020;35(6):994–1001. https://doi.org/10.1093/ndt/gfy293.
89. Aliferis K, Hellé S, Gyapay G, Duchatelet S, Stoetzel C, Mandel JL, Dollfus H. Differentiating Alström from Bardet-Biedl syndrome (BBS) using systematic ciliopathy genes sequencing. Ophthalmic Genet. 2012;33(1):18–22. https://doi.org/10.3109/13816810.2011.620055. Epub 2011 Oct 17.
90. Guimaraes TAC, Arram E, Shakarchi AF, Georgiou M, Michaelides M. Inherited causes of combined vision and hearing loss: clinical features and molecular genetics. Br J Ophthalmol. 2022;107:1403. https://doi.org/10.1136/bjo-2022-321790. Epub ahead of print.
91. Ben-Avi R, Rivera A, Hendler K, Sharon D, Banin E, Khateb S, Yahalom C. Prevalence and associated factors of cystoid macular edema in children with early onset inherited retinal dystrophies. Eur J Ophthalmol. 2022;33(2):1109. https://doi.org/10.1177/11206721221136318. Epub ahead of print.
92. Fanconi G, Hanhart E, von Albertini A, Uhlinger E, Dolivo G, Prader A. Die familiäre juvenile Nephronophthise (die idiopathische parenchymatöse Schrumpfniere) [Familial, juvenile nephronophthisis (idiopathic parenchymal contracted kidney)]. Helv Paediatr Acta. 1951;6(1):1–49. Undetermined Language.
93. Senior B, Friedmann AI, Braudo JL. Juvenile familial nephropathy with tapetoretinal degeneration. A new oculorenal dystrophy. Am J Ophthalmol. 1961;52:625–33. https://doi.org/10.1016/0002-9394(61)90147-7.
94. Loken AC, Hanssen O, Halvorsen S, Jolster NJ. Hereditary renal dysplasia and blindness. Acta Paediatr (Stockh). 1961;50:177–84. https://doi.org/10.1111/j.1651-2227.1961.tb08037.x.
95. Ronquillo CC, Bernstein PS, Baehr W. Senior-Løken syndrome: a syndromic form of retinal dystrophy associated with nephronophthisis. Vis Res. 2012;75:88–97. https://doi.org/10.1016/j.visres.2012.07.003. Epub 2012 Jul 20.
96. Joubert M, Eisenring JJ, Robb JP, Andermann F. Familial agenesis of the cerebellar vermis. A syndrome of episodic hyperpnea, abnormal eye movements, ataxia, and retardation. Neurology. 1969;19(9):813–25. https://doi.org/10.1212/wnl.19.9.813.
97. Wang SF, Kowal TJ, Ning K, Koo EB, Wu AY, Mahajan VB, Sun Y. Review of ocular manifestations of Joubert syndrome. Genes (Basel). 2018;9(12):605. https://doi.org/10.3390/genes9120605.
98. Zhang J, Wang L, Chen W, Duan J, Meng Y, Yang H, Guo Q. Whole exome sequencing facilitated the diagnosis in four Chinese pediatric cases of Joubert syndrome related disorders. Am J Transl Res. 2022;14(7):5088–97.
99. Hartill V, Szymanska K, Sharif SM, Wheway G, Johnson CA. Meckel-Gruber syndrome: an update on diagnosis, clinical management, and research advances. Front Pediatr. 2017;5:244. https://doi.org/10.3389/fped.2017.00244.
100. Spiteri Cornish K, Ho J, Downes S, Scott NW, Bainbridge J, Lois N. The epidemiology of Stargardt disease in the United Kingdom. Ophthalmol Retina. 2017;1(6):508–13. https://doi.org/10.1016/j.oret.2017.03.001. Epub 2017 Apr 21.
101. Huang D, Heath Jeffery RC, Aung-Htut MT, McLenachan S, Fletcher S, Wilton SD, Chen FK. Stargardt disease and progress in therapeutic strategies. Ophthalmic Genet. 2022;43(1):1–26. https://doi.org/10.1080/13816810.2021.1966053. Epub 2021 Aug 29.
102. Strauss RW, Muñoz B, Ho A, Jha A, Michaelides M, Mohand-Said S, Cideciyan AV, Birch D, Hariri AH, Nittala MG, Sadda S, Scholl HPN, ProgStar Study Group. Incidence of atrophic lesions in Stargardt disease in the progression of atrophy secondary to Stargardt disease (ProgStar) study: report no. 5. JAMA Ophthalmol. 2017;135(7):687–95. https://doi.org/10.1001/jamaophthalmol.2017.1121.
103. Klufas MA, Tsui I, Sadda SR, Hosseini H, Schwartz SD. Ultrawidefield autofluorescence in ABCA4 Stargardt disease. Retina. 2018;38(2):403–15. https://doi.org/10.1097/IAE.0000000000001567.
104. Roborel de Climens A, Tugaut B, Dias Barbosa C, Buggage R, Brun-Strang C. Living with Stargardt disease: insights from patients and their parents. Ophthalmic Genet. 2021;42(2):150–60. https://doi.org/10.1080/13816810.2020.1855663. Epub 2020 Dec 11.
105. Kubota R, Birch DG, Gregory JK, Koester JM. Randomised study evaluating the pharmacodynamics of emixustat hydrochloride in subjects with macular atrophy secondary to Stargardt disease. Br J Ophthalmol. 2022;106(3):403–8. https://doi.org/10.1136/bjophthalmol-2020-317712. Epub 2020 Nov 19.
106. Radu RA, Mata NL, Nusinowitz S, Liu X, Sieving PA, Travis GH. Treatment with isotretinoin inhibits lipofuscin accumulation in a mouse model of recessive Stargardt's macular degeneration. Proc Natl Acad Sci U S A. 2003;100(8):4742–7. https://doi.org/10.1073/pnas.0737855100. Epub 2003 Apr 1.
107. Wang Y, Ma X, Muthuraman P, Raja A, Jayaraman A, Petrukhin K, Cioffi CL, Ma JX, Moiseyev G. The novel visual cycle inhibitor (±)-RPE65-61 protects retinal photoreceptors from light-induced degenera-

tion. PLoS One. 2022;17(10):e0269437. https://doi.org/10.1371/journal.pone.0269437.

108. Mehat MS, Sundaram V, Ripamonti C, Robson AG, Smith AJ, Borooah S, Robinson M, Rosenthal AN, Innes W, Weleber RG, Lee RWJ, Crossland M, Rubin GS, Dhillon B, Steel DHW, Anglade E, Lanza RP, Ali RR, Michaelides M, Bainbridge JWB. Transplantation of human embryonic stem cell-derived retinal pigment epithelial cells in macular degeneration. Ophthalmology. 2018;125(11):1765–75. https://doi.org/10.1016/j.ophtha.2018.04.037. Epub 2018 Jun 5.
109. Gullapalli VK, Zarbin MA. New prospects for retinal pigment epithelium transplantation. Asia Pac J Ophthalmol (Phila). 2022;11(4):302–13. https://doi.org/10.1097/APO.0000000000000521. Epub 2022 Aug 30.
110. Johnson AA, Guziewicz KE, Lee CJ, Kalathur RC, Pulido JS, Marmorstein LY, Marmorstein AD. Bestrophin 1 and retinal disease. Prog Retin Eye Res. 2017;58:45–69. https://doi.org/10.1016/j.preteyeres.2017.01.006. Epub 2017 Jan 30.
111. Vedantham V, Ramasamy K. Optical coherence tomography in Best's disease: an observational case report. Am J Ophthalmol. 2005;139(2):351–3. https://doi.org/10.1016/j.ajo.2004.07.039.
112. O'Gorman S, Flaherty WA, Fishman GA, Berson EL. Histopathologic findings in Best's vitelliform macular dystrophy. Arch Ophthalmol. 1988;106(9):1261–8. https://doi.org/10.1001/archopht.1988.01060140421045.
113. Battaglia Parodi M, Iacono P, Romano F, Bandello F. Spectral domain optical coherence tomography features in different stages of best vitelliform macular dystrophy. Retina. 2018;38(5):1041–6. https://doi.org/10.1097/IAE.0000000000001634.
114. Qian CX, Charran D, Strong CR, Steffens TJ, Jayasundera T, Heckenlively JR. Optical coherence tomography examination of the retinal pigment epithelium in best vitelliform macular dystrophy. Ophthalmology. 2017;124(4):456–63. https://doi.org/10.1016/j.ophtha.2016.11.022. Epub 2017 Feb 7.
115. Burgess R, Millar ID, Leroy BP, Urquhart JE, Fearon IM, De Baere E, Brown PD, Robson AG, Wright GA, Kestelyn P, Holder GE, Webster AR, Manson FD, Black GC. Biallelic mutation of BEST1 causes a distinct retinopathy in humans. Am J Hum Genet. 2008;82(1):19–31. https://doi.org/10.1016/j.ajhg.2007.08.004.
116. Tsunoda K, Hanazono G. Microstructural changes of photoreceptor layers detected by ultrahigh-resolution SD-OCT in patients with autosomal recessive bestrophinopathy. Am J Ophthalmol Case Rep. 2022;28:101706. https://doi.org/10.1016/j.ajoc.2022.101706.
117. Brecher R, Bird AC. Adult vitelliform macular dystrophy. Eye (Lond). 1990;4(Pt 1):210–5. https://doi.org/10.1038/eye.1990.28.
118. Querques G, Forte R, Querques L, Massamba N, Souied EH. Natural course of adult-onset foveomacular vitelliform dystrophy: a spectral-domain optical coherence tomography analysis. Am J Ophthalmol. 2011;152(2):304–13. https://doi.org/10.1016/j.ajo.2011.01.047. Epub 2011 Jun 12.
119. Gass JD. A clinicopathologic study of a peculiar foveomacular dystrophy. Trans Am Ophthalmol Soc. 1974;72:139–56.
120. Patrinely JR, Lewis RA, Font RL. Foveomacular vitelliform dystrophy, adult type. A clinicopathologic study including electron microscopic observations. Ophthalmology. 1985;92(12):1712–8. https://doi.org/10.1016/s0161-6420(85)34097-6.
121. Bansal R, Yangzes S, Singh R, Katoch D, Dogra MR, Gupta V, Gupta A. Retinal pigment epithelium aperture: a late-onset complication in adult-onset foveomacular vitelliform dystrophy. Indian J Ophthalmol. 2018;66(1):83–8. https://doi.org/10.4103/ijo.IJO_676_17.
122. Birtel J, von Landenberg C, Gliem M, Gliem C, Reimann J, Kunz WS, Herrmann P, Betz C, Caswell R, Nesbitt V, Kornblum C, Charbel IP. Mitochondrial retinopathy. Ophthalmol Retina. 2022;6(1):65–79. https://doi.org/10.1016/j.oret.2021.02.017. Epub 2021 Jul 10.
123. Mustafi D, Bharathan SP, Calderon R, Nagiel A. Human cellular models for retinal disease: from induced pluripotent stem cells to organoids. Retina. 2022;42(10):1829–35. https://doi.org/10.1097/IAE.0000000000003571.
124. Burnight ER, Gupta M, Wiley LA, Anfinson KR, Tran A, Triboulet R, Hoffmann JM, Klaahsen DL, Andorf JL, Jiao C, Sohn EH, Adur MK, Ross JW, Mullins RF, Daley GQ, Schlaeger TM, Stone EM, Tucker BA. Using CRISPR-Cas9 to generate gene-corrected autologous iPSCs for the treatment of inherited retinal degeneration. Mol Ther. 2017;25(9):1999–2013. https://doi.org/10.1016/j.ymthe.2017.05.015. Epub 2017 Jun 12.
125. Garafalo AV, Cideciyan AV, Héon E, Sheplock R, Pearson A, WeiYang YC, Sumaroka A, Aguirre GD, Jacobson SG. Progress in treating inherited retinal diseases: early subretinal gene therapy clinical trials and candidates for future initiatives. Prog Retin Eye Res. 2020;77:100827. https://doi.org/10.1016/j.preteyeres.2019.100827. Epub 2019 Dec 30.
126. Maguire AM, Russell S, Wellman JA, Chung DC, Yu ZF, Tillman A, Wittes J, Pappas J, Elci O, Marshall KA, McCague S, Reichert H, Davis M, Simonelli F, Leroy BP, Wright JF, High KA, Bennett J. Efficacy, safety, and durability of voretigene neparvovec-rzyl in RPE65 mutation-associated inherited retinal dystrophy: results of phase 1 and 3 trials. Ophthalmology. 2019;126(9):1273–85. https://doi.org/10.1016/j.ophtha.2019.06.017. Epub 2019 Jun 22.
127. Pennesi ME, Schlecther CL. The evolution of retinal gene therapy: from clinical trials to clinical prac-

tice. Ophthalmology. 2020;127(2):148–50. https://doi.org/10.1016/j.ophtha.2019.12.003. Erratum in: Ophthalmology. 2020;127(4):557.

128. Testa F, Melillo P, Di Iorio V, Iovino C, Farinaro F, Karali M, Banfi S, Rossi S, Della Corte M, Simonelli F. Visual function and retinal changes after voretigene neparvovec treatment in children with biallelic RPE65-related inherited retinal dystrophy. Sci Rep. 2022;12(1):17637. https://doi.org/10.1038/s41598-022-22180-6.
129. Gange WS, Sisk RA, Besirli CG, Lee TC, Havunjian M, Schwartz H, Borchert M, Sengillo JD, Mendoza C, Berrocal AM, Nagiel A. Perifoveal chorioretinal atrophy after subretinal voretigene neparvovec-rzyl for RPE65-mediated Leber congenital amaurosis. Ophthalmol Retina. 2022;6(1):58–64. https://doi.org/10.1016/j.oret.2021.03.016. Epub 2021 Apr 8.
130. Deng C, Zhao PY, Branham K, Schlegel D, Fahim AT, Jayasundera TK, Khan N, Besirli CG. Real-world outcomes of voretigene neparvovec treatment in pediatric patients with RPE65-associated Leber congenital amaurosis. Graefes Arch Clin Exp Ophthalmol. 2022;260(5):1543–50. https://doi.org/10.1007/s00417-021-05508-2. Epub 2022 Jan 10.
131. Parker MA, Erker LR, Audo I, Choi D, Mohand-Said S, Sestakauskas K, Benoit P, Appelqvist T, Krahmer M, Ségaut-Prévost C, Lujan BJ, Faridi A, Chegarnov EN, Steinkamp PN, Ku C, da Palma MM, Barale PO, Ayelo-Scheer S, Lauer A, Stout T, Wilson DJ, Weleber RG, Pennesi ME, Sahel JA, Yang P. Three-year safety results of SAR422459 (EIAV-ABCA4) gene therapy in patients with ABCA4-associated Stargardt disease: an open-label dose-escalation phase I/IIa clinical trial, cohorts 1-5. Am J Ophthalmol. 2022;240:285–301. https://doi.org/10.1016/j.ajo.2022.02.013. Epub 2022 Mar 4.
132. Pennesi ME, Yang P, Birch DG, Weng CY, Moore AT, Iannaccone A, Comander JI, Jayasundera T, Chulay J, XLRS-001 Study Group. Intravitreal delivery of rAAV2tYF-CB-hRS1 vector for gene augmentation therapy in patients with X-linked retinoschisis: 1-year clinical results. Ophthalmol Retina. 2022;6(12):1130–44. https://doi.org/10.1016/j.oret.2022.06.013. Epub 2022 Jun 30.
133. Santos A, Humayun MS, de Juan E Jr, Greenburg RJ, Marsh MJ, Klock IB, Milam AH. Preservation of the inner retina in retinitis pigmentosa. A morphometric analysis. Arch Ophthalmol. 1997;115(4):511–5. https://doi.org/10.1001/archopht.1997.01100150513011.
134. De Silva SR, Moore AT. Optogenetic approaches to therapy for inherited retinal degenerations. J Physiol. 2022;600(21):4623–32. https://doi.org/10.1113/JP282076. Epub 2022 Aug 17.
135. Sahel JA, Boulanger-Scemama E, Pagot C, Arleo A, Galluppi F, Martel JN, Esposti SD, Delaux A, de Saint Aubert JB, de Montleau C, Gutman E, Audo I, Duebel J, Picaud S, Dalkara D, Blouin L, Taiel M, Roska B. Partial recovery of visual function in a blind patient after optogenetic therapy. Nat Med. 2021;27(7):1223–9.https://doi.org/10.1038/s41591--021-01351-4. Epub 2021 May 24.
136. Fujinami K, Yang L, Joo K, Tsunoda K, Kameya S, Hanazono G, Fujinami-Yokokawa Y, Arno G, Kondo M, Nakamura N, Kurihara T, Tsubota K, Zou X, Li H, Park KH, Iwata T, Miyake Y, Woo SJ, Sui R, East Asia Inherited Retinal Disease Society Study Group. Clinical and genetic characteristics of east Asian patients with occult macular dystrophy (Miyake disease): east Asia occult macular dystrophy studies report number 1. Ophthalmology. 2019;126(10):1432–44. https://doi.org/10.1016/j.ophtha.2019.04.032. Epub 2019 Apr 25.
137. Yahya S, Smith CEL, Poulter JA, McKibbin M, Arno G, Ellingford J, Kämpjärvi K, Khan MI, Cremers FPM, Hardcastle AJ, Castle B, Steel DHW, Webster AR, Black GC, El-Asrag ME, Ali M, Toomes C, Inglehearn CF, UK Inherited Retinal Dystrophy Consortium, Genomics England Research Consortium. Late-onset autosomal dominant macular degeneration caused by deletion of the CRX gene. Ophthalmology. 2023;130(1):68–76. https://doi.org/10.1016/j.ophtha.2022.07.023. Epub 2022 Aug 5.
138. Sohocki MM, Sullivan LS, Mintz-Hittner HA, Birch D, Heckenlively JR, Freund CL, McInnes RR, Daiger SP. A range of clinical phenotypes associated with mutations in CRX, a photoreceptor transcription-factor gene. Am J Hum Genet. 1998;63(5):1307–15. https://doi.org/10.1086/302101.
139. Spaide RF. Treatment of Sorsby fundus dystrophy with anti-tumor necrosis factor-alpha medication. Eye (Lond). 2022;36(9):1810–2. https://doi.org/10.1038/s41433-021-01735-3. Epub 2021 Aug 10.
140. Bryan JM, Rojas CN, Mirza RG. Macular findings expedite accurate diagnosis of MIDD in a young female patient with newly diagnosed diabetes. Am J Ophthalmol Case Rep. 2022;27:101578. https://doi.org/10.1016/j.ajoc.2022.101578.
141. Ambonville C, Meas T, Lecleire-Collet A, Laloi-Michelin M, Virally M, Kevorkian JP, Paques M, Massin P, Guillausseau PJ. Macular pattern dystrophy in MIDD: long-term follow-up. Diabetes Metab. 2008;34(4 Pt 1):389–91. https://doi.org/10.1016/j.diabet.2008.05.002. Epub 2008 Jun 30.
142. Agarwal A, editor. Gass' atlas of macular diseases, vol. 1. 5th ed. Saunders/Elsevier; 2012. p. 240–436.

14 Vascular Malformations, Childhood Cancer Predisposition Syndromes and Their Systemic Associations

14.1 Introduction

Retinal vascular malformations and tumours arising in the various structures of the eye are rare and benign in their course. However, they compromise the vision of the affected eye to varying degrees. More importantly, however, these have strong genetic implications and systemic associations. Complications and morbidity arising from these can be anticipated by ophthalmic examination long before these manifest clinically. Retinoblastoma (RB), retinal capillary hemangioblastoma, retinal astrocytoma, Neurofibromatosis type1 and type 2, and Ciliary body medulloepithelioma are some of the childhood cancer predisposition syndromes that have significant ocular manifestations. Neurofibromatosis type 1 is associated with optic pathway glioma. These patients may develop high-grade glioma in the brain and malignant peripheral nerve sheath tumours. Detection of highly characteristic retinal astrocytomas associated with tuberous sclerosis can help to timely detect subependymal giant cell astrocytoma. Retinoblastoma, arising from the primitive retina, is one of the most common intraocular malignant tumours in infancy and early childhood. It is locally invasive if not detected in time, leading to distant metastasis and fatal outcomes. External beam radiation therapy and chemotherapy for retinoblastoma are associated with the late development of osteogenic sarcomas and other cancers. The most common intraocular malignant tumour in adulthood is malignant uveal melanoma, which may have distant metastasis before it gets detected. Discussion on this cancer is beyond the scope of this chapter and is not discussed hereafter. The following retinal vascular malformations and retinal astrocytoma have strong systemic associations and will be discussed in some detail.

1. Retinal capillary hemangioblastoma (von Hippel-Lindau's disease).
2. Capillary hemangioma of the choroid (Sturge-Weber syndrome).
3. Arteriovenous malformation (Wyburn Mason syndrome).
4. Congenital retinal macrovessels.
5. Cavernous hemangioma of the retina.
6. Retinal astrocytoma.
7. Neurofibromatosis type 1.
8. Neurofibromatosis type 2.
9. Retinoblastoma.

A. Gupta et al., *Ophthalmic Signs in Practice of Medicine*,
https://doi.org/10.1007/978-981-99-7923-3_14

14.2 Retinal Capillary Hemangioblastoma

14.2.1 Retinal Capillary Hemangioblastoma—Historical Aspects

Retinal capillary hemangioblastoma, more popularly called retinal angioma, is not rare, with a point prevalence of heterozygotes in 1:54,000 and an estimated rate of 1:36,000 in live births [1]. It is a multisystem disorder, but patients in their mid-twenties usually present to their ophthalmologist with visual complaints. In large tertiary care centres, these patients may receive ocular screening from other disciplines. First described by von Hippel in 1904 as a rare retinal angioma, its association with a cerebellar hemangioblastoma was first described as Lindau's disease in 1927, and only about a decade later, it got the name von Hippel Lindau's (VHL) disease, a name that has stuck. https://eyewiki.org/w/index.php?title=Retinal_Capillary_Hemangioblastoma_and_von_Hippel-Lindau_Disease&oldid=81219

14.2.2 Retinal Capillary Hemangioblastoma—Genetic Aspects

Germline mutations in a tumour suppressor gene located on the short arm of chromosome 3 in the region 3p25-26 cause VHL disease [2]. In most patients, the VHL disease is autosomal dominant with a high degree of penetrance, but in about 20%, it is seen as a sporadic tumour. The tumour suppressor genes typically control and regulate the unbridled proliferation of cells, and the inactivation of both gene copies leads to cancer formation. It is a prime example of Knudson's two-hit theory regarding the tumour suppressor genes (antioncogenes) [3]. People born with a single copy of the abnormal gene and develop, post-conception, a somatic mutation at random (by loss, mutation, or methylation) in the wild-type allele in a single cell develop a sporadic single organ disease not transmittable to the offspring [4, 5]. Typically, the VHL protein is responsible for the degradation of Hypoxia-inducible factor under normoxic conditions. The mutant VHL protein cannot carry out this degradation and hence cannot control the transcription of the VEGF and PDGF mRNA, leading to the formation of hemangioblastoma [6]. The other cancers caused by tumour suppressor genes are seen in sporadic and inherited forms; the prime examples, among several others, are retinoblastoma, neuroblastoma, and the Wilms' tumour [3]. Patients born with complete deletion were less likely to develop retinal lesions than those born with partial deletion, missense, or nonsense mutations [7].

14.2.3 Retinal Capillary Hemangioblastoma—Systemic Associations

The inherited VHL disease develops multiple tumours and cysts in several organs at varying intervals. The most common among the affected organs are the kidneys, cerebellum, spinal cord, pancreas, adrenal glands (pheochromocytoma), and epididymis in males and broad ligament in females (Fig. 14.1) [8]. Before the institution of screening programs, mortality before the age of 50 years was common, mainly from cerebellar hemangioblastoma and clear cell RCC [9, 10].

The RCC develops in up to 70% of patients with VHL disease [9]. Patients who develop RCC (44 ± 10.9 years) are much older than those who develop cerebellar hemangioblastoma (29 ± 10 years) or retinal hemangioblastoma

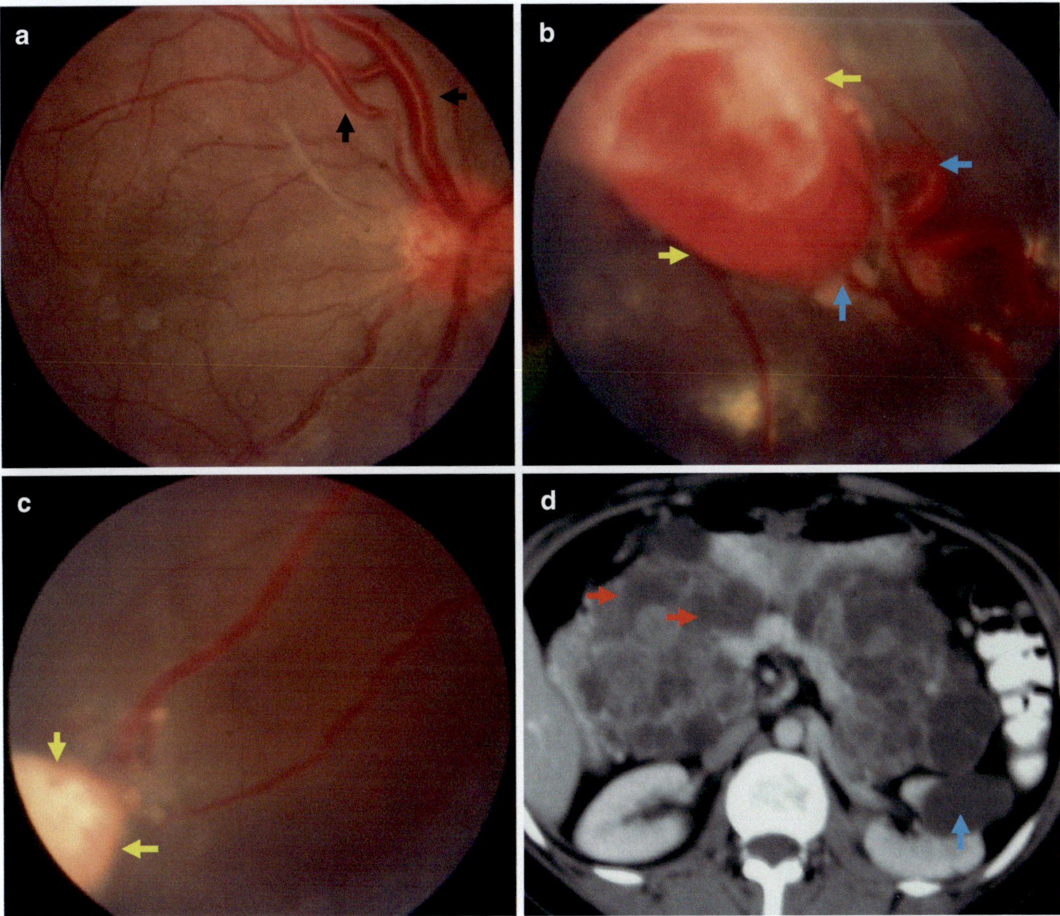

Fig. 14.1 Dilated, tortuous vessels in the right eye of a patient with VHL disease (**a**), especially of the superotemporal quadrant (black arrows), being the feeder vessels (blue arrow) of the retinal capillary haemangioma (yellow arrows) in the superotemporal periphery (**b**). The inferotemporal periphery also shows a retinal angioma (yellow arrow) (**c**). Axial CECT abdomen shows multiple cysts of varying sizes in the pancreas (red arrows) along with a simple cyst in visualized left kidney (blue arrow). Interpretation of image (**d**) by Dr. Chirag Ahuja, Department of Radiodiagnosis and imaging, Post Graduate Institute of Medical Education and Research, Chandigarh, India

(25.4 ± 12.7 years), with median survival being 49 years [4, 5]. Clustering of clinical features of VHL in different affected families may occur due to different mutations in the complex VHL locus on chromosome 3p25-26 [11]. More than 50% of inherited VHL may show only one systemic feature [4, 5]. The clinical diagnosis of VHL can be made in patients with a positive family history in the presence of even a single hemangioblastoma in the retina, nervous system, pheochromocytoma, RCC, or multiple pancreatic cysts (Fig. 14.1). Renal and epididymal cysts are too common to qualify for a diagnosis of VHL on their own [9, 10]. (See Box 14.1).

Box 14.1 Familial Phenotypes in von Hippel-Lindau Disease

Type	Ocular component	Systemic associations
Type 1	Retinal hemangioblastoma	Reduced risk of pheochromocytoma CNS hemangioblastoma; Pancreatic cysts and neoplasm; ccRCC
Type 2A	Retinal hemangioblastoma	Pheochromocytoma CNS hemangioblastoma No ccRCC
Type 2B	Retinal hemangioblastoma	Pheochromocytoma; CNS hemangioblastoma ccRCC
Type 2C	None	Pheochromocytoma alone

Abbreviations: *CNS* central nervous system; *cc* clear cell; *RCC* renal cell carcinoma.

Adapted with permission of the publishers from Lonser et al. [10].

The nervous system hemangioblastoma is a thin-walled, encapsulated benign tumour that is most common in the spinal cord and cerebellum and least common in the brain stem. These have variable periods of growth alternating with periods of growth arrest. These become symptomatic depending upon the availability of space to expand, most of the expansion occurring in the cysts rather than the solid tumours. Thus, the spinal cord and brain stem hemangioblastoma present earlier than the cerebellar tumours/cysts. Detected well in time, surgery can safely excise these [12]. Because of the pleomorphic nature of the VHL disease, a detailed family history, genetic testing and counselling, and comprehensive screening and care are required by a multidisciplinary team [10]. The kidneys have multiple cysts and solid tumours. Nearly 40% of the partial nephrectomy samples in VHL disease had clear cell renal carcinoma (RCC). Most solid lesions and 21% of the renal cysts harboured RCC [13]. The VHL is the commonest cause of inherited RCC. It is a major malignant lesion with variable periods of growth. It may be seen in up to 45% of patients with VHL. Renal cysts are often bilateral and multiple and remain asymptomatic. Detection of these cysts and tumours, before they become symptomatic in a screening program, improves the outcome of these tumours (Box 14.2).

Box 14.2 Screening Guidelines for von Hippel-Lindau Disease

	Beginning age in years for the tests					
Exam/Test/Labs	<5	5	11	15	30	65 and >
History and physical exam	Annual from the age of 1 year					
BP and pulse	Annual from the age of 2 years					
Dilated fundus exam	From <1 till 30 years every 6–12 months				Annual after 30 throughout life	
Blood metanephrine 24-hour urine catecholamines		Annual from 5 to 65 years of age				Skip routine after 65
MRI brain and spine			Every 2 years from 11 to 65 years of age			Skip routine after 65
MRI abdomen				Every 2 years from 15 to 65 years of age		Skip routine after 65
Audiogram			Every 2 years from 11 to 65 years of age			Skip routine after 65
MRI internal auditory canal				Once		

Adapted with permission from: https://www.vhl.org/patients/clinical-care/screening/.

14.2.4 Retinal Capillary Hemangioblastoma (Angiomas)

Retinal hemangioblastoma (angiomas) is a common lesion in patients with VHL disease and may occur in 50–60% of the patients. Although the usual age of presentation is mid-twenties, retinal screening of their offspring may discover retinal hemangioblastoma (RH) as early as one year. This red-coloured RH in the inherited VHL is

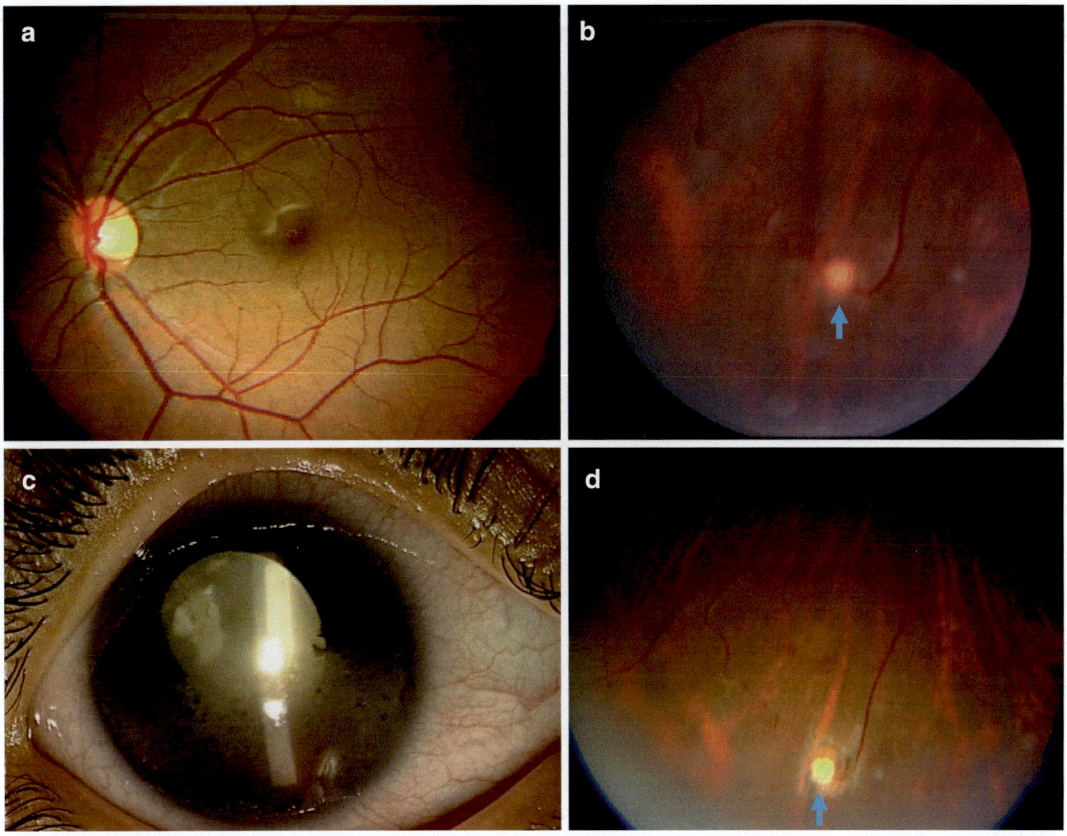

Fig. 14.2 Left eye (**a**) of a 12-year-old male, with a solitary retinal angioma (blue arrow) in inferior periphery (**b**). At 5 years follow-up, while the right eye failed treatment (**c**), the left eye remained stable (blue arrow) after laser photocoagulation (**d**)

often bilateral and multiple and is seen in the retinal periphery (Figs. 14.2 and 14.3). On OCT, these angiomas are seen as hyperreflective mass lesions in the inner retina, and as they grow, they push the retina outwards [14]. The sessile retinal angiomas may be seen on the optic disc or the juxtapapillary area Figs. 14.4 and 14.5). A single unilateral RH may be seen sporadically. However, in the presence of positive family history or any of the systemic lesions of VHL discussed above, the diagnosis of inherited VHL should be made. Notably, new RH may keep appearing over time in the young offspring. The RH may vary from the very small detected on screening of the offspring to the large symptomatic. As the peripheral RH lesions grow, they tend to develop a

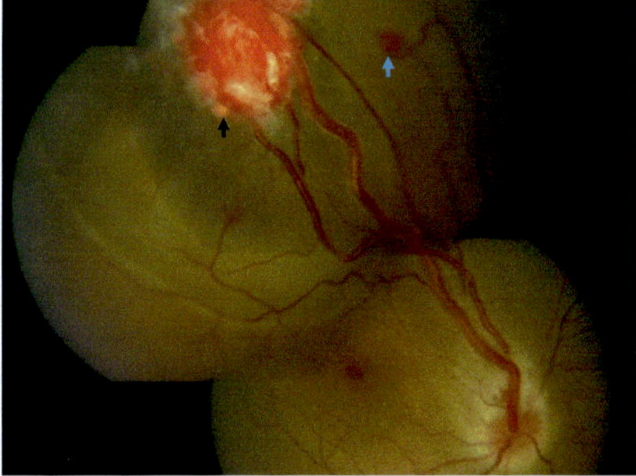

Fig. 14.3 A 24-year-old male with a family history of VHL presented with diminution of vison in right eye due to exudative retinal detachment. A large retinal angioma (black arrow) was seen in upper temporal periphery, along with a small angioma (blue arrow)

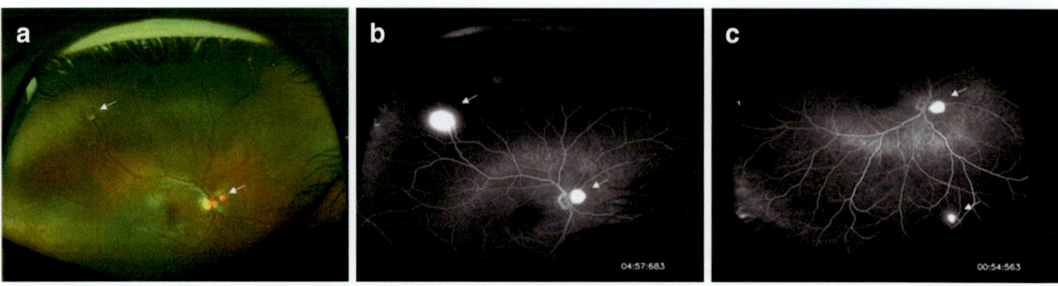

Fig. 14.4 A 29-year-old male presented with episodes of sweating, palpitations, headache, and breathlessness on exertion for 3 months. Detected to have paroxysmal hypertension, he was diagnosed with pheochromocytoma. Wide field fundus photograph (**a**) of right eye showed retinal angiomas (white arrows) nasal to optic disc and in superior periphery, suggestive of VHL disease. Fluorescein angiography showed hyperfluorescent lesions nasal to optic disc, in superior (**b**) and inferior (**c**) periphery

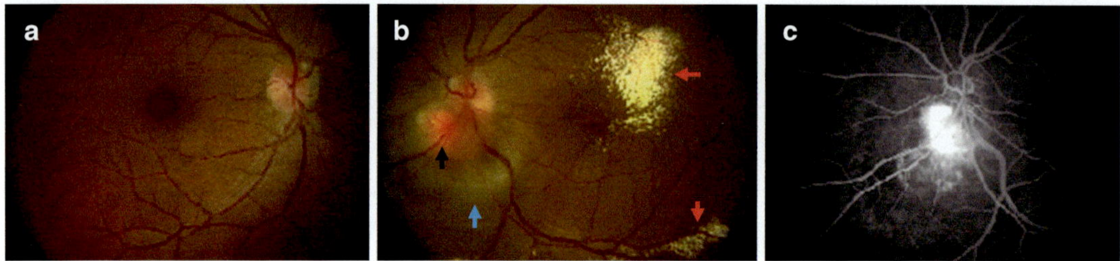

Fig. 14.5 A 37-year-old woman had loss of vision in left eye for 2 years, with vision 6/60. Right eye was normal (**a**). Left eye (**b**) had a juxtapapillary retinal capillary hemangioma (black arrow), peripapillary exudative retinal detachment (blue arrows), and retinal exudates (red arrows). There were no apparent feeder vessels. Fluorescein angiography showed the retinal angioma on the optic disc (**c**)

markedly dilated and tortuous feeder arteriole and a draining vein, a characteristic VHL feature (Figs. 14.1 and 14.3). The RH are highly permeable, and irrespective of the site, the leaking fluid, and exudates, accumulate in the macula as massive hard exudates and submacular fluid (Fig. 14.3). In the advanced stages, there may be a massive exudative retinal detachment. As the RH grow large, they develop fibrous proliferation on their surface, firmly adherent to the posterior vitreous face. The contracting scar tissue may pull the RH and the retina anteriorly, leading to a tractional retinal detachment. Fundus fluorescein angiography (FFA) is a sensitive tool for the early detection of even small angiomas, as these show early hyperfluorescence and late staining (Fig. 14.4) [14]. Ultrawide field FFA is helpful as most RH lesions are in the peripheral retina. It has been found to be more sensitive than ophthalmoscopy and the conventional FFA [15]. Further, on wide angle FFA, besides staining of the hemangioblastoma, nearly 1/3rd of the patients with larger peripheral retinal hemangioblastoma may show extensive non-perfusion of the peripheral retina, which may be associated with retinal neovascularization on the tumour surface [16].

The pathology of the cerebellar and retinal hemangioblastoma is similar and consists of a network of thin-walled capillary vessels, 8–14 μm in diameter and lined with flat endothelium. The capillary network is separated by vacuolated foamy (phospholipids-filled) stromal cells and collagenous fibres [17]. These stromal cells show heterozygosity for the VHL gene, but not the vascular cells and thus qualify for the label of a neoplasm. The overexpression of the VEGF is responsible for the massive new vessels in these tumours and increased permeability [6].

14.2.5 Treatment of von Hippel-Lindau's Disease

Various treatment strategies have been used, including plaque, external beam radiation, and photodynamic therapy, with mixed results. Except for laser photocoagulation for very small RH and Pars plana vitreous surgery for large tumours, no other strategy has been able to eradicate the RH tumour masses. Small RH (<1.5 mm) with or without exudation can be successfully treated with laser photocoagulation [18]. Peripheral angiomas >1.5 to <4 mm are more challenging to treat with laser photocoagulation and may require multiple treatment sessions (Fig. 14.6). The peripheral large RH lesions are treated with triple freeze-thaw cryotherapy applied either trans-conjunctival or trans-scleral after making a conjunctival incision. Cryotherapy runs the risk of increasing fibrous contraction and formation of tractional retinal detachment. Occasionally, the retina may develop tears leading to a combined tractional and rhegmatogenous retinal detachment. Pars plana vitreous (PPV) surgery to excise the tumour has the highest success rate for eradicating large RH tumours [18]. The PPV is often combined with scleral buckling. Doing laser photocoagulation preoperatively to the feeder vessels and the tumour mass may be helpful. The posterior vitreous hyaloid membrane is rather firmly adherent to the retina in young people, which poses a challenge to remove. Postoperative fibrous proliferation may necessitate more than one procedure [19, 20]. During vitreous surgery, a trans-vitreal ligation of the feeder vessel can be done before the enblock dissection of the tumour [21]. Although the fundamental molecular mechanisms in VHL are well known, there have been mixed results with antibodies against these growth factors [22]. Combining ranibizumab with an anti-PDGF therapy in a phase1/2 trial did not yield a positive outcome [23].

14.2.6 Active Surveillance in VHL

Since it is not known when the lesions will start or progress, all patients with a VHL tumour, a family history, or a genetic test positive for VHL should remain under active surveillance of a multidisciplinary team. See Box 14.2 (https://www.vhl.org/clinicians/surveillance/).

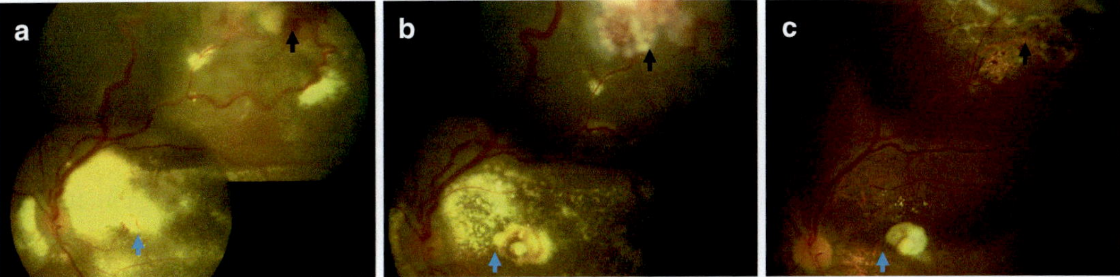

Fig. 14.6 A large peripheral retinal angioma (black arrow) with extensive exudation (blue arrows) was treated with multiple sessions of laser photocoagulation treatment (**a**). At 3 months (**b**), there was a decrease in the size of the angioma along with reduction of exudation. At 16 months (**c**), there was near-complete regression of the angioma and exudation

14.3 Sturge-Weber Syndrome

Sturge-Weber syndrome (SWS) is an uncommon neuro-ocular-cutaneous syndrome classified as one phakomatosis. A phakomatosis is a group of neuro-cutaneous hamartomas that are essentially non-cancerous, disorganized, self-limiting abnormal growth of the native tissues (including connective and vascular) in a specific body region. There are four components of the SWS, a congenital port-wine stain (PWS) (Fig. 14.7), capillary hemangioma of the choroid, glaucoma, and leptomeningeal angiomas. Secondary glaucoma complicates nearly 2/3rd of the children with facial PWS who develop ocular-neurological signs and is a major cause of childhood glaucoma leading to buphthalmos and blindness. Adolescent patients may have late-onset glaucoma [24]. Whole genome sequencing of tissue samples led to the discovery of a somatic mosaic single nucleotide mutation (c.548G → A, p.Arg183Gln) in the Guanine nucleotide-binding protein G (q) subunit α (GNAQ) gene in 88% of the SWS and 92% of the non-syndromic PWS. The severity and the extent of the clinical manifestation depend upon the time of the somatic mutations [25]. This mutation has been found in the episcleral and scleral tissue of all patients with SWS and glaucoma [26, 27].

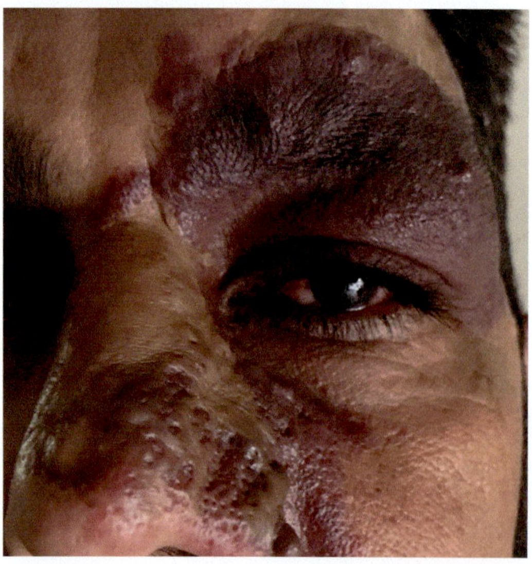

Fig. 14.7 Congenital port-wine stain (PWS) in a 40-year-old male patient of Sturge-Weber syndrome (SWS)

14.3.1 Sturge-Weber Syndrome—Port-Wine Stain

Port-wine stain (PWS), a birthmark seen in 0.3% of all newborns, is present mainly in the head and neck, but can be present in any part of the body. Nearly 8–10% of patients with PWS have ocular (glaucoma) and neurological complications (epilepsy) that constitute the SWS. However, the most prominent feature of the SWS is the presence of the PWS in the distribution of the first division of the trigeminal nerve-the dermatome V1 [24]. PWS may also accompany these in the distribution of the V2 and V3. Notably, the PWS not involving the V1 is not associated with the SWS. Nearly 32–65% of patients with PWS in the V1 dermatome have ocular and/or neurological associations [28]. Although in the past, the PWS has been described in the context of the trigeminal nerve dermatomes, it is now known that these are purely vascular lesions and have nothing to do with nerves and hence need to be described in the context of location rather than dermatome [29].

The PWS, red or darker in colour and called naevus flammeus, consists of permanently dilated, malformed dermal vessels. The PWS appears to follow the distribution of the trigeminal nerve dermatomes and is generally restricted to the skin of one-half of the forehead, face, and the ipsilateral lids (Fig. 14.7). The presence of the PWS on the upper or the lower lid carries a lifelong risk of developing glaucoma [29]. However, bilateral lesions of PWS can be seen in 10–20% of patients [28]. The PWS should be treated with a pulsed dye laser in infancy[29]. The PWS must be differentiated from benign periocular capillary hemangiomas present at birth or in infancy in nearly 10% of newborns. These may be strawberry nevi in the superficial dermis, which may also be combined with a subcutaneous component, or subcutaneous nevi may be associated with orbital hemangioma [30]. The superficial periocular hemangiomas may appear as small macular lesions of telangiectatic vessels that may grow during infancy. However, a large majority will spontaneously involute with time by 4–7 years of age. In the past, ultrasonography or

MRI scans were used to define the site of these hemangiomas. More recently, using a Swept source Doppler Optical coherence tomography, the malformed vessels of the PWS were found to be 114 ± 92 μ in diameter, increasing in diameter with their depth in the dermis compared to 39 ± 19 μ seen in the capillary hemangioma. Although highly variable, both were seen at an almost similar mean depth of about 300 μ. The large cavitary lesions of the PWS also showed blood flow on Doppler. While nearly 3/4th of vessels in the hemangioma were capillaries, only 1/3rd of the vessels in the PWS were capillaries [31]. It has been shown that compared to the non-involved skin, vessels in the PWS are poorly innervated by the autonomic nerve fibres that regulate the vessel diameter. Hence, the absence of these fibres leads to uncontrolled dilatation/ectasia of these vessels [32].

14.3.2 Sturge-Weber Syndrome—Diffuse Choroidal Hemangioma

Diffuse choroidal hemangioma (DCH) is a common association of SWS and may be seen in up to 55% of cases [33]. The fundus in diffuse hemangioma appears 'tomato ketchup' coloured due to the expansion of the choroidal vasculature that has no well-defined borders (Fig. 14.8). The clinical diagnosis of diffuse choroidal hemangioma

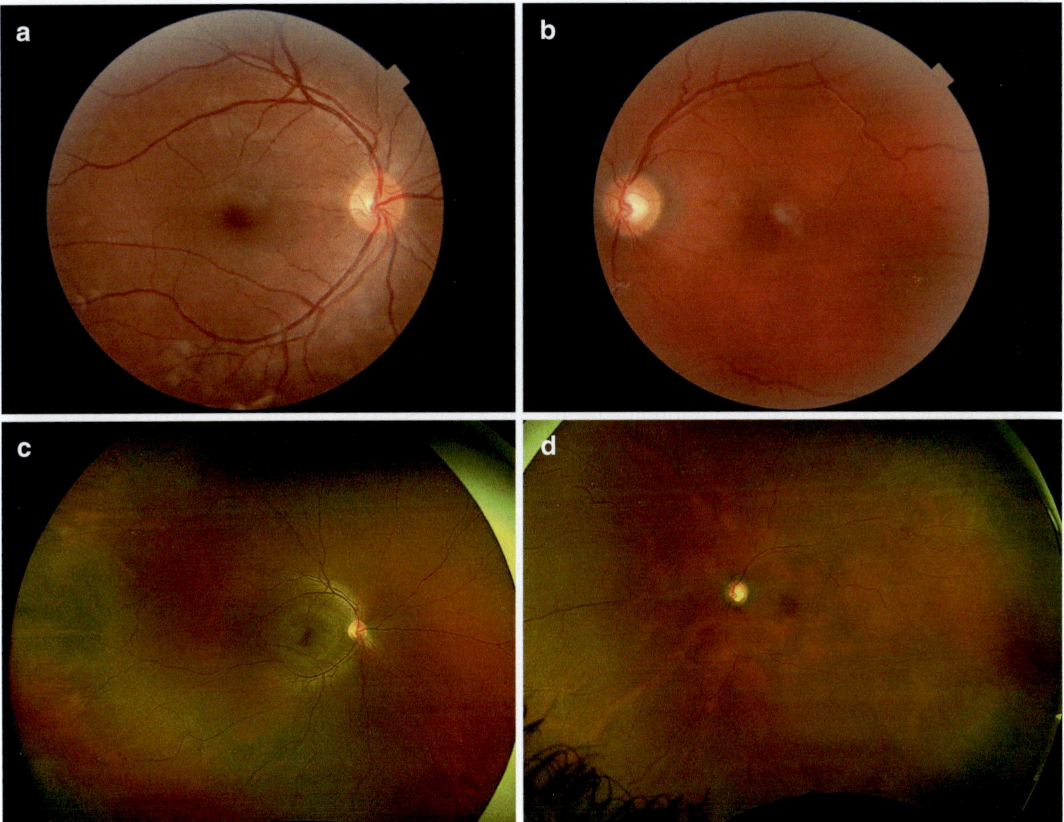

Fig. 14.8 Diffuse choroidal haemangioma. Conventional camera fundus photographs of right (**a**) and left (**b**) eyes of the patient in Fig. 14.7, and ultrawide field fundus photographs of right (**c**) and left (**d**) eyes of the same patient. The fundus in diffuse haemangioma (left eye in this case) appears 'tomato ketchup' coloured due to the expansion of the choroidal vasculature that has no well-defined borders. The clinical diagnosis of diffuse choroidal haemangioma can be a challenge and is best noted by quickly comparing the colour of the fundus in the affected eye (left eye in this case) with the contralateral normal eye (right eye in this case)

can be challenging and is best noted by quickly comparing the colour of the fundus in the affected eye with the contralateral eye. Diffuse choroidal hemangioma may be bilateral in nearly 20% of the patients with SWS, compounding the clinical diagnosis. DCH is very commonly associated with leptomeningeal angiomas. Thus, patients who have PWS must undergo a retina exam to detect it. On optical coherence tomography (OCT), there is a loss of the usual pattern of the choroidal vasculature, thickening of the choroid, and loss of the choroido-scleral interface [34]. There is anecdotal evidence that photodynamic therapy (PDT) with verteporfin for diffuse choroidal hemangioma may improve vision and stabilize the hemangioma [35]. In the past, diffuse choroidal hemangioma with symptomatic exudation was subjected to external beam radiotherapy over 4 weeks. More recently, plaque therapy for 4 days has been found highly successful for quick resolution of the subretinal fluid in these hemangiomas [36].

14.3.3 Circumscribed Choroidal Hemangiomas Are Not Associated with SWS

Diffuse hemangiomas must also be differentiated from circumscribed choroidal hemangiomas (CCH). While DCH may be asymptomatic, both may cause localized or diffuse exudative retinal detachment. However, it is unusual for a CCH to be associated with SWS. In more than 1/3rd of the patients, CCH may be mistaken for metastatic deposits or an amelanotic choroidal melanoma [37]. The CCH are always a unilateral, orange-coloured solitary lesion, often located in the posterior pole. The lesion may have a pigmented outline and some punctate white spots on the surface, both occurring due to alterations in the overlying RPE. Early hyperfluorescence during indocyanine green angiography and fundus fluorescein angiography, and late fluorescence are highly characteristic (Fig. 14.9) [38]. On OCT angiography, a distinct pattern of abnormal vessels can be seen in the choriocapillaris slab with clear demarcation between the normal and the affected area [39]. These are associated with serous detachment of the retina (Fig. 14.9). In the past, the long-term visual outcome of treatment with external beam radiation, plaque therapy, or laser photocoagulation remained poor in most eyes [37, 40]. Introducing photodynamic therapy (PDT) with intravenous verteporfin has vastly improved the visual outcome in circumscribed choroidal hemangiomas ([41]). Adding anti-VEGF therapy to PDT may improve the visual outcome [42].

14.3.4 Sturge-Weber Syndrome—Glaucoma

Unilateral glaucoma is commonly associated with SWS and may be seen in up to 71% of the patients with this syndrome [33]. Glaucoma in SWS has a bimodal presentation, nearly 2/3rd presenting early in infancy or up to 2 years of age with raised intraocular pressure, open-angle, and even buphthalmos due to enlargement of the globe and cornea and corneal edema. Anterior chamber anomalies are likely responsible for this type of glaucoma. Nearly 1/3rd of patients with glaucoma may present after 5 years of age or in young adolescents. The raised episcleral venous pressure is likely responsible for raised intra-ocular pressure in such patients. The conjunctival and episcleral involvement is seen as dilated, and tortuous vessels are seen in up to 70% of the cases with SWS. Electron microscopy studies in a 20-year-old woman with SWS revealed the presence of a cluster of abnormal vessels and the accumulation of granular extracellular matrix in the trabecular meshwork [43]. The raised episcleral venous pressure in patients presenting late may be due to intrascleral or episcleral hemangioma. The veins draining from the canal of Schelmm may likely be draining into the hemangioma, or even the canal of Schelmm may be a part of the hemangioma [44]. The episcleral venous pressure in SWS-associated glaucoma is significantly higher than in the normal contralateral eye [45]. Patients with PWS remain at risk for developing glaucoma throughout life and should have an annual checkup of their eyes [46]. Medical management of SWS glaucoma includes timolol maleate, and latanoprost may be effective in a small number of cases,

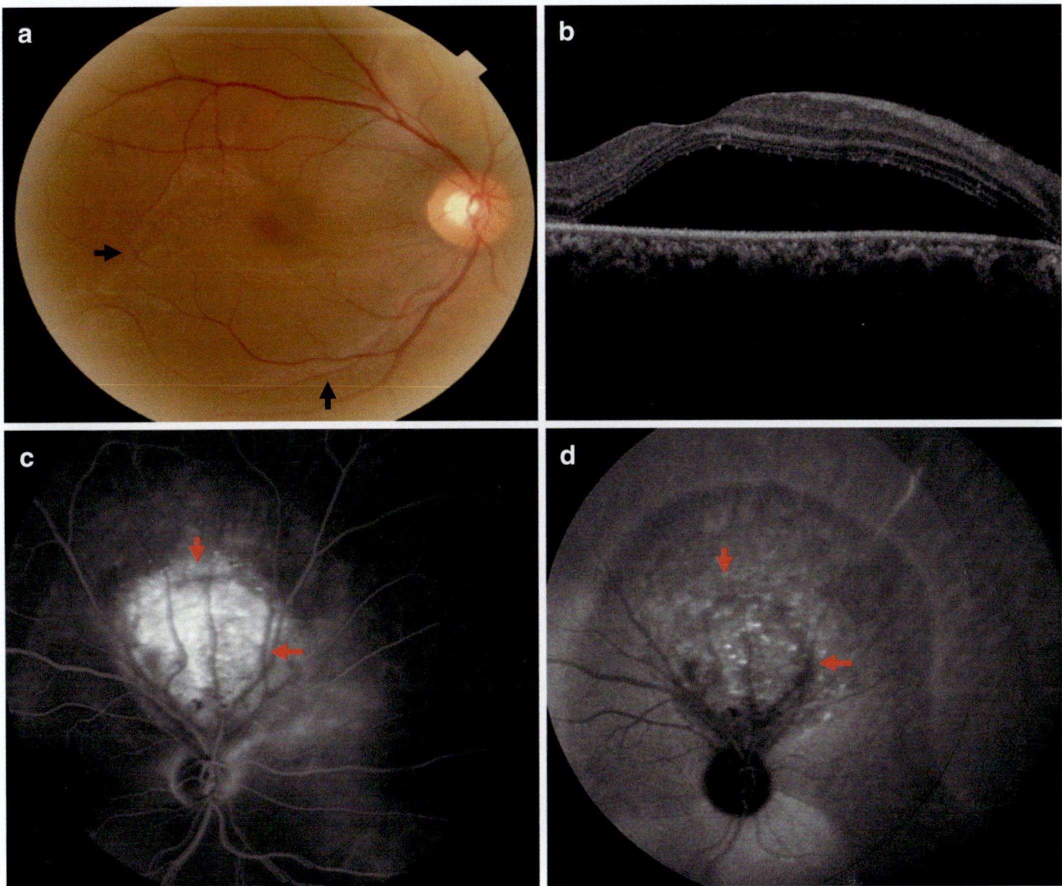

Fig. 14.9 Circumscribed choroidal haemangioma: fundus photograph (**a**) showing exudative retinal detachment (black arrows) in right eye due to a circumscribed choroidal haemangioma along the upper temporal vessels (blue arrow). OCT through macula shows serous retinal detachment (**b**). Fluorescein and ICG angiography show the hyperfluorescence due to the choroidal haemangioma (**c**, **d**)

a majority requiring an Ahmed glaucoma valve (AGV) drainage implant to normalize the pressure. Exudative and even haemorrhagic choroidal detachments are frequent in the presence of diffuse choroidal hemangioma. Preoperative use of oral propranolol has been found highly effective in preventing and treating these sight-threatening complications [47, 48].

14.3.5 Sturge-Weber Syndrome—Neurological Associations

Nearly 80% of children with SWS develop seizures, and 75% get them before one year. Patients with PWS in trigeminal nerve dermatomes V1 and V2 are likelier to have these than those with PWS elsewhere. More than half of the patients also suffer from delayed development [49]. The delayed development may be linked to a deficiency of growth hormones in SWS [50]. In neuroimaging studies, a leptomeningeal angioma is seen in the parieto-occipital area, which is seen as ipsilateral to the PWS and has a strong association with diffuse choroidal hemangioma also on the same side. A CT scan may reveal an S-shaped calcification associated with cortical atrophy [28]. However, the contrast-enhanced MRI scan is superior to a CT scan for evaluating patients with SWS [51, 52], especially for demonstrating the cortical atrophy and also the patency and extent of the leptomeningeal angioma. In the past, it was recommended that children with SWS should have neuroimaging done from 6 to 12 months of age and, if positive, should have an FDG-PET scan for initiating prophylactic anti-epileptic therapy [28]. However, recently there has been a change in the recommendations for neuroimaging. Routine screening for neuroimaging is not recommended in infants and newborns with high-risk PWS but no history of seizures or neurological symptoms. It should be done only in select cases if prophylactic therapy is being considered [53].

14.4 Arteriovenous Malformation of the Retina (AVM)—Wyburn-Mason Syndrome

Arteriovenous malformations of the retina (AVM) are rare congenital unilateral disorders of the retinal vessels which are part of an oculo-cutaneous-neurological syndrome now named after Wyburn-Mason after a critical and detailed analysis of several anecdotal reports available; till then was the first to synthesize a detailed clinical account of the AVM occurring in the midbrain where these were most symptomatic by way of squint and intracranial haemorrhage and were seen simultaneously in the ipsilateral retina and facial vascular nevi and mental changes. In many cases, these were fatal and discovered only in autopsy studies [54]. In his review series, nearly 80% of the patients had intracranial AVM, many of whom also had subarachnoid haemorrhage. This information is likely skewed as carotid angiography was rarely done in his era. AVM of the retina is likely seen only in about 8% of patients with CNS AVM [55]. The AVMs may occasionally be seen in other brain areas and even the orbit producing a pulsatile proptosis [56]. Rarely, an AVM may occur in the suprasellar region and the orbit without retinal involvement [57]. or with retinal involvement [58]. Magnetic resonance angiography may reveal a direct communication of facial vascular nevus with the retinal AVM and has serious visual implications for any interventions, including embolization, sclerotherapy, laser photocoagulation, or even the proton beam irradiations for the communicating facial naevi [59]. Unlike VHL disease, which has a strong autosomal inheritance pattern, there is no evidence that AVMs are inherited.

Moreover, there is no angioma or tumour formation. The retinal AVM arise on the optic disc and extends into the macular area or the peripheral retina. At least three patterns were recognized by Archer et al. [60]. Type 1 AVM is seen either in one or more than one quadrant, most often in the macula. It has a dilated capillary network between the dilated arterioles and the draining veins. It is difficult to tell the difference between the arteriole and the vein except on FFA, which also shows the site of AV communication. These do not show any extravasation of the fluorescein dye and remain stable over the long term. Type 2 AVM are high flow AV malformations without intervening capillary bed. These are high-flow AVM, and arteries and veins dilate more than in type 1. Not uncommonly, the high flow in the retinal veins may cause endothelial damage from shear stress and cause thrombosis [61–64].

Thrombosis may also cause spontaneous resolution of the AVM [65]. These arterioles may develop macroanuerysmal dilatations, and some decompensation may be seen. Although these seem stable, the macroaneurysms may cause exudation and rupture years later with sub-retinal haemorrhage. These may finally resolve [66]. These involute spontaneously, but in those causing exudation or haemorrhage, laser photocoagulation, or even the use of intravitreal anti-VEGF agents may help [67, 68]. In the event of type 2 AVM in the macular area with macular edema, anti-VEGF agents may have an inadequate response and laser photocoagulation may help resolve the macular edema [69, 70]. In type 3 AVM, the vessels are hugely dilated and may be decompensated. It is difficult to tell the difference between the arteries and the veins. This type has malformations originally described by Wyburn-Mason and has a strong component of AVM in the midbrain [60]. By and large, Wyburn-Mason syndrome is an asymptomatic disorder and is detected on routine examination. However, it is vital to recognize these malformations as nearly 30% of the patients may have associated AVM in the midbrain. Unlike the AVM in the retina, which may remain unaltered for decades, the ones in the brain usually cause cerebral haemorrhage and may be fatal. All patients with

Archer's type 3 AVM in the retina should be evaluated by MR/CT angiography to rule out intracranial involvement.

14.5 Congenital Retinal Macrovessel

Congenital retinal macrovessel (CRM) is a rare retinal vascular anomaly characterized by a large retinal vein that crosses the horizontal raphe in the macula and receives blood from above and below the horizontal raphe. Jensen drew detailed fundus drawings of the left eye of 100 patients to study the distribution pattern of the retinal arterioles and veins. He found a strict quadrant-wise territorial distribution of both the retinal arterioles and the corresponding veins except in one patient where a normal retinal arteriole crossed the horizontal raphe [71]. The CRM vessel may even cross the foveal avascular zone. While CRM was first described in the German literature in the nineteenth century, in more recent years, it was described by Archer et al. in 1973 as group 1 arteriovenous malformations [60].

A detailed description of these abnormal vessels was provided by Brown et al. [72], who noted small arteriovenous anastomosis around the fovea. Although group 1 AVM of Archer et al. [60] had arteriovenous anastomosis between the larger than capillary vessels, not all patients with CRM have these arteriovenous anastomoses. While the large, dilated veins of the CRM may be explained by the AV anastomosis communicating high-pressure arterial blood into these vessels and early filling of the CRM, not all patients with CRM show obvious anastomosis and hence dilated retinal vein appears to be a standalone characteristic feature of the CRM. Remarkably delayed dye clearance in the FFA's late frames is seen in these vessels. There may be perivenous capillary non-perfusion surrounding the CRM [72]. There is no dye leakage from these vessels, and they appear stable [73]. Systemic associations were not known earlier as non-invasive neuroimaging studies were unavailable, and invasive arteriography was not done in the asymptomatic patients. Compared to the general population who show venous malformations of the brain in 0.2–6%, a review of the 10-year data from multiple centres worldwide has shown that 24% of the patients with CRM on MRI scans had venous malformations in the brain. Seventy–five per cent of the venous malformations associated with CRM were in the frontal lobe, and most of these were ipsilateral to the CRM. MRI scans are recommended for all patients with CRM based on this data. Instead of the CRM, these should be labelled as retinal venous malformations, given their close association with cerebral venous malformations [74].

14.5.1 Retinal Cavernous Hemangioma—Clinical Presentations

Retinal cavernous hemangioma (RCH) is a rare, benign, unilateral retinal angioma characterized by a cluster of sac-like or dark-red grape-like aneurysmal dilatations along a major retinal vein. Rarely, the RCH may be seen on the optic disc [75, 76]. Most RCH cases are asymptomatic and discovered on routine examination in young adults. The RCH has no feeder vessels unlike the retinal capillary hemangioma associated with VHL disease, which has highly characteristic dilated and tortuous feeder vessels. Moreover, RCH is stationary and has no potential to grow or leak fluid in the retinal interstitial tissues. However, they develop fibrous scar tissue on the surface or rarely even a phlebolith [77]. The RCH may get thrombosed or fibrosed over time [78]. Fundus fluorescein angiography (FFA) is highly characteristic as there is a delay in the venous filling in the affected quadrant. There is a delayed filling of aneurysmal sacs with the fluorescein dye with late fluorescence of the supernatant plasma and blocking of the fluorescence of the bottom of the sac due to sedimented red blood cells. These features suggest stagnant venous blood in these cavernous sacs [75]. The optical coherence tomography shows thin-walled large cystic cavities with a thin epiretinal membrane stretched over these cystic lesions [79].

14.5.2 Retinal Cavernous Hemangioma—Systemic Associations and Genetics

The RCH is a part of the neuro-oculo-cutaneous syndrome (phakomatosis) and may occur in sporadic and inherited forms. Of the three patients, Gass [75] described a female patient presented with RCH and multiple cutaneous angiomas. Her father had RCH, a history of seizures, and ultimately died of a cerebral haemorrhage. His autopsy revealed cavernous hemangioma of the midbrain and the cerebellum. [75]. While the cavernous hemangiomas of the skin are relatively common because of their occurrence in association with brain stem and cerebellar cavernous hemangioma and RCH, cavernous skin hemangiomas are likely a component of the neuro-oculo-cutaneous syndrome, as has also been noted in a 4-generation pedigree of 90 members with an autosomal dominant transmission of this syndrome [80] and another, a 3-generation pedigree [81]. Mutations in at least three cerebral cavernous hemangiomas (CCH) genes, a point mutation within exon 5 of KRIT19 (7q21.2), a large deletion in MGC4607 (7p13), and complete deletion of PDCD10 (3q26.1) have also been noted in patients with RCH [82, 83]. Nearly, 5% of the patients with familial cavernous hemangioma of the brain have RCH [83], whereas 14% of all the RCH patients had CCH, most of whom were asymptomatic [84]. Compared to computerized tomography, magnetic resonance imaging (MRI) of the brain is far more sensitive in detecting these malformations. Multiple lesions may be seen in the familial forms of the CCH, compared to the sporadic variety, which has a solitary lesion [85]. Moreover, various MR imaging techniques have been used to improve the localization of these lesions [86].

14.5.3 Retinal Cavernous Hemangioma—Complications

By and large, the RCH remains unchanged over decades. Occasionally, however, they may develop vitreous haemorrhage. As noted above, the OCT shows a fibrous membrane stretched over the surface of the thin-walled RCH cystic lesions. Contraction of this membrane may explain why a vitreous haemorrhage occurs spontaneously or following a minor trauma [79]. However, spontaneous or birth trauma-related vitreous haemorrhages are rarely reported [79, 87–89]. A unique case of RCH was followed up from birth to the age of 52 with recurrent vitreous haemorrhages, and hyphema, ultimately leading to a painful blind eye. The eye was ultimately removed and subjected to histopathology. The RCH consisted of large endothelial cell-lined vascular channels typically seen in cavernous hemangioma. The RCH was seen extending into the ciliary body and was responsible for recurrent hyphema in this patient [90].

14.5.4 Retinal Cavernous Hemangioma—Treatment

A majority of the RCH do not require any treatment. However, in patients with recurrent vitreous haemorrhages, one may consider either cryotherapy, PDT, or plaque radiation (https://retinatoday.com/pdfs/0715RT_Mini_Shields.pdf). However, patients with RCH should undergo MRI to rule out any asymptomatic or symptomatic CCH [91]. The CCH are circumscribed and can be excised by neurosurgeons, and those located in deep inaccessible areas can be treated with stereotactic radiosurgery.

14.6 Retinal Astrocytoma

14.6.1 Hamartomas-Tuberous Sclerosis Complex—Introduction

Hamartomas are uncommon congenital benign growths of a mixture of various cells and tissues found in their normal place. The tuberous sclerosis complex (TSC) is a neuro-oculo-cutaneous autosomal dominant disorder (9q34.13 mutation in the gene TSC1/2) with the development of hamartomatous growths in multiple organs, the symptoms showing a wide variation in severity depending upon the organs involved. Nearly half of the patients with TSC have retinal or optic nerve astrocytoma, a hamartoma arising from the retinal glial cells [92]. Other significant lesions in TSC include cortical tubers, triangular-shaped hamartomatous lesions, the apex pointing towards the ventricles and located at the grey-white matter junction in frontal and parietal lobes. These may cause seizures in infants, causing repetitive spasms of the head and legs. The children may have a learning disability (Mental retardation in ~30%). Other major neurological complications include raised intracranial pressure, cranial nerve palsies, and cortical visual defects [93]. More than 90% of patients of TSC have ash-leaf hypo-pigmented patches on their skin, acne-like angiofibroma growth on the face (adenoma sebaceum), and periungual fibromas (Fig. 14.10a). Major organs such as the heart (rhabdomyoma), lungs (Lymphangiomyomatosis), and kidneys (angiomyolipoma) may have

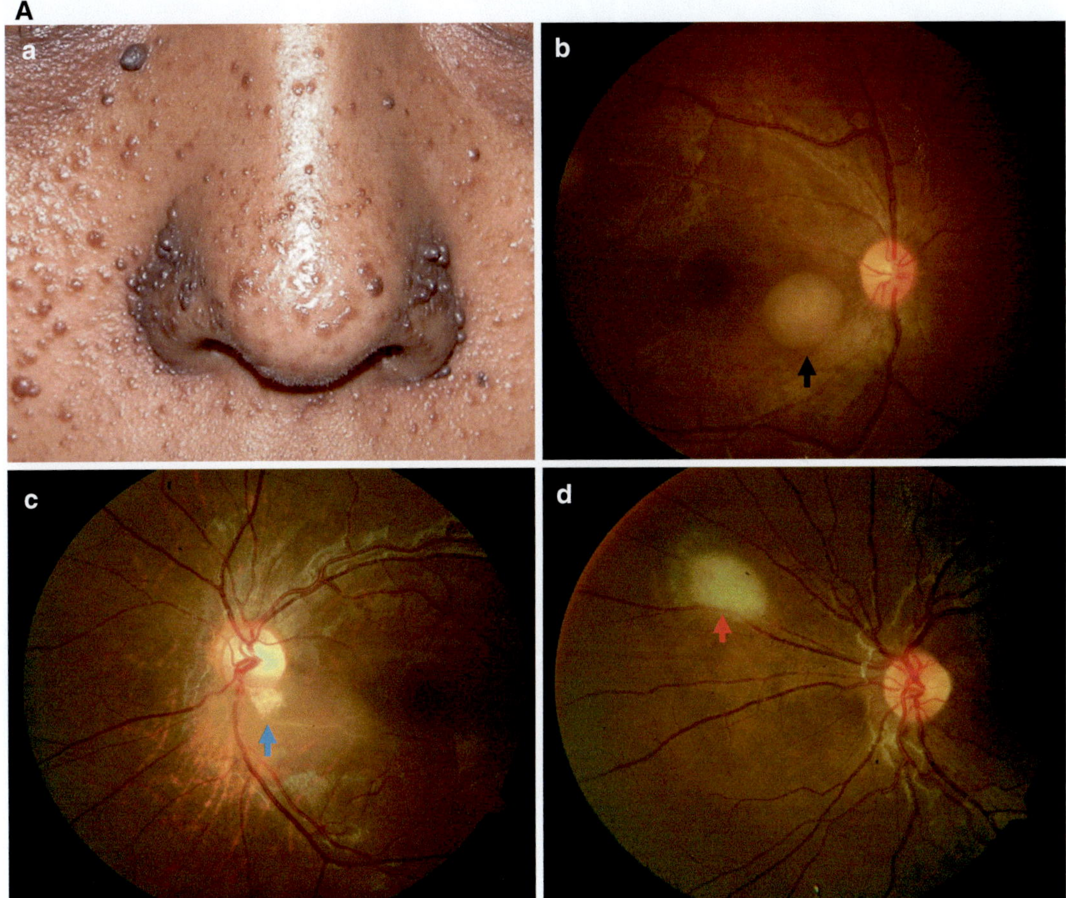

Fig. 14.10 (**A**) Adenoma sebaceum in tuberous sclerosis complex: Ash-leaf hypo-pigmented patches on skin, acne-like angiofibroma growth on the face (**a**). Various clinical phenotypes of retinal astrocytomas are recognized; (**b**) translucent flat, slightly elevated, oval salmon patch with gradually merging borders with the normal retina (black arrow); (**c**) an elevated, grey-white, multinodular lesion with a mulberry-type surface, located near the optic disc margins (blue arrow). The lesions are calcified and detectable on an X-ray. There is a characteristic 'moth-eaten' appearance on OCT due to multiple cavities; (**d**) a nodular lesion located in the centre of a flat salmon-coloured flat patch (red arrow). (**B**) A 6/12 months female child was seen with bilateral multifocal translucent retinal astrocytomas (**a**, **b**). An antenatal diagnosis of tuberous sclerosis was made based on T2-weighted MRI scans which showed an angiomyolipoma of the kidney (**c**, red arrow). At 6 months of age, angiomyolipoma of the heart right ventricle (**d**, red arrow) and multiple subependymal astrocytomas were seen on a CT scan (**e**, **f** red arrows)

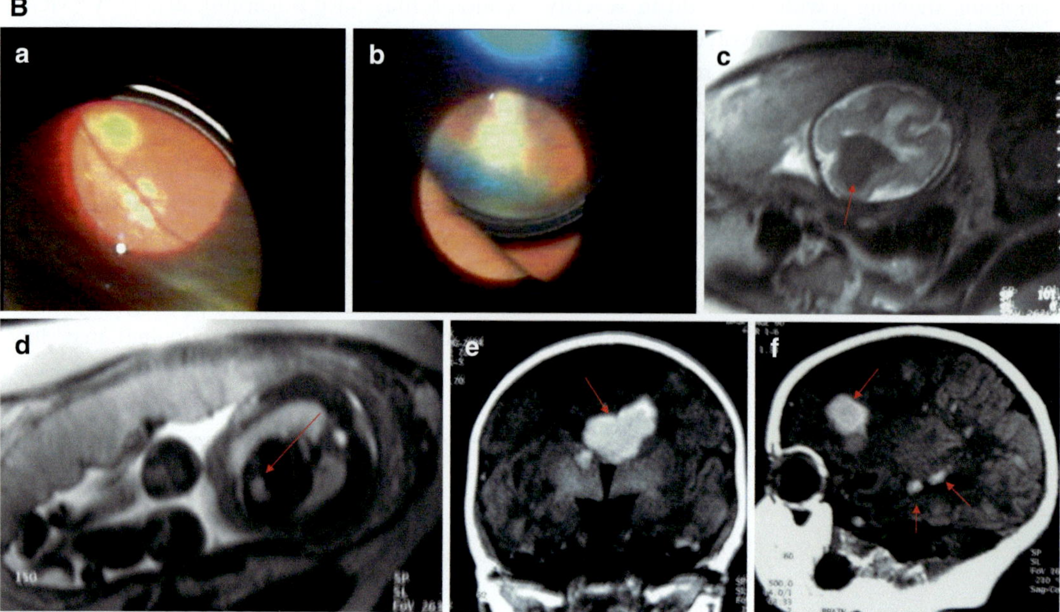

Fig. 14.10 (continued)

tubers. X-ray or CT scan of the brain may show calcification. Online Mendelian Inheritance in Man database developed by Johns Hopkins University School MIM *605284/191092. https://omim.org/entry/

14.6.2 Tuberous Sclerosis Complex—Genetics

TSC is an autosomal dominant disorder with mutations in either TSC1, located on chromosome 9, which encodes for hamartin, or the TSC2 gene, located on chromosome 16, which encodes for tuberin, tumour suppressor proteins. In a large cohort of diagnosed or suspected TSC patients, nearly 74% had pathological mutations in either of the two genes, with a detection rate of 85% in confirmed cases of TSC. The TSC2 mutations were at least 3 X more common than in the TSC1 gene [94].

14.6.3 Retinal Astrocytoma—Clinical Signs

In a population-based study in the Wessex counties of the UK, the prevalence of TSC was 4.9 per 100,000 population. Of the 100 patients of TSC thoroughly examined, 44 had retinal astrocytoma, one-third of which were bilateral [95]. Patients with either multiple lesions or bilateral cases are likely to be inherited disorders versus monofocal lesions, which are likely to be sporadic. Unless the fovea is involved, the vision in the affected remains normal. At least three clinical phenotypes are recognized. The most common phenotype is a single or multiple translucent flat, slightly elevated, oval salmon patch with gradually merging borders with the normal retina (Fig. 14.10b–d). It may be easily missed unless one is looking for it. If one follows a retinal arteriole from the optic disc to the retinal periphery, sudden haziness of the vessels may lead to the detection of an overlying plaque-like lesion. These are best imaged with blue and green reflectance imaging. On fundus autofluorescence, these lesions appear hypofluorescent. On the structural OCT, these appear uniformly hyperreflective lesions in the nerve fibre layer [96, 97]. The second phenotype is more easily recognizable and near the optic disc margins. It is an elevated, grey-white, multinodular with a mulberry-type surface. The lesions are calcified and detectable on an X-ray. There is a characteristic 'moth-eaten' appearance on OCT due to multiple cavities [98]. The third phenotype, transitional astrocytoma, is much less common and seen as a multinodular lesion in the centre of a flat salmon-coloured flat patch. Multiple types may present in the same eye [92]. Generally, the retinal astrocytomas remain stable. However, rarely these may start growing and lead to exudative retinal detachment and a painful blind eye. They may show an endophytic or exophytic growth pattern [99]. Because of possible growth, although rare, the astrocytomas should be imaged and regularly followed up for any increase. Only the lesions close to the optic disc were seen to grow in size, and the other associated lesions in the periphery did not show any progression [99].

The histopathology of the retinal astrocytoma shows glial astrocytic proliferation in the retinal nerve fibre layer, and the tumour overlies the retinal vessels. The larger lesions may show cystic changes, haemorrhages, and calcification [92]. The enucleated eyeballs of patients blind from the massive growth of the astrocytomas have shown the lesions to be predominantly composed of giant glial astrocytes not different from those seen in the subependymal giant cell astrocytomas of the brain seen in TSC. The immunohistochemical staining of the tumour showed features consistent with a glioneuronal phenotype tumour composed of both the neuronal and glial cells. The tumour showed extensive necrosis varying from 50 to 95% of the tumour size and was filled with blood. Multicentric calcification was seen [99].

14.6.4 Retinal Astrocytoma—Treatment

The inherited retinal astrocytomas, in general, are fairly stable and, apart from multidisciplinary screening for any other associated organ involvement, do not require any active intervention except for observation and documentation on fundus imaging for any possible growth in the eye. Sight-threatening growing lesions with exudation have been treated with oral inhibitors of the mechanistic target of rapamycin (mTORis), such as Sirolimus and Everolimus. The treatment was well tolerated, the size of the growing tumour was reduced or stabilized, and there was a good improvement in exudation [26, 27]. Previously, oral rapamycin has been successfully used in subependymal giant astrocytic hamartoma [100] and renal angiomyolipoma associated with TSC [101].

An acquired progressive astrocytic hamartoma in an old lady was successfully treated with intravitreal bevacizumab [98]. A fine needle biopsy-proven acquired retinal astrocytoma associated with retinal exudation was successfully treated with photodynamic therapy [102]. Similar cases have also been reported earlier [103].

14.7 Glioma of the Optic Pathways and Neurofibromatosis

The optic pathway gliomas develop in 15–20% of type 1 neurofibromatosis (NF) or peripheral von Recklinghausen disease. Lisch nodules and hypertelorism are other ocular signs in type 1 NF. It is an autosomal dominant disorder resulting from deletion or mutations in any of the nearly 1000 alleles at the 17q11.2 band in the NF1 gene which is family-specific. The systemic phenotype is characterized by the development of cutaneous or subcutaneous neurofibromas (76%), Plexiform neurofibroma (76%), Cafe-au-lait spots (93%), spinal neurofibroma, facial asymmetry; coarse features; macrocephaly, bone cysts; Joint laxity; delayed cognition, and speech difficulty and attention deficit. For more details, the readers may see MIM # 613675 https://omim.org/entry, the Online Mendelian Inheritance in Man database developed by Johns Hopkins University School.

Type 2 neurofibromatosis is a distinct adult-onset autosomal dominant disorder resulting from mutations in the 22q11.2 band in the NF2 gene. The ocular lesions include cataracts, epiretinal membrane, and retinal hamartomas. The systemic phenotype is characterized by bilateral vestibular schwannomas or acoustic neuromas (90–95%), which develop in all by 30 years. These are benign but highly disabling tumours. Other systemic phenotypes include intracranial meningiomas (45–58%) and other cranial nerve neuromas (24–51%), spinal ependymoma, spinal cord astrocytoma (63–90%), skin peripheral nerve tumours, plaques, and peripheral neuropathy (66%) [104]. The presence of bilateral vestibular schwannomas does not require any additional findings for diagnosing NF 2. However, in unilateral vestibular schwannoma, positive family history or, in its absence, two of the other NF2 lesions—meningiomas, neurofibroma, schwannoma, glioma, or cataract—are required to reach a diagnosis. In multiple meningiomas, unilateral vestibular schwannoma and any of the two other signs are required to diagnose NF2 [104].

14.7.1 Retinoblastoma–Clinical Presentations

Retinoblastoma (RB) is a childhood cancer of the primitive retina seen in nearly 1:15,000–20,000 live births. It is invariably fatal if left untreated. The major challenge in RB care is its early detection. In the Western world, more than 80% of RB cases are detected by parents/relatives when they notice a white reflex in the pupillary area of the eye (leukocoria). The white reflex may be caused by several sight-threatening conditions such as congenital cataracts, retinopathy of prematurity, Coats' disease (Fig. 14.11), and the life-threatening RB. The other presentations of RB may include squinting eyes. There is often a delay of several weeks between noting a white reflex and seeking an ophthalmological consultation and referral to a multidisciplinary oncology unit to provide comprehensive care to these babies.

Compared to sporadic unilateral RB cases, familial RB is diagnosed early because of the opportunity to examine the newborn babies within 1–2 weeks of the birth. The early tumours are round single, or multiple grey-white translucent and grow rapidly, sometimes within a matter of days (Fig. 14.12). The colour becomes more opaque and pinkish as the tumour gets vascularized from the retina, which can be confirmed on FFA. As the lesions progress, the non-cohesive tumour cells may be released into the subretinal space or the vitreous cavity. There may be an accumulation of the subretinal fluid [105]. The tumour may show exophytic or endophytic growth. Very rarely, a diffuse infiltrative variety may present as a pearly-white iris deposit/hypopyon in the anterior chamber. Advanced cases

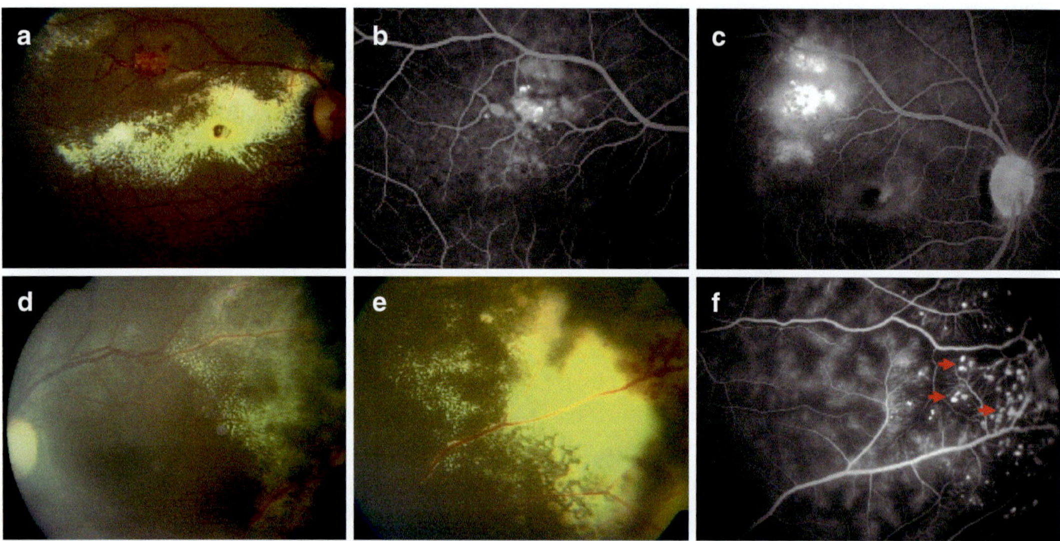

Fig. 14.11 Coats disease in a 21-year-old male with macroaneurysms and massive exudation in right eye (**a**). Fluorescein angiography shows hyperfluorescence of the macroaneurysms (**b**) and leakage from the telangiectatic vessels (**c**). Coats disease in a 22-year-old female in the left eye with massive exudation (**d**) and telangiectatic vessels in periphery (**e**). Fluorescein angiography shows hyperfluorescence of the aneurysms (red arrows) with light bulb appearance (**f**)

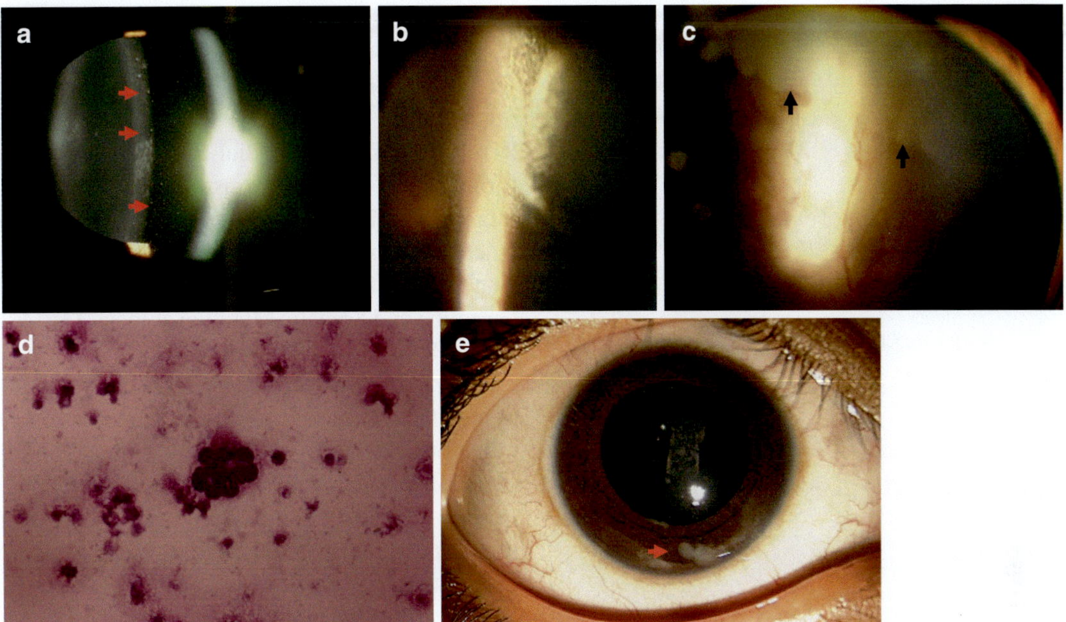

Fig. 14.12 An 8-year-old female child presented with anterior chamber inflammation. Anterior segment photograph showing large white coloured cells (red arrows) in the anterior chamber (**a**). Ophthalmoscopy revealed dense vitreous cellular infiltrates (**b**) and large, white-coloured vitreous deposits (black arrows) from a rapidly growing retinoblastoma (**c**). The colour becomes opaquer and more pinkish as the tumour gets vascularized. Vitreous tap revealed retinoblastoma on histopathology (**d**). The next day, pearly white deposits (red arrow) appeared in the anterior chamber (**e**). Reproduced with permission of the publishers from Gupta A and Gupta V (2009) Paediatric uveitis in Gupta A, Gupta V, Herbort C, Khairallah M (eds) Uveitis: Text and Imaging 1st Edn. Jaypee Brothers Medical Publishers (P) Ltd., New Delhi. P. 518

may present with iris neovascularization and neovascular glaucoma. In the late stages, the RB infiltrates the optic nerve, choroid, and sclera and extends into the orbit to present as a proptosis or as an orbital fungating mass in highly neglected cases. Until the mid-90 s, the standard of care was using fractionated external beam radiation therapy, which is now reserved only for the eyes that have shown failure with conservative treatment. The introduction of chemo reduction of the tumours using six cycles of intravenous vincristine, etoposide, and carboplatin followed by destructive tumour therapy for each tumour with laser photocoagulation, thermotherapy, brachytherapy, or cryopexy has changed the outlook for a successful outcome. The need to closely follow up the tumour following chemo reduction has led to developing of a new staging classification of the RB (Box 14.3) [106]. More advanced tumours in unilateral RB (Group D or >) and the eye with the more advanced tumour in bilateral RB are usually enucleated. Group E eyes are generally non-salvageable and should be enucleated. The patient may be given chemo reduction therapy before enucleation to reduce the chances of metastasis. During surgery, the eye should be handled gently to prevent any hematogenous spread of the RB cells. At least 10 mm of the optic nerve should be removed with the globe. The eye should be examined by histopathology for any infiltration of the optic nerve, choroid or sclera. Before preserving the eye in formalin, fresh tumour tissue should be taken and sent for RB1 gene mutations. The subject of comprehensive screening and management of RB children has been extensively reviewed [107], and we strongly recommend that readers interested in the subject go through it.

Box 14.3 International Classification of Retinoblastoma and Outcome of Treatment

Group	Subgroup	Clinical features	Number treated (Success rate)
A	Small	RB ≤ 3 mm in size (base or thickness) outside the fovea	23 (100%)
B	Large Macular Juxtapapillary SRF	RB > 3 mm ≤ 3 mm to the foveal Centre or ≤ 1.5 mm to optic disc or Clear SRF ≤ 3 mm from the tumour margin	96 (93%)
C1	Focal subretinal seeds	≤ 3 mm from RB	6 (100%)
C2	Focal vitreous seeds	≤ 3 mm from the RB	14 (93%)
C3	Both subretinal and vitreous seeds	≤ 3 mm from the RB	1 (0%)
D1	Diffuse subretinal seeds	>3 mm from the RB	82 (57%)
D2	Diffuse vitreous seeds	>3 mm from the RB	10 (30%)
D3	Diffuse both subretinal and vitreous seeds	>3 mm from the RB	17 (6%)
E	Extensive	RB >50% of the globe; opaque media due to vitreous seeds; hemorrhage; NVG; Infiltration of optic nerve >2 mm, sclera, anterior chamber, orbit	Excluded from the trial and hence no outcome reported

Abbreviations: *RB* retinoblastoma; *SRF* subretinal fluid.

Reproduced with permission of the publishers from Shields CL, Mashayekhi A, Au AK, Czyz C, Leahey A, Meadows AT, Shields JA. The International Classification of Retinoblastoma predicts chemoreduction success. Ophthalmology. 2006 Dec;113(12):2276–80. doi: 10.1016/j.ophtha.2006.06.018. Epub 2006 Sep 25. PMID: 16996605.

14.7.2 Retinoblastoma—Genetics in Brief and Implications of Testing

RB is seen in both familial forms and sporadic forms. In the familial forms, it appears early in infancy, is bilateral, and often multifocal. The inactivation of both alleles of a tumour suppression gene RB1(RB1/p105-Rb) causes it. Both Germline and Somatic Mutation at locus 13q14.2 lead to RB.

Nearly 40% of the RB patients are familial/bilateral and carry germline (constitutional) mutation inherited from either parent. Familial cases of RB have major systemic associations, namely Trilateral retinoblastoma, Osteogenic sarcoma, Bladder cancer, and Small cell cancer of intestine.

All cells of the body in these patients carry the germline mutation. RB develops when there is a somatic mutation in the second allele of the RB1 gene in the primitive retinal tissue. Unilateral RB is seen in nearly 60% of the cases who develop RB from a somatic mutation in both alleles in the primitive retina and are unlikely to transmit the RB in their offspring. In a country-wide cohort, 92% of bilateral RB/familial patients and 10% of the unilateral/non-familial cases in the Netherlands had mutations in the RB1 gene [108]. In another study, nearly 86% of the unilateral RB cases had no germline RB1 mutations, but 12–14% had a germline mutation. Thus, patients with unilateral RB risk transmitting RB to their offspring unless tested by highly sensitive techniques such as allele-specific PCR or next-generation sequencing to detect the germline mutation [109]. Unilateral RB patients advised enucleation and detected negative in the blood for the RB1 gene mutation found in their tumour need not be under surveillance in the oncology clinic [107]. A major concern in the heritable RB survivors is the development of second cancers, namely osteosarcomas, soft tissue sarcomas, skin cancer, lung cancer, and various other cancers in different time frames. Radiation therapy and Systemic chemotherapy for RB increase the risk of such cancers by 3.0X and 1.8X, respectively, and necessitates life-long cancer surveillance [110].

References

1. Maher ER, Iselius L, Yates JR, Littler M, Benjamin C, Harris R, Sampson J, Williams A, Ferguson-Smith MA, Morton N. Von Hippel-Lindau disease: a genetic study. J Med Genet. 1991;28(7):443–7. https://doi.org/10.1136/jmg.28.7.443. PMID: 1895313; PMCID: PMC1016952.
2. Latif F, Tory K, Gnarra J, Yao M, Duh FM, Orcutt ML, Stackhouse T, Kuzmin I, Modi W, Geil L, et al. Identification of the von Hippel-Lindau disease tumor suppressor gene. Science. 1993;260(5112):1317–20. https://doi.org/10.1126/science.8493574. PMID: 8493574.
3. Knudson AG Jr. Hereditary cancer, oncogenes, and antioncogenes. Cancer Res. 1985;45(4):1437–43. PMID: 2983882.
4. Maher ER, Yates JR, Ferguson-Smith MA. Statistical analysis of the two stage mutation model in von Hippel-Lindau disease, and in sporadic cerebellar haemangioblastoma and renal cell carcinoma. J Med Genet. 1990;27(5):311–4. https://doi.org/10.1136/jmg.27.5.311. PMID: 2352258; PMCID: PMC1017082.
5. Maher ER, Yates JR, Harries R, Benjamin C, Harris R, Moore AT, Ferguson-Smith MA. Clinical features and natural history of von Hippel-Lindau disease. Q J Med. 1990;77(283):1151–63. https://doi.org/10.1093/qjmed/77.2.1151. PMID: 2274658.
6. Chan CC, Vortmeyer AO, Chew EY, Green WR, Matteson DM, Shen DF, Linehan WM, Lubensky IA, Zhuang Z. VHL gene deletion and enhanced VEGF gene expression detected in the stromal cells of retinal angioma. Arch Ophthalmol. 1999;117(5):625–30. https://doi.org/10.1001/archopht.117.5.625. PMID: 10326959.
7. Chew EY. Ocular manifestations of von Hippel-Lindau disease: clinical and genetic investigations. Trans Am Ophthalmol Soc. 2005;103:495–511. PMID: 17057815; PMCID: PMC1447586.
8. Linehan WM, Lerman MI, Zbar B. Identification of the von Hippel-Lindau (VHL) gene. Its role in renal cancer. JAMA. 1995;273(7):564–70. PMID: 7837390.
9. Friedrich CA. Von Hippel-Lindau syndrome. A pleomorphic condition. Cancer. 1999;86(11 Suppl):2478–82. PMID: 10630173.
10. Lonser RR, Glenn GM, Walther M, Chew EY, Libutti SK, Linehan WM, Oldfield EH. von Hippel-Lindau disease. Lancet. 2003;361(9374):2059–67. https://doi.org/10.1016/S0140-6736(03)13643-4. PMID: 12814730.
11. Neumann HP, Wiestler OD. Clustering of features of von Hippel-Lindau syndrome: evidence for a complex genetic locus. Lancet. 1991;337(8749):1052–4. https://doi.org/10.1016/0140-6736(91)91705-y. PMID: 1673491.
12. Wanebo JE, Lonser RR, Glenn GM, Oldfield EH. The natural history of hemangioblastomas of the central nervous system in patients with von Hippel-Lindau disease. J Neurosurg. 2003;98(1):82–94. https://doi.org/10.3171/jns.2003.98.1.0082. PMID: 12546356.
13. Poston CD, Jaffe GS, Lubensky IA, Solomon D, Zbar B, Linehan WM, Walther MM. Characterization of the renal pathology of a familial form of renal cell carcinoma associated with von Hippel-Lindau disease: clinical and molecular genetic implications. J Urol. 1995;153(1):22–6. https://doi.org/10.1097/00005392-199501000-00009. PMID: 7966777.
14. Schoen MA, Shields CL, Say EAT, Douglass AM, Shields JA, Jampol LM. Clinically invisible retinal hemangioblastomas detected by spectral domain optical coherence tomography and fluorescein angiography in twins. Retin Cases Brief Rep. 2018;12(1):12–6. https://doi.org/10.1097/ICB.0000000000000382. PMID: 27533642. PMID: 8433820.
15. Chen X, Sanfilippo CJ, Nagiel A, Hosseini H, Mitchell D, McCannel CA, Schwartz SD, McCannel TA. Early detection of retinal hemangioblastomas in von Hippel-Lindau disease using ultra-widefield fluorescein angiography. Retina. 2018;38(4):748–54. https://doi.org/10.1097/IAE.0000000000001601. PMID: 28368975.
16. Dalvin LA, Yu MD, Ancona-Lezama DA, Pulido JS, Olsen TW, Shields CL. Retinal haemangioblastoma associated with peripheral non-perfusion: widefield fluorescein angiography analysis of 41 cases. Br J Ophthalmol. 2020;104(2):167–72. https://doi.org/10.1136/bjophthalmol-2019-314021. Epub 2019 May 16. PMID: 31097435.
17. Nicholson DH, Green WR, Kenyon KR. Light and electron microscopic study of early lesions in angiomatosis retinae. Am J Ophthalmol. 1976;82(2):193–204. https://doi.org/10.1016/0002-9394(76)90418-9. PMID: 986118.
18. Hajjaj A, van Overdam KA, Gishti O, Ramdas WD, Kiliç E. Efficacy and safety of current treatment options for peripheral retinal haemangioblastomas: a systematic review. Acta Ophthalmol. 2022;100(1):e38–46. https://doi.org/10.1111/aos.14865. Epub 2021 Apr 8. PMID: 33834636.
19. Gaudric A, Krivosic V, Duguid G, Massin P, Giraud S, Richard S. Vitreoretinal surgery for severe retinal capillary hemangiomas in von Hippel-Lindau disease. Ophthalmology. 2011;118(1):142–9. https://doi.org/10.1016/j.ophtha.2010.04.031. PMID: 20801520.
20. Wiley HE, Krivosic V, Gaudric A, Gorin MB, Shields C, Shields J, Aronow ME, Chew EY. Management of retinal hemangioblastoma in von Hippel-Lindau disease. Retina. 2019;39(12):2254–63. https://doi.org/10.1097/IAE.0000000000002572. PMID: 31259811; PMCID: PMC6878154.

21. Weng CY. Transvitreal feeder vessel ligation and en bloc resection of a retinal capillary hemangioblastoma. Am J Ophthalmol. 2022;237:e3–5. https://doi.org/10.1016/j.ajo.2022.01.007. Epub 2022 Jan 14. PMID: 31611094.
22. Wong WT, Liang KJ, Hammel K, Coleman HR, Chew EY. Intravitreal ranibizumab therapy for retinal capillary hemangioblastoma related to von Hippel-Lindau disease. Ophthalmology. 2008;115(11):1957–64. https://doi.org/10.1016/j.ophtha.2008.04.033. Epub 2008 Sep 11. PMID: 18789534; PMCID: PMC3034164.
23. Hwang CK, Chew EY, Cukras CA, Keenan TDL, Wong WT, Linehan WM, Chittiboina P, Pacak K, Wiley HE. Intravitreous treatment of severe ocular von Hippel-Lindau disease using a combination of the VEGF inhibitor, ranibizumab and PDGF inhibitor, E10030: results from a phase 1/2 clinical trial. Clin Exp Ophthalmol. 2021;49(9):1048–59. https://doi.org/10.1111/ceo.14001. Epub 2021 Oct 26. PMID: 34549489.
24. Ch'ng S, Tan ST. Facial port-wine stains—clinical stratification and risks of neuro-ocular involvement. J Plast Reconstr Aesthet Surg. 2008;61(8):889–93. https://doi.org/10.1016/j.bjps.2007.05.011. Epub 2007 Jul 2. PMID: 17604243.
25. Shirley MD, Tang H, Gallione CJ, Baugher JD, Frelin LP, Cohen B, North PE, Marchuk DA, Comi AM, Pevsner J. Sturge-Weber syndrome and port-wine stains caused by somatic mutation in GNAQ. N Engl J Med. 2013;368(21):1971–9. https://doi.org/10.1056/NEJMoa1213507. Epub 2013 May 8. PMID: 23656586; PMCID: PMC3749068.
26. Wu Y, Peng C, Huang L, Xu L, Ding X, Liu Y, Zeng C, Sun H, Guo W. Somatic GNAQ R183Q mutation is located within the sclera and episclera in patients with Sturge-Weber syndrome. Br J Ophthalmol. 2022;106(7):1006–11. https://doi.org/10.1136/bjophthalmol-2020-317287. Epub 2021 Mar 11. PMID: 33707187; PMCID: PMC9234408
27. Wu F, McGarrey MP, Geenen KR, Skalet AH, Guillot FH, Wilson JL, Shah AS, Gonzalez E, Thiele EA, Kim IK, Aronow ME. Treatment of aggressive retinal astrocytic hamartoma with oral mechanistic target of rapamycin inhibition. Ophthalmol Retina. 2022;6(5):411–20. https://doi.org/10.1016/j.oret.2022.01.003. Epub 2022 Jan 8. PMID: 35007768.
28. Baselga E. Sturge-Weber syndrome. Semin Cutan Med Surg. 2004;23(2):87–98. https://doi.org/10.1016/j.sder.2004.01.002. PMID: 15295918.
29. Poliner A, Fernandez Faith E, Blieden L, Kelly KM, Metry D. Port-wine birthmarks: update on diagnosis, risk assessment for Sturge-Weber syndrome, and management. Pediatr Rev. 2022;43(9):507–16. https://doi.org/10.1542/pir.2021-005437. PMID: 36045161.
30. Bang GM, Setabutr P. Periocular capillary hemangiomas: indications and options for treatment. Middle East Afr J Ophthalmol. 2010;17(2):121–8. https://doi.org/10.4103/0974-9233.63071. PMID: 20616917; PMCID: PMC2892126.
31. Latrive A, Teixeira LR, Gomes AS, Zezell DM. Characterization of skin Port-Wine Stain and Hemangioma vascular lesions using Doppler OCT. Skin Res Technol. 2016;22(2):223–9. https://doi.org/10.1111/srt.12253. Epub 2015 Sep 3. PMID: 27060596.
32. Rosen S, Smoller BR. Port-wine stains: a new hypothesis. J Am Acad Dermatol. 1987;17(1):164–6. https://doi.org/10.1016/s0190-9622(87)70186-8. PMID: 3611452.
33. Sullivan TJ, Clarke MP, Morin JD. The ocular manifestations of the Sturge-Weber syndrome. J Pediatr Ophthalmol Strabismus. 1992;29(6):349–56. https://doi.org/10.3928/0191-3913-19921101-05. PMID: 1287171.
34. Surve A, Azad S, Venkatesh P, Kumar V, Chawla R, Gupta V, Vohra R. Choroidal vascular pattern in cases of Sturge-Weber syndrome. Ophthalmol Retina. 2019;3(12):1091–7. https://doi.org/10.1016/j.oret.2019.07.009. Epub 2019 Jul 22. PMID: 31523035.
35. Anaya-Pava EJ, Saenz-Bocanegra CH, Flores-Trejo A, Castro-Santana NA. In a Sturge-Weber syndrome case, there is diffuse choroidal hemangioma associated with exudative retinal detachment: photodynamic therapy and intravitreous bevacizumab. Photodiagn Photodyn Ther. 2015;12(1):136–9. https://doi.org/10.1016/j.pdpdt.2014.12.002. Epub 2015 Jan 3. PMID: 25560419.
36. Arepalli S, Shields CL, Kaliki S, Emrich J, Komarnicky L, Shields JA. Diffuse choroidal hemangioma management with plaque radiotherapy in 5 cases. Ophthalmology. 2013;120(11):2358–9, 2359.e1-2. PMID: 24182566. https://doi.org/10.1016/j.ophtha.2013.07.058.
37. Shields CL, Honavar SG, Shields JA, Cater J, Demirci H. Circumscribed choroidal hemangioma: clinical manifestations and factors predictive of visual outcome in 200 consecutive cases. Ophthalmology. 2001;108(12):2237–48. https://doi.org/10.1016/s0161-6420(01)00812-0. Erratum in: Ophthalmology 2002 Feb;109(2):222. PMID: 11733265.
38. Arevalo JF, Shields CL, Shields JA, Hykin PG, De Potter P. Circumscribed choroidal hemangioma: characteristic features with indocyanine green video angiography. Ophthalmology. 2000;107(2):344–50. https://doi.org/10.1016/s0161-6420(99)00051-2. PMID: 10690837.
39. Shanmugam PM, Sagar P. OCT angiography in identification of subtle choroidal hemangioma. Ophthalmol Retina. 2020;4(12):1195. https://doi.org/10.1016/j.oret.2020.05.013. PMID: 33279011.
40. Di Nicola M, Williams BK Jr, Srinivasan A, Al-Dahmash S, Mashayekhi A, Shields JA, Shields CL. Photodynamic therapy for circumscribed choroidal hemangioma in 79 consecutive patients: comparative analysis of factors predictive of visual

outcome. Ophthalmol Retina. 2020;4(10):1024–33. https://doi.org/10.1016/j.oret.2020.04.018. Epub 2020 Apr 25. PMID: 32344158.

41. Shields CL, Dalvin LA, Lim LS, Chang M, Udyaver S, Mazloumi M, Vichitvejpaisal P, Su GL, Florakis E, Mashayekhi A, Shields JA. Circumscribed choroidal hemangioma: visual outcome in the pre-photodynamic therapy era versus photodynamic therapy era in 458 cases. Ophthalmol Retina. 2020;4(1):100–10. https://doi.org/10.1016/j.oret.2019.08.004. Epub 2019 Aug 22. PMID: 31611094.
42. Durrani AF, Zhou Y, Musch DC, Demirci H. Treatment of choroidal hemangioma with photodynamic therapy and bevacizumab. Ophthalmol Retina. 2022;6(6):533–5. https://doi.org/10.1016/j.oret.2022.01.015. Epub 2022 Feb 1. PMID: 35114415.
43. Mwinula JH, Sagawa T, Tawara A, Inomata H. Anterior chamber angle vascularization in Sturge-Weber syndrome. Report of a case. Graefes Arch Clin Exp Ophthalmol. 1994;232(7):387–91. https://doi.org/10.1007/BF00186578. PMID: 7523256
44. Phelps CD. The pathogenesis of glaucoma in Sturge-Weber syndrome. Ophthalmology. 1978;85(3):276–86. https://doi.org/10.1016/s0161-6420(78)35667-0. PMID: 662281.
45. Shiau T, Armogan N, Yan DB, Thomson HG, Levin AV. The role of episcleral venous pressure in glaucoma associated with Sturge-Weber syndrome. J AAPOS. 2012;16(1):61–4. https://doi.org/10.1016/j.jaapos.2011.09.014. PMID: 22370668.
46. Thavikulwat AT, Edward DP, AlDarrab A, Vajaranant TS. Pathophysiology and management of glaucoma associated with phakomatoses. J Neurosci Res. 2019;97(1):57–69. https://doi.org/10.1002/jnr.24241. Epub 2018 Apr 1. PMID: 29607552.
47. Alhayaza R, Khan SA, Semidey VA, Owaidhah O. The effectiveness of propranolol in managing hemorrhagic choroidal and exudative retinal detachment following Ahmed glaucoma valve implantation in Sturge-Weber syndrome: case report and literature review. Case Rep Ophthalmol. 2021;12(3):859–69. https://doi.org/10.1159/000518805. PMID: 34899259; PMCID: PMC8613549.
48. Kaushik S, Kataria P, Joshi G, Singh R, Handa S, Pandav SS, Ram J, Gupta A. Perioperative propranolol: a useful adjunct for glaucoma surgery in Sturge-Weber syndrome. Ophthalmol Glaucoma. 2019;2(4):267–74. https://doi.org/10.1016/j.ogla.2019.03.006. Epub 2019 Mar 28. PMID: 32672550.
49. Sujansky E, Conradi S. Sturge-Weber syndrome: age of onset of seizures and glaucoma and the prognosis for affected children. J Child Neurol. 1995;10(1):49–58. https://doi.org/10.1177/088307389501000113. PMID: 7769179.
50. Miller RS, Ball KL, Comi AM, Germain-Lee EL. Growth hormone deficiency in Sturge-weber syndrome. Arch Dis Child. 2006;91(4):340–1. https://doi.org/10.1136/adc.2005.082578. PMID: 16551788; PMCID: PMC2065976.
51. Martí-Bonmatí L, Menor F, Poyatos C, Cortina H. Diagnosis of Sturge-Weber syndrome: comparison of the efficacy of CT and MR imaging in 14 cases. AJR Am J Roentgenol. 1992;158(4):867–71. https://doi.org/10.2214/ajr.158.4.1546607. PMID: 1546607.
52. Tournut P, Turjman F, Guibal AL, Revol M, Gilly R, Lapras C, Froment JC. MRI in Sturge-Weber syndrome. J Neuroradiol. 1992;19(4):285–92. English, French. PMID: 1464780.
53. Sabeti S, Ball KL, Bhattacharya SK, Bitrian E, Blieden LS, Brandt JD, Burkhart C, Chugani HT, Falchek SJ, Jain BG, Juhasz C, Loeb JA, Luat A, Pinto A, Segal E, Salvin J, Kelly KM. Consensus statement for the management and treatment of Sturge-Weber syndrome: neurology, neuroimaging, and ophthalmology recommendations. Pediatr Neurol. 2021;121:59–66. https://doi.org/10.1016/j.pediatrneurol.2021.04.013. Epub 2021 May 6. PMID: 34153815; PMCID: PMC9107097.
54. Wyburn-Mason R. Arteriovenous aneurysm of mid-brain and retina, facial nævi and mental changes. Brain. 1943;66(3):163–203. https://doi.org/10.1093/brain/66.3.163.
55. Bech K, Jensen OA. On the frequency of co-existing racemose haemangiomata of the retina and brain. Acta Psychiatr Scand. 1961;36(1):47–56. https://doi.org/10.1111/j.1600-0447.1961.tb01756.x. PMID: 13688352.
56. Dayani PN, Sadun AA. A case report of Wyburn-Mason syndrome and review of the literature. Neuroradiology. 2007;49(5):445–56. https://doi.org/10.1007/s00234-006-0205-x. Epub 2007 Jan 18. PMID: 17235577.
57. Ponce FA, Han PP, Spetzler RF, Canady A, Feiz-Erfan I. Associated arteriovenous malformation of the orbit and brain: a case of Wyburn-Mason syndrome without retinal involvement. Case report. J Neurosurg. 2001;95(2):346–9. https://doi.org/10.3171/jns.2001.95.2.0346. PMID: 11780909.
58. Hopen G, Smith JL, Hoff JT, Quencer R. The Wyburn-Mason syndrome. Concomitant chiasmal and fundus vascular malformations. J Clin Neuroophthalmol. 1983;3(1):53–62. PMID: 6222080.
59. Goh D, Malik NN, Gilvarry A. Retinal racemose haemangioma directly communicating with a intramuscular facial cavernous haemangioma. Br J Ophthalmol. 2004;88(6):840–2. https://doi.org/10.1136/bjo.2003.028191. PMID: 15148230; PMCID: PMC1772200.
60. Archer DB, Deutman A, Ernest JT, Krill AE. Arteriovenous communications of the retina. Am J Ophthalmol. 1973;75(2):224–41. https://doi.org/10.1016/0002-9394(73)91018-0. PMID: 4697179.
61. Hardy TG, O'Day J. Retinal arteriovenous malformation with fluctuating vision and ischemic central retinal vein occlusion and its sequelae:

25-year follow-up of a case. J Neuroophthalmol. 1998;18(4):233–6. PMID: 9858001.

62. Nadal J, Delás B. Temporal branch retinal vein occlusion secondary to a racemose hemangioma. Retin Cases Brief Rep. 2010;4(4):323–5. https://doi.org/10.1097/ICB.0b013e3181af7b57. PMID: 25390909.
63. Schatz H, Chang LF, Ober RR, McDonald HR, Johnson RN. Central retinal vein occlusion associated with retinal arteriovenous malformation. Ophthalmology. 1993;100(1):24–30. https://doi.org/10.1016/s0161-6420(93)31701-x.
64. Wester ST, Murray TG. Retinal arteriovenous malformation presenting with retinal vein occlusion during pregnancy. Retin Cases Brief Rep. 2010;4(2):112–5. https://doi.org/10.1097/ICB.0b013e318196b36b. PMID: 25390378.
65. Elizalde J, Vasquez L. Spontaneous regression in a case of racemose haemangioma archer's type 2. Retin Cases Brief Rep. 2011;5(4):294–6. https://doi.org/10.1097/ICB.0b013e3181f66a97. PMID: 25390417.
66. Yamauchi K, Suzuki Y, Tanaka-Gonome T, Adachi K, Maeda N, Nakazawa M. Racemose hemangioma complicated with macular macroaneurysm rupture. Am J Ophthalmol Case Rep. 2021;22:101053. https://doi.org/10.1016/j.ajoc.2021.101053. PMID: 33786403; PMCID: PMC7994723.
67. Pichi F, Morara M, Torrazza C, Manzi G, Alkabes M, Balducci N, Vitale L, Lembo A, Ciardella AP, Nucci P. Intravitreal bevacizumab for macular complications from retinal arterial macroaneurysms. Am J Ophthalmol. 2013;155(2):287–294.e1. https://doi.org/10.1016/j.ajo.2012.07.029. Epub 2012 Oct 27. PMID: 23111179.
68. Vishal R, Avadesh O, Srinivas R, Taraprasad D. Retinal racemose hemangioma with retinal artery macroaneurysm: optical coherence tomography angiography (OCTA) findings. Am J Ophthalmol Case Rep. 2018;21(11):98–100. https://doi.org/10.1016/j.ajoc.2018.06.018. PMID: 29998207; PMCID: PMC6038827.
69. Janetos T, Cicinelli MV, Mirza RG, Jampol LM. Photocoagulation of transudative type 2 retinal arteriovenous malformation. JAMA Ophthalmol. 2021;139(7):805–7. https://doi.org/10.1001/jamaophthalmol.2021.1436. PMID: 34014273.
70. Wolff B, Tick S, Cohen SY. Photocoagulation therapy of leaking Archer's type 2 retinal arteriovenous communication. Retin Cases Brief Rep. 2013;7(1):95–7. https://doi.org/10.1097/ICB.0b013e31826f0927. PMID: 25390534.
71. Jensen VA. X: studies on the branchings of the retinal blood vessels. Acta Ophthalmol. 1936;14:100–9. https://doi.org/10.1111/j.1755-3768.1936.tb07311.x.
72. Brown GC, Donoso LA, Magargal LE, Goldberg RE, Sarin LK. Congenital retinal macrovessels. Arch Ophthalmol. 1982;100(9):1430–6. https://doi.org/10.1001/archopht.1982.01030040408006. PMID: 7115168.
73. Polk TD, Park D, Sindt CW, Heffron ET. Congenital retinal macrovessel. Arch Ophthalmol. 1997;115(2):290–1. https://doi.org/10.1001/archopht.1997.01100150292030. PMID: 9046273.
74. Pichi F, Freund KB, Ciardella A, Morara M, Abboud EB, Ghazi N, Dackiw C, Choudhry N, Souza EC, Cunha LP, Arevalo JF, Liu TYA, Wenick A, He L, Villarreal G Jr, Neri P, Sarraf D. Congenital retinal macrovessel and the association of retinal venous malformations with venous malformations of the brain. JAMA Ophthalmol. 2018;136(4):372–9. https://doi.org/10.1001/jamaophthalmol.2018.0150. Erratum in: JAMA Ophthalmol. 2018 Oct 1;136(10):1208. PMID: 29494725; PMCID: PMC5876911.
75. Gass JD. Cavernous hemangioma of the retina. A neuro-oculo-cutaneous syndrome. Am J Ophthalmol. 1971;71(4):799–814. https://doi.org/10.1016/0002-9394(71)90245-5. PMID: 5553009.
76. Patikulsila D, Visaetsilpanonta S, Sinclair SH, Shields JA. Cavernous hemangioma of the optic disk. Retina. 2007;27(3):391–2. https://doi.org/10.1097/01.iae.0000239415.16669.47. PMID: 17460599.
77. Yu MD, Dalvin LA, Shields CL. Retinal cavernous hemangioma with intralesional phleboliths. Retin Cases Brief Rep. 2020;14(4):301–4. https://doi.org/10.1097/ICB.0000000000000724. PMID: 29505489.
78. Messmer E, Laqua H, Wessing A, Spitznas M, Weidle E, Ruprecht K, Naumann GO. Nine cases of cavernous hemangioma of the retina. Am J Ophthalmol. 1983;95(3):383–90. https://doi.org/10.1016/s0002-9394(14)78309-6. PMID: 6829684.
79. Pringle E, Chen S, Rubinstein A, Patel CK, Downes S. Optical coherence tomography in retinal cavernous haemangioma may explain the mechanism of vitreous haemorrhage. Eye (Lond). 2009;23(5):1242–3. https://doi.org/10.1038/eye.2008.156. Epub 2008 Jun 6. PMID: 18535599.
80. Goldberg RE, Pheasant TR, Shields JA. Cavernous hemangioma of the retina. A four-generation pedigree with neurocutaneous manifestations and an example of bilateral retinal involvement. Arch Ophthalmol. 1979;97(12):2321–4. https://doi.org/10.1001/archopht.1979.01020020537005. PMID: 229814.
81. Sarraf D, Payne AM, Kitchen ND, Sehmi KS, Downes SM, Bird AC. Familial cavernous hemangioma: an expanding ocular spectrum. Arch Ophthalmol. 2000;118(7):969–73. PMID: 1090011200.
82. Labauge P, Denier C, Bergametti F, Tournier-Lasserve E. Genetics of cavernous angiomas. Lancet Neurol. 2007;6(3):237–44. https://doi.org/10.1016/S1474-4422(07)70053-4. PMID: 17303530.
83. Labauge P, Krivosic V, Denier C, Tournier-Lasserve E, Gaudric A. Frequency of retinal cavernomas in 60 patients with familial cerebral cavernomas: a clinical and genetic study. Arch Ophthalmol. 2006;124(6):885–6. https://doi.org/10.1001/archopht.124.6.885. PMID: 16769843.

84. Wang W, Chen L. Cavernous hemangioma of the retina: a comprehensive review of the literature (1934–2015). Retina. 2017;37(4):611–21. https://doi.org/10.1097/IAE.0000000000001374. PMID: 27820777.
85. Rigamonti D, Hadley MN, Drayer BP, Johnson PC, Hoenig-Rigamonti K, Knight JT, Spetzler RF. Cerebral cavernous malformations. Incidence and familial occurrence. N Engl J Med. 1988;319(6):343–7. https://doi.org/10.1056/NEJM198808113190605. PMID: 3393196.
86. Mouchtouris N, Chalouhi N, Chitale A, Starke RM, Tjoumakaris SI, Rosenwasser RH, Jabbour PM. Management of cerebral cavernous malformations: from diagnosis to treatment. ScientificWorldJournal. 2015;2015:808314. https://doi.org/10.1155/2015/808314. Epub 2015 Jan 5. PMID: 25629087; PMCID: PMC4300037.
87. Fowler BJ, Simon L, Scott NL, Negron CI, Berrocal AM. Case report: vitreous hemorrhage as the presenting sign of retinal cavernous hemangioma in a newborn. Am J Ophthalmol Case Rep. 2021;22(23):101174. https://doi.org/10.1016/j.ajoc.2021.101174. PMID: 34381923; PMCID: PMC8332665.
88. Hasanpour H, Ramezani A, Karimi S. Recurrent vitreous hemorrhage in a case of retinal cavernous hemangioma: a rare presentation. J Ophthalmic Vis Res. 2016;11(3):333–5. https://doi.org/10.4103/2008-322X.188398. PMID: 27621796; PMCID: PMC5000541.
89. Karpe A, Suganeswari G. Spontaneous vitreous hemorrhage in a case of retinal cavernous hemangioma: a rare presentation. JAMA Ophthalmol. 2013;131(7):897. https://doi.org/10.1001/jamaophthalmol.2013.1424. PMID: 23846203.
90. Shields JA, Eagle RC Jr, Ewing MQ, Lally SE, Shields CL. Retinal cavernous hemangioma: fifty-two years of clinical follow-up with clinicopathologic correlation. Retina. 2014;34(6):1253–7. https://doi.org/10.1097/IAE.0000000000000232. PMID: 24849703.
91. Sakano LY, Neufeld CR, Aihara T. Medical monitoring of patient with cavernous hemangioma of the retina and intracranial involvement. Am J Ophthalmol Case Rep. 2020;27(17):100602. https://doi.org/10.1016/j.ajoc.2020.100602. PMID: 32083222; PMCID: PMC7019121.
92. Robertson DM. Ophthalmic manifestations of tuberous sclerosis. Ann N Y Acad Sci. 1991;615:17–25. https://doi.org/10.1111/j.1749-6632.1991.tb37744.x. PMID: 2039142.
93. Wan MJ, Chan KL, Jastrzembski BG, Ali A. Neuro-ophthalmological manifestations of tuberous sclerosis: current perspectives. Eye Brain. 2019;11:13–23. https://doi.org/10.2147/EB.S186306. PMID: 31417327; PMCID: PMC65920650.
94. Sancak O, Nellist M, Goedbloed M, Elfferich P, Wouters C, Maat-Kievit A, Zonnenberg B, Verhoef S, Halley D, van den Ouweland A. Mutational analysis of the TSC1 and TSC2 genes in a diagnostic setting: genotype--phenotype correlations and comparison of diagnostic DNA techniques in Tuberous Sclerosis Complex. Eur J Hum Genet. 2005;13(6):731–41. https://doi.org/10.1038/sj.ejhg.5201402. PMID: 15798777.
95. Rowley SA, O'Callaghan FJ, Osborne JP. Ophthalmic manifestations of tuberous sclerosis: a population based study. Br J Ophthalmol. 2001;85(4):420–3. https://doi.org/10.1136/bjo.85.4.420. PMID: 11264130; PMCID: PMC1723924.
96. Mutolo MG, Marciano S, Benassi F, Pardini M, Curatolo P, Gialloreti LE. Optical coherence tomography and infrared images of astrocytic hamartomas not revealed by FUNDUSCOPY in tuberous sclerosis complex. Retina. 2017;37(7):1383–92. https://doi.org/10.1097/IAE.0000000000001373. PMID: 27787447.
97. Venkatesh R, Reddy NG, Jayadev C, Bhatt A, Agrawal R, Yadav NK. Utility of multimodal ocular imaging in tuberous sclerosis complex—review of literature along with a case illustration. Indian J Ophthalmol. 2022;70(7):2720–4. https://doi.org/10.4103/ijo.IJO_2920_21. PMID: 35791221; PMCID: PMC9426122.
98. Allan KC, Hua HU, Singh AD, Yuan A. Rapid symptomatic and structural improvement of a retinal astrocytic hamartoma in response to anti-VEGF therapy: a case report. Am J Ophthalmol Case Rep. 2022;27:101606. https://doi.org/10.1016/j.ajoc.2022.101606. PMID: 35692434; PMCID: PMC9184888.
99. Shields JA, Eagle RC Jr, Shields CL, Marr BP. Aggressive retinal astrocytomas in four patients with tuberous sclerosis complex. Trans Am Ophthalmol Soc. 2004;102:139–47; discussion 147-8. PMID: 15747752; PMCID: PMC1280094.
100. Franz DN, Leonard J, Tudor C, Chuck G, Care M, Sethuraman G, Dinopoulos A, Thomas G, Crone KR. Rapamycin causes regression of astrocytomas in tuberous sclerosis complex. Ann Neurol. 2006;59(3):490–8. https://doi.org/10.1002/ana.20784. PMID: 16453317
101. Li M, Zhou Y, Chen C, et al. Efficacy and safety of mTOR inhibitors (rapamycin and its analogues) for tuberous sclerosis complex: a meta-analysis. Orphanet J Rare Dis. 2019;14:39. https://doi.org/10.1186/s13023-019-1012-x.
102. House RJ, Mashayekhi A, Shields JA, Shields CL. Total regression of acquired retinal astrocytoma using photodynamic therapy. Retin Cases Brief Rep. 2016;10(1):41–3. https://doi.org/10.1097/ICB.0000000000000169. PMID: 26164044.
103. Eskelin S, Tommila P, Palosaari T, Kivelä T. Photodynamic therapy with verteporfin to induce regression of aggressive retinal astrocytomas. Acta Ophthalmol. 2008;86(7):794–9. https://doi.org/10.1111/j.1755-3768.2007.01151.x. Epub 2008 Aug 27. PMID: 18759802.

104. Asthagiri AR, Parry DM, Butman JA, Kim HJ, Tsilou ET, Zhuang Z, Lonser RR. Neurofibromatosis type 2. Lancet. 2009;373(9679):1974–86. https://doi.org/10.1016/S0140-6736(09)60259-2. Epub 2009 May 22. PMID: 19476995; PMCID: PMC4748851.
105. Linn Murphree A. Intraocular retinoblastoma: the case for a new group classification. Ophthalmol Clin N Am. 2005;18(1):41–53. https://doi.org/10.1016/j.ohc.2004.11.003, viii. PMID: 15763190.
106. Shields CL, Mashayekhi A, Au AK, Czyz C, Leahey A, Meadows AT, Shields JA. The international classification of retinoblastoma predicts chemoreduction success. Ophthalmology. 2006;113(12):2276–80. https://doi.org/10.1016/j.ophtha.2006.06.018. Epub 2006 Sep 25. PMID: 16996605.
107. Canadian Retinoblastoma Society. National Retinoblastoma Strategy Canadian Guidelines for Care: Stratégie thérapeutique du rétinoblastome guide clinique canadien. Can J Ophthalmol. 2009;44(Suppl 2):S1–88. https://doi.org/10.3129/i09-194. PMID: 20237571.
108. Dommering CJ, Mol BM, Moll AC, Burton M, Cloos J, Dorsman JC, Meijers-Heijboer H, van der Hout AH. RB1 mutation spectrum in a comprehensive nationwide cohort of retinoblastoma patients. J Med Genet. 2014;51(6):366–74. https://doi.org/10.1136/jmedgenet-2014-102264. Epub 2014 Mar 31. PMID: 24688104.
109. Rushlow D, Piovesan B, Zhang K, Prigoda-Lee NL, Marchong MN, Clark RD, Gallie BL. Detection of mosaic RB1 mutations in families with retinoblastoma. Hum Mutat. 2009;30(5):842–51. https://doi.org/10.1002/humu.20940. PMID: 19280657.
110. Temming P, Arendt M, Viehmann A, Eisele L, Le Guin CH, Schündeln MM, Biewald E, Astrahantseff K, Wieland R, Bornfeld N, Sauerwein W, Eggert A, Jöckel KH, Lohmann DR. Incidence of second cancers after radiotherapy and systemic chemotherapy in heritable retinoblastoma survivors: a report from the German reference center. Pediatr Blood Cancer. 2017;64(1):71–80. https://doi.org/10.1002/pbc.26193. Epub 2016 Aug 27. PMID: 27567086.

Optic Disc Signs—Cupping, Swelling, Inflammation, and Pallor

15

15.1 Anatomical Considerations

Nearly 1.2 million retinal ganglion cells (RGCs) axons exit at the back of the eye through fine fenestrations in the sclera termed lamina cribrosa. These RGC axons, also called the retinal nerve fibre (RNF), form the anteriormost layer of the neurosensory retina (NSR). The RGCs are the thickest at the fovea and 7-cell thick; in the retinal periphery, they are barely one cell thick. Glial septa separate the RNF layer (RNFL) bundles and converge at the optic disc to exit the eye as the optic nerve, the second cranial nerve. The RGC axons turn 90° over the Bruch's membrane and retinal pigment epithelium (RPE) at the border of the scleral canal to exit the eye through the fine fenestrations in the lamina cribrosa.

Till they exit the eye, the RGC axons are unmyelinated. The RGC axons are arranged in a laminar fashion. The most peripheral axons lie deepest in the RNFL and enter the optic disc in the most peripheral part. The retinal fibres from the posterior retina enter the more central part of the optic disc. Nearly 90% of the axons leaving the eye arise from the macula [1]. Each axon receives inputs from nearly 100 rod photoreceptors and 4–5 cone photoreceptors. These RGC axons are also accompanied by glial cells, including astrocytes (provide nutrition), microglia (phagocytic), and oligodendrocytes seen only posterior to the lamina cribrosa (myelination). The optic disc, also known as the optic nerve head (ONH), marks the beginning of the optic nerve, which courses through the orbit and finally exits the orbit through the optic canal to enter the cranial cavity. As the optic nerve exits the sclera, it gets myelinated by the oligodendrocytes and becomes ~twice the thickness of the ONH (~3 mm). The pia mater and the arachnoid cover the optic nerve. The pia mater is a fibrovascular covering of the nerve which sends delicate fibrovascular septa and segregates the axons into fascicles or bundles. It provides blood supply to the core of the optic nerve. The arachnoid layer is a loose web-like syncytial fibro cellular layer that covers the optic nerve. The dura mater is the outermost tough fibrous sheath, also called the optic nerve sheath, which gets fused with the sclera anteriorly and, through the optic canal, continues posteriorly with the dural lining of the brain. The subarachnoid space around the optic nerve contains cerebrospinal fluid (CSF) right up to the sclera and is continuous with the CSF in the brain.

The intraocular part of the ONH is ~1 mm and has four parts, superficial nerve fibre layer, prelaminar, laminar, and retrolaminar. The internal limiting membrane of the retina continues over the ONH as Elschnig's membrane. The centre of the ONH has a gliotic central meniscus of Kuhnt, a remnant of the hyaloid artery. The axons in the ONH are separated from the NSR, RPE, Bruch's membrane, choroid, and sclera by an astrocytic

A. Gupta et al., *Ophthalmic Signs in Practice of Medicine*,
https://doi.org/10.1007/978-981-99-7923-3_15

ring of connective tissue, the intermediary tissue of Kuhnt, the border tissue of Jacoby, and the border tissue of Elschnig, respectively.

In the intraocular course, the macular fibres lie temporally, and the nasal fibres lie nasally. However, the macular fibres lie in the optic nerve's centre as they course through the orbit. The optic nerve has a sinuous course in orbit of ~25 to 30 mm (for the eye's movement in orbit). It runs for about ~10 mm in the optic canal and is firmly anchored to the optic canal. The optic nerve is surrounded by the pia mater, the arachnoid, and the dura mater extending from behind the globe into the optic canal.

The intracranial part of the optic nerve, also termed the cisternal segment, is covered with only the pia mater. As the optic nerves emerge from the optic foramen, they extend posteriorly, rise by about 45°, and converge to form the optic chiasm at the base of the brain (Fig. 15.1). The optic chiasm lies in a suprasellar cistern, ~10 mm above the pituitary gland in the sella turcica. The anterior part of the third ventricle lies just above the optic chiasm.

In the chiasm, the fibres from the nasal half of the retina from both eyes decussate (cross in 'X') to the opposite side, while the temporal fibres remain uncrossed. Therefore, the optic tracts that diverge from the optic chiasm carry fibres for the opposite half of the field of vision, i.e. the right optic tract projects to the left hemifield and vice versa for the left optic tract. Nearly 53% of the retinal fibres cross over to the opposite side.

In the chiasm, the crossing nasal axons and the uncrossed temporal axons from the inferior retina cross anteriorly on the ventral aspect of the optic

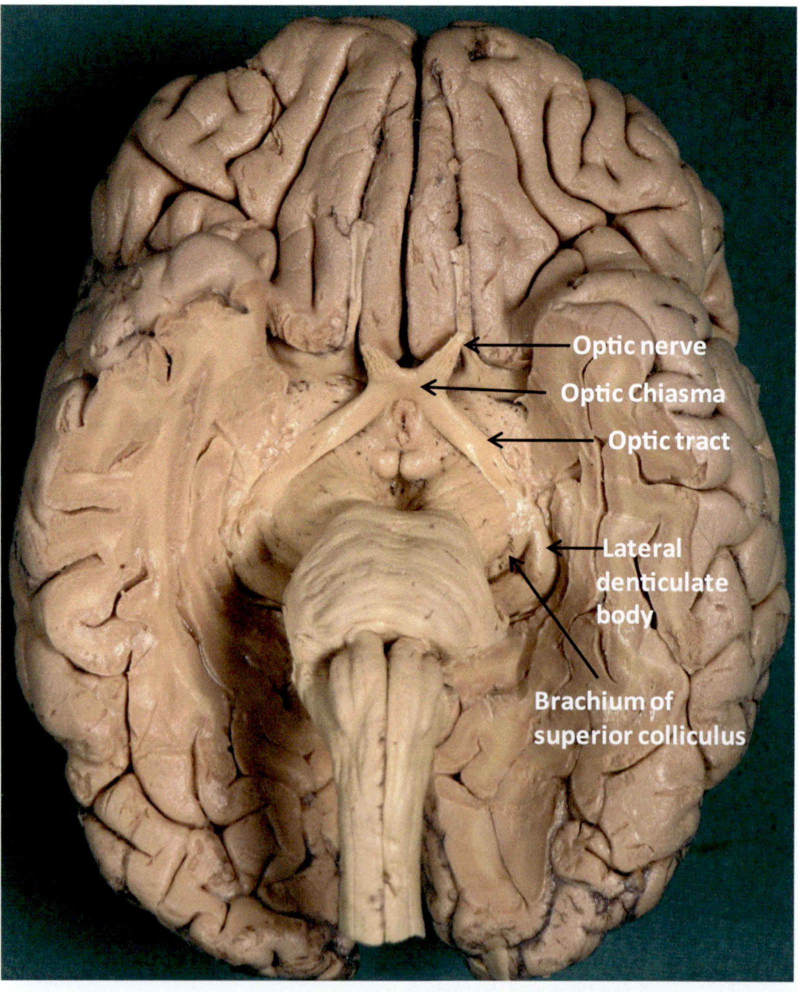

Fig. 15.1 Inferior aspect of the human brain showing some of the components of the visual pathway. Image courtesy of Prof Daisy Sahni (Ex-Professor) and Prof Anjali Aggarwal (Head), Department of Anatomy, Post Graduate Institute of Medical Education and Research, Chandigarh, India

chiasm, while the superior axons cross on the chiasma's dorsal aspect. These axons become vulnerable to an enlarging pituitary tumour producing initially a bitemporal quadrantanopia that progresses to a bitemporal hemianopia. The crossing axons from the nasal macula cross in the posterior part of the chiasma. Nearly 85–90% of axons proceed to the lateral geniculate nucleus (LGN) located on the posteroinferior aspect of the thalamus; the rest go to the pretectal nucleus. The lower nasal crossing axons from the left eye and uncrossed lower temporal axons from the right eye synapse in the lateral third of the right LGN. The lateral third of the right LGN projects to the left-sided upper temporal quadrant of the homonymous field of vision. The upper nasal crossing axons from the left eye and the uncrossed upper temporal axons from the right eye end up in the medial third of the right LGN. These project to the left-sided lower temporal quadrant of the homonymous field of vision. The crossing axons from the nasal retina synapse in the LGN in layers 1, 4, and 6 and the uncrossed temporal fibres synapse in layers 2, 3, and 5. The macular axons synapse in LGN in its upper and posterior portions, and the post-synaptic axons extend into the optic radiation in the central third. The superior and inferior axons extend posteriorly in the optic radiation's superior and inferior third, respectively. The inferior axons form Meyer's loop. In the visual cortex, the axons from the inferior retina synapse in the inferior bank of the calcarine fissure and the axons from the superior retina synapse in the superior bank of the calcarine fissure. The macular fibres synapse in the caudal visual cortex, where they are most vulnerable to the trauma sustained during a fall on the occiput. [2].

15.2 Blood Supply of the Visual Pathways

15.2.1 Blood Supply of the Optic Chiasm

The optic chiasm gets its blood supply from the anterior cerebral arteries, anterior communicating arteries on its dorsal and anterior aspect and the basilar artery, posterior communicating arteries, and the posterior cerebral arteries from below. This network of arteries is called the arterial circle of Willis. The internal carotid arteries flank the chiasm, and the cavernous sinus lies below and lateral.

LGN gets its blood supply from the anterior and posterior choroidal arteries. The optic tracts do so from the anterior choroidal and middle cerebral arteries. The visual cortex in the calcarine sulcus gets its blood supply from the posterior cerebral artery.

15.2.2 Blood Supply of the Optic Nerve

The ophthalmic artery is the first branch that arises from the intradural part of the internal carotid artery, and the diameter varies from 2.16 mm to 2.25 mm at its origin. It courses anteriorly through the floor of the optic canal ensheathed with the optic nerve and, just before entering the orbital apex, penetrates the dura mater again to exit the optic foramen from the lateral aspect of the optic nerve [3]. The intracranial part of the optic nerve is supplied by the superior hypophyseal arteries, 1–4 in number and 0.1–0.5 mm in size. These arise from the internal carotid artery and the posterior communicating artery. The intracanalicular part is supplied by the subpial and the intraneural branches of the superior hypophyseal arteries, and some may come from the intracranial (one, <0.1 mm) or the intraorbital (2–5, 0.1–0.4 mm) part of the ophthalmic artery. Because of the rigid canal with a small diameter, the vessels are vulnerable to rupture by trauma and cause compression of the optic nerve by swelling or haemorrhage in the subdural space [4]. The intraorbital part of the optic nerve is supplied by branches from the short and long posterior ciliary arteries which enter the dura, cross the dural space, and form a subpial and intraneural plexus [4]. The central retina artery enters the dural sheath about 12 mm behind the globe, runs in the subarachnoid space, and then runs an intraneural course to enter the eye.

15.2.3 Blood Supply of the Optic Nerve Head

The superficial nerve fibre layer gets blood supply through the capillary network drawn from the retinal arterial supply (Fig. 15.2). The prelaminar part of the optic disc gets its blood supply from the peripapillary choroid, which in turn gets its supply from 2–3 posterior ciliary arteries, varying from 1 to 5. There is no supply from the choriocapillaris or the central retina artery in the prelaminar part. The laminar part of the ONH gets supplied from the arterial circle of Zinn and Haller (ZHAC) and, when present (~50%), is formed by branches of the posterior ciliary arteries. Thus, individuals' arterial supply to the laminar ONH is highly variable [5]. The ZHAC is located in the posterior sclera surrounding the ONH at the junction of the dura mater with the sclera [6]. The ZHAC has strict distribution in the superior and inferior parts of the ONH. This part of the ONH has a rich capillary plexus. The laminar part of the ONH is packed with 1.2 million fibres in a very narrow and confined space. It is highly vulnerable to the pressure differential between the intraocular and cerebrospinal fluid pressure in the optic nerve sheath. Notably, the posterior ciliary arteries are strictly end-arterial under autonomic control, making the ONH's laminar part highly vulnerable to developing ischaemic events due to a fall in perfusion pressure. The fundus fluorescein angiography often reveals a watershed zone between the blood supply from the lateral and medial ciliary arteries [5]. The retrolaminar part gets supply from the centripetal pial branches, some branches from the central retinal artery or the rich plexus formed by the recurrent branches from the circle of Zinn-Haller (Fig. 15.2). Longitudinal vessels have also been demonstrated to extend from the retrolaminar optic nerve to the anterior surface of the ONH. These are seen to anastomose with the transverse system drawn from the ciliary circulation [7].

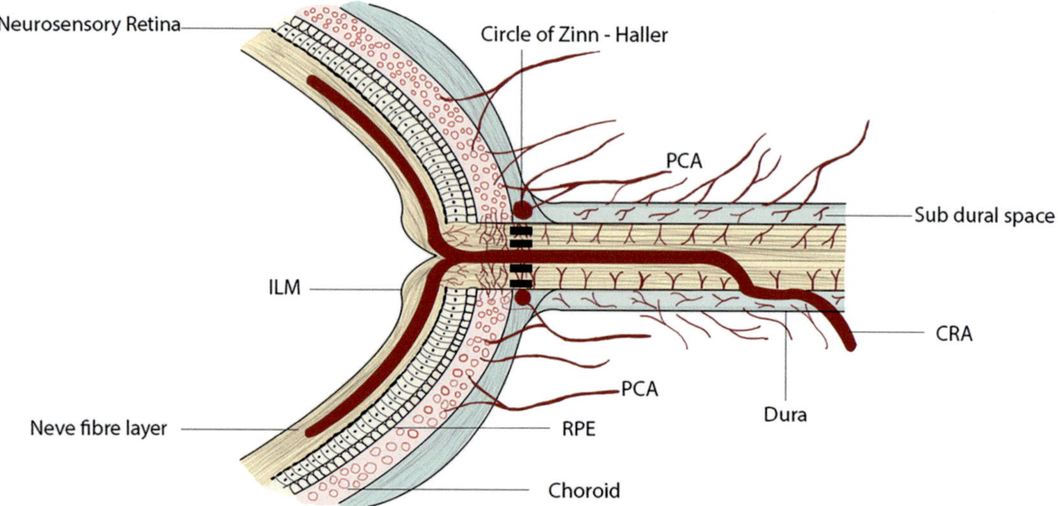

Fig. 15.2 Highly schematic representation of the blood supply of the optic nerve head. (CRA = Centra Retinal Artery; ILM = Internal limiting membrane; PCA = Posterior ciliary artery; RPE = Retinal pigment epithelium). Note that the laminar optic nerve head receives blood supply from the branches of the posterior ciliary arteries. In contrast, the prelaminar optic nerve head gets supply from the peripapillary choroid. The superficial optic nerve head gets its supply from the capillaries drawn from the retinal artery branches. The central retinal artery does not supply blood to the retrolaminar optic nerve, which is served by the pial branches of the posterior ciliary arteries. Graphic by Kritika Thakur

15.3 Evaluation of the Optic Disc

The anterior end of the optic nerve is visible in the eye on ophthalmoscopy. It is called the ONH or the optic disc (OD). It is a pink, vertically oval disc-like structure. The ONH/OD size measured on histopathological examination in eye bank eyes is 1.88 mm vertical and 1.77 mm horizontal, irrespective of the axial length of the eyeballs. It is larger than the diameter measured with imaging techniques. The vertical diameter in blacks is significantly greater than that in whites. Women have a narrower horizontal diameter than men [8].

15.3.1 Clinical Assessment of the Optic Disc Size

The optic disc size can be easily estimated using the middle viewing aperture on a direct ophthalmoscope which projects a 1.5 mm diameter (5°) of the light spot on the retina and about covers the entire extent of the ONH. The optic disc size can also be measured using high + biconvex lenses, 60D, 78D, or 90D, during the biomicroscopic examination of the optic disc. A narrow slit-lamp beam is projected to measure the horizontal or vertical diameter; the beam height is shortened until it covers the optic disc edge to edge. A correction must be applied to the beam length (beam height scale shown on the slit-lamp) 1.0X, 1.1X, and 1.3X, respectively, for the 60, 78, and 90 D lenses. The same technique can measure the optic disc cup (ODC) height and width.

15.3.2 Optic Disc Cup (ODC) and Glaucoma

A normal-sized ONH shows a small round or slight vertical oval depression centred a little to the temporal side called the physiological cup (Fig. 15.3a). The central retinal artery and the central retinal vein usually emerge from the nasal side of the cup. The area between the margins of the cup and the scleral rim is packed with exiting RGC neurons called the neuroretinal rim (NRR). The cup is covered with a remnant gliotic membrane of Kuhnt. There are wide variations in the ONH size depending on the size of the scleral canal. Irrespective of the size of the ONH, almost 1.2 million axons get packed; thus, a small ONH crowded with axons may not show any physiological cup. Such eyes are at risk of developing non-arteritic anterior ischaemic optic neuropathy (ni-AION).

On the other hand, a large-sized ONH carries the same number of axons and is still left with a large cup (Fig. 15.3b). The space between the lamina cribrosa and the surface of the ONH is filled with prelaminar tissue. The cup is usually assessed for its vertical and horizontal diameter. The cup diameter is compared to the diameter of the ONH and is expressed as a fraction termed cup-to-disc ratio, the C/D ratio, or CDR. Enlarging optic disc cup (ODC) is a critical sign of the progression of open-angle glaucoma (OAG) (Fig. 15.3 c, d). OAG is now believed to be an optic neuropathy resulting in progressive, irreversible RGC axons loss (Fig. 15.4). The significant risk factors for OAG are higher than normal intraocular pressure (IOP), myopia, age, and race. Nearly 1/3rd of the patients with OAG may show normal or lower than-normal IOP (Fig. 15.4). The loss of RGC axons is reflected in their attrition from the ONH, with a consequent increase in the size of the ODC. A uniform enlargement of the ODC may be mistaken for a large physiological cup unless a smaller cup has been imaged previously in the same eye. The median CDR is 0.3. Usually, the CDR < 0.7 is normal if the optic disc size is average. CDR ≥ 0.8 is highly suspicious of OAG, irrespective of the disc size. Asymmetric enlargement of the ODC, especially when seen at the ONH's upper or lower pole as a focal notch, is almost always acquired and pathognomonic of OAG (Fig. 15.4). ONH smaller than average often has no ODC. Thus, ODC of any size in such eyes highly suggests OAG. Notably, the ODC in the two eyes are symmetrical, and variation of C/D Raito ≥ 1 between the two eyes should raise suspicion of glaucoma.

The loss of the RGC axons is reflected in visual field defects called scotomas (Fig. 15.4c). OAG is an asymptomatic disorder and is a sig-

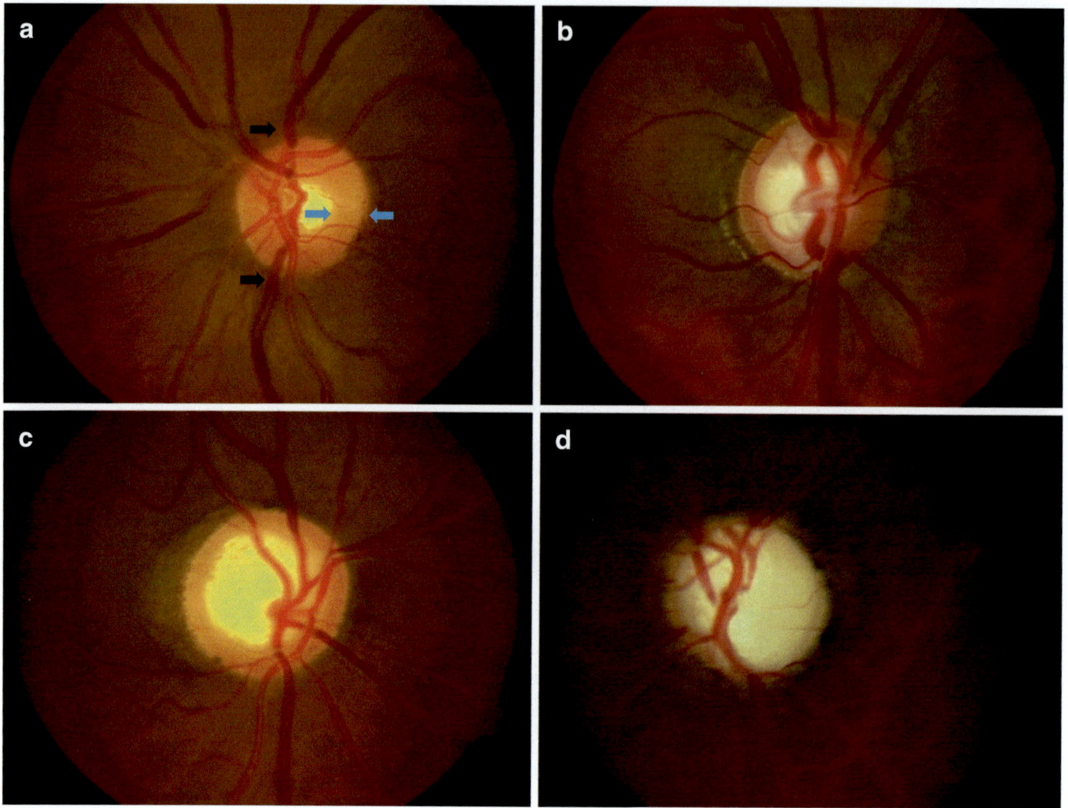

Fig. 15.3 ONH evaluation and glaucoma: A normal-sized ONH shows a small round or slight vertical oval depression centred a little to the temporal (T) side called the physiological cup (**a**). The central retinal artery and the central retinal vein usually emerge (black arrows) from the cup's nasal (N) side. The area between the margins of the cup and the scleral rim is packed with exiting RGC neurons called the neuroretinal rim (blue arrows). A large-sized ONH carries the same number of axons and is still left with a large cup (**b**). An enlarged optic disc cup (ODC) is a critical sign of the progression of open-angle glaucoma (OAG) (**c**, **d**). Images courtesy of Prof SS Pandav, Professor and Head, Advanced Eye Centre, Post Graduate Institute of Medical Education and Research, Chandigarh, India

nificant cause of blindness. ODC evaluation during a screening visit is the most critical sign in suspecting and preventing blindness from OAG. A visual field examination confirms the loss of RGC axons (Fig. 15.4c). Since IOP is a significant risk factor for OAG, the only known intervention reducing the risk of further damage is lowering IOP using local therapy or filtration surgical procedures. While a higher-than-normal IOP may provide a clue to OAG, many such patients may not show glaucomatous ODC or visual field changes and are labelled ocular hypertension. Given the uncertainty of the IOP as a diagnostic sign and the logistic and time constraints of doing visual field testing in a screening program, evaluation of the optic disc for glaucomatous cupping either on the ophthalmoscopy or remote evaluation from the optic disc imaging remains the most favoured technique.

Using enhanced depth imaging with spectral domain optical coherence tomography (EDI-OCT), the depth of the physiological cup can be measured and the volume can be calculated.

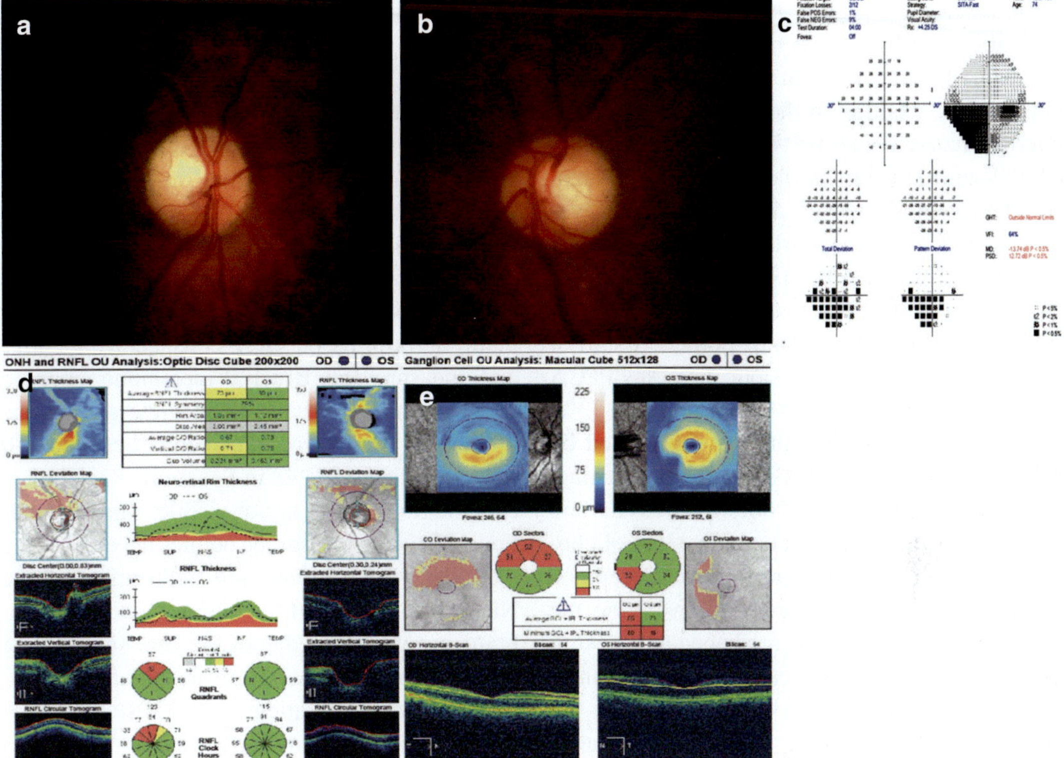

Fig. 15.4 A 77- year-old man was referred as a case of open-angle glaucoma. He had a history of sudden blurring of vision. His visual acuity was 6/12 in the right eye and 6/6 in the left eye. The intraocular pressures were 12mmHg in both eyes. The superior half of the neuroretinal rim of the right optic disc showed pallor (**a**). The left optic disc appeared normal (**b**). A 24.2 visual field in the right eye showed an inferior altitudinal defect corresponding to the rim pallor(**c**). SD-OCT showed thinning of the superior peripapillary RNFL in the right eye (**d**). There was significant thinning of the macular ganglion cells in the superior half of the right eye and some thinning of the lower nasal sector in the left eye (**e**). Images courtesy of Prof SS Pandav, Professor and Head, Advanced Eye Centre, Post Graduate Institute of Medical Education and Research, Chandigarh, India

15.3.3 Challenges of Evaluation of the Optic Disc Cupping

Typically, the optic disc is slightly vertically oval, and the margins are finely blurred as the bundles of RGC axons cross over the edge. The vertical diameter is the maximum diameter, and the horizontal diameter is the minimum, with a difference of about 7%. In a normal population study, the horizontal diameter was 1.76 ± 0.31 mm (0.91–2.61 mm), and the vertical 1.92 ± 0.29 mm. A shallow cup, if present, is slightly horizontally oval. The mean horizontal cup diameter was 0.83 ± 0.58 mm (0.00–2.08 mm), and the mean vertical diameter was 0.77 ± 0.55 mm (0.00–2.13 mm) [9]. This appearance is due to the usual direct entry of the optic nerve into the eye. However, the nerve may enter the eye obliquely, producing the appearance of either a vertical or horizontally tilted disc. These are more often seen in eyes with myopia. The vertical tilt most often results in the temporally tilted disc and shows parapapillary atrophy temporally to the optic disc. In a temporally tilted disc, the temporal NRR is thinned out, and the horizontal boundary of the cup may be difficult to define.

On the other hand, the horizontal tilt results in an inferior tilted disc with parapapillary atrophy below the disc. Since these eyes also have an axial elongation, the IOP exerts maximum pressure on the axons passing through the disc's upper and lower poles, resulting in the loss of superior and inferior arcuate retinal nerve fibres. The horizontal tilt leads to the loss of the inferior retinal arcuate fibres [10]. Moreover, the optic disc tilt eyes show significant corneal astigmatism, the steeper axis aligned with the tilt axis [11]. There is frequently a parapapillary chorioretinal atrophy (PPCA) beyond the scleral border tissue of Elschnig that surrounds the optic disc. Any PPCA is seen in 59%, zone α in 58% and zone β in 13%. The zone β, a greyish-white area, is caused by RPE falling short of Bruch's membrane opening, exposing the underlying choroidal vessels and sclera. In zone β, there is a complete loss of choriocapillaris, RPE, and overlying photoreceptors. Large choroidal vessels are seen overlying the sclera. It is seen as a crescent-shaped area next to the optic disc. It can be measured in histopathology as the distance between the RPE and the Bruch's membrane ending. Beyond the zone β, RPE hypo and hyper pigmentary are labelled Zone α. It has no significance. The presence of zone β is three times more likely to be present in patients with POAG [12]. PPCA is most frequent temporal to the optic disc and is infrequent in the nasal sector. In patients with early POAG, zone α (23%) and β are seen (42%) [13]. Zone γ is the bare peripapillary scleral flange in axial myopia without overlying choriocapillaris, BM, or RPE and is seen in the juxtapapillary area. The zone within the zone γ, which lacks blood vessels larger than 50μm, is labelled zone *δ*. Zone *δ* is seen in very high axial myopia [14].

15.3.4 OCT Evaluation of the Glaucomatous Optic Neuropathy (GON)

In recent years, remarkable progress has been made in evaluating the optic disc, RNFL, and macular parameters in the early detection and progression of glaucoma damage. All three measurements complement each other, and the sensitivity to detect changes varies with the specificity required. Several OCT machines and different algorithms are currently used to evaluate these parameters. The data are not transferrable between the machines [15].

The earliest measured cRNFL thickness at a fixed 3.5 mm circle centred on the optic disc remains the gold standard in diagnosing glaucoma [15].

In contrast to a rough estimation of the optic disc size (within the white scleral ring), automatic algorithms on OCT consistently identify and measure the Bruch's membrane opening (BMO) which currently defines the size of the optic disc. It measures the vectors between 180 points in Cirrus and 48 in Spectralis. On clinical examination, BMO is not visible. The termination of Bruch's membrane defines the edge of the disc. The ILM defines the delineation of the NRR. Termination of the internal limiting membrane provides the edge of the cup, and the size of the opening gives the diameter of the ODC [16]. Clinical estimation of the CDR on stereoscopic fundus pictures consistently underestimates the CDR. Although the clinical examination may provide a quick clue for suspecting OAG, the SD-OCT provides a more objective measurement of glaucoma damage progression [16].

15.3.5 Bruch's Membrane Opening—Minimum Rim Width in GON

On Spectralis OCT (Heidelberg Engineering, Inc., Heidelberg, Germany), 24 radial line B-scans (48 points on the BMO) can automatically measure the distance between the BMO and the ILM to give the rim width in sectors. The minimum rim width (MRW) parameter in the lower temporal sector is highly sensitive in detecting early glaucoma in younger people compared to the older, as this sector shows age-related MRW.

However, the cRNFL thickness has the highest sensitivity in detecting perimetric glaucoma [17, 18]. Guided progression analysis of the cRNFL provides the highest accuracy in detecting glaucoma progression [15].

15.3.6 Macular OCT in Glaucoma

Nearly 50% of the retinal ganglion cells are in the macula in a multilayered fashion. Although histopathological studies have shown the loss of RGC, the advent of OCT technology's ability to measure the RGC consistently has focused on the thickness of the RGC to diagnose early glaucoma. Notably, the RGC layer, the IPL, and the INL show an age-related decline by 2.8%, 2.1%, and 0.78% per decade of life [19]. So do the cRNFL thickness and the minimum neuroretinal width, but at half the rate making the RGC layer measurements attractive [19]. There is significant thinning of the GCL with increasing the axial length of the eyeball. The Cirrus HD-OCT (Carl Zeiss Meditec, Dublin, CA) provides high-speed acquisition, and a cube scan is done measuring 6 × 6 × 2 mm to provide 512 × 128 A-scans centred on the fovea. It provides a macula GCIPL thickness map of an oval 4.5 × 4 mm with the central 1.2 × 1 mm of the foveal centre removed. The thickness map is provided for six sectors, three above and three below the horizontal raphe (Fig. 15.4e). A meta-analysis of 150 studies comparing the cRNFL thickness and ganglion cell inner plexiform layer (GCIPL) found the former slightly more accurate in diagnosing early or pre-perimetric glaucoma. However, they performed equally well with moderate or advanced glaucoma. All five OCT machines performed equally well [20]. A vertical asymmetry in the inner retinal thickness is a highly valued tool in diagnosing early glaucoma [21]. Notably, the GCIPL thickness has ethnic variations, and there is a need for normative data for different ethnic groups [22].

15.3.7 Horizontal Raphe Hemifield Test in Glaucoma

The nasal step in visual fields in OAG is a pathognomonic test of perimetric OAG. In OAG, the loss of ganglion cells and their axons is asymmetric above and below the horizontal raphe. It is responsible for the step-like difference in the GCIPL above and below the horizontal raphe. It is highly discriminatory in patients with perimetric or pre-perimetric OAG, even when the optic disc signs are equivocal. For the hemifield test to be positive, the horizontal line from the temporal inner and outer annulus should be detectable for at least over half of the distance; if the thickness difference of the ganglion cells-inner plexiform layer (GCIPL) is ≥5μm and if the colour is blue in one half and red/yellow or white in the other half [23]. In older adults with a large CDR, a positive hemifield test predicted the development of normal tension glaucoma years later [24].

15.3.8 OCT Angiography

OCT angiography detects non-invasive movement of red blood cells (RBCs) in the blood vessels. In patients with glaucoma, it shows decreased superficial capillary vessel density in the peripapillary and the macular area. It also shows a lack of choriocapillaris in the parapapillary areas of chorioretinal atrophy [25].

15.3.9 Artificial Intelligence for Automatic Diagnosis of Glaucomatous Optic Neuropathy (GON)

Given the limited expertise available for interpreting the various OCT parameters for detecting OAG, attempts have been made to validate 3-D deep learning techniques for the automatic detection of OAG. The features used for deep learning were the same as those used by physicians. The accuracy reached >85%, with high sensitivity (78–90%) and specificity (79–86%) [26].

15.3.10 Myopia and GON

Myopia frequently accompanies OAG. Myopic eyes tend to have a shallow temporal rim, a shelving cup, a myopic crescent, and zone β of parapapillary chorioretinal atrophy. Zone γ is seen due to axial elongation of the eyeball in axial myopia. The fundus is tessellated, and there is overall thinning and shifting of the double hump of RNFL. In a multi-task 3-D model of deep learning, all the information was gathered about the presence or absence of myopia features and the SD-OCT findings in GON. It will simplify the classification of GON yes or no and myopic features yes or no and is likely to be useful in primary care settings [27].

15.4 Choosing a Tool for Fundus Examination in Neuro-Ophthalmological Disorders

A direct ophthalmoscope is a favourite tool of general physicians for fundus examination (Fig. 15.5A). A large aperture illuminates a 10° retina view at 15X magnification. Apart from the raised intracranial pressure, several other pathologies, including vascular and inflammatory, cause swelling of the ONH (Fig. 15.5A–C). To get a broader view, the examiner has to illuminate

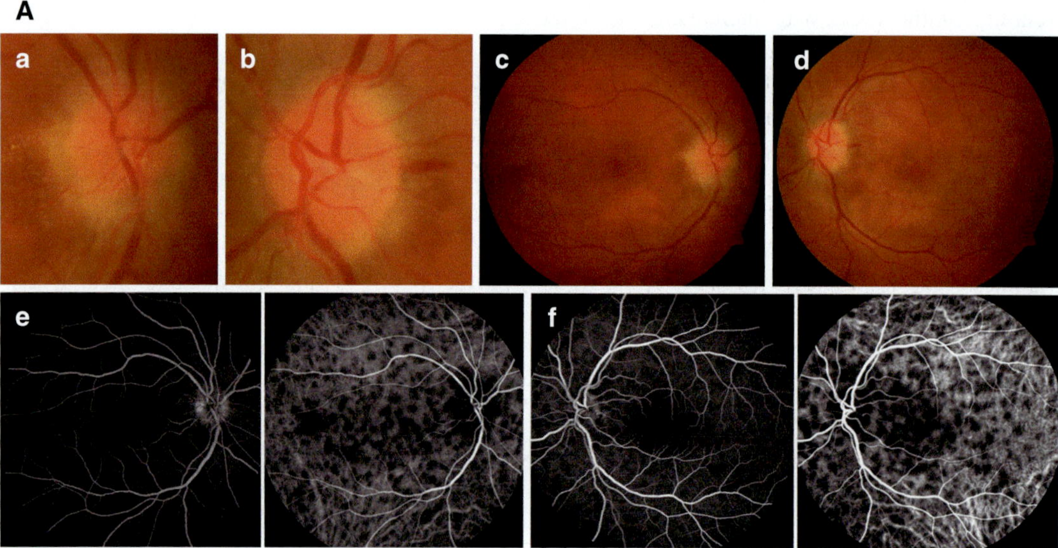

Fig. 15.5 (**A**) Direct ophthalmoscope view of right (**a**) and left (**b**) eyes, allowing direct 15X but only 5–10° field of examination. This patient was referred to as papilledema with a diminution of vision in both eyes for 10 days; the visual acuity was 6/24 and 6/12 in the right and left eyes, respectively. When examined on a + 90 D slit lamp indirect ophthalmoscopy and captured on fundus camera (**c**, **d**) it showed macular edema as the main reason for vision loss. Further ancillary investigations with combined FFA and ICG angiography (**e**, **f**) revealed the presence of bilateral multifocal choroidal granulomas producing hypofluorescent lesions ICG and FFA suggestive of Vogt Koyanagi Harada (VKH) disease, an immune-mediated panuveitis. These patients have signs of meningismus and tinnitus during prodrome and present to neurologists. A careful fundus examination can prevent unnecessary neuroimaging and invasive CSF taps. (**B**) A 34-year-old man presented with vision loss in both eyes and bilateral optic disc edema (**a**, **b**). Fundus fluorescein angiography confirmed optic disc edema (**c**–**f**). Note subtle hypofluorescent discreet lesions in the background show late hyper fluorescence (White arrows in (**d**, (**e**), **f**). A slit lamp exam shows keratic precipitates (red arrows in **g**, **h**), ruling out a primary neurological disease. This prompted a search for inflammatory pathology. The tuberculin skin test was negative. His angiotensin-converting enzyme levels were elevated. The CT scan chest showed multiple enlarged hilar and mediastinal lymph nodes (Not shown here). Endobronchial ultrasound-guided lymph node biopsy revealed epithelioid cell granulomas with lymphoid aggregation and non-necrotizing inflammation suggestive of Sarcoidosis. (**C**) A 40-year-old woman presented with bilateral optic disc edema (**a**–**d**). Note the presence of fine new vessels on the optic disc in both eyes, more marked in the red-free images (**b**, **d**) and are silhouetted against a white background in late frames of fluorescein angiography (**e**, **f**). This patient was also proven to have sarcoidosis and was treated on oral corticosteroids with a resolution of the new vessels and optic disc edema at a one-year follow-up (**g**, **h**)

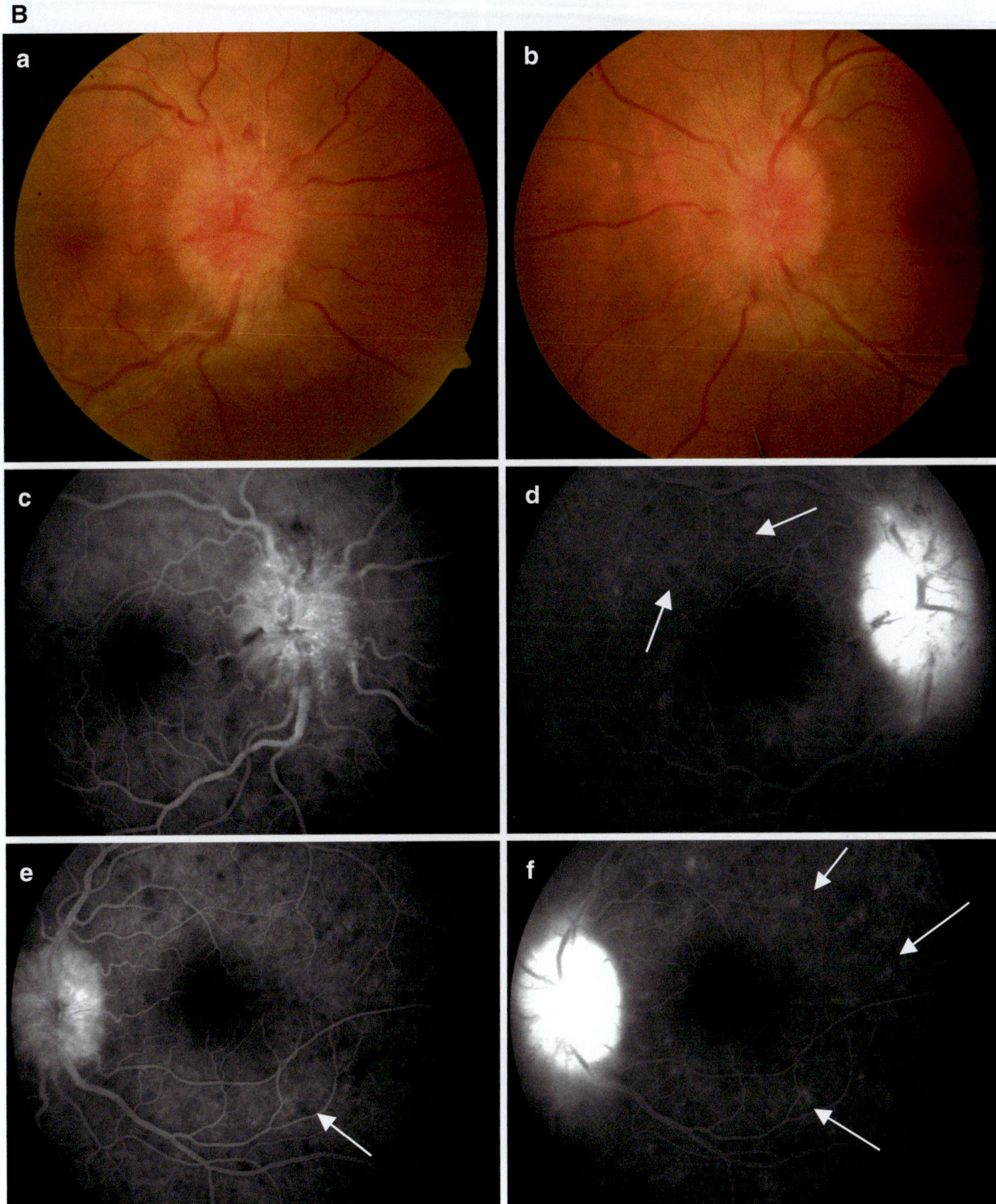

Fig. 15.5 (continued)

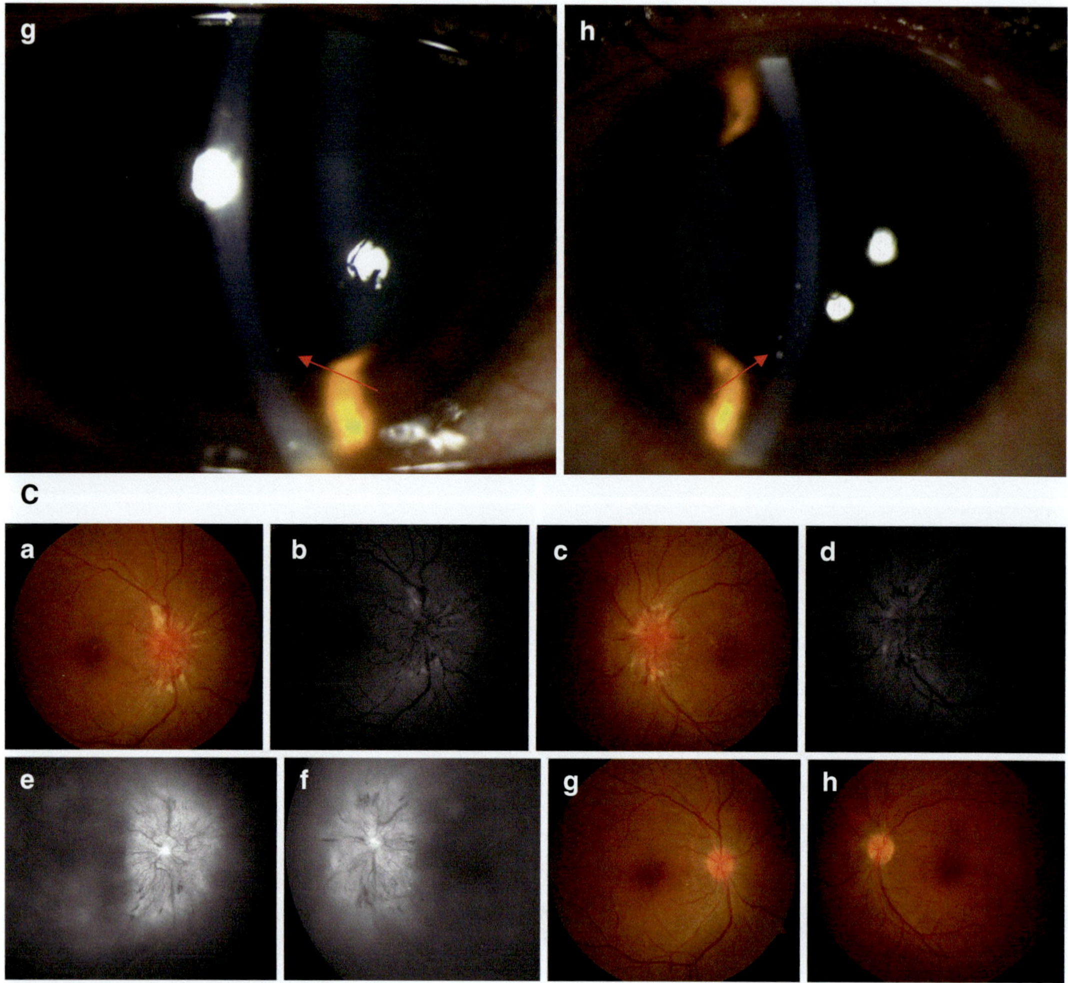

Fig. 15.5 (continued)

various parts of the retina and mentally create a montage of the retina. There is always a chance of missing a forest for a tree. The main challenge in evaluating ONH swelling is determining whether it is due to an ophthalmological or neurological pathology. Thus, doing a binocular biomicroscopic indirect ophthalmoscopy of the retina and slit lamp evaluation whenever one encounters an ONH swelling is advisable especially if the neurological signs are subtle or absent (Fig. 15.5A–C).

Fundus examination is an important step in the neurological examination. Fundus signs provide significant diagnostic clues to the physician before ordering neuroimaging or invasive procedures. In patients with headaches, the absence of papilledema rules out increased intracranial pressure secondary to intracranial space-occupying lesions or idiopathic intracranial hypertension (IIH). On the other hand, visual symptoms with optic disc pallor may indicate an SOL compressing on the anterior visual pathways.

The retinal signs of hypertension, such as focal arteriolar narrowing, AV changes, or the signs of diabetic retinopathy, are related to prevalent stroke, incident stroke, or mortality from stroke. Retinal arteriolar emboli are related to stroke mortality (Fig. 15.6) [28]. In a series of patients referred to the neuro-ophthalmology clinic, nearly 40% of patients referred with a

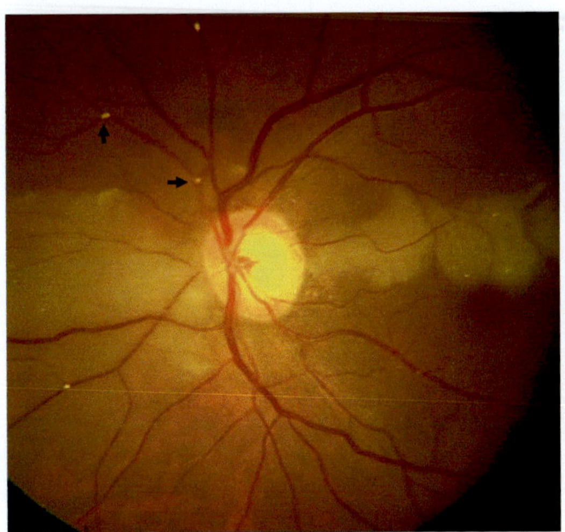

Fig. 15.6 Multiple emboli (black arrows) seen as shiny refractile cholesterol emboli embedded at the bifurcation of arterioles in a patient with BRAO

diagnosis of IIH did not have IIH. The majority had already received treatment for IIH. Most of these patients had abnormal ophthalmoscopy pictures, and all had been subjected to unnecessary neuro-imaging and spinal taps simply because they failed to evaluate the optic disc on ophthalmoscopy [29]. Ophthalmoscopy of the over-diagnosed IIH revealed pseudo papilledema, ONH drusen, optic atrophy, optic neuritis, sequential anterior ischaemic optic neuropathy, and optic nerve hypoplasia [29].

Using a hand-held direct ophthalmoscope is a significant challenge for non-initiated resident doctors. In general, physicians need more confidence in doing fundus examinations. Very few emergency department physicians (14%) perform direct ophthalmoscopy on patients presenting to the emergency department with neurological symptoms. Under those circumstances, looking at the 45° digital images of the fundus taken by a non-mydriatic camera is an appropriate alternative. Thirteen per cent of patients had significant positive findings, detected on 45° fundus images taken by a non-mydriatic camera, relevant to the immediate care of the patients. These included papilledema, optic atrophy, and changes in malignant hypertension [30]. ED physicians are likelier to look at non-mydriatic camera fundus pictures than direct ophthalmoscopy [31].

The non-mydriatic camera has been found superior to direct ophthalmoscopy in neurological patients. Digital images of the fundus also facilitate a remote consultation with an ophthalmologist [32]. Moreover, digital fundus images are an excellent tool for teaching neurology residents about detecting and interpreting various retinal signs crucial to diagnosing and managing their patients [33].

15.4.1 Optic Nerve Head Edema and Papilledema-Clinical Evaluation

Swelling of the ONH is termed 'papilledema' when it results from raised intracranial pressure (ICP) due to space-occupying lesions, intracranial haemorrhage, central venous thrombosis, or IIH (Fig. 15.7). Any pathology that leads to either increased production of CSF or decreased absorption leads to a rise in ICP. In adults, the normal ICP in the supine position ranges from 7 to 15 mm of Hg. The subarachnoid space of the brain is continuous with subarachnoid space around the optic nerve up to the fusion of the dura mater with the sclera. Thus, any rise in ICP is transmitted to the subarachnoid space around the optic nerve compressing the axons pass as they pass through the lamina cribrosa. At the lamina cribrosa, posteriorly, the axons are subjected to pressure in the subarachnoid space and anteriorly to the IOP. This results in stasis of the retrograde axoplasmic flow in the axons anterior to the lamina cribrosa. The increased pressure in the ONH leads to fluid leakage from the dilated capillaries, further compromising the axoplasmic flow.

The timely diagnosis of papilledema is life-saving. Usually, papilledema is symmetrical in both eyes. However, occasionally due to small-sized optic canals, ONH swelling may be asymmetric on one side [34]. Notably, atrophic optic nerves do not show papilledema even in the presence of raised ICP. The raised ICP may not manifest as papilledema in infants with as-yet open fontanelles.

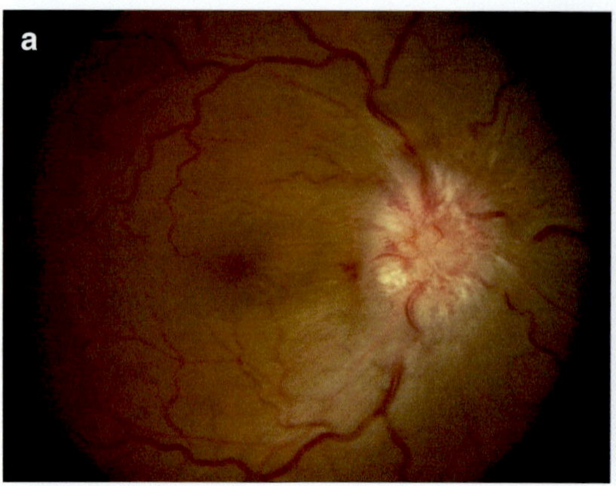

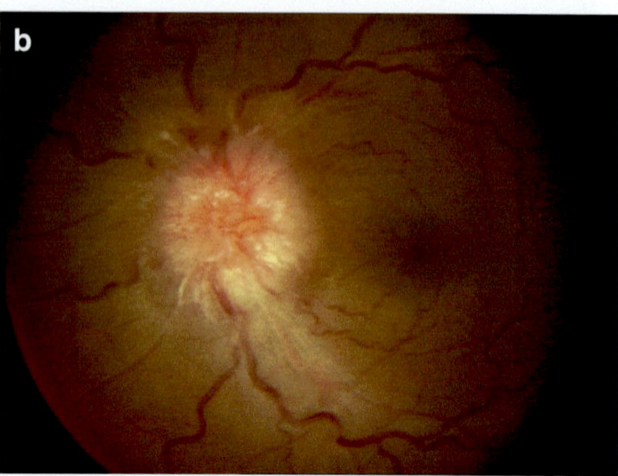

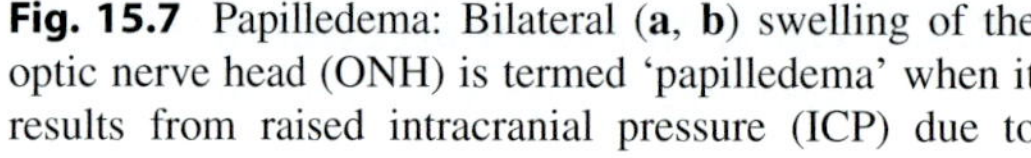

Fig. 15.7 Papilledema: Bilateral (**a**, **b**) swelling of the optic nerve head (ONH) is termed 'papilledema' when it results from raised intracranial pressure (ICP) due to space-occupying lesions, intracranial hemorrhage, central venous thrombosis, or idiopathic intracranial hypertension

Patients with raised ICP often complain of morning headaches that worsen during coughing or Valsalva manoeuvre. Headache may be accompanied by vomiting. They may also complain of diplopia due to sixth nerve paresis as a non-localizing sign of raised ICP. Although the visual acuity may remain normal for a long time, they may complain of transient obscurations of vision, especially with a change in posture. Patients may complain of tinnitus as well.

15.4.2 Ocular Causes of ONH Swelling

Several pathologies in the eye lead to the swelling of the ONH, including central retinal vein occlusion, malignant hypertension, optic neuritis, non-arteritic ischaemic optic neuropathy, diabetes, hypotony, posterior scleritis, thyroid ophthalmopathy, inflammatory and infiltrative diseases of the ONH by Sarcoidosis, leukemia, lymphoma, metastatic lesions, or orbital pathologies. Diagnosis of ONH swelling in ocular diseases does not pose as much of a challenge as in early cases of papilledema.

15.4.3 Signs of Papilledema

The first manifestation of papilledema is blurring of ONH margins (Fig. 15.7). The margins of the normal optic disc are finely blurred as the RNF bundles enter the disc. These fibres are best seen in red-free light. The normal blurring of the optic disc needs to be distinguished from the incipient papilledema due to raised ICP. In nearly 80% of normal people, spontaneous venous pulsations are visible on the optic disc. These spontaneous pulsations are abolished if the ICP exceeds 20 mm of Hg. The presence of these pulsations rules out raised ICP. Notably, venous pulsations may be absent in 20% of normal people, but can be elicited by lightly pressing the globe with a finger. Next is the obscuration of the physiological cup due to axonal swelling. The disc margins' blurring is exaggerated in small optic discs that are otherwise normal, called pseudo papilledema. In both instances, the optic disc cup is full/absent. In optic neuritis, the RNFL may also be seen as coarse, and the ODC may be absent or partially obliterated (Figs. 15.8, 15.9, and 15.10).

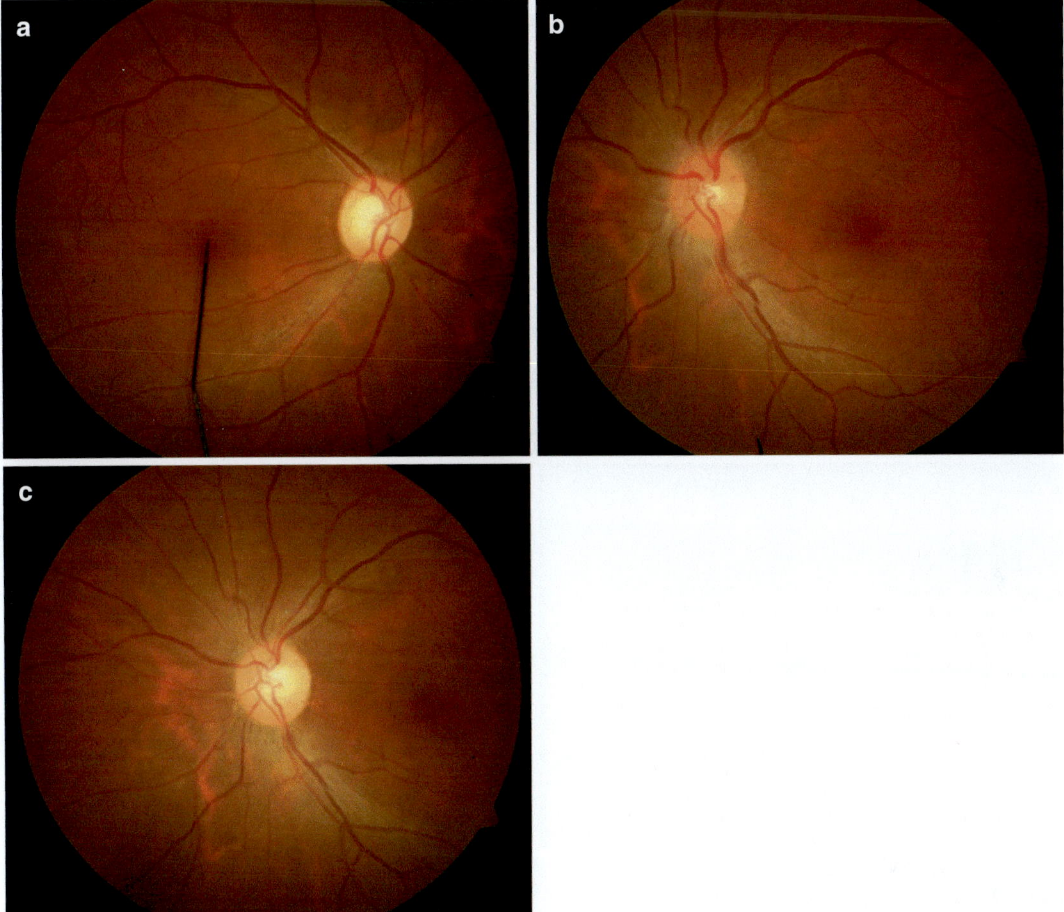

Fig. 15.8 Right eye optic disc is normal (**a**), while left eye optic disc shows hyperemia, edema, obliteration of physiological cup, and tortuous vessels (**b**). Following treatment with systemic steroids, the optic disc edema resolved at 2 weeks with mild pallor of optic nerve head (**c**)

In eyes with pseudopapilledema, the bright reflexes from the large retinal vessels and retina are seen. Normal RNFL striations are also visible.

In true papilledema, on the other hand, the reflexes from the large vessels are lost, which appear dark and dull. The RNFL striations appear coarse and obliterated [35]. The swelling of the neuronal axons first appears in the inferior and superior poles of the ONH. On stereoscopic examination, the ONH is seen elevated. The height of this elevation can be measured by first focusing on the peripapillary retina and followed by the surface of the ONH with a direct ophthalmoscope. A + 3D elevation approximates 1 mm of elevation of the ONH.

Persistence of papilledema also leads to congestion of the retinal capillaries, giving the ONH a hyperemic appearance. The central retinal vein and its branches appear full and congested. Linear haemorrhages may be seen on the optic disc margins (Fig. 15.7). Circumferential folds around the ONH, termed Paton's lines, are due to either retinal wrinkles in the RNFL temporal to the ONH; outer retina folds when associated with subretinal fluid or, less commonly, choroidal folds [36]. These are mechanical stress lines which may be radial, circumferential, or spiral.

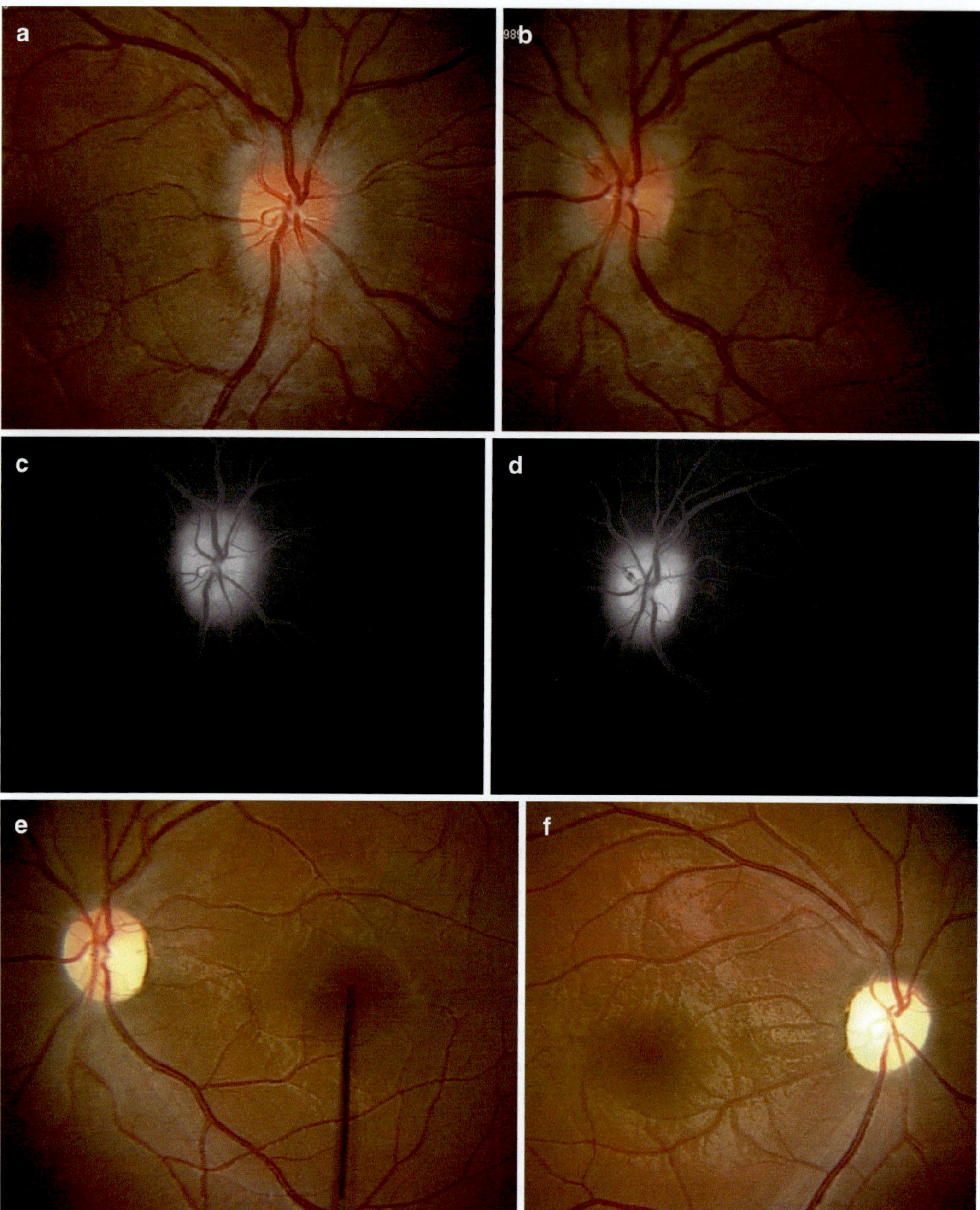

Fig. 15.9 (**a**–**d**) A 20-Y-O female presented with 3 days of headache, pain, and loss of vision in BE. Visual acuity was only the perception of hand motions in the right eye and counting fingers at 2 meters in the left eye. The right showed a RAPD. There was significant opacification of circumpapillary RNFL R > L. MRI WNL. She was treated with IV Methylprednisolone. Her vision improved to 6/9 within a week in the left eye. (**f**–**h**). Nine months later, both optic discs showed pallor R > L (**e**, **f**). Corresponding visual fields showed a superior relative paracentral scotoma in the left eye (**g**) and an inferior Centro-cecal scotoma in the right eye

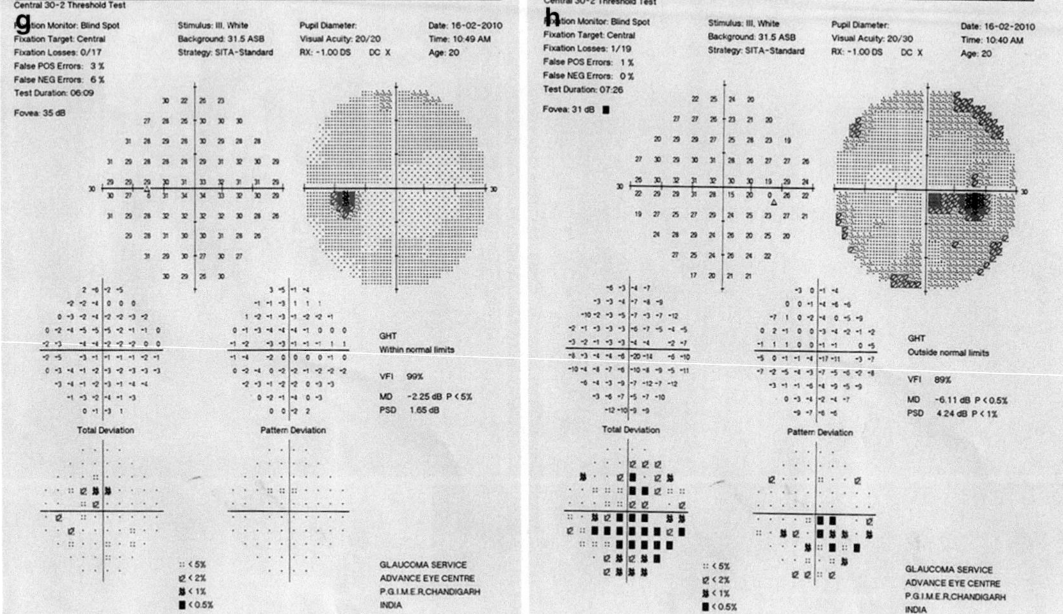

Fig. 15.9 (continued)

Choroidal folds are often seen in patients with peripapillary scleritis or orbital pathologies. The subretinal fluid can be seen on SD-OCT in the juxtapapillary area. Cotton wool spots and hard exudates may be seen in the late stages, forming a macular fan. Chronically persistent raised ICP may ultimately lead to secondary optic atrophy with the pallor of the ONH and astrocytic proliferation on the surface of the ONH, which may also develop shiny pseudo-drusen-like deposits from the extruded axoplasm.

Central visual acuity is normal in early papilledema, but if it persists for several months, there may be a significant decline in visual acuity, ultimately leading to blindness. In the early stages, the visual fields show an enlargement of the blind spot, but in chronic cases, the visual field starts showing constricted visual fields.

On fundus fluorescein angiography, there is an initial delay in filling the retinal arterioles but marked by capillary dilatation in the arteriovenous phase and leakage of the dye in the late stages. Microaneurysmal dilations may be seen on the optic disc surface.

15.4.3.1 Clinical Grading of Papilledema

Changes in the ONH occur progressively depending upon the severity of the ICP and the duration of the sustained rise in ICP. Scott et al. [37] used a modified Frisén scale to grade papilledema. Under this scale, grade 0 is a normal disc in which the RNFL follows the ISNT rule, whereby the RNFL striations are thickest in the inferior sector, followed by the superior, nasal, and temporal sectors. In larger optic discs, these RNFL striations tend to be thinner. In grade 1, there is minimal optic disc edema, and the temporal disc margin is normal; a subtle halo obscures the underlying retina around the rest of the disc. In grade 2, this halo surrounds the optic disc; the nasal disc margins are thickened but without obscuring emerging vessels from the disc. In grade 3, the circumferential halo is significant, and the disc margins are elevated. The blood vessels are obscure in ≥1 quadrant. In grade 4, there is obscuration of the retinal vessel segments; the cup is full, and the disc is elevated with a marked circumferential halo. In grade 5, all the vessels on the disc are obscured [37].

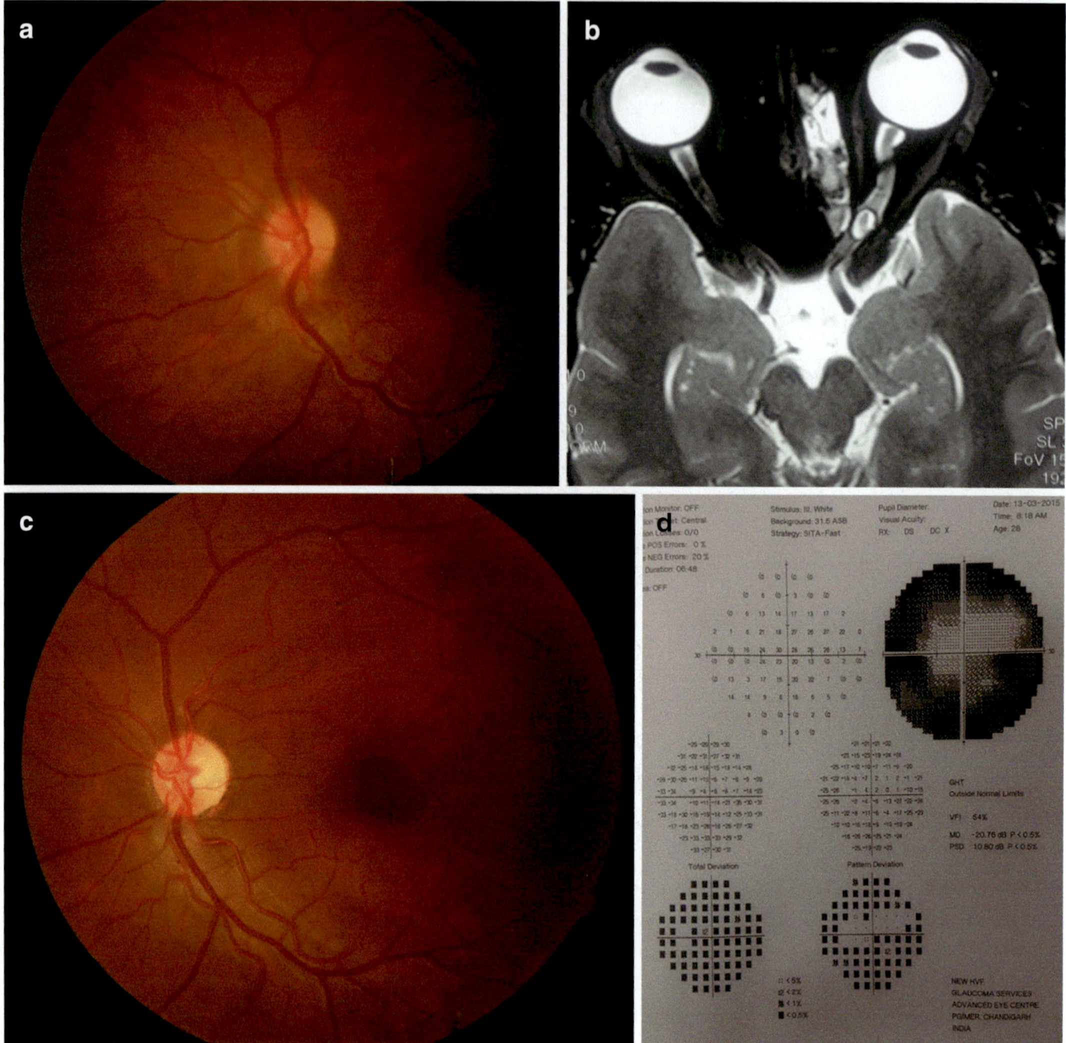

Fig. 15.10 A 28-year-old woman presented with blurred vision in her left eye for one-day duration. Her visual acuity was 6/6 in the right eye and 6/12 in the left eye. There was no RAPD in the left eye. Mild optic disc edema was noted in the left eye (**a**). Contrast-enhanced MRI orbit showed a single lesion in the left optic nerve near the orbital apex, hypointense on T2 showing ring enhancement (**b**). A diagnosis of left intraorbital neurocysticercosis with optic neuritis was made. Endoscopic excision of the cysticercosis was followed by immediate worsening of vision and disc edema. She was treated on oral albendazole and intravenous followed by oral corticosteroids. She recovered normal vision and was left with a mild optic disc pallor (**c**) and contracted visual fields (**d**)

15.4.4 Role of OCT in Papilledema

Peripapillary RNFL (pRNFL) thickness is increased in raised ICP. The measurement of pRNFL in patients with papilledema correlates with the CSF tap's opening pressure. Although the pRNFL thickness is decreased after the control of ICP, its interpretation as a measure of control of ICP needs caution as secondary optic atrophy due to papilledema also leads to the loss of RNFL. Thinning of the macular GCIPL layer is a better indicator for assessing secondary atrophy, as this layer does not show an increase in thickness with the raised ICP. EDI-OCT can help differentiate pseudo from true papilledema, especially in eyes with buried optic disc drusen (ODD) [38].

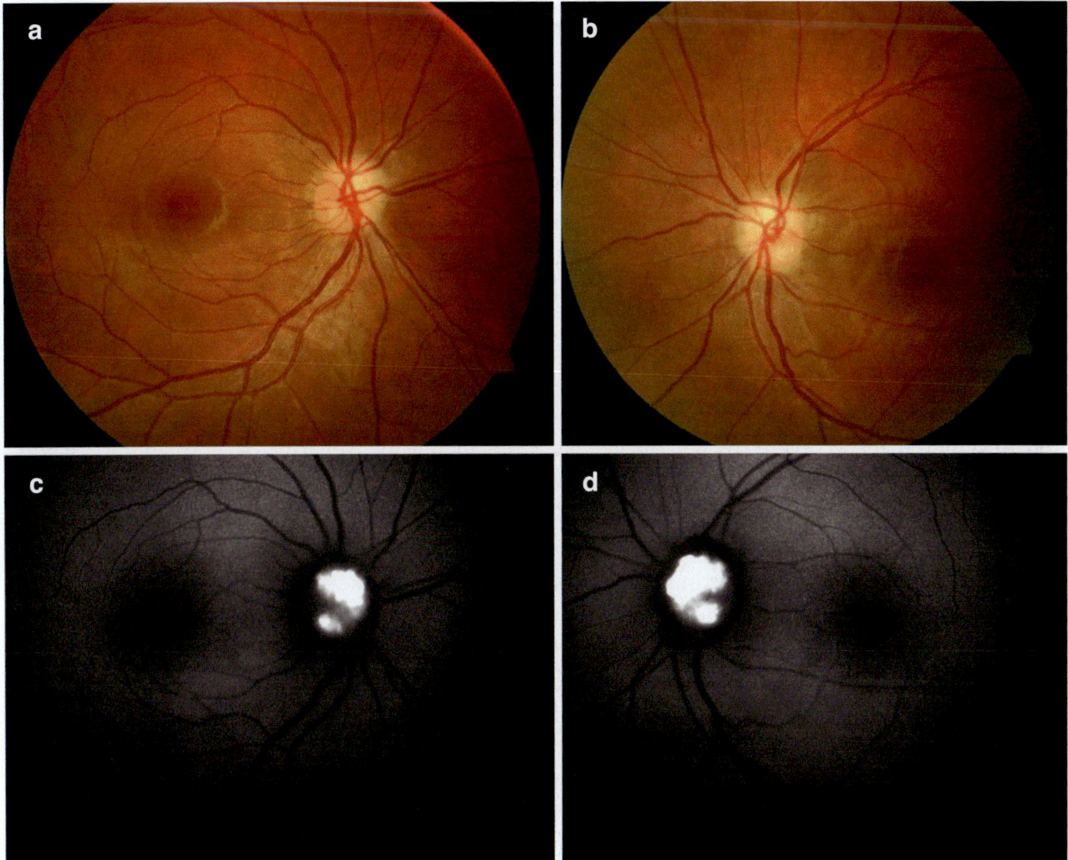

Fig. 15.11 A 21-year-old woman with blurred optic disc margins and the absence of a cup in both eyes (**a**, **b**) was suspected of having raised intracranial pressure. Fundus autofluorescence reveals intensely hyperautofluorescent buried drusen (**c**, **d**). Without neurological symptoms/signs, buried drusen should be ruled out before ordering neuroimaging

15.4.5 Psudopapilledema Due to Optic Disc Drusen

Before ordering neuroimaging in a patient with suspected papilledema, getting a fundus autofluorescence imaging of the fundus is worthwhile. At times, buried ODD in the ONH may also obliterate the ODC and have blurring of the disc margin. These are calcific deposits and can also be detected on ultrasonography by their high reflectivity from their surface and shadowing. These ODDs are highly hyperautofluorescent (Fig. 15.11). The ODD is often buried in children but becomes apparent with advancing age. More superficial drusen may appear as lumpy, bumpy nodular lesions on the ONH. The buried drusen predispose the eyes to RNFL defects, retinal vascular occlusions, and acute AION at a young age [39]. In patients under 50 years with Non-arteritic AION, nearly 50% have buried ODD. On OCT, these appear as hyperreflective ovoid mass-like structures [40]. They may show progressive visual field defects or develop choroidal neovascular membranes [41].

15.4.6 Papilledema in Idiopathic Intracranial Hypertension

Idiopathic intracranial hypertension (IIH) is not an uncommon cause of papilledema due to raised ICP without a known cause. Before making this diagnosis, both intracranial space-occupying lesions and non-tumour causes of raised ICP, like central venous thrombosis and meningitis, must be ruled out. It is a progressively blinding disorder most often seen in obese women. Patients with mild-to-moderate IIH may be asymptomatic, diagnosed during a routine clinical examination, or symptomatic in severe IIH with headache, diplopia, and pulsatile or non-pulsatile tinnitus. Headaches in IIH may be due to increased ICP with features like early morning worsening, association with nausea and vomiting, transient obscuration of vision, and a change in posture or Valsalva precipitates symptoms. Imaging in IIH should include an MRI of the brain and optic nerves with venography. Specific MRI signs of raised ICP include empty(or partially empty) sella turcica, venous sinus stenosis, narrowing of ventricles (slit ventricles), prominence of peri optic nerve sheath, vertical tortuosity of the optic nerves, scleral indentation, and posterior flattening of the globe [42]. Other lesser common signs include narrowing Meckel's cave and cavernous sinuses. Meckel's cave is a recess in the dura mater containing the CN V and its ganglion. In any case, MRI/CT scans are mandatory to rule out ICSOL. MR or CT venography is required to rule out venous thrombosis (Fig. 15.12A and B). Without any secondary cause of raised ICP, CSF opening pressure of 250 mm of water on lumbar puncture in adults and 280 mm in children is diagnostic of IIH. Care should be taken while recording CSF pressure, and it should be recorded in a lateral decubitus position with legs relaxed. CSF pressure should not be recorded in isolation, and the patient's clinical status should be given priority while making the diagnosis. In the presence of at least one of the following criteria, pulse synchronous tinnitus, bilateral VI nerve paresis, Frišen grade 2 optic disc edema (Box 15.2), collapse, or narrowing of lateral sinus on MRV, even 200–250 mm of water may be considered positive for diagnosing IIH [43].

As evaluated on the Frišen scale, the papilledema severity correlates with the circumpapillary RNFL thickness (cRFNL) [37].

IIH carries a higher risk of poor outcomes in very severe papilledema in men, black men, and those with additional risk factors like hypertension, anaemia, and obesity [44, 45]. The increasing severity of papilledema is accompanied by the increasing severity of peripapillary RNFL, subretinal, or preretinal haemorrhages and the increasing severity of the cotton wool spots on and around the optic disc. The severity of papilledema is a marker for a poor visual outcome, but haemorrhages and cotton wool spots are not independent markers for the final visual outcome [44, 45]. Few patients of IIH who present with an early, rapidly progressive visual loss within 4 weeks of the onset of initial clinical symptoms are referred to as having Fulminant IIH, which requires aggressive management.

The standard of care has been oral acetazolamide, as it reduces the production of CSF. Other drugs used in IIH are topiramate, furosemide, etc. Patients are encouraged to lose weight. Headaches in IIH must be managed with prophylaxis of migraine, tension-type headache, or mixed headaches. In refractory cases, CSF diversion procedures like optic nerve sheath fenestration can be done with an attendant risk of blindness and progression of the disease. Alternatively, shunt procedures (The lumboperitoneal or ventriculoperitoneal shunt) to divert CSF have also successfully controlled the symptoms and papilledema. Neurovascular stenting has a controversial role in the management of IIH. Patients with IIH need to be monitored on fundus pictures for the resolution of papilledema. On OCT, the measurement of the GCIPL complex can provide an accurate evaluation of secondary optic atrophy [46].

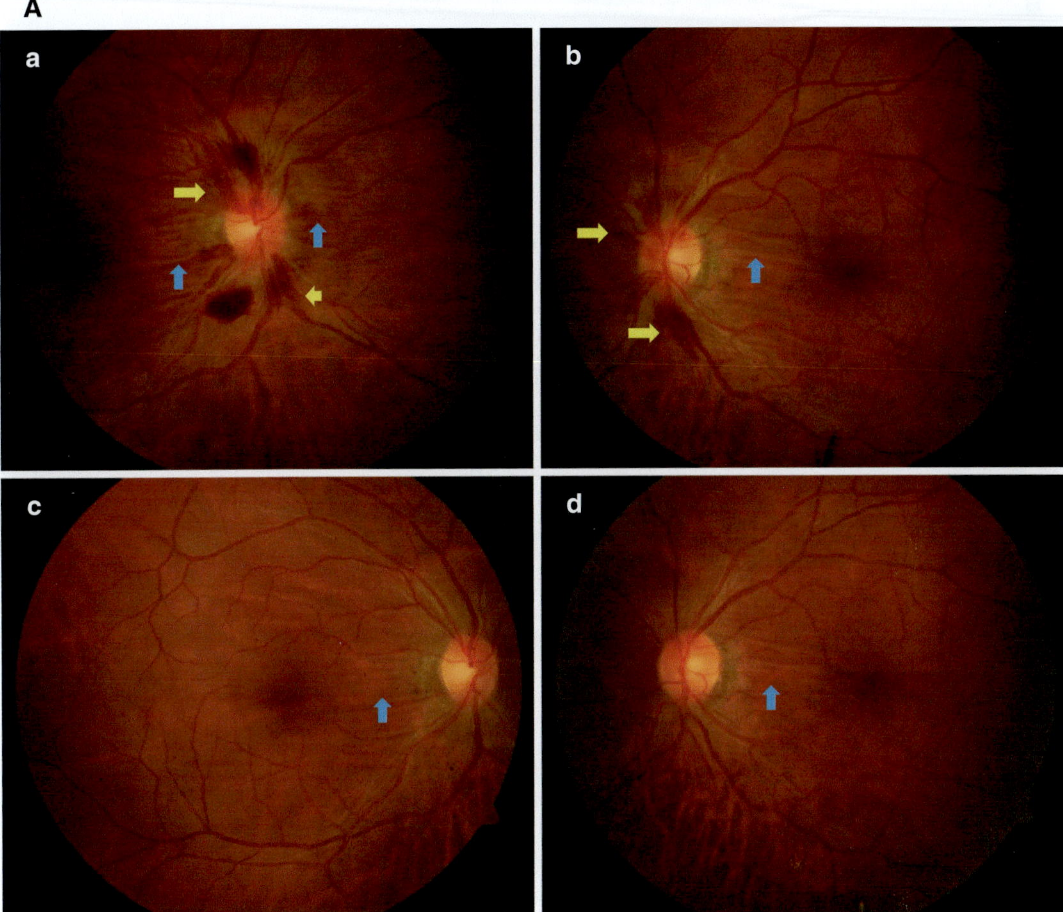

Fig. 15.12 (**A**) A 49-year-old man with subdural hemorrhage presented with bilateral papilledema with peripapillary linear hemorrhages (yellow arrows) (**a**, **b**). Note the peripapillary radial folds (blue arrows), a sign of raised ICP. The radial folds have persisted (blue arrows) even after 15 months, although the papilledema has resolved (**c**, **d**). (**B**) In a patient with Terson Syndrome due to venous sinus thrombosis, (**a**) MRI brain (non-contrast T1-weighted sequence) showing acute left temporal hemorrhagic infarct, and (**b**) filling defect in the superior sagittal sinus (arrow) on Gadolinium-enhanced T1 sequence; (**c**) MR Venography showing left-sided sigmoid and transverse sinus thrombosis. Baseline fundus photograph shows optic disc hemorrhage in right eye (**d**) and a large premacular sub–internal limiting membrane and subhyaloid bleed in the left eye (**e**). Follow-up fundus photographs (**f**, **g**) show substantial resolution. Reproduced with permission of the publishers from: Takkar A, Kesav P, Lal V, Gupta A. Teaching NeuroImages: Terson syndrome in cortical venous sinus thrombosis. Neurology. 2013 Aug 6;81(6):e40–1. doi: 10.1212/WNL.0b013e31829e6f13. PMID: 23918868

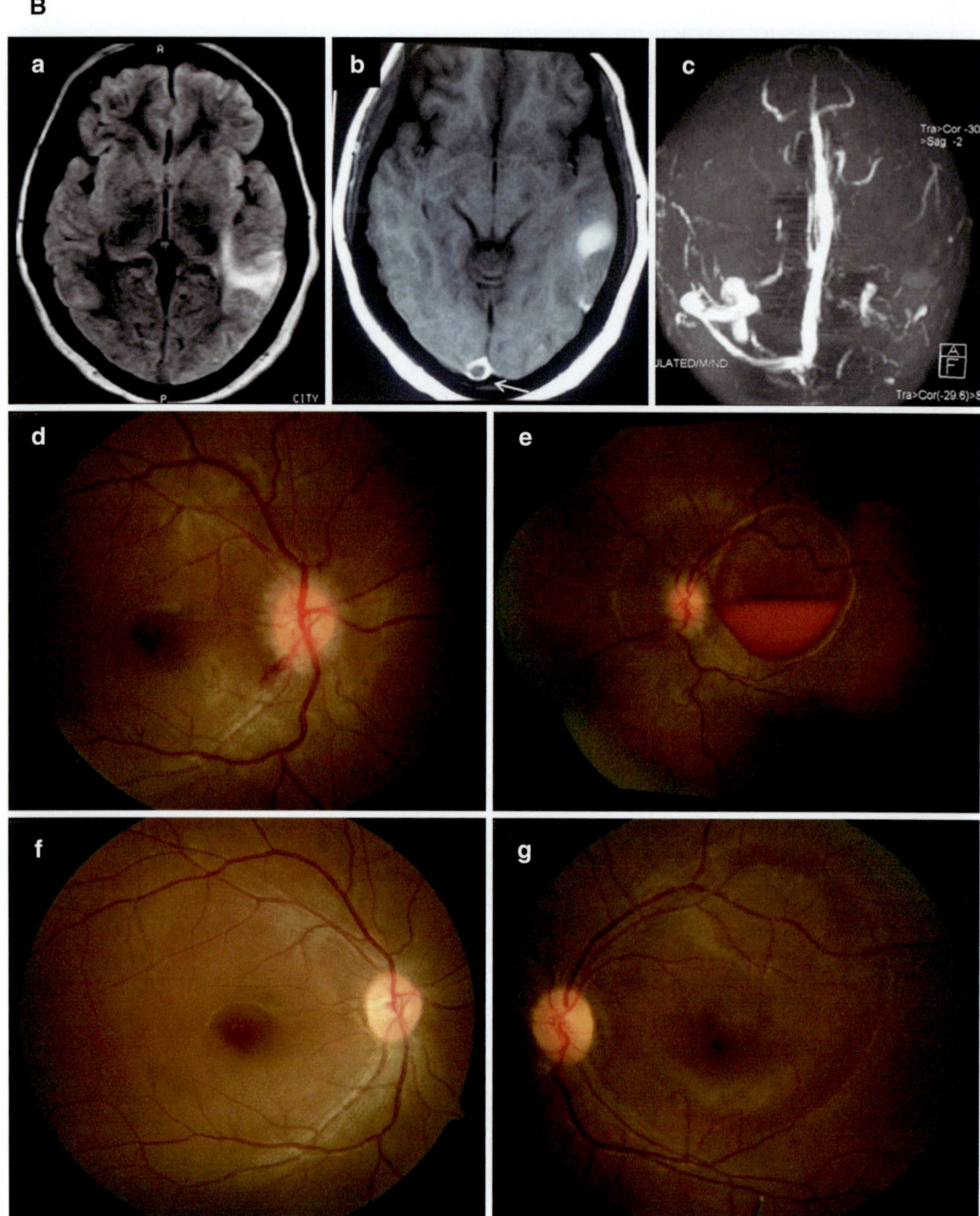

Fig. 15.12 (continued)

15.5 Optic Neuritis—Inflammation of the Optic Nerve

Several diseases including infections—bacterial, viral, parasitic, or systemic inflammatory diseases, may lead to secondary optic neuritis and the most common are listed in Box 15.1. This chapter will not focus on secondary optic neuritis but autoimmune Optic neuritis (ON). ON is an optic nerve inflammation, including the ganglion cell axons, intradural space, or the optic nerve meningeal sheaths. It is a common manifestation of multiple sclerosis and the first manifestation in 25% of the patients. ON may occur as isolated, monophasic, relapsing or chronic relapsing, and progressive. Isolated ON is defined when it is not accompanied by pathological brain or spinal cord lesions and does not show any potentially pathogenic antibody [47].

Etiologically, ON may be broadly divided into three basic groups, (1) Autoimmune ON, which is often relapsing and is associated with multiple sclerosis (MS), Aquaporin4 IgG antibodies-associated neuromyelitis optica spectrum disorder (NMOSD) or Anti-myelin oligodendrocytes glycoprotein antibody-associated disease (MOGAD); (2) Post-infectious or post-vaccination ON, which are typically monophasic. See Box 15.1; and (3) idiopathic. A forme fruste of ON is defined when CSF IgG oligoclonal bands or antibodies are present in isolated monophasic ON [47].

The optic nerve may be affected in the intracranial, intraorbital, retrolaminar, laminar, or prelaminar compartment. It may affect the young <17 years, 18–40 or > 40. ON is characterized by acute or subacute vision loss, generally described as fading of objects, affecting low-contrast vision more frequently than high-contrast vision. In the optic neuritis treatment trial (ONTT), the presenting high contrast visual acuity varied from 6/6 to no light perception (NLP), with only 3% of the patients having NLP [48]. These patients frequently complain of the dullness of colour vision (acquired dyschromatopsia) and have retro-ocular pain in the movement of the eyes. It may be unilateral or bilateral. It may be monophasic, relapsing, sequential, or chronic. [47].

Box 15.1 Secondary Causes of Optic Neuritis- Infectious and Systemic Diseases

Post-infectious causes of optic neuritis	Systemic diseases associated with optic neuritis
Bacterial infections Brucella spp. Cat scratch disease (Bartonella henselae) Lyme disease (Borrelia burgdorferi) Syphilis (Treponema pallidum) Tuberculosis (mycobacterium tuberculosis) Typhus fever (rickettsia prowazekii) Whipple disease (Tropheryma whipplei) Streptococcal infection *Viral infections* Chikungunya, Cytomegalovirus, Coronavirus HIV Hepatitis- B and C Herpes simplex Human herpes virus-6 Varicella zoster virus, West Nile virus Zika virus *Parasitic infestations* Toxoplasmosis, Neurocysticercosis Neurotoxocariasis *Post-vaccination optic neuritis*	Systemic vasculitis and inflammatory diseases Giant cell arteritis Polyarteritis nodosa Takayasu's arteritis ANCA-associated vasculitis Systemic lupus erythematosus Kawasaki disease Behçet's disease Sarcoidosis Sjögren syndrome Antiphospholipid antibodies syndrome Ankylosing spondylitis

Adapted with permission of publishers from: Petzold et al. Diagnosis and classification of optic neuritis. Lancet Neurol. 2022 Dec;21(12):1120–1134. doi: 10.1016/S1474-4422(22)00200-9. Epub 2022 Sep 27. PMID: 36179757.

15.5.1 Epidemiology of Optic Neuritis

In the past, all patients with autoimmune optic neuritis (ON) were considered due to multiple sclerosis. In the present era, when pathogenic antibodies have been identified in some ON cases, population-based ON data from a predominantly white population county in the US found the annual incidence of ON to be 3.9/per 100,000 population. The most common cause of ON remains multiple sclerosis (MS-ON), accounting for 57%, followed by MOG-IgG+ ON (MOG-ON) in 5%, AQP4-IgG-positive ON (AQP4-ON) in 3%, infectious 2%, Sarcoidosis in 2%, and 29% remained idiopathic [49]. Significant ethnic variations in the proportion of ON cases due to AQP4-ON and MOG-ON have been seen. In the ONTT, none of the patients had AQP4-ON. More recent data show that only 2.9% of ON in the USA have AQP4-ON. However, in the Chinese population, AQP4-ON varies from 29.8 to 40.2% among unilateral and 19.4–45.6% in bilateral cases. While MOG-ON was seen in 1.7% of all ON patients in the US, it was 10.7–27.6% in the Japanese population. In the Chinese population, 17.7–20.2% of unilateral and 26.3–28.1% of bilateral cases had MOG-ON [50].

15.5.2 Evaluation of Optic Neuritis in the Clinic

The most important clinical test in the evaluation of ON is the swinging flashlight test to detect the conduction defect in the optic nerve, termed the relative afferent pupil defect (RAPD) in unilateral or grossly asymmetric bilateral cases. Briefly, in a semi-dark room, bright pen torch light is shone swinging (not more than four times) alternately between the eyes. If both eyes are normal, when light is shone on one eye, the pupil constricts in both eyes. However, if there is a conduction defect in one eye, on swinging the light from the normal eye (the pupils in both eyes get constricted) to the abnormal eye, the pupil of the abnormal eye starts dilating. On fundus examination, there is hyperemia and swelling of the ONH, depending upon the site of inflammation (Figs. 15.13 and 15.14). Inflammation of the optic nerve posterior to the globe may not show any optic disc swelling or hyperemia. Such patients are often labelled as retrobulbar neuritis.

15.5.2.1 Paraclinical Tests

(a). *OCT*: In acute cases (up to 3 months), ONH swelling and thickening of the ganglion cell inner plexiform complex (GCIPL) > 4μm

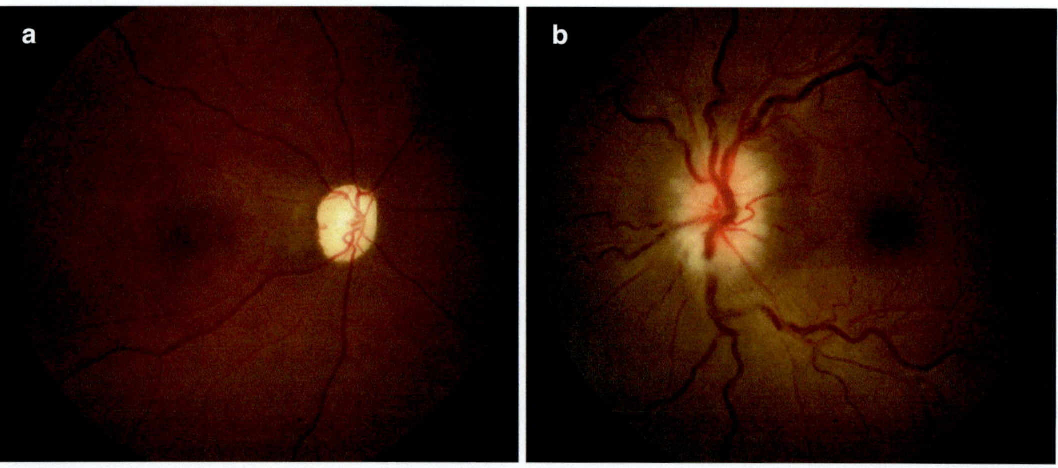

Fig. 15.13 Complete pallor of the optic disc with arterial attenuation as seen in optic atrophy (**a**), in contrast to disc blurring and dilated tortuous vessels in optic disc edema (**b**)

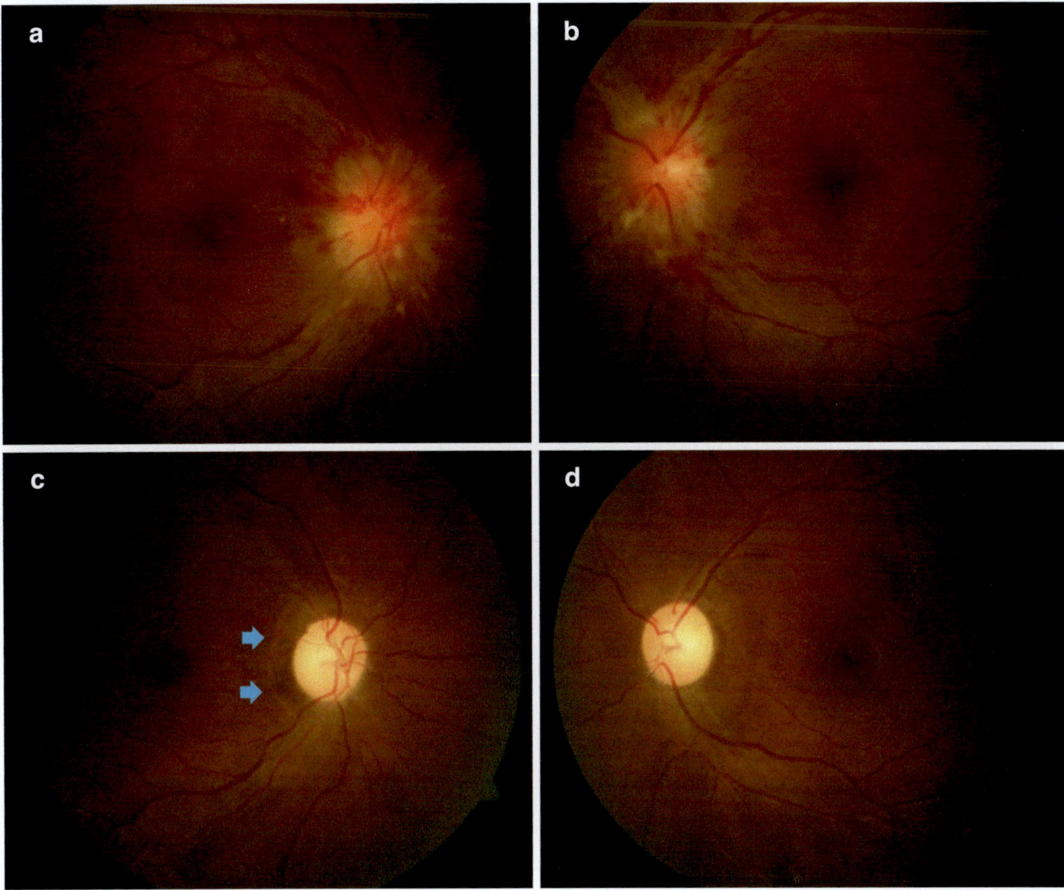

Fig. 15.14 A 32-year-old woman with simultaneous bilateral neuro-retinitis shows optic disc edema, radial folds, very prominent swelling of peripapillary nerve fibres, linear hemorrhages, and very subtle hard exudates in the papillomacular area (**a**, **b**). Two months later, the swelling resolved with the pallor of the optic discs (**c**, **d**). The peripapillary Paton line (blue arrow) is appreciable in the right eye (**c**)

can be elicited. The average GCIPL thickness is 100μm. The peripapillary RNFL (pRNFL) thickness > 5μm persists for several months after the onset of optic neuritis.

(b). *MRI*: Another commonly performed imaging test is MRI which may show contrast enhancement of the affected optic nerve or its sheaths.

(c). *Laboratory tests* for biomarkers include antibodies for Aquaporin 4 (AQP4) to rule out NMOSD, myelin oligodendrocyte glycoprotein (MOG) to rule out MOG-antibody disease, collapsing response mediator protein 5 (CRMP5) to rule out cancer-associated paraneoplastic optic neuritis, retinitis and vitritis, and CSF oligoclonal bands for IgG.

Role of Optical Coherence Tomography in Optic Neuritis

The introduction of Optical coherence tomography (OCT) is akin to the profound changes in the practice of medicine brought about by the development of imaging technologies like ultrasonography, computerized tomography (CT scan), and magnetic resonance imaging (MRI). It has become an important imaging tool in neurology, neuro-ophthalmology, and ophthalmology clinics worldwide. Huang et al. [51] developed OCT technology to examine non-invasively the cross-sectional details of biological tissues. The basic principle of the use of OCT is like the use of ultrasonography. Like the sound waves, the reflected light signals are detected as a low-coherence light beam passes through the retina, which either gets reflected or transmitted. The initial time-domain technology has been replaced by spectral-domain (SD) technology. It uses a broad-band near-infrared superluminescent diode as a light source and a spectrometer to detect the Fourier transformation of the reflected light from the tissue interfaces. The axial resolution has improved to 1–3μ. There has been a tremendous change in the acquisition time to obtain information from each point of the retinal structures enabling a 3-D construct of the retina. Apart from the cross-sectional image of the various microstructures, a layer by retinal layer information is obtained as en-face imaging.

On the other hand, the swept-source OCT (SS-OCT) uses a narrow band of a tunable laser source. The higher acquisition speed with SS-OCT to 100,000 scans/s compared to 50,000 scans/s with the SD-OCT has allowed a 12 × 12 mm wider scan line compared to a 6 × 6 mm line scan with SD-OCT. Using a higher wavelength of 1050 nm than the SD-OCT (840 nm), SS-OCT gives higher resolution images (1μ) of the deeper retinal structures [52].

Because of the relatively consistent and reproducible measurements, it has become common to use OCT to study the thickness and microstructure of circumpapillary RNFL (cRNFL) and the thickness of the ganglion cell-inner plexiform complex and inner nuclear layer. In patients with MS, besides the demyelination of the optic nerve fibres, there is a loss of neuronal axons, which can be measured around the optic nerve head (a 3.4 mm diameter circle from the optic disc centre) as cRNFL thickness in various sectors. Various layers of the neurosensory retina can be segmented, and their thickness measured. Of interest in patients of optic neuritis is the thickness of the ganglion cells layer (GCL), GCL-inner plexiform layer (GCIPL) layer, and the inner nuclear layer. Notably, in patients with MS-ON, the cRNFL may show swelling of the axons, which may be present even without clinical swelling of the ONH. Following an acute episode of ON, the earliest thinning of the temporal RNFL is appreciable at 2 months from the onset, and the loss of fibres is stabilized by 6–7 months. Thus, measuring the cRNFL in the short term may give erroneous information on the loss of axons [53]. On the other hand, there is no swelling of the ganglion cells even in the acute ON; the first thinning of the GCIPL is seen by the end of 1 month after an acute episode [54]. Hence, monitoring the GCIPL thickness accurately estimates the neuronal damage and progressive stage of MS-ON.

Microcystic macular edema (MME) is seen in 4.7–6% of the patients with MS-ON. An increased inner nuclear layer (INL) thickness is also noted without a demonstrable leakage from the retinal capillaries. MME is more often seen in AQP4-ON than the MS-ON. It may also be seen in severe isolated ON. The increased INL thickness was associated with increased disease severity scores, development of contrast-enhancing lesions, expanded disability status scale, and more relapses in a relapsing-remitting MS [47, 55, 56].

Although MME has been believed to predict the severity of MS-ON in the past, it has been seen in other hereditary optic neuropathies that do not have either inflammation or breakdown of the blood-retinal barrier. The only constant feature of all the eyes showing MME is the thinning of the GCIPL layer [57]. Oral acetazolamide is effective in treating MME associated with optic neuropathies; it reduces the INL thickness but has no impact on the visual function [58].

A significant challenge is a delayed diagnosis in many patients. As many as 3 years may elapse for the conversion of relapsing-remitting MS (RRMS) to secondary progressive MS (SPMS). Before the conversion, faster thinning rates of cRNFL and GCIPL can be reliable biomarkers for the appropriate management of these patients [59, 60].

The thinning of the cRNFL is first seen in the optic disc's temporal sector, and thickness < 75μm is associated with permanent visual field loss [61]. In MS-ON, the cRNFL loss is less severe. It preferentially affects the temporal sector (papillomacular bundle) compared to AQP4-ON, which has severer and more diffuse damage and affects the upper and lower sector of the cRNFL [62].

Magnetic Resonance Imaging in Optic Neuritis

Imaging in ON should include gadolinium-enhanced MRI of brain and optic nerves with T1/ T2-weighted, FLAIR, contrast-enhanced, and fat-suppressed images to delineate the lesion better. On MRI, acute ON shows T2-weighted hyperintensities and gadolinium contrast enhancement in T1-weighted images. Patients with MS-ON show only focal and limited longitudinal enhancement (usually anterior predominant) in the intracanalicular or intraorbital segments of the optic nerve. In contrast, the AQP4-ON is associated with extensive longitudinal and posterior predominant lesions of the optic nerve, and at times, may involve the optic chiasma as well. MOG-AD-associated ON shows bilateral enhancement. Perineuritic fat enhancement is uncommon in MS-ON and AQP4-ON compared to MOG-ON [63]. The MOG-ON affects the intraorbital, intracanalicular, and intracranial optic nerve segments. However, the AQP4-ON most commonly affects the intracranial segments, including the optic tracts).

15.5.3 Diagnosis of Optic Neuritis

The diagnosis of definitive optic neuritis can be made if the patient has the classical presentation of acute/subacute visual loss, RAPD, loss of colour vision, and painful eye movements with at least one imaging or biomarker-positive. In the event a patient does not have pain, two paraclinical tests are required to make a diagnosis of definitive optic neuritis. If the patient has bilateral eye involvement with or without pain, at least two tests are required, including positive findings on the MRI [47].

The optic nerve length involvement is predictive of the loss of GCIPL thinning at 12 months; the longer the optic nerve involvement, the more significant the loss of GCIPL thickness and volume. There is a compensatory thickening of the INL. The cause of the optic disc edema and the cRNFL thickening in the acute phase of optic neuritis is confusing as the optic disc edema and thickening of the cRNFL recovers, but no loss of the cRNFL may be noted at 12 months [64].

15.5.4 Multiple Sclerosis-Associated Optic Neuritis (MS-ON)

Multiple sclerosis is a demyelinating disease, an autoimmune inflammatory reaction to the myelin sheath of the neuronal axons, ultimately destroying the myelin sheath. For diagnosing MS, McDonald's criteria revised in 2017 are applied [65]. The criteria are typically used to diagnose MS in a clinically isolated syndrome. The demyelinating lesions are disseminated in the CNS in different parts of the CNS (space), and dissemination occurs at different periods (time). The lesions must affect two of the four regions of the brain, namely periventricular, juxtacortical or cortical, infratentorial, and the spinal cord. MS can be formally diagnosed if there are ≥2 relapses with evidence of damage in ≥2 areas of the CNS on T2-weighted MRI scans. However, if there have been ≥2 relapses and damage only in one area, MRI should demonstrate symptomatic or asymptomatic typical T2 lesions in ≥2 areas. If there is only one relapse and damage in two areas, either wait for a new relapse or demonstrate evidence of a new diseased area on MRI or the presence of oligoclonal bands in the CSF. The new criteria require a demonstration of the oligoclonal band if a new area of damage cannot be demonstrated. Primary progressive MS is diagnosed if the disability worsens over 1 year. They must have at least two signs: one brain lesion, two spinal cord lesions, or a positive oligoclonal band in CSF.

Notably, ON is not included in the imaging criteria for diagnosing MS. In the optic neuritis treatment trial, 50% of the patients with ON went on to develop MS by 15 years of follow-up. Twenty five percent of those with no associated CNS lesions on MRI and 75% with at least one CNS lesion developed MS. The absence of MRI findings, male sex, optic disc swelling, and atypical ON carries a low risk of progression [66].

Until recently, all autoimmune optic neuritis, especially in young women, was considered due to multiple sclerosis (MS) until pathogenic antibody-associated optic neuritis was discovered with a different course, systemic associations, and outcome. Optic neuritis is a presenting sign of MS in 25% and 75% of the disease. Multiple sclerosis-associated Optic neuritis (MS-ON) is seen twice more commonly in women than men at a median age of 29 years and is unilateral in ~75% of patients. They do not show any ONH swelling and primarily affect the retrolaminar and intracanalicular segments of the optic nerve. It does not affect either the chiasma or the optic tract. The oligoclonal bands are + in the CSF in most MS-ON patients. Evoked potentials (both visual and brainstem) are prolonged in MS.

15.5.4.1 Treatment of MS-ON

In the optic neuritis treatment trial, high-dose intravenous methylprednisolone (3 days) (IVMP) followed by oral steroids (11 days) hastened the recovery of vision. However, there was no difference in the outcome at 6 months or one-year follow-up compared to the placebo group. On the other hand, oral corticosteroids led to increased recurrences and were not recommended. Definitive MS developed in 8% of the IVMP group versus 17% in the placebo group. The beneficial effect of IVMP was apparent for up to 2 years and none after 5 years [67]. Ninety percent of the patients in the ONTT recovered ≥6/12 at the end of 5 years of follow-ups [48]. Disease-modifying therapies should be initiated at the earliest to prevent further relapses.

15.5.5 Pathogenic Antibody-Associated Optic Neuritis Syndromes

Two significant glial antibody-associated optic neuritis syndromes are associated with the AQP4 IgG-positive neuromyelitis optica spectrum disorder (NMOSD) and the myelin oligodendrocyte glycoprotein IgG- (MOG-IgG) associated ON. These were erroneously labelled as MS in the past, but had a different disease course from MS. These two antibodies are not detected in patients with MS-ON [68].

15.5.5.1 Aquaporin-4 Antibody Associated with Neuromyelitis Optica Spectrum Disorder

Till 2004, neuromyelitis Optica (NMO), optic neuritis with myelitis syndrome, was considered a part of multiple sclerosis when the antibodies to aquaporin 4 IgG antibodies (AQP-4), an astrocyte water channel, were discovered in patients of optic neuritis with transverse myelitis also known as Devic's disease. AQP4-ON is often seen in adults than children; most patients are women. Most present with a severe vision loss ≤6/60; bilateral in 20%. Nearly half the patients have pain in the movement of the eyes. Mild ONH swelling may be seen [69]. Myelitis is characterized by loss of sensations in the legs, weakness (paraparesis), and incontinence. Isolated ON or isolated transverse myelitis (TM) with AQP4 IgG+ is called NMO spectrum disorder. More than 50% progress to the definitive NMO within the first year. The definitive NMO consists of ON, TM, and two of the three criteria (1). MRI shows extensive longitudinal myelitis in at least three segments; (2). MRI is not suggestive of MS, and (3). AQP-4 IgG+ [70].

In the inner retina, the AQP4 channels are expressed in the Muller cells but not in the non-myelinated axons in the retina and the prelaminar optic nerve. The astrocytes separate the axons from the pial septa in the retrolaminar optic nerve. AQP4 is expressed in the footplates of these astrocytes.

The NMO spectrum disorder includes patients with optic neuritis, transverse myelitis (TM), or extensive longitudinal myelitis. Patients with bilateral optic neuritis who are AQP4-positive are also part of the spectrum of the disease. Most often, it affects women at the median age of 39 years. Compared to good visual recovery in MS-ON, visual recovery in patients with AQP4-ON is poor. Thirty percent have ≤6/60 high contrast visual acuity and 70% of patients with a relapsing disease have this level of blindness [69].

Earlier, NMO was considered a monophasic disorder, but now relapsing cases are known [71]. The lesions in NMO are far more extensive and may involve the optic chiasma and even the thalamus. The vision loss in NMO is very severe, and visual recovery is poor. The damage in NMOSD is irreversible.

The AQP4 antibodies, once they enter the CNS tissue, bind with AQP4 at the footplates of the astrocytes, and activate complement, form a membrane attack complex, initiate an inflammatory reaction, and lead to the destruction of the neural tissue. Thus, recovery from NMO lesions is minimal [72].

Treatment of AQP4-ON and NMOSD

Patients with NMOSD do not respond as well to intravenous corticosteroids as MS-ON. One may consider plasmapheresis followed by intravenous corticosteroids or immunoglobulins, especially in refractory cases. Various immunomodulators are used for the prevention of relapses in NMOSD. Azathioprine, mycophenolate mofetil, and methotrexate are some of them. Of the US FDA-approved biological agents in treating NMOSD, rituximab is the most commonly used. The other agents are eculizumab, inebilizumab, and satralizumab. Eculizumab prevents the splitting of Complement 5 into C5a and C5b and thus prevents the formation of the membrane attack complex. Inebilizumab destroys AQP4 IgG-producing plasmablast cells. Satralizumab is a humanized antibody against IL-6. A recent network meta-analysis showed that of the three agents, eculizumab was more effective in preventing relapses of NMOSD than the other two suggesting that blocking specifically Complement 5 was more effective in preventing relapses of NMOSD than a more non-specific blockage [73].

15.5.5.2 Myelin Oligodendrocyte Glycoprotein Antibody-Associated Optic Neuritis

The MOG-antibody associated with ON (MOG-ON) runs a relapsing course, which is painful and associated with ONH swelling. There is no gender predilection. The median age of presentation is 31 years. Nearly 40% are bilateral. Most have retroocular pain in the movement of the eyes. Severe visual loss <6/60 is seen in most. They show moderate to severe ONH swelling. The visual field loss is central but may show more diffuse field loss. Isolated optic chiasm or optic tract involvement is more common in MOG-ON than in other etiologies [69]. They may have heterogeneous clinical manifestations of encephalomyelitis and resemble NMOSD, but the AQP4 antibodies are absent. The MRI shows perineural enhancement and extensive longitudinal involvement [74].

Recurrences of MOG-antibody associated with ON may or may not be accompanied by CNS inflammation. The vision at presentation is mostly poor, but unlike AQP4-ON, visual recovery is good in most, and the average visual acuity in the short term may improve to 20/30 [74]. Since it is a chronic relapsing disorder with cumulative damage to the neural axons, high contrast visual acuity recovery in short-term follow-up obtained in clinical settings may not reflect the actual outcome of MOG-IgG+ ON.

The recurrences are more frequent in MOG-ON compared to the AQP4-ON patients. In comparison, the AQP4-ON leads to severe damage in a single attack and relapsing attacks in MOG-ON cause cumulative damage in the pRNFL and the GCIPL thickness [75].

Treatment of MOG-ON

These patients show good responses to corticosteroids. They also show good recovery compared to the AQP4-ON. During the acute attack, MOG-ON patients require intravenous methylprednisolone or plasma exchange to minimize neuronal damage. Since it is a relapsing disease, these patients require long-term immunosuppressive therapy.

15.5.5.3 Collapsin-Response Mediator Protein-5- (CRMP-5) Associated Optic Neuritis

Collapsin-response mediator protein-5 (CRMP-5) IgG antibodies were first discovered in cancer patients as a marker of the paraneoplastic syndrome [76]. In the first large series of CRMP-5-positive paraneoplastic syndromes, optic neuritis was seen in only 7% of patients [77]. More recently, 38% of the CRMP-5-positive patients had neuro-ophthalmic manifestations. Of these,

62% had associated cancer, primarily small cell lung cancers. Women were more commonly affected. In nearly 3/4th of patients, the eye manifestations preceded cancer diagnosis. More than 80% had optic neuritis with ONH swelling, retinitis, vitritis, or uveitis. Less than 20% had retinitis or uveitis without optic neuritis. None of the patients had optic nerve enhancement on MRI. Nearly 40% of patients may show ocular motility disorders and diplopia [78].

15.6 Optic Disc Pallor (Atrophy)

The normal optic disc is pink due to blood capillaries and shows finely blurred disc margins. It transmits nearly 1.2 million ganglion cell axons. However, following several optic nerve disorders such as optic neuritis, chiasmatic compressive tumours, ischaemic optic neuropathy, trauma, papilledema, drugs, and toxins, the axons degenerate, leaving behind a complete or sectoral pallor of the optic disc (Figs. 15.13, 15.14, and 15.15). As the axons degenerate, these get replaced by glial tissue, and the capillaries attenuate, causing disc pallor. Pathologically, the antegrade or ascending optic atrophy is caused by degeneration of the ganglion cells in the retina seen in open-angle glaucoma, inherited retinal degenerations, and drug toxicities. Retrograde or descending optic atrophy is classically caused by chiasmal compression by pituitary tumours and proceeds towards the eye. There is often a trans-synaptic degeneration of axons which can be

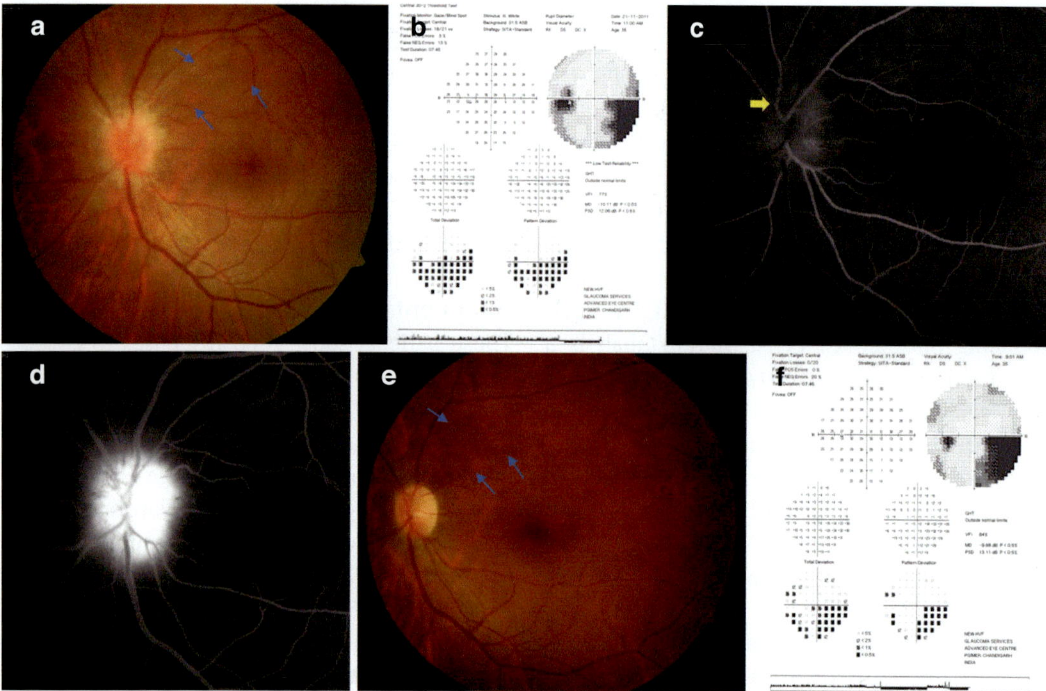

Fig. 15.15 A 35-year-old woman presented with visual loss in the left eye for 2 weeks. She had received Tacrolimus 1 mg twice daily for nephrotic syndrome for 2 years. Visual acuity was 6/6 in both eyes. She had a relative afferent pupillary defect in the left eye. The left eye had optic disc swelling, more remarkable in the upper pole (**a**). Humphrey's visual field analysis using the 30.2 strategy showed an inferior altitudinal field defect (**b**); On FFA, there was delayed filling (yellow arrow) of the upper half of the disc (**c**) with late diffuse staining (**d**). Tacrolimus was discontinued, and she was treated with oral corticosteroids. She maintained RAPD and 6/6 visual acuity in this eye. There was a loss of retinal nerve fibres along the upper temporal arcade (arrows, **e**). The visual field continued to show an inferior altitudinal defect (**f**) Reproduced with permission of the publishers from Gupta M, Bansal R, Beke N, Gupta A. Tacrolimus-induced unilateral ischaemic optic neuropathy in a non-transplant patient. BMJ Case Rep. 2012 Aug 21;2012:bcr2012006718. doi: 10.1136/bcr-2012-006718. PMID: 22914240; PMCID: PMC4544422

antegrade when the pathology in the photoreceptors can lead to changes in the visual cortex or retrograde when a pathology in the visual cortex results in atrophy of the axons in the eye [79].

Clinically, the optic disc pallor is called primary when the axonal degeneration leaves behind a pale optic disc with sharp margins. Primary optic atrophy is usually seen in pituitary tumours, traumatic optic atrophy, or post-optic neuritis. Secondary optic atrophy results from optic disc papilledema or papillitis and is marked by exuberant glial tissue proliferation and indistinct disc margins. Consecutive optic atrophy results from retinal pathology like retinal arterial occlusion, retinitis pigmentosa, and chorioretinal inflammations. Of all the etiologies, we shall briefly discuss hereditary optic atrophy, Leber's hereditary optic neuropathy, dominant hereditary optic atrophy, and chiasmal compression syndromes.

15.6.1 Inherited Optic Neuropathies

Inherited optic neuropathies lead to slow and symmetrical degeneration of the ganglion cells in the retina. Unlike other causes of optic atrophy, they do not show RAPD. Neuroimaging is normal. A Canadian cohort of 97 patients with bilateral optic atrophy, where all the known causes of optic atrophy had been excluded, was subjected to 22 nuclear panel NGS and complete mtDNA sequencing; 20% had a nuclear variant, most of which were in the OPA1 gene. A nuclear variant is likely positive in patients with a family history [74]. Leber's hereditary optic neuropathy (LHON) is the most important phenotype of mtDNA mutation, and autosomal dominant optic atrophy is the most common phenotype of nuclear mutation, OPA1, which encodes for a mitochondrial protein. Mitochondria play a crucial role in maintaining the health of the optic nerve.

15.6.1.1 Leber's Hereditary Optic Neuropathy

Leber's hereditary optic neuropathy (LHON) is one of the most frequently maternally inherited mitochondrial genetic disorders seen in 1 per 25,000. It manifests with simultaneous or sequential (within 1–2 months) painless subacute loss of central vision with dyschromatopsia from 10 to 70, mostly in people under 50. A history of similar vision loss can be elicited in the maternal relatives. The optic disc may be normal on fundoscopy or show prominent RNFL and peripapillary telangiectatic vessels. The retinal vessels appear tortuous. Pupillary reactions are normal. The FFA is normal. The visual evoked potential and the ERG are normal. Neuroimaging is normal. On perimetry, they show central or centrocecal visual field defects (Fig. 15.16). On OCT, the GCL shows atrophy. By 6 months, the optic discs are pale. The visual outcome is poor [80]. There may be extraocular associations such as MS, parkinsonism, and myelopathy without evidence of CNS involvement [81]. On OCT, in the early LHON (< 6 months from onset), the RNFL is thickened, but in the late atrophic stage of LHON, there is marked thinning of the RNFL. The temporal fibres of the papillomacular bundle are the first and most severely affected compared to the nasal fibres of the papillomacular fibres (Figs. 15.16 and 15.17) [82].

In LHON, the full field ERG is normal, but the flash Visual evoked potentials (VEP) and Pattern ERG are abnormal and consistent with optic nerve conduction defects. There may be variably reduced amplitude in the cone ERG and the flicker ERG suggestive of photoreceptor pathology in some patients with LHON. The SD-OCT is however, normal [83].

LHON results from point mutations in mitochondrial DNA. The most common mtDNA mutations are G11778A, T14484C, or G3460A. In a large cohort of suspected LHON, 29.4% were positive for these three targeted mutations [84, 85]. Nearly 50% of men and 10% of women ever get LHON. Most LHON patients carry homoplasmic, i.e. the mutant alleles; 10–15% may have heteroplasmy with a mixture of mutant and wild-type alleles. The clinical manifestations develop depending on when the mutant allele becomes more dominant. Since not all people who carry the mutation develop LHON, environmental factors such as nutritional factors, smoking, alcohol, and vitamin B deficiency may play a role [80]. Despite using vita-

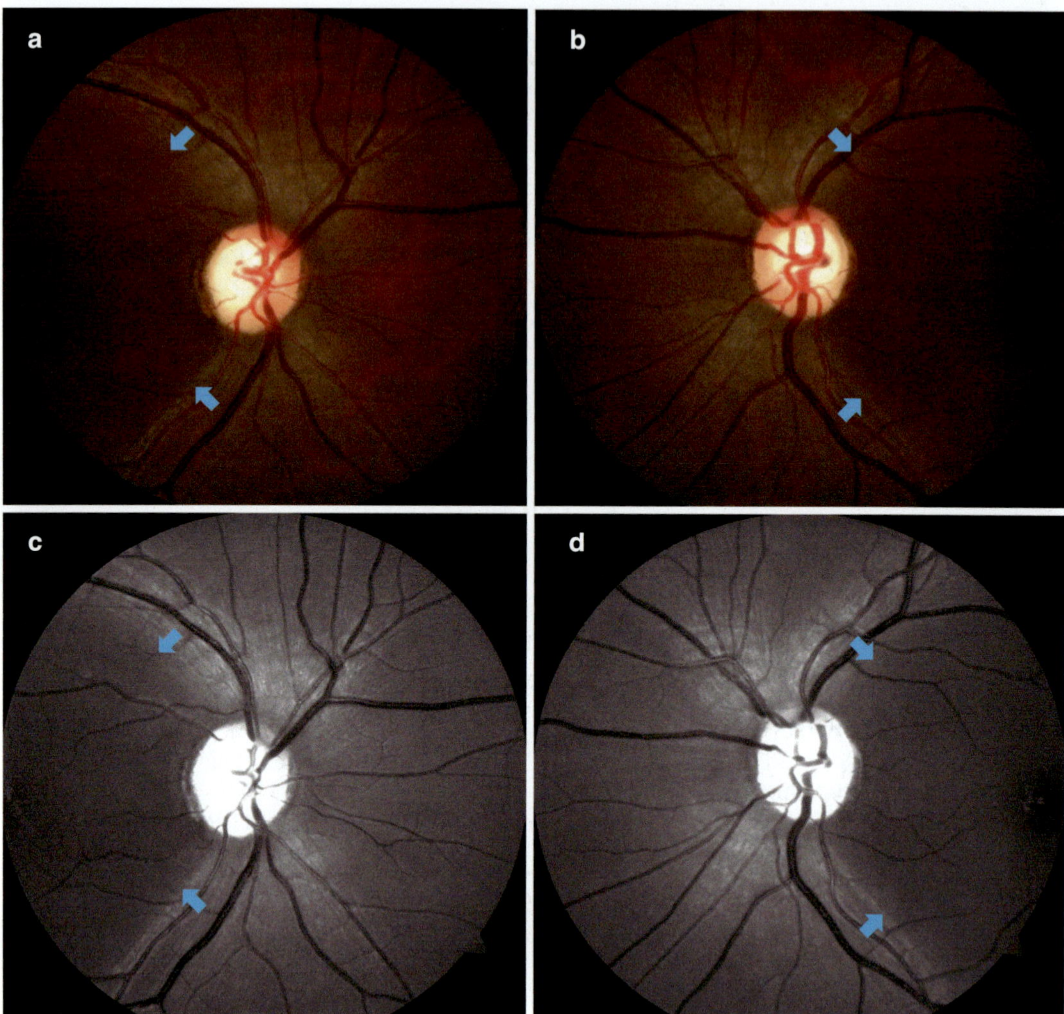

Fig. 15.16 (**a**–**d**) A case of Leber's hereditary optic neuropathy (LHON) (**a**, **b**), with the temporal fibres of the papillomacular bundle being the first and most severely affected (blue arrows) compared to the nasal fibres, better appreciated on red-free fundus photographs (**c**, **d**). (**e**, **h**) OCT (**e**, **f**) shows RNFL is thickened in the early LHON (<6 months from onset). Visual fields (**g**, **h**) show central or centrocecal visual field defects. Images courtesy of Dr. SS Pandav, Professor and Head, Advanced Eye Centre, Post Graduate Institute of Medical Education and Research, Chandigarh, India

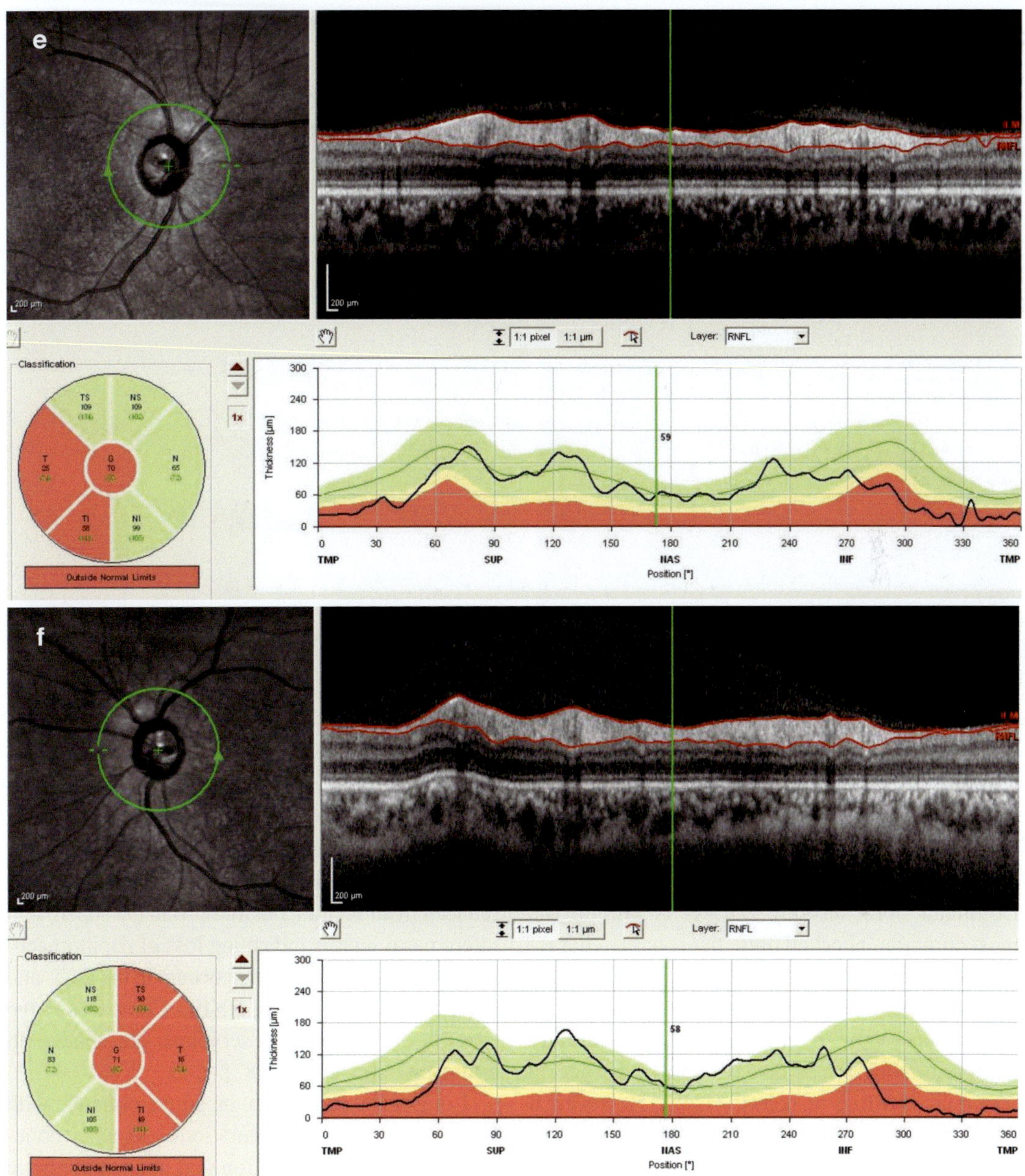

Fig. 15.16 (continued)

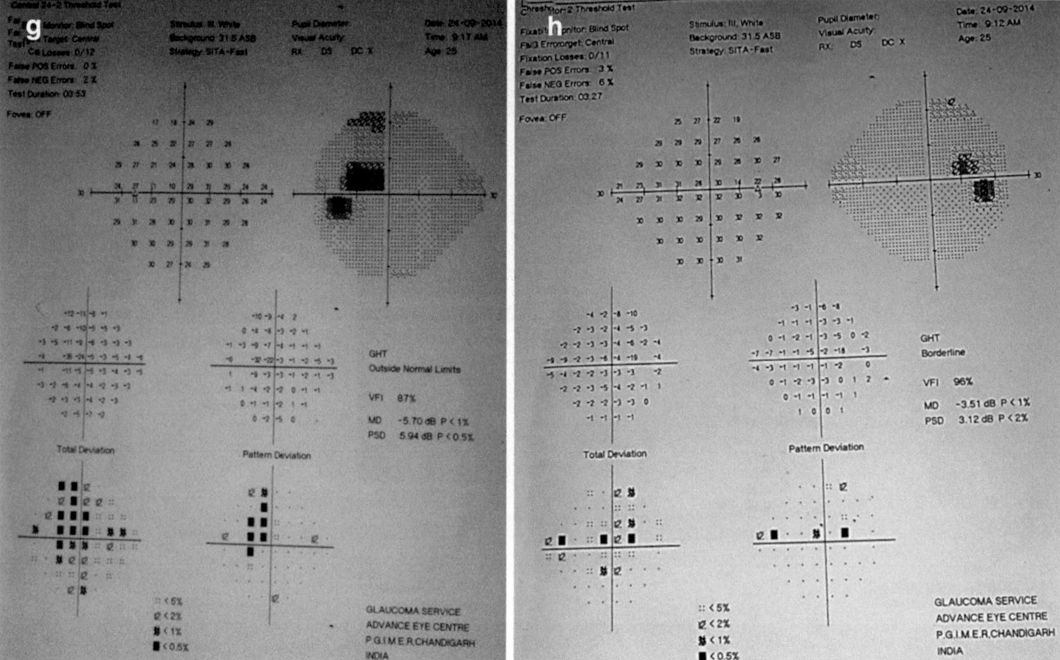

Fig. 15.16 (continued)

min cocktails, there has been no proven therapy for LHON. Gene therapy has reached the stage of conducting clinical trials [84, 85].

15.6.1.2 Dominant Optic Atrophy

Dominant optic atrophy (DOA) is among the most common inherited optic neuropathy characterized by the progressive loss of ganglion cells, ultimately leading to temporal optic atrophy. It starts insidiously in childhood and eventually leads to blindness. The patients show centrocecal scotomas and loss of colour vision. However, it runs a variable course even in the same families. Most cases are reported with a mutation in OPA1 located on 3q28-q29. This gene encodes for a mitochondrial protein. This gene is involved in oxidative phosphorylation and maintenance of mtDNA. All cells express OPA1 genes, but the mutation in this gene affects only the RGC and interferes with the transmission of signals. The small cell RGCs in the papillomacular bundles get affected due to low energy reserves in these cells. A mutation results in oxidative stress resulting in apoptosis of the RGCs [86].

On OCT, it preferentially involves the small fibres of papillomacular bundles. On SD-OCT, there was a significant decrease in the overall cRNFL thickness and more so in the temporal and inferior sectors. The macular GCIPL thickness is reduced in all sectors, but more so in the supero and infero nasal sectors indicating loss of papillomacular bundles. The first change occurs in the GCL and is followed by the loss of RNFL. Compared to the LHON, the centrocecal scotomas are smaller in dominant optic atrophy [87].

Long-term follow-up in some patients with DOA with OPA1 mutations shows cone-photoreceptor degeneration and abnormal photic cone response ERG. However, outer photoreceptor degeneration is more evident in patients of DOA with optic atrophy type 13 mediated by a mutation in SSBP1 [83].

There is no proven treatment in DOA. The treatment options are vitamins B12 and C, lutein supplements that reduce the optic nerve's oxidative stress, and idebenone- a ubiquinone analogue. Gene therapy is a promising option in the future.

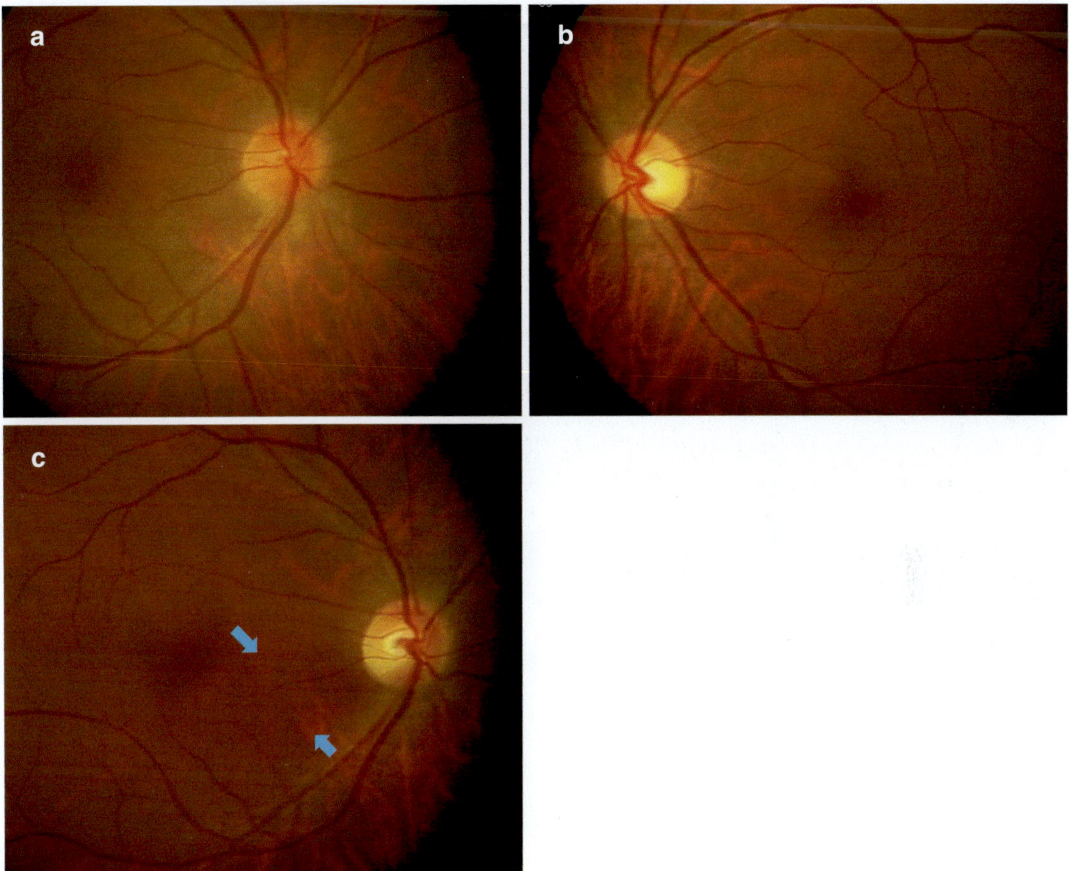

Fig. 15.17 A 44-year-old man presented with a blurring of vision in the right eye three days following an attack of a migraine. Visual acuity was 6/18. The right eye showed mild optic disc edema with obscuration of the cup (**a**). The left eye was normal with a normal cup (**b**). Two months later, the optic disc edema in the right eye resolved, and the optic cup became visible (**c**). Note loss of the inferotemporal papillomacular nerve fibres (blue arrows in c). The corresponding central scotoma (**d**) in the upper temporal quadrant did not improve (**e**). He was not tested for mtDNA mutations. The clinical picture was highly suggestive of Leber's hereditary optic neuropathy. Image courtesy of Dr. SS Pandav, Professor and Head, Advanced Eye Centre, Post Graduate Institute of Medical Education and Research, Chandigarh, India

15.6.2 Chiasmal Compression Syndrome

The optic chiasm lies above the sella turcica, harbouring the pituitary gland. The anterior part of the third ventricle lies above the chiasm. Nearly 53% of the axons from the nasal half of each retina, projecting to the temporal field of vision, decussate in the chiasm. The pathologies affecting the chiasm most commonly produce visual symptoms. Several pathologies can cause chiasmal syndrome by (1). intrinsic pathologies involving the chiasm's substance include demyelinating disorders like MS, inflammatory or infiltrative disorders, neurofibromatosis, syphilis, tuberculosis, or Sarcoidosis; (2). The most common extrinsic lesions that cause compression are pituitary adenoma, craniopharyngioma, parasellar meningioma, and parasellar internal carotid artery aneurysm.

15.6.2.1 Pituitary Adenomas

Pituitary adenomas are the most common cause of the chiasmal syndrome. They need to grow to a large size before they can compress the chiasm from below. If the chiasm is placed normally, the

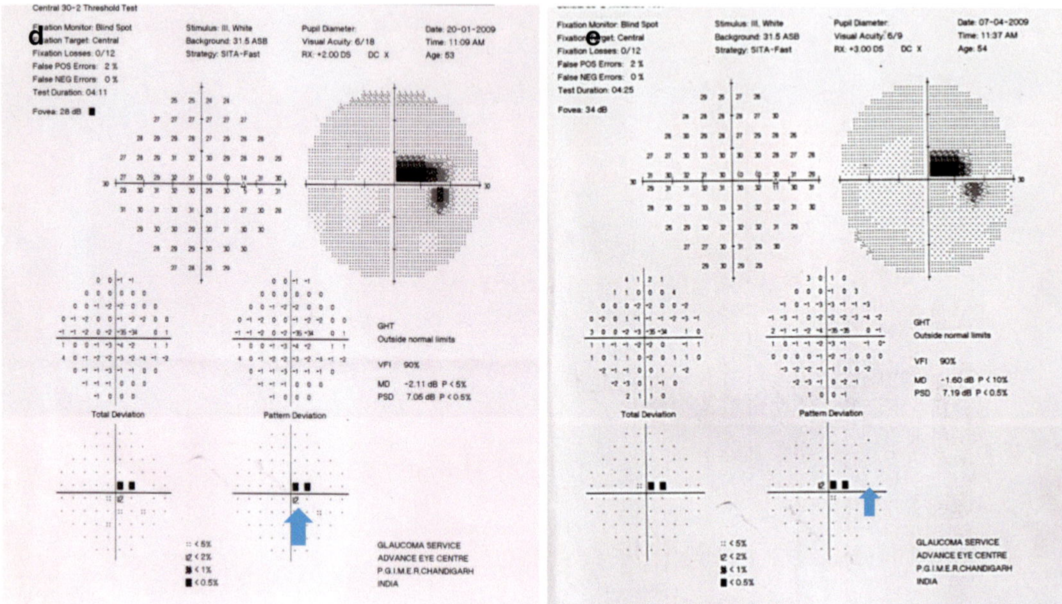

Fig. 15.17 (continued)

crossing fibres from the retina (projecting to the temporal field in both eyes) are affected. As the fibres from the lower nasal sector cross on the undersurface of the chiasm, these are affected first and produce bitemporal superior field defects, which progress clockwise in the right temporal field and anticlockwise in the left temporal field. Patients suffer from blindness temporal to the point of fixation, and the earliest symptom may be bumping into objects. The visual field is charted on Humphrey's VF 24.2. The earliest defect may be depression of the sensitivity by ≥2Dbs. Depending upon the fixation of the chiasm, the optic nerves or even the optic tracts may be affected.

On OCT, there is a characteristic binasal loss of the fibres in the papillomacular bundle (between the foveal centre and the optic disc) with preservation of the upper and lower temporal arcuate fibres, which do not cross in the chiasma and remain preserved for a long time. The OCT may detect loss of crossing axons even before the perimetric changes can be demonstrated [44, 45]. RNFL thinning is a prognosis marker for visual recovery following the decompression of pituitary tumours. More than 97.5% recovered ≥6/12 visual acuity at 9–15 months of follow-up compared to 88% with RNFL loss. Maximum improvement occurs between 6 and 10 weeks of surgery [88]. Moreover, the binasal GCIPL thinning may precede the onset of visual fields, which appears to be a less sensitive tool than OCT [89–91].

15.6.2.2 Craniopharyngiomas

Craniopharyngiomas are either cystic or solid benign tumours of childhood between the age of 5 and 14 years and account for 10–15% of all pituitary tumours and ~ 6% of all childhood intracranial space-occupying lesions. In adults, these may arise from 50 to 74 years. These tumours arise from the epithelial remnants of the Rathke's pouch (craniopharyngeal duct) and may have intrasellar or suprasellar growth. The craniopharyngiomas may be adamantinomatous (ACP) or papillary (PCP); the former are primarily cystic and may be seen in childhood or later, and the latter is solid and seen only in adults [92]. The diagnosis is often delayed. The common symptoms include headache, imbalance, slow growth, symptoms of diabetes insipidus, and vision defects. The symptoms arise from the compression of the pituitary gland. https://rarediseases.org/rare-diseases/craniopharyngioma/

These do not usually cause erosion of the sella turcica. In children, these may produce raised ICP and papilledema. In adults, these are slow-growing, solid tumours that compress the optic chiasm from above and behind and present with optic atrophy. These tend to produce bitemporal field defects that initiate in the lower temporal quadrants and are asymmetric. On CT scans, 90% of ACP show calcification. MRI shows these as cauliflower-type lesions, enhancement in 90%, and cystic in 90% [92]. Apart from neuroimaging, the functioning of the pituitary gland is evaluated by testing for growth hormone, insulin-like growth factor-1, prolactin, cortisol, follicle-stimulating hormone, luteinizing hormone, thyroid stimulating hormone, cortisol, testosterone, and estradiol. The extent of hypothalamus damage is predictive of hypothalamic obesity in these patients [93].

15.6.2.3 Meningiomas

Meningiomas are the dura mater's most common, slow-growing primary CNS tumours. These tumours affect women, most commonly between 35 and 60 years. These may involve afferent and efferent visual pathways. The symptoms depend upon the site of involvement. Meningiomas from tuberculum sellae, anterior clinoid, dorsum clivus, and the parasellar dura often affect the chiasm and the optic nerve and produce asymmetric perimetry changes. Patients usually complain of progressive loss of vision and present with chronic papilledema or optic atrophy. (Fig. 15.18). The presence of refractile bodies in the ONH in these patients indicates prolonged optic disc edema. The most common differential diagnosis is optic neuritis. Any patient with suspected optic neuritis who does not improve vision by 2 weeks should be strongly suspected of harbouring suprasellar meningioma. The meningiomas arising from the inner third of the sphenoidal ridge produce visual symptoms and paresis of extraocular muscles by compressing on the structures passing through the superior orbital fissure. The meningiomas may present with primary optic atrophy if involving the optic nerve, optic chiasm, or papilledema from raised ICP. Opto-ciliary shunt vessels on an atrophic optic disc highly suggest a long-standing perioptic meningioma [94, 95]. There are no specific tests for meningiomas, and they need to undergo a complete neuro-ophthalmic examination, including recording of pupil reactions, visual acuity, colour vision, perimetry, and OCT. Neuroimaging provides the diagnosis (Fig. 15.18).

15.6.3 Ischaemic Optic Neuropathies (ION)

Sudden loss of vision in an older adult (> 50 years) due to optic nerve ischaemia is not uncommon who report to the eye emergency. These are broadly classified into: (1). arteritic anterior ischaemic optic neuropathy (A-AION); (2). Non-arteritic ischaemic optic neuropathy is further divided into (a). anterior and (b). posterior. The ION must be differentiated from demyelinating optic neuropathies (multiple sclerosis) seen primarily in young women (<50) who also present with sudden acute or subacute vision loss associated with pain in the movement of eyes. The MS-ON runs a relapsing-remitting course, showing disseminated CNS and Spinal involvement in space and time.

15.6.3.1 Nonarteritic Anterior Ischaemic Optic Neuropathy

NAION accounts for nearly 90% of all optic neuropathies. It is seen more commonly in apparently healthy-looking men >50 years.

15.6.3.2 Risk Factors for NAION

The significant risk factors are hypertension (50%), diabetes mellitus (25%), coronary artery disease, dyslipidemia, and smoking [96]. The relative risk of obstructive sleep apnea in patients with NAION is 4.9 compared to the normal population [97, 98]. Non-compliance with continuous positive airway pressure increases the risk of developing NAION in the fellow eye. Notably, there is a significant association between OSA, glaucoma, and stroke [99]. OSA should be considered in all patients with NAION, especially

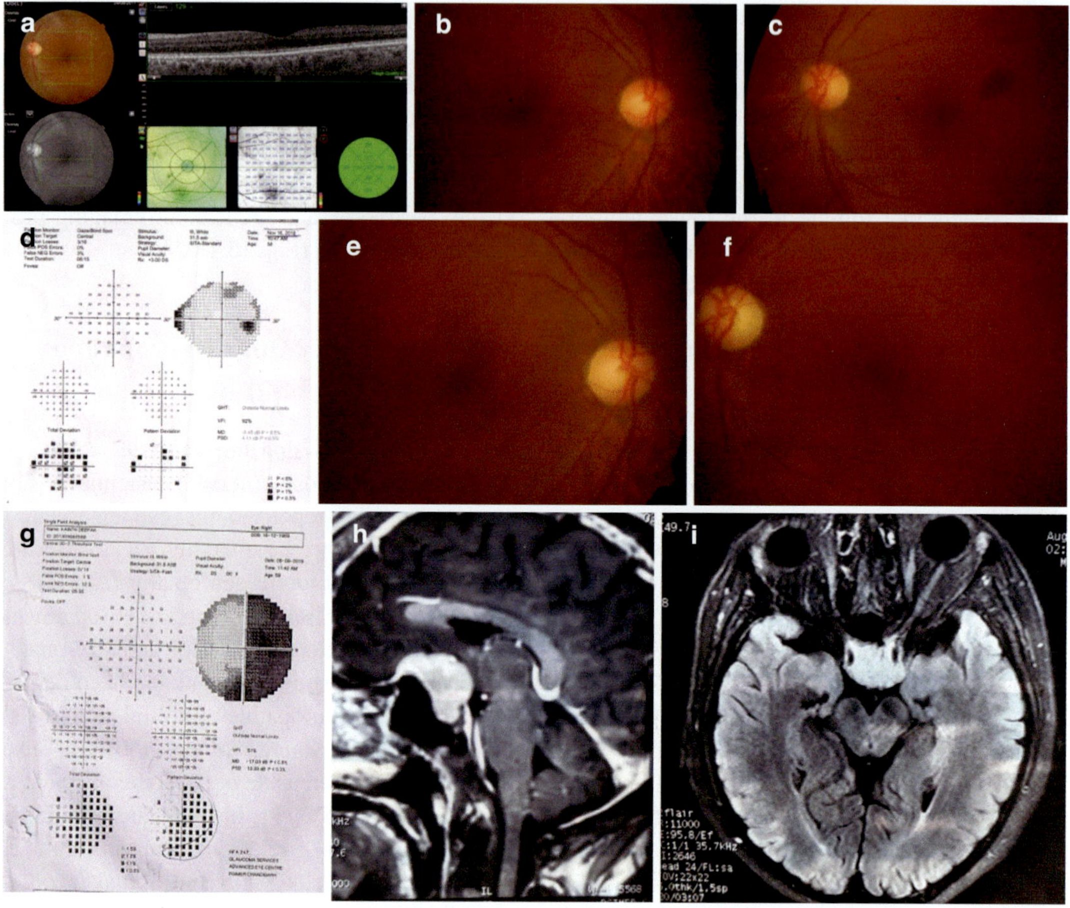

Fig. 15.18 A 28-year-old man with ankylosing spondylitis remained under active follow-up for 31 years with recurrent acute anterior uveitis in both eyes, which remitted and returned to normal vision after each attack. He maintained a visual acuity of 6/6 in both eyes. At the age of 59 years, he complained of visual loss in the left eye without concurrent uveitis. His visual acuity was 6/6 and 6/12 in the right and left eyes, respectively. The OCT examination of the left eye ruled out a suspected cystoid macular edema (**a**). He returned 1 year later with a normal-looking optic disc (**b** and **c**), although there was a further decline in visual acuity in the left eye. VA in the left eye had dropped to finger counting at 2.5 m. Six months later, he had no light perception in the left eye. The visual field was possible only in the right eye, but a superior temporal quadrantanopia was overlooked (**d**). He returned after 1 year when temporal optic disc pallor L > R was noted (**e** and **f**). The Visual Field showed a right-eye temporal hemianopic defect that progressed into the lower nasal quadrant (**g**, cf. **d**). MRI revealed a large suprasellar meningioma that extended into the sella turcica (**h** and **i**)

the young [100]. The possible mechanism of NAION on OSA is cerebral venous dilatation and increased ICP.

The blood supply in the prelaminar ONH is drawn from the peripapillary short ciliary vessels. The ciliary supply is strictly an end-arterial supply. On FFA, the optic disc can be frequently seen in the watershed zone, making them vulnerable to hemodynamic variations. Patients on oral anti-hypertensive drugs have a dip in their nocturnal blood pressure, which affects optic disc perfusion in patients who are already at risk [101]. NAION patients with multifactorial risk factors also risk developing cerebrovascular accidents [102]. A low perfusion pressure during sleep at night in patients at risk precipitates an attack of NAION. Other risk factors include vasoconstrictors used as nasal decongestants [103], amiodarone [104], and phosphodiesterase type5 inhibitors [105].

15.6.3.3 The Clinical Course of NAION

On waking up in the morning, the patients usually complain of sudden painless vision loss from one eye. The vision loss may progress over the next several hours or even days. The visual acuity may vary from 6/6 to 6/60.

On examination, they show RAPD in the affected eye. The ONH is swollen and hyperemic. It may also show linear haemorrhages. A small optic disc with no cup is considered a 'disc at risk' (Fig. 15.19). Since a swollen ONH in the affected eye does not reveal the presence of a preexisting cup, examination of the fellow eye may reveal a disc at risk or even sectoral pallor from a previous attack of the NAION. If the fellow eye shows a normal cup, the possibility of an A-AION should always be considered. More recent data suggest that instead of crowding the axons in a smaller optic disc, the cup's smaller size is significantly associated with NAION [106]. On the confrontation field (CF) testing, the affected eye shows an altitudinal field defect, most often in the lower nasal quadrant or a central scotoma. Standard automatic perimetry (SAP) should be done to document the field defect. On Goldmann perimetry in NAION, absolute inferior nasal quadrantic defects were found in 22.4% versus 8% altitudinal fields. The most common was a combination of inferior altitudinal with an absolute defect in the lower nasal quadrant (Fig. 15.4) [107]. The absolute inferior nasal defect is due to the vulnerable blood supply of the upper temporal aspect of the optic disc. When looking for an altitudinal field or central defects, CF testing is 75–100% sensitive

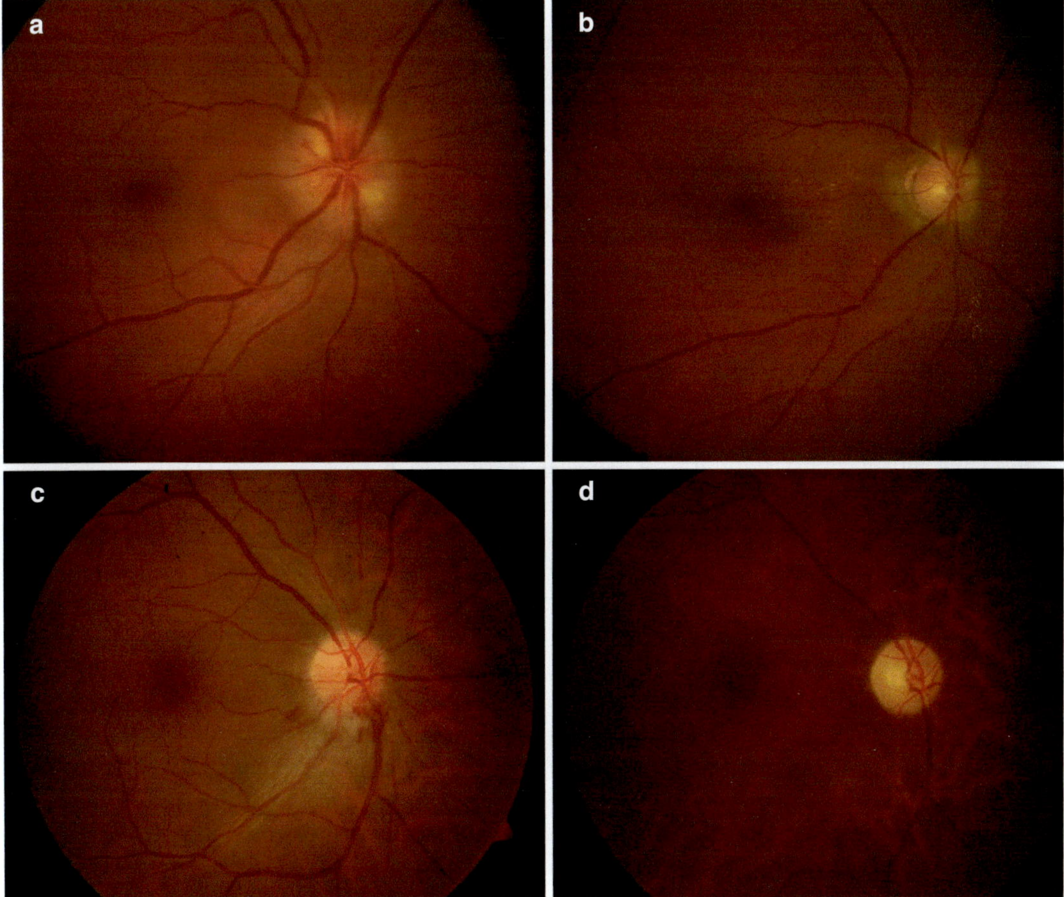

Fig. 15.19 A swollen and hyperemic optic nerve head (**a**). A small optic disc with no cup is considered a 'disc at risk' for developing anterior ischemic optic neuropathy. Three weeks later, the ODE resolved (**b**). Another case of AION, with splinter peripapillary hemorrhages and ODE (**c**). Three years later, there was optic atrophy (**d**)

and has >70% positive predictive value compared to automated perimetry [108].

The MRI of the optic nerves is usually normal, and diffusion restriction of the optic nerves can be observed in a few if MRI is done very early in the course. However, if the diagnosis of NAION is in doubt, contrast-enhanced and fat-suppressed MRI of the brain and orbit should be done to rule out compressive optic neuropathy and inflammatory optic neuritis [109]. MRI Brain may show micro-angiopathic changes in addition to implicating vascular involvement at other sites in the brain.

The ONH swelling may take several weeks for resolution and leaves behind a sectoral pallor of the optic disc [110]. In the natural course, significant improvement in visual acuity may be seen in up to 30% of eyes. Twenty per cent of eyes may show progressive deterioration in visual acuity over the next 3 months [111]. There is a 12–15% risk of the fellow eye suffering from NAION in the next 5 years. The same eye may show recurrence in 5% [109].

15.6.3.4 Treatment of NAION

There is no definitive treatment for NAION. Patients who present with poor vision, have persistent ONH edema, any suspicion of A-AION, or show progressive deterioration of vision may be treated with oral corticosteroids. Recognizing the underlying risk factors and minimizing those with appropriate interventions is important [109].

In a large patient choice study, 70% of patients with ≥20/70 visual acuity who received oral corticosteroids showed significant improvement in vision compared to 40% who did not. The visual fields improved in 40% of the treatment group versus 20% in the non-treated group [112].

Recognizing that NAION is a compartment syndrome, an optic nerve decompression trial was carried out, which showed that 31% in the careful follow-up group and 29.4% in the optic nerve decompression group improved visual acuity by three lines. Moreover, 21.8% in the control group versus 20% in the treatment group suffered from significant vision loss [111]. The trial was prematurely terminated on detecting that by 6 months of follow-up, more patients lost vision due to intervention than careful follow-up [113]. Intravitreal injections of anti-vascular endothelial growth factors or corticosteroids have been used, and although they hasten the recovery of ONH edema, there is no beneficial effect on visual recovery [114].

15.6.4 Posterior Ischaemic Optic Neuropathy (PION)

Posterior ischaemic optic neuropathy is uncommon and challenging to diagnose as it does not have ONH edema or haemorrhages associated with sudden painless vision loss and visual field loss. There are three types. The most common is perioperative, and the less common are non-arteritic and arteritic. These patients mimic retrobulbar neuritis. It is important to rule out MS and infiltrative and compressive optic neuropathies by contrast-enhanced MR studies. They have the same risk factors as NAION except that they do not have structural characteristics of the ONH, as seen in NAION. It may not be easy to differentiate a posterior non-arteritic from an arteritic ischaemic optic neuropathy. In a study of 53 eyes of 42 patients with PION, 12 suffered from an arteritic PION due to giant cell arteritis [115]. In elderly patients in the non-surgical setting who present with bilateral PION with headache, it is critical to rule out the arteritic type. ION in non-ocular surgeries is extremely rare, and only 1 case per 125,000 was reported in non-cardiac surgeries at the Mayo Clinic and 0.06% in coronary artery bypass surgeries [116].

On the other hand, ION is more frequent following cardiac surgeries than percutaneous cardiac interventions and spine surgeries [117]. Following spine surgeries, 0.028% developed ION. Prone position during surgery is a risk factor [118]. An advisory was issued by the American Society of Anesthesiologists to rule out high-risk patients for ION and to warn the patients of such a complication (American Society of Anesthesiologists Task Force on Perioperative Visual Loss; North American Neuro-Ophthalmology Society; Society for Neuroscience in Anesthesiology and Critical Care. Practice Advisory for Perioperative Visual Loss Associated with Spine Surgery 2019: An Updated Report by the American Society of Anesthesiologists Task

Force on Perioperative Visual Loss, the North American Neuro-Ophthalmology Society, and the Society for Neuroscience in Anesthesiology and Critical Care, [119]).

15.6.5 Arteritic Anterior Ischaemic Optic Neuropathy

Arteritic anterior ischaemic optic neuropathy (A-AION) is a devastating complication of small vessel vasculitis, most commonly giant cell arteritis (GCA). See Box 15.2 for the current diagnostic criteria of GCA. Rarely ANCA-associated vasculitis (AAV) may cause A-AION and erroneously point towards GCA because of temporal artery involvement in AAV. The two must be differentiated, as the GCA is a granulomatous inflammation involving small vessels. On the other hand, AAV is a necrotizing vasculitis of small and medium vessels, and the two have vastly different courses and treatment strategies. Mononeuritis multiplex and pauci-immune glomerulonephritis in AAV will help differentiate the two.

Box 15.2 ACR and EULAR Classification of Giant Cell Arteritis (2022)

Score	Criteria
Absolute requirement -age > 50 years	
Additional clinical criteria	
2	Morning stiffness in shoulders and neck
3	Sudden onset loss of vision
2	Jaw or tongue claudication
2	New temporal headache
2	Scalp tenderness
2	Temporal artery -tenderness, cord-like appearance, or decreased pulsation
Laboratory, imaging, and biopsy criteria	
3	Max. ESR >50 mm/h or max. CRP >10 mg/L
5	Positive temporal artery biopsy or + halo sign on USG of temporal artery
2	Bilateral axillary artery involvement -stenosis on angiography, increased uptake on FDG-PET, or halo sign on USG.

A sum of scores of ≥ 6 is deemed + for GCA. These criteria classify med-large vessel GCA after excluding other pathologies.

A-AION accounts for about 10% of all ischaemic optic neuropathies. Other manifestations in the eye include central retinal artery occlusion and the occlusion of posterior ciliary arteries leading to infarcts of the choroid [120]. Primarily seen in older women of North European descent, it causes a sudden painless loss of vision accompanied by headache, jaw claudication, and temporal tenderness. The patients may have a history of low-grade fever, weight loss, myalgias, and other constitutional symptoms. In diagnosing GCA, limb and jaw claudication are more sensitive symptoms than temporal tenderness, temporal artery thickness, or loss of pulsations in the temporal artery [121]. Patients may have symptoms only in the eye without any systemic features in ~20% of the patients and are labelled 'Occult giant cell arteritis' [120]. The A-AION has ethnic variations, with the highest incidence reported from the south of Norway at 32.8 per 100,000 population versus 0.4 per 100,000 African Americans in a US county [122]. In the Asian -Indian population, an earlier age of onset, male predominance, and more frequent ocular involvement were observed [123].

The presenting visual acuity is less than 6/60, and nearly 20% may have no light perception. A-AION is an Ophthalmic emergency, and a quick diagnosis must be reached as the other eye may get involved within days [124]. Urgent C-reactive proteins and ESR should be ordered. In an older person with A-AION, jaw claudication, C-reactive proteins >2.45 mg/dl, and ESR > 47 mm/h are highly sensitive and specific to reaching a diagnosis of GCA [125]. A temporal artery biopsy should be ordered to confirm the diagnosis. On USG, the inflamed artery shows a hypoechoic 'halo sign' indicating the inflamma-

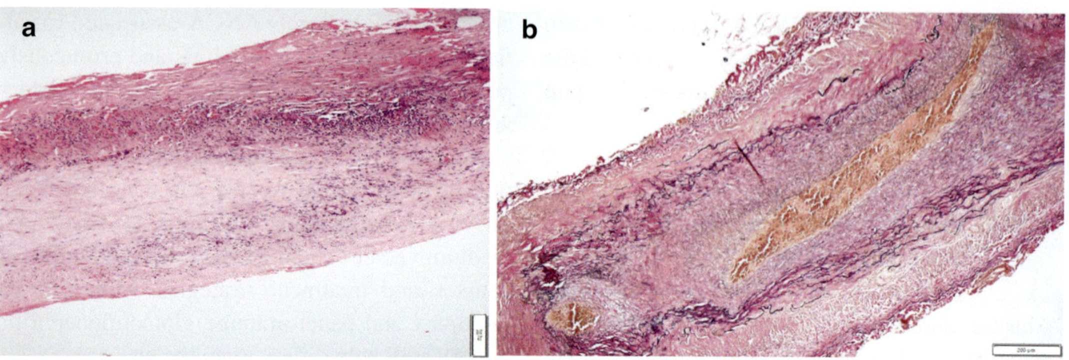

Fig. 15.20 Photomicrograph of temporal artery biopsy shows (**a**) granulomatous inflammation of media of artery with intimal fibrous luminal occlusion (**a**) EVG break of internal and external elastic lamina (**b**). (H&E a, EVG- b.a ×10, b ×40original magnification). Images courtesy of Prof Rithambra Nada, Professor of Pathology, Post Graduate Institute of Medical Education and Research, Chandigarh, India

tory thickening of the temporal artery wall. USG helps determine the biopsy site to avoid skip areas of arteritis in the temporal artery (Fig. 15.20). Skip areas in the temporal artery biopsy of patients with proven GCA may occasionally show areas that lack either the giant cells, epithelioid cells, or any inflammatory cells) [126]. Preferably, the USG and the biopsy should be done before starting intravenous corticosteroids. Once the steroids are started, the wall thickness disappears within 2–3 days [127]. In A-AION, the chances of a positive temporal artery biopsy were nine times higher in the presence of jaw claudication, 3.4 times with neck pain, two times higher with an ESR of 47–107 mm/h, 3.2 times with C-reactive protein >2.45 mg/dl, and two times higher with age 75 years or higher [125].

On clinical examination, these patients show RAPD, a chalky-white optic disc, and may show an area of retinal opacification due to a cilioretinal or a branch artery occlusion. More than 50% of the eyes show either a counting finger vision or no light perception. Although the visual field examination is critical in diagnosing ischaemic optic neuropathy, in A-AION, because of poor visual acuity, it may not be possible to carry out a visual field examination on a Goldmann or Humphrey's visual field analyzer (HFA). A carefully performed confrontation field testing can provide a valuable clue to the nature of field defects. A sectoral defect or an island of vision is encountered on visual field examination. The field defects respect the horizontal meridian, unlike the chiasmal syndromes that respect the vertical meridian [128]. Compared to the Goldmann perimeter, both HFA3 and the Octopus 900 kinetic perimeter with the target moving 5° per second provide equivalent results [129].

15.6.5.1 Treatment of A-AION

Time is of the essence in initiating treatment in A-AION primarily to prevent involvement of the other eye. A-AION must be suspected in elderly patients with profound vision loss with a temporal headache. GCA is highly sensitive to corticosteroids and shows a response with improved temporal headache, tenderness, jaw claudication, and myalgia. The treatment is initiated with intravenous methylprednisolone 1–2 g/day for 2–3 days, followed by oral prednisolone at 1–2 mg/kg/day.

Visual function in A-AION may improve in 4% and worsen in 4% of eyes [130, 131].

To minimize the side effects of high corticosteroids, steroid-sparing disease-modifying antirheumatic drugs such as methotrexate have been used. More recently, recurrences are often seen on tapering of steroids. A controlled recently reported sustained remission with every week or every other week treatment with tocilizumab with a 6-month course of corticosteroids [132].

C-reactive proteins and ESR are the two most sensitive parameters for patients with GCA [131]. In large series of patients with A-AION, they could achieve remission with normal ESR and C-reactive proteins without corticosteroids only in 7% of patients. GCA flares may cause permanent visual loss, cerebral ischaemia, or aortic aneurysms [133]. Methotrexate and tocilizumab are the only two FDA-approved therapies, although several drugs are currently under trial [133].

References

1. Salazar JJ, Ramírez AI, De Hoz R, Salobrar-Garcia E, Rojas P, Fernández-Albarral JA, López-Cuenca I, Blanca Rojas B, Triviño A, Ramírez JM. Anatomy of the human optic nerve: structure and function. In: Ferreri FM, editor. Optic nerve [Internet]. London: IntechOpen; 2018. [cited 2022 Dec 28]. Available from: https://www.intechopen.com/chapters/62850. https://doi.org/10.5772/intechopen.79827.
2. Freddo TF, Chaum E. Chapter 15: The optic nerve and visual pathways. In: Anatomy of the eye and orbit: the clinical essentials. Philadelphia: Lippincott Williams & Wilkins; 2018. p. 241–58.
3. Erdogmus S, Govsa F. Anatomic features of the intracranial and intracanalicular portions of ophthalmic artery: for the surgical procedures. Neurosurg Rev. 2006;29(3):213–8. https://doi.org/10.1007/s10143-006-0028-6. Epub 2006 May 31. PMID: 16775743.
4. van Overbeeke J, Sekhar L. Microanatomy of the blood supply to the optic nerve. Orbit. 2003;22(2):81–8. https://doi.org/10.1076/orbi.22.2.81.14316. PMID: 12789588
5. Hayreh SS. Inter-individual variation in blood supply of the optic nerve head. Its importance in various ischemic disorders of the optic nerve head, and glaucoma, low-tension glaucoma and allied disorders. Doc Ophthalmol. 1985;59(3):217–46. https://doi.org/10.1007/BF00159262. PMID: 4006669.
6. Jonas JB, Holbach L, Panda-Jonas S. Peripapillary arterial circle of Zinn-Haller: location and spatial relationships with myopia. PLoS One. 2013;8(11):e78867. https://doi.org/10.1371/journal.pone.0078867. PMID: 24223862; PMCID: PMC3815204.
7. Lieberman MF, Maumenee AE, Green WR. Histologic studies of the vasculature of the anterior optic nerve. Am J Ophthalmol. 1976;82(3):405–23. https://doi.org/10.1016/0002-9394(76)90489-x. PMID: 961792.
8. Quigley HA, Brown AE, Morrison JD, Drance SM. The size and shape of the optic disc in normal human eyes. Arch Ophthalmol. 1990;108(1):51–7. https://doi.org/10.1001/archopht.1990.01070030057028. PMID: 2297333.
9. Jonas JB, Gusek GC, Naumann GO. Optic disc, cup and neuroretinal rim size, configuration and correlations in normal eyes. Invvest Ophthalmol Vis Sci. 1988;29(7):1151–8. Erratum in: Invest Ophthalmol Vis Sci 1991 May;32(6):1893. Erratum in: Invest Ophthalmol Vis Sci 1992 Feb;32(2):474-5. PMID: 3417404.
10. Lee KM, Lee EJ, Kim TW. Lamina cribrosa configuration in tilted optic discs with different tilt axes: a new hypothesis regarding optic disc tilt and torsion. Invest Ophthalmol Vis Sci. 2015;56(5):2958–67. https://doi.org/10.1167/iovs.14-15953. PMID: 25788647.
11. Jonas JB, Kling F, Gründler AE. Optic disc shape, corneal astigmatism, and amblyopia. Ophthalmology. 1997;104(11):1934–7. https://doi.org/10.1016/s0161-6420(97)30004-9. PMID: 9373129.
12. Ramrattan RS, Wolfs RC, Jonas JB, Hofman A, de Jong PT. Determinants of optic disc characteristics in a general population: the Rotterdam Study. Ophthalmology. 1999;106(8):1588–96. https://doi.org/10.1016/S0161-6420(99)90457-8. PMID: 10442908.
13. Jonas JB, Nguyen XN, Gusek GC, Naumann GO. Parapapillary chorioretinal atrophy in normal and glaucoma eyes. I. Morphometric data. Invest Ophthalmol Vis Sci. 1989;30(5):908–18. PMID: 2722447.
14. Jonas JB, Jonas SB, Jonas RA, Holbach L, Dai Y, Sun X, Panda-Jonas S. Parapapillary atrophy: histological gamma zone and delta zone. PLoS One. 2012;7(10):e47237. https://doi.org/10.1371/journal.pone.0047237. Epub 2012 Oct 18. PMID: 23094040; PMCID: PMC3475708.
15. Vazquez LE, Bye A, Aref AA. Recent developments in the use of optical coherence tomography for glaucoma. Curr Opin Ophthalmol. 2021;32(2):98–104. https://doi.org/10.1097/ICU.0000000000000733. PMID: 33332883
16. Mwanza JC, Huang LY, Budenz DL, Shi W, Huang G, Lee RK. Differences in optical coherence tomography assessment of Bruch membrane opening compared to stereoscopic photography for estimating cup-to-disc ratio. Am J Ophthalmol. 2017;184:34–41. https://doi.org/10.1016/j.ajo.2017.09.024. Epub 2017 Sep 28. PMID: 28964804.
17. McCann P, Hogg RE, Wright DM, McGuinness B, Young IS, Kee F, Azuara-Blanco A. Diagnostic accuracy of spectral-domain OCT circumpapillary, optic nerve head, and macular parameters in the detection of perimetric glaucoma. Ophthalmol Glaucoma. 2019;2(5):336–45. https://doi.

org/10.1016/j.ogla.2019.06.003. Epub 2019 Jun 27. PMID: 32672676.

18. Oddone F, Lucenteforte E, Michelessi M, Rizzo S, Donati S, Parravano M, Virgili G. Macular versus retinal nerve fiber layer parameters for diagnosing manifest glaucoma: a systematic review of diagnostic accuracy studies. Ophthalmology. 2016;123(5):939–49. https://doi.org/10.1016/j.ophtha.2015.12.041. Epub 2016 Feb 15. PMID: 26891880.
19. Chauhan BC, Vianna JR, Sharpe GP, Demirel S, Girkin CA, Mardin CY, Scheuerle AF, Burgoyne CF. Differential effects of aging in the macular retinal layers, neuroretinal rim, and peripapillary retinal nerve fiber layer. Ophthalmology. 2020;127(2):177–85. https://doi.org/10.1016/j.ophtha.2019.09.013. Epub 2019 Sep 21. PMID: 31668716; PMCID: PMC6982591.
20. Kansal V, Armstrong JJ, Pintwala R, Hutnik C. Optical coherence tomography for glaucoma diagnosis: an evidence based meta-analysis. PLoS One. 2018;13(1):e0190621. https://doi.org/10.1371/journal.pone.0190621. PMID: 29300765; PMCID: PMC5754143.
21. Mohammadzadeh V, Fatehi N, Yarmohammadi A, Lee JW, Sharifipour F, Daneshvar R, Caprioli J, Nouri-Mahdavi K. Macular imaging with optical coherence tomography in glaucoma. Surv Ophthalmol. 2020;65(6):597–638. https://doi.org/10.1016/j.survophthal.2020.03.002. Epub 2020 Mar 19. PMID: 32199939; PMCID: PMC7423773.
22. Tham YC, Chee ML, Dai W, Lim ZW, Majithia S, Siantar R, Thakur S, Rim T, Cheung CY, Sabanayagam C, Aung T, Wong TY, Cheng CY. Profiles of ganglion cell-inner Plexiform layer thickness in a multi-ethnic Asian population: the Singapore epidemiology of eye diseases study. Ophthalmology. 2020;127(8):1064–76. https://doi.org/10.1016/j.ophtha.2020.01.055. Epub 2020 Feb 8. PMID: 32197910.
23. Kim YK, Yoo BW, Kim HC, Park KH. Automated detection of hemifield difference across horizontal raphe on ganglion cell—inner plexiform layer thickness map. Ophthalmology. 2015;122(11):2252–60. https://doi.org/10.1016/j.ophtha.2015.07.013. Epub 2015 Aug 13. PMID: 26278860.
24. Ha A, Kim YK, Kim JS, Jeoung JW, Park KH. Temporal raphe sign in elderly patients with large Optic disc cupping: its evaluation as a predictive factor for glaucoma conversion. Am J Ophthalmol. 2020;219:205–14. https://doi.org/10.1016/j.ajo.2020.07.001. Epub 2020 Jul 8. PMID: 32652053.
25. Rao HL, Pradhan ZS, Suh MH, Moghimi S, Mansouri K, Weinreb RN. Optical coherence tomography angiography in glaucoma. J Glaucoma. 2020;29(4):312–21. https://doi.org/10.1097/IJG.0000000000001463. PMID: 32053551; PMCID: PMC7117982.
26. Ran AR, Cheung CY, Wang X, Chen H, Luo LY, Chan PP, Wong MOM, Chang RT, Mannil SS, Young AL, Yung HW, Pang CP, Heng PA, Tham CC. Detection of glaucomatous optic neuropathy with spectral-domain optical coherence tomography: a retrospective training and validation deep-learning analysis. Lancet Digit Health. 2019;1(4):e172–82. https://doi.org/10.1016/S2589-7500(19)30085-8. Epub 2019 Aug 9. PMID: 33323187.
27. Ran AR, Wang X, Chan PP, Chan NC, Yip W, Young AL, Wong MOM, Yung HW, Chang RT, Mannil SS, Tham YC, Cheng CY, Chen H, Li F, Zhang X, Heng PA, Tham CC, Cheung CY. Three-dimensional multi-task deep learning model to detect glaucomatous Optic neuropathy and myopic features from optical coherence tomography scans: a retrospective multi-Centre study. Front Med (Lausanne). 2022;9:860574. https://doi.org/10.3389/fmed.2022.860574. PMID: 35783623; PMCID: PMC9240220.
28. Baker ML, Hand PJ, Wang JJ, Wong TY. Retinal signs and stroke: revisiting the link between the eye and brain. Stroke. 2008;39(4):1371–9. https://doi.org/10.1161/STROKEAHA.107.496091. Epub 2008 Feb 28. PMID: 18309171.
29. Fisayo A, Bruce BB, Newman NJ, Biousse V. Overdiagnosis of idiopathic intracranial hypertension. Neurology. 2016;86(4):341–50. https://doi.org/10.1212/WNL.0000000000002318. Epub 2015 Dec 30. PMID: 26718577; PMCID: PMC4776085.
30. Bruce BB, Thulasi P, Fraser CL, Keadey MT, Ward A, Heilpern KL, Wright DW, Newman NJ, Biousse V. Diagnostic accuracy and use of nonmydriatic ocular fundus photography by emergency physicians: phase II of the FOTO-ED study. Ann Emerg Med. 2013;62(1):28–33.e1. https://doi.org/10.1016/j.annemergmed.2013.01.010. Epub 2013 Feb 21. PMID: 23433654; PMCID: PMC3722897.
31. Bruce BB, Biousse V, Newman NJ. Nonmydriatic ocular fundus photography in neurologic emergencies. JAMA Neurol. 2015;72(4):455–9. https://doi.org/10.1001/jamaneurol.2014.4053. PMID: 25665183.
32. Alm M, Hautala N, Bloigu R, Huhtakangas J. Comparison of optic disc evaluation methods in neurology emergency patients. Acta Neurol Scand. 2019;140(6):449–51. https://doi.org/10.1111/ane.13167. Epub 2019 Oct 2. PMID: 31518442.
33. Pyatka N, Banks MK, Fotedar N, DeLozier SJ, Morgan M, Preston DC. Nonmydriatic retinal photography in the outpatient neurology resident clinic. J Neuroophthalmol. 2022;42(1):68–72. https://doi.org/10.1097/WNO.0000000000001236. Epub 2022 Jan 5. PMID: 34999652.
34. Bidot S, Bruce BB, Saindane AM, Newman NJ, Biousse V. Asymmetric papilledema in idiopathic intracranial hypertension. J Neuroophthalmol. 2015;35(1):31–6. https://doi.org/10.1097/WNO.0000000000000205. PMID: 25494197; PMCID: PMC4326590.

35. Hoyt WF, Knight CL. Comparison of congenital disc blurring and incipient papilledema in red-free light—a photographic study. Investig Ophthalmol. 1973;12(4):241–7. PMID: 4694185.
36. Sibony PA, Kupersmith MJ, OCT Substudy Group of the NORDIC Idiopathic Intracranial Hypertension Treatment Trial. "Paton's Folds" revisited: peripapillary wrinkles, folds, and creases in papilledema. Ophthalmology. 2016;123(6):1397–9. https://doi.org/10.1016/j.ophtha.2015.12.017. Epub 2016 Jan 14. PMID: 26778344; PMCID: PMC4877233.
37. Scott CJ, Kardon RH, Lee AG, Frisén L, Wall M. Diagnosis and grading of papilledema in patients with raised intracranial pressure using optical coherence tomography vs clinical expert assessment using a clinical staging scale. Arch Ophthalmol. 2010;128(6):705–11. https://doi.org/10.1001/archophthalmol.2010.94. PMID: 20547947.
38. Biousse V, Danesh-Meyer HV, Saindane AM, Lamirel C, Newman NJ. Imaging of the optic nerve: technological advances and future prospects. Lancet Neurol. 2022;21(12):1135–50. https://doi.org/10.1016/S1474-4422(22)00173-9. Epub 2022 Sep 22. PMID: 36155662.
39. Purvin V, King R, Kawasaki A, Yee R. Anterior ischemic optic neuropathy in eyes with optic disc drusen. Arch Ophthalmol. 2004;122(1):48–53. https://doi.org/10.1001/archopht.122.1.48. PMID: 14718294.
40. Hamann S, Malmqvist L, Wegener M, Fard MA, Biousse V, Bursztyn L, Citirak G, Costello F, Crum AV, Digre K, Fraser JA, Huna-Baron R, Katz B, Lawlor M, Newman NJ, Peragallo JH, Petzold A, Sibony PA, Subramanian PS, Warner JEA, Wong SH, Fraser CL, Optic Disc Drusen Studies Consortium. Young adults with anterior ischemic optic neuropathy: a multicenter optic disc Drusen study. Am J Ophthalmol. 2020;217:174–81. https://doi.org/10.1016/j.ajo.2020.03.052. Epub 2020 Apr 13. PMID: 32298654.
41. Lam BL, Morais CG Jr, Pasol J. Drusen of the optic disc. Curr Neurol Neurosci Rep. 2008;8(5):404–8. https://doi.org/10.1007/s11910-008-0062-6. PMID: 18713576.
42. Barkatullah AF, Leishangthem L, Moss HE. MRI findings as markers of idiopathic intracranial hypertension. Curr Opin Neurol. 2021;34(1):75–83. https://doi.org/10.1097/WCO.0000000000000885. PMID: 33230036; PMCID: PMC7856277.
43. Friedman DI, McDermott MP, Kieburtz K, Kupersmith M, Stoutenburg A, Keltner JL, Feldon SE, Schron E, Corbett JJ, Wall M, NORDIC IIHTT Study Group. The idiopathic intracranial hypertension treatment trial: design considerations and methods. J Neuroophthalmol. 2014;34(2):107–17. https://doi.org/10.1097/WNO.0000000000000114. PMID: 24739993.
44. Micieli JA, Bruce BB, Vasseneix C, Blanch RJ, Berezovsky DE, Peragallo JH, Newman NJ, Biousse V. Optic nerve appearance as a predictor of visual outcome in patients with idiopathic intracranial hypertension. Br J Ophthalmol. 2019;103(10):1429–35. https://doi.org/10.1136/bjophthalmol-2018-313329. Epub 2018 Dec 8. PMID: 30530819.
45. Micieli JA, Newman NJ, Biousse V. The role of optical coherence tomography in the evaluation of compressive optic neuropathies. Curr Opin Neurol. 2019;32(1):115–23. https://doi.org/10.1097/WCO.0000000000000636. PMID: 30418197.
46. Ahmad SR, Moss HE. Update on the diagnosis and treatment of idiopathic intracranial hypertension. Semin Neurol. 2019;39(6):682–91. https://doi.org/10.1055/s-0039-1698744. Epub 2019 Dec 17. PMID: 31847039; PMCID: PMC7713505.
47. Petzold A, Fraser CL, Abegg M, Alroughani R, Alshowaeir D, Alvarenga R, Andris C, Asgari N, Barnett Y, Battistella R, Behbehani R, Berger T, Bikbov MM, Biotti D, Biousse V, Boschi A, Brazdil M, Brezhnev A, Calabresi PA, Cordonnier M, Costello F, Cruz FM, Cunha LP, Daoudi S, Deschamps R, de Seze J, Diem R, Etemadifar M, Flores-Rivera J, Fonseca P, Frederiksen J, Frohman E, Frohman T, Tilikete CF, Fujihara K, Gálvez A, Gouider R, Gracia F, Grigoriadis N, Guajardo JM, Habek M, Hawlina M, Martínez-Lapiscina EH, Hooker J, Hor JY, Howlett W, Huang-Link Y, Idrissova Z, Illes Z, Jancic J, Jindahra P, Karussis D, Kerty E, Kim HJ, Lagrèze W, Leocani L, Levin N, Liskova P, Liu Y, Maiga Y, Marignier R, McGuigan C, Meira D, Merle H, Monteiro MLR, Moodley A, Moura F, Muñoz S, Mustafa S, Nakashima I, Noval S, Oehninger C, Ogun O, Omoti A, Pandit L, Paul F, Rebolleda G, Reddel S, Rejdak K, Rejdak R, Rodriguez-Morales AJ, Rougier MB, Sa MJ, Sanchez-Dalmau B, Saylor D, Shatriah I, Siva A, Stiebel-Kalish H, Szatmary G, Ta L, Tenembaum S, Tran H, Trufanov Y, van Pesch V, Wang AG, Wattjes MP, Willoughby E, Zakaria M, Zvornicanin J, Balcer L, Plant GT. Diagnosis and classification of optic neuritis. Lancet Neurol. 2022;21(12):1120–34. https://doi.org/10.1016/S1474-4422(22)00200-9. Epub 2022 Sep 27. PMID: 36179757.
48. Beck RW, Cleary PA, Anderson MM Jr, Keltner JL, Shults WT, Kaufman DI, Buckley EG, Corbett JJ, Kupersmith MJ, Miller NR, et al. A randomized, controlled trial of corticosteroids in the treatment of acute optic neuritis. The Optic Neuritis Study Group. N Engl J Med. 1992;326(9):581–8. https://doi.org/10.1056/NEJM199202273260901. PMID: 1734247.
49. Hassan MB, Stern C, Flanagan EP, Pittock SJ, Kunchok A, Foster RC, Jitprapaikulsan J, Hodge DO, Bhatti MT, Chen JJ. Population-based incidence of optic neuritis in the era of aquaporin-4 and myelin oligodendrocyte glycoprotein antibodies. Am J Ophthalmol. 2020;220:110–4. https://doi.org/10.1016/j.ajo.2020.07.014. Epub 2020 Jul 21. PMID: 32707199; PMCID: PMC8491771.
50. Hickman SJ, Petzold A. Update on optic neuritis: an international view. Neuroophthalmology. 2021;46(1):1–18. https://doi.org/10.1080/01658

107.2021.1964541. PMID: 35095131; PMCID: PMC8794242.

51. Huang D, Swanson EA, Lin CP, Schuman JS, Stinson WG, Chang W, Hee MR, Flotte T, Gregory K, Puliafito CA, et al. Optical coherence tomography. Science. 1991;254(5035):1178–81. https://doi.org/10.1126/science.1957169. PMID: 1957169; PMCID: PMC4638169.
52. Tan CS, Sadda SVR. Swept-source optical coherence tomography. In: Meyer SS, Sadda SVR, editors. Spectral domain optical coherence tomography in macular diseases Carsten H. Springer India; 2017. p. 59–77.
53. Costello F, Hodge W, Pan YI, Eggenberger E, Coupland S, Kardon RH. Tracking retinal nerve fiber layer loss after optic neuritis: a prospective study using optical coherence tomography. Mult Scler. 2008;14(7):893–905. https://doi.org/10.1177/1352458508091367. Epub 2008 Jun 23. PMID: 18573837.
54. Kupersmith MJ. Optical imaging of the optic nerve: beyond demonstration of retinal nerve fiber layer loss. J Neuroophthalmol. 2015;35(2):210–9. https://doi.org/10.1097/WNO.0000000000000248. PMID: 25893873.
55. Gelfand JM, Nolan R, Schwartz DM, Graves J, Green AJ. Microcystic macular oedema in multiple sclerosis is associated with disease severity. Brain. 2012;135(Pt 6):1786–93. https://doi.org/10.1093/brain/aws098. Epub 2012 Apr 25. PMID: 22539259; PMCID: PMC3359753.
56. Saidha S, Sotirchos ES, Ibrahim MA, Crainiceanu CM, Gelfand JM, Sepah YJ, Ratchford JN, Oh J, Seigo MA, Newsome SD, Balcer LJ, Frohman EM, Green AJ, Nguyen QD, Calabresi PA. Microcystic macular oedema, thickness of the inner nuclear layer of the retina, and disease characteristics in multiple sclerosis: a retrospective study. Lancet Neurol. 2012;11(11):963–72. https://doi.org/10.1016/S1474-4422(12)70213-2. Epub 2012 Oct 4. Erratum in: Lancet Neurol. 2012 Dec;11(12):1021. PMID: 23041237; PMCID: PMC3533139.
57. Barboni P, Carelli V, Savini G, Carbonelli M, La Morgia C, Sadun AA. Microcystic macular degeneration from optic neuropathy: not inflammatory, not trans-synaptic degeneration. Brain. 2013;136(Pt 7):e239. https://doi.org/10.1093/brain/awt014. Epub 2013 Feb 8. PMID: 23396580.
58. Borruat FX, Dysli M, Voide N, Abegg M. Acetazolamide reduces retinal inner nuclear layer thickness in microcystic macular edema secondary to optic neuropathy. Eur Neurol. 2018;79(3–4):150–3. https://doi.org/10.1159/000487665. Epub 2018 Mar 7. PMID: 29514169.
59. El Ayoubi NK, Sabbagh HM, Bou Rjeily N, Hannoun S, Khoury SJ. Rate of retinal layer thinning as a biomarker for conversion to progressive disease in multiple sclerosis. Neurol Neuroimmunol Neuroinflamm. 2022;9(6):e200030. https://doi.org/10.1212/NXI.0000000000200030. PMID: 36229190; PMCID: PMC9562042.
60. Sotirchos ES, Gonzalez Caldito N, Filippatou A, Fitzgerald KC, Murphy OC, Lambe J, Nguyen J, Button J, Ogbuokiri E, Crainiceanu CM, Prince JL, Calabresi PA, Saidha S, International Multiple Sclerosis Visual System (IMSVISUAL) Consortium. Progressive multiple sclerosis is associated with faster and specific retinal layer atrophy. Ann Neurol. 2020;87(6):885–96. https://doi.org/10.1002/ana.25738. Epub 2020 Apr 28. PMID: 32285484; PMCID: PMC8682917.
61. Costello F, Coupland S, Hodge W, Lorello GR, Koroluk J, Pan YI, Freedman MS, Zackon DH, Kardon RH. Quantifying axonal loss after optic neuritis with optical coherence tomography. Ann Neurol. 2006;59(6):963–9. https://doi.org/10.1002/ana.20851. PMID: 16718705.
62. Green AJ, Cree BA. Distinctive retinal nerve fibre layer and vascular changes in neuromyelitis optica following optic neuritis. J Neurol Neurosurg Psychiatry. 2009;80(9):1002–5. https://doi.org/10.1136/jnnp.2008.166207. Epub 2009 May 21. PMID: 19465415.
63. Ramanathan S, Prelog K, Barnes EH, Tantsis EM, Reddel SW, Henderson AP, Vucic S, Gorman MP, Benson LA, Alper G, Riney CJ, Barnett M, Parratt JD, Hardy TA, Leventer RJ, Merheb V, Nosadini M, Fung VS, Brilot F, Dale RC. Radiological differentiation of optic neuritis with myelin oligodendrocyte glycoprotein antibodies, aquaporin-4 antibodies, and multiple sclerosis. Mult Scler. 2016;22(4):470–82. https://doi.org/10.1177/1352458515593406. Epub 2015 Jul 10. PMID: 26163068.
64. Denis M, Woillez JP, Smirnov VM, Drumez E, Lannoy J, Boucher J, Zedet M, Pruvo JP, Labreuche J, Zephir H, Leclerc X, Outteryck O. Optic nerve lesion length at the acute phase of optic neuritis is predictive of retinal neuronal loss. Neurol Neuroimmunol Neuroinflamm. 2022;9(2):e1135. https://doi.org/10.1212/NXI.0000000000001135. PMID: 35091465; PMCID: PMC8802684.
65. Thompson AJ, Banwell BL, Barkhof F, Carroll WM, Coetzee T, Comi G, Correale J, Fazekas F, Filippi M, Freedman MS, Fujihara K, Galetta SL, Hartung HP, Kappos L, Lublin FD, Marrie RA, Miller AE, Miller DH, Montalban X, Mowry EM, Sorensen PS, Tintoré M, Traboulsee AL, Trojano M, Uitdehaag BMJ, Vukusic S, Waubant E, Weinshenker BG, Reingold SC, Cohen JA. Diagnosis of multiple sclerosis: 2017 revisions of the McDonald criteria. Lancet Neurol. 2018;17(2):162–73. https://doi.org/10.1016/S1474-4422(17)30470-2. Epub 2017 Dec 21. PMID: 29275977.
66. Optic Neuritis Study Group. Multiple sclerosis risk after optic neuritis: final optic neuritis treatment trial follow-up. Arch Neurol. 2008;65(6):727–32. https://doi.org/10.1001/archneur.65.6.727. PMID: 18541792; PMCID: PMC2440583.

67. Beck RW, Gal RL. Treatment of acute optic neuritis: a summary of findings from the optic neuritis treatment trial. Arch Ophthalmol. 2008;126(7):994–5. https://doi.org/10.1001/archopht.126.7.994. PMID: 18625951; PMCID: PMC9353544.
68. Chen JJ, Flanagan EP, Jitprapaikulsan J, López-Chiriboga ASS, Fryer JP, Leavitt JA, Weinshenker BG, McKeon A, Tillema JM, Lennon VA, Tobin WO, Keegan BM, Lucchinetti CF, Kantarci OH, McClelland CM, Lee MS, Bennett JL, Pelak VS, Chen Y, VanStavern G, Adesina OO, Eggenberger ER, Acierno MD, Wingerchuk DM, Brazis PW, Sagen J, Pittock SJ. Myelin oligodendrocyte glycoprotein antibody-positive optic neuritis: clinical characteristics, radiologic clues, and outcome. Am J Ophthalmol. 2018;195:8–15. https://doi.org/10.1016/j.ajo.2018.07.020. Epub 2018 Jul 26. PMID: 30055153; PMCID: PMC6371779.
69. Bennett JL, Costello F, Chen JJ, Petzold A, Biousse V, Newman NJ, Galetta SL. Optic neuritis and autoimmune optic neuropathies: advances in diagnosis and treatment. Lancet Neurol. 2023;22(1):89–100. https://doi.org/10.1016/S1474-4422(22)00187-9. Epub 2022 Sep 22. PMID: 36155661.
70. Wingerchuk DM, Banwell B, Bennett JL, Cabre P, Carroll W, Chitnis T, de Seze J, Fujihara K, Greenberg B, Jacob A, Jarius S, Lana-Peixoto M, Levy M, Simon JH, Tenembaum S, Traboulsee AL, Waters P, Wellik KE, Weinshenker BG, International Panel for NMO Diagnosis. International consensus diagnostic criteria for neuromyelitis optica spectrum disorders. Neurology. 2015;85(2):177–89. 10.1212/WNL.0000000000001729. Epub 2015 Jun 19. PMID: 26092914; PMCID: PMC4515040.
71. Levin MH, Bennett JL, Verkman AS. Optic neuritis in neuromyelitis optica. Prog Retin Eye Res. 2013;36:159–71. https://doi.org/10.1016/j.preteyeres.2013.03.001. Epub 2013 Mar 30. PMID: 23545439; PMCID: PMC3770284.
72. Papadopoulos MC, Verkman AS. Aquaporin 4 and neuromyelitis optica. Lancet Neurol. 2012;11(6):535–44. https://doi.org/10.1016/S1474--4422(12)70133-3. Epub 2012 May 16. PMID: 22608667; PMCID: PMC3678971.
73. Wingerchuk DM, Zhang I, Kielhorn A, Royston M, Levy M, Fujihara K, Nakashima I, Tanvir I, Paul F, Pittock SJ. Network meta-analysis of food and drug administration-approved treatment options for adults with Aquaporin-4 immunoglobulin G-positive neuromyelitis Optica spectrum disorder. Neurol Ther. 2022;11(1):123–35.https://doi.org/10.1007/s40120--021-00295-8. Epub 2021 Nov 13. PMID: 34773597; PMCID: PMC8857350.
74. Chen AT, Brady L, Bulman DE, Sundaram ANE, Rodriguez AR, Margolin E, Waye JS, Tarnopolsky MA. An evaluation of genetic causes and environmental risks for bilateral optic atrophy. PLoS One. 2019;14(11):e0225656. https://doi.org/10.1371/journal.pone.0225656. PMID: 31765440; PMCID: PMC6876833.
75. Pache F, Zimmermann H, Mikolajczak J, Schumacher S, Lacheta A, Oertel FC, Bellmann-Strobl J, Jarius S, Wildemann B, Reindl M, Waldman A, Soelberg K, Asgari N, Ringelstein M, Aktas O, Gross N, Buttmann M, Ach T, Ruprecht K, Paul F, Brandt AU, in cooperation with the Neuromyelitis Optica Study Group (NEMOS). MOG-IgG in NMO and related disorders: a multicenter study of 50 patients. Part 4: afferent visual system damage after optic neuritis in MOG-IgG-seropositive versus AQP4-IgG-seropositive patients. J Neuroinflammation. 2016;13(1):282. https://doi.org/10.1186/s12974-016-0720-6. PMID: 27802824; PMCID: PMC5088645.
76. Dalmau J, Rosenfeld MR. Paraneoplastic syndromes of the CNS. Lancet Neurol. 2008;7(4):327–40. https://doi.org/10.1016/S1474-4422(08)70060-7. PMID: 18339348; PMCID: PMC2367117.
77. Yu Z, Kryzer TJ, Griesmann GE, Kim K, Benarroch EE, Lennon VA. CRMP-5 neuronal autoantibody: marker of lung cancer and thymoma-related autoimmunity. Ann Neurol. 2001;49(2):146–54. PMID: 11220734.
78. Cohen DA, Bhatti MT, Pulido JS, Lennon VA, Dubey D, Flanagan EP, Pittock SJ, Klein CJ, Chen JJ. Collapsin response-mediator protein 5-associated retinitis, vitritis, and optic disc edema. Ophthalmology. 2020;127(2):221–9. https://doi.org/10.1016/j.ophtha.2019.09.012. Epub 2019 Sep 20. PMID: 31676123.
79. Sharma S, Chitranshi N, Wall RV, Basavarajappa D, Gupta V, Mirzaei M, Graham SL, Klistorner A, You Y. Trans-synaptic degeneration in the visual pathway: neural connectivity, pathophysiology, and clinical implications in neurodegenerative disorders. Surv Ophthalmol. 2022;67(2):411–26. https://doi.org/10.1016/j.survophthal.2021.06.001. Epub 2021 Jun 17. PMID: 34146577.
80. Yu-Wai-Man P, Turnbull DM, Chinnery PF. Leber hereditary optic neuropathy. J Med Genet. 2002;39(3):162–9. https://doi.org/10.1136/jmg.39.3.162. PMID: 11897814; PMCID: PMC1735056.
81. Martikainen MH, Suomela M, Majamaa K. Magnetic resonance imaging negative myelopathy in Leber's hereditary optic neuropathy: a case report. BMC Neurol. 2022;22(1):487. https://doi.org/10.1186/s12883-022-03007-3. PMID: 36522697; PMCID: PMC9753244.
82. Barboni P, Savini G, Valentino ML, Montagna P, Cortelli P, De Negri AM, Sadun F, Bianchi S, Longanesi L, Zanini M, de Vivo A, Carelli V. Retinal nerve fiber layer evaluation by optical coherence tomography in Leber's hereditary optic neuropathy. Ophthalmology. 2005;112(1):120–6. https://doi.org/10.1016/j.ophtha.2004.06.034. PMID: 15629831.

83. Chang YH, Kang EY, Liu PK, Levi SR, Wang HH, Tseng YJ, Seo GH, Lee H, Yeh LK, Chen KJ, Wu WC, Lai CC, Liu L, Wang NK. Photoreceptor manifestations of primary mitochondrial optic nerve disorders. Invest Ophthalmol Vis Sci. 2022;63(5):5. https://doi.org/10.1167/iovs.63.5.5. PMID: 35506936; PMCID: PMC9078049.
84. Sundaramurthy S, SelvaKumar A, Ching J, Dharani V, Sarangapani S, Yu-Wai-Man P. Leber hereditary optic neuropathy-new insights and old challenges. Graefes Arch Clin Exp Ophthalmol. 2021;259(9):2461–72. https://doi.org/10.1007/s00417-020-04993-1. Epub 2020 Nov 13. PMID: 33185731.
85. Sundaramurthy S, Selvakumar A, Dharani V, Soumittra N, Mani J, Thirumalai K, Periyasamy P, Mathavan S, Sripriya S. Prevalence of primary mutations in Leber hereditary optic neuropathy: a five-year report from a tertiary eye care center in India. Mol Vis. 2021;11(27):718–24. PMID: 35035206; PMCID: PMC8711579
86. Chun BY, Rizzo JF 3rd. Dominant optic atrophy: updates on the pathophysiology and clinical manifestations of the optic atrophy 1 mutation. Curr Opin Ophthalmol. 2016;27(6):475–80. https://doi.org/10.1097/ICU.0000000000000314. PMID: 27585216.
87. Barboni P, Savini G, Cascavilla ML, Caporali L, Milesi J, Borrelli E, La Morgia C, Valentino ML, Triolo G, Lembo A, Carta A, De Negri A, Sadun F, Rizzo G, Parisi V, Pierro L, Bianchi Marzoli S, Zeviani M, Sadun AA, Bandello F, Carelli V. Early macular retinal ganglion cell loss in dominant optic atrophy: genotype-phenotype correlation. Am J Ophthalmol. 2014;158(3):628–36.e3. https://doi.org/10.1016/j.ajo.2014.05.034. Epub 2014 Jun 5. PMID: 24907432.
88. Danesh-Meyer HV, Wong A, Papchenko T, Matheos K, Stylli S, Nichols A, Frampton C, Daniell M, Savino PJ, Kaye AH. Optical coherence tomography predicts visual outcome for pituitary tumors. J Clin Neurosci. 2015;22(7):1098–104. https://doi.org/10.1016/j.jocn.2015.02.001. Epub 2015 Apr 16. PMID: 25891894.
89. Blanch RJ, Micieli JA, Oyesiku NM, Newman NJ, Biousse V. Optical coherence tomography retinal ganglion cell complex analysis for the detection of early chiasmal compression. Pituitary. 2018;21(5):515–23.https://doi.org/10.1007/s11102--018-0906-2. PMID: 30097827.
90. Monteiro MLR. Macular ganglion cell complex reduction preceding visual field loss in a patient with chiasmal compression with a 21-month follow-up. J Neuroophthalmol. 2018;38(1):124–7. https://doi.org/10.1097/WNO.0000000000000625. PMID: 29319560.
91. Vuong LN, Hedges TR 3rd. Ganglion cell layer complex measurements in compressive optic neuropathy. Curr Opin Ophthalmol. 2017;28(6):573–8. https://doi.org/10.1097/ICU.0000000000000428. PMID: 28984725
92. Müller HL, Merchant TE, Warmuth-Metz M, Martinez-Barbera JP, Puget S. Craniopharyngioma. Nat Rev Dis Primers. 2019;5(1):75. https://doi.org/10.1038/s41572-019-0125-9. PMID: 31699993.
93. Roth CL, Eslamy H, Werny D, Elfers C, Shaffer ML, Pihoker C, Ojemann J, Dobyns WB. Semiquantitative analysis of hypothalamic damage on MRI predicts risk for hypothalamic obesity. Obesity (Silver Spring). 2015;23(6):1226–33. https://doi.org/10.1002/oby.21067. Epub 2015 Apr 17. PMID: 25884561; PMCID: PMC5029599.
94. Ellenberger C, Perioptic meningiomas. Syndrome of long-standing visual loss, pale disk edema, and optociliary veins. Arch Neurol. 1976;33(10):671–4. https://doi.org/10.1001/archneur.1976.00500100005004. PMID: 973803.
95. Rodrigues MM, Savino PJ, Schatz NJ. Spheno-orbital meningioma with optociliary veins. Am J Ophthalmol. 1976;81(5):666–70. https://doi.org/10.1016/0002-9394(76)90135-5. PMID: 1275046.
96. Hayreh SS. Anterior ischemic optic neuropathy. Clin Neurosci. 1997;4(5):251–63. PMID: 9292252.
97. Archer EL, Pepin S. Obstructive sleep apnea and non-arteritic anterior ischemic optic neuropathy: evidence for an association. J Clin Sleep Med. 2013;9(6):613–8. https://doi.org/10.5664/jcsm.2766. PMID: 23772197; PMCID: PMC3659384.
98. Yang HK, Park SJ, Byun SJ, Park KH, Kim JW, Hwang JM. Obstructive sleep apnoea and increased risk of non-arteritic anterior ischaemic optic neuropathy. Br J Ophthalmol. 2019;103(8):1123–8. https://doi.org/10.1136/bjophthalmol-2018-312910. Epub 2018 Nov 9. PMID: 30413419.
99. Farahvash A, Micieli JA. Neuro-ophthalmological manifestations of obstructive sleep apnea: current perspectives. Eye Brain. 2020;12:61–71. https://doi.org/10.2147/EB.S247121. PMID: 32753994; PMCID: PMC7353992.
100. Lei S, Micieli JA. Severe obstructive sleep apnea diagnosed after non-arteritic anterior ischaemic optic neuropathy in a young man. BMJ Case Rep. 2019;12(11):e232512. https://doi.org/10.1136/bcr-2019-232512. PMID: 31791996; PMCID: PMC6887377.
101. Hayreh SS, Podhajsky P, Zimmerman MB. Role of nocturnal arterial hypotension in optic nerve head ischemic disorders. Ophthalmologica. 1999;213(2):76–96. https://doi.org/10.1159/000027399. PMID: 9885384.
102. Hayreh SS, Joos KM, Podhajsky PA, Long CR. Systemic diseases associated with nonarteritic anterior ischemic optic neuropathy. Am J Ophthalmol. 1994;118(6):766–80. https://doi.org/10.1016/s0002-9394(14)72557-7. PMID: 7977604.

103. Fivgas GD, Newman NJ. Anterior ischemic optic neuropathy following the use of a nasal decongestant. Am J Ophthalmol. 1999;127(1):104–6. https://doi.org/10.1016/s0002-9394(98)00312-2. PMID: 9933016.
104. Murphy MA, Murphy JF. Amiodarone and optic neuropathy: the heart of the matter. J Neuroophthalmol. 2005;25(3):232–6. https://doi.org/10.1097/01.wno.0000177290.09649.38. PMID: 16148635.
105. Campbell UB, Walker AM, Gaffney M, Petronis KR, Creanga D, Quinn S, Klein BE, Laties AM, Lewis M, Sharlip ID, Kolitsopoulos F, Klee BJ, Mo J, Reynolds RF. Acute nonarteritic anterior ischemic optic neuropathy and exposure to phosphodiesterase type 5 inhibitors. J Sex Med. 2015;12(1):139–51. https://doi.org/10.1111/jsm.12726. Epub 2014 Oct 31. PMID: 25358826.
106. González Martín-Moro J, Contreras I, Gutierrez-Ortiz C, Gómez-Sanz F, Castro-Rebollo M, Fernández-Hortelano A, Pilo-De-La-Fuente B. Disc configuration as a risk and prognostic factor in NAION: the impact of cup to disc ratio, disc diameter, and crowding index. Semin Ophthalmol. 2019;34(3):177–81. https://doi.org/10.1080/08820538.2019.1620792. Epub 2019 Jun 4. PMID: 31162995.
107. Hayreh SS, Zimmerman B. Visual field abnormalities in nonarteritic anterior ischemic optic neuropathy: their pattern and prevalence at initial examination. Arch Ophthalmol. 2005;123(11):1554–62. https://doi.org/10.1001/archopht.123.11.1554. PMID: 16286618.
108. Johnson LN, Baloh FG. The accuracy of confrontation visual field test in comparison with automated perimetry. J Natl Med Assoc. 1991;83(10):895–8. PMID: 1800764; PMCID: PMC2571584.
109. Biousse V, Newman NJ. Ischemic optic neuropathies. N Engl J Med. 2015;372(25):2428–36. https://doi.org/10.1056/NEJMra1413352. Erratum in: N Engl J Med. 2015 Dec 10;373(24):2390. PMID: 26083207.
110. Hayreh SS. Ischemic optic neuropathies - where are we now? Graefes Arch Clin Exp Ophthalmol. 2013;251(8):1873–84. https://doi.org/10.1007/s00417-013-2399-z. Epub 2013 Jul 3. PMID: 23821118.
111. Ischemic Optic Neuropathy Decompression Trial. Twenty-four-month update. Arch Ophthalmol. 2000;118(6):793–8. PMID: 10865316.
112. Hayreh SS, Zimmerman MB. Non-arteritic anterior ischemic optic neuropathy: role of systemic corticosteroid therapy. Graefes Arch Clin Exp Ophthalmol. 2008;246(7):1029–46. https://doi.org/10.1007/s00417-008-0805-8. Epub 2008 Apr 11. PMID: 18404273; PMCID: PMC2712323.
113. Optic nerve decompression surgery for nonarteritic anterior ischemic optic neuropathy (NAION) is not effective and may be harmful. The Ischemic Optic Neuropathy Decompression Trial Research Group. JAMA. 1995;273(8):625–32. PMID: 7844872.
114. Atkins EJ, Bruce BB, Newman NJ, Biousse V. Treatment of nonarteritic anterior ischemic optic neuropathy. Surv Ophthalmol. 2010;55(1):47–63. https://doi.org/10.1016/j.survophthal.2009.06.008. PMID: 20006051; PMCID: PMC3721361.
115. Hayreh SS. Posterior ischaemic optic neuropathy: clinical features, pathogenesis, and management. Eye (Lond). 2004;18(11):1188–206. https://doi.org/10.1038/sj.eye.6701562. PMID: 15534605.
116. Nuttall GA, Garrity JA, Dearani JA, Abel MD, Schroeder DR, Mullany CJ. Risk factors for ischemic optic neuropathy after cardiopulmonary bypass: a matched case/control study. Anesth Analg. 2001;93(6):1410–6, table of contents. https://doi.org/10.1097/00000539-200112000-00012. PMID: 11726415.
117. Rubin DS, Matsumoto MM, Moss HE, Joslin CE, Tung A, Roth S. Ischemic optic neuropathy in cardiac surgery: incidence and risk factors in the United States from the National Inpatient Sample 1998 to 2013. Anesthesiology. 2017;126(5):810–21. https://doi.org/10.1097/ALN.0000000000001533. PMID: 28244936; PMCID: PMC5395417.
118. Chang SH, Miller NR. The incidence of vision loss due to perioperative ischemic optic neuropathy associated with spine surgery: the Johns Hopkins Hospital Experience. Spine (Phila Pa 1976). 2005;30(11):1299–302. https://doi.org/10.1097/01.brs.0000163884.11476.25. PMID: 15928556.
119. American Society of Anesthesiologists Task Force on Perioperative Visual Loss; North American Neuro-Ophthalmology Society; Society for Neuroscience in Anesthesiology and Critical Care. Practice advisory for perioperative visual loss associated with spine surgery 2019: an updated report by the American Society of Anesthesiologists Task Force on Perioperative Visual Loss, the North American Neuro-Ophthalmology Society, and the Society for Neuroscience in Anesthesiology and Critical Care. Anesthesiology. 2019;130(1):12–30. https://doi.org/10.1097/ALN.0000000000002503. PMID: 30531555; PMCID: PMC9556164.
120. Hayreh SS, Podhajsky PA, Zimmerman B. Ocular manifestations of giant cell arteritis. Am J Ophthalmol. 1998;125(4):509–20. https://doi.org/10.1016/s0002-9394(99)80192-5. PMID: 9559737
121. van der Geest KSM, Sandovici M, Brouwer E, Mackie SL. Diagnostic accuracy of symptoms, physical signs, and laboratory tests for Giant cell arteritis: a systematic review and meta-analysis. JAMA Intern Med. 2020;180(10):1295–304. https://doi.org/10.1001/jamainternmed.2020.3050. PMID: 32804186; PMCID: PMC7432275.
122. Skanchy DF, Vickers A, Ponce CMP, Lee AG. Ocular manifestations of giant cell arteritis. Expert Rev Ophthalmol. 2019;14(1):23–32. https://doi.org/10.1080/17469899.2018.1560265.
123. Sharma A, Sagar V, Prakash M, Gupta V, Khaire N, Pinto B, Dhir V, Bal A, Aggarwal A, Kumar

S, Sharma K, Rathi M, Das A, Singh R, Singh S, Gupta A. Giant cell arteritis in India: report from a tertiary care center along with total published experience from India. Neurol India. 2015;63(5):681–6. https://doi.org/10.4103/0028-3886.166543. PMID: 26448225.

124. Mohan K, Gupta A, Jain IS, Banerjee CK. Bilateral central retinal artery occlusion in occult temporal arteritis. J Clin Neuroophthalmol. 1989;9(4):270–2. PMID: 2531166.

125. Hayreh SS, Podhajsky PA, Raman R, Zimmerman B. Giant cell arteritis: validity and reliability of various diagnostic criteria. Am J Ophthalmol. 1997;123(3):285–96.https://doi.org/10.1016/s0002--9394(14)70123-0. PMID: 9063237.

126. Albert DM, Ruchman MC, Keltner JL. Skip areas in temporal arteritis. Arch Ophthalmol. 1976;94(12):2072–7. https://doi.org/10.1001/archopht.1976.03910040732006. PMID: 999553.

127. Schmidt WA. Role of ultrasound in the understanding and management of vasculitis. Ther Adv Musculoskelet Dis. 2014;6(2):39–47. https://doi.org/10.1177/1759720X13512256. PMID: 24688604; PMCID: PMC3956137.

128. Fakin A, Kerin V, Hawlina M. Visual fields in giant cell arteritis (Horton's disease). Translat Neurosci. 2011;2:325–30. https://doi.org/10.2478/s13380-011-0034-1.

129. Bevers C, Blanckaert G, Van Keer K, Fils JF, Vandewalle E, Stalmans I. Semi-automated kinetic perimetry: comparison of the octopus 900 and Humphrey visual field analyzer 3 versus Goldmann perimetry. Acta Ophthalmol. 2019;97(4):e499–505. https://doi.org/10.1111/aos.13940. Epub 2018 Oct 21. PMID: 30345638.

130. Hayreh SS, Zimmerman B. Management of giant cell arteritis. Our 27-year clinical study: new light on old controversies. Ophthalmologica. 2003;217(4):239–59. https://doi.org/10.1159/000070631. PMID: 12792130.

131. Hayreh SS, Zimmerman B, Kardon RH. Visual improvement with corticosteroid therapy in giant cell arteritis. Report of a large study and review of literature. Acta Ophthalmol Scand. 2002;80(4):355–67. https://doi.org/10.1034/j.1600-0420.2002.800403.x. Erratum in: Acta Ophthalmol Scand. 2002 Dec;80(6):688. PMID: 12190776.

132. Stone JH, Tuckwell K, Dimonaco S, Klearman M, Aringer M, Blockmans D, Brouwer E, Cid MC, Dasgupta B, Rech J, Salvarani C, Schett G, Schulze-Koops H, Spiera R, Unizony SH, Collinson N. Trial of tocilizumab in giant-cell arteritis. N Engl J Med. 2017;377(4):317–28. https://doi.org/10.1056/NEJMoa1613849. PMID: 28745999.

133. Szekeres D, Al Othman B. Current developments in the diagnosis and treatment of giant cell arteritis. Front Med (Lausanne). 2022;13(9):1066503. https://doi.org/10.3389/fmed.2022.1066503. PMID: 36582285; PMCID: PMC9792614.

Part II

Extraocular Signs

16 Pupillary Signs

16.1 Anatomical Considerations

The pupil is an aperture in the iris diaphragm that regulates light entry into the eye to optimize image formation on the retina. It constricts in bright light and dilates in dim light. The pupil size is controlled by two autonomic muscles, the sphincter pupillae and the dilator pupillae, under parasympathetic and sympathetic control, respectively.

16.1.1 The Sphincter Pupillae

The sphincter pupillae is a 1-mm wide circumferentially oriented smooth muscle located in the iris stroma at the pupillary border just in front of the anterior pigmented iris epithelium and is covered with melanocytes and fibroblasts. It is innervated by the postganglionic fibres of the short ciliary nerves arising from the ciliary ganglion.

16.1.2 The Dilator Pupillae

The dilator muscle fibres are radially oriented myoepithelial cells embedded in the pigmented iris epithelium and run from the sphincter pupillae to the peripheral iris, where these end up as a circumferentially oriented sphincter bundle. It is connected to the elastic fibromuscular ciliary mesh with tent-like iridial strands anterior to the ciliary muscle [1].

16.1.3 The Ciliary Ganglion

The ciliary ganglion is a 1–2 mm parasympathetic ganglion lying medial to the lateral rectus in the posterior orbit. It contains, on average, 2500 neurons, fewer in women [2]. The ciliary ganglia receive three types of neural fibres: (1) somatic motor fibres from the inferior division of the oculomotor cranial nerve (CN III), (2) postganglionic sympathetic fibres, and (3) parasympathetic fibres projecting from the Edinger-Westphal nucleus. Only the parasympathetic fibres synapse in the ciliary ganglion. The postganglionic parasympathetic fibres leave the ganglion with short posterior ciliary nerves. Only 5% of the fibres innervate the sphincter pupillae, and the rest innervate the ciliary muscles located in the ciliary body. The postganglionic sympathetic fibres course along the long ciliary nerves (branches of the nasociliary nerve, itself a branch of CN V1) and innervate the dilator muscle.

A. Gupta et al., *Ophthalmic Signs in Practice of Medicine*,
https://doi.org/10.1007/978-981-99-7923-3_16

16.1.4 Pupil Size

In mesopic light conditions, neither too bright nor too dark, the size of the pupil varies from 2 to 4 mm. There is a progressive decrease in pupil size with each decade. The pupils do not remain constant in size, but show rhythmic oscillations called Hippus (pupillary athetosis) at a rate of ~1 Hz. The Hippus may get exaggerated in aconitine (a plant alkaloid) poisoning, trauma, renal disease, and altered sensorium, generally indicating a frontal lobe dysfunction. The hippus originates from the parasympathetic system [3]. It may also indicate non-convulsive status epilepticus [4] and early mortality in hospitalized patients [5].

16.2 Pathway for the Pupil Light Reflex

The afferent limb of the pupil light reflex (PLR) arc starts in the melanopsin-containing intrinsic photosensitive retinal ganglion cells(ipRGC) (Fig. 16.1). The ipRGC are few and constitute less than 1.5% of all the RGC, distributed mainly in the perifoveal retina. Nearly half of the ipRGC are found in the ganglion cell layer, and the rest in the inner or outer border of the inner plexiform layer. The ipRGC show decline with ageing [6] and, notably, in Alzheimer's and Parkinson's disease [7]. Although intrinsically photosensitive, the ipRGC also receive inputs from the rod and cone photoreceptors [8, 9].

The ipRGC are resistant to degeneration in Leber's hereditary optic neuropathy and dominant optic atrophy. [10]. PLR may be elicited in these patients, even in total blindness.

The spectral sensitivity of the ipRGC peaks in the blue region of the light spectrum, consistent with their role in the non-visual tasks, especially the circadian rhythm (day-night cycle by suppression of melatonin), cognition, heart rate, fight, or flight response [11]. On the other hand, the spectral sensitivity of the rods and cones mediated PLR peaks in the red light. PLR mediated by red light is short-duration and ill-sustained; the pupil dilates even while the light is on. Pupil constriction in PLR mediated by blue light sustains so long the light is on. The ipRGC represent the retinohypothalamic tract. Patients with multiple sclerosis (MS) who show

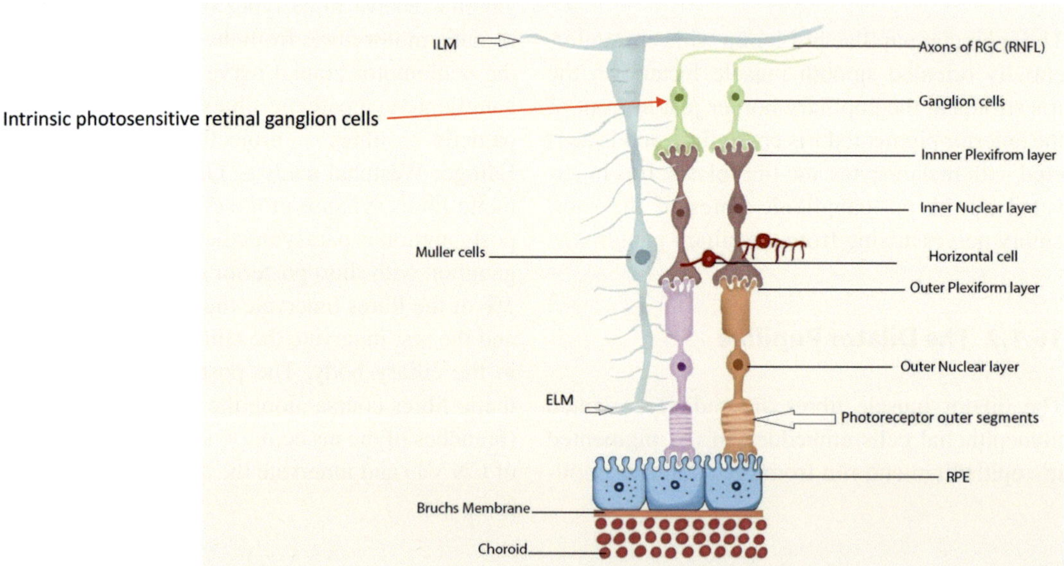

Fig. 16.1 Ultrastructure of the retina. Reproduced with permission from the publishers from Gupta, A. (2022). Bench-to-Bedside Research in Ophthalmology. In: Sobti, R., Ganju, A. K. (eds) Biomedical Translational Research. Springer, Singapore. https://doi.org/10.1007/978-981-16-8845-4_5

thinning of the Ganglion cell-inner plexiform layer show a significant decline in pupillary constriction response to blue light compared to MS patients who do not have thinning of the GCL-IPL layers [12]. Thus, in MS, the attenuation of the retinohypothalamic pathway, as determined by blue light pupillometry, may be responsible for disturbed circadian rhythm and the perception of fatigue experienced by MS patients [13].

Nasally arising axons from the RGCs and the ipRGCs cross in the optic chiasm, while the temporal axons pass uncrossed through the chiasm and proceed along the optic tracts (Fig. 16.2). However, instead of ending up in the lateral geniculate nucleus, these fibres from the ipRGCs project to the ipsilateral pretectal nucleus in the oculomotor complex in the rostrodorsal midbrain in front of the superior colliculus. The pretectal nucleus sends projections to the ipsilateral and contralateral Edinger-Westphal (EW) nuclei which lie medial to the oculomotor nuclei in the midbrain (Fig. 16.3).

The efferent path of the PLR starts as preganglionic fibres from the EW nuclei and course

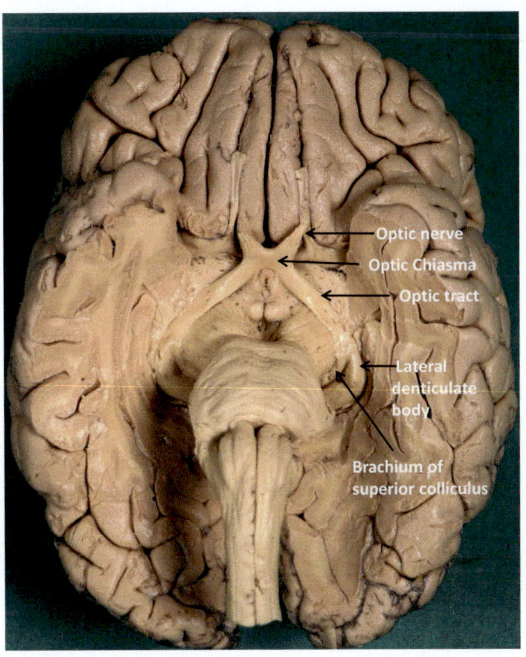

Fig. 16.2 Inferior aspect of the human brain showing some of the components of the visual pathway. Image courtesy of Prof Daisy Sahni (Ex-Professor) and Prof Anjali Aggarwal (Head), Department of Anatomy, Post Graduate Institute of Medical Education and Research, Chandigarh, India

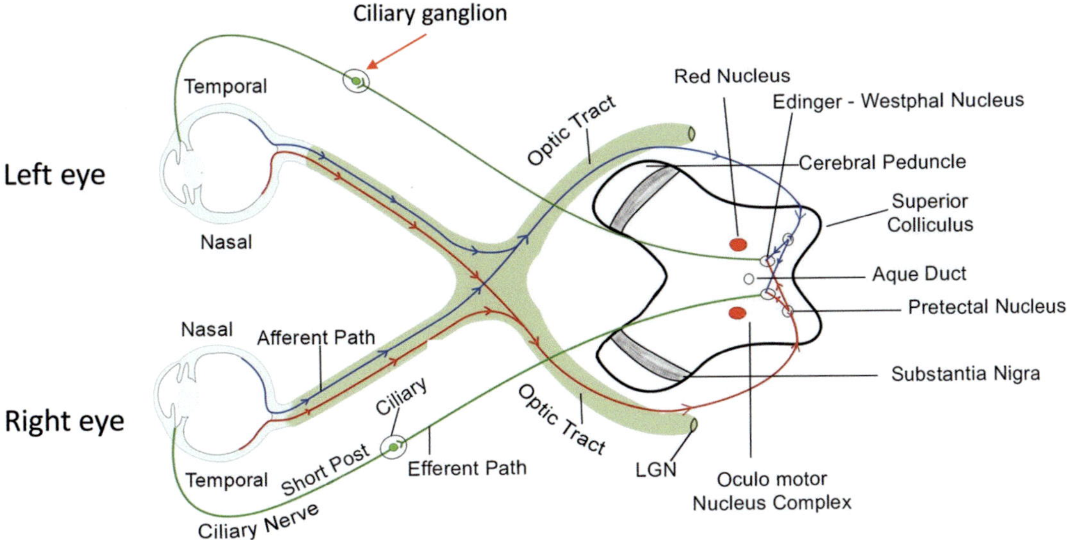

Fig. 16.3 Highly schematic pupillary light reflex (PLR) pathway, midbrain, optic tracts, chiasma, and optic nerves. The afferent pupillomotor fibres from the nasal retina (blue from the right eye and red from the left eye) cross in the optic chiasma, travel in the optic tracts, but instead of ending up in the lateral geniculate nucleus like the visual fibres, proceed to the ipsilateral and the contralateral pretectal nucleus and end up in the Edinger-Westphal (E-W) nucleus. The efferent PLR fibres (shown in green) start from the E-W nucleus and reach the ciliary ganglion along the inferior division of the 3rd cranial nerve, from where the postganglionic fibres accompany the short posterior ciliary nerves to the iris and the ciliary body. Abbreviations; LGN, lateral geniculate nucleus. Graphics by Kritka Thakur

along the oculomotor nerve and synapse in the ciliary ganglion. The postganglionic fibres innervate the iris and ciliary muscles.

16.2.1 Sympathetic Pathway

The first neuron of the sympathetic pathway is located in the hypothalamus, where the fibres descend in the brain stem, run in the periphery of the anterolateral funiculus of the spinal cord, and cross to the intermediolateral grey matter (ciliospinal centre of Budge) synapse here. They also cross over the contralateral ciliospinal centre at the level of C8 to T2 [14]. The second neuron, preganglionic fibres, emerges along the ventral roots of the spinal cord and ascends in the thorax to end in the superior cervical ganglion, which lies in the adventitial wall of the carotid artery at its bifurcation. The postganglionic pupillomotor sympathetic fibres travel along the periarterial plexus along the internal carotid artery, while the vasomotor sympathetic fibres pass along the external carotid artery. The oculomotor-sympathetic fibres pass through the superior orbital fissure and the ciliary ganglion to travel with the long posterior ciliary nerves and innervate the dilator pupillae [15] (Fig. 16.4). The sympathetic fibres also innervate the thin Muller muscle fibres that lie under the levator palpebrae superiors in the upper lid and the retractor fibres of the lower lid.

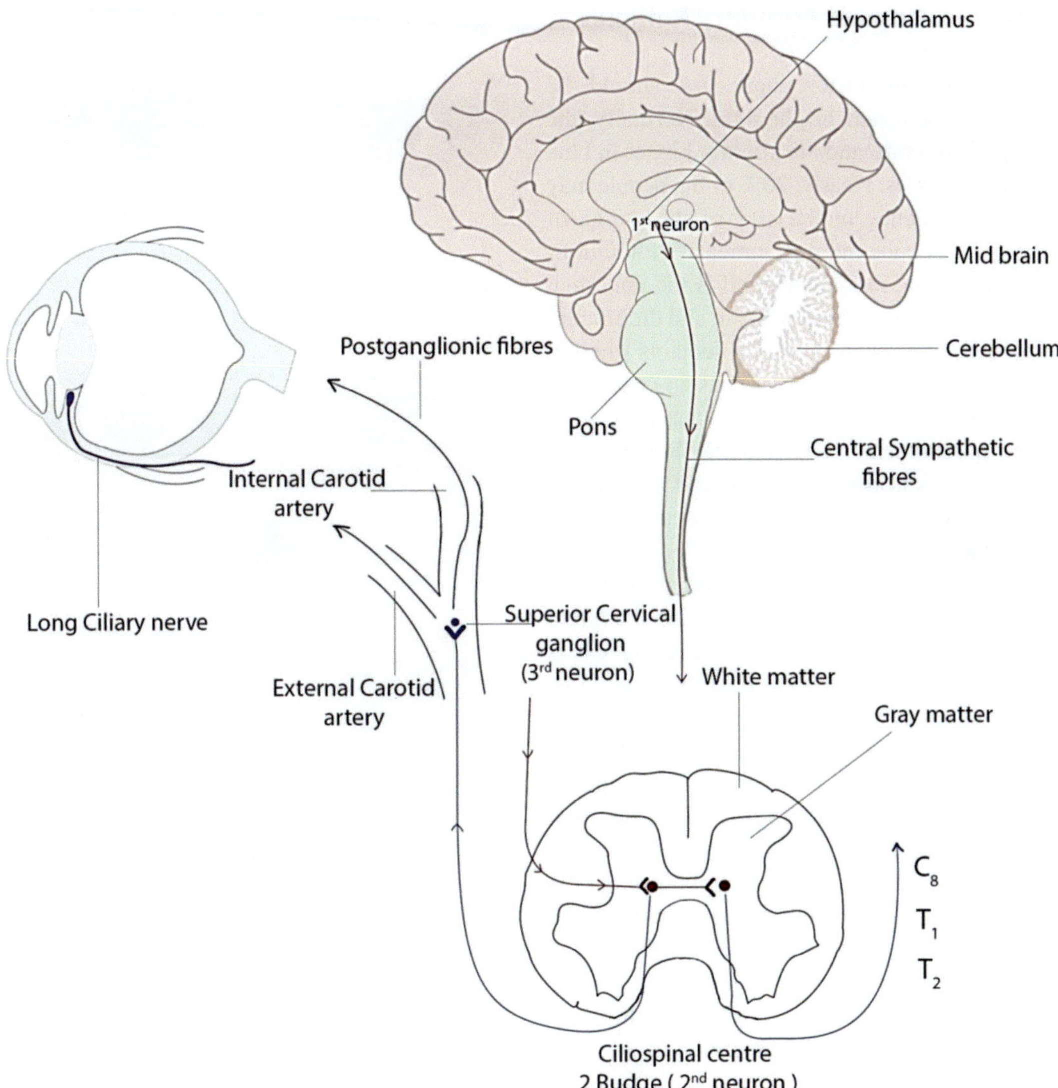

Fig. 16.4 A highly schematic diagram of the sympathetic pathway. The first neuron of the sympathetic pathway is in the hypothalamus, from where the fibres descend along the brain stem, medulla oblongata, and reach the ciliospinal centre of Budge, where the 2nd neuron is located. Here the interneurons are located in the grey matter at the level of T2 to C8. The preganglionic fibres emerge along the ventral roots of the spinal cord. These fibres ascend in the thorax to reach the superior cervical ganglion located in the adventitia of the carotid artery at the level of its bifurcation. The fibres synapse in the superior cervical ganglion, where the 3rd neuron is located. The postganglionic fibres travel along the internal carotid artery, enter the orbit along the branches of the ophthalmic branch, and travel with the long ciliary nerves to reach the dilator pupillae muscle. Graphics by Kritika Thakur

16.3 Testing for Pupillary Reflexes

Before eliciting PLR, pupil size should be checked in dim and bright light. Normally, the pupils are isocoric and are slightly bigger in blue vs the dark irides. Nearly, 20% of the people may show a difference in the size of the pupils of <0.3 mm. In encountering patients with significant anisocoria, the larger pupil is the abnormal pupil if it remains dilated in light, and the smaller pupil is the abnormal pupil if it remains small in the dark. The colour of the iris has no bearing on the pupil light reflex (PLR) when tested by automated pupillometry [16]. If the PLR is normal, the near reflex is always normal, so it need not be tested. However, if the PLR is absent, the near reflex must be tested.

Pupil constriction in the ipsilateral eye when the light is shown into the eye is called the direct reflex, and constriction of the contralateral eye is called the consensual reflex. Each eye should be tested individually. Lack of direct reflex indicates either an afferent or an efferent defect in the ipsilateral eye. For instance, if shining light into the right eye does not elicit constriction of the right pupil, it could either be an afferent or an efferent defect. However, if shining the light through the left eye still does not elicit constriction of the right pupil, it indicates an efferent defect in the right eye. If, however, shining the light into the left eye elicits a pupillary constriction of the right pupil, it indicates an afferent defect in the right eye (Fig. 16.5).

Bilateral absent pupillary responses generally indicate unfavourable outcomes in patients with severe brain injury and coma. Occasionally, false positive absent pupillary responses may be seen up to 3 days in traumatic or infective brain injury, but not in ischaemic encephalopathy beyond which no false positive tests are seen [17].

Notably, pupillary reflexes are absent in preterm babies with less than 30 weeks of gestation; they develop gradually beyond this age, and by 35 weeks, the reflex is present in all babies [18].

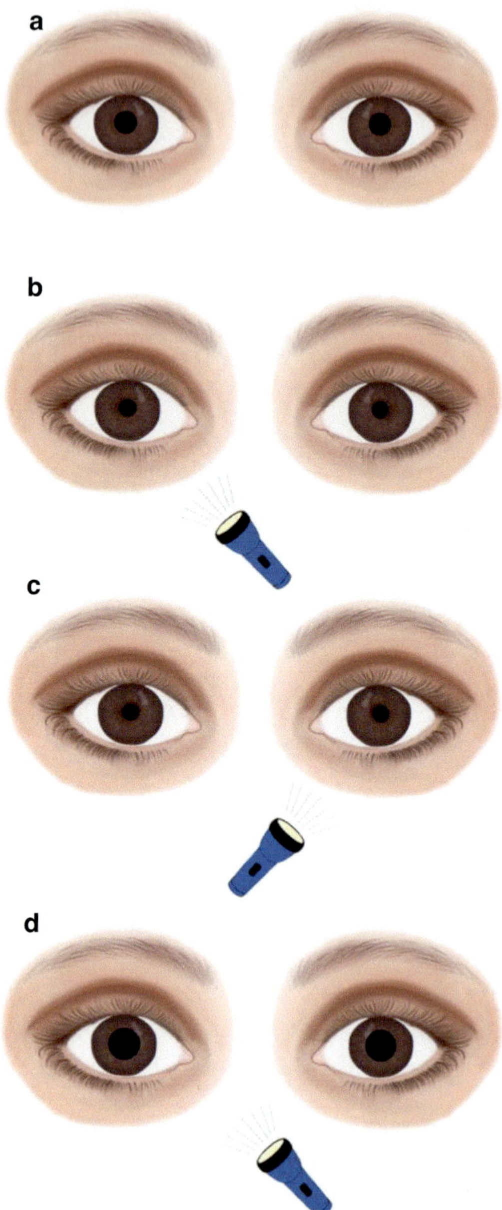

Fig. 16.5 Relative afferent pupil defect in the right eye. In ambient light, pupil size is equal in both eyes (**a**). When the light is shone in the right eye, the pupil constricts in both the right and left eyes (**b**). When the light is shone into the left eye, the pupil constricts in both eyes (**c**). When light is swung back into the RE, the pupils in the right and left eyes start dilating (**d**). Graphics by Kritika Thakur

16.3.1 Swinging Flashlight Test

The swinging flashlight test is the most critical subjective clinical test to detect conduction defects in the optic nerve in unilateral or bilateral asymmetric cases and is termed the relative afferent pupil defect (RAPD). Although first described by Marcus Gunn as a response to darkness, Levatin [19] described the RAPD test as a pupillary escape phenomenon due to unequal light sense in the two eyes due to gross retinal or optic nerve disorders.

In a semi-dark room, bright pen torch light (Halogen 3.5v) is shone from 45° below the optic axis for 2 s or a count of two, swinging (not more than four times with a pause time of 3 s) alternately between the eyes. If both eyes are normal, when light is shone on one eye, the pupil constricts in both eyes. However, if there is a conduction defect in one eye, on swinging the light from the normal eye (the pupils in both eyes get constricted) to the abnormal eye, the pupil of the abnormal and the normal eye starts dilating (Fig. 16.5). The RAPD can be measured by putting a series of neutral density filters (0.3–1.6 log units) in front of the good eye till the pupil constriction becomes equal in both eyes [20]. However, the major disadvantage of using neutral density filters is the poor visibility of the pupil by the examiner. Clinical grading of RAPD has also been done in the past [21].

16.3.2 Phases of Pupil Light Reflex

Once stimulated with light, there is a latent period before the pupil starts constricting, attains maximum constriction velocity, and achieves max constriction, followed by pupillary escape in which the pupil dilates to some extent and on switching off the stimulus, it gets back to the prestimulus size [22]. These phases of pupil reaction can be reproducibly captured on an automated pupillometer.

16.3.3 Causes of RAPD

The RAPD is not seen in refractive errors, media opacities, or feigned blindness. In patients with amblyopia, the diagnosis of RPAD should be made with caution as it rarely exceeds 0.3 log units [23]. However, RAPD can be elicited if there is an asymmetric conduction defect in the optic nerve or the optic chiasm [23]. Lesions in the optic tracts and superior colliculus show a contralateral RAPD. However, the latter is without concurrent homonymous hemianopia [24, 25].

The most common cause of RAPD is conduction defect, as seen in optic neuritis, ischaemic optic neuropathy, asymmetric glaucoma, traumatic optic atrophy, optic nerve gliomas, and optic nerve sheath meningiomas. RAPD is also present in diffuse and extensive retinal disorders like retinal ischaemia, central retinal artery occlusion, ischaemic central retinal vein occlusion, rhegmatogenous retinal detachment, and destruction and scarring of the retina in extensive chorioretinitis.

16.4 Pupillary Changes in Lesions of Parasympathetic Pathways

The efferent fibres of the parasympathetic pathways travel from the Edinger -Westphal nucleus and course along the oculomotor nerve (Cranial nerve III), lying superficially on the dorsal aspect of the nerve. The CN III emerges from the ventral aspect of the midbrain into the interpeduncular fossa and lies below the posterior cerebral artery and above the superior cerebellar artery. At this location, it is vulnerable to compression by a posterior communicating artery (PCA) aneurysm. As it proceeds to enter the cavernous sinus, it lies on the edge of the tentorium cerebelli. It becomes vulnerable to brain herniation in an acute rise in ICP due to subarachnoid haemorrhage. It pierces the dura mater to lie in the upper part of the lateral wall of the cavernous sinus, where it is vulnerable to compression by internal carotid artery aneurysms, the carotid-cavernous fistula, and tumours.

Involvement of the preganglionic parasympathetic fibres leads to pupillary dilation, which is almost always accompanied by compressive lesions of CN III and needs surgical care. While PCA aneurysms mainly cause fixed dilated pupils with ophthalmoplegia, occasionally isolated pupil dilation may be seen with accompanying headaches.

On the other hand, CN III paresis/palsy without pupillary involvement is caused by ischaemia in patients with diabetes, hypertension, and atherosclerosis. Most of these have painless onset of CN III palsy and are managed by medical means. Notably, the superficial nerve fibres have a rich collateral supply; hence, the parasympathetic fibres escape ischaemia. Hence, it is termed pupil-sparing CN III palsy.

Although uncommon, hemianopic pupil reaction (Wernicke's pupil sign) is seen typically in optic tract lesions. Optic tract lesions are rare and are characterized by highly incongruous homonymous hemianopic visual field defects. When the light is shone from the blind side of the field, there is no PLR, but it reacts normally when the light is shone from the seeing half [26].

On encountering a patient with anisocoria, the cause must be ascertained. It could be physiological (PLR in both pupils is normal), the smaller pupil may be the abnormal pupil (in the dark, it remains small), or the larger pupil may be abnormal (remains large in lighted conditions). Isolated pupil dilatation with poor PLR without ptosis or extraocular muscle paresis/palsy is unusual due to intracranial pathology [27].

Patients with evidence of CN III paresis with pupillary dilation need urgent imaging studies to rule out a PCA aneurysm in the cistern, pathology in the cavernous sinus, or the superior orbital fissure. Patients with PCA aneurysms have a history of acute-onset headaches and diplopia.

An isolated dilated pupil may be caused by blunt trauma with rupture of the sphincter pupillae, acute glaucoma, or accidental atropinization. An atropinized pupil is non-reactive to light reflex and near objects (accommodation reflex). It also does not constrict with dilute pilocarpine. The most frequent cause of isolated, unilateral dilated pupils is Adie's tonic pupil, seen commonly in young women. It is caused by damage to the postganglionic parasympathetic fibres in the ciliary ganglion or the short ciliary nerves in orbit or the eye. It may be caused by a viral infection of the ciliary ganglion, trauma or tumour in orbit, or photocoagulation in the eye. Bilateral cases of Adie's pupil may be due to diabetes, amyloidosis, autonomic neuropathy, and paraneoplastic syndrome [25]. The cause of Adie's pupil remains largely idiopathic. It results in a dilated, non-reacting pupil and blurred vision due to accommodation paralysis. There may be only segmental involvement of the sphincter muscle fibres. Iris transillumination defects have been reported using infrared videography in the denervated segments of the iris [28]. The most characteristic feature of Adie's pupil is denervation hypersensitivity to a diluted 0.0625% pilocarpine. Constriction of the pupil by $\geq$0.5 mm is a highly sensitive and specific test [29]. Some patients with Adie's pupil have a benign decrease in deep tendon reflexes. The treatment of Adie's pupil includes prescribing plus lenses to facilitate reading. Over several years, the pupil size may assume to the normal size.

Episodic unilateral dilated pupil lasting a few minutes to a day has been reported in migraine [30].

16.5 Argyll Robertson Pupil

The Argyll Robertson pupil is rare and classically seen in patients with tertiary syphilis. It is characterized by bilateral small tonic pupils that do not react to light but maintain near reflexes (Fig. 16.6). The pupils dilate when the patient is asked to look far distance. The pupils may be irregular. The AR pupil results from a lesion in the dorsal midbrain in the pretectal area where the light fibres are interrupted, the near reflex fibres being more ventral escape damage and

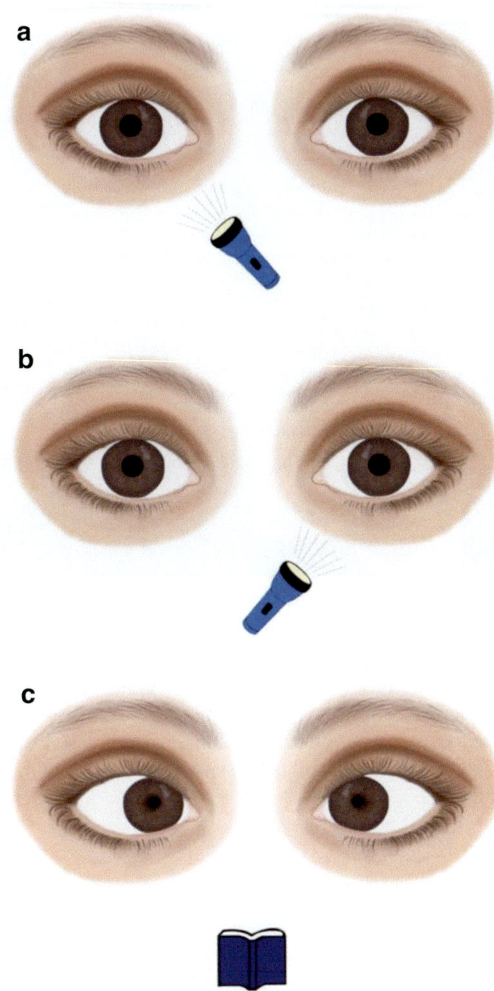

Fig. 16.6 Light near dissociation. Pupils are small and tonic and do not react when light is shone on the eyes (**a**, **b**). However, when prompted to accommodate by looking at a near target, the pupils contract promptly (**c**). The near reflex fibres are more ventral in the dorsal midbrain to pupillary light reflex fibres, which are interrupted. Near reflex fibres escape in pretectal pathologies in the midbrain. Note that the eyes converge when a near reflex is initiated (**c**). Graphics by Kritika Thakur

hence the intact near reflex. A similar pupil can be seen in old age and diabetes, neurosarcoidosis [31], multiple sclerosis, and Lyme disease. The absent light reflexes in normal looking person should prompt neuroimaging to rule out tumours dorsolateral to the superior colliculi [32]. The light near dissociation is also seen in Parinaud's syndrome and Adie's pupil, which in contrast to small pupils in AR, has dilated pupils. Misdirected regenerating fibres in CN III palsy may also produce pseudo-AR pupil wherein the fibres meant for the medial rectus innervate the sphincter pupillae. Unlike the AR pupil, these are unilateral cases.

16.5.1 Automated Pupillometry

Estimating the pupil size and PLR, when tested by healthcare providers with different levels of competence, may show inconsistent results that may have a bearing on the appropriate care of the patients [33]. Critical care and neurosurgical nurses underestimate pupils' size and reactions, necessitating automation in recording pupil reactions [34]. Automated pupillometry is a more reliable tool than manual pupillary assessment in detecting early neurological deterioration of stroke patients [35]. It is a critical ICU tool [36] (Fig. 16.7). Contrary to these observations, a single-centre study of patients admitted to a neuroscience intensive care unit found no significant difference between manual and automated pupil reactions and size [37].

The automated pupillometer measures pupil diameters, latency, constriction ratio, constriction, and dilation velocity in a reliable and reproducible manner [38]. In a critical care setting, compared to 39% interobserver variability in manual pupillometry, it was reduced to 1% with portable automated pupillometers [39]. More importantly, automated pupillometry can reproducibly measure the various phases of PLR, as mentioned above, which serve as important parameters in pupillary evaluation in intensive care settings. The phases of PLR cannot be measured in manual pupillometry.

In one of the early studies in healthy volunteers, the mean pupil diameter was 4.1 mm, and after stimulation, it decreased to a minimum of 2.7 mm. The constriction velocity was 1.48 ± 0.33 mm/s. The changes were symmetrical in both eyes in healthy volunteers, irrespective of the refractive error [40]. There is no significant difference in the various pupil parameters from 1 to 18 years. The adult data can also be extrapolated to the children [41].

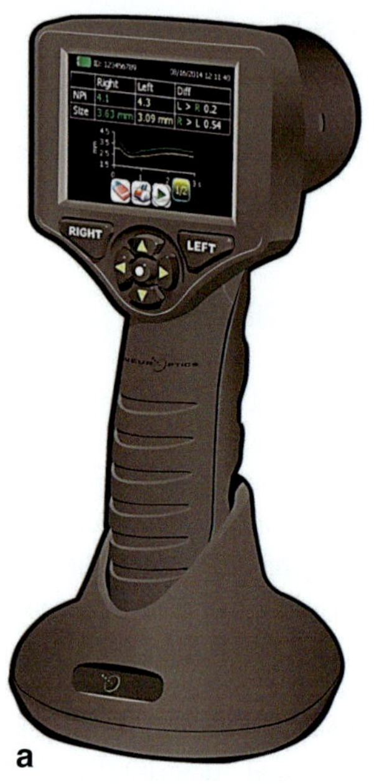

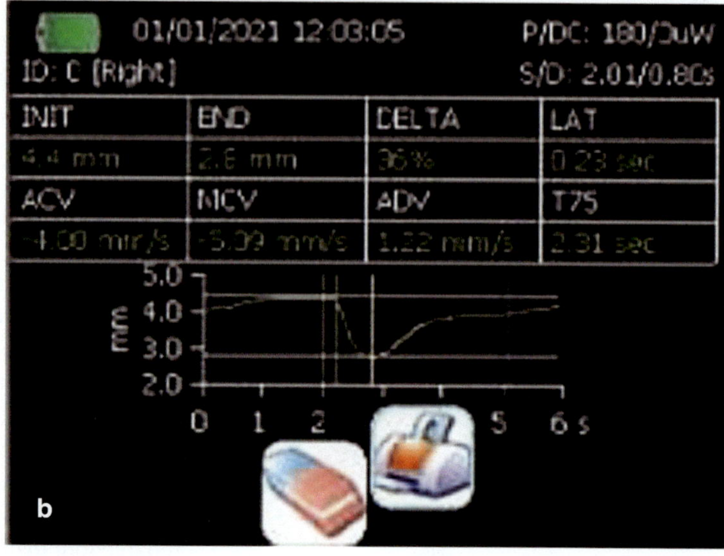

Fig. 16.7 Portable automated infrared pupillometer PLR-3000 from NeurOptics, inc. (Irvine, CA 92612, USA) (**a**). A typical data output chart of this portable automated infrared pupillometer (**b**). Abbreviations; NPi, neurological pupillary index; INIT, Maximum diameter; End, Minimum diameter; Delta, % age change from Maximum to minimum pupil diameter; Lat, latency; ACV, the average velocity of pupil constriction; MCV, maximum constriction velocity; ADV, average dilatation velocity; T 75, time to reach 75% of the baseline diameter after peak constriction. Published with permission of the manufacturers

16.5.2 Neurological Pupil Index

Neurological pupillary index (NPi) is a proprietary pupil reactivity assessment scale developed by NeurOptics, inc. (Irvine, CA 92612, USA), one of the manufacturers of US-FDA-approved infrared pupillometers (Fig. 16.7). The NPi considers various parameters of pupil size and PLR and grades on a scale of 0–5; values above three are considered normal [42]. A score difference of ≥0.7 between the two eyes is considered abnormal. The NPi provides reproducible information using a non-invasive tool. It is now a part of the routine clinical examination and follow-up of patients in neuroscience intensive care and emergency departments. The recent American Heart Association guidelines for neuro prognostication of patients who recover from cardiac arrest include monitoring the patient's pupillary responses at 72 h with an automated pupillometer. Bilateral absent PLR 72 h after cardiac arrest indicates poor neurological outcomes [43].

A "0" score on the NPi must be confirmed with manual PLR. Occasionally, slowly reacting pupils may give a false no reaction on automated pupillometry [44].

Sometimes differentiating optic neuritis (ON) from ischaemic optic neuropathy (ION) can be challenging. Using automated pupillometry, while delayed pupil constriction latency and decreased constriction velocity and constriction ratio are lower than normal, the pupil constriction latency is significantly delayed in ON compared to ION. All the parameters recover in ON but not in ION [45].

At high altitudes, exposure to hypobaric hypoxia leads to significant slowing of pupil latency and constriction velocity that gets reversed during acclimatization [46]. Measuring NPi on an automated pupillometer can be a potential surrogate tool to diagnose space flight-associated neuro ocular syndrome, in which raised ICP plays a major role [47].

16.6 Effect of Head Injury on Pupillary Parameters

In patients with an acute head injury and raised intracranial pressure (ICP) (>20 mm Hg) but without significant midline shift, there was no change in pupillometry. However, if there was a midline shift >3 mm and the ICP remained above 20 mm, there was a significant reduction in constriction velocity to <0.6 mm/s on the side of the mass effect [40].

Coma varies from drowsiness to brain death and is scored on the Glasgow coma scale (GCS), which has three major components: eye-opening, response to verbal commands, and motor response. It should be noted that pupil reactions are not a component of the severity scale of coma because of inconsistencies, and only 2/third of the patients with non-reacting pupils have a low score [48].

However, among patients admitted to neuroscience intensive care, even one episode of NPi difference $\geq$ 0.7 between the two eyes had a modified Rankin disability score at the discharge of 3.9 for stroke and 4.1 for traumatic brain injury. Those with NPi of <0.7 scored 2.7 and 2.9, respectively [49]. A modified Rankin score of 4 indicates moderately severe disability, inability to walk, and needing assistance for bodily functions. Information from both GCS and pupil reactions should be combined for prognostication. Patients in a coma from traumatic brain injury with a GCS of 3 with intact pupil reactions have a survival chance of 33% and a 0% chance of survival of non-reacting pupils at a GCS of 3 [50].

In children admitted with encephalopathy or brain injury, elevated intracranial pressure (ICP) negatively correlated with NPi, pupil size, constriction, and dilation velocity compared to when the ICP was normal [51]. In shaken baby syndrome, who present with extensive intraocular haemorrhages, vision loss is usually due to brain injury. Good initial PLR is a prognostic marker for visual recovery and good neurological outcomes in these babies [52].

Testing pupillary reactions using an automated pupillometer in comatose patients is a challenge. Hence, an infrared pupillometer technique has been tested for PLR through closed lids [53].

16.6.1 Hutchinson Pupil

Hutchinson's dilated pupil due to lateral shift (or herniation) of the midbrain by an acute rise in ICP is seen in patients with a rapidly developing subdural haematoma. Ipsilateral pupil dilatation with absent PLR is an early sign before the onset of CN III paralysis. There may be a phase of ipsilateral pupil constriction in the first few minutes. In the later stages, the contralateral cerebral peduncle compression gives rise to a false localizing sign of ipsilateral hemiplegia. A dilated pupil indicates poor head injury outcomes [54]. Likely, reduced blood flow to the midbrain rather than its mechanical lateral shift is responsible for the pupillary signs [55]. In a systematic review of bilateral fixed pupils in tentorial herniation, 2/3rd of patients underwent decompression surgery within 2 h of noting the bilateral dilated fixed pupils. Of these, 67% died. Of the survivors, half had a good outcome (17% of the entire cohort), while the other half had severe disabilities [56].

16.6.2 Parinaud' Syndrome

Parinaud's dorsal brain stem syndrome is most often seen due to tumours of the pineal gland and MS in the young, haemorrhage, and ischaemia in the old. Nearly 1/3rd of the cases are caused by pineal gland tumours. The pineal gland is a midline structure between the two cerebral hemispheres just above and posterior to the dorsal aspect of the superior colliculus. It is attached to the posterior wall of the third ventricle floor. Tumours from the pineal gland compress several surrounding structures, the cerebellum, and the Sylvian aqueduct resulting in hydrocephalus, and compress on the rostral interstitial nucleus of the medial fascicular bundle, pretectal, and the Edinger-Westphal nucleus. The resulting Parinaud's syndrome consists of a constellation of signs. The most constant feature is supranuclear vertical gaze palsy due to damage to the interstitial nuclei of the MLF; the fibres for the up gaze lie more laterally and more susceptible to compression than the more medial fibres for the downgaze that lie more medially. The PLR afferent fibres are present more dorsally than the near reflex; hence, the light reflex is lost in compressive lesions. The near reflex remains intact, an example of light-near dissociation seen in nearly 2/3rd of the patients. The upper lid retraction is seen in nearly 1/3rd. However, the eyes can move up on the doll's eye movements. There is a convergence nystagmus [57] (Fig. 16.8).

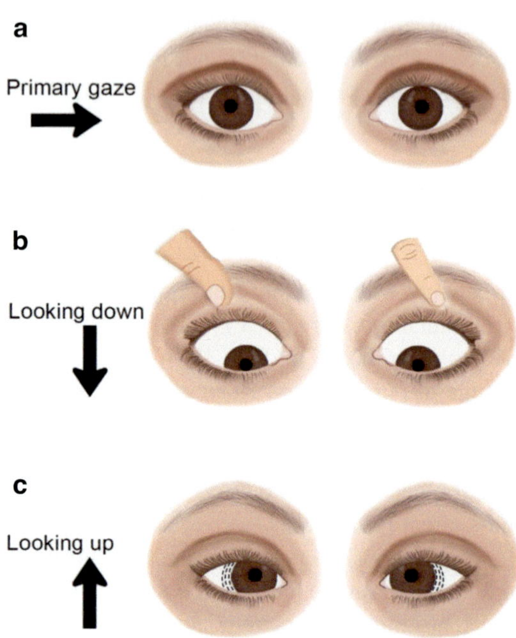

Fig. 16.8 Highly Schematic representation of supranuclear gaze palsy seen in pineal tumours in young age and haemorrhage and ischaemic events in old age. Compressive lesions affect the rostral interstitial nucleus of the medial longitudinal fasciculus, pretectal area, and the Edinger-Westphal nucleus. The fibres for the upgaze lie more laterally and are prone to compression than the downgaze fibres. The eyes are normal in primary gaze (**a**) and looking down (**b**). But when asked to look up, there is vertical gaze palsy; the eyes converge and retract and have nystagmus (**c**). Near reflex is normal in most patients as these fibres being more ventral escape the pathology. The vestibulo-ocular reflexes are intact and hence the eyes can move up in Doll's head manoeuvre. Graphics by Kritika Thakur

16.6.3 Horner's Syndrome

Compared to the parasympathetic oculomotor pathway, the 3-neuron sympathetic fibres run a much longer and tortuous path and are hence prone to interruption of its fibres at multiple sites; the first neuron at the level of the hypothalamus and brain stem or the second neuronal fibres emerge from the spinal cord at the level of C8 to T1(ciliospinal centre of Budge) and ascend in the thorax or the third neuron postganglionic fibres from the superior cervical ganglion as they travel in the wall of the internal carotid artery to the cavernous sinus.

The triad of Horner syndrome includes small pupil, mild ptosis of the upper lid (<2 mm), and anhidrosis (Fig. 16.9). Ptosis of the lower lid is caused by loss of the innervation of the retractors, and thus the lower lid appears slightly elevated and is also called reverse ptosis. The apraclonidine (alpha 2-adrenergic agonist) test confirms the diagnosis of Horner's syndrome by demonstrating sympathetic denervation hypersensitivity. It may be negative in very early cases till degeneration of the nerves has set in. Within 30–40 min of the apraclonidine 0.5% eyedrop, there is dilatation of the affected pupil and elevation of the ptotic lid.

Other ocular signs of Horner's syndrome include lower intraocular pressure in the ipsilateral eye. In the congenital Horner syndrome, the affected eyes have a lighter-coloured iris.

The central and preganglionic Horner syndrome produces significant anhidrosis of the face. The postganglionic Horner's syndrome does not cause anhidrosis as the sympathetic fibres meant for the sweat glands of the face leave the superior cervical ganglion along the branches of the external carotid artery (https://eyewiki.aao.org/Horner_Syndrome).

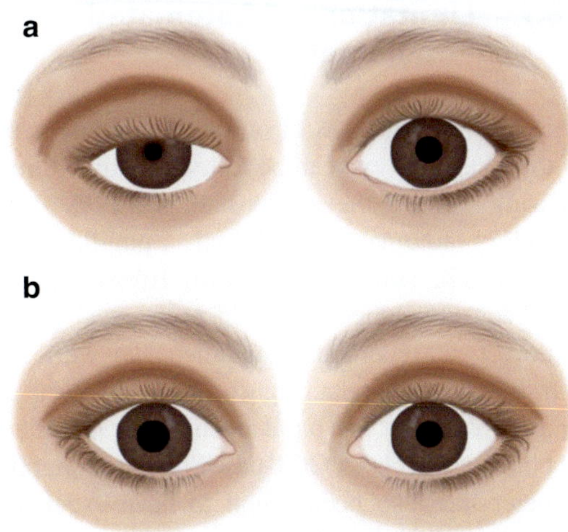

Fig. 16.9 Right eye Horner's syndrome: The right eye shows ptosis of both upper and lower lids. Note that in ptosis of the lower lid, the lower lid moves down. The pupil is miotic. (right eye, **a**)The left eye is normal. The upper lid margin covers 0.5–1.5 mm of the upper limbus, while the lower lid just touches the limbus (left eye, **a**). Thirty minutes after the instillation of apraclonidine 0.5% eyedrops in both eyes, there is a remarkable improvement in ptosis of both lids in the right eye, and the pupil is dilated (right, **b**). This phenomenon is a sympathetic denervation hypersensitivity response seen in the right eye with Horner's syndrome. There is no change in the lids or the pupil in the left normal eye (left eye, **b**). The sympathetic pathway for ocular innervation is shown in Fig. 16.4. Graphics by Kritika Thakur

The constellation of signs and the investigations to establish the cause depends on the level of injury and the cause of the Horner syndrome.

The most common cause of first neuron injury (central Horner's syndrome) is haemorrhagic stroke, demyelination, ischaemia, syringomyelia (fluid-filled cysts in the spinal cord), arteriovenous malformations, meningitis, arachnoiditis, or cervical spinal injury.

The second neuronal Horner's syndrome results from interruption of preganglionic fibres due to lung cancer above the first rib (Pancoast tumour, most of which are non-small cell adenocarcinomas and produce pain in the arm), cervical rib, supraclavicular nodes, aneurysm of the subclavian artery, injury to the brachial plexus, or thoracic injury during surgical procedures.

The third neuronal postganglionic Horner's syndrome is caused by dissection of the internal carotid artery, skull-base fracture, herpes zoster, middle ear infections, migraine, cavernous sinus thrombosis, and temporal arteritis. Nearly 1/3rd of the cases of Horner syndrome remain idiopathic.

The cause of Horner's syndrome may vary depending on where the patient first reports. Thus, most patients reporting first to Ophthalmology may be idiopathic, followed by surgical procedures and 3% due to undetected cancers [58]. A definitive cause was recognized in 61% of 159 apraclonidine-confirmed Horner syndrome cases. The most common cause was neck, chest, skull, or paraspinal procedures, followed by cervical carotid dissection. In the pharmacologically unconfirmed cohort, tumours were next common to the procedures. In most cases, the cause of Horner's syndrome is known at presentation. If the cause is unknown before its diagnosis, a tumour or dissection of the aorta must be ruled out by appropriate imaging, CT angiography, and CT chest [59].

16.6.4 Adie's Tonic Pupil

Adie's tonic pupil is dilated due to damage to the parasympathetic fibres in the ciliary ganglion due to trauma, inflammation, and viral infections and is more often unilateral than bilateral. The patient complains of difficulty in near vision with the affected eye. The pupil is non-reactive to light, but may react and constrict in near reflex due to aberrant regeneration of the parasympathetic fibres. The parasympathetic supply to the ciliary body is 30 times higher than the iris (https://eyewiki.aao.org/Adie_Pupil). The pupil may be irregular in shape due to patchy atrophy of the sphincter pupillae. The diagnosis is confirmed by using a diluted cholinergic drop like diluted pilocarpine (0.0625%) which causes marked constriction of the affected pupil due to super sensitivity of the post-ganglionic parasympathetic receptors. There is no effect on the normal pupil of such diluted pilocarpine [60] (Fig. 16.10).

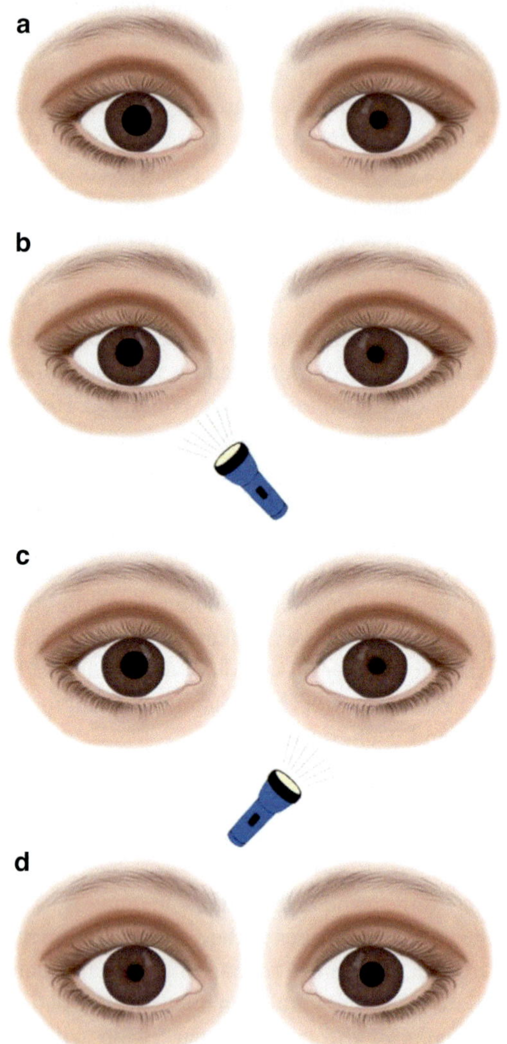

Fig. 16.10 Right eye Adie's pupil. Adie's pupil is a tonic pupil resulting from damage to the ciliary ganglion due to various insults that cause loss of the parasympathetic ganglion cells. Therefore, the pupil gets dilated due to the unopposed action of the dilator muscle (**a**). When the light is shone into the right eye, the right pupil does not constrict, but the left constricts due to consensual light reflex as the afferent path is intact (**b**). On shining light into the left eye, the left pupil constricts, but the right pupil stays dilated (**c**). Instillation of diluted pilocarpine drops (0.0625%) in both eyes leads to constriction of the right pupil in 30 min due to supersensitivity of post-ganglionic receptors to highly diluted cholinergic drops, but does not affect the normal left pupil (**d**). Graphics by Kritika Thakur

16.7 Limitations of Automated Pupillometry

One of the limitations of portable pupillometers is that only one eye can be tested at a time, thus missing out on the consensual reflex. A new mobile automated infrared pupillometer (Hitomiru®, Hitomiru Co., Ltd. Tokyo, Japan) has been developed in which both eyes' pupil diameter is recorded simultaneously with an infrared video camera. Light stimulus is given to one eye at a time. The pupil reactions are recorded in both eyes [61]. An OCT-based binocular pupillometer has also been found to have excellent test-retest reliability [62].

16.8 Effect of Drugs on Pupillary Parameters

Intravenous diazepam, midazolam, and morphine lead to a transient symmetric decrease in constriction velocity. Another opioid, tramadol, leads to a dose-dependent decrease in latency, amplitude, and constriction velocity [63]. Calcium channel blockers and the neuromuscular blocking drugs used in anaesthesia (pancuronium and vencuronium) do not affect the pupillometer parameters [40, 64]. Except for an increased latency of pupillary constriction in patients with positive urine drug screening for opioids, there was no difference in the NPi from the controls [65].

16.9 Pupillometry in Psychological Evaluation

It is well known that pupils dilate under cognitive overload, tasks demanding more attention or memory use, emotional stress, or interpretation of difficult tasks [66]. A sustained continuous cognitive demand leads to sustained pupillary dilatation. The afferent pathways project from the dorsolateral prefrontal cortex areas involved in cognition and emotional control to limbic areas, the amygdala, and the midbrain striate cortex. These areas send efferent fibres to the oculomotor nuclei [67, 68]. Moreover, dynamic pupillary changes reflect dynamic conscious information processing and mind wandering [69]. The pupillary responses are more useful in young people than the old, who are less sensitive to memory load [70].

References

1. Flügel-Koch CM, Tektas OY, Kaufman PL, Paulsen FP, Lütjen-Drecoll E. Morphological alterations within the peripheral fixation of the iris dilator muscle in eyes with pigmentary glaucoma. Invest Ophthalmol Vis Sci. 2014;55(7):4541–51. https://doi.org/10.1167/iovs.13-13765. PMID: 24938519; PMCID: PMC4453212.
2. Perez GM, Keyser RB. Cell body counts in human ciliary ganglia. Invest Ophthalmol Vis Sci. 1986;27(9):1428–31. PMID: 3744735.
3. Turnbull PR, Irani N, Lim N, Phillips JR. Origins of pupillary hippus in the autonomic nervous system. Invest Ophthalmol Vis Sci. 2017;58(1):197–203. https://doi.org/10.1167/iovs.16-20785. PMID: 28114580.
4. Fernández-Torre JL, Paramio-Paz A, Lorda-de Los Ríos I, Martín-García M, Hernández-Hernández MA. Pupillary hippus as clinical manifestation of refractory autonomic nonconvulsive status epilepticus: pathophysiological implications. Seizure. 2018;63:102–4. https://doi.org/10.1016/j.seizure.2018.11.006. Epub 2018 Nov 15. PMID: 30527343.
5. Denny JC, Arndt FV, Dupont WD, Neilson EG. Increased hospital mortality in patients with bedside hippus. Am J Med. 2008;121(3):239–45. https://doi.org/10.1016/j.amjmed.2007.09.014. PMID: 18328309.
6. Esquiva G, Lax P, Pérez-Santonja JJ, García-Fernández JM, Cuenca N. Loss of melanopsin-expressing ganglion cell subtypes and dendritic degeneration in the aging human retina. Front Aging Neurosci. 2017;9:79. https://doi.org/10.3389/fnagi.2017.00079. PMID: 28420980; PMCID: PMC5378720.
7. La Morgia C, Ross-Cisneros FN, Sadun AA, Carelli V. Retinal ganglion cells and circadian rhythms in Alzheimer's disease, Parkinson's disease, and beyond. Front Neurol. 2017;8:162. https://doi.org/10.3389/fneur.2017.00162. PMID: 28522986; PMCID: PMC5415575.
8. Hannibal J, Christiansen AT, Heegaard S, Fahrenkrug J, Kiilgaard JF. Melanopsin expressing human retinal ganglion cells: subtypes, distribution, and intraretinal connectivity. J Comp Neurol. 2017;525(8):1934–61. https://doi.org/10.1002/cne.24181. Epub 2017 Mar 10. PMID: 28160289.
9. Hannibal J, Hindersson P, Ostergaard J, Georg B, Heegaard S, Larsen PJ, Fahrenkrug J. Melanopsin is expressed in PACAP-containing retinal ganglion cells of the human retinohypothalamic tract. Invest Ophthalmol Vis Sci. 2004;45(11):4202–9. https://doi.org/10.1167/iovs.04-0313. PMID: 15505076.
10. La Morgia C, Ross-Cisneros FN, Hannibal J, Montagna P, Sadun AA, Carelli V. Melanopsin-expressing retinal ganglion cells: implications for human diseases. Vis Res. 2011;51(2):296–302. https://doi.org/10.1016/j.visres.2010.07.023. Epub 2010 Aug 4. PMID: 20691201.
11. Mure LS. Intrinsically photosensitive retinal ganglion cells of the human retina. Front Neurol. 2021;12:636330. https://doi.org/10.3389/fneur.2021.636330. PMID: 33841306; PMCID: PMC8027232.
12. Meltzer E, Sguigna PV, Subei A, Beh S, Kildebeck E, Conger D, Conger A, Lucero M, Frohman BS, Frohman AN, Saidha S, Galetta S, Calabresi PA, Rennaker R, Frohman TC, Kardon RH, Balcer LJ, Frohman EM. Retinal architecture and Melanopsin-mediated pupillary response characteristics: a putative pathophysiologic signature for the Retino-hypothalamic tract in multiple sclerosis. JAMA Neurol. 2017;74(5):574–82. https://doi.org/10.1001/jamaneurol.2016.5131. PMID: 28135360; PMCID: PMC5822208.
13. White OB, Costello F. Melanopsin effects on pupil responses: is the eye the window to the weary soul? JAMA Neurol. 2017;74(5):506–8. https://doi.org/10.1001/jamaneurol.2016.5385. PMID: 28135345.
14. Kerr RW, Brown JA. Pupillomotor pathways in the spinal cord. Arch Neurol. 1964;10:262–70. https://doi.org/10.1001/archneur.1964.00460150032003. PMID: 14106982.
15. Lykstad J, Reddy V, Hanna A. Neuroanatomy, pupillary dilation pathway. In: StatPearls [Internet]. Treasure Island (FL): StatPearls Publishing; 2022. [Updated 2022 Aug 8]. Available from: https://www.ncbi.nlm.nih.gov/books/NBK535421/.
16. Al-Obaidi S, Atem F, Stutzman SE, Aiyagari V, Olson DM. Investigating the association between eye colour and the neurological pupil index. Aust Crit Care. 2020;33(5):436–40. https://doi.org/10.1016/j.aucc.2019.10.001. Epub 2019 Nov 20. PMID: 31759859.
17. Carter BG, Butt W, Taylor A. Bilaterally absent pupillary responses: not always a bad sign. Anaesth Intensive Care. 2007;35(6):984–7. https://doi.org/10.1177/0310057X0703500623. PMID: 18084996.
18. Robinson J, Fielder AR. Pupillary diameter and reaction to light in preterm neonates. Arch Dis Child. 1990;65(1 Spec No):35–8. https://doi.org/10.1136/adc.65.1_spec_no.35. PMID: 2306132; PMCID: PMC1590160.

19. Levatin P. Pupillary escape in disease of the retina or optic nerve. Arch Ophthalmol. 1959;62:768–79. https://doi.org/10.1001/archopht.1959.04220050030005. PMID: 14416133.
20. Thompson HS, Corbett JJ, Cox TA. How to measure the relative afferent pupillary defect. Surv Ophthalmol. 1981;26(1):39–42. https://doi.org/10.1016/0039-6257(81)90124-7. PMID: 7280994.
21. Bell RA, Waggoner PM, Boyd WM, Akers RE, Yee CE. Clinical grading of relative afferent pupillary defects. Arch Ophthalmol. 1993;111(7):938–42. https://doi.org/10.1001/archopht.1993.01090070056019. PMID: 8328935.
22. Hall CA, Chilcott RP. Eyeing up the future of the pupillary light reflex in neurodiagnostics. Diagnostics (Basel). 2018;8(1):19. https://doi.org/10.3390/diagnostics8010019. PMID: 29534018; PMCID: PMC5872002.
23. Wilhelm H. Neuro-ophthalmology of pupillary function—practical guidelines. J Neurol. 1998;245(9):573–83. https://doi.org/10.1007/s004150050248. PMID: 9758294.
24. Girkin CA, Perry JD, Miller NR. A relative afferent pupillary defect without any visual sensory deficit. Arch Ophthalmol. 1998;116(11):1544–5. https://doi.org/10.1001/archopht.116.11.1544. PMID: 9823369.
25. Kawasaki A. Physiology, assessment, and pupil disorders. Curr Opin Ophthalmol. 1999;10(6):394–400. https://doi.org/10.1097/00055735-199912000-00005. PMID: 10662243.
26. Savino PJ, Paris M, Schatz NJ, Orr LS, Corbett JJ. Optic tract syndrome. A review of 21 patients. Arch Ophthalmol. 1978;96(4):656–63. https://doi.org/10.1001/archopht.1978.03910050352011. PMID: 646693.
27. Lee AG, Taber KH, Hayman LA, Tang RA. A guide to the isolated dilated pupil. Arch Fam Med. 1997;6(4):385–8. https://doi.org/10.1001/archfami.6.4.385. PMID: 9225713.
28. Kardon RH, Corbett JJ, Thompson HS. Segmental denervation and reinnervation of the iris sphincter as shown by infrared videographic transillumination. Ophthalmology. 1998;105(2):313–21. https://doi.org/10.1016/s0161-6420(98)93328-0. PMID: 9479293.
29. Yoo YJ, Hwang JM, Yang HK. Dilute pilocarpine test for diagnosis of Adie's tonic pupil. Sci Rep. 2021;11(1):10089. https://doi.org/10.1038/s41598-021-89148-w. PMID: 33980910; PMCID: PMC8115311.
30. Woods D, O'Connor PS, Fleming R. Episodic unilateral mydriasis and migraine. Am J Ophthalmol. 1984;98(2):229–34. https://doi.org/10.1016/0002-9394(87)90359-x. PMID: 6476048.
31. Poole CJ. Argyll Robertson pupils due to neurosarcoidosis: evidence for site of lesion. Br Med J (Clin Res Ed). 1984;289(6441):356. https://doi.org/10.1136/bmj.289.6441.356. PMID: 6432097; PMCID: PMC1442382.
32. Dacso CC, Bortz DL. Significance of the Argyll Robertson pupil in clinical medicine. Am J Med. 1989;86(2):199–202. https://doi.org/10.1016/0002-9343(89)90269-6. PMID: 2643871.
33. Clark A, Clarke TN, Gregson B, Hooker PN, Chambers IR. Variability in pupil size estimation. Emerg Med J. 2006;23(6):440–1. https://doi.org/10.1136/emj.2005.030247. PMID: 16714502; PMCID: PMC2564337.
34. Kerr RG, Bacon AM, Baker LL, Gehrke JS, Hahn KD, Lillegraven CL, Renner CH, Spilman SK. Underestimation of pupil size by critical care and neurosurgical nurses. Am J Crit Care. 2016;25(3):213–9. https://doi.org/10.4037/ajcc2016554. PMID: 27134226.
35. Marshall M, Deo R, Childs C, Ali A. Feasibility and variability of automated pupillometry among stroke patients and healthy participants: potential implications for clinical practice. J Neurosci Nurs. 2019;51(2):84–8. https://doi.org/10.1097/JNN.0000000000000416. PMID: 30489422.
36. Zafar SF, Suarez JI. Automated pupillometer for monitoring the critically ill patient: a critical appraisal. J Crit Care. 2014;29(4):599–603. https://doi.org/10.1016/j.jcrc.2014.01.012. Epub 2014 Jan 29. PMID: 24613394.
37. Smith J, Flower O, Tracey A, Johnson P. A comparison of manual pupil examination versus an automated pupillometer in a specialised neurosciences intensive care unit. Aust Crit Care. 2020;33(2):162–6. https://doi.org/10.1016/j.aucc.2019.04.005. Epub 2019 May 31. PMID: 31160216.
38. Fountas KN, Kapsalaki EZ, Machinis TG, Boev AN, Robinson JS, Troup EC. Clinical implications of quantitative infrared pupillometry in neurosurgical patients. Neurocrit Care. 2006;5(1):55–60. https://doi.org/10.1385/NCC:5:1:55. PMID: 16960298.
39. Meeker M, Du R, Bacchetti P, Privitera CM, Larson MD, Holland MC, Manley G. Pupil examination: validity and clinical utility of an automated pupillometer. J Neurosci Nurs. 2005 Feb;37(1):34–40.
40. Taylor WR, Chen JW, Meltzer H, Gennarelli TA, Kelbch C, Knowlton S, Richardson J, Lutch MJ, Farin A, Hults KN, Marshall LF. Quantitative pupillometry, a new technology: normative data and preliminary observations in patients with acute head injury. Technical note. J Neurosurg. 2003;98(1):205–13. https://doi.org/10.3171/jns.2003.98.1.0205. PMID: 12546375.
41. Brown JT, Connelly M, Nickols C, Neville KA. Developmental changes of normal pupil size and reactivity in children. J Pediatr Ophthalmol Strabismus. 2015;52(3):147–51. https://doi.org/10.3928/01913913-20150317-11. PMID: 26225382.
42. Chen JW, Vakil-Gilani K, Williamson KL, Cecil S. Infrared pupillometry, the Neurological Pupil index and unilateral pupillary dilation after traumatic brain injury: implications for treatment

paradigms. Springerplus. 2014;3:548. https://doi.org/10.1186/2193-1801-3-548. PMID: 25332854; PMCID: PMC4190183.

43. Panchal AR, Bartos JA, Cabañas JG, Donnino MW, Drennan IR, Hirsch KG, Kudenchuk PJ, Kurz MC, Lavonas EJ, Morley PT, O'Neil BJ, Peberdy MA, Rittenberger JC, Rodriguez AJ, Sawyer KN, Berg KM. Adult basic and advanced life support writing group. Part 3: adult basic and advanced life support: 2020 American Heart Association guidelines for cardiopulmonary resuscitation and emergency cardiovascular care. Circulation. 2020;142(16_suppl_2):S366–468. https://doi.org/10.1161/CIR.0000000000000916. Epub 2020 Oct 21. PMID: 33081529.
44. Kramer CL, Rabinstein AA, Wijdicks EF, Hocker SE. Neurologist versus machine: is the pupillometer better than the naked eye in detecting pupillary reactivity. Neurocrit Care. 2014;21(2):309–11. https://doi.org/10.1007/s12028-014-9988-5. PMID: 24865269.
45. Yoo YJ, Hwang JM, Yang HK. Differences in pupillary light reflex between optic neuritis and ischemic optic neuropathy. PLoS One. 2017;12(10):e0186741. https://doi.org/10.1371/journal.pone.0186741. PMID: 29049405; PMCID: PMC5648212.
46. Wilson MH, Edsell M, Imray C, Wright A, Birmingham Medical Research Expeditionary Society. Changes in pupil dynamics at high altitude—an observational study using a handheld pupillometer. High Alt Med Biol. 2008;9(4):319–25. https://doi.org/10.1089/ham.2008.1026. PMID: 19115917.
47. Shirah BH, Sen J, Naaman NK, Pandya S. Automated pupillometry in space neuroscience. Life Sci Space Res. 2023;37:1–2. https://doi.org/10.1016/j.lssr.2023.01.004.
48. Jennett B, Teasdale G. Aspects of coma after severe head injury. Lancet. 1977;1(8017):878–81. https://doi.org/10.1016/s0140-6736(77)91201-6. PMID: 67287.
49. Privitera CM, Neerukonda SV, Aiyagari V, Yokobori S, Puccio AM, Schneider NJ, Stutzman SE, Olson DM, END PANIC Investigators. A differential of the left eye and right eye neurological pupil index is associated with discharge modified Rankin scores in neurologically injured patients. BMC Neurol. 2022;22(1):273. https://doi.org/10.1186/s12883-022-02801-3. PMID: 35869429; PMCID: PMC9306158.
50. Lieberman JD, Pasquale MD, Garcia R, Cipolle MD, Mark Li P, Wasser TE. Use of admission Glasgow Coma Score, pupil size, and pupil reactivity to determine outcome for trauma patients. J Trauma. 2003;55(3):437–42; discussion 442-3. https://doi.org/10.1097/01.TA.0000081882.79587.17. PMID: 14501883.
51. Freeman AD, McCracken CE, Stockwell JA. Automated pupillary measurements inversely correlate with increased intracranial pressure in pediatric patients with acute brain injury or encephalopathy. Pediatr Crit Care Med. 2020;21(8):753–9. https://doi.org/10.1097/PCC.0000000000002327. PMID: 32195898.
52. Kivlin JD, Simons KB, Lazoritz S, Ruttum MS. Shaken baby syndrome. Ophthalmology. 2000;107(7):1246–54. https://doi.org/10.1016/s0161-6420(00)00161-5. PMID: 10889093.
53. Farraj Y, Buxboim A, Cohen JE, Kan-Tor Y, Glasner Hagege S, Weiss D, Goldman V, Beatus T. Measuring pupil size and light response through closed eyelids. Biomed Opt Express. 2021;12(10):6485–95. https://doi.org/10.1364/BOE.435508. PMID: 34745751; PMCID: PMC8548001.
54. Fisher CM. Brain herniation: a revision of classical concepts. Can J Neurol Sci. 1995;22(2):83–91. https://doi.org/10.1017/s0317167100040142. PMID: 7627921.
55. Ritter AM, Muizelaar JP, Barnes T, Choi S, Fatouros P, Ward J, Bullock MR. Brain stem blood flow, pupillary response, and outcome in patients with severe head injuries. Neurosurgery. 1999;44(5):941–8. https://doi.org/10.1097/00006123-199905000-00005. PMID: 10232526.
56. Griepp DW, Miller A, Sorek S, Rahme R. Are bilaterally fixed and dilated pupils the kiss of death in patients with transtentorial herniation? Systematic review and pooled analysis. World Neurosurg. 2022;164:e427–35. https://doi.org/10.1016/j.wneu.2022.04.118. Epub 2022 May 2. PMID: 35513282.
57. Feroze KB, Patel BC. Parinaud syndrome. In: StatPearls [Internet]. Treasure Island (FL): StatPearls Publishing; 2019. [Updated 2019 Jan 13]. Available from: https://www.ncbi.nlm.nih.gov/books/NBK441892/.
58. Maloney WF, Younge BR, Moyer NJ. Evaluation of the causes and accuracy of pharmacologic localization in Horner's syndrome. Am J Ophthalmol. 1980;90(3):394–402. https://doi.org/10.1016/s0002-9394(14)74924-4. PMID: 7425056.
59. Sabbagh MA, De Lott LB, Trobe JD. Causes of Horner syndrome: a study of 318 patients. J Neuroophthalmol. 2020;40(3):362–9. https://doi.org/10.1097/WNO.0000000000000844. PMID: 31609831; PMCID: PMC7148177.
60. Leavitt JA, Wayman LL, Hodge DO, Brubaker RF. Pupillary response to four concentrations of pilocarpine in normal subjects: application to testing for Adie tonic pupil. Am J Ophthalmol. 2002;133(3):333–6. https://doi.org/10.1016/s0002-9394(01)01420-9. PMID: 11860969.
61. Kotani J, Nakao H, Yamada I, Miyawaki A, Mambo N, Ono Y. A novel method for measuring the pupil diameter and pupillary light reflex of healthy volunteers and patients with intracranial lesions using a newly developed Pupilometer. Front Med (Lausanne). 2021;8:598791. https://doi.org/10.3389/fmed.2021.598791. PMID: 34557496; PMCID: PMC8452878.

62. Chopra R, Mulholland PJ, Petzold A, Ogunbowale L, Gazzard G, Bremner FD, Anderson RS, Keane PA. Automated pupillometry using a prototype binocular optical coherence tomography system. Am J Ophthalmol. 2020;214:21–31. https://doi.org/10.1016/j.ajo.2020.02.013. Epub 2020 Feb 28. PMID: 32114180.
63. Fliegert F, Kurth B, Göhler K. The effects of tramadol on static and dynamic pupillometry in healthy subjects—the relationship between pharmacodynamics, pharmacokinetics and CYP2D6 metaboliser status. Eur J Clin Pharmacol. 2005;61(4):257–66. https://doi.org/10.1007/s00228-005-0920-y. Epub 2005 May 20. PMID: 15906019.
64. Gray AT, Krejci ST, Larson MD. Neuromuscular blocking drugs do not alter the pupillary light reflex of anesthetized humans. Arch Neurol. 1997;54(5):579–84. https://doi.org/10.1001/archneur.1997.00550170055014. PMID: 9152114.
65. Jolkovsky EL, Fernandez-Penny FE, Alexis M, Benson LN, Wang BH, Abella BS. Impact of acute intoxication on quantitative pupillometry assessment in the emergency department. J Am Coll Emerg Physicians Open. 2022;3(5):e12825. https://doi.org/10.1002/emp2.12825. PMID: 36311337; PMCID: PMC9601771.
66. Franzen PL, Buysse DJ, Dahl RE, Thompson W, Siegle GJ. Sleep deprivation alters pupillary reactivity to emotional stimuli in healthy young adults. Biol Psychol. 2009;80(3):300–5. https://doi.org/10.1016/j.biopsycho.2008.10.010. Epub 2008 Nov 11. PMID: 19041689; PMCID: PMC3107827.
67. Siegle GJ, Steinhauer SR, Stenger VA, Konecky R, Carter CS. Use of concurrent pupil dilation assessment to inform interpretation and analysis of fMRI data. NeuroImage. 2003;20(1):114–24. https://doi.org/10.1016/s1053-8119(03)00298-2. PMID: 14527574.
68. Urry HL, van Reekum CM, Johnstone T, Kalin NH, Thurow ME, Schaefer HS, Jackson CA, Frye CJ, Greischar LL, Alexander AL, Davidson RJ. Amygdala and ventromedial prefrontal cortex are inversely coupled during regulation of negative affect and predict the diurnal pattern of cortisol secretion among older adults. J Neurosci. 2006;26(16):4415–25. https://doi.org/10.1523/JNEUROSCI.3215-05.2006. PMID: 16624961; PMCID: PMC6673990.
69. Kang OE, Huffer KE, Wheatley TP. Pupil dilation dynamics track attention to high-level information. PLoS One. 2014;9(8):e102463. https://doi.org/10.1371/journal.pone.0102463. PMID: 25162597; PMCID: PMC4146469.
70. Van Gerven PW, Paas F, Van Merriënboer JJ, Schmidt HG. Memory load and the cognitive pupillary response in aging. Psychophysiology. 2004;41(2):167–74. https://doi.org/10.1111/j.1469-8986.2003.00148.x. PMID: 15032982.

17 Red Eyes—Conjunctivitis, Corneal Ulcers, Dry Eye Disease, and Acute Uveitis

17.1 Anatomy of the Conjunctiva

Conjunctiva is a thin, non-keratinized, multilayered mucus membrane comprising a columnar and cuboidal epithelial cellular layer (3–5 cells), an adenoid layer, and a thin fibrous tissue layer. It is a transparent, vascularized membrane that starts at the lid margin and covers the posterior (inner) surface of the upper and the lower lids, where it is termed palpebral or tarsal conjunctiva. There are three parts; the first part is up to 2 mm from the lid margin marginal conjunctiva, the second part is the tarsal conjunctiva, and the third part is the orbital part that extends posteriorly up to the fornices, from where it reflects and lines the anterior sclera's surface till the cornea's limbus. It is termed bulbar conjunctiva when it covers the sclera. The junction of the marginal and the tarsal conjunctiva is marked by a sulcus, sulcus subtarsalis. The fornices are the line of reflection from the palpebral to the bulbar conjunctiva. While the tarsal conjunctiva is firmly adherent to the underlying tarsal plate, the bulbar conjunctiva is loosely adherent to the sclera to facilitate free eye movement except anteriorly in the perilimbal 3 mm, where the conjunctiva is fused with the tenon's capsule and the episclera. The tenon's capsule and episcleral fibres separate the bulbar conjunctiva from the sclera. Redundancy of conjunctiva in the fornices allows for its stretching in extreme eyeball movements. The superior fornix is deeper than the inferior, the medial being the shallowest. The superior fornix, a deep recess, is also a favourite site for lodging foreign bodies irritating the eye. The other site for the lodgement of foreign bodies is sulcus subtarsalis. The superior fornix cannot be examined unless double-everted with a lid retractor. https://www.eophtha.com/posts/anatomy-of-conjunctiva

The conjunctival sac is a pouch in the fornices and opens anteriorly between the upper and lower lids, termed the palpebral fissure. The conjunctival sac contains lacrimal fluid secreted by the accessory and the main lacrimal glands. The maximum volume that can be held in the conjunctival sac is 30 μl and significantly decreased if the conjunctiva is swollen (chemosis), frequently seen in postoperative patients [1]. Thus, any eyedrop instilled into the conjunctival sac more than 30 μL flows over the lids. On histology, the conjunctiva consists of an epithelial layer (stratified epithelial cells) and a lymphoid stroma containing an adenoid layer and a fibrous layer. Accessory lacrimal glands lie in the stroma. The epithelial cells also have mucin-secreting goblet cells.

17.1.1 Blood Supply of the Conjunctiva

The blood supply of the conjunctiva is drawn mainly from the penetrating branches of the arterial arcades located at the margin of the lids. The

A. Gupta et al., *Ophthalmic Signs in Practice of Medicine*,
https://doi.org/10.1007/978-981-99-7923-3_17

medial aspects of the upper and lower lids get their supply from the medial palpebral artery (MPA), a branch of the Ophthalmic artery. The MPA runs under the medial tarsal ligament and divides into two branches. The superior MPA branches run laterally between the tarsus and the orbicularis muscle at the lid margin to form the upper eyelid's marginal arcade and above the tarsal plate to form the peripheral arcade. The inferior MPA is the main branch and runs laterally at the lower lid margin to form the inferior marginal and the peripheral arcades. The lateral aspect of the lids is supplied by the terminal branches of the lacrimal artery, which divides into a superior and inferior lateral palpebral artery to join the respective branches of the MPA to complete the marginal and peripheral arcades [2]. Smaller branches from the marginal and peripheral arcades ascend or descend in the upper and lower lids to form superficial and deep plexus to supply the muscle and skin. Other branches penetrate the tarsus plate to provide arterial blood to the palpebral conjunctiva.

The external carotid artery branches, the superficial temporal artery and angular artery, a branch of the facial artery laterally and branches of the internal carotid artery, the supraorbital and supratrochlear medially anastomose with the arcades. The upper palpebral conjunctiva receives its main supply anteriorly from the penetrating branches from the marginal arcade, which penetrate the tarsus at the level of sulcus subtarsalis and posteriorly from the descending branches from the peripheral arcade. The ascending branches from the peripheral arcade supply the conjunctival fornix and the peripheral bulbar conjunctiva [3, 4].

Muscular branches of the Ophthalmic artery give rise to seven anterior ciliary arteries, two of which run along each rectus muscle except the lateral rectus, which has a single artery. Just before the muscular arteries penetrate the sclera to form the major arterial circle with long posterior ciliary arteries at the root of the iris, they give off anterior ciliary arteries that run anteriorly in the episclera to form an epiciliary plexus around the limbus from where they penetrate the conjunctiva and form recurrent conjunctival arteries that supply 3–6 mm of para limbal conjunctiva. The other vessels form marginal loops and palisades of Vogt [5].

The veins from the palpebral conjunctiva drain into the respective venous plexuses in the lids and drain out of the orbit along the superior and inferior ophthalmic veins. Veins from the bulbar conjunctiva drain into the anterior ciliary veins.

17.1.2 Nerve Supply of the Conjunctiva

The palpebral conjunctiva has a rich nerve supply from the supratrochlear, supraorbital, lacrimal (branches of the Ophthalmic division of the CN V), and infraorbital nerves (a branch of the Maxillary division of CN V).

Branches from the long ciliary nerves supply the anterior bulbar conjunctiva. These nerves also supply the cornea. The sensory nerves form a rich plexus under the conjunctival epithelial cells and around the blood vessels.

17.1.3 Lymphatic Drainage of the Conjunctiva

The lymphatic system maintains extravascular tissue homeostasis by removing proteins and other macromolecules from the interstitial tissues. It plays a critical role in the trafficking of leukocytes. These channels are unidirectional; many are blind-ended and carry the lymph to the regional lymph nodes from where it enters the circulation. In recent years, the availability of lymphatic endothelial cell immunohistochemical markers has enabled the study of the lymphatic system in greater detail. The lymphatic channels lie under the epithelial layer of the conjunctiva, and progressively larger valved pre-collector channels lie in the sub-tenon's space [6]. These channels likely play a role in aqueous outflow as well. The lymphatic collector channels from the conjunctiva and the lateral aspects of the lids drain into the preauricular glands, while that from the medial aspect drains into the submandibular glands. However, recent scintigraphy studies in patients with lid tumours have shown preauricular lymph nodes to be the primary site of lymphatic drainage from the lids [7].

17.2 Brief Anatomy of the Cornea

The cornea is the anterior transparent continuation of the sclera and is the primary lens for transmitting light into the eye. It consists of five layers. The anterior-most is the 5–6 layered stratified epithelial layer followed by the Bowman's membrane—condensation of the anterior stromal fibres, corneal stroma, Descemet's membrane-the basement membrane, and the innermost is the single layer of post-mitotic endothelial cells. The stromal layer consists of densely packed parallel small collagen fibrils extending across the cornea. The small size and the lamellar arrangement provide for the transparency of the cornea. This layer also has extracellular matrix proteins, the proteoglycans, which provide structural stability and watch glass shape to the cornea. The cornea is avascular, but has a rich nerve ending under the epithelial layer and intercellular junctions. Stroma also contains keratocytes that continuously constitute proteoglycans [8].

17.3 Red Eyes

Compared to the palpebral conjunctiva, the bulbar conjunctiva is almost transparent, with hardly visible vessels. Many insults, from trivial to sight-threatening infections, lead to conjunctival congestion and redness. These include corneal/conjunctival sac foreign bodies, corneal abrasions (epithelial defects), trauma (Fig. 17.1), allergies, and infections caused by viral, bacterial, fungi, parasites, or foreign bodies (Fig. 17.2). Abnormalities of the tear film, dry eye disease (DED), and either deficient secretion or excessive evaporation led to inflammation of the conjunctiva. Inflammations of the episclera, sclera or uvea, and acute rise in intraocular pressure also led to conjunctival congestion.

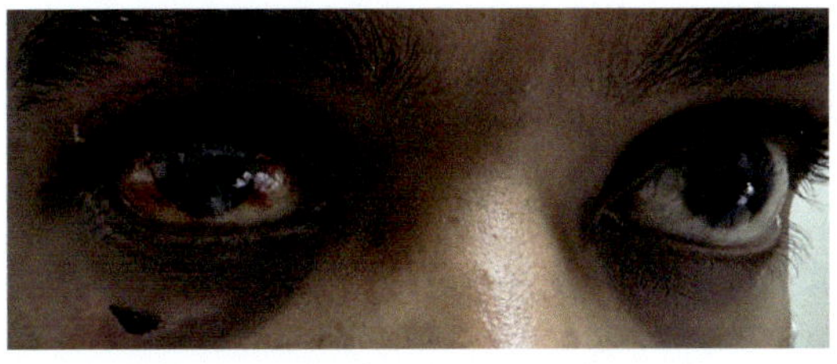

Fig. 17.1 Red eye due to subconjunctival hemorrhage following blunt trauma to the right eye

17.3.1 Allergic Conjunctivitis—Clinical Features and Pathogenetic Mechanisms in Brief

Allergies are the commonest cause of conjunctival congestion associated with congested eyes, intense itching, and lacrimation. Seasonal allergic conjunctivitis is associated with environmental allergens (pollens), while perennial is often due to household dust and dander shed by pets. Conjunctival vasodilation occurs due to the release of preformed histamine from the binding of IgE to the mast cells. The mast cells are abundant in the conjunctival stroma and, in sensitized individuals, within minutes of exposure to the allergen, these cells release preformed histamine, a potent vasodilator molecule [9]. Acute phase hypersensitivity type 1 response is seen in patients already sensitized to the offending allergen. Usually, the tight junctions between the conjunctival epithelial cells do not allow the allergens to reach the mast cells. In people prone to allergies, these junctional proteins are downregulated; moreover, contact with these allergens disrupts the epithelial barriers allowing the allergen to reach the mast cells. The antigen-specific IgE binds the receptors on the mast cells to prompt degranulation of the mast cells and the release of histamine and other amines.

During the sensitization phase, the dendritic cells and the antigen-presenting cells phagocytose and process the allergen. The peptides are presented with the HLA class II antigens to the naïve helper T-cells, which express antigen-specific receptors and finally differentiate into the effector Th1 and Th2 cells and memory T cells. The Th2 cells are involved in IgE-mediated

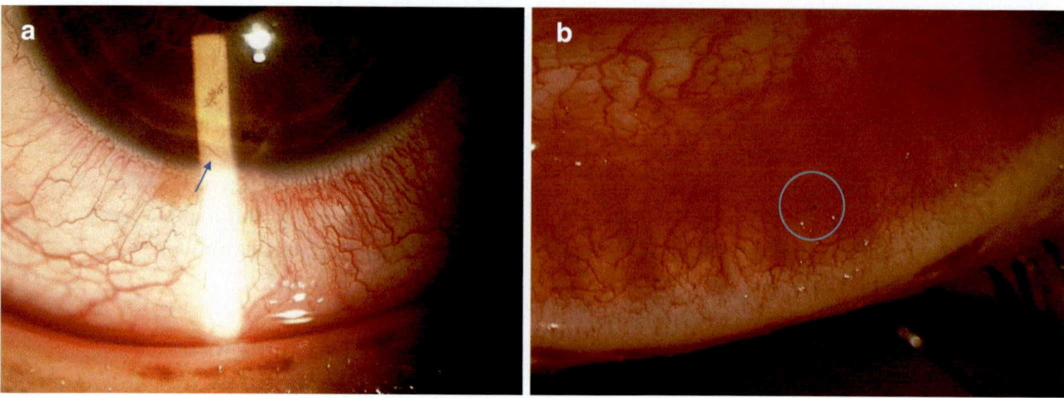

Fig. 17.2 Red eye due to caterpillar hair in the corneal stroma (arrow, **a**) and palpebral conjunctiva (circle, **b**)

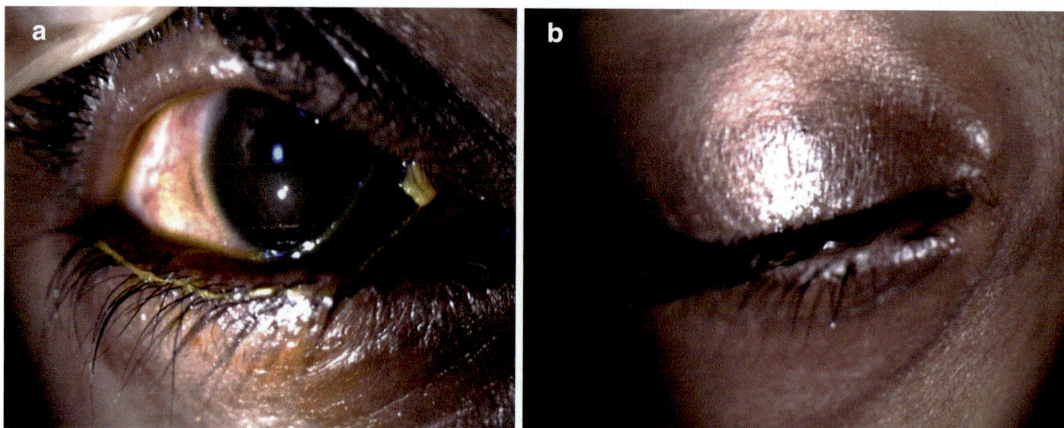

Fig. 17.3 Ropy discharge (**a**) and allergic shiners (**b**) in vernal keratoconjunctivitis. Images courtesy of Dr. Chintan Malhotra, Professor, Cornea, Lens and Refractive Surgery Services, Advanced Eye Centre, Post Graduate Institute of Medical Education and Research, Chandigarh, India

allergic response and release several cytokines, which prompt B cells to produce IgE [9, 10].

Several hours after the initial response, the mast cells release prostaglandins, leukotrienes, and chemotactic factors, which lead to increased permeability and vasodilation of the conjunctival vessels and attract leucocytes, including eosinophils and neutrophils, and set up a chronic inflammatory reaction. These are responsible for the chronic allergic response seen in vernal keratoconjunctivitis (VKC). Th2 T lymphocytes are mainly involved in the IgE-mediated allergic response activating the conjunctival and corneal epithelial cells, mast cells, and fibroblasts, expressing several inflammatory cytokines and adhesion molecules that recruit inflammatory cells, eosinophil accumulation, and mucus production [9, 11].

17.3.2 Vernal Keratoconjunctivitis

Vernal keratoconjunctivitis (VKC) is a seasonal or chronic allergic conjunctivitis most often seen in young boys and adolescents. It has a worldwide distribution, usually seen in warm climates. It is characterized by itching, intense foreign body sensation, watering, ropy thread formation, and photophobia (Fig. 17.3). It has three clinical phenotypes: giant papillary conjunctivitis (GPC) on the upper lid (Fig. 17.4), gelatinous limbal hypertrophy, and mixed type. The limbal form is

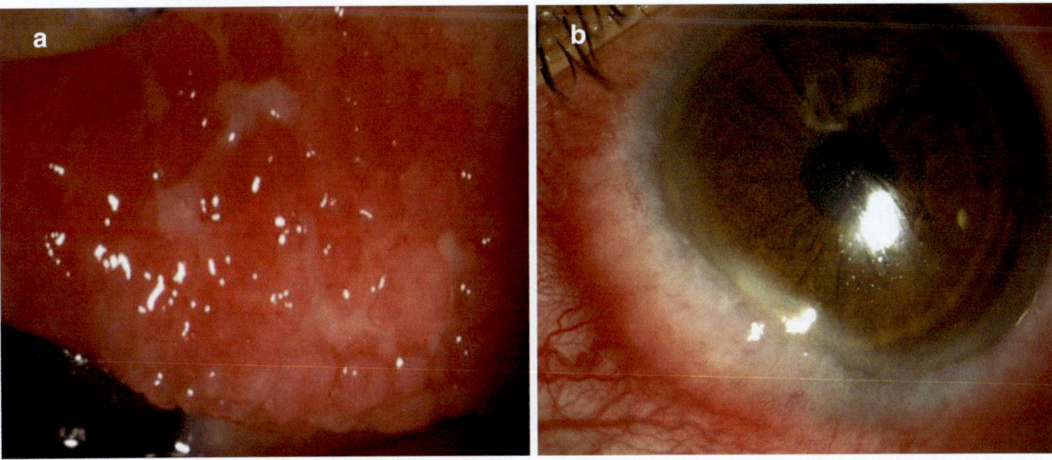

Fig. 17.4 Giant papillary conjunctivitis (**a**) and gelatinous thickening at the limbus with pseudogerontoxon (**b**) in vernal keratoconjunctivitis.Images courtesy of Dr. Chintan Malhotra, Professor, Cornea, Lens and Refractive Surgery Services, Advanced Eye Centre, Post Graduate Institute of Medical Education and Research, Chandigarh, India

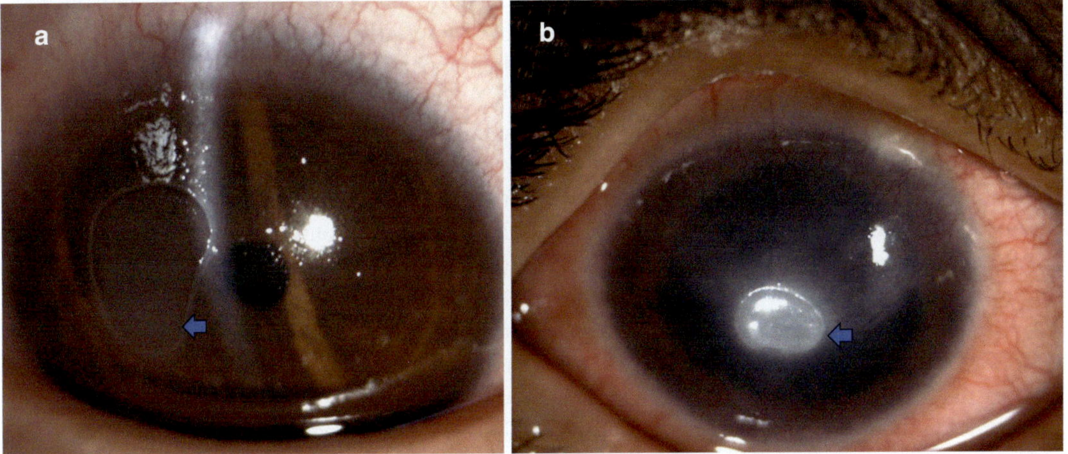

Fig. 17.5 Shield ulcers (arrows, **a**, **b**) in vernal keratoconjunctivitis are typically oval or pentagonal, superficial, and often superiorly located. Images courtesy of Dr. Chintan Malhotra, Professor, Cornea, Lens and Refractive Surgery Services, Advanced Eye Centre, Post Graduate Institute of Medical Education and Research, Chandigarh, India

seen more frequently than the GPC [12]. The formation of shield ulcers complicates VKC (Fig. 17.5). Nearly 50% of the affected children do not have a family history of allergies or show any atopic diathesis or IgE sensitization; most of those testing negative have limbal VKC. The disease is significantly more common in males (2–4:1). It spontaneously resolves after the onset of puberty, indicating a role of sex hormones [11, 13].

VKC is driven by a Th2 immune response, IL4, IL9, and IL13 prompting the B cells to produce IgE. Overexpression of IL5 and GM-CSF drives the overproduction of eosinophils and IL3 from the mast cells. Cells in the VKC patients' tears may go up to 45%. One of the most characteristic findings in the palpebral conjunctiva is excessive connective tissue growth in the substantia propria and the formation of sessile papilliform growths (Fig. 17.4). These are accompanied by capillary proliferation to support the papillae. It is due to increased growth factors, namely the epidermal growth factor, TGFb-1and fibroblastic growth factor detectable in the tissue supernatants as well tears of these patients [12]. Moreover, there is almost a 5X increase in the goblet cell density in the conjunctival epithelium with the overproduction of ropey mucus (Fig. 17.3).

The treatment of VKC follows the severity of symptoms. In mild cases, topical mast cell stabilizers, sodium cromoglycate 2–4%, lodoxamide 0.1%, or dual action (anti-histamine receptor and mast cell stabilizer) Olopatadine 0.1% have been effective. Preservative-free tear drops should be frequently instilled to dilute the inflammatory cytokines. While corticosteroids are most effective in VKC, these run the risk of causing glaucoma and are reserved for exacerbations of VKC. Immunomodulatory drugs, topical cyclosporine A 2% (CsA) or tacrolimus 0.1% ointment, are the drugs of choice in patients with GPC for long-term use [14]. More recently, CsA in cationic emulsion 0.1% four times daily improved quality of life and ameliorated symptoms in VKC children over 12 months of follow-up [15, 16]. For more detailed information, the readers may refer to detailed guidelines provided by the UK and European groups [17, 18].

17.4 Infectious Conjunctivitis

Patients with infectious conjunctivitis frequently present to primary care physicians. Most of these may be caused by bacteria, viruses, or chlamydia. Among the children, infectious conjunctivitis was bacterial in 71% and viral in 16%. On the other hand, in adults, viral conjunctivitis was seen in 78% and bacterial in 16%. In children, mucopurulent discharge associated with otitis media is more frequently seen due to bacterial infections, whereas viral conjunctivitis is common among adults. Contact with another person with conjunctivitis, preauricular lymph nodes, and pharyngitis favour diagnosis of viral conjunctivitis [19].

17.4.1 Viral Conjunctivitis

It is important to note that different viruses, such as adenovirus, herpes simplex, and enterovirus, can cause viral conjunctivitis. The clinical features may vary depending on the specific virus causing the infection. Adenoviruses cause 65–90% of viral conjunctivitis [20, 21].

17.4.1.1 Epidemic Keratoconjunctivitis

The epidemic keratoconjunctivitis (EKC) is often caused by highly contagious human adenovirus (HAdV) serotypes 8, 19, 37,53, and 54 [22]. HAdV serotypes 1, 2, 3, 4, 5, and 7 cause children's pharyngoconjunctival fever (PCF). The PCF infection is contracted by swimming in contaminated water. On the other hand, the EKC virus is usually contracted in eye clinics, contaminated surfaces, solutions, or instruments. If one family member contracts EKC, it rapidly spreads to the other family members. The HAdV enters the epithelial cells by adhering to the two receptors, the coxsackie adenovirus receptor (CAR) and the junction-adhesion molecule [23], followed by endocytosis of the virus. The virus initially elicits an innate immune response mediated by natural killer cells and type 1 interferon; later, the body mounts an adaptive immune response by the CD 8+ T cells and Th1 cells mediated by interferon-gamma (IFN).

In children, PCF is characterized by fever, pharyngitis, follicular conjunctivitis, and preauricular lymphadenopathy. There is an overlap between the clinical manifestations of the PCF and the EKC.

The EKC is the more severe of the two [22]. The symptoms of EKC usually appear suddenly and can be severe. Both eyes are usually affected, and the symptoms are often worse in one eye. The conjunctiva appears intensely red, and the small blood vessels are visible on its surface and

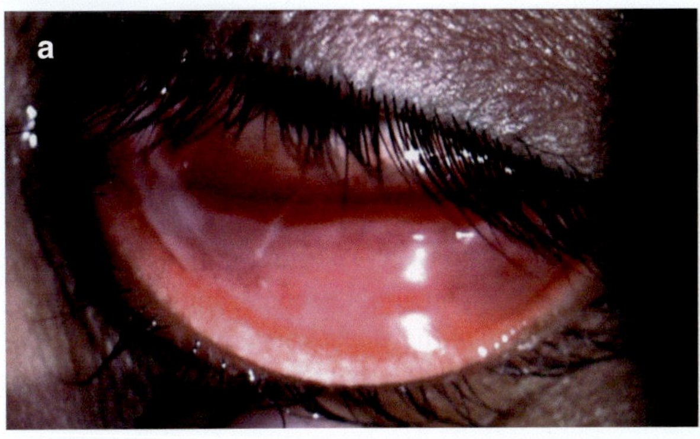

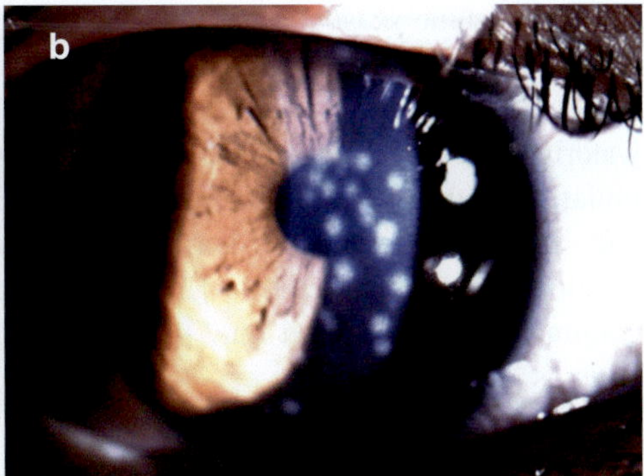

Fig. 17.6 Pseudomembrane in the inferior fornix (**a**) in Epidemic Keratoconjunctivitis and subepithelial infiltrates (**b**) in Adenoviral conjunctivitis. Images courtesy of Dr. Chintan Malhotra, Professor, Cornea, Lens and Refractive Surgery Services, Advanced Eye Centre, Post Graduate Institute of Medical Education and Research, Chandigarh, India

may be accompanied by varying amounts of petechial or subconjunctival hemorrhages. There is conjunctival and eyelid edema. The eyes have a gritty sensation and have sand in them feeling. There may be a copious amount of thick, stringy discharge from the eyes. In severe cases, a pseudo membrane may form on the conjunctiva, which can be peeled off to reveal a raw surface underneath. It is a collection of necrotic material, fibrin, and leucocytes (Fig. 17.6a).

The eyes become sensitive to light, and bright light can cause pain. Swollen lymph nodes may be present in front of the ear (preauricular lymphadenopathy). Two to three days after the onset, subepithelial infiltrates (SEI) appear in the cornea as small, raised bumps that may cause blurred vision (Fig. 17.6b). These are caused by viral replication in the corneal epithelium and the stroma. While PCF is self-limiting in 2–3 weeks, EKC can have a prolonged course, with symptoms lasting several weeks or even months.

One of the most serious, although infrequent systemic complications of EKC is the development of Guillain-Barre syndrome (GBS). This rare but serious neurological disorder can occur after an infection or vaccination. There have been reports of GBS occurring after viral infections, including the adenovirus infections (1:1,000,000) that cause epidemic viral conjunctivitis (EKC). Symptoms of GBS can include weakness or tingling in the legs or arms, difficulty walking or standing, and difficulty moving the eyes or facial muscles. Urgent medical attention is required if a patient experiences these symptoms after a viral infection.

It is important to note that EKC is highly contagious, and proper hygiene measures such as frequent handwashing and avoiding touching the eyes can help prevent its spread. The treatment includes irrigation with povidone-iodine 5%. It is a broad-spectrum antiseptic and effective against extracellular viruses; eliminating the shed virus may decrease the infectivity of the individuals. Topical corticosteroids effectively relieve the symptoms and the SEI, but the latter return soon after stopping the treatment. Moreover, using corticosteroids in herpetic keratitis with a mistaken diagnosis of EKC could result in blindness [24]. Combining povidone-iodine 1% and dexamethasone 0.1% led to a rapid improvement in 5–7 days [25]. Tacrolimus 0.03% ointment applied twice daily for 22 weeks significantly relieved symptoms and resolved the SEI [26]. However, there needs to be a higher certainty level of any treatment protocols for EKC [20].

17.4.1.2 Herpes Simplex Virus Conjunctivitis

It is clinically difficult to differentiate between Herpes simplex virus (HSV) follicular conjunctivitis and the EKC. In a series of viral conjunctivitis in Japan, 4.8% were positive for HSV type1 by cell culture, 80.3% for HAdV, and 5.7% for chlamydia trachomatis [27]. HSV conjunctivitis shows the same seasonal variation from June to August as with HAdV. Most patients complained of discharge, itching, foreign body sensation, and watering. Most cases of HSV conjunctivitis were unilateral and resolved in 8–9 days. Nearly 30% had superficial punctate keratitis, but none developed dendritic keratitis [27]. HSV type 2 conjunctivitis is rare and may be seen in HIV+ patients [28].

17.4.2 Bacterial Conjunctivitis

Bacterial conjunctivitis is commonly seen in children under 12 and may be associated with otitis media. Gram-positive more than gram-negative organisms cause bacterial conjunctivitis. Usually, it has an abrupt onset and spreads to the other eye within a day. The patient may complain of watering, redness, and mucopurulent discharge. Diagnosis of bacterial conjunctivitis is not a challenge, and cultures from the secretions may be done if the patient does not respond to initial therapy. Bacterial conjunctivitis is usually treated with frequent application of broad-spectrum fluoroquinolones. Unlike HAdV infection, lymphadenopathy is uncommon in bacterial conjunctivitis except those caused by methicillin-resistant Staphylococcus aureus and Neisseria Gonorrhea. The latter causes the exuberant purulent discharge. Gonococcal conjunctivitis is hyperacute and seen in sexually active young adults. It spreads rapidly to the cornea and may perforate the eye and hence needs to be seen urgently by an ophthalmologist for systemic and local aggressive therapy with fluoroquinolones [29] HM.

Current recommendations include giving a single dose of intramuscular ceftriaxone 500 mg. If chlamydial infection has not been ruled out, doxycycline 100 mg twice daily for 7 days is recommended [30].

17.4.2.1 Ophthalmia Neonatorum

Ophthalmia neonatorum is conjunctivitis in newborns within the first month of life. It is typically caused by bacterial or viral infections, although chemical irritants or other factors can also cause it.

With the introduction of routine prophylactic eye drops or ointment containing antibiotics such as erythromycin or tetracycline, the incidence of bacterial ophthalmia neonatorum has significantly decreased in developed countries. However, ophthalmia neonatorum is still seen in some parts of the world where prophylactic measures may not be routinely implemented, such as in developing countries or where there is inadequate or absent prenatal care.

The most common bacterial cause of ophthalmia neonatorum is Neisseria gonorrhoeae, which is a sexually transmitted infection that can be transmitted from an infected mother to her baby during delivery. The incubation period for gonococcal infection is 24–48 h, while that for chlamydial infection is 5–14 days. If the mother has gonorrhoea, but the baby does not yet show any signs of infection, ceftriaxone 20–50 mg/kg body weight not to exceed 250 mg be administered as a single intramuscular or intravenous dose [30].

Other bacteria that can cause ophthalmia neonatorum include Chlamydia trachomatis, Streptococcus pneumoniae, and Haemophilus influenzae. Viral infections that can cause ophthalmia neonatorum include herpes simplex, varicella-zoster, and adenovirus. Chemical irritants such as silver nitrate, other topical antiseptics, and trauma during delivery can also cause ophthalmia neonatorum, which usually manifests within hours.

Prompt diagnosis and treatment of ophthalmia neonatorum are essential to prevent complications such as corneal ulceration, scarring, and blindness. Treatment typically involves topical antibiotics or antiviral medications, depending on the cause of the infection.

17.4.2.2 Chlamydial Infection of Conjunctiva

Trachoma

Trachoma is a bacterial eye infection in young preschool children caused by Chlamydia trachomatis, serotypes A-C. It is a leading cause of irreversible but preventable blindness in at least 42 countries, particularly in areas with poor sanitation, water shortage, crowded families, and limited access to healthcare. According to the World Health Organization, trachoma is estimated to be responsible for blindness or visual impairment in around 1.9 million people worldwide and 1.4% of all blindness. As of June 2022, 125 million people live in the areas at risk for developing trachoma (https://www.who.int/news-room/fact-sheets/detail/trachoma).

The acute infection with chlamydia trachomatis typically presents as follicular conjunctivitis, characterized by small, white, or yellow bumps on the inner surface of the eyelids. Direct fluorescent antibody testing from the everted upper lid is the only FDA-approved test for chlamydial conjunctival infections [30]. Other tell-tale signs of trachoma include an Arlt's line (of scarring) at the junction of anterior one-third and posterior two-thirds of the upper palpebral conjunctiva. Herbert's pits are formed at the upper limbus by scarring of the limbal follicles and a trachomatous pannus with corneal haze in the superior cornea. Repeated infections lead to inflammation and scarring of the conjunctiva, which can result in the development of trichiasis (inward turning of the eyelashes) and entropion (inward turning of the eyelid margin). Trichiasis can cause the eyelashes to rub against the cornea, leading to corneal ulceration, opacity, scarring, and blindness. Trachoma sequelae are seen in patients with frequent superadded bacterial co-infections and manifest by the time the person is 30–40 years old. Women are affected four times more often than men because of proximity to their infected children.

The infection spreads from person to person by the hand and by sharing clothes and bedding. House flies are a major carrier of infection from one child to the other. The house flies feed on the overflow of conjunctival discharge and spread the infection to the other children.

Treatment of trachoma typically involves a combination of antibiotics, such as azithromycin (single dose 20 mg/kg of body weight), or doxycycline (100 mg twice a day for 3–4 weeks) to clear the infection, along with surgery to correct any eyelid abnormalities such as trichiasis or entropion. In addition to treatment, prevention is a critical component of trachoma control programs, including improving sanitation and hygiene, promoting facial cleanliness, and implementing community-wide mass drug administration programs to distribute antibiotics to at-risk populations.

The WHO recommended a SAFE strategy; S for the surgical treatment of trachomatous trichiasis, A for antibiotics for mass administration (azithromycin), F for facial cleanliness, and E for environmental improvement, especially the availability of water and sanitation.

The World Health Organization had set a goal of eliminating trachoma as a public health problem by 2020, which involves reducing the prevalence of trachomatous inflammation-follicular (TF) to less than 5% in children aged 1–9 years and reducing the prevalence of trachomatous trichiasis (TT) to less than 1 case per 1000 population. Till October 2022, 15 countries in Africa, Asia, and the Middle East had been declared trachoma-free (https://www.who.int/news-room/fact-sheets/detail/trachoma).

Inclusion Conjunctivitis

Chlamydia trachomatis (*C. trachomatis*) serotypes D-K is among the most common sexually transmitted infections. It may manifest as painful urination or pelvic pain, pain during sexual intercourse or vaginal discharge. Women are more commonly infected. Infected women can pass on the chlamydial infection to their babies, resulting in ophthalmia neonatorum. It may remain asymptomatic in many infected patients adding to the pool of infected individuals in society. Inclusion conjunctivitis (IC) due to *C. trachomatis* is seen in sexually active persons and is transmitted to the eyes by hand from the infected genitalia. It often results in unilateral mild follicular conjunctivitis with or without mucopurulent discharge and preauricular lymphadenopathy. Unlike trachoma, which infects the upper palpebral conjunctiva, genital IC predominantly affects the lower lid. There are no cicatricial sequelae of IC.

The chlamydial infection is diagnosed by doing a nucleic acid amplification test from the vaginal discharge in women and urine in men. Direct fluorescent antibody testing from the everted upper lid is the only FDA-approved test for chlamydial conjunctival infections [30]. CDC recommends annual screening for sexually active women less than <25 years of age or older women with multiple sex partners. IC can be diagnosed by demonstrating basophilic cytoplasmic inclusion bodies on Giemsa stain or immunofluorescence staining of the conjunctival smears. Oral treatment with doxycycline 100 mg twice a day for 7 days, erythromycin 250 mg four times a day for 7 days, or a single dose of oral azithromycin 1 gm or levofloxacin 500 mg twice a day for 7 days is recommended for chlamydial infections.

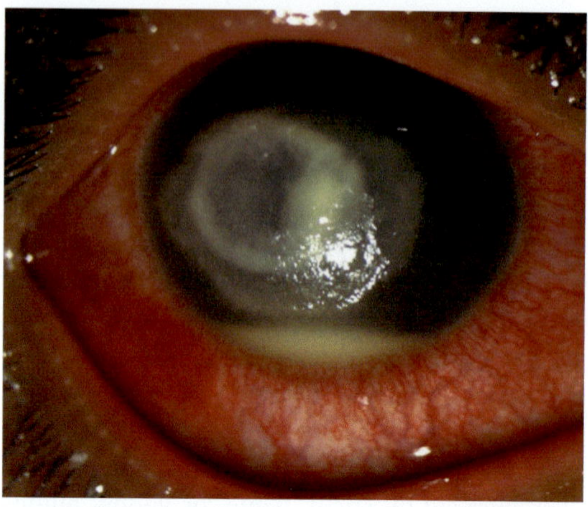

Fig. 17.7 Fungal keratitis due to *Fusarium Solanii.* Image courtesy of Dr. Chintan Malhotra, Professor, Cornea, Lens and Refractive Surgery Services, Advanced Eye Centre, Post Graduate Institute of Medical Education and Research, Chandigarh, India

17.5 Corneal Ulcers

Corneal ulcers are the leading cause of corneal blindness in developing and economically weaker countries of Asia and sub-Saharan Africa. A corneal epithelium defect and stroma infiltration with inflammatory cells and necrosis characterize corneal ulcers. Many infections, trauma, dry eye, contact lens wear, autoimmune disorders, and systemic diseases can cause them. They constitute an eye emergency and lead to corneal perforation, endophthalmitis, and permanent loss of vision if not timely treated. Bacteria, viruses, fungi, or parasites cause these. Even if treated adequately and timely, it leaves behind corneal scars (opacities) that interfere with vision if located in the visual axis and may require corneal grafts.

Gross regional and geographical differences exist in the prevalence of the various types of corneal ulcers. Epidemiological data are available from tertiary care referral centres, which the patient reaches after unsuccessful attempts to treat these at primary or secondary care facilities or even after self-treatments. Fungal keratitis is the most common cause of microbial keratitis in tropical and subtropical countries, especially in low-income countries (Fig. 17.7).

While bacterial infections were more predominant in the past (Fig. 17.8), filamentous fungal infections have become a significant challenge worldwide, especially in extended-wear contact lens users among the economically poorer segments, even in developed countries [31]. Contaminated contact lens solutions have led to outbreaks of fusarium keratitis even in the developed world [32].

There is a delay in diagnosis as the ophthalmologists are unfamiliar with fungal keratitis as it has been traditionally considered a disease of tropical and subtropical countries [33].

17.5.1 Microbiological Profile of Corneal Ulcers

The yield using traditional microbiological methods for diagnosing corneal ulcers, such as smears and cultures, is poor as most patients have been exposed to broad-spectrum antibiotics.

In recent microbiological studies of corneal ulcers treated at tertiary referral centres in South and West India, culture positivity was only 37.5% (n = 312) and 27% (n = 100), respectively [34, 35]. Almost similar culture positivity rates (37.7%) were seen in infectious keratitis in

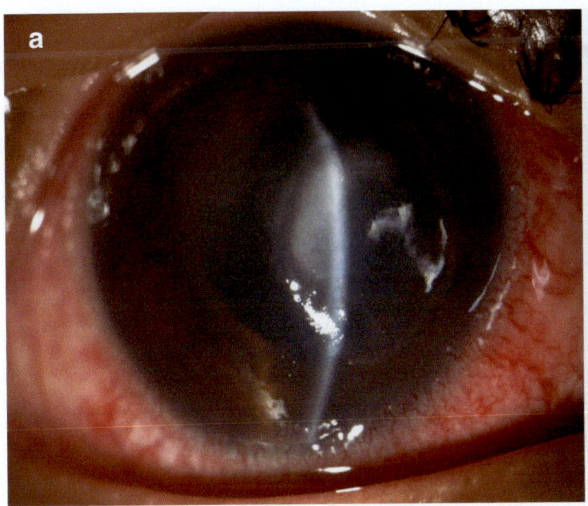

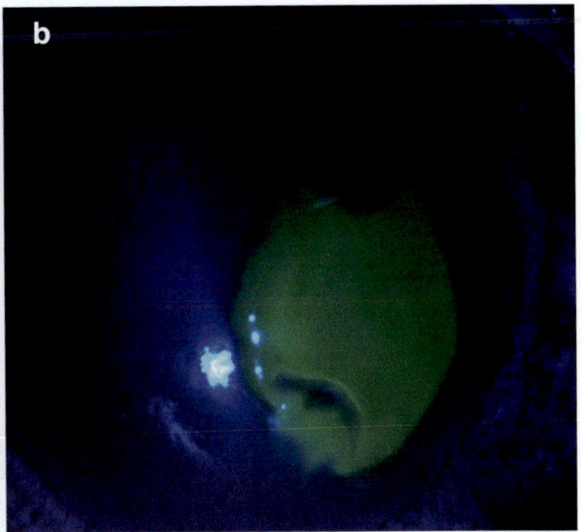

Fig. 17.8 Contact lens induced Pseudomonas keratitis in a young female patient, with crescent-shaped infiltrate surrounded by large area of stromal lysis (**a**). Fluorescein staining reveals a large epithelial defect (**b**). Images courtesy of Dr. Chintan Malhotra, Professor, Cornea, Lens and Refractive Surgery Services, Advanced Eye Centre, Post Graduate Institute of Medical Education and Research, Chandigarh, India

the UK [36]. There are wide variations in the microbial profile of corneal ulcers in various parts of the world. Of the culture-positive cases, 44.5–48% were bacterial, and 49.5–52% were fungal in India [34, 35], while in the UK, bacterial corneal ulcers were seen in 98.2%, acanthamoeba in 4.2%, and fungal in 3% [36]. Herpes simplex virus (HSV) is one of the commonest causes of keratitis in the industrialized world. They have a characteristic clinical picture, and effective antiviral therapy is available; recurrences constitute a significant challenge as the HSV remains latent in the trigeminal ganglion.

17.5.2 Predisposing Factors for Corneal Ulcers

Viral corneal ulcers are the commonest cause of corneal ulceration and pose a significant challenge because of the frequent recurrences throughout a person's life. Dry eye and atopic disease are risk factors for recurrences of HSV keratitis. Stress induced by physical, psychological, hormonal, fever, surgery, contact lens wear, or injury may cause a recurrence of HSV keratitis. Alpha-adrenergic drugs and steroids increase viral replication. HIV infection, immunosuppressive therapy, and corticosteroids decrease the immune response to the viral infection [37].

On the other hand, local factors such as corneal foreign bodies, corneal abrasion from trichiasis, dry eyes, sleeping overnight with contact lenses, use of corticosteroid eye drops for trivial trauma, and diabetes are some of the major predisposing factors that compromise the corneal epithelial barrier and predispose to the development of bacterial or fungal corneal ulcers. Corneal ulcers are a preventable cause of blindness even if only rudimentary health care is available, especially in rural areas. In a prospective study, using chloramphenicol eye drops three times a day in patients with corneal abrasions prevented infection in 96% and none who presented within 18 h developed corneal ulcers [38]. Using contaminated contact lens solutions or swimming in contaminated pools predisposes *Acanthamoeba* keratitis (Figs. 17.9 and 17.10), a parasitic corneal infection. In predominant agricultural economies, trauma sustained during agricultural activities, especially harvesting, is a significant risk for fungal keratitis (Fig. 17.7).

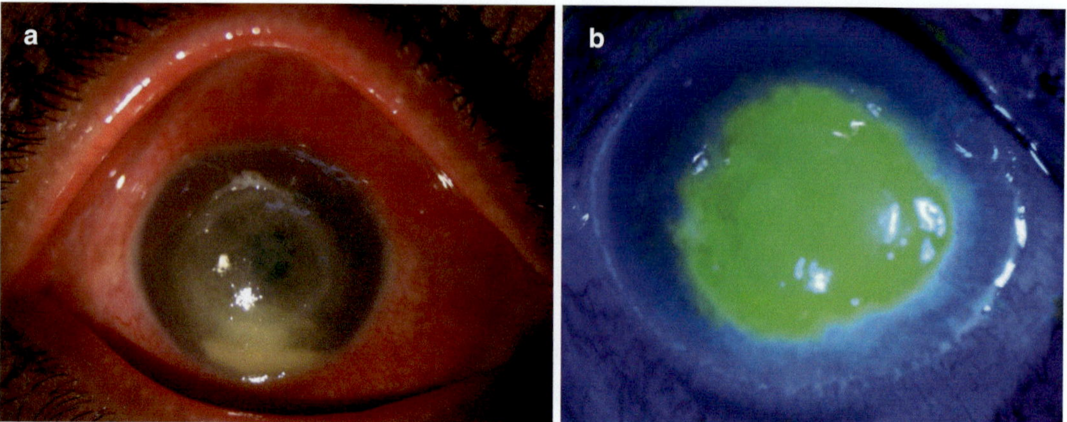

Fig. 17.9 Ring infiltrates with hypopyon in a case of acanthamoeba keratitis (**a**) and fluorescein staining (**b**), revealing the extent of the ulcer. Images courtesy of Dr. Chintan Malhotra, Professor, Cornea, Lens and Refractive Surgery Services, Advanced Eye Centre, Post Graduate Institute of Medical Education and Research, Chandigarh, India

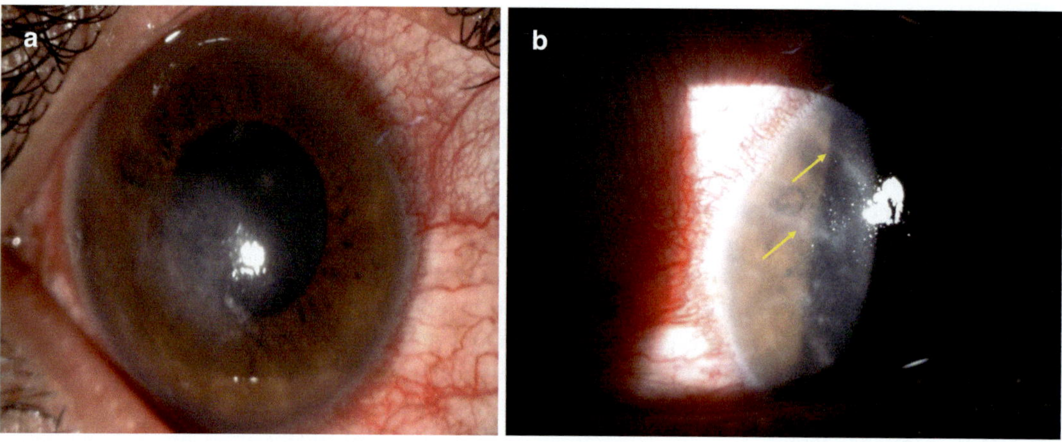

Fig. 17.10 Another case of Acanthamoeba keratitis (**a**) with radial keratoneuritis (arrows) seen in the peripheral cornea (**b**). Images courtesy of Dr. Chintan Malhotra, Professor, Cornea, Lens and Refractive Surgery Services, Advanced Eye Centre, Post Graduate Institute of Medical Education and Research, Chandigarh, India

17.5.3 Clinical Features of Corneal Ulcers

17.5.3.1 Viral Ulcers

Herpes Simplex and Varicella-zoster are the two major causes of viral corneal ulcers. Herpetic corneal ulcers typically present with a dendritic pattern on the cornea, a branching ulcer with distinct edges. Patients may report a history of recurrent episodes of eye pain, redness, and watering. Vision may be impaired if the ulcer involves the visual axis.

Herpes Simplex Virus Keratitis

Dendritic corneal ulcers are a typical manifestation of the Herpes simplex virus (HSV) infection and are the commonest cause of corneal ulcers in the world's developed economies. These account for nearly 66% of all HSV keratitis patients [39].

The global incidence is 1.5 million cases, of whom 40,000 go blind or have severe visual impairment yearly [40]. It is a largely unilateral disease. The dendrites appear in the corneal epithelium as a dead-tree branching pattern and cause redness and irritation of the eye, blurred

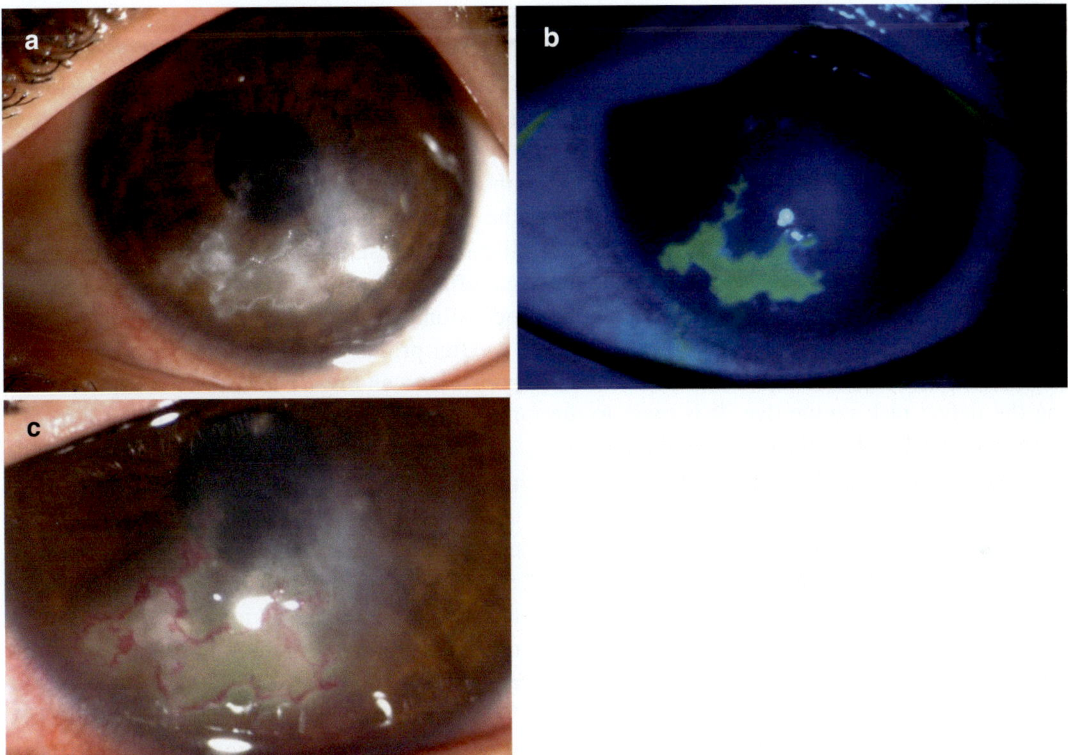

Fig. 17.11 Slit lamp photo of the dendro-geographic lesion due to HSV Keratitis in diffuse illumination (**a**), fluorescein staining of the base of the ulcer (**b**), and Rose Bengal staining of the edges containing the viral laden cells (**c**). Images courtesy of Dr. Chintan Malhotra, Professor, Cornea, Lens and Refractive Surgery Services, Advanced Eye Centre, Post Graduate Institute of Medical Education and Research, Chandigarh, India

vision, foreign body sensation, watery eyes, and photophobia [37]. Superficial punctate keratitis may precede the development of dendrites (Fig. 17.11). Corneal sensations are dull. These need to be differentiated from other causes of keratitis and promptly treated. Delayed treatment or exposure to corticosteroids can lead to an extension of the lesions into the corneal stroma. The HSV dendrites are best diagnosed on the slit-lamp after staining with fluorescein dye (Fig. 17.11). The HSV dendrites need to be differentiated from the VZV dendrites.

Herpes Zoster Ophthalmicus

Following a subclinical infection or a Chickenpox (varicella) attack, the primary varicella-zoster virus (VZV) infection becomes latent in the dorsal sensory ganglia. VZV-specific cell-mediated immunity keeps the virus from getting reactivated. In old age and with decreased immunity, the virus may reactivate and travel along the neurons to manifest as a recurrent infection called herpes zoster (shingles). The risk of herpes zoster (HZ) is 15 X more in HIV than the non-HIV patients. Thus, the varicella vaccine is recommended for people above the age of 50 years and those who are likely to be immunosuppressed.

When it involves the trigeminal nerve's ophthalmic branch, it leads to a painful eruption of skin vesicles—herpes zoster Ophthalmicus in the dermatome served by the Ophthalmic division of CN V. When the nasociliary branch is affected, it may manifest as VZV keratitis as well as uveitis. The eruptions are often preceded by pain in the affected dermatome [41]. Nearly 2.5% of all HZ patients develop ocular complications, including keratitis (76%), uveitis (46%), and conjunctivitis (35%). Recurrences were seen in ~7% each of keratitis and uveitis [42]. The HZO lesions in the cornea appear as SPK or micro dendrites with epithelial defects and raised edges or as stromal keratitis associated with severe pain.

Differentiating HSV and VZV Keratitis

The HSV dendrites are typically thin with linear branching and terminal bulbs. The epithelial defect allows the fluorescein dye to diffuse and stain the corneal tissue. The rose bengal dye stains the HSV dendrites poorly and may appear punctate as the devitalized epithelial cells bordering the defect pick up the dye. It is toxic to the normal corneal and conjunctival epithelium, so its use is discouraged. In the VZV Keratitis (VZK), the dendrites are fewer, short, and stumpy and do not show terminal bulbs. These are seen in the peripheral cornea. The VZK dendrites stain better with rose bengal than fluorescein.

Other Clinical Manifestations of HSV and VZV

Exposure to corticosteroids or confluence of several dendrites may progress to a geographic lesion. The periphery of these geographic lesions shows branching dendrites to differentiate them from non-epithelizing geographic lesions that develop into meta herpetic lesions. The floor and border of the meta herpetic lesions are covered with devitalized heaped-up epithelial cells, which stain with rose bengal. The base of the geographic lesions does not stain with rose bengal stain. The immune response to the HSV and VZV causes an inflammatory reaction in the stroma, leading to edema, neovascularization, and scarring. The immune response can also cause damage to the corneal nerves, leading to decreased corneal sensitivity. Even in one eye, damage to the sensory corneal nerves can reduce brainstem signals to the lacrimal gland in both eyes, reduce the reflex secretion of tears, and cause dry eye disease. The other clinical manifestation includes stromal keratitis with or, more often, without ulceration with yellowish-white infiltrates. An immune-mediated clinical manifestation is disc-shaped corneal stromal edema, the disciform keratitis associated with keratic precipitates confined to the area of the stromal edema.

Pathogenesis of HSV and VZV Keratitis

The primary HSV infection is asymptomatic. Ninety percent of the world's population is infected. Seroprevalence in the US is 27% in the younger age group, increasing up to 60% above the age of 50 years [43]. The HSV and the VZV viruses are unique as they establish a life-long presence/latency in the cranial nerve ganglia's neuronal cells and get activated occasionally.

After primary infection, the virus enters sensory nerve endings and travels along axons to the sensory ganglia, establishing latent infection in a subset of neurons. During the latent phase, the virus does not actively replicate. The HSV evades immune recognition by producing non-coding microRNA that suppresses lytic gene expression and limits the expression of proteins, thus disabling the host's innate immune mechanisms to eliminate the infected host cells. The reactivation of the VZV is kept in check by VZV-specific T cell-mediated response. HSV shows frequent reactivation, and the virus is shed regularly. However, since not all the infected cells show activation simultaneously, clinical disease may not become apparent every time the virus is shed [44]. HSV causes frequent recurrences of epithelial keratitis and anterior uveitis. The shed virus remains subclinical. However, if they cross a threshold number, they can cause necrosis of epithelial cells. The virus spreads from cell to cell and clinically appears as branches of a dead tree.

Recurrences of HSV Keratitis

HSV keratitis is a recurrent disease and the frequency and severity increase with the duration of the disease. There are individual variations. 30–50% show recurrences in the first year.

Diagnosis of HSV and VZV Keratitis

Diagnosis of dendritic HSV and VZV (when accompanied by HZO) is mainly clinical. Real-time PCR can confirm the diagnosis of HSV keratitis in cases of endotheliitis with feathery stromal keratitis that poses a diagnostic challenge [45].

Treatment of HSV and VZV Keratitis

For the dendritic HSK or VZV keratitis, the treatment of choice is acyclovir 3% ointment five times daily, trifluridine 1% every 2 hourly (maximum nine times daily), or ganciclovir 0.15% five times daily until the lesions are healed. Alternately, oral valacyclovir 500 mg twice daily or acyclovir 400 mg five times daily can be used. Scraping of lesions hastens the healing of the epithelial lesions. For stromal HSK or VZK, topical therapy has poor penetration. They are treated with oral antivirals as listed above except in cases of concomitant HZO, when the dose of valacyclovir is increased to 1000 mg/three times daily or acyclovir 800 mg five times daily for 7–10 days. Topical corticosteroids can be started after initiating oral antivirals only if there is no ulceration. Disciform keratitis is treated with topical steroids [37].

Prevention of Recurrences of HSV Keratitis

If there are more than three attacks of dendritic keratitis or more than two attacks of stromal keratitis, oral acyclovir 400 mg twice a day or valacyclovir 500 mg daily may be given for 6–12 months. Topical steroids or cyclosporine/tacrolimus may be considered if there are frequent relapses despite oral antivirals [37]. In patients who undergo corneal grafting, oral acyclovir may reduce the incidence of HSV keratitis [46].

17.5.3.2 Bacterial Corneal Ulcers

Bacterial infection is the most common cause of corneal ulcers in developing countries. *Staphylococcus aureus, Pseudomonas aeruginosa,* and *Streptococcus pneumoniae* are the most common bacterial pathogens responsible for corneal ulcers. *Pseudomonas aeruginosa* (26%), *Staph aureus* (11%), and coagulase-negative Staph species (11%) were isolated in a West India series [34]. *Staph aureus* (18%), *Pseudomonas aeruginosa* (8.5%), *Strep. pneumonia* (8%), coagulase-negative Staph spp. (7%), and other gram-negative bacilli (6%) were isolated in the South India series [35]. In the UK, Gram-positive organisms were isolated most commonly (53.8%) and Gram-negative in 39% [36].

It is critical to differentiate between the various types of infective corneal ulcers. Patients with bacterial corneal ulcers usually present with eye pain, redness, photophobia, diminution of vision, and a discharge that can be purulent or mucopurulent. The ulcer appears as a white, grey, yellowish opacification of the cornea, surrounded by infiltrates or satellite lesions (Fig. 17.8). The eye is severely congested, with mucopurulent discharge sticking to the corneal ulcer. Vision is reduced due to corneal edema and infiltrates in the cornea. There is often a ground glass appearance of the rest of the cornea in rapidly progressive bacterial ulcers due to Pseudomonas aeruginosa infection. A hypopyon (layered collection of leukocytes and fibrin) in the anterior chamber frequently accompanies bacterial corneal ulcers.

17.5.3.3 Fungal Corneal Ulcers

Fungal infections can also cause corneal ulcers, especially in patients with a weakened immune system, contact lens wearers, or those who have experienced trauma with vegetable matter to the eye. The most common fungal pathogens are *Aspergillus* and *Fusarium* species (spp.). Mixed infection may also be seen. Among the fungal corneal ulcers, *Fusarium* spp. was the most isolated (36%), followed by aspergillus spp. (11%) in the South India series [35], while in the West India series, *Aspergillus flavus* (30%) and *Aspergillus niger* (22%) were isolated [34].

Fungal corneal ulcers can have a similar clinical appearance to bacterial ulcers. They are usually dry looking, elevated above the surface and with little discharge. Fungal ulcers tend to have satellite lesions. They tend to progress more slowly and can be associated with a feathery or filamentous appearance. Hypopyon in fungal ulcers tends to be disproportionate to the extent of the corneal ulcers and appears convex (Fig. 17.7). Often there is a plaque on the posterior surface of the cornea. Vision loss is common. Treating fungal keratitis is a major challenge because of delayed diagnosis, non-availability of trained human laboratory resources or point-of-care testing and non-efficacy of the known antifungal agents or non-availability.

17.5.3.4 Management of Corneal Ulcers

There is often a challenge in telling the fungal from bacterial keratitis. In the management of corneal ulcers, not only is the detection of the offending microbe important, but it is also critical to note the response to treatment and the healing or worsening of the lesion. Manual drawings or photography are thus essential to document the lesion. Location, size and depth of the lesion, any areas of thinning or impending perforation, intracorneal hemorrhage, corneal vascularization, corneal sensations in the unaffected part of the cornea and associated signs such as the size of the hypopyon are essential to document. Staining with fluorescein sodium can show the characteristic staining pattern seen in HSV dendritic or geographical keratitis. The size of the epithelial defect, as noted after staining with fluorescein sodium, can be a good indicator for recording the response to treatment.

After clearing the discharge and debris, multiple scrapings are taken from the base and the progressive edge of the ulcer. Smears are prepared for microscopic examination after staining with the Gram and Giemsa stains and KOH 10% + calcofluor white (CFW) staining. Culture media, blood agar, chocolate agar, MacConkey agar for the bacterial, and Sabouraud's dextrose agar for fungi are inoculated for culture and sensitivity. In one of the largest series of fungal keratitis (n = 1354), smear examination alone led to the fungal etiology in >95% of the cases [47]. The positivity of smears is higher in advanced cases of keratitis than in early cases. The Gram stain detected bacteria in 36% of early vs 41% of advanced cases of bacterial keratitis. KOH + CFW detected 61% of the early vs 81% of advanced fungal keratitis [48]. The authors recommended initiating antifungal therapy based on smear examination [47, 48].

The major challenge in bacterial corneal ulcers is the inability to obtain positive cultures at the most in only 40% of the patients. All bacteria have 16S ribosomal DNA with highly conserved nucleotide sequences and nine variable regions. Following broad amplifications, sequences can be compared with the database to identify the genus and species [49]. Pathogen-specific polymerase chain reactions (PCR) are more sensitive than cultures, but less specific in detecting bacteria from bacterial corneal ulcers. Moreover, the treating physician has to provide a list of likely pathogens based on their geographic location and profile of bacterial infections. The results can be available in hours. Antimicrobial resistance can be checked as well. However, there is always the risk of getting positive commensal results [50]. Metagenomic deep sequencing in an unbiased, hypothesis-free manner provides diagnostic results in under 48 h [51]. However, it is yet to be available in the clinics. For detailed information on bacterial ulcers, the reader may refer to a major review [52].

17.5.3.5 Treatment of Bacterial Corneal Ulcers

Apart from gross variability in the microbial profile in different parts of the world, the major challenge in treating bacterial corneal ulcers is the rising incidence of methicillin-resistant *Staphylococcus aureus* (MRSA) from 0.5% [53] to 36.6% for *Staphylococuus aureus* and 48.8% for coagulase-negative. *Staph* spp in a US study. [54].

Cephalosporins are beta-lactam antibiotics active against a broad range of bacteria. In a susceptible study in the UK, 100% of Gram-positive organisms were sensitive to cephalosporin, 81.3% to fluoroquinolones, and 92% to aminoglycosides. For the gram-negative bacteria, respective sensitivities were 98%, 95%, and 98% [36]. It is recommended to start frequent dual combination therapy with topical cephalosporin/aminoglycoside or fluoroquinolone monotherapy. Cefazolin, the first-generation cephalosporin, is non-toxic to the epithelium and is used in a 50–100 mg/mL concentration. If a subconjunctival injection is required, 200 mg/mL can be injected. Commercially available aminoglycosides gentamycin and tobramycin eye drops are available in 0.3% (3 mg/mL) concentration, which must be fortified to 14 mg/mL using the injectable version (40 mg/mL). Amikacin eye drops are available as a 1% solution. The drops are instilled every 5–10 min for the first hour, and then the frequency is 30–60 min until the epithelium is healed. The antibiotics must be continued for at least a week after complete healing to prevent recurrences. If two antibiotics are being used, these are instilled alternately. If monotherapy is used, it is preferable to use Levofloxacin (5-15 mg/mL), Gatifloxacin (3 mg/mL), Moxifloxacin (5 mg/mL), or Basifloxacin, a fourth-generation fluoroquinolone rather than ciprofloxacin (3 mg/ml) or Ofloxacin (3 mg/mL). Concerns are being raised about the rising incidence of antibiotic resistance with the prior use of fluoroquinolones [55].

Adjunctive therapy with topical steroids, if started within 3 days of antibiotics, has led to a gain of one line over 3 months of follow-up. Before starting corticosteroids, one must ensure the culture's positivity and a positive response to antibiotics in the first 48 h. The patient should not suffer from Herpes, fungal, Nocardia, or atypical mycobacteria infection [56]. Corneal cross-linking is used as an adjunct for quicker reepithelialization and prevention of stromal thinning [57–59].

17.5.3.6 Treatment of Filamentous Fungal Keratitis

The treatment of filamentous fungal keratitis remains challenging, prolonged, and fraught with poor outcomes. Patients may continue progressing despite treatment, and nearly 25% of eyes perforate [31]. Intracameral injections of antifungal agents have been given in cases resistant to natamycin with favourable outcomes [60]. It led to faster healing in recalcitrant fungal corneal ulcers [61, 62], but other studies did not find any advantage over conventional treatment [63]. The standard of care for filamentous fungal keratitis remains using Natamycin 5% administered one-hourly for the first 48 h, followed by every 2 h till the ulcer epithelializes and then four times a day for 3 weeks [61]. It is superior or equal in efficacy to topical voriconazole 1%. Supplementation with oral voriconazole does not appear to add any benefit [64]. Chlorhexidine 0.2%, an antiseptic commonly used as an oral mouthwash, compared to Natamycin 5%, gave favourable outcomes [65].

Eyes that perforate or do not respond may require penetrating corneal grafting [61].

17.5.4 Parasitic Corneal Ulcers

Acanthamoeba keratitis accounts for 1–2.4% of all ulcers [66, 67]. The other parasitic infections that can cause corneal ulcers include Microsporidia. *Acanthamoeba* is a freshwater amoeba and may contaminate homemade soft contact lens solutions. *Acanthamoeba* keratitis is characterized by extreme pain due to radial neuritis disproportionate to the corneal infiltrates. The patient may complain of redness, photophobia, foreign body, blurred vision, and tearing. On corneal examination, there are white infiltrative epitheliopathy and pseudo dendrites with a peripheral ring-shaped lesion with a surrounding halo (Figs. 17.9 and 17.10). It may be confused with HSV dendritic keratitis. However, the pain in *Acanthamoeba* keratitis is disproportionately more. The diagnosis may be delayed in patients who do not wear contact lenses. In extreme cases, corneal melting and perforation may be seen.

17.5.4.1 Diagnosis of *Acanthamoeba* Keratitis

Acanthamoeba keratitis can be diagnosed on in vivo confocal microscopy (IVCM), which provides non-invasive magnification of corneal structures at 200–500 X. The cysts of the *Acanthamoeba* can be visualized as 12–25 μm double-walled hyper refractile structures with a bright centre, signet rings, or hyperreflective spots [68]. Cultures from the corneal scrapings have a long incubation period and are positive in only 1/3rd of the cases compared to the IVCM, which is 100% sensitive. Polymerase chain reaction (PCR) to detect the presence of *Acanthamoeba* is nearly 70% sensitive [69].

Prevention of *Acanthamoeba* Keratitis

Acanthamoeba keratitis is a preventable disease. Good hand hygiene and contact lens care are essential in preventing *Acanthamoeba* keratitis. The use of single-use disposable contact lenses should be encouraged. Avoid swimming with contact lenses or should wear protective eyeglasses during swimming. Non-sterile water should not be used for cleaning contact lenses [70].

Treatment of Acanthamoeba Keratitis

Acanthamoeba keratitis is challenging and requires long-term treatment with antiparasitic medications such as chlorhexidine 0.05%, polyhexamethylene biguanide (PHMB) 0.02% eye drops, or pentamidine isethionate 1% eye drops. Eye drops are used frequently. It takes several weeks before the response is seen. Long-term therapy lasting 6–12 months is often required [71] combined with an antibiotic or anti-inflammatory agent. In severe cases, surgical intervention may be necessary to prevent corneal perforation. Treatment should be continued for an extended period to prevent a recurrence. Nearly 90% of patients presenting with epithelial dendriform or peri-neuritic form recover 20/30 or better vision. However, those with ring ulcers or stromal keratitis have a poor outcome [72].

17.5.4.2 Microsporidial Keratitis

Various species of the phylum microsporidia, 1–40 μm size spores, are intracellular obligate parasites and have emerged as a cause of chronic keratoconjunctivitis in immunocompromised patients (Fig. 17.12). In recent years, deep stro-

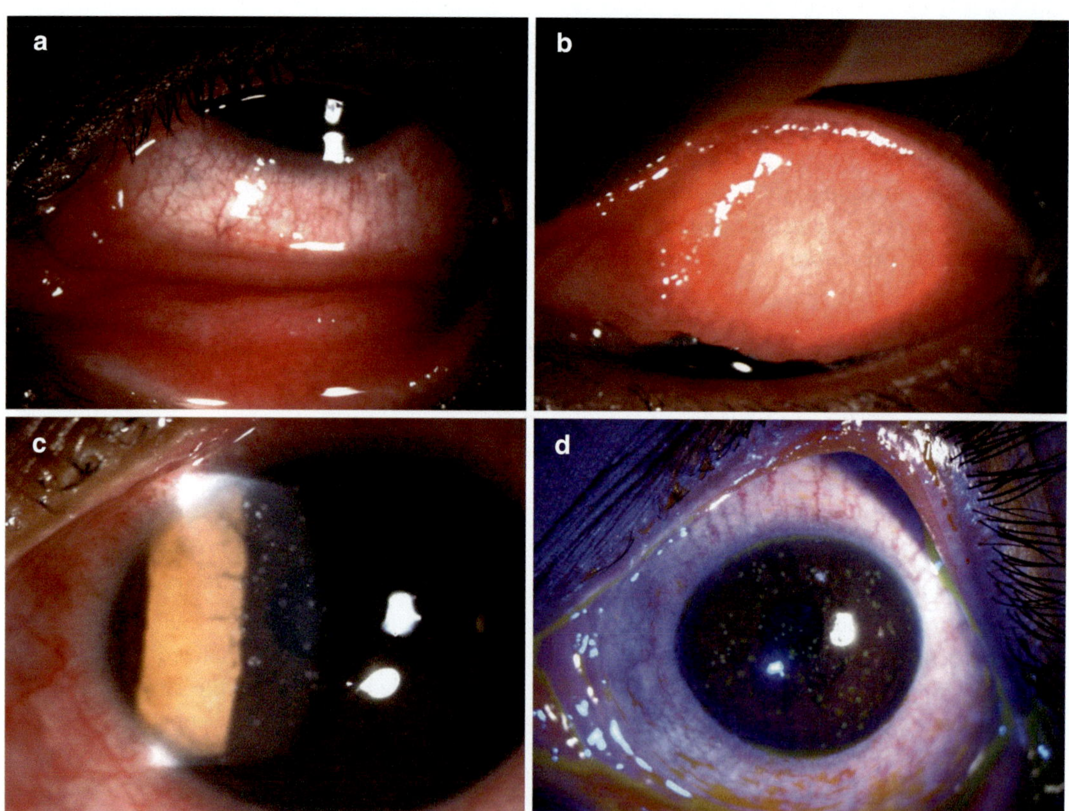

Fig. 17.12 Microsporidial keratoconjunctivitis with follicles on inferior palpebral conjunctiva (**a**), and Papillary reaction in the upper lid (**b**). Coarse epitheliopathy is characterized by '*stuck on appearance*' seen clinically (**c**) and on fluorescein staining (**d**). Images courtesy of Dr. Chintan Malhotra, Professor, Cornea, Lens and Refractive Surgery Services, Advanced Eye Centre, Post Graduate Institute of Medical Education and Research, Chandigarh, India

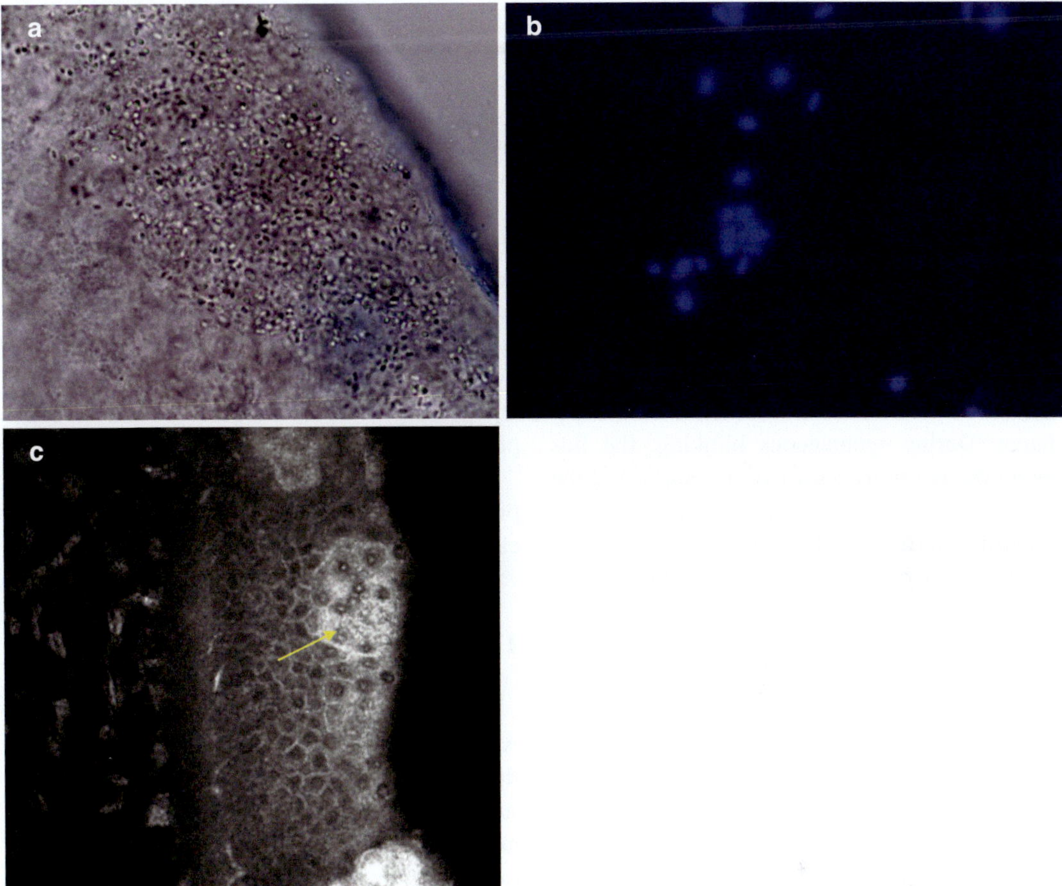

Fig. 17.13 Oval spores of Microsporidia on KOH wet mount (**a**), on calcofluor white (**b**). Confocal microscopy shows multiple ovoid pinpoint 'spore-like' structures (yellow arrow) in oblique view (**c**). Images courtesy of Dr. Chintan Malhotra, Professor, Cornea, Lens and Refractive Surgery Services, Advanced Eye Centre, Post Graduate Institute of Medical Education and Research, Chandigarh, India

mal keratitis with crystalline keratopathy has been recognized even in immunocompetent individuals, especially in the rainy season. Some risk factors include exposure to muddy water, contact lens wear, exposure to corticosteroids, and minor trauma. Definitive diagnosis can be made on electronic and in vivo confocal microscopy (Fig. 17.13). Modified Ziehl-Neelsen and Gram chromo trope stain can demonstrate the microsporidia. Propamidine isethionate 0.1%, given six times daily, is effective in microsporidial keratoconjunctivitis. Oral albendazole has been tried. Penetrating keratoplasty is needed to completely rid the eye of the microsporidia in deep stromal keratitis [73].

17.6 Dry Eye Disorders

17.6.1 Physiological Considerations of Tears in Brief

The eye's outer surface is constantly washed with a three-layer tear film (4–5 μm thick), the major components of which are the innermost layer of mucin adsorbed on the outer surface epithelium of the external eye, the middle aqueous layer, and the outermost lipid layer. The mucin is produced by the conjunctiva's goblet cells (gel-forming Muc5AC) and the lacrimal glands' acinar cells; the accessory lacrimal glands produce the aqueous layer, which is supplemented by a reflex secretion from the main lacrimal gland. The lipid is produced in the meibomian glands present in the tarsal plates. The lipid layer paints a thin layer on the aqueous tears with each upstroke of the blink. The lipid layer minimizes the evaporation of tears and provides surface tension to stabilize the tear film during the open phase of the blink. The gel-forming mucus layer binds the aqueous layer. It has an increasing gradient towards the surface, adsorbed on the surface epithelial surface, which provides stability to the film. It traps debris, the shed epithelial cells, and foreign particles and collects these as thread-like mucus discharge. During spontaneous blinking, the lids spread the tear film evenly over the surface of the exposed eye, much like the wipers of a car.

During the relaxed blinking phase, the tears exit the ocular surface via the lacrimal puncta on the lid margins at the medial end of the lids. Women blink more frequently than men, 19 vs 11 in a minute; the upper lid excursion's blink rate, velocity, and completeness decrease with age [74]. The total volume of the tears is 7 μl, and the secretory rate of 1.03 ± 0.39 μL/min [75, 76]. Tears pool at the lower and upper meniscus to provide the tear reserve. The average height of the lower meniscus is 0.2 mm, < 0.1 mm is the lower cut-off value, and the upper limit is 0.25 mm; anything above would indicate reflex tearing [77].

The tear film provides a smooth first refractive surface of the eye. The tears provide oxygen and micronutrients to the avascular cornea. It is the first line of defence against foreign particles and microbes which get washed away with each blink. Moreover, it defends the outer surface with several antimicrobial enzymes, lysozymes, lactoferrin, and immunoglobulins. The tears' proteome differs from the blood; more than 2000 proteins have been detected in tears. In dry eye disease, there is an increase in tear proinflammatory proteins [78].

17.6.2 Dry Eye Disease

Dry eye disease (DED) is the most common eye disorder in elderly post-menopausal women and causes a variable degree of ocular discomfort, irritation, and redness and affects vision. It is caused by either a deficient tear production, as seen in Sjogren syndrome (SS) -associated dry eye syndromes or non-SS keratoconjunctivitis sicca. The other main reason is the excessive evaporation of tears. The DED has been recently redefined by the tear film and ocular surface society as "Dry eye is a multifactorial disease of the ocular surface characterized by a loss of homeostasis of the tear film, and accompanied by ocular symptoms, in which tear film instability and hyperosmolarity, ocular surface inflammation and damage, and neurosensory abnormalities play etiological roles." [79, 80].

Drugs like antihistamines or diuretics, antidepressants, antianxiety, and corticosteroids may cause dry eye [81].

17.6.3 Systemic Diseases and Other Factors Associated with DED

Autoimmune disorders like Sjogren's syndrome, rheumatoid arthritis, systemic lupus erythematosus, and sarcoidosis cause inflammation of the main and the accessory lacrimal glands and lead to a deficiency of the aqueous layer (Fig. 17.14A). By the time patients develop keratolysis, they have advanced RA (Fig. 17.14B). Nearly 10% of all DED may be associated with primary Sjogren's syndrome [82, 83], leading to a severe DED and dry mouth.

It is important to know that primary Sjogren syndrome patients have a high risk (18.8%) of developing non-Hodgkin lymphoma [84].

Diabetes and thyroid disorders may also lead to dry eye. Environmental factors like excessive air conditioning, low humidity, hot climate, windy conditions, and staring long hours at the computer screens and video display terminal users disturb the normal tear film [85].

17.6.4 Pathogenesis of Dry Eye Disorder (DED)

DED is an inflammatory ocular surface disorder. The key event in the DED is the tear hyperosmolarity caused by an aqueous deficiency or evapo-

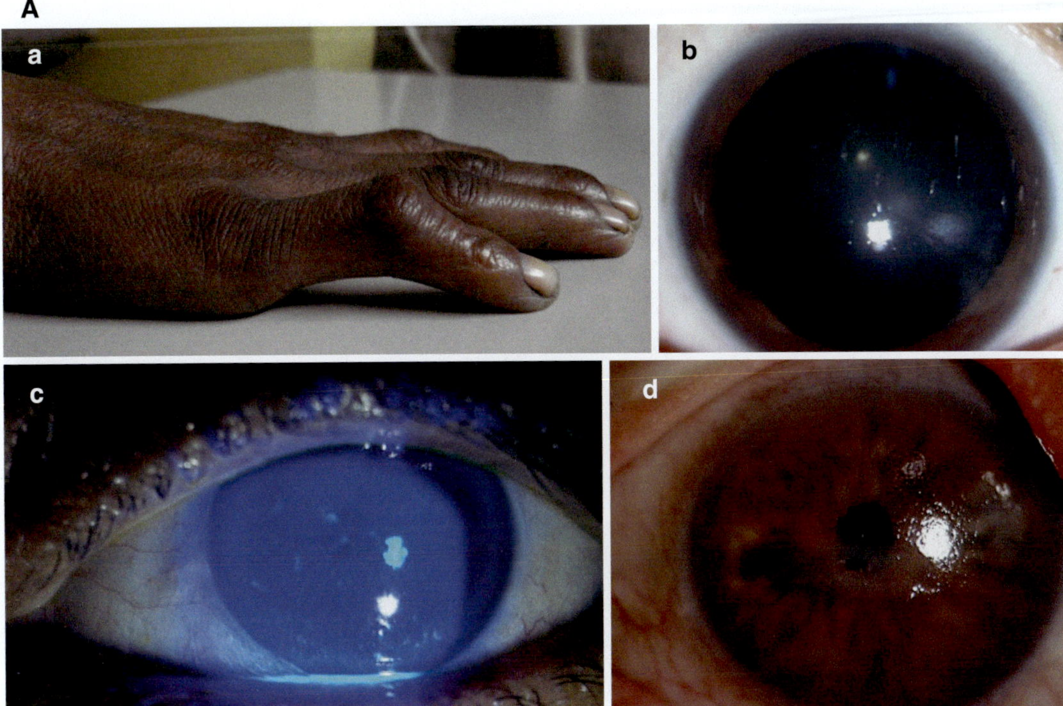

Fig. 17.14 (**A**) Dry eye in rheumatoid arthritis. Boutonniere deformity in a patient with rheumatoid arthritis (**a**). Complications of Keratoconjunctivitis sicca as filamentary keratitis (**b**), fluorescein stain of filamentary keratitis (**c**), and paracentral corneal thinning (**d**). Figure 'a' reproduced with permission of the publishers from Bambery P, Sharma A, Gupta A and Gupta V (2009) Systemic examination and imaging in Gupta A, Gupta V, Herbort C, Khairallah M (eds) Uveitis: Text and Imaging 1st Edn. Jaypee Brothers Medical Publishers (P) Ltd., New Delhi. P 288. Figures b-d courtesy of Prof Amit Gupta, Advanced Eye Centre, Post Graduate Institute of Medical Education and Research, Chandigarh, India. (**B**) Advanced Rheumatoid arthritis bilateral wrist and hands with bilaterally symmetric carpal erosions and collapse of carpal arcs and carpometacarpal and metacarpophalangeal subluxations. Image courtesy of Dr. Anandita Sinha. Department of Radiodiagnosis and Imaging, Post Graduate Institute of Medical Education and Research, Chandigarh, India

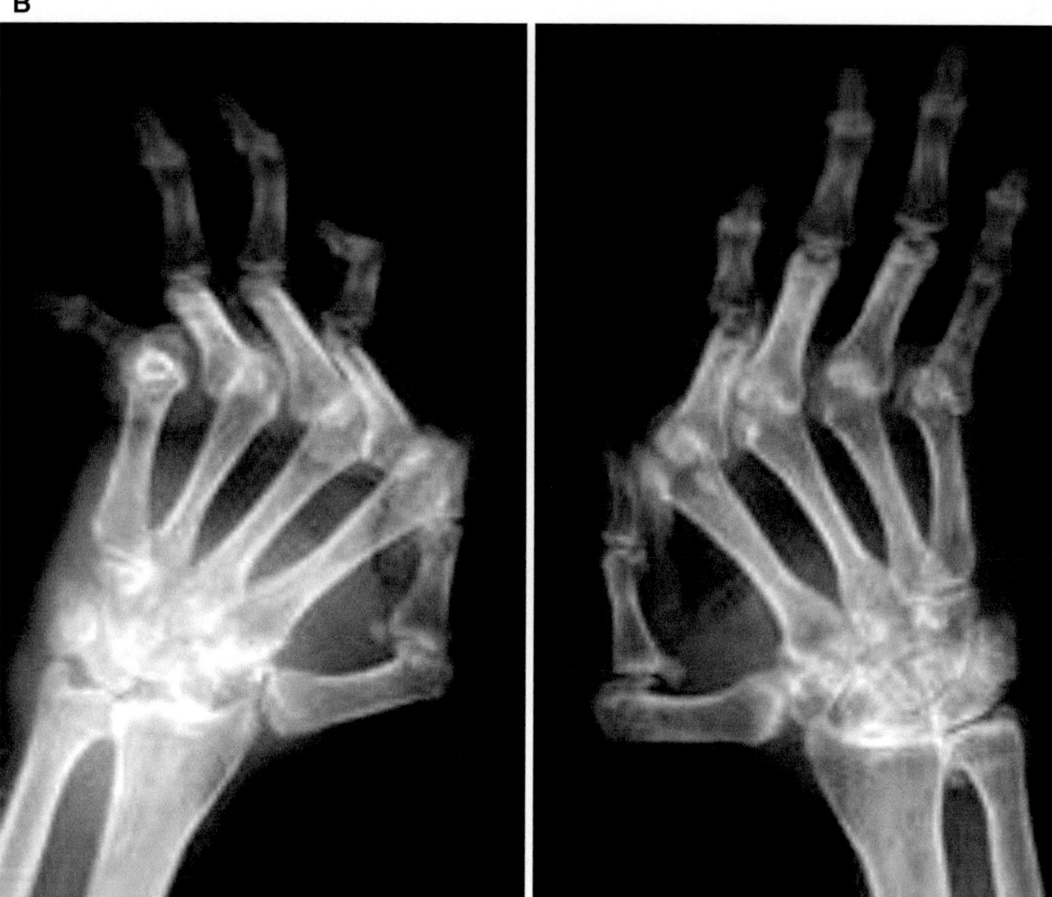

Fig. 17.14 (continued)

ration of the aqueous layer due to an unstable tear film leading to activation of the conjunctival and corneal epithelial mitogen-activated protein kinase (MAPK) and NFkB pathways. These set the stage for releasing inflammatory cytokines, matrix metalloproteinases (MMPs), and the recruitment of inflammatory cells. The net result of these is the loss of both the epithelial and the goblet cells, compounding the insult, and setting up a vicious cycle of chronic inflammation and dry eye. Apart from the tear deficiency per se, the tear film becomes unstable due to meibomian gland disease (MGD), blepharitis, contact lens wear, vitamin A deficiency, and preservatives in the eye drops, which also leads to hyperosmolarity of tears setting up the vicious cycle [86].

17.6.5 Diagnosis of Dry Eye Disease

The diagnosis of the DED is made in the clinic by a comprehensive eye examination on the slit lamp. It includes measurement of tear production, tear film stability, examination of the ocular surface after staining with vital dyes (fluorescein, rose bengal, and lissamine green), examination of the lid margins, meibomian glands plugging, scarring and telangiectasia, and detailed questioning on the symptomatology in the eye as well as the systemic disorders. (See Boxes 17.1 and 17.2).

Box 17.1 Tests in Dry Eye Disorder (DED) in the Clinic

Ocular tests	
Schirmer's test A 5 × 35 mm Whatman filter paper # 41 strip is folded 5 mm from one end and placed in the lower eyelid between the bulbar and palpebral conjunctiva. Wetness is measured after 5 min. Eyes are lightly closed.	A value >10 mm at 5 min indicates normal tear formation. < 5 mm is suggestive of DED
Tear strip meniscometry! Using an 85 mm × 7 mm × 0.3 mm SM tube. One end is kept at the lower lid margin for 5 s. Blue colouration read from the scale on the strip	≥ 5 mm is normal < 5 mm is suggestive of DED
Tear film break up time In the absence of a non-invasive technique, tears are stained with a fluorescein dye strip. The patient is seated on the slit lamp and asked to keep their eyes open. Examined under the broad beam of cobalt blue light for the appearance of dry spots after the last blink.	Normal break-up time is ≥10 s Suspicious of DED 5 to < 10 s Suggestive of DED <5 s Punctate staining of the cornea indicates the epithelial disease
*Tear osmolarity**	Normal 302.2 ± 8.3 mOsm/L Mild-moderate (315.0 ± 11.4 mOsm/L Severe (336.4 ± 22.3 mOsm/L >308 mOsm/L indicates OSD Inter eye difference > 8 mOsm/L OSD
*Tear matrix metalloprotein-ase-9*** (InflammaDry 4 POC). The test collector dabs the inferior conjunctiva; assembles the cassette; dipped into buffer for 20 s; and results read at 10 min.	Designed to give + result if MMP-9 level is >40 ng/mL. One blue line is negative. Test One blue and one red line is positive
Cornea and conjunctiva staining score# Fluorescein 2% for corneal stain (cobalt blue filter) Lissamine green 1% (red filter) for conjunctiva Rose bengal stain is discouraged	Corneal stain graded from 0–3 severity based on number of spots, o, 1–5, 6–30 and > 30 Conjunctival staining spots 0–3 severity based on number of spots 0, 1–9, 10–32, 33–100, >100
Lipiview interferometry$ To measure the thickness of the lipid layer	≤ 75 nm MGD, S, 65.8%; Sp, 63.4% ≤ 60 nm MGD, S, 47.9%; Sp, 90.2
Meibography for the morphology of meibomian glands, density, and tortuosity $$ LipiView II, Johnson and Johnson vision, CA	Grade 0, no atrophy; grade 1, ≤ 25%; grade 2, 26–50% grade3, 51–75, grade 4,>75% Tortuosity is graded into three grades.

! [87]; *[88]; **[89]; # [90]; $[91]; $$[92].

Box 17.2 Laboratory Investigations for Detecting Systemic Diseases Associated with the Dry Eye Disorder

Primary Sjögren's syndrome or secondary Sjögren's syndrome	ESR; CRP ANA Rh factor Anti-SS-A antibodies Anti-SS-B antibodies Anti-SP1; Anti-CA6; Anti-PSP antibodies* Complete blood chemistry
Thyroid eye disease	Anti-TPO antibodies Antithyroglobulin antibodies CT/MRI orbit
Sarcoidosis	Serum lysozyme; CT chest; Biopsy from available tissue, lymph node, skin, or conjunctival follicle.
SLE	*Antiphospholipid antibodies* Anti-cardiolipin antibodies *OR* Anti-β2GP1 antibodies *OR* Lupus anticoagulant Anti-dsDNA antibody or Anti-smith antibody

SSA Sjogren's syndrome A antibodies; *SSB*, Sjogren's syndrome B antibodies; *ANA* antinuclear antibodies; *Rh factor* rheumatoid factor; *SP1* salivary protein 1; *CA6* carbonic anhydrase 6; PSP, parotid secretory protein; Anti-TPO, anti-thyroid peroxidase.

*[93].

17.6.6 Management of dry eye Disorders

Management depends on whether the DED is symptomatic and the severity of the ocular surface severity index. It is important to determine the causative factors and identify whether it is an aqueous deficiency or evaporative due to MGD, blepharitis, or the lids' parasitic infestation (demodex). Nearly 60% of DED are caused by meibomian gland dysfunctioning. Warm compresses are advised to the lids for improving lipid flow from meibomian glands. Oral tetracyclines or doxycycline may be required for lid inflammation and blepharitis. In patients with deficient meibomian glands, intense pulsed light with an expression of the meibomian glands has been found to be an effective strategy [94]. For a detailed review of the guidelines for managing patients with MGD, the readers may refer to an exhaustive review [95].

Mild to moderate DED can be managed with frequent instillation of artificial tear substitutes. When possible, modifications in environmental factors that exacerbate DED symptoms should be identified and avoided to the extent possible.

Local or systemic drugs that cause or aggravate symptoms of DED should be avoided, and alternative drugs should be sought. Oral omega-3 supplements are useful in patients with MGD and blepharitis in improving the ocular surface disease index [96, 97].

17.6.7 Newer Agents in DED

Use of topical secretagogue, diquafosol eye drops 3% (Diquas®), six times a day, has been found non-inferior to 0.1% sodium hyaluronate in improving the corneal and conjunctival dye staining scores. It improves the secretion of aqueous and mucin [98], increases tear film break-up time [99] and other clinical parameters of DED, but not the ocular surface disease index [100]. Topical secretagogues Diquas® and Mucosta® (rebamipide) are available in Japan only.

Anti-inflammatory drugs like topical cyclosporin 0.05% (Restasis®, Ikervis®) or lifitegrast 5% (Xiidra®) are available in the US and European markets. Topical cyclosporin is effective in reducing the T-cell infiltration of the conjunctiva. Lifitegrast is an antiinflammatory agent that blocks the binding of intercellular adhesion molecule-1 (ICAM-1) to the lymphocyte function-associated molecule-1. It has been found effective in improving the symptoms of DED [101].

The autologous serum has been used for persistent epithelial defects in DED for nearly four decades as it contains epidermal growth factors, lactoferrin, retinoic acid, and proteins that favour healing. More recently, selenoprotein P has been isolated from serum, which promotes healing by reducing oxidative stress in DED [102]. It is an effective and safe therapy in DED [103].

Other alternatives when nothing seems to work include therapeutic contact lenses (especially in filamentary keratitis), amniotic membrane grafting, tarsorrhaphy, punctal plugs, and occlusion and lacrimal duct grafting [79, 80].

17.7 Anterior Uveitis

17.7.1 Anatomical, Physiological, and Immunological Considerations of the Anterior Segment

Anatomically, the eye is divided into an anterior segment comprising the anterior chamber (AC) and a posterior chamber (PC); and a posterior segment comprising the vitreous cavity, retina, and choroid. The cornea, iris, and anterior part of the ciliary body enclose the AC. The PC is bound anteriorly by the iris, laterally by the pars ciliaris, and posteriorly by the crystalline lens and the zonular fibres. The AC and PC are filled with a transparent fluid, the aqueous humour, continuously secreted by the ciliary epithelium into the PC. A pressure gradient moves it through the pupil into the AC. It exits the eye through trabecular meshwork at the angle of the anterior chamber. The cornea is lined with a single layer of hexagonal cells, the endothelial cells arranged in a honeycomb pattern. The uvea is the middle vascular pigmented eye layer consisting of the choroid posteriorly, which continues anteriorly into the ciliary body and iris.

Like the brain and testes, the eye is an immune-privileged site. This means there will be no inflammatory reaction in the ocular tissues under ordinary circumstances.

The immune privilege in the anterior segment is maintained via a blood-aqueous barrier through the tight junctions of the pigmented epithelial cells that line the iris up to the pupillary border; the non-pigmented ciliary epithelium of the ciliary body and the tight endothelial cell junctions of the iris vessels. Notably, the aqueous humour secreted from the ciliary epithelium in the AC contains 1% of the plasma proteins, even without the breakdown of the blood-aqueous barrier [104]. It is now believed that plasma proteins that leak from the ciliary body capillaries into the ciliary body stroma (which contains 74% of the proteins) also have some of these leaked into the AC at the root of the iris stroma, close to the exit channels of the AC [105]. The pupil's valve-like apposition with the crystalline lens's anterior capsule ensures that these leaked proteins remain in the AC only. Thus, a flare in the AC is not always pathological. Moreover, pathologies that cause iris pigment atrophy allow the AC's proteins (and the growth factors) to move into the PC and are responsible for the formation of complicated cataracts.

The iris comprises a discontinuous anterior border layer of fibroblasts, melanocytes, and collagen fibrils. Most iris stroma comprises collagen fibres containing fibroblasts, macrophages, dendritic, and mast cells. While occasional T cells may be present, B or plasma cells are absent. Posteriorly, the iris is lined by a myoepithelial layer and a posterior pigmented epithelial layer up to the pupillary border. All the cells in the iris, including the melanocytes and iris-pigmented epithelium layer, play a role in immune reactions. The latter likely plays a role in the immune privilege by a contact inhibition of the T cell activation [106].

The ciliary body (CB) is continuous, with the iris anteriorly and the choroid posteriorly. The CB is divided into an anterior pars plicata and a posterior pars plana. The CB is covered with double epithelial layers, the inner non-pigmented ciliary epithelium, continuous posteriorly with the neurosensory retina (secretes aqueous humour), and the outer pigmented layer continuous anteriorly with the myoepithelial layer of the iris and posteriorly with the RPE. The CB stroma has almost the same type of cells as the iris. The pigmented epithelial cells of the CB also play an immune regulatory role. The major function of the dendritic cells in the iris and CB stroma is antigen presentation, of macrophages cytokine production and antigen presentation, that of melanocytes recognition of pathogen associate molecular patterns (PAMPS), and of the mast cells an immediate response to pathogens [106].

17.7.2 Immunology of Uveitis in Brief

One of the major strategies to maintain the eye's immune privilege is the phenomenon of anterior chamber-associated immune deviation (ACAID). In the absence of lymphatics within the eye, the antigen-presenting cells that capture an offensive antigen are carried to the spleen, which induces antigen-specific Tregs. This mechanism plays a key role in preventing corneal allograft rejection [107]. Moreover, the aqueous humour contains a number of anti-inflammatory and immunosuppressive molecules which prevent damage to the ocular tissues.

The blood ocular barriers ensure that no noxious agents or cellular elements can enter AC or PC under normal circumstances. There are no formal lymphatic channels in the intraocular tissues. The blood ocular barriers ensure that the ocular antigens remain sequestrated and are not exposed to the body's immune system.

Most high-affinity ocular antigen-specific T-cells formed during development in the thymus are exposed to their cognate antigens in the thymus medulla during maturation and eliminated by apoptotic mechanisms. Some antigen-specific T-cells with intermediate affinity develop into natural Tregs, which provide peripheral tolerance. A few T cells, however, escape and carry ocular antigen-specific receptors, which can become pathogenic on exposure to the target antigen through gut microbial mimicry or direct exposure to the target antigens during trauma. Such escapee self-antigen-specific T cells (in the non-immune privileged sites) develop tolerance on exposure to self-antigens in the other organs. But in the case of the eye, these do not have access to the self-antigen (ocular-specific) because of the blood-retinal barrier. The naïve self-reactive T cells cannot enter the eye on their own and need to be activated before entering the ocular tissues. The gut-eye axis activates these ocular antigen-specific T cells [108].

Overall, the unique immunology of the eye's anterior segment can maintain the eye's immune homeostasis that prevents infections and inflammation. However, the immune system's dysregulation leads to anterior uveitis. The most favoured view for immune dysregulation is dysbiosis in the intestine.

The most common cause of anterior uveitis is an autoimmune reaction. The activated ocular antigen-specific T cells enter the eye and mount an immune response against the ocular antigens.

The activated ocular antigen-specific T-cells recognize ocular antigens as foreign, releasing pro-inflammatory cytokines such as interferon-gamma (IFN-γ) and tumour necrosis factor-alpha (TNF-α). Activated T cells and other immune cells such as macrophages, dendritic cells, and B cells infiltrate the iris and ciliary body. Pro-inflammatory cytokines such as IFN-γ, TNF-α, interleukin-1 beta (IL-1β), and interleukin-6 (IL-6) are released by immune cells and contribute to the inflammation and tissue damage in anterior uveitis. Upregulation of the adhesion molecules in the iris and ciliary body, such as intercellular adhesion molecule-1 (ICAM-1) and vascular cell adhesion molecule-1 (VCAM-1), promotes the infiltration of immune cells into the tissue. Activation of complement pathways further amplifies the inflammatory reaction.

17.7.3 Mediators of Inflammation

The discovery of interferons by Issacs and Lindenmann in 1957 [109] brought in a revolution in cell biology. These molecules blocked and interfered with the replication of viruses. It was followed by the discovery of interleukins (IL) and a host of similar molecules called cytokines that were abbreviated IL. As more of these were discovered, they were sequentially numbered as IL-1 and onwards [110]. Cytokines are short-lived cell surface proteins that cannot enter the cells but dictate the activation of a host of intracellular signalling pathways involved in normal physiological and pathological pathways. The cells interact with each other via cytokines. The cytokines control the behavior of cells, including their activation, differentiation, and proliferation and even decide if the cells should die or produce more cytokines. Cytokines are further subdivided into interferons (prevent viral replication), interleukins (the largest cytokine family), chemokines (proteins that control trafficking and migration of cells), and Tumour necrosis factor-α (TNF-α, cytokine produced by macrophages, lymphocytes, granulocytes responsible for acute inflammation, cell death, and apoptosis).

The macrophages and B lymphocytes produce IL-1, a proinflammatory cytokine that activates the T-helper cells. The IL-2, also a proinflammatory cytokine, activates Th-1 helper cells and further the proliferation of T cells. IL-6 helps differentiate B lymphocytes into plasma cells and produce antibodies, hence a critical player in inflammation. There is a lot of redundancy and pleiotropy in the functioning of the cytokines. More than one cell type can produce multiple cytokines, interacting with several different cells [111].

Briefly, IL-1 is produced by macrophages and B cells, stimulates T-helper cells, and plays a role in inflammation; IL-2 is produced by the Th1 cells and causes proliferation and differentiation of T cells; IL-6 is produced by a variety of cells such as B cells, Th2, macrophages, and endothelial cells and helps in differentiation of B cells into plasma cells and antibody production and is a key regulator of inflammation; IL-17 is secreted by the Th17 cells. TNF-α, an acute phase reactant, is produced by macrophages, monocytes, lymphocytes, and granulocytes and is responsible for acute inflammation [111].

In their functions, the cytokines are either proinflammatory or anti-inflammatory; e.g. in acute inflammation, IL-1 and TNF-α act together to worsen the inflammatory response. Once the infection is controlled, these stop expressing themselves, and the inflammation dies. The IL-10 and TGF-β are anti-inflammatory and get upregulated in the ocular fluids once the inflammation is controlled. In people predisposed to autoimmune disorders, the genes expressing the proinflammatory cytokines never shut down entirely, thus perpetuating the autoimmune inflammatory response [112]. Among the cytokines detected in the intraocular fluids and serum of patients with endogenous uveitis include TNF- α, IL-1β, IL-6, IL-10, and IL-17 [113–115]. Developing antibodies to block these cytokines has revolutionized the treatment of systemic autoimmune disorders, including endogenous uveitis [116].

17.7.4 Anterior Uveitis-Epidemiology

In anterior uveitis (AU), the major site of inflammatory reaction is the eye's anterior chamber. There are three major causes of AU- non-infectious anterior uveitis, less commonly infectious AU, and least common masquerades due to malignancies. In a large retrospective claims database in the US, the prevalence of non-infectious uveitis (NIU) was 121/100,000 in adults vs 29/100,000 in children. Anterior NIU accounted for 81% of all NIU in adults and 75% of all NIU in children. The prevalence of NIU causing intermediate, posterior, and panuveitis accounted for just 1, 10, and 12 per 100,000 adults and 0.3 and 4 per 100,000 children population [117]. The NIU tends to be recurrent (24 per person-year), especially in younger patients [118]. NIU associated with HLA B27 tends to be more recurrent, with wide intervals between the recurrences [119].

17.7.4.1 Anterior Uveitis (AU)—Clinical Characteristics

In AU (iritis, iridocyclitis), inflammation is limited to the anterior chamber, characterized by cells and flare with some spillover inflammatory cells in the vitreous cavity. The most common causes include Acute AU (AAU) associated with systemic diseases such as spondyloarthropathies and positive HLA B 27 and, less commonly, sarcoidosis. Infectious causes such as viral uveitis, syphilis, tuberculosis, and Posner-Schlossman syndrome must be differentiated from non-infectious causes for appropriate treatment [120].

Nearly, 60% of AAU patients are associated with HLA-B27, most often seen in young men. The AAU in these patients has an abrupt onset of painful anterior uveitis and runs a remitting and

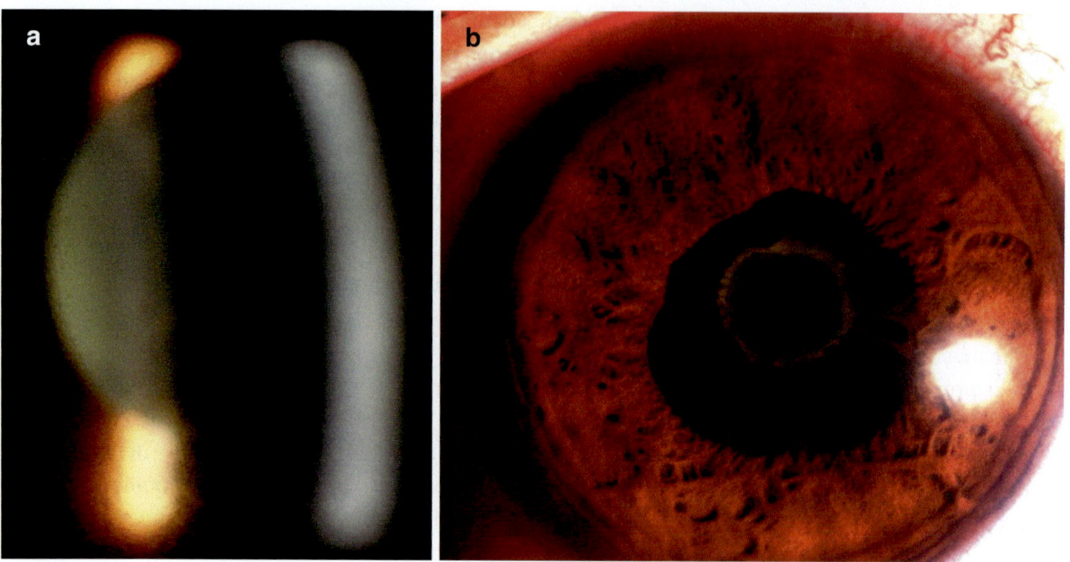

Fig. 17.15 Sudden onset pain, redness, and dimness of vision in the left eye of a patient with a history of morning stiffness of the lower back, with cellular reaction in the anterior chamber as acute anterior uveitis (**a**). Formation of filiform posterior synechiae and anterior lens opacity (**b**)

recurring course. The inflammation is active in one eye at a time and alternates between the two. The inflammation is marked by marked circumciliary injection, intense flare, fibrinous exudates in the anterior chamber, and the formation of filiform posterior synechiae (Figs. 17.15, 17.16, and 17.17). The intraocular pressure is low. The eye may become tender to touch a day or two before the onset of the acute attack (prodrome). The patient in prodrome may complain of pain without any signs of eye inflammation. An ultrasonic biomicroscopy (UBM) examination reveals a swollen ciliary body with blunting of the ciliary processes at this stage (Fig. 17.18).

There is a strong association between HLA B27-associated AAU and spondyloarthropathies. However, two-thirds of the patients presenting with acute uveitis may not be aware of the arthropathy [121]. Several diseases cause uveitis and arthritis, including spondylarthritis (SpA) group, Blau's syndrome, Juvenile idiopathic arthritis, Kawasaki disease, sarcoidosis, and relapsing polychondritis [122]. SpA is a group of inflammatory diseases which involve the joints, skin, gut, and eyes and include Ankylosing spondylitis (AS) (Fig. 17.16), reactive arthritis (ReA), psoriatic arthritis (PsA), non-radiographic spondyloarthropathy, and undifferentiated spondyloarthropathy. The absence of auto-reactive antibodies characterizes the SpA [123]. The lifetime risk of developing uveitis in AS is 33.2% [124].

Criteria for SpA

The All Assessment of Spondyloarthritis International Society (ASAS) criteria for axial spondyloarthropathies included two arms, one imaging arm (sacroiliitis on radiography or MRI) and the other a clinical arm (HLA B27+). The imaging arm required one criterion, and the clinical arm required two additional criteria. The criteria included dactylitis (sausage-shaped inflammation of a finger), inflammatory bowel disease, inflammatory back pain, HLA B27 +, elevated CRP, response to non-steroid anti-inflammatory agents, and family history of SpA [125].

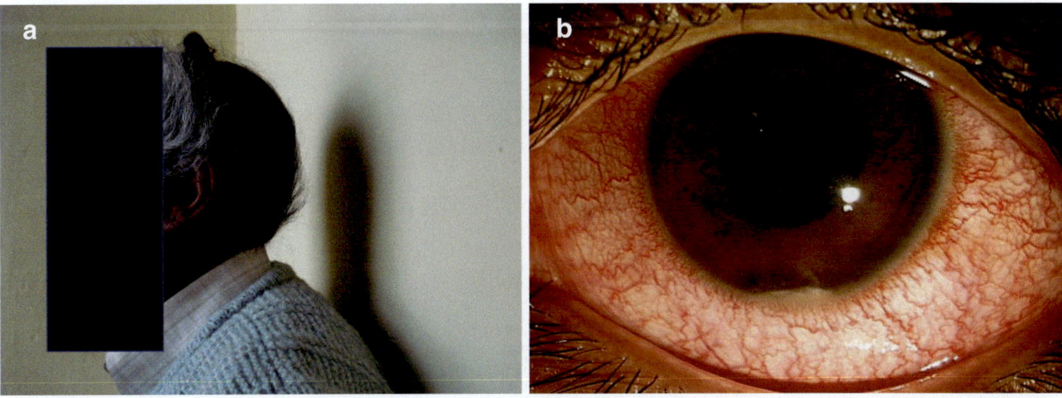

Fig. 17.16 Increasing head-to-wall distance in ankylosing spondylitis (**a**). Fibrinous hypopyon in acute anterior uveitis (**b**). Figure 'a' reproduced with permission of the publishers from Bambery P, Sharma A, Gupta A and Gupta V (2009) Systemic examination and imaging in Gupta A, Gupta V, Herbort C, Khairallah M (eds) Uveitis: Text and Imaging 1st Edn. Jaypee Brothers Medical Publishers (P) Ltd., New Delhi. P 282

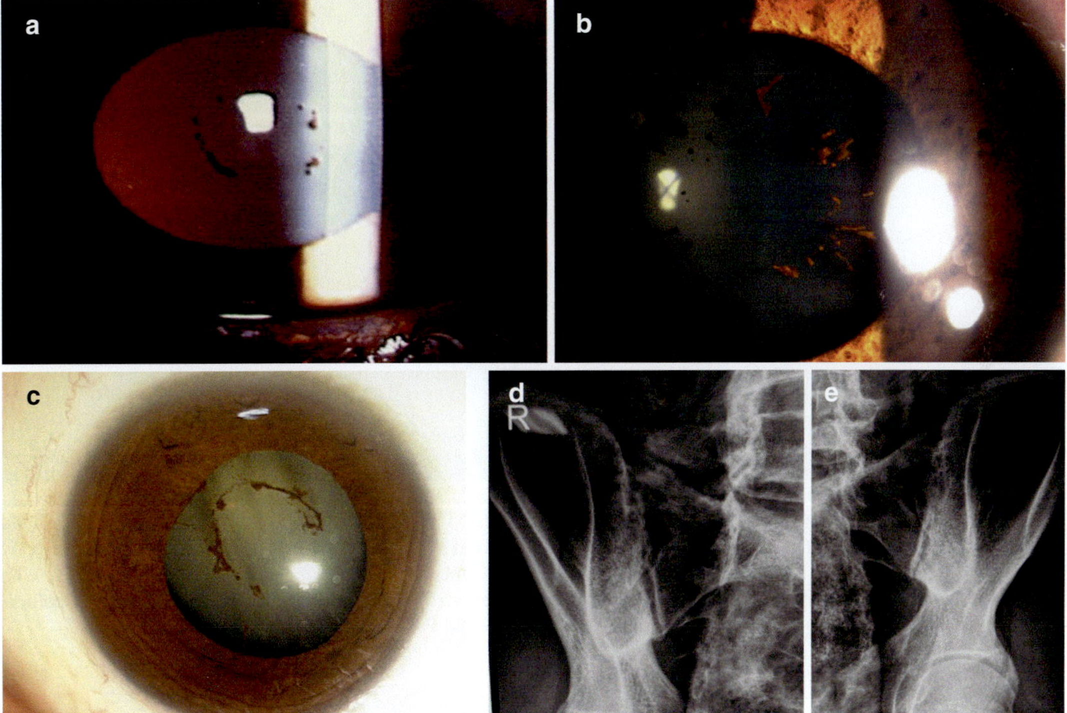

Fig. 17.17 Pigment on anterior lens surface in acute anterior uveitis (AAU) (**a**–**c**) quiescence stage in three different patients. X-ray Sacro-iliac joints in a patient with AAU show enthesopathy right iliolumbar ligament with erosions in the sacroiliac joint (**d**, **e**). (Images courtesy of Dr Anandita Sinha. Department of Radiodiagnosis and imaging, Post Graduate Institute of Medical Education and Research, Chandigarh, India)

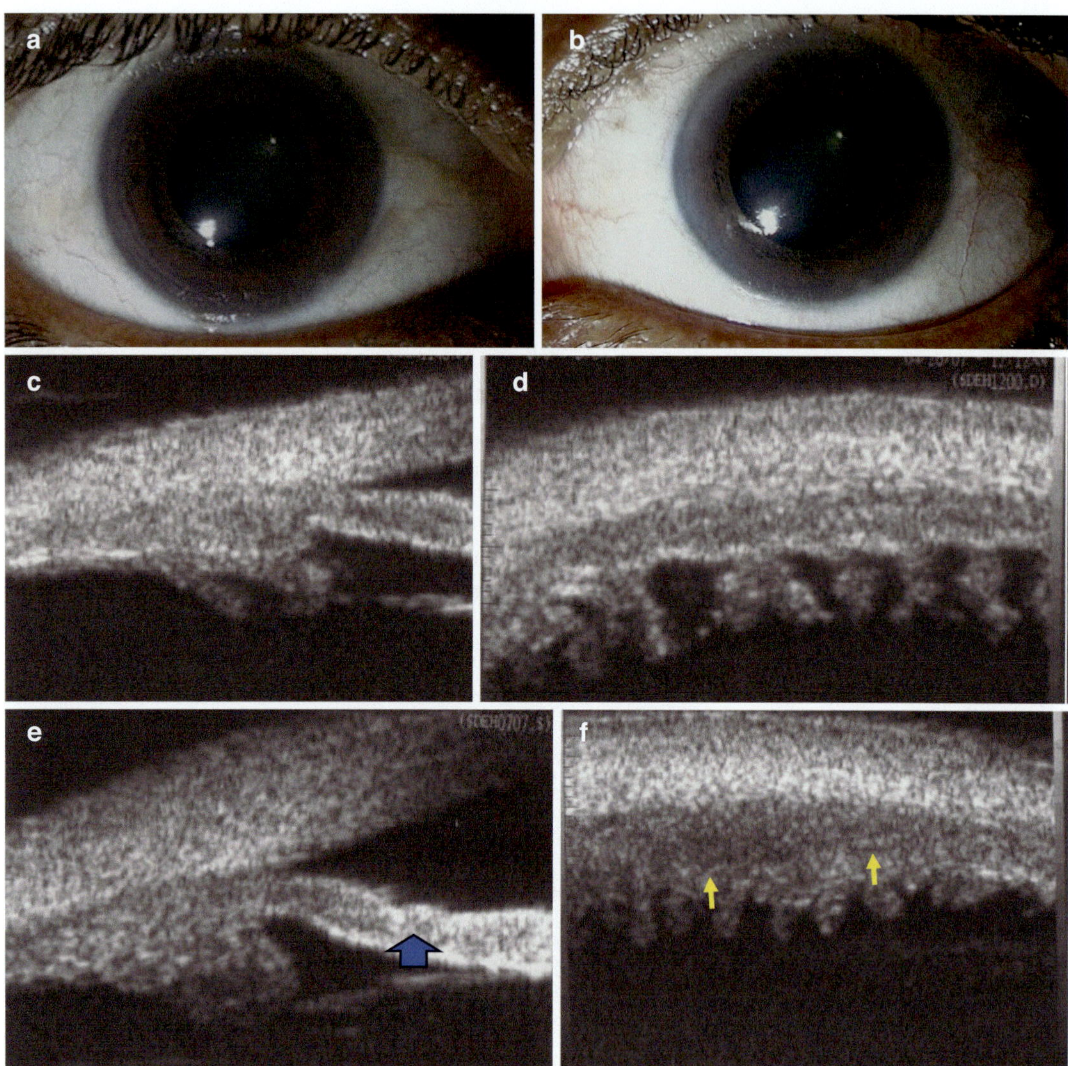

Fig. 17.18 A 57-year-old male, HLA B27-positive, presented with the normal right eye (**a**) and anterior uveitis with cells and flare 2+ (**b**) in the left eye. UBM revealed a normal iris and ciliary body in the right eye (**c**, **d**), while the left eye showed swelling of the iris (blue arrow) and ciliary body (yellow arrows) (**e**, **f**). Reproduced with permission of the publishers from Gupta A, Singh R, Gupta V, Tran VT, Herbort CP (2009) Ultrasound biomicroscopy in Gupta A, Gupta V, Herbort C, Khairallah M (eds) Uveitis: Text and Imaging 1st Edn. Jaypee Brothers Medical Publishers (P) Ltd., New Delhi. P 172

For the peripheral SpA, criteria include "peripheral arthritis and/or enthesitis and/or dactylitis with one or more of the criteria A, psoriasis, inflammatory bowel disease, preceding infection, HLA B27, uveitis, sacroiliitis on imaging, or B, two or more other parameters: arthritis, enthesitis, dactylitis, inflammatory back pain in the past, family history of SpA." [126].

SpA and Acute Anterior Uveitis

In a prospective study of AAU, all of whom had MRI of the sacroiliac joints, 56% had SpA, of whom 93% had axial SpA. Only 7% had peripheral SpA. Seventy percent of the patients were unaware of the SpA at the time of AAU and recommended that all patients with AAU undergo rheumatological examination ([127]).

In a multicentric, prospective study of arthritis with AU (798 patients), 59% were men at a mean age of 45. Sixty percent were HLA B27-positive. Of the positive HLA B27 and AU, 69.8% had axial SpA vs 27.3% in negative HLA B27 and AU. Peripheral SpA was seen in 29.1% vs 11.1% of the positive and negative HLA B27 patients, respectively [128].

HLA B 27 and AAU

HLA B27 positivity increases the risk of spondyloarthritis by 100-fold [129]. HLA B locus genes are highly polymorphic, and even for the B27 locus, more than 25 gene variants are known, of which HLA B*2705 and HLA B*2702 are the most frequently associated with the HLA B 27-associated AAU. The outcome in terms of complications of AAU in B27-positive cases is worse than the B27-negative cases. The risk of cystoid macular oedema is 5X more in the B27-positive cases [119].

Gut-Eye Axis and AAU

Experimental studies reveal an increasing role of alteration of the gut microbiome by HLA B27 in the causation of AU, ankylosing arthritis, and reactive arthritis [129, 130]. A number of mechanisms have been proposed for the gut-eye axis, some or all of which may be involved. (1) The gut microbiota may disturb the immune homeostasis between the regulatory and effector responses, (2) there may be molecular mimicry between the self-antigen and the microbial antigens in the gut, mounting an adaptive immune response in the eye and the joints, (3) microbial products may reach the eye through the breakdown of the intestinal epithelium and act as an adjuvant in the immune reaction in the eye, or (4) the gut microbiota may regulate the extraintestinal movement of the gut immune cells to reach the eye and participate in the immune reaction in the eye [131].

Treatment of AAU

Timely treatment with frequent topical corticosteroids, mydriatics, and cycloplegics often breaks the synechiae and relieves pain by attenuating the ciliary body spasm. Pigment clumps on the surface of the crystalline lens distributed on the lens indicate a past attack of AAU. An occasional patient may require a short course of oral corticosteroids.

Sulfasalazine treatment appears to reduce the number of AU recurrences [132].

17.7.4.2 Anterior Uveitis and Psoriatic Arthritis

AU is a well-known, although uncommon, association with psoriatic arthritis (Fig. 17.19). Seven percent of psoriatic arthritis had AU [133]. AU in psoriatic arthritis is often bilateral, has an insidious onset, and runs a chronic course [134]. Half the patients in the above series had axial arthritis, and most were HLA B 27-positive. Psoriatic arthritis in children ≤4 years, although less common, tends to have a higher prevalence of AU than in those arising after four years (18.8% vs 8.8%) ([135] The AU tends to be severe and persistent in younger children [136]. In a primary care cohort, patients with psoriatic arthritis had a significant risk of developing uveitis and Crohn's disease, but not ulcerative colitis [137].

17.7.4.3 Inflammatory Bowel Disease and Anterior Uveitis

AU may precede the development of Inflammatory bowel disease (IBD). Patients with uveitis are at higher risk of developing Crohn's disease. In a population cohort-based study, the incidence of IBD in uveitis patients was 4.13% vs 1.48% in normal controls [138]. Most suffer from Crohn's disease. Among Crohn's disease, 3.5–6.8% may develop ocular inflammation. There does not appear to be any relation between intestinal activity and uveitis. Uveitis is bilateral, insidious in onset, persistent, and seen more often in women. Less than 50% of them may be HLA B27-positive. However, most IBD patients are associated with SpA [139, 140].

17.7.4.4 Reactive Arthritis and Uveitis (Reiter's Syndrome)

Two- to four weeks following urinary or gastrointestinal tract infection, HLA B27-positive young adults may develop pain and redness in the eyes due to bilateral conjunctivitis and acute

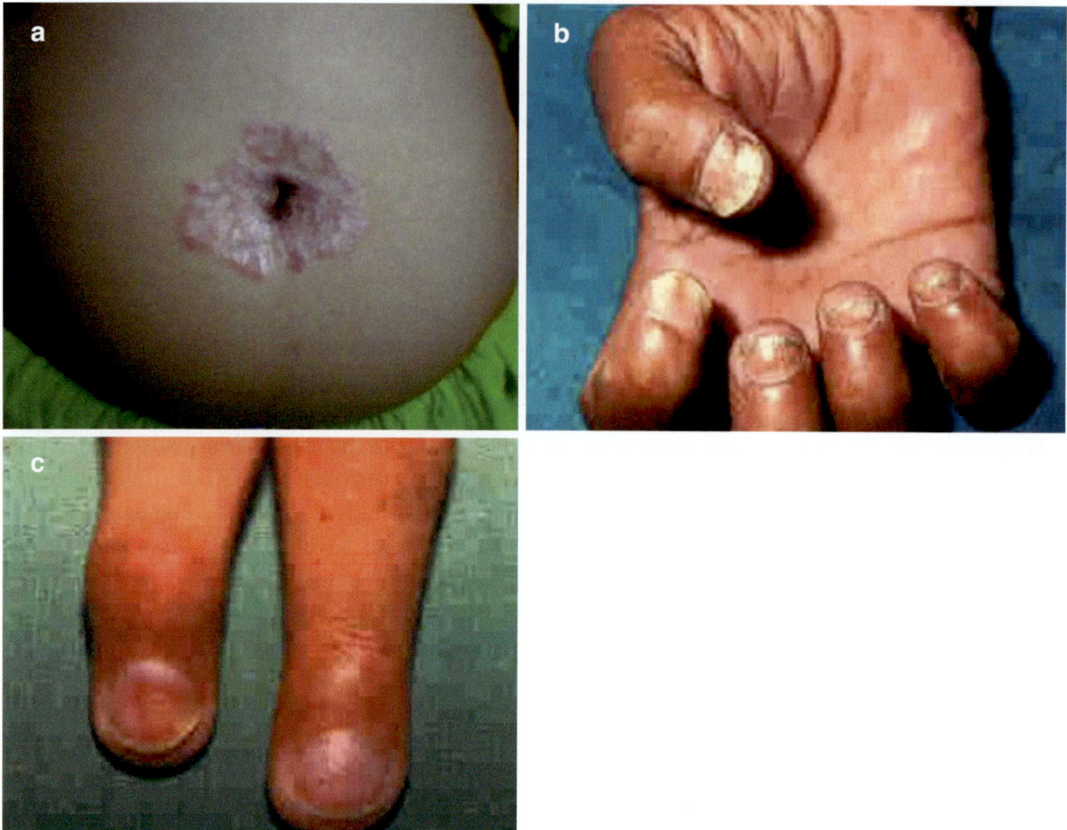

Fig. 17.19 Psoriasis skin lesions (**a**) on abdomen. Hand of the patient with psoriasis and arthritis showing extensive nail changes due to this disease (**b** and **c**). Figures a–c reproduced with permission of the publishers from Bambery P, Sharma A, Gupta A and Gupta V (2009) Systemic examination and imaging in Gupta A, Gupta V, Herbort C, Khairallah M (eds) Uveitis: Text and Imaging 1st Edn. Jaypee Brothers Medical Publishers (P) Ltd., New Delhi. P 287–288

uveitis (Fig. 17.20). Both sexes are equally affected, except more men are affected by ReA following chlamydia trachomatis urinary infection [141]. Unlike unilateral AAU seen in patients with AS, the involvement in Reiter's syndrome is bilateral. Rarely, episcleritis, scleritis, optic disc edema, cystoid macular edema, and retinal vasculitis may also be seen. Recurrent attacks may lead to extensive posterior and anterior synechiae.

Major criteria for diagnosis include oligoarthritis of the large joint of lower limbs, ocular involvement (conjunctivitis, acute uveitis), urogenital (urethritis, prostatitis, or cystitis), and skin (keratoderma blennorrhagica, circinate balanitis) [142]. Corneal involvement as disciform/stromal keratitis or corneal ulcer may be seen, especially in recurrent cases [143, 144]. The treatment requires antibiotics for the triggering infection and the use of nonsteroidal anti-inflammatory drugs. Sulfasalazine is effective if started within 3 months of the onset of ReA [141].

17.7.5 Tubulointerstitial Nephritis and Uveitis (TINU)

Tubulointerstitial nephritis (TIN) is a frequent cause of acute kidney injury which may evolve

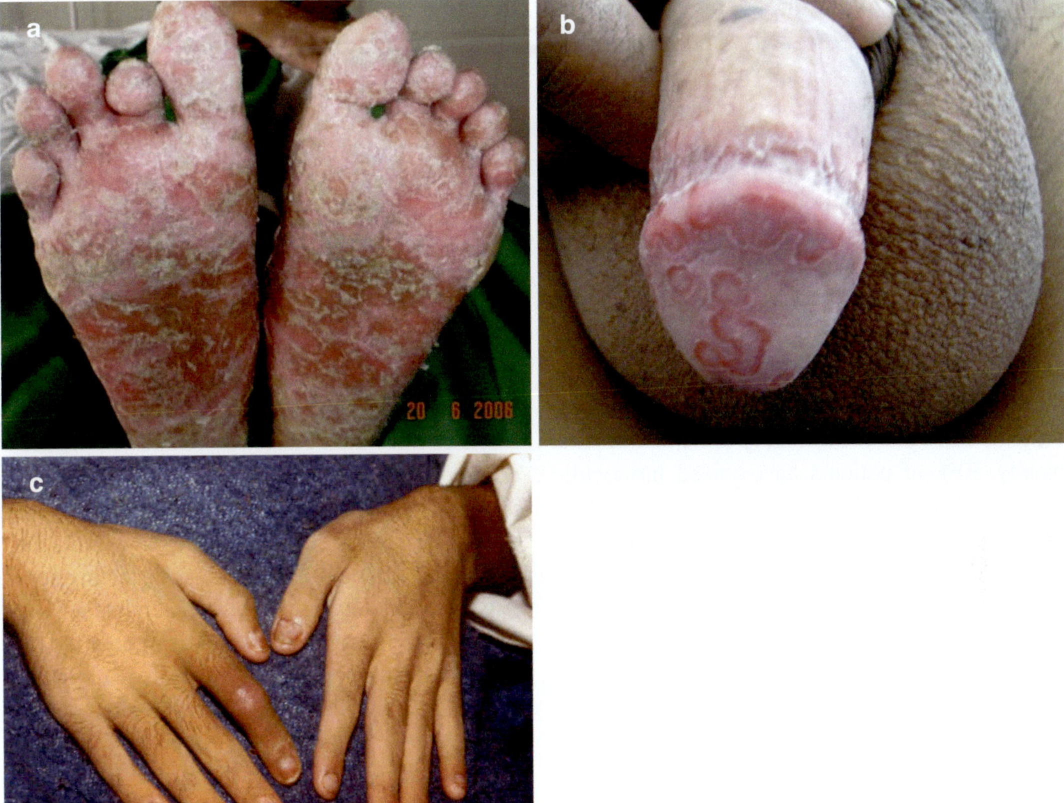

Fig. 17.20 Reactive arthritis (Reiter's disease). Keratoderma blennorrhagica in Reiter's syndrome (**a**). Circinate balanitis in reactive arthritis (**b**) Asymmetric involvement of the proximal interphalangeal joints of the right hand in Reiter's Syndrome (**c**). Figures a-c reproduced with permission of the publishers from Bambery P, Sharma A, Gupta A, and Gupta V (2009) Systemic examination and imaging in Gupta A, Gupta V, Herbort C, Khairallah M (eds) Uveitis: Text and Imaging 1st Edn. Jaypee Brothers Medical Publishers (P) Ltd., New Delhi. P 285

into chronic kidney disease. It is an immune-mediated inflammation of the renal tubules, most often resulting from drug reactions to NSAIDs, aspirin, penicillin, and diuretics, among others, but may also result from infections or as a part of systemic inflammatory disorders or IgG4-associated immune complex multiorgan autoimmune disease [145].

The symptoms of chronic TIN are fatigue, loss of appetite, weight loss, fever, and nausea, while acute TIN may present with pain in the flanks, hematuria, and oliguria. The diagnosis is often made by renal biopsy, which shows lymphocytic and eosinophilic infiltration. In children, the cause of TIN remains unclear. In a prospective study of TIN in children below 18 years who underwent ophthalmological examination at diagnosis and at 3- and 6-month follow-ups, 16 of the 19 patients were found to have uveitis. TIN uveitis (TINU) may also be seen in adults; 71% of adult TIN may be associated with bilateral uveitis, and nearly one-third progressed to chronic kidney disease despite corticosteroids. [146].

All patients with TIN need to be evaluated for uveitis as 25–50% of the patients of TINU run a chronic course and may be asymptomatic [147, 148].

It is one of the most overlooked uveitis entities because of the nonfamiliarity with the systemic symptomatology of this disease by ophthalmologists. While TINU is rare and accounted for only 1.7% of all uveitis patients in a tertiary uveitis centre, it accounted for 32% of patients with sudden onset of bilateral painful acute uveitis in patients under 20 years [149]. A minority of patients may develop uveitis before the onset of TIN, simultaneously or months after the onset of TIN [148]. In some series, TINU was seen predominantly in women [150].

Patients may complain of photophobia, pain, and redness. Ophthalmological examination reveals flare and cells, fine keratic precipitates, vitreous cells, and occasionally optic disc edema. Nearly 50% of patients have raised intraocular pressure. Rarely, TINU patients may also show evidence of posterior uveitis [151]. On ultra-widefield fundus fluorescein angiography, 65% of eyes showed peripheral retinal vascular, 25% optic disc, and 30% showed macular leaks [152].

The positive laboratory investigations include raised ESR, elevated serum creatinine, low molecular weight proteinuria (α1- or β2-microglobulin), and glucosuria [148, 153]. In the standardization of uveitis nomenclature (SUN), classification, inflammation in the anterior chamber with either a positive renal biopsy or nephritis evidenced by elevated serum creatinine, and/or abnormal urine analysis and elevated urine β-2 microglobulin were highly sensitive and specific for diagnosing TINU syndrome [154].

Despite corticosteroid treatment, half the patients had renal sequelae and required long-term monitoring [147]. There is no correlation between the systemic activity of TIN and uveitis. Uveitis is often difficult to control and may recur despite corticosteroids.

17.7.6 Juvenile Idiopathic Arthritis (JIA) -Associated Uveitis

Uveitis is the most common extraarticular complication of Juvenile Idiopathic Arthritis (JIA-AU) and accounts for nearly three-fourths of all uveitis seen in children. Several arthritic diseases have their onset before age 16; the most common variant associated with uveitis is oligo-articular arthritis, characterized by non-deforming arthritis involving 1–4 joints during the first 6 months of the disease lasting for at least 6weeks. It can be either persistent if $\leq$4 joints continue to be affected throughout the disease course or extended if $\geq$4 joints get affected. For diagnosing JIA-AU, it is important to rule out a history of psoriasis in the patient or any first-degree relative, arthritis in an HLA B27-positive patient beginning after the 6th birthday, AAU enthesitis-related arthritis or IBD or Reiter's syndrome in the patient or a first-degree relative (Fig. 17.21), positive IgM Rh factor twice at least 3 months apart, or systemic JIA [155].

In a large multicentric cohort, the mean age of the JIA-AU was 5 years, and 81% were females. Eighty-one per cent of those tested were positive for antinuclear antibodies. The uveitis was

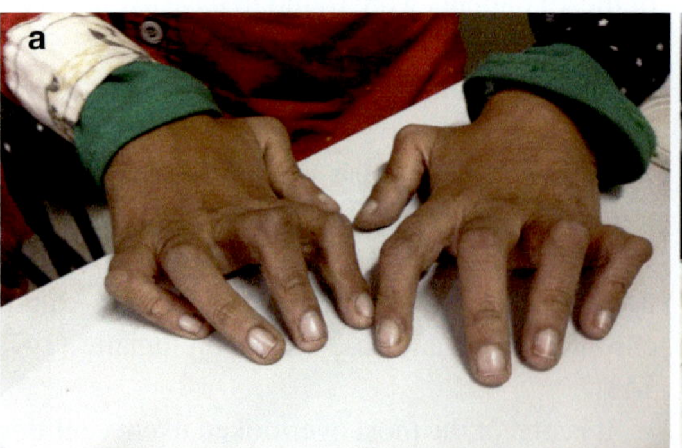

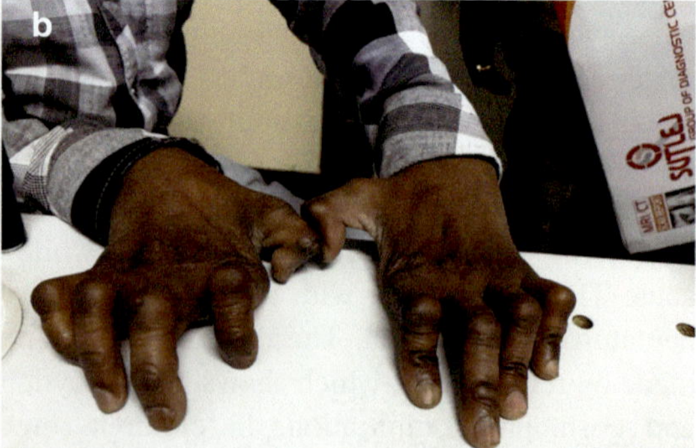

Fig. 17.21 Hand deformities in patient of JIA (**a**) and his father (**b**)

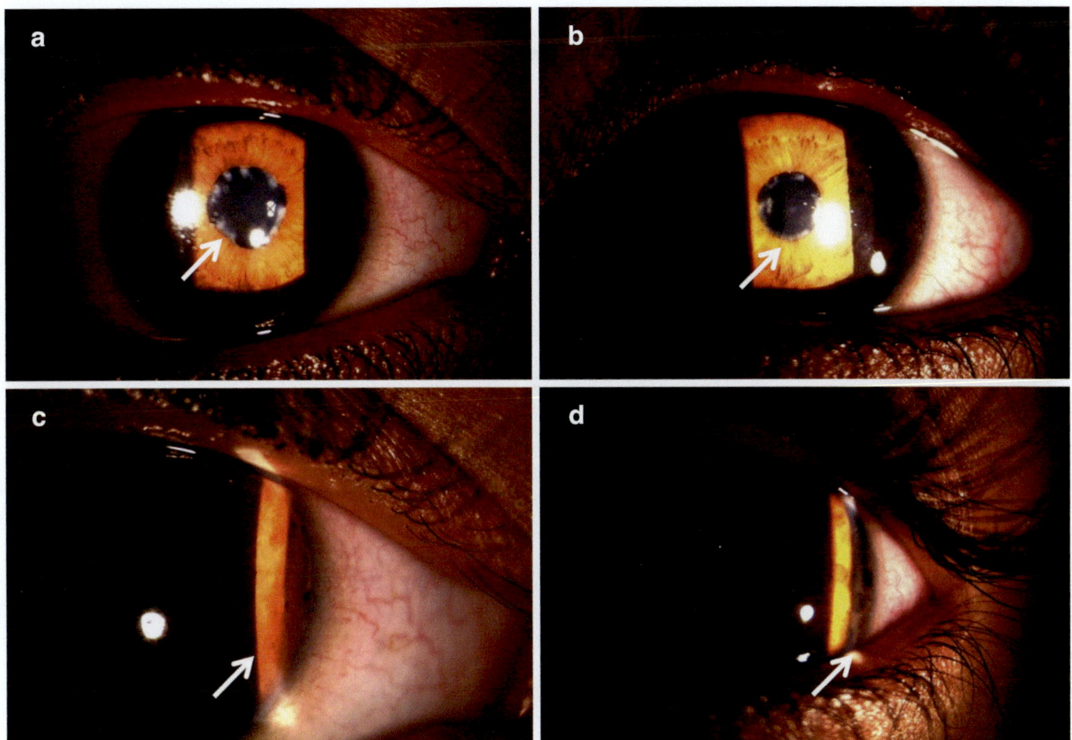

Fig. 17.22 Bilateral chronic anterior uveitis and posterior synechiae in a child with JIA (**a**, **b**), with peripheral band-shaped keratopathy (**c**, **d**)

chronic, and most had bilateral disease (66%) (Fig. 17.22). Cornea was normal in 72%, while band-shaped keratopathy was noted in 28%. Fine keratic precipitates were seen in 22%. The majority had one to three + cells in the anterior chamber. The majority showed no cells in the vitreous cavity and none or up to 2+ flare. Posterior synechiae were seen in 29% [156].

Nearly 24% of patients with JIA and up to 30–40% of ANA-positive patients develop chronic anterior uveitis [157]. Uveitis is asymptomatic in >90% of patients. It is frequently called "white uveitis" [158]. Being asymptomatic, patients often present late when complications like cataracts, band-shaped keratopathy (Fig. 17.22), glaucoma, or hypotony (Fig. 17.23) have already occurred.

Ninety percent of JIA-AU present within 8 years of the onset of arthritis, most within 4 years. However, in 10%, uveitis may precede the onset of arthritis [159].

17.7.6.1 Screening, Monitoring, and Treatment for JIA-AU

Patients at high risk of developing chronic anterior uveitis include those who are ANA-positive, have oligoarthritis, rheumatoid factor negative polyarthritis, psoriatic arthritis, or undifferentiated arthritis, and are <7 years at onset, and have had JIA arthritis for ≤4 years [160]. These patients should be screened every 3 months on a slit lamp till 8 years after the onset of arthritis. Those at low risk for developing uveitis, age of onset ≥7 years, ANA-negative, and duration of JIA > 4 years, should be screened every 6–12 months [160].

Those with uveitis should be monitored for response to treatment targeting <1+ cells in the anterior chamber. Laser flaremeter is preferred to measure flare severity. Look for complications such as posterior synechiae, cataracts, raised intraocular pressure or hypotony, and posterior segment evaluation for cystoid macular edema.

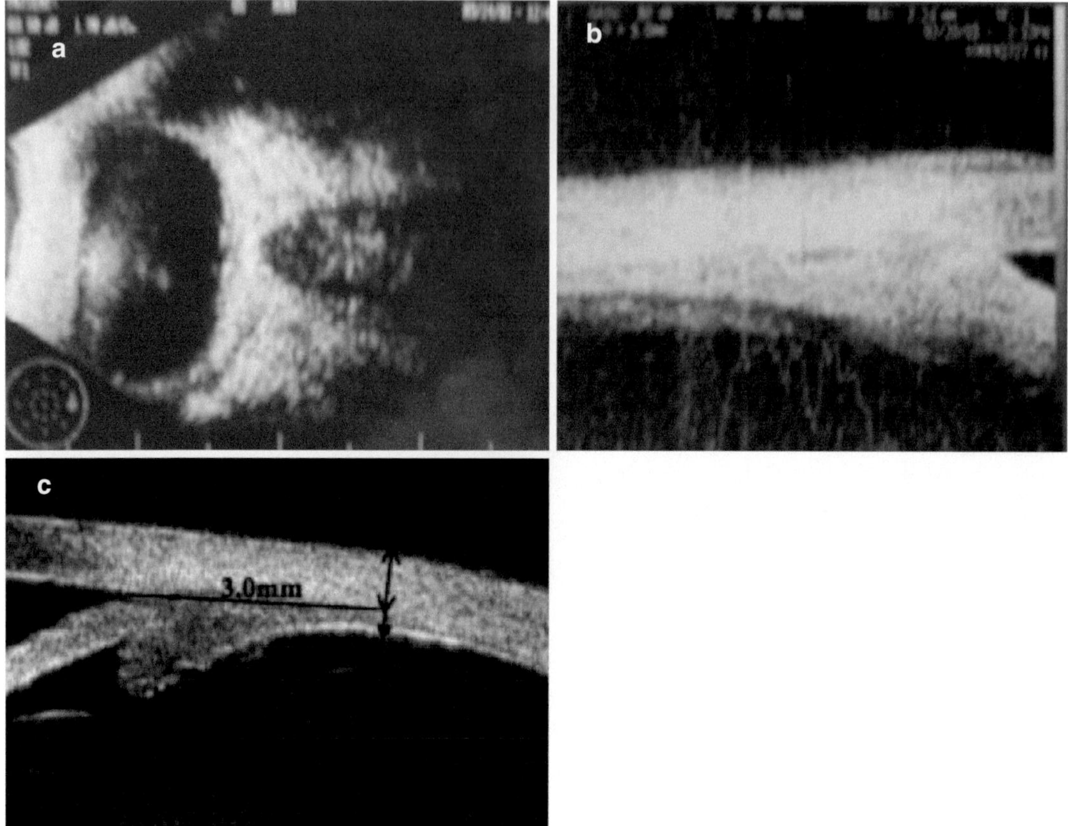

Fig. 17.23 A 22-year-old girl with light perception vision and IOP 4 mm Hg developed complicated cataract and hypotony. Note prephithisical eye on ultrasonography (**a**) in JIA-uveitis due to ciliary body atrophy (**b**, **c**) seen on UBM

Stable patients on treatment should be examined every 3 months.

Active uveitis should be treated with topical corticosteroids. Systemic immunosuppression is indicated if there is no remission within 3 months of topical treatment. The first drug of choice is weekly methotrexate. If it is not tolerated, the patient should be switched to biologicals, and adalimumab is the drug of choice. Other alternatives are infliximab or golimumab. Etanercept is best avoided. In case of the refractory disease to one anti-TNF-α agent, one could switch to another agent [161].

Topical treatment should be tapered first before systemic therapy. For those who remain on 1–2 drops of prednisolone acetate, systemic therapy should be tapered only after the disease has remained quiescent for at least 2 years. When the topical treatment is tapered, the patient should be examined within 1 month, and when stopping systemic therapy within 5 months [160].

17.7.7 Autoinflammatory Syndromes and Uveitis

Monogenic mutations in the innate immune pathways have been increasingly recognized in childhood-onset, familial, often recurrent, multisystem inflammatory disorders. These are termed autoinflammatory disorders and sharply contrast with autoimmune disorders, which result from autoantigen-specific adaptive immune diseases resulting from loss of autoantigen tolerance.

Non-specific infections drive autoinflammatory disorders due to dysregulated innate immune responses caused by genetic mutations in the major players of the innate immune pathways.

Autoinflammatory disorders arise spontaneously, involving recurrent skin or mucosal ulcerations, fever, and childhood-onset uveitis.

17.7.7.1 Mechanism of Innate Immunity and its Dysregulation

Pathogen-recognition receptors (PRR) on the cells of innate immunity, namely the macrophages and dendritic cells, recognize microbes by their pathogen-associated molecular patterns (PAMP), the danger signals. The PRR also recognize the molecules released by the damaged cells (the danger signals), which are the damage-associated molecular patterns (DAMPs). The microbes and damaged cell contents must be eliminated from the body to maintain homeostasis. The encounter of innate cells with the PAMP activates the PRRs and initiates inflammatory response pathways to eliminate the infected cell. The dead cell products, the DAMPs, further activate the PRR setting up a vicious cycle to eliminate the microbes and protect the tissues [162].

Sensing the PAMPs/DAMPS (danger signals) by the toll-like receptors leads mRNA transcription into proproteins, pro-IL1β and IL-18. The danger signals also inhibit Rho A, an inhibitory molecule for activating intracellular inflammasomes Pyrin, NLRP3 (nucleotide-binding domain, leucine-rich–containing family, pyrin domain–containing-3), NLRC4 (NLR Family CARD Domain Containing 4), and PSTPIP1(Proline-Serine-Threonine Phosphatase Interacting Protein 1). The activated inflammasomes cleave pro-Caspase-1 to Caspase −1. Caspase-1 cleaves the proproteins pro-IL-1β and pro-IL-18 to their active forms. The cytokines IL1-β and IL18 are secreted from the cell to activate the immune cells and set up inflammation ([163]).

Inflammasomopathies result from a gain of function mutations in the genes for Pyrin, NLRP3, NLRC4, and PSTPIP1 and result in familial Mediterranean fever (FMF), cryopyrin-associated periodic fever (CAPS), familial cold autoinflammatory syndrome-4 (FCAS4), and pyogenic arthritis and pyoderma gangrenosum (PAPA), respectively. Inflammasomopathies may also result from loss of function mutations in the regulatory proteins XIAP (X-linked inhibitor of Apoptosis), resulting in X-linked proliferative disease (XLP-2) and CDC 42 (cell division control 42), resulting in Neonatal-onset multi-system inflammatory disease [163].

In addition to inflammasomopathies, at least four other categories of autoinflammatory disorders, including interferonopathies, unfolded protein response/endoplasmic reticulum stress disorders, relopathies, and uncharacterized syndromes, have been described. Readers interested in details of these disorders should refer to an extensive review [163].

17.7.7.2 Autoinflammatory Disorders and Uveitis

Many autoinflammatory syndromes, namely FMF, Muckle-Wells syndrome, CAPS, NOMID (Neonatal onset multisystem inflammatory syndrome), and Blau syndrome, are associated with uveitis [164].

A triad of arthritis, dermatitis, and panuveitis characterizes Blau syndrome. It results from a gain of function single nucleotide mutation in the NOD2 (Nucleotide-binding oligomerization domain protein) gene, also known as CARD15, an intracellular receptor mainly in the monocytes and macrophages responsible for recognizing and eliminating bacterial antigens via activation of the caspase pathway. This syndrome is often mistaken for JIA-associated uveitis, which is strictly an anterior uveitis, while uveitis in Blau syndrome is a panuveitis. [165]. The functioning of the protein encoded by the NOD2 gene is well known. However, it is not known how mutations in the NOD2 gene in the uvea lead to uveitis [165]. In a prospective worldwide study, of the 50 cases with Blau's syndrome, the median age of onset was 5 years. Seventy eight percent of patients had uveitis, which was almost always bilateral, and more than half of patients had panuveitis, with characteristic chorioretinitis lesions, peripapillary nodules, and optic atrophy. Anterior segment inflammation was noted in 40% of eyes. Controlling ocular morbidity was a major challenge [166]. In a single-centre experience from

North India, ten of the elven patients were children at a mean age of 4 years. Six had a positive family history. There was a significant delay in diagnosis varying from 0.8 to 20 years in diagnosis. The frequency of arthritis, dermatitis, and panuveitis was 100%, 81.8%, and 81.8%, respectively. All patients had swelling of wrist and ankle joints. Contractures and deformities of small joints were seen. All had R334W variants in the NOD2 gene. Control of uveitis required the use of adalimumab. [167]. A triad of fever with rash and panuveitis in children, positive family history of arthritis, contractures of small joints, camptodactyly (digital flexion deformity), and refractory uveitis should raise suspicion of Blau syndrome [167].

17.7.7.3 Blau Syndrome and Sarcoidosis

Blau syndrome has been previously labelled as early onset sarcoidosis because of several similarities between the two, including soft tissue non-caseating granulomas. Despite several similarities in the histopathology of granulomas of the two diseases, in Blau's, a characteristic feature is the emperipolesis (cell within a cell) of lymphocytes within the multinucleated giant cells, which is not observed in the sarcoid granulomas. While Blau is an autosomal dominant inherited childhood-onset disorder, sarcoidosis is typically seen in adults or sometimes in adolescents and is not inherited. However, there is likely a genetic predisposition for sarcoidosis. While Blau is a dysregulated innate immune response to non-specific microbes, environmental exposure to *Mycobacterium tuberculosis* and *Propionibacterium acnes* is believed to result in sarcoidosis in genetically predisposed patients. Systemic multiorgan involvement in Blau may appear like sarcoidosis, but lung involvement is seen in 90% of sarcoidosis patients, while interstitial lung disease is rare in Blau [168].

17.7.8 Infective Anterior Uveitis—Viral Uveitis

Viruses of the Herpesviridae family are the most common cause of anterior uveitis worldwide. The herpes simplex virus (HSV) is the most frequent, followed by the varicella-zoster virus (VZV) (Figs. 17.24 and 17.25). Cytomegalovirus-AU is frequently seen in Asian countries. Most of the data are available from tertiary care uveitis centres. The prevalence of herpes anterior uveitis, proven or suspected in these reports, has varied from a low of 4.6% in Finland to 11.6% in the US [169]. The highest incidence (31%) of

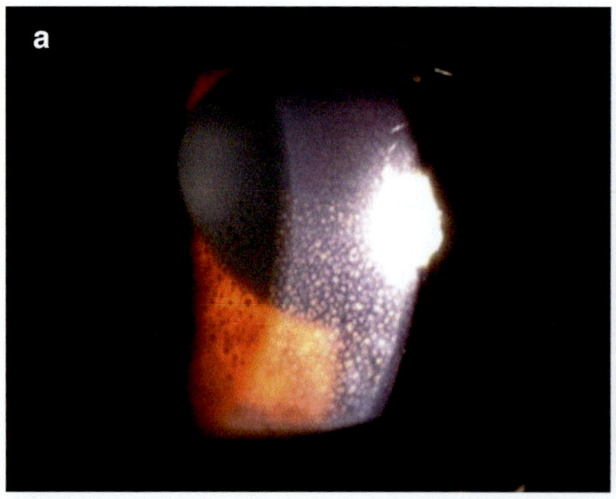

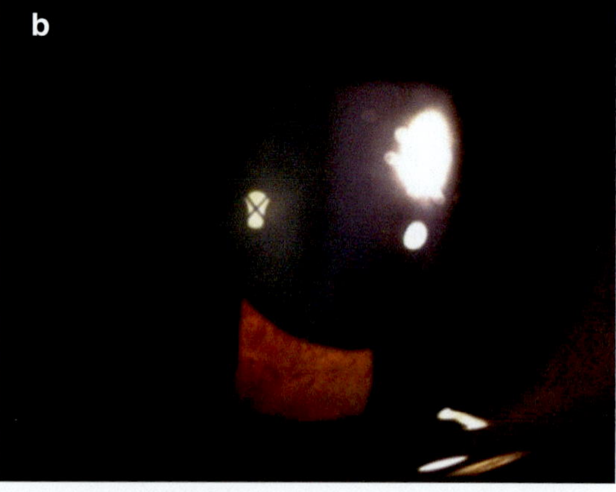

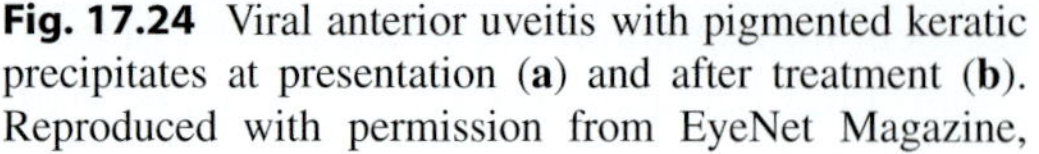

Fig. 17.24 Viral anterior uveitis with pigmented keratic precipitates at presentation (**a**) and after treatment (**b**). Reproduced with permission from EyeNet Magazine, Agarwal AK et al., Pigmented Keratic Precipitates in Herpes Simplex Virus Anterior Uveitis November 2018

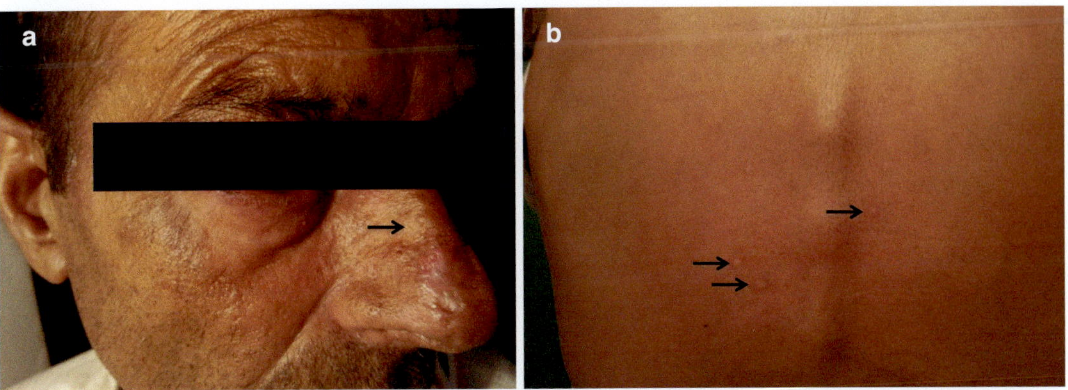

Fig. 17.25 Nose (**a**) and back (**b**) lesions (arrows) in a patient who presented with VZV anterior uveitis

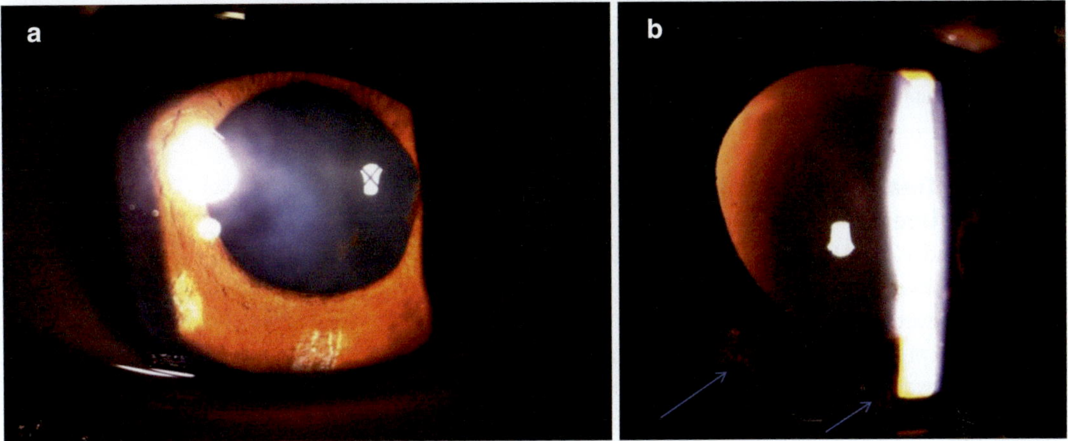

Fig. 17.26 Sectoral iris atrophy (**a**), seen in iris transillumination (arrows, **b**)

viral anterior uveitis is reported in France [170]. Twelve per cent of anterior uveitis in people over 60 years is caused by herpes viruses [171]. The unilateral anterior uveitis caused by HSV, VZV, and CMV shares many similarities with some differences in clinical signs. Comparing the three viral AU, HSV-AU was seen predominantly in women compared to VZV-AU and CMV-AU, which were seen more frequently in men. The mean age of patients with VZV was the highest at 61 years, compared to 50 years for the HSV and 54 years for the CMV. CMV-AU is seen in two clinical phenotypes, (1) acute onset of the Posner Schlossman syndrome with a few moderate to large keratic precipitates and high intraocular pressure or (2) the chronic, insidious onset type. The frequency of the two clinical variants may differ in different ethnic populations [172]. AU in HSV and VZV is more acute and abrupt in onset.

The inflammation is more severe in VZV-AU and the HSV-AU and is marked by pain, redness, and blurring of vision. The keratic precipitates are medium to large in VZV and HSV-AU, while these may be large/small or coin-shaped in CMV-AU. Raised intraocular pressure is seen in all, but is maximum in the CMV-AU. Sector iris atrophy and posterior synechiae were seen in VZV and HSV (Fig. 17.26). Diffuse iris atrophy may be seen in CMV AU [173, 174].

Diagnosing viral AU requires PCR for all three viruses [175–177].

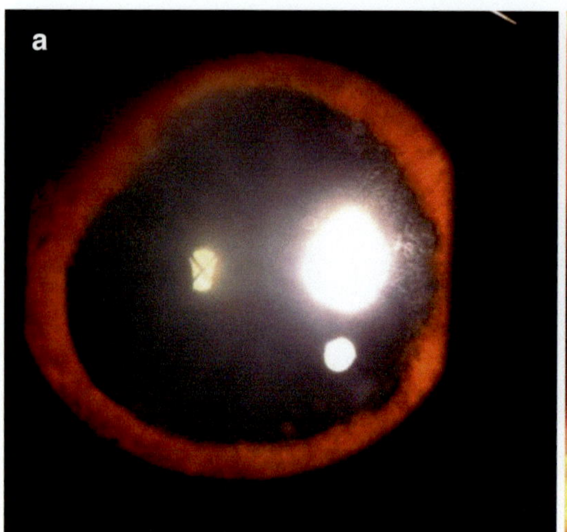

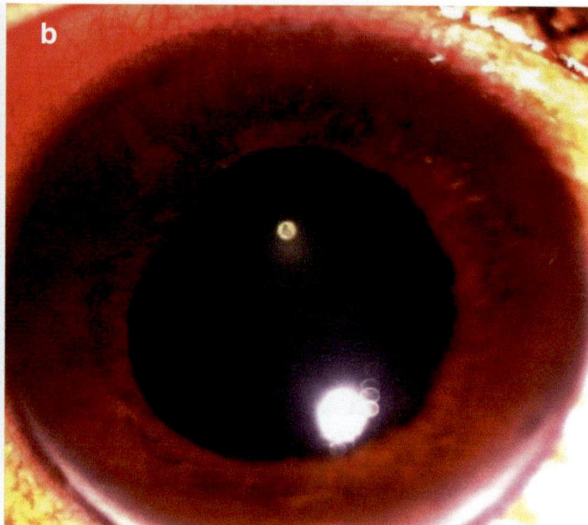

Fig. 17.27 Following treatment of viral anterior uveitis, corneal edema (**a**) with raised intraocular pressure cleared (**b**) after instituting antiviral therapy. Reproduced with permission From EyeNet Magazine, Gupta AK, et al., Infectious uveitis-New challenges Emerge, September 2014

17.7.8.1 Treatment of Viral Anterior Uveitis

The HSV and VZV-AU respond well to oral antiviral agents like acyclovir or valacyclovir. HSV uveitis, however, is a recurrent disease and needs oral antiviral prophylaxis, as discussed in the section on viral keratitis. Acyclovir is ineffective in CMV-AU, which responds best to ganciclovir or its prodrug valganciclovir. Oral valganciclovir 900 mg twice daily for 3 weeks, followed by valganciclovir 450 mg twice daily for another 4 weeks [172], has been the standard of care (Fig. 17.27). Topical ganciclovir 0.15 has been used as a long-term therapy to prevent recurrences [172, 178, 179]. Topical corticosteroids are administered under antiviral cover. Antiglaucoma medicines are needed for most of the CMV-AU. Although the CMV-AU responds in 75% of the patients, recurrences are common. Topical ganciclovir can be used long-term without fear of systemic side effects. However, long-term therapy risks developing resistance [180].

References

1. Kang YK, Im JC, Shin JP, Kim IT, Park DH. Short-term analysis of the residual volume of an eye drop following 23-gauge microincision vitrectomy surgery. Korean J Ophthalmol. 2017;31(5):439–45. https://doi.org/10.3341/kjo.2016.0090. Epub 2017 Jul 6. PMID: 28682023; PMCID: PMC5636720.
2. Erdogmus S, Govsa F. The arterial anatomy of the eyelid: importance for reconstructive and aesthetic surgery. J Plast Reconstr Aesthet Surg. 2007;60(3):241–5. https://doi.org/10.1016/j.bjps.2006.01.056. Epub 2006 Nov 20. PMID: 17293279.
3. Lopez R, Lauwers F, Paoli JR, Boutault F, Guitard J. The vascular system of the upper eyelid. Anatomical study and clinical interest. Surg Radiol Anat. 2008;30(3):265–9. https://doi.org/10.1007/s00276-008-0323-8. Epub 2008 Feb 21. PMID: 18288439.
4. Tucker SM, Linberg JV. Vascular anatomy of the eyelids. Ophthalmology. 1994;101(6):1118–21. https://doi.org/10.1016/s0161-6420(94)31212-7. PMID: 28932076; PMCID: PMC5583569. PMID: 8008353
5. Goldberg MF, Bron AJ. Limbal palisades of vogt. Trans Am Ophthalmol Soc. 1982;80:155–71. PMID: 7182957; PMCID: PMC1312261.
6. Subileau M, Vittet D. Lymphatics in eye fluid homeostasis: minor contributors or significant actors? Biology (Basel). 2021;10(7):582. https://doi.org/10.3390/biology10070582. PMID: 34201989; PMCID: PMC8301034.
7. Echegoyen JC, Hirabayashi KE, Lin KY, Tao JP. Imaging of eyelid lymphatic drainage. Saudi J Ophthalmol. 2012;26(4):441–3. https://doi.org/10.1016/j.sjopt.2012.08.003. PMID: 23961030; PMCID: PMC3729830.
8. Riordan-Eva P. Chapter 1. Anatomy & embryology of the eye. In: Riordan-Eva P, Cunningham Jr ET, editors. Vaughan & Asbury's general ophthalmol-

ogy, 18e. McGraw Hill; 2011. Accessed March 04, 2023. https://accessmedicine.mhmedical.com/content.aspx?bookid=387§ionid=40229318.

9. Irkec MT, Bozkurt B. Molecular immunology of allergic conjunctivitis. Curr Opin Allergy Clin Immunol. 2012;12(5):534–9. https://doi.org/10.1097/ACI.0b013e328357a21b. PMID: 22885886.
10. Elieh Ali Komi D, Rambasek T, Bielory L. Clinical implications of mast cell involvement in allergic conjunctivitis. Allergy. 2018;73(3):528–39. https://doi.org/10.1111/all.13334. Epub 2017 Nov 20. PMID: 29105783.
11. Bonini S, Lambiase A, Sgrulletta R, Bonini S. Allergic chronic inflammation of the ocular surface in vernal keratoconjunctivitis. Curr Opin Allergy Clin Immunol. 2003;3(5):381–7. https://doi.org/10.1097/00130832-200310000-00011. PMID: 14501439.
12. Leonardi A. Vernal keratoconjunctivitis: pathogenesis and treatment. Prog Retin Eye Res. 2002;21(3):319–39. https://doi.org/10.1016/s1350-9462(02)00006-x. PMID: 12052387.
13. Bonini S, Lambiase A, Schiavone M, Centofanti M, Palma LA, Bonini S. Estrogen and progesterone receptors in vernal keratoconjunctivitis. Ophthalmology. 1995;102(9):1374–9. https://doi.org/10.1016/s0161-6420(95)30861-5. PMID: 9097776.
14. Vichyanond P, Kosrirukvongs P. Use of cyclosporine A and tacrolimus in treatment of vernal keratoconjunctivitis. Curr Allergy Asthma Rep. 2013;13(3):308–14.https://doi.org/10.1007/s11882--013-0345-0. PMID: 23625179.
15. Bremond-Gignac D, Doan S, Amrane M, Ismail D, Montero J, Németh J, Aragona P, Leonardi A, VEKTIS Study Group. Twelve-month results of cyclosporine a cationic emulsion in a randomized study in patients with pediatric vernal keratoconjunctivitis. Am J Ophthalmol. 2020;212:116–26. https://doi.org/10.1016/j.ajo.2019.11.020. Epub 2019 Nov 23. PMID: 31770513.
16. Leonardi A, Doan S, Amrane M, Ismail D, Montero J, Németh J, Aragona P, Bremond-Gignac D, VEKTIS Study Group. A randomized, controlled trial of cyclosporine a cationic emulsion in pediatric vernal keratoconjunctivitis: the VEKTIS study. Ophthalmology. 2019;126(5):671–81. https://doi.org/10.1016/j.ophtha.2018.12.027. Epub 2018 Dec 27. PMID: 30593775.
17. Dahlmann-Noor A, Bonini S, Bremond-Gignac D, Heegaard S, Leonardi A, Montero J, Silva ED, EUR-VKC Group. Novel insights in the management of vernal keratoconjunctivitis (VKC): European Expert Consensus using a modified nominal group technique. Ophthalmol Ther. 2023;12:1207. https://doi.org/10.1007/s40123-023-00665-5. Epub ahead of print. PMID: 36790673.
18. Ghauri AJ, Biswas S, Manzouri B, Barua A, Sharma V, Hoole J, Dahlmann-Noor A. Management of vernal keratoconjunctivitis in children in the United Kingdom: a review of the literature and current best practice across six large United Kingdom centers. J Pediatr Ophthalmol Strabismus. 2023;60(1):6–17. https://doi.org/10.3928/01913913-20220328-01. Epub 2022 May 25. PMID: 35611818.
19. Johnson D, Liu D, Simel D. Does this patient with acute infectious conjunctivitis have a bacterial infection?: The rational clinical examination systematic review. JAMA. 2022;327(22):2231–7. https://doi.org/10.1001/jama.2022.7687. PMID: 35699701.
20. Liu SH, Hawkins BS, Ng SM, Ren M, Leslie L, Han G, Kuo IC. Topical pharmacologic interventions versus placebo for epidemic keratoconjunctivitis. Cochrane Database Syst Rev. 2022;3(3):CD013520. https://doi.org/10.1002/14651858.CD013520.pub2. PMID: 35238405; PMCID: PMC8892837.
21. O'Brien TP, Jeng BH, McDonald M, Raizman MB. Acute conjunctivitis: truth and misconceptions. Curr Med Res Opin. 2009;25(8):1953–61. https://doi.org/10.1185/03007990903038269. PMID: 19552618.
22. Chigbu DI, Labib BA. Pathogenesis and management of adenoviral keratoconjunctivitis. Infect Drug Resist. 2018;17(11):981–93. https://doi.org/10.2147/IDR.S162669. PMID: 30046247; PMCID: PMC6054290.
23. Bomsel M, Alfsen A. Entry of viruses through the epithelial barrier: pathogenic trickery. Nat Rev Mol Cell Biol. 2003;4(1):57–68. https://doi.org/10.1038/nrm1005. PMID: 12511869; PMCID: PMC7097689.
24. Kaufman HE. Adenovirus advances: new diagnostic and therapeutic options. Curr Opin Ophthalmol. 2011;22(4):290–3. https://doi.org/10.1097/ICU.0b013e3283477cb5. PMID: 21537185.
25. Kovalyuk N, Kaiserman I, Mimouni M, Cohen O, Levartovsky S, Sherbany H, Mandelboim M. Treatment of adenoviral keratoconjunctivitis with a combination of povidone-iodine 1.0% and dexamethasone 0.1% drops: a clinical prospective controlled randomized study. Acta Ophthalmol. 2017;95(8):e686–92. https://doi.org/10.1111/aos.13416. Epub 2017 Mar 25. PMID: 28342227.
26. Levinger E, Trivizki O, Shachar Y, Levinger S, Verssano D. Topical 0.03% tacrolimus for subepithelial infiltrates secondary to adenoviral keratoconjunctivitis. Graefes Arch Clin Exp Ophthalmol. 2014;252(5):811–6.https://doi.org/10.1007/s00417--014-2611-9. Epub 2014 Apr 4. PMID: 24696044.
27. Uchio E, Takeuchi S, Itoh N, Matsuura N, Ohno S, Aoki K. Clinical and epidemiological features of acute follicular conjunctivitis with special reference to that caused by herpes simplex virus type 1. Br J Ophthalmol. 2000;84(9):968–72. https://doi.org/10.1136/bjo.84.9.968. PMID: 10966946; PMCID: PMC1723617.
28. Esra N, Hollhumer R. Herpes simplex virus-related conjunctivitis resistant to aciclovir: a case report and review of the literature. Cornea. 2021;40(8):1055–8.

https://doi.org/10.1097/ICO.0000000000002613. PMID: 33264148.

29. Leibowitz HM. The red eye. N Engl J Med. 2000;343(5):345–51. https://doi.org/10.1056/NEJM200008033430507. PMID: 10922425.
30. Workowski KA, Bachmann LH, Chan PA, Johnston CM, Muzny CA, Park I, Reno H, Zenilman JM, Bolan GA. Sexually transmitted infections treatment guidelines, 2021. MMWR Recomm Rep. 2021;70(4):1–187. https://doi.org/10.15585/mmwr.rr7004a1. PMID: 34292926; PMCID: PMC8344968.
31. Hoffman JJ, Burton MJ, Leck A. Mycotic keratitis-a global threat from the filamentous fungi. J Fungi (Basel). 2021;7(4):273. https://doi.org/10.3390/jof7040273. PMID: 33916767; PMCID: PMC8066744.
32. Chang DC, Grant GB, O'Donnell K, Wannemuehler KA, Noble-Wang J, Rao CY, Jacobson LM, Crowell CS, Sneed RS, Lewis FM, Schaffzin JK, Kainer MA, Genese CA, Alfonso EC, Jones DB, Srinivasan A, Fridkin SK, Park BJ, Fusarium Keratitis Investigation Team. Multistate outbreak of Fusarium keratitis associated with use of a contact lens solution. JAMA. 2006;296(8):953–63. https://doi.org/10.1001/jama.296.8.953. PMID: 16926355.
33. Bernal MD, Acharya NR, Lietman TM, Strauss EC, McLeod SD, Hwang DG. Outbreak of Fusarium keratitis in soft contact lens wearers in San Francisco. Arch Ophthalmol. 2006;124(7):1051–3. https://doi.org/10.1001/archopht.124.7.ecr60006. Epub 2006 Jun 12. PMID: 16769826.
34. Assudani HJ, Pandya JM, Sarvan RR, Sapre AM, Gupta AR, Mehta SJ. Etiological diagnosis of microbial keratitis in a tertiary care hospital in Gujarat. Natl J Med Res. 2013;3(01):60–2. Retrieved from https://njmr.in/index.php/file/article/view/576.
35. Ranjini CY, Waddepally VV. Microbial profile of corneal ulcers in a tertiary care hospital in South India. J Ophthalmic Vis Res. 2016;11(4):363–7. https://doi.org/10.4103/2008-322X.194071. PMID: 27994804; PMCID: PMC5139547.
36. Ting DSJ, Ho CS, Cairns J, Elsahn A, Al-Aqaba M, Boswell T, Said DG, Dua HS. 12-year analysis of incidence, microbiological profiles and in vitro antimicrobial susceptibility of infectious keratitis: the Nottingham Infectious Keratitis Study. Br J Ophthalmol. 2021;105(3):328–33. https://doi.org/10.1136/bjophthalmol-2020-316128. Epub 2020 Jun 24. PMID: 32580955; PMCID: PMC7907586.
37. Labetoulle M, Boutolleau D, Burrel S, Haigh O, Rousseau A. Herpes simplex virus, varicella-zoster virus and cytomegalovirus keratitis: facts for the clinician. Ocul Surf. 2021;28:336–50. https://doi.org/10.1016/j.jtos.2021.07.002. Epub ahead of print. PMID: 34314898.
38. Upadhyay MP, Karmacharya PC, Koirala S, Shah DN, Shakya S, Shrestha JK, Bajracharya H, Gurung CK, Whitcher JP. The Bhaktapur eye study: ocular trauma and antibiotic prophylaxis for the prevention of corneal ulceration in Nepal. Br J Ophthalmol. 2001;85(4):388–92. https://doi.org/10.1136/bjo.85.4.388. PMID: 11264124; PMCID: PMC1723912.
39. Labetoulle M, Auquier P, Conrad H, Crochard A, Daniloski M, Bouée S, El Hasnaoui A, Colin J. Incidence of herpes simplex virus keratitis in France. Ophthalmology. 2005;112(5):888–95. https://doi.org/10.1016/j.ophtha.2004.11.052. PMID: 15878072.
40. Farooq AV, Shukla D. Herpes simplex epithelial and stromal keratitis: an epidemiologic update. Surv Ophthalmol. 2012;57(5):448–62. https://doi.org/10.1016/j.survophthal.2012.01.005. Epub 2012 Apr 28. PMID: 22542912; PMCID: PMC3652623
41. Liesegang TJ. Herpes zoster ophthalmicus natural history, risk factors, clinical presentation, and morbidity. Ophthalmology. 2008;115(2 Suppl):S3–12. https://doi.org/10.1016/j.ophtha.2007.10.009. PMID: 18243930.
42. Yawn BP, Wollan PC, St Sauver JL, Butterfield LC. Herpes zoster eye complications: rates and trends. Mayo Clin Proc. 2013;88(6):562–70. https://doi.org/10.1016/j.mayocp.2013.03.014. Epub 2013 May 9. Erratum in: Mayo Clin Proc. 2017 Sep;92(9):1458. PMID: 23664666; PMCID: PMC3788821.
43. McQuillan G, Kruszon-Moran D, Flagg EW, Paulose-Ram R. Prevalence of herpes simplex virus type 1 and type 2 in persons aged 14–49: United States, 2015–2016. NCHS Data Brief. 2018;304:1–8. PMID: 29442994.
44. Cohen JI. Herpesvirus latency. J Clin Invest. 2020;130(7):3361–9. https://doi.org/10.1172/JCI136225. PMID: 32364538; PMCID: PMC7324166.
45. Todokoro D, Hosogai M, Nakano S, Akiyama H. Effective diagnosis by real-time PCR of herpes simplex diffuse endotheliitis that is similar in appearance to fungal keratitis: case series. J Ophthalmic Inflamm Infect. 2021;11(1):20. https://doi.org/10.1186/s12348-021-00250-6. PMID: 34250547; PMCID: PMC8273046
46. Bhatt UK, Abdul Karim MN, Prydal JI, Maharajan SV, Fares U. Oral antivirals for preventing recurrent herpes simplex keratitis in people with corneal grafts. Cochrane Database Syst Rev. 2016;11:CD007824. https://doi.org/10.1002/14651858.CD007824.pub2. Accessed 10 March 2023.
47. Gopinathan U, Garg P, Fernandes M, Sharma S, Athmanathan S, Rao GN. The epidemiological features and laboratory results of fungal keratitis: a 10-year review at a referral eye care center in South India. Cornea. 2002;21(6):555–9. https://doi.org/10.1097/00003226-200208000-00004. PMID: 12131029.
48. Sharma S, Kunimoto DY, Gopinathan U, Athmanathan S, Garg P, Rao GN. Evaluation of corneal scraping smear examination methods in the diagnosis of bacterial and fungal keratitis: a survey of eight years of laboratory

experience. Cornea. 2002;21(7):643–7. https://doi.org/10.1097/00003226-200210000-00002. PMID: 12352078.

49. Cabrera-Aguas M, Khoo P, Watson SL. Infectious keratitis: a review. Clin Exp Ophthalmol. 2022;50(5):543–62. https://doi.org/10.1111/ceo.14113. Epub 2022 Jun 3. PMID: 35610943; PMCID: PMC9542356

50. Liu HY, Hopping GC, Vaidyanathan U, Ronquillo YC, Hoopes PC, Moshirfar M. Polymerase chain reaction and its application in the diagnosis of infectious keratitis. Med Hypothesis Discov Innov Ophthalmol. 2019;8(3):152–5. PMID: 31598517; PMCID: PMC6778471.

51. Borroni D, Romano V, Kaye SB, Somerville T, Napoli L, Fasolo A, Gallon P, Ponzin D, Esposito A, Ferrari S. Metagenomics in ophthalmology: current findings and future prospectives. BMJ Open Ophthalmol. 2019;4(1):e000248. https://doi.org/10.1136/bmjophth-2018-000248. Erratum in: BMJ Open Ophthalmol 2019 Jun 27;4(1):e000248corr1. PMID: 31276030; PMCID: PMC6557081.

52. Ung L, Chodosh J. Urgent unmet needs in the care of bacterial keratitis: an evidence-based synthesis. Ocul Surf. 2021;28:378–400. https://doi.org/10.1016/j.jtos.2021.08.013. Epub ahead of print. PMID: 34461290.

53. Ting DSJ, Settle C, Morgan SJ, Baylis O, Ghosh S. A 10-year analysis of microbiological profiles of microbial keratitis: the North East England Study. Eye (Lond). 2018;32(8):1416–7. https://doi.org/10.1038/s41433-018-0085-4. Epub 2018 Apr 3. PMID: 29610521; PMCID: PMC6085375.

54. Thomas RK, Melton R, Asbell PA. Antibiotic resistance among ocular pathogens: current trends from the ARMOR surveillance study (2009–2016). Clin Optom (Auckl). 2019;11:15–26. https://doi.org/10.2147/OPTO.S189115. PMID: 30881168; PMCID: PMC6419597.

55. Ray KJ, Prajna L, Srinivasan M, Geetha M, Karpagam R, Glidden D, Oldenburg CE, Sun CQ, McLeod SD, Acharya NR, Lietman TM. Fluoroquinolone treatment and susceptibility of isolates from bacterial keratitis. JAMA Ophthalmol. 2013;131(3):310–3. https://doi.org/10.1001/jamaophthalmol.2013.1718. PMID: 23307105; PMCID: PMC3833086.

56. Tallab RT, Stone DU. Corticosteroids as a therapy for bacterial keratitis: an evidence-based review of 'who, when and why'. Br J Ophthalmol. 2016;100(6):731–5. https://doi.org/10.1136/bjophthalmol-2015-307955. Epub 2016 Jan 7. PMID: 26743622.

57. Davis SA, Bovelle R, Han G, Kwagyan J. Corneal collagen cross-linking for bacterial infectious keratitis. Cochrane Database Syst Rev. 2020;6(6):CD013001. https://doi.org/10.1002/14651858.CD013001.pub2. PMID: 32557558; PMCID: PMC7389372.

58. Said DG, Elalfy MS, Gatzioufas Z, El-Zakzouk ES, Hassan MA, Saif MY, Zaki AA, Dua HS, Hafezi F. Collagen cross-linking with photoactivated riboflavin (PACK-CXL) for the treatment of advanced infectious keratitis with corneal melting. Ophthalmology. 2014;121(7):1377–82. https://doi.org/10.1016/j.ophtha.2014.01.011. Epub 2014 Feb 25. PMID: 24576886.

59. Ting DSJ, Henein C, Said DG, Dua HS. Photoactivated chromophore for infectious keratitis - corneal cross-linking (PACK-CXL): A systematic review and meta-analysis. Ocul Surf. 2019;17(4):624–34. https://doi.org/10.1016/j.jtos.2019.08.006. Epub 2019 Aug 8. PMID: 31401338.

60. Kaushik S, Ram J, Brar GS, Jain AK, Chakraborti A, Gupta A. Intracameral amphotericin B: initial experience in severe keratomycosis. Cornea. 2001;20(7):715–9. https://doi.org/10.1097/00003226-200110000-00009. PMID: 11588423.

61. Hoffman JJ, Arunga S, Mohamed Ahmed AHA, Hu VH, Burton MJ. Management of filamentous fungal keratitis: a pragmatic approach. J Fungi (Basel). 2022;8(10):1067. https://doi.org/10.3390/jof8101067. PMID: 36294633; PMCID: PMC9605596.

62. Shao Y, Yu Y, Pei CG, Tan YH, Zhou Q, Yi JL, Gao GP. Therapeutic efficacy of intracameral amphotericin B injection for 60 patients with keratomycosis. Int J Ophthalmol. 2010;3(3):257–60. https://doi.org/10.3980/j.issn.2222-3959.2010.03.18. Epub 2010 Sep 18. PMID: 22553567; PMCID: PMC3340624.

63. Sharma N, Sankaran P, Agarwal T, Arora T, Chawla B, Titiyal JS, Tandon R, Satapathy G, Vajpayee RB. Evaluation of intracameral amphotericin B in the management of fungal keratitis: randomized controlled trial. Ocul Immunol Inflamm. 2016;24(5):493–7. https://doi.org/10.3109/09273948.2015.1057597. Epub 2015 Sep 23. PMID: 26400628.

64. Prajna NV, Krishnan T, Rajaraman R, Patel S, Srinivasan M, Das M, Ray KJ, O'Brien KS, Oldenburg CE, McLeod SD, Zegans ME, Porco TC, Acharya NR, Lietman TM, Rose-Nussbaumer J, Mycotic Ulcer Treatment Trial II Group. Effect of oral voriconazole on fungal keratitis in the mycotic ulcer treatment trial II (MUTT II): a randomized clinical trial. JAMA Ophthalmol. 2016;134(12):1365–72. https://doi.org/10.1001/jamaophthalmol.2016.4096. PMID: 27787540; PMCID: PMC6044431.

65. Rahman MR, Minassian DC, Srinivasan M, Martin MJ, Johnson GJ. Trial of chlorhexidine gluconate for fungal corneal ulcers. Ophthalmic Epidemiol. 1997;4(3):141–9. https://doi.org/10.3109/09286589709115721. PMID: 9377282.

66. Gopinathan U, Sharma S, Garg P, Rao GN. Review of epidemiological features, microbiological diagnosis and treatment outcome of microbial keratitis: experience of over a decade. Indian J Ophthalmol. 2009;57(4):273–9. https://doi.org/10.4103/0301-4738.53051. PMID: 19574694; PMCID: PMC2712695.

67. Srinivasan M, Gonzales CA, George C, Cevallos V, Mascarenhas JM, Asokan B, Wilkins J, Smolin G, Whitcher JP. Epidemiology and aetiological diagnosis of corneal ulceration in Madurai, south India. Br J Ophthalmol. 1997;81(11):965–71. https://doi.org/10.1136/bjo.81.11.965. PMID: 9505820; PMCID: PMC1722056.
68. Vaddavalli PK, Garg P, Sharma S, Sangwan VS, Rao GN, Thomas R. Role of confocal microscopy in the diagnosis of fungal and acanthamoeba keratitis. Ophthalmology. 2011;118(1):29–35. https://doi.org/10.1016/j.ophtha.2010.05.018. PMID: 20801515.
69. Goh JWY, Harrison R, Hau S, Alexander CL, Tole DM, Avadhanam VS. Comparison of in vivo confocal microscopy, PCR and culture of corneal scrapes in the diagnosis of acanthamoeba keratitis. Cornea. 2018;37(4):480–5. https://doi.org/10.1097/ICO.0000000000001497. PMID: 29256983.
70. Carnt N, Hoffman JJ, Verma S, Hau S, Radford CF, Minassian DC, Dart JKG. *Acanthamoeba* keratitis: confirmation of the UK outbreak and a prospective case-control study identifying contributing risk factors. Br J Ophthalmol. 2018;102(12):1621–8. https://doi.org/10.1136/bjophthalmol-2018-312544. Epub 2018 Sep 19. PMID: 30232172.
71. Carrijo-Carvalho LC, Sant'ana VP, Foronda AS, de Freitas D, de Souza Carvalho FR. Therapeutic agents and biocides for ocular infections by free-living amoebae of Acanthamoeba genus. Surv Ophthalmol. 2017;62(2):203–18. https://doi.org/10.1016/j.survophthal.2016.10.009. Epub 2016 Nov 9. PMID: 27836717.
72. Thebpatiphat N, Hammersmith KM, Rocha FN, Rapuano CJ, Ayres BD, Laibson PR, Eagle RC Jr, Cohen EJ. Acanthamoeba keratitis: a parasite on the rise. Cornea. 2007;26(6):701–6. https://doi.org/10.1097/ICO.0b013e31805b7e63. PMID: 17592320.
73. Sharma S, Das S, Joseph J, Vemuganti GK, Murthy S. Microsporidial keratitis: need for increased awareness. Surv Ophthalmol. 2011;56(1):1–22. https://doi.org/10.1016/j.survophthal.2010.03.006. Epub 2010 Nov 11. PMID: 21071051.
74. Sforza C, Rango M, Galante D, Bresolin N, Ferrario VF. Spontaneous blinking in healthy persons: an optoelectronic study of eyelid motion. Ophthalmic Physiol Opt. 2008;28(4):345–53. https://doi.org/10.1111/j.1475-1313.2008.00577.x. PMID: 18565090.
75. Mishima S. Some physiological aspects of the precorneal tear film. Arch Ophthalmol. 1965;73:233–41. https://doi.org/10.1001/archopht.1965.00970030235017. PMID: 14237794.
76. Tomlinson A, Doane MG, McFadyen A. Inputs and outputs of the lacrimal system: review of production and evaporative loss. Ocul Surf. 2009;7(4):186–98. https://doi.org/10.1016/s1542-0124(12)70186-6. PMID: 19948102.
77. Doughty MJ, Laiquzzaman M, Oblak E, Button N. The tear (lacrimal) meniscus height in human eyes: a useful clinical measure or an unusable variable sign? Cont Lens Anterior Eye. 2002;25(2):57–65. https://doi.org/10.1016/s1367-0484(01)00005-4. PMID: 16303478.
78. Zhou L, Beuerman RW. The power of tears: how tear proteomics research could revolutionize the clinic. Expert Rev Proteomics. 2017;14(3):189–91. https://doi.org/10.1080/14789450.2017.1285703. Epub 2017 Feb 1. PMID: 28117610.
79. Craig JP, Nelson JD, Azar DT, Belmonte C, Bron AJ, Chauhan SK, de Paiva CS, Gomes JAP, Hammitt KM, Jones L, Nichols JJ, Nichols KK, Novack GD, Stapleton FJ, Willcox MDP, Wolffsohn JS, Sullivan DA. TFOS DEWS II report executive summary. Ocul Surf. 2017;15(4):802–12. https://doi.org/10.1016/j.jtos.2017.08.003. Epub 2017 Aug 8. PMID: 28797892.
80. Craig JP, Nichols KK, Akpek EK, Caffery B, Dua HS, Joo CK, Liu Z, Nelson JD, Nichols JJ, Tsubota K, Stapleton F. TFOS DEWS II definition and classification report. Ocul Surf. 2017;15(3):276–83. https://doi.org/10.1016/j.jtos.2017.05.008. Epub 2017 Jul 20. PMID: 28736335.
81. Moss SE, Klein R, Klein BE. Long-term incidence of dry eye in an older population. Optom Vis Sci. 2008;85(8):668–74. https://doi.org/10.1097/OPX.0b013e318181a947. PMID: 18677233.
82. Akpek EK, Klimava A, Thorne JE, Martin D, Lekhanont K, Ostrovsky A. Evaluation of patients with dry eye for presence of underlying Sjögren syndrome. Cornea. 2009;28(5):493–7. https://doi.org/10.1097/ICO.0b013e31818d3846. PMID: 19421051; PMCID: PMC2693267.
83. Liew MS, Zhang M, Kim E, Akpek EK. Prevalence and predictors of Sjogren's syndrome in a prospective cohort of patients with aqueous-deficient dry eye. Br J Ophthalmol. 2012;96(12):1498–503. https://doi.org/10.1136/bjophthalmol-2012-301767. Epub 2012 Sep 21. PMID: 23001257.
84. Zintzaras E, Voulgarelis M, Moutsopoulos HM. The risk of lymphoma development in autoimmune diseases: a meta-analysis. Arch Intern Med. 2005;165(20):2337–44. https://doi.org/10.1001/archinte.165.20.2337. PMID: 16287762.
85. Uchino M, Schaumberg DA, Dogru M, Uchino Y, Fukagawa K, Shimmura S, Satoh T, Takebayashi T, Tsubota K. Prevalence of dry eye disease among Japanese visual display terminal users. Ophthalmology. 2008;115(11):1982–8. https://doi.org/10.1016/j.ophtha.2008.06.022. Epub 2008 Aug 16. PMID: 18708259.
86. Bron AJ, de Paiva CS, Chauhan SK, Bonini S, Gabison EE, Jain S, Knop E, Markoulli M, Ogawa Y, Perez V, Uchino Y, Yokoi N, Zoukhri D, Sullivan DA. TFOS DEWS II pathophysiology report. Ocul Surf. 2017;15(3):438–510. https://doi.org/10.1016/j.jtos.2017.05.011. Epub 2017 Jul 20. Erratum in: Ocul Surf. 2019 Oct;17(4):842. PMID: 28736340.

87. Wu Y, Wang C, Wang X, Mou Y, Yuan K, Huang X, Jin X. Advances in dry eye disease examination techniques. Front Med (Lausanne). 2022;8:826530. https://doi.org/10.3389/fmed.2021.826530. PMID: 35145982; PMCID: PMC8823697.
88. Keech A, Senchyna M, Jones L. Impact of time between collection and collection method on human tear fluid osmolarity. Curr Eye Res. 2013;38(4):428–36. https://doi.org/10.3109/02713683.2013.763987. Epub 2013 Feb 12. PMID: 23402632.
89. Sambursky R, Davitt WF 3rd, Latkany R, Tauber S, Starr C, Friedberg M, Dirks MS, McDonald M. Sensitivity and specificity of a point-of-care matrix metalloproteinase 9 immunoassay for diagnosing inflammation related to dry eye. JAMA Ophthalmol. 2013;131(1):24–8. https://doi.org/10.1001/jamaophthalmol.2013.561. Erratum in: JAMA Ophthalmol 2013 Mar 1;131(3):364. PMID: 23307206.
90. Whitcher JP, Shiboski CH, Shiboski SC, Heidenreich AM, Kitagawa K, Zhang S, Hamann S, Larkin G, McNamara NA, Greenspan JS, Daniels TE, Sjögren's International Collaborative Clinical Alliance Research Groups. A simplified quantitative method for assessing keratoconjunctivitis sicca from the Sjögren's Syndrome International Registry. Am J Ophthalmol. 2010;149(3):405–15. https://doi.org/10.1016/j.ajo.2009.09.013. Epub 2009 Dec 29. PMID: 20035924; PMCID: PMC3459675.
91. Finis D, Pischel N, Schrader S, Geerling G. Evaluation of lipid layer thickness measurement of the tear film as a diagnostic tool for Meibomian gland dysfunction. Cornea. 2013;32(12):1549–53. https://doi.org/10.1097/ICO.0b013e3182a7f3e1. PMID: 24097185.
92. Brooks CC, Gupta PK. Meibomian gland morphology among patients presenting for refractive surgery evaluation. Clin Ophthalmol. 2021;15:315–21. https://doi.org/10.2147/OPTH.S292919. PMID: 33542616; PMCID: PMC7851383.
93. Jin Y, Li J, Chen J, Shao M, Zhang R, Liang Y, Zhang X, Zhang X, Zhang Q, Li F, Cheng Y, Sun X, He J, Li Z. Tissue-specific autoantibodies improve diagnosis of primary Sjögren's Syndrome in the early stage and indicate localized salivary injury. J Immunol Res. 2019;2019:3642937. https://doi.org/10.1155/2019/3642937. PMID: 31205955; PMCID: PMC6530237.
94. Ren X, Chou Y, Wang Y, Chen Y, Liu Z, Li X. Comparison of intense pulsed light and near-infrared light in the treatment of dry eye disease: a prospective randomized study. Acta Ophthalmol. 2021;99(8):e1307–14. https://doi.org/10.1111/aos.14833. Epub 2021 Apr 25. PMID: 33899331.
95. Geerling G, Tauber J, Baudouin C, Goto E, Matsumoto Y, O'Brien T, Rolando M, Tsubota K, Nichols KK. The international workshop on meibomian gland dysfunction: report of the subcommittee on management and treatment of meibomian gland dysfunction. Invest Ophthalmol Vis Sci. 2011;52(4):2050–64. https://doi.org/10.1167/iovs.10-6997g. PMID: 21450919; PMCID: PMC3072163.
96. Liu K, Chan YK, Peng X, Yuan R, Liao M, Liang J, Tang X, Xu Y, Cai Y, Li Q, Wang H. Improved dry eye symptoms and signs of patients with meibomian gland dysfunction by a dietary supplement. Front Med (Lausanne). 2021;8:769132. https://doi.org/10.3389/fmed.2021.769132. PMID: 34869485; PMCID: PMC8632949.
97. Macsai MS. The role of omega-3 dietary supplementation in blepharitis and meibomian gland dysfunction (an AOS thesis). Trans Am Ophthalmol Soc. 2008;106:336–56. PMID: 19277245.
98. Nakamura M, Imanaka T, Sakamoto A. Diquafosol ophthalmic solution for dry eye treatment. Adv Ther. 2012;29(7):579–89. https://doi.org/10.1007/s12325-012-0033-9. Epub 2012 Jul 27. PMID: 22843206.
99. Nam KT, Ahn SM, Eom Y, Kim HM, Song JS. Immediate effects of 3% diquafosol and 0.1% hyaluronic acid ophthalmic solution on tear break-up time in normal human eyes. J Ocul Pharmacol Ther. 2015;31(10):631–5. https://doi.org/10.1089/jop.2015.0062. Epub 2015 Aug 20. PMID: 26630617.
100. Shigeyasu C, Yamada M, Akune Y, Tsubota K. Diquafosol sodium ophthalmic solution for the treatment of dry eye: clinical evaluation and biochemical analysis of tear composition. Jpn J Ophthalmol. 2015;59(6):415–20. https://doi.org/10.1007/s10384-015-0408-y. Epub 2015 Aug 27. PMID: 26310103.
101. Keating GM. Lifitegrast ophthalmic solution 5%: a review in dry eye disease. Drugs. 2017;77(2):201–8. https://doi.org/10.1007/s40265-016-0681-1. PMID: 28058622.
102. Higuchi A. Autologous serum and serum components. Invest Ophthalmol Vis Sci. 2018;59(14):DES121–9. https://doi.org/10.1167/iovs.17-23760. PMID: 30481816.
103. Cui D, Li G, Akpek EK. Autologous serum eye drops for ocular surface disorders. Curr Opin Allergy Clin Immunol. 2021;21(5):493–9. https://doi.org/10.1097/ACI.0000000000000770. PMID: 34261888.
104. Tripathi RC, Millard CB, Tripathi BJ. Protein composition of human aqueous humor: SDS-PAGE analysis of surgical and post-mortem samples. Exp Eye Res. 1989;48(1):117–30. https://doi.org/10.1016/0014--4835(89)90025-0. PMID: 2920779.
105. Freddo TF. A contemporary concept of the blood-aqueous barrier. Prog Retin Eye Res. 2013;32:181–95. https://doi.org/10.1016/j.preteyeres.2012.10.004. Epub 2012 Nov 2. PMID: 23128417; PMCID: PMC3544162.
106. Reekie IR, Sharma S, Foers A, Sherlock J, Coles MC, Dick AD, Denniston AK, Buckley CD. The cellular composition of the uveal immune environment. Front Med (Lausanne). 2021;8:721953. https://doi.

org/10.3389/fmed.2021.721953. PMID: 34778287; PMCID: PMC8586083.
107. Niederkor JY, Ligocki AJ. 2016. https://utsouthwestern.pure.elsevier.com/en/publications/immunology-of-the-eye.
108. Gery I, Caspi RR. Tolerance induction in relation to the eye. Front Immunol. 2018;9:2304. https://doi.org/10.3389/fimmu.2018.02304. PMID: 30356688; PMCID: PMC6189330.
109. Isaacs A, Lindenmann J, Valentine RC. Virus interference. II. Some properties of interferon. Proc R Soc Lond B Biol Sci. 1957;147(927):268–73. https://doi.org/10.1098/rspb.1957.0049. PMID: 13465721; Burke DC 2009. (http://www.brainimmune.com/the-discovery-of-interferon-the-first-cytokine-by-alick-isaacs-and-jean-lindenmann-in-1957/).
110. di Giovine FS, Duff GW. Interleukin 1: the first interleukin. Immunol Today. 1990;11(1):13–20. https://doi.org/10.1016/0167-5699(90)90005-t. PMID: 2405873.
111. Ferreira VL, Borba HH, Bonetti A d F, Leonart LP, Pontarolo R. Cytokines and interferons: types and functions. In: Khan WA, editor. Autoantibodies and cytokines [Internet]. London: IntechOpen; 2018. [cited 2022 Oct 19]. Available from: https://www.intechopen.com/chapters/59914. https://doi.org/10.5772/intechopen.74550.
112. Gupta A. In: Sobti RC, Ganju AK, editors. Bench to bedside research in ophthalmology in biomedical translational research: from disease diagnosis to treatment. Vol II. Springer Nature; 2022. p. 67–124.
113. Jawad S, Liu B, Agron E, Nussenblatt RB, Sen HN. Elevated serum levels of interleukin-17A in uveitis patients. Ocul Immunol Inflamm. 2013;21(6):434–9. https://doi.org/10.3109/09273948.2013.815786. Epub 2013 Aug 19. PMID: 23957503; PMCID: PMC5569243.
114. Kuiper JJ, Mutis T, de Jager W, de Groot-Mijnes JD, Rothova A. Intraocular interleukin-17 and proinflammatory cytokines in HLA-A29-associated birdshot chorioretinopathy. Am J Ophthalmol. 2011;152(2):177–182.e1. https://doi.org/10.1016/j.ajo.2011.01.031. Epub 2011 May 13. PMID: 21570674.
115. Ooi KG, Galatowicz G, Calder VL, Lightman SL. Cytokines and chemokines in uveitis: is there a correlation with clinical phenotype? Clin Med Res. 2006;4(4):294–309. https://doi.org/10.3121/cmr.4.4.294. PMID: 17210978; PMCID: PMC1764804.
116. Dinarello CA. Historical insights into cytokines. Eur J Immunol. 2007;37(Suppl 1(Suppl 1)):S34–45. https://doi.org/10.1002/eji.200737772. PMID: 17972343; PMCID: PMC3140102.
117. Thorne JE, Suhler E, Skup M, Tari S, Macaulay D, Chao J, Ganguli A. Prevalence of noninfectious uveitis in the United States: a claims-based analysis. JAMA Ophthalmol. 2016;134(11):1237–45. https://doi.org/10.1001/jamaophthalmol.2016.3229. PMID: 27608193.
118. Grunwald L, Newcomb CW, Daniel E, Kaçmaz RO, Jabs DA, Levy-Clarke GA, Nussenblatt RB, Rosenbaum JT, Suhler EB, Thorne JE, Foster CS, Kempen JH. Systemic immunosuppressive therapy for eye diseases cohort study. Risk of relapse in primary acute anterior uveitis. Ophthalmology. 2011;118(10):1911–5. https://doi.org/10.1016/j.ophtha.2011.02.044. Epub 2011 Jun 16. PMID: 21680024; PMCID: PMC3179829.
119. Chang JH, McCluskey PJ, Wakefield D. Acute anterior uveitis and HLA-B27. Surv Ophthalmol. 2005;50(4):364–88. https://doi.org/10.1016/j.survophthal.2005.04.003. PMID: 15967191.
120. Karaconji T, Maconochie Z, McCluskey P. Acute anterior uveitis in Sydney. Ocul Immunol Inflamm. 2013;21(2):108–14. https://doi.org/10.3109/09273948.2012.745882. Epub 2012 Dec 19. PMID: 23252660.
121. Rosenbaum JT. Characterization of uveitis associated with spondyloarthritis. J Rheumatol. 1989;16(6):792–6. PMID: 2778762.
122. Rosenbaum JT. The eye in spondyloarthritis. Semin Arthritis Rheum. 2019;49(3S):S29–31. https://doi.org/10.1016/j.semarthrit.2019.09.014. PMID: 31779847; PMCID: PMC6981236.
123. Taams LS, Steel KJA, Srenathan U, Burns LA, Kirkham BW. IL-17 in the immunopathogenesis of spondyloarthritis. Nat Rev Rheumatol. 2018;14(8):453–66.https://doi.org/10.1038/s41584--018-0044-2. PMID: 30006601.
124. Zeboulon N, Dougados M, Gossec L. Prevalence and characteristics of uveitis in the spondyloarthropathies: a systematic literature review. Ann Rheum Dis. 2008;67(7):955–9. https://doi.org/10.1136/ard.2007.075754. Epub 2007 Oct 25. PMID: 17962239.
125. Rudwaleit M, van der Heijde D, Landewé R, Listing J, Akkoc N, Brandt J, Braun J, Chou CT, Collantes-Estevez E, Dougados M, Huang F, Gu J, Khan MA, Kirazli Y, Maksymowych WP, Mielants H, Sørensen IJ, Ozgocmen S, Roussou E, Valle-Oñate R, Weber U, Wei J, Sieper J. The development of Assessment of SpondyloArthritis international Society classification criteria for axial spondyloarthritis (part II): validation and final selection. Ann Rheum Dis. 2009;68(6):777–83. https://doi.org/10.1136/ard.2009.108233. Epub 2009 Mar 17. Erratum in: Ann Rheum Dis 2019 Jun;78(6):e59. PMID: 19297344.
126. Rudwaleit M, van der Heijde D, Landewé R, Akkoc N, Brandt J, Chou CT, Dougados M, Huang F, Gu J, Kirazli Y, Van den Bosch F, Olivieri I, Roussou E, Scarpato S, Sørensen IJ, Valle-Oñate R, Weber U, Wei J, Sieper J. The Assessment of SpondyloArthritis

International Society classification criteria for peripheral spondyloarthritis and for spondyloarthritis in general. Ann Rheum Dis. 2011;70(1):25–31. https://doi.org/10.1136/ard.2010.133645. Epub 2010 Nov 24. PMID: 21109520.
127. Rademacher J, Müllner H, Diekhoff T, Haibel H, Igel S, Pohlmann D, Proft F, Protopopov M, Rios Rodriguez V, Torgutalp M, Pleyer U, Poddubnyy D. Keep an eye on the back: spondyloarthritis in patients with acute anterior uveitis. Arthritis Rheum. 2023;75(2):210–9. https://doi.org/10.1002/art.42315. Epub 2022 Dec 23. PMID: 35905288.
128. Juanola X, Loza Santamaría E, Cordero-Coma M, SENTINEL Working Group. Description and prevalence of spondyloarthritis in patients with anterior uveitis: The SENTINEL interdisciplinary collaborative project. Ophthalmology. 2016;123(8):1632–6. https://doi.org/10.1016/j.ophtha.2016.03.010. Epub 2016 Apr 12. PMID: 27084561.
129. Rosenbaum JT. Why HLA-B27? My thirty-year quest: the Friedenwald lecture. Invest Ophthalmol Vis Sci. 2011;52(10):7712–5, 7711. https://doi.org/10.1167/iovs.11-8247. PMID: 21960642; PMCID: PMC3183985.
130. Wakefield D, Clarke D, McCluskey P. Recent developments in HLA B27 anterior uveitis. Front Immunol. 2021;5(11):608134. https://doi.org/10.3389/fimmu.2020.608134. PMID: 33469457; PMCID: PMC7813675.
131. Rosenbaum JT, Asquith M. The microbiome and HLA-B27-associated acute anterior uveitis. Nat Rev Rheumatol. 2018;14(12):704–13. https://doi.org/10.1038/s41584-018-0097-2. PMID: 30301938; PMCID: PMC6597169.
132. Muñoz-Fernández S, Hidalgo V, Fernández-Melón J, Schlincker A, Bonilla G, Ruiz-Sancho D, Fonseca A, Gijón-Baños J, Martín-Mola E. Sulfasalazine reduces the number of flares of acute anterior uveitis over a one-year period. J Rheumatol. 2003;30(6):1277–9. PMID: 12784403.
133. Lambert JR, Wright V. Eye inflammation in psoriatic arthritis. Ann Rheum Dis. 1976;35(4):354–6. https://doi.org/10.1136/ard.35.4.354. PMID: 970993; PMCID: PMC1007395.
134. Paiva ES, Macaluso DC, Edwards A, Rosenbaum JT. Characterisation of uveitis in patients with psoriatic arthritis. Ann Rheum Dis. 2000;59(1):67–70. https://doi.org/10.1136/ard.59.1.67. PMID: 10627431; PMCID: PMC1752985.
135. Zisman D, Gladman DD, Stoll ML, Strand V, Lavi I, Hsu JJ, Mellins ED, CARRA Legacy Registry Investigators. The juvenile psoriatic arthritis cohort in the CARRA registry: clinical characteristics, classification, and outcomes. J Rheumatol. 2017;44(3):342–51. https://doi.org/10.3899/jrheum.160717. Epub 2017 Feb 1. PMID: 28148698.
136. Salek SS, Pradeep A, Guly C, Ramanan AV, Rosenbaum JT. Uveitis and juvenile psoriatic arthritis or psoriasis. Am J Ophthalmol. 2018;185:68–74. https://doi.org/10.1016/j.ajo.2017.10.018. Epub 2017 Oct 31. PMID: 29101009; PMCID: PMC5819354.
137. Charlton R, Green A, Shaddick G, Snowball J, Nightingale A, Tillett W, Smith CH, McHugh N, PROMPT study group. Risk of uveitis and inflammatory bowel disease in people with psoriatic arthritis: a population-based cohort study. Ann Rheum Dis. 2018;77(2):277–80. https://doi.org/10.1136/annrheumdis-2017-212328. Epub 2017 Nov 1. PMID: 29092855.
138. Lo TC, Chen YY, Chen HH. Risk of inflammatory bowel disease in uveitis patients: a population-based cohort study. Eye (Lond). 2022;36(6):1288–93. https://doi.org/10.1038/s41433-021-01645-4. Epub 2021 Jun 21. PMID: 34155367; PMCID: PMC9151650.
139. Lyons JL, Rosenbaum JT. Uveitis associated with inflammatory bowel disease compared with uveitis associated with spondyloarthropathy. Arch Ophthalmol. 1997;115(1):61–4. https://doi.org/10.1001/archopht.1997.01100150063010. PMID: 9006426.
140. Troncoso LL, Biancardi AL, de Moraes HV, Zaltman C Jr. Ophthalmic manifestations in patients with inflammatory bowel disease: a review. World J Gastroenterol. 2017;23(32):5836–48. https://doi.org/10.3748/wjg.v23.i32.5836. PMID: 28932076; PMCID: PMC5583569.
141. Selmi C, Gershwin ME. Diagnosis and classification of reactive arthritis. Autoimmun Rev. 2014;13(4–5):546–9. https://doi.org/10.1016/j.autrev.2014.01.005. Epub 2014 Jan 10. PMID: 24418301.
142. Yang P. Uveitis associated with reactive arthritis. In: Atlas of uveitis. Singapore: Springer; 2021. https://doi.org/10.1007/978-981-15-3726-4_16.
143. Behera G, Madhuri C, Panicker GJ, Thabah MM. Corneal ulcer in reactive arthritis. J R Coll Physicians Edinb. 2021;51(3):258–61. https://doi.org/10.4997/JRCPE.2021.310. PMID: 34528614.
144. Suresh PS. Bilateral disciform keratitis in Reiter's syndrome. Indian J Ophthalmol. 2016;64(9):685–7. https://doi.org/10.4103/0301-4738.97088. PMID: 27853023; PMCID: PMC5151165.
145. Joyce E, Glasner P, Ranganathan S, Swiatecka-Urban A. Tubulointerstitial nephritis: diagnosis, treatment, and monitoring. Pediatr Nephrol. 2017;32(4):577–87.https://doi.org/10.1007/s00467--016-3394-5. Epub 2016 May 7. PMID: 27155873; PMCID: PMC5099107.
146. Legendre M, Devilliers H, Perard L, Groh M, Nefti H, Dussol B, Trad S, Touré F, Abad S, Boffa JJ, Frimat L, Torner S, Seidowsky A, Massy ZA, Saadoun D, Rieu V, Schoindre Y, Heron E, Frouget T, Lionet A, Glowacki F, Arnaud L, Mousson C, Besancenot JF, Rebibou JM, Bielefeld P. Clinicopathologic char-

acteristics, treatment, and outcomes of tubulointerstitial nephritis and uveitis syndrome in adults: a national retrospective strobe-compliant study. Medicine (Baltimore). 2016;95(26):e3964. https://doi.org/10.1097/MD.0000000000003964. PMID: 27367994; PMCID: PMC4937908.

147. Chevalier A, Duflos C, Clave S, Boyer O, Hogan J, Lahoche A, Decramer S, Broux F, Vrillon I, Allain-Launay E, Bacchetta J, Tanne C, Allard L, Cloarec S, Pietrement C, Bourdat-Michel G, Djeddi D, Dunand O, Faudeux C, Nobili F, Taque S, Ulinski T, Zaloszyc A, Morin D, Fila M. Renal prognosis in children with tubulointerstitial nephritis and uveitis syndrome. Kidney Int Rep. 2021;6(12):3045–53. https://doi.org/10.1016/j.ekir.2021.09.017. PMID: 34901573; PMCID: PMC8640547.

148. Saarela V, Nuutinen M, Ala-Houhala M, Arikoski P, Rönnholm K, Jahnukainen T. Tubulointerstitial nephritis and uveitis syndrome in children: a prospective multicenter study. Ophthalmology. 2013;120(7):1476–81. https://doi.org/10.1016/j.ophtha.2012.12.039. Epub 2013 Mar 16. PMID: 23511116.

149. Mackensen F, Smith JR, Rosenbaum JT. Enhanced recognition, treatment, and prognosis of tubulointerstitial nephritis and uveitis syndrome. Ophthalmology. 2007;114(5):995–9. https://doi.org/10.1016/j.ophtha.2007.01.002. Epub 2007 Mar 26. PMID: 17383731.

150. Paroli MP, Cappiello D, Staccini D, Caccavale R, Paroli M. Tubulointerstitial nephritis and uveitis syndrome (TINU): a case series in a tertiary care uveitis setting. J Clin Med. 2022;11(17):4995. https://doi.org/10.3390/jcm11174995. PMID: 36078924; PMCID: PMC9457268.

151. Ali A, Rosenbaum JT. TINU (tubulointerstitial nephritis uveitis) can be associated with chorioretinal scars. Ocul Immunol Inflamm. 2014;22(3):213–7. https://doi.org/10.3109/09273948.2013.841624. Epub 2013 Oct 21. PMID: 24143861.

152. Cao JL, Srivastava SK, Venkat A, Lowder CY, Sharma S. Ultra-widefield fluorescein angiography and OCT findings in tubulointerstitial nephritis and uveitis syndrome. Ophthalmol Retina. 2020;4(2):189–97. https://doi.org/10.1016/j.oret.2019.08.012. Epub 2019 Sep 20. PMID: 31708486.

153. Hettinga YM, Scheerlinck LM, Lilien MR, Rothova A, de Boer JH. The value of measuring urinary β2-microglobulin and serum creatinine for detecting tubulointerstitial nephritis and uveitis syndrome in young patients with uveitis. JAMA Ophthalmol. 2015;133(2):140–5. https://doi.org/10.1001/jamaophthalmol.2014.4301. PMID: 25356569.

154. Standardization of Uveitis Nomenclature (SUN) Working Group. Classification criteria for tubulointerstitial nephritis with uveitis syndrome. Am J Ophthalmol. 2021;228:255–61. https://doi.org/10.1016/j.ajo.2021.03.041. Epub 2021 May 11. PMID: 33845023; PMCID: PMC8634781.

155. Petty RE, Southwood TR, Manners P, Baum J, Glass DN, Goldenberg J, He X, Maldonado-Cocco J, Orozco-Alcala J, Prieur AM, Suarez-Almazor ME, Woo P, International League of Associations for Rheumatology. International League of Associations for Rheumatology classification of juvenile idiopathic arthritis: second revision, Edmonton, 2001. J Rheumatol. 2004;31(2):390–2. PMID: 14760812.

156. Standardization of Uveitis Nomenclature (SUN) Working Group. Classification criteria for juvenile idiopathic arthritis-associated chronic anterior uveitis. Am J Ophthalmol. 2021;228:192–7. https://doi.org/10.1016/j.ajo.2021.03.055. Epub 2021 May 11. PMID: 33845021; PMCID: PMC8594759.

157. Ravelli A, Felici E, Magni-Manzoni S, Pistorio A, Novarini C, Bozzola E, Viola S, Martini A. Patients with antinuclear antibody-positive juvenile idiopathic arthritis constitute a homogeneous subgroup irrespective of the course of joint disease. Arthritis Rheum. 2005;52(3):826–32. https://doi.org/10.1002/art.20945. PMID: 15751057.

158. Kotaniemi K, Kautiainen H, Karma A, Aho K. Occurrence of uveitis in recently diagnosed juvenile chronic arthritis: a prospective study. Ophthalmology. 2001;108(11):2071–5. https://doi.org/10.1016/s0161-6420(01)00773-4. PMID: 11713082.

159. Rypdal V, Glerup M, Songstad NT, Bertelsen G, Christoffersen T, Arnstad ED, Aalto K, Berntson L, Fasth A, Herlin T, Ekelund M, Peltoniemi S, Toftedal P, Nielsen S, Leinonen S, Bangsgaard R, Nielsen R, Rygg M, Nordal E, Nordic Study Group of Pediatric Rheumatology. Uveitis in juvenile idiopathic arthritis: 18-year outcome in the population-based Nordic Cohort Study. Ophthalmology. 2021;128(4):598–608. https://doi.org/10.1016/j.ophtha.2020.08.024. Epub 2020 Aug 29. PMID: 32866542.

160. Angeles-Han ST, Ringold S, Beukelman T, Lovell D, Cuello CA, Becker ML, Colbert RA, Feldman BM, Holland GN, Ferguson PJ, Gewanter H, Guzman J, Horonjeff J, Nigrovic PA, Ombrello MJ, Passo MH, Stoll ML, Rabinovich CE, Sen HN, Schneider R, Halyabar O, Hays K, Shah AA, Sullivan N, Szymanski AM, Turgunbaev M, Turner A, Reston J. 2019 American College of Rheumatology/Arthritis Foundation guideline for the screening, monitoring, and treatment of juvenile idiopathic arthritis-associated uveitis. Arthritis Care Res. 2019;71(6):703–16. https://doi.org/10.1002/acr.23871. Epub 2019 Apr 25. PMID: 31021540; PMCID: PMC6777949.

161. Constantin T, Foeldvari I, Anton J, de Boer J, Czitrom-Guillaume S, Edelsten C, Gepstein R, Heiligenhaus A, Pilkington CA, Simonini G,

Uziel Y, Vastert SJ, Wulffraat NM, Haasnoot AM, Walscheid K, Pálinkás A, Pattani R, Györgyi Z, Kozma R, Boom V, Ponyi A, Ravelli A, Ramanan AV. Consensus-based recommendations for the management of uveitis associated with juvenile idiopathic arthritis: the SHARE initiative. Ann Rheum Dis. 2018;77(8):1107–17. https://doi.org/10.1136/annrheumdis-2018-213131. Epub 2018 Mar 28. PMID: 29592918; PMCID: PMC6059050.

162. Amarante-Mendes GP, Adjemian S, Branco LM, Zanetti LC, Weinlich R, Bortoluci KR. Pattern recognition receptors and the host cell death molecular machinery. Front Immunol. 2018;9:2379. https://doi.org/10.3389/fimmu.2018.02379. PMID: 30459758; PMCID: PMC6232773.

163. Rood JE, Behrens EM. Inherited autoinflammatory syndromes. Annu Rev Pathol. 2022;17:227–49. https://doi.org/10.1146/annurev--pathmechdis-030121-041528. Epub 2021 Oct 26. PMID: 34699263.

164. Forrester JV, Kuffova L, Dick AD. Autoimmunity, autoinflammation, and infection in uveitis. Am J Ophthalmol. 2018;189:77–85. https://doi.org/10.1016/j.ajo.2018.02.019. Epub 2018 Mar 2. PMID: 29505775.

165. Holland GN, Rosenbaum JT. The challenge of Blau syndrome. Am J Ophthalmol. 2018;187:xviii–xix. https://doi.org/10.1016/j.ajo.2017.12.006. Epub 2018 Jan 12. PMID: 29338849.

166. Sarens IL, Casteels I, Anton J, Bader-Meunier B, Brissaud P, Chédeville G, Cimaz R, Dick AD, Espada G, Fernandez-Martin J, Guly CM, Hachulla E, Harjacek M, Khubchandani R, Mackensen F, Merino R, Modesto C, Naranjo A, Oliveira-Knupp S, Özen S, Pajot C, Ramanan AV, Russo R, Susic G, Thatayatikom A, Thomée C, Vastert S, Bertin J, Arostegui JI, Rose CD, Wouters CH. Blau syndrome-associated uveitis: preliminary results from an international prospective interventional case series. Am J Ophthalmol. 2018;187:158–66. https://doi.org/10.1016/j.ajo.2017.08.017. Epub 2017 Sep 6. PMID: 28887115.

167. Kumrah R, Pilania RK, Menia NK, Rawat A, Sharma J, Gupta A, Vignesh P, Jindal AK, Rikhi R, Agarwal A, Gupta V, Singh S, Suri D. Blau syndrome: lessons learned in a tertiary care centre at Chandigarh, North India. Front Immunol. 2022;13:932919. https://doi.org/10.3389/fimmu.2022.932919. PMID: 36189202; PMCID: PMC9521334.

168. Kaufman KP, Becker ML. Distinguishing Blau syndrome from systemic sarcoidosis. Curr Allergy Asthma Rep. 2021;21(2):10. https://doi.org/10.1007/s11882-021-00991-3. PMID: 33560445; PMCID: PMC9762981.

169. Radosavljevic A, Agarwal M, Chee SP, Zierhut M. Epidemiology of viral induced anterior uveitis. Ocul Immunol Inflamm. 2022;30(2):297–309. https://doi.org/10.1080/09273948.2020.1853177. Epub 2021 Feb 22. PMID: 33617392.

170. Bodaghi B, Cassoux N, Wechsler B, Hannouche D, Fardeau C, Papo T, Huong DL, Piette JC, LeHoang P. Chronic severe uveitis: etiology and visual outcome in 927 patients from a single center. Medicine (Baltimore). 2001;80(4):263–70. https://doi.org/10.1097/00005792-200107000-00005. PMID: 11470987.

171. Rathinam SR, Namperumalsamy P. Global variation and pattern changes in epidemiology of uveitis. Indian J Ophthalmol. 2007;55(3):173–83. https://doi.org/10.4103/0301-4738.31936. PMID: 17456933.

172. Touhami S, Qu L, Angi M, Bojanova M, Touitou V, Lehoang P, Rozenberg F, Bodaghi B. Cytomegalovirus anterior uveitis: clinical characteristics and long-term outcomes in a French series. Am J Ophthalmol. 2018;194:134–42. https://doi.org/10.1016/j.ajo.2018.07.021. Epub 2018 Jul 26. PMID: 30055154.

173. Takase H, Kubono R, Terada Y, Imai A, Fukuda S, Tomita M, Miyanaga M, Kamoi K, Sugita S, Miyata K, Mochizuki M. Comparison of the ocular characteristics of anterior uveitis caused by herpes simplex virus, varicella-zoster virus, and cytomegalovirus. Jpn J Ophthalmol. 2014;58(6):473–82. https://doi.org/10.1007/s10384-014-0340-6. Epub 2014 Aug 16. PMID: 25124341.

174. Terada Y, Kaburaki T, Takase H, Goto H, Nakano S, Inoue Y, Maruyama K, Miyata K, Namba K, Sonoda KH, Kaneko Y, Numaga J, Fukushima M, Horiguchi N, Ide M, Ehara F, Miyazaki D, Hasegawa E, Mochizuki M. Distinguishing features of anterior uveitis caused by herpes simplex virus, varicella-zoster virus, and cytomegalovirus. Am J Ophthalmol. 2021;227:191–200. https://doi.org/10.1016/j.ajo.2021.03.020. Epub 2021 Mar 25. PMID: 33773985.

175. Standardization of Uveitis Nomenclature (SUN) Working Group. Classification criteria for herpes simplex virus anterior uveitis. Am J Ophthalmol. 2021;228:231–6. https://doi.org/10.1016/j.ajo.2021.03.053. Epub 2021 Apr 9. PMID: 33845009; PMCID: PMC8501150.

176. Standardization of Uveitis Nomenclature (SUN) Working Group. Classification criteria for varicella zoster virus anterior uveitis. Am J Ophthalmol. 2021;228:165–73. https://doi.org/10.1016/j.ajo.2021.03.037. Epub 2021 Apr 15. PMID: 33845010; PMCID: PMC8594747.

177. Standardization of Uveitis Nomenclature (SUN) Working Group. Classification criteria for cytomegalovirus anterior uveitis. Am J Ophthalmol. 2021;228:89–95. https://doi.org/10.1016/j.ajo.2021.03.060. Epub 2021 Apr 9. PMID: 33845019; PMCID: PMC8501153.

178. La Distia NR, Putera I, Mayasari YD, Hikmahwati W, Pertiwi AM, Ridwan AS, Sitompul R, Westcott M, Chee SP, Pavesio C, Thng ZX, Gupta V, Agrawal R. Clinical characteristics and treatment outcomes of cytomegalovirus anterior uveitis and endotheliitis: a systematic review and meta-analysis. Surv Ophthalmol. 2022;67(4):1014–30. https://doi.org/10.1016/j.survophthal.2021.12.006. Epub 2021 Dec 23. PMID: 34954093.
179. Wong JX, Agrawal R, Wong EP, Teoh SC. Efficacy and safety of topical ganciclovir in the management of cytomegalovirus (CMV)-related anterior uveitis. J Ophthalmic Inflamm Infect. 2016;6(1):10. https://doi.org/10.1186/s12348-016-0078-z. Epub 2016 Mar 15. PMID: 26976016; PMCID: PMC4791412.
180. Jap A, Chee SP. Viral anterior uveitis. Curr Opin Ophthalmol. 2011;22(6):483–8. https://doi.org/10.1097/ICU.0b013e32834be021. PMID: 21918442.

Episcleritis, Scleritis, and Peripheral Corneal Ulceration

18

18.1 Sclera and Episclera-Anatomical Considerations

Sclera is the outer white fibrous coat of the eyeball, which continues anteriorly with the transparent cornea. Posteriorly, the sclera has perforations, the lamina cribrosa, that allow the retinal nerve fibres to exit the eye and form the optic nerve. The dura mater lining the optic nerve is continuous with the sclera. The anterior sclera is covered with a thin layer of elastic tissue, the episclera. The episclera has a rich vascular supply and sends penetrating vessels into the sclera. Six extraocular muscles (four recti and two obliques) are inserted into the sclera at variable distances from the limbus. Posteriorly, the sclera is perforated by the short and long ciliary nerves, short (15–20) and long ciliary arteries (two), and four vortex veins. The sclera is 0.3 mm thick at the insertion site of the extraocular muscle tendons; elsewhere, it is 0.6 mm [1]. The sclera provides the outer hard structural support to the eye's contents and resists distortion of the eyeball during eyeball movement by the extraocular muscles. Like tendons, which it mimics in its properties, it is relatively avascular and rich in collagen-fibrous proteins in its extracellular matrix [2]. Most of the cells in the scleral stroma are fibrocytes capable of transforming into fibroblasts. Besides, the episclera has a rich population of macrophages that act as antigen-presenting cells (APC) [3]. These cells' density is much higher in the episclera than in the sclera. There are no lymphatic vessels in the sclera. The upregulation of antiangiogenic factors and downregulation of pro-angiogenic factors maintain the avascularity of the sclera. The antiangiogenic factors highly expressed in the sclera include fibulin 5, pigment epithelial-derived growth factor, and tissue inhibitor of metalloproteinase 2 (TIMP2). At the same time, several proangiogenic factors are downregulated. Scleral homogenate does not promote the proliferation of blood or lymphatic endothelial cells [4].

18.2 Episcleritis and Scleritis

Episcleritis and scleritis are among the most common extraarticular complications of rheumatoid arthritis, an autoimmune inflammatory disorder of the synovial membrane and the cartilage of the joints. The human sclera consists mainly of type I collagen versus type II collagen in the cartilage. However, the human sclera and cartilage share common evolutionary development. Several species, except for mammals, have cartilage and small ossicles to support the sclera of their eyes [5]. Although strictly speaking, the sclera is not cartilage; it has several similarities with the latter. The primary component of the human sclera is a type I collagen secreted by the

A. Gupta et al., *Ophthalmic Signs in Practice of Medicine*,
https://doi.org/10.1007/978-981-99-7923-3_18

scleral fibrocytes. Scleral cells isolated from guinea pigs have pluripotent stem cell properties. They can be differentiated into adipocytes, chondrocytes, and osteocytes [6]. In culture media, the scleral cells can be induced to produce type II collagen and aggrecan, a proteoglycan characteristic of chondrocytes indicating a common origin of the cartilage, synovial membrane and sclera. It explains the common occurrence of episcleral and scleral inflammation in patients who have rheumatoid arthritis [7].

18.2.1 Epidemiology of Episcleritis and Scleritis

Episcleritis is a common cause of painful red eyes, showing a sectoral inflammation of the episcleral tissue (Figs. 18.1 and 18.2). In the majority, the inflammation does not cause elevation of the episcleral tissues. It is termed simple and is most often sectoral than diffuse. In one-third of the eyes, it may be nodular. In a US county-based population study (mostly Caucasians) over 10 years, the incidence of episcleritis was 15.4 per 100,000 population per year. It was seen at least three times more often than scleritis. The average age of episcleritis was 40 years, and there was a 3:2 ratio in favour of women. Nearly, 95% of episcleritis patients did not have an associated systemic disease. Those with systemic diseases were more likely to have more recurrences than those with idiopathic episcleritis [8]. The incidence may vary from 21/100,000 person-years [9] to 41/100,000 person-years [10], depending on the composition of the population. Systemic inflammatory diseases were seen only in 5% of episcleritis patients, including SLE, rheumatoid arthritis, Crohn's disease, Ankylosing spondylitis, and reactive arthritis [8].

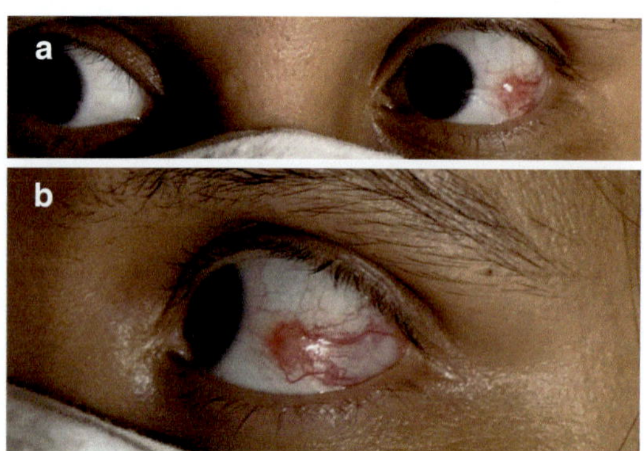

Fig. 18.1 Episcleritis seen as sectoral inflammation of the episcleral tissue in the left eye (**a**). The engorged vessels are seen prominently in right lateral gaze (**b**)

18.2.2 Etiology of Non-infectious Scleritis

Scleritis most often results from autoimmune inflammation or seldom from an infective process. In the Intelligent Research in Sight (IRIS) registry of the American Academy of Ophthalmology, 111,314 scleritis patients were registered between 2013 and 2019 who made at least three office visits. Of these, only 5% of scleritis patients were noted to have associated systemic diseases [11]. This data reflects the community-level practice and is likely underreporting the systemic associations. On the other hand, data from tertiary care centres, reflecting more complicated cases, shows a much higher association with systemic diseases. Nearly 30% of patients with scleritis may have associated systemic inflammatory diseases, most commonly rheumatoid arthritis (RA), granulomatosis with polyangiitis (GPA), ankylosing spondylitis, primary Sjogren syndrome, relapsing polychondritis, systemic lupus erythematosus (SLE), polyarteritis nodosa (PAN), Gout and inflammatory bowel disease (Figs. 18.2 and 18.3) [12, 13]. RA precedes the onset of scleritis in most patients. Rarely, recurrent isolated scleritis has been reported in asymptomatic Takayasu's arteritis [14]. Rarely, paraneoplastic syndrome may present as scleritis [15]. Although episcleritis may be the first manifestation of IgA nephropathy, it may rarely manifest even as posterior scleritis [16].

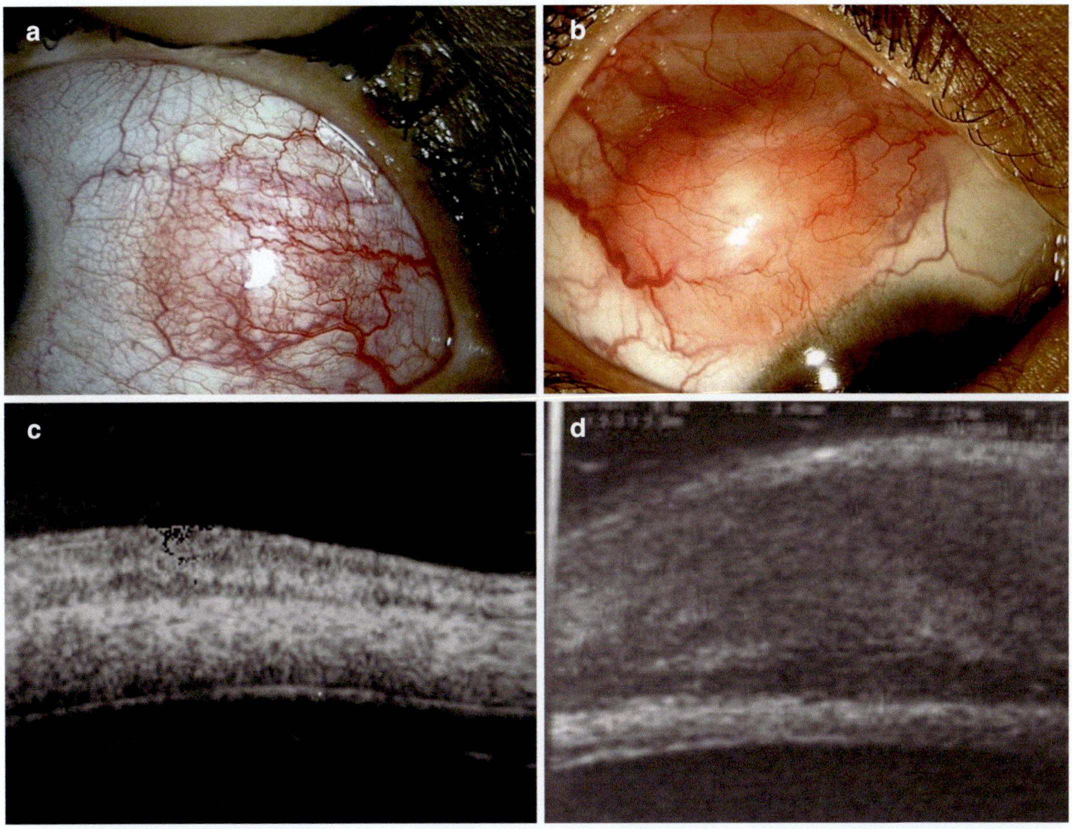

Fig. 18.2 Episcleritis (**a**) and anterior nodular scleritis (**b**). Ultrasound bio-microscopy (UBM) shows a preserved, normal scleral structure in episcleritis (**c**), while the whole of sclera gets involved in scleritis (**d**)

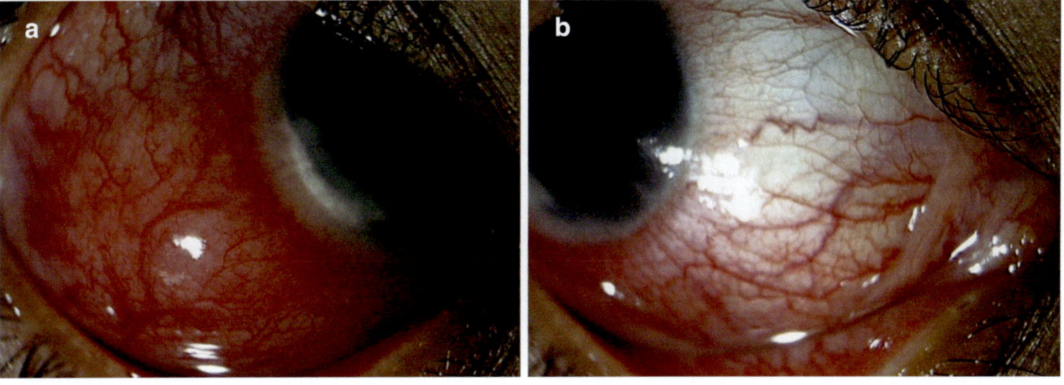

Fig. 18.3 Diffuse scleritis with peripheral corneal involvement in the right eye, seen in medial gaze (**a**) and lateral gaze (**b**)

18.2.3 Etiology of Infectious Scleritis

Infections by herpes zoster virus, mycobacterium tuberculosis, pseudomonas aeruginosa, or fungi may be responsible for 5–10% of all scleritis cases [17–20]. In large series, 7% of all scleritis was caused by herpes viruses. Herpetic scleritis tends to be unilateral and painful. Most have diffuse anterior scleritis and are less commonly nodular or necrotizing. Conjunctival sensations are often lost over the site of scleritis. A clue to the possible viral etiology of scleritis is the loss of conjunctival sensations in areas other than those affected by scleritis [21]. Vision may be lost in nearly 34% of viral scleritis cases [17].

Most cases of tubercular scleritis are reported from TB-endemic regions of the world (Fig. 18.4). However, TB-nonendemic regions have isolated disease and are rarely associated with miliary TB, TB lymphadenitis or pulmonary disease. Non-contributory chest imaging in over half the patients may cause considerable delay in initiating a definitive treatment. Vision is adversely affected in older patients, those with posterior scleritis and by delayed initiating definitive treatment and using corticosteroids before anti-TB treatment [22].

Syphilis is making a comeback. Syphilis may present as nodular scleritis [23, 24] or even as necrotizing nodular scleritis [25]. Uveitis and focal retinal vasculitis may accompany syphilitic scleritis [26].

18.2.4 Clinical Characteristics of Episcleritis

Episcleritis is characterized by localized or diffuse hyperemia with mild pain or discomfort (Figs. 18.1 and 18.2). In a large referral clinic cohort, episcleritis was diffuse in 84% and nodular in 16% [27, 28]. This hyperemia gets blanched with the use of topical phenylephrine. There is no corneal involvement or anterior uveitis. Most of the cases are benign and resolve spontaneously. Unless associated with a systemic inflammatory disease, episcleritis is usually non-recurrent and does not require any investigations. Laboratory investigations should be done in recurrent cases as done for scleritis (Box 18.1).

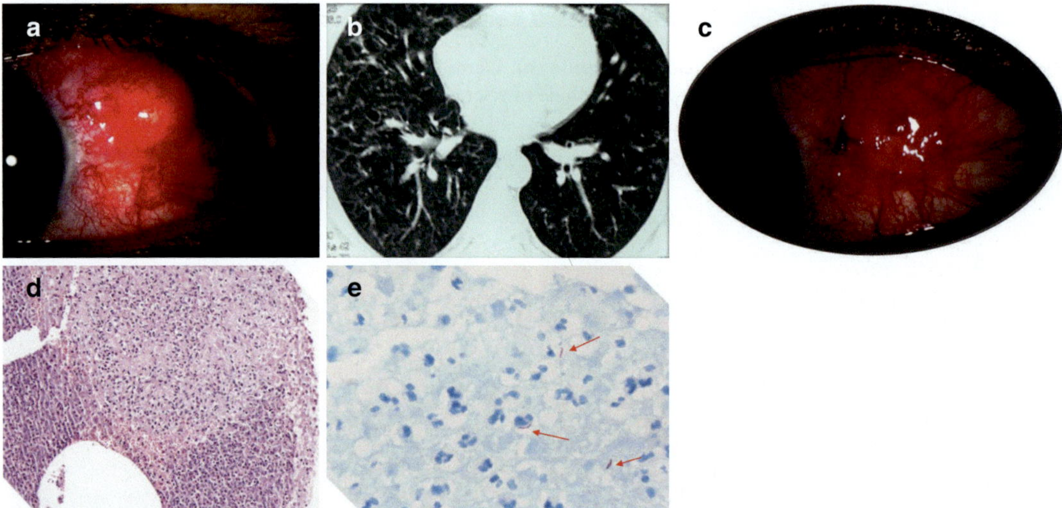

Fig. 18.4 (**a**–**e**) Anterior nodular scleritis (**a**) in a patient with multiple discrete mediastinal lymph nodes and retroperitoneal lymphadenopathy on CECT chest/abdomen (**b**). He underwent scleral biopsy (**c**) which revealed multiple epithelioid cell granulomas (**d**). ZN staining showed acid-fast bacilli (AFB), suggestive of *Mycobacterium tuberculosis* (red arrows, **e**). Anti-tubercular therapy (ATT) was initiated. (**f**, **g**) One month after starting ATT, scleritis showed healing (**f**), and was completely healed at 3 months (**g**)

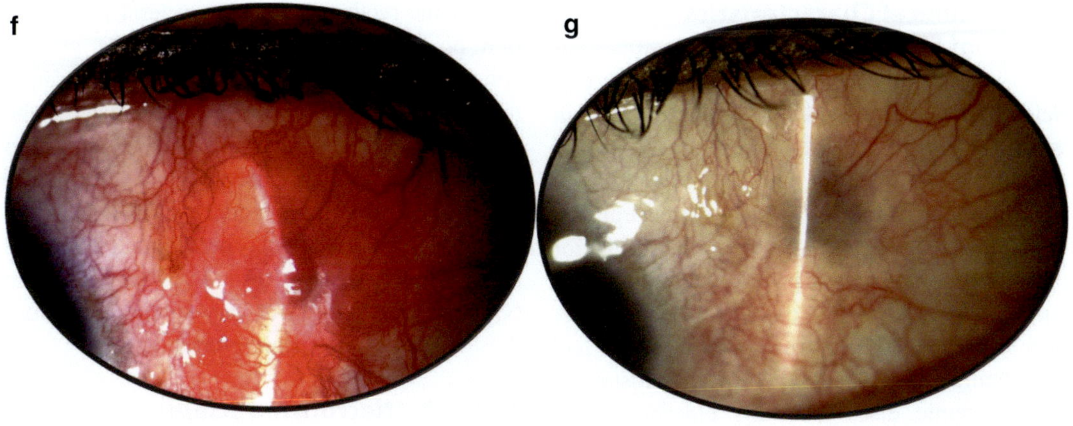

Fig. 18.4 (continued)

Box 18.1 Key Local and Systemic Lab Investigations in Necrotising Scleritis and Peripheral Ulcerative Keratitis

Local or systemic disorder	Lab tests
RA	RF; anti-CCP antibodies; ANCA; CBC; ESR, CRP Imaging X-rays
Primary Sjogren syndrome	Anti-SS-A antibodies; anti-SS-B antibodies; ANA; CRP; ESR; CBC; complements; Schirmer's test; ocular surface staining with vital dyes; salivary gland function tests; salivary gland imaging; sialometry; labial gland biopsy; urine analysis; S. immunoglobulin levels
SLE*	ANA; anti-dsDNA antibodies; anti-Smith antibodies; anti-SS-A antibodies; anti-SS-B antibodies; anti-PLs antibodies; CBC; RFT; LFT; urine analysis; antibodies to histone; tissue biopsy
Relapsing poly-chondritis	ESR; CRP; echocardiography; FDG-PET-CT scan
Granulomatosis with polyangiitis	ANCA-PR3; ANCA-MPO; CRP; ESR; TLC; urine analysis; CT chest
Polyarteritis nodosa	HBV serology; LFT; ANCA-ve; CRP; renal functions; CT/MR arteriography to detect microaneurysms and focal narrowing of medium arteries; biopsy. ADA2 gene mutation and ADA2 levels in monogenic variant DADA2
Bacterial keratitis/infectious scleritis	Corneal/scleral scrapping for smear and culture/sensitivity

Abbreviations: *RA* rheumatoid arthritis; *RF* rheumatoid factor; *A-CCP* anti-cyclic citrullinated peptide; *ANCA* anti-neutrophil cytoplasmic antibodies; *CBC* complete blood counts; *ESR* erythrocyte sedimentation rate; *CRP* c-reactive proteins; *MRI* magnetic resonance imaging; *SS* Sjogren syndrome; *ANA* antinuclear antibodies; *anti-PLs antibodies* anti-phospholipids antibodies; *RFT* renal function tests; *LFT* liver function tests; *ESR* erythrocyte sedimentation rate; *CRP* c-reactive protein; *MRI* magnetic resonance imaging; *FDG PET-CT* fluorodeoxyglucose positron emission tomography-computerized tomography; *ANCA-PR3* anti-neutrophil cytoplasmic antibody-proteinase 3; *ANCA-MPO* anti-neutrophil cytoplasmic antibody-myeloperoxidase; *HBV* hepatitis B virus; *CT/MR* computerized tomography/magnetic resonance imaging; *ADA2* adenosine deaminase2; *DADA2* deficiency of adenosine deaminase2.

*source: https://www.lupus.org/resources/glossary-of-lupus-blood-tests.

18.2.5 Clinical Characteristics of Scleritis

Scleral inflammations are seen more often in women (65–70%) and are bilateral in 30–40% of the cases (Fig. 18.3) [11, 27, 28]. Patients with scleritis are older (mean 53.7 years) than episcleritis (mean 47.4 years). Scleritis presenting for the first time above 60 appears uncommon and accounted for only 3% of cases in a referral practice. While 65% had diffuse scleritis, 35% had necrotizing scleritis, and GPA was the most common systemic disease in this elderly cohort. Nodular scleritis in the elderly was significantly less common. However, necrotizing scleritis was significantly more common in the elderly than those younger than 60 [29].

Inflammation of the sclera is characterized by eye redness with extreme radiating pain that wakes the patient at night and improves during the daytime. Pain is often referred to the face and jaw as the nerve fibres of CN V are primarily affected [27, 28]. Pain is worsened by eye movements. The purplish hue of the congested scleral vessels is best seen in daylight or slit-lamp. The redness of scleritis cannot be blanched with phenylephrine.

18.2.5.1 Classification of Scleritis

The classification of immune-mediated scleritis has remained almost the same as first described [30]. Anterior scleritis is inflammation of the sclera that extends from the limbus to the insertion of the recti muscles. Any scleral inflammation posterior to the insertion of the recti is considered posterior scleritis. The most common is non-necrotizing anterior scleritis which may be diffuse or nodular and is most often unilateral. In a large cohort in a US-based referral centre, scleritis was diffuse (75%), nodular (14%), necrotizing (4%), scleromalacia perforans (1%), and posterior uveitis (6%) (Fig. 18.5) [27, 28]. The types of scleritis did not vary significantly from those seen in a European referral centre.

18.2.5.2 Necrotizing Scleritis

While necrotizing scleritis is less common, it tends to be bilateral, may involve the peripheral cornea, and is a sight-threatening disease. Clinically, the necrotic area appears as an avascular area of the sclera, with brown or black uvea showing through a thin sclera surrounded by dilated vessels (Fig. 18.5b). The avascular necrotic sequestrum gives a white-glazed porcelain-like appearance [31]. The sequestrum formation may be seen in necrotizing scleritis with inflammation (41%) and without inflammation (77%) [31]. The sequestrum may shed off without warning in scleromalacia perforans. The diagnosis of scleromalacia perforans is often delayed due to a lack of symptoms. The avascularity of the lesion can be best evaluated by anterior segment ICG angiography or, presently, with enface OCT and OCT angiography. There is no inflammation in scleromalacia perforans, and it is painless (Fig. 18.5b). It is caused by vasculitis

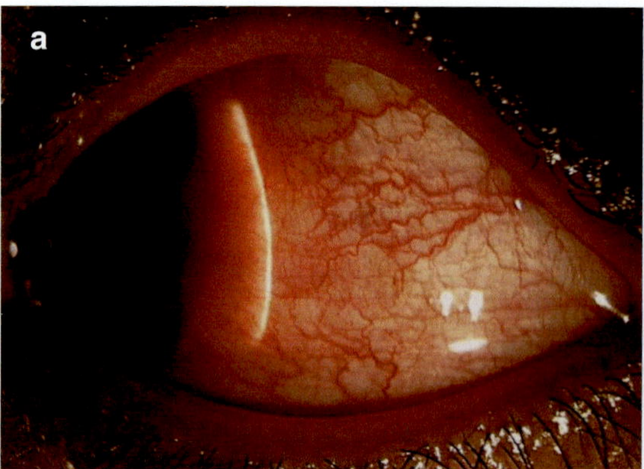

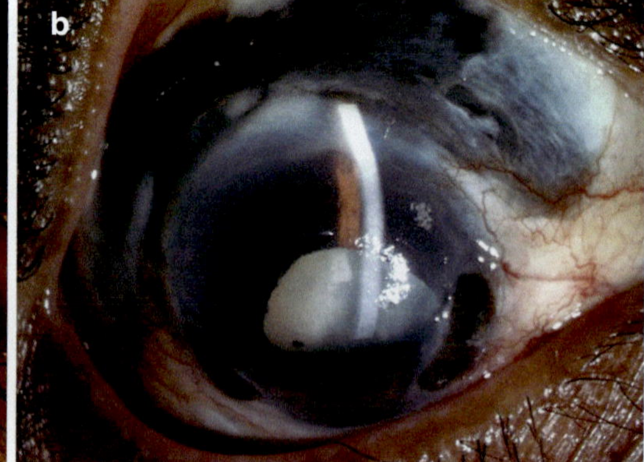

Fig. 18.5 Diffuse anterior scleritis (**a**) and scleromalacia perforans (**b**). Images courtesy of Prof Amit Gupta, Advanced Eye Centre, Post Graduate Institute of Medical Education and Research, Chandigarh

and looks like dead white tissue. It is always associated with life-threatening systemic inflammatory disorders like granulomatosis with polyangiitis (GPA) (Figs. 18.6, 18.7 and 18.8) and rheumatoid arthritis (RA). The painless necrotizing scleritis without obvious signs of inflammation (scleromalacia perforans) indicates the onset of vasculitic complications of RA.

In contrast to the slow onset and benign course of non-necrotizing anterior scleritis, necrotizing scleritis has an acute onset and follows a rapidly progressive course [32]. The presence of bilateral diffuse anterior scleritis, necrosis, and corneal involvement is highly suggestive of underlying GPA [33]. The character of scleritis remains the same in recurrent scleritis. The conversion of non-necrotizing to necrotizing scleritis may occur in 12% of the cases and is always seen in patients with associated systemic disease [32].

18.2.5.3 Posterior Scleritis

Among all the phenotypes of scleritis, posterior scleritis is uncommon and may manifest as a diffuse or a nodular form. In a large series of posterior scleritis, the majority were women at a mean age of 45. Bilaterality was seen in 16%. Systemic

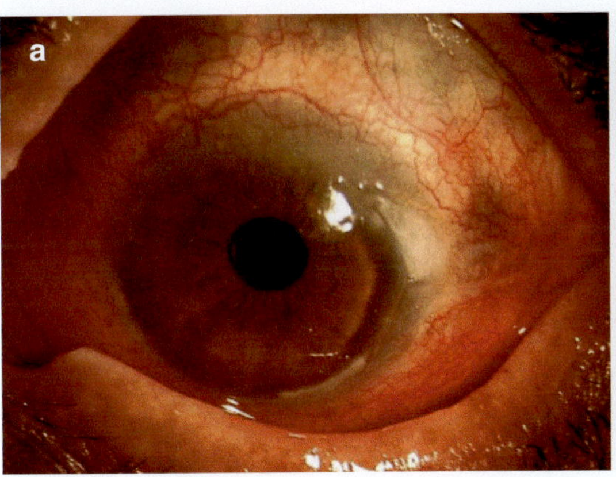

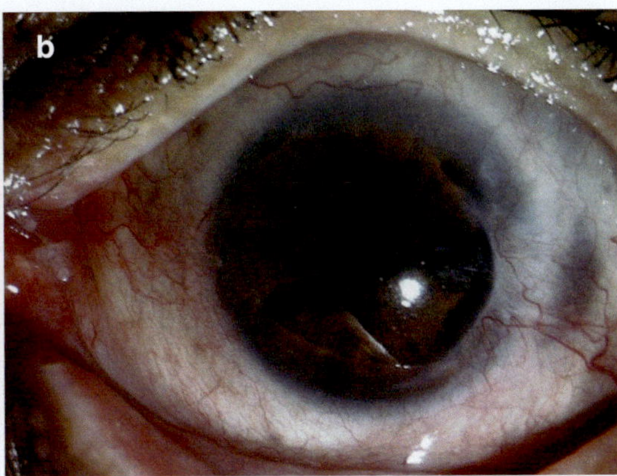

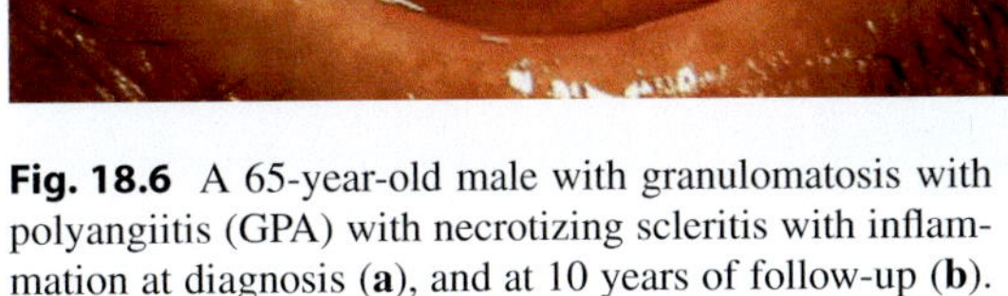

Fig. 18.6 A 65-year-old male with granulomatosis with polyangiitis (GPA) with necrotizing scleritis with inflammation at diagnosis (**a**), and at 10 years of follow-up (**b**). Images courtesy of Prof Amit Gupta, Advanced Eye Centre, Post Graduate Institute of Medical Education and Research, Chandigarh, India

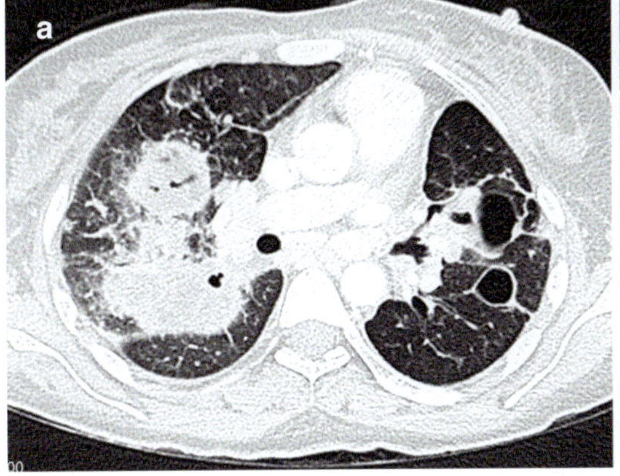

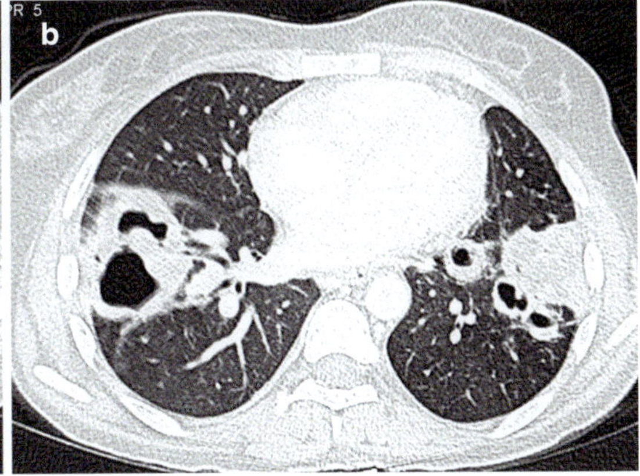

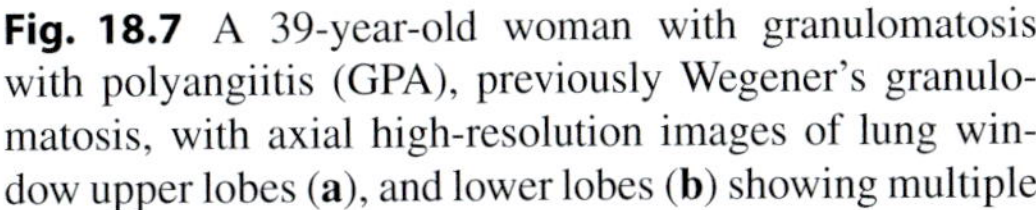

Fig. 18.7 A 39-year-old woman with granulomatosis with polyangiitis (GPA), previously Wegener's granulomatosis, with axial high-resolution images of lung window upper lobes (**a**), and lower lobes (**b**) showing multiple nodules with many having cavitations. Images courtesy of Dr Manphool Singhal, Department of Radiodiagnosis, Post Graduate Institute of Medical Education and Research, Chandigarh

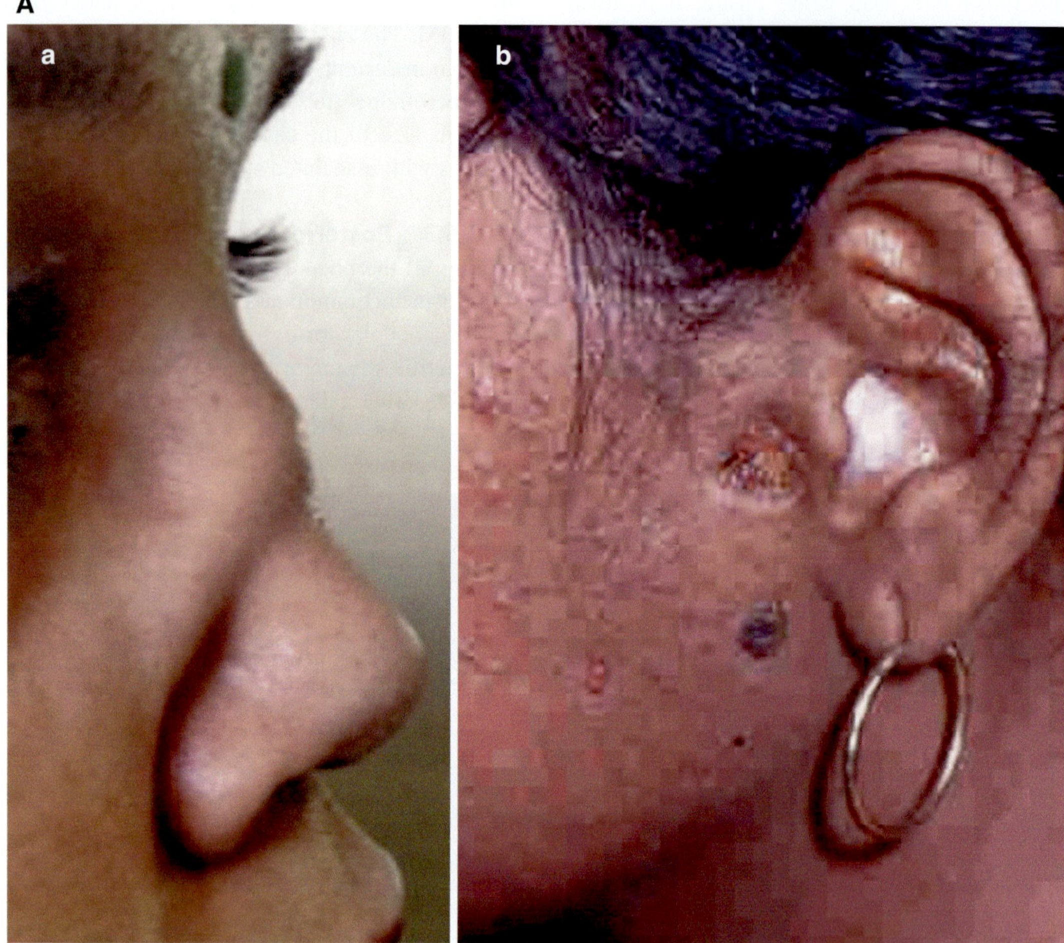

Fig. 18.8 (**A**) Collapse of the nasal bridge (**a**) in a patient with granulomatosis with polyangiitis (GPA). Reproduced with permission of the publishers from Sharma A, Bambery P. (2015) Relapsing Polychondritis. In: (Sharma A (ed).Textbook of Systemic Vasculitis, 1st Edn. Jaypee Brothers Medical Publishers (P) Ltd., New Delhi. P. 292. A biopsy-positive sinus in front of the tragus in another patient with GPA (**b**). Figure 'b' reproduced with permission of the publishers from Bambery P, Sharma A, Gupta A and Gupta V (2009) Systemic examination and imaging in Gupta A, Gupta V, Herbort C, Khairallah M (eds) Uveitis: Text and Imaging 1st Edn. Jaypee Brothers Medical Publishers (P) Ltd., New Delhi. P. 290. (**B**) Granulomatosis with polyangiitis. Photomicrograph of skin biopsy shows fibrinoid necroses of the dermal artery with perivascular granulomatous inflammation (**a**) b Martius Scarlet Blue (MSB) confirms fibrinoid necroses of the artery (**b**) (H&E a, 4X; MSB, b × 40 original). Small vessel vasculitis; Photomicrograph of skin biopsy shows leukocytoclastic vasculitis of dermal capillaries (**c**) (H&E c, ×40 original). Images courtesy of Dr. Rithambra Nada, Prof of Pathology, Post Graduate Institute of Medical Education and Research, Chandigarh, India

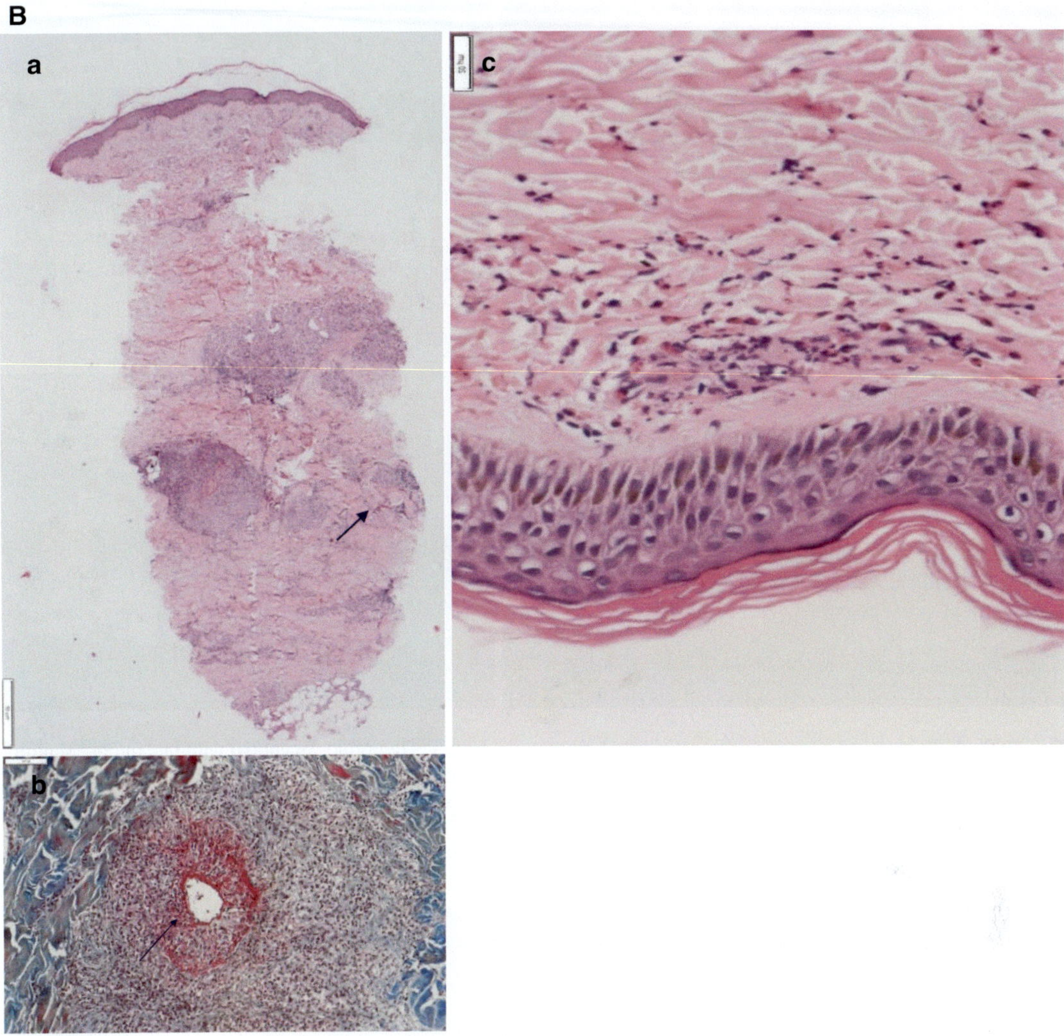

Fig. 18.8 (continued)

inflammatory diseases were noted in 40% of cases [34]. Posterior scleritis presents with painful vision loss due to an exudative retinal detachment, choroidal folds, optic disc edema, and occasional choroidal detachment (Figs. 18.9 and 18.10). The FFA shows pinpoint dye leakage with pooling in late frames (Fig. 18.9). Very often, there is an associated anterior scleritis and inflammatory cells in the anterior chamber. It is the most common scleritis phenotype in children. On ultrasonography, scleral thickness > 2 mm was seen in more than half of the patients, and T-sign could be observed in nearly 40% of the affected eyes [34].

Recurrences were seen in one-third of the patients at a rate of 15.8 per person/year ([34]. Nodular posterior scleritis may present as a mass lesion in the fundus associated with exudative retinal detachment [35]. It may not always be painful [36], and at times, it can present a diagnostic challenge [37]. The eye may be enucleated for a mistaken diagnosis of malignancy in a necrotizing nodular posterior scleritis [38].

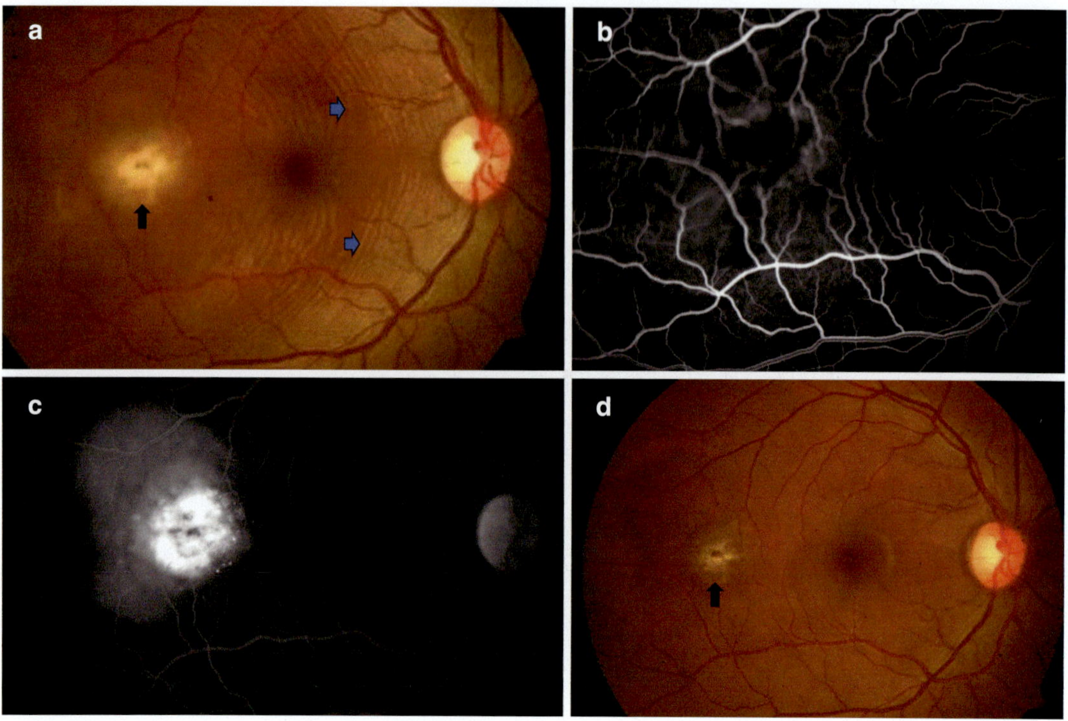

Fig. 18.9 A 26-year-old woman with posterior scleritis, having circumlinear-oriented retinal folds (blue arrows), intense white choroiditis lesion (black arrow) with surrounding subretinal fluid (**a**). On fluorescein angiography, the lesion is hypofluorescent (**b**) with late intense staining and staining of subretinal fluid (**c**). Six months later, fundus showed a healed pigmented scar (**d**)

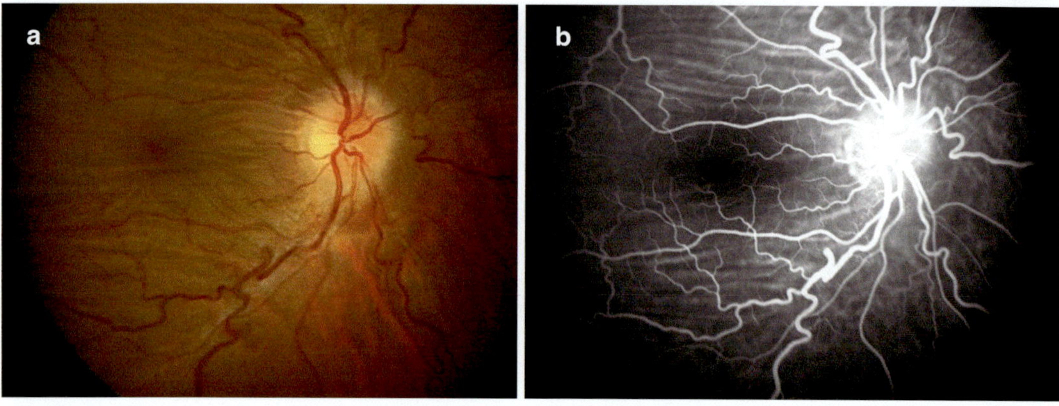

Fig. 18.10 Choroidal folds in posterior scleritis as seen clinically (**a**), and on fundus fluorescein angiography (**b**)

18.2.5.4 Scleritis in Relapsing Polychondritis

Relapsing polychondritis (RP) is a recurrent inflammation of the soft cartilaginous structures rich in proteoglycans, such as auricles, nasal septa, and sclera (Fig. 18.11). In a large scleritis series associated with systemic inflammatory diseases, 10% were caused by RP. Nearly, 70% of patients with RP may have an additional systemic inflammatory disease [39]. From 10 to 40% of

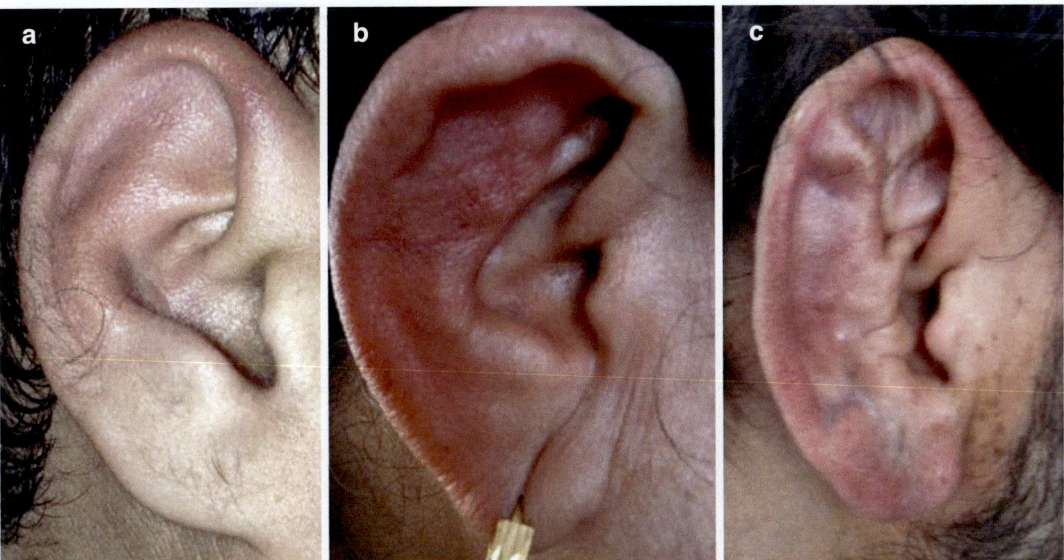

Fig. 18.11 Relapsing polychondritis. (**a**–**c**) Different stages of auricular cartilage involvement: (**a**) Redness of the cartilaginous area characteristically sparing the ear lobule; (**b**) Thickening and redness of the ear with sparing of lobule in a patient with the disease for 3 years; (**c**) Mutilating involvement of the ear in the later stages after 10 years of illness. Reproduced with permission of the publishers from Sharma A, Law AD, Sharma K, Handa R (2015) Relapsing Polychondritis. In: (Sharma A (ed). Textbook of Systemic Vasculitis, 1st Edn. Jaypee Brothers Medical Publishers (P) Ltd., New Delhi. p. 345

patients with RP may first present with ocular involvement, including conjunctivitis, episcleritis, scleritis, or peripheral ulcerative keratitis (PUK) and less frequently with orbital inflammation, perioptic neuritis or ocular nerve palsies. Nearly, 60% of all RP may eventually develop ocular complications [40]. It is a potentially fatal disease and affects multiple systems. The inflammation of the auricles appearing as red ears and nasal cartilage resulting in saddle nose deformity and laryngotracheal collapse are seen most frequently (Figs. 18.11 and 18.12). Other less common involvements include the joints, heart valves, coronary arteries, cranial nerves, and kidneys [40]. Scleritis in RP is often bilateral, diffuse, and recurrent. It may be associated with PUK, anterior uveitis, raised intraocular pressure, and diminution of vision [39].

18.2.5.5 Scleritis in the Paediatric Age Group

Scleritis in the paediatric age group is distinctly less common than the adults, and the diagnosis may be delayed because of a low index of suspicion. In a series of 1658 patients seen over 10 years in a tertiary referral centre in India, only 20 (1.2%) were ≤ 16 years [41]. Most often, the scleritis was unilateral with equal gender distribution. In this series, posterior scleritis was the most common presentation seen in 40%, unlike in adults, where it is rare. Because of the severity of pain, and orbital and adnexal signs, posterior scleritis in children is likely to be mistaken for orbital inflammation [42]. Granulomatosis with polyangiitis is extremely uncommon in children but may present with scleritis, dacryoadenitis, orbital inflammation, limitation of movements, lid edema, or even iritis [43]. There is no associated inflammatory systemic disease in paediatric scleritis except for the association of tuberculosis in 15% of the affected children in one series from India [41]. The anterior scleritis was nodular in 33% and was associated with inflammatory cells in the aqueous and anterior vitreous. Necrotizing scleritis was seen only in two of the 20 patients in this series. Posterior scleritis manifested as optic disc edema, subretinal fluid,

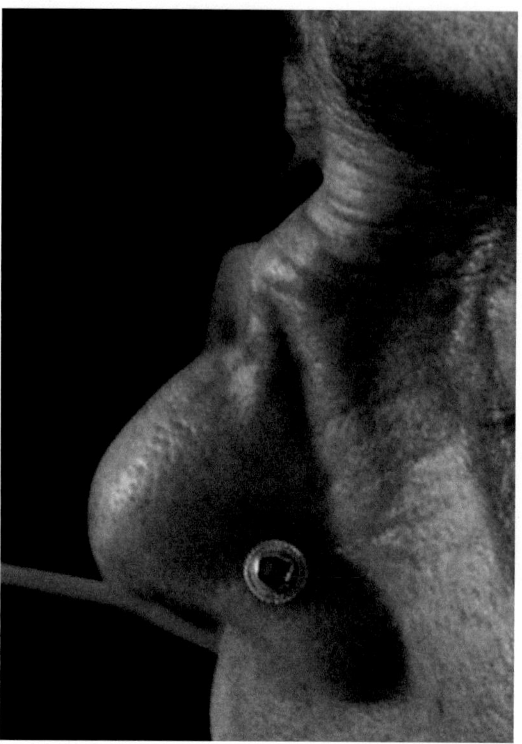

Fig. 18.12 Saddle-nose deformity in relapsing polychondritis. Reproduced with permission of the publishers from Sharma A, Law AD, Sharma K, Handa R (2015) Relapsing Polychondritis. In: (Sharma A (ed).Textbook of Systemic Vasculitis, 1st Edn. Jaypee Brothers Medical Publishers (P) Ltd., New Delhi. p. 346

and ILM striae [41, 44]. Demonstration of a T sign on USG was helpful in making a diagnosis of posterior uveitis [44, 45]. There was no association with systemic inflammatory disease in the Cheung and Chee series of 20 eyes of 13 children with posterior scleritis. Ocular pain, diminution of vision, and exudative retinal detachment are characteristic features of posterior scleritis. The fundus fluorescein angiography shows pinpoint leakage [45]. Anterior scleritis with marginal keratitis, loss of corneal sensations, anterior uveitis, and raised intraocular pressure has been described in a child following live varicella vaccination [46]. For greater details, the readers may refer to a recent review on scleritis in the paediatric age group [47].

18.2.5.6 Severity of Scleritis

A simple scoring system for measuring the severity of scleritis was proposed based on the area of scleral inflammation, tenderness, presence of nodules, scleral necrosis, corneal involvement, cells in the anterior chamber, vitreous cells, and presence of retinal detachment [48] and has been used ever since in the scleritis treatment trials.

18.2.6 Surgically Induced Necrotizing Scleritis

Surgical trauma, most often following cataract surgery and only rarely the pterygium, squint, or vitreous surgery, may lead to necrotizing scleritis, termed Surgically induced necrotizing scleritis or SINS. It is often seen following cataract surgery in patients predisposed or already suffering from autoimmune disorders. It must be differentiated from necrotizing scleritis that may follow years after using β-radiation or antimetabolites in pterygium surgery. It must also be differentiated from infectious scleritis, which often complicates pterygium and scleral buckle surgery [49]. Purulent discharge and hypopyon with necrotizing scleritis in the post-operative setting suggest an infectious etiology rather than SINS [49]. The most common cause of postoperative infectious scleritis is Pseudomonas spp. followed by Staphylococcus spp. [49].

18.2.7 Complications of Episcleritis and Scleritis

Ocular complications in nearly 45% of scleritis include anterior uveitis, decreased vision, PUK, and raised intraocular pressure. Complications are significantly more in necrotizing scleritis. Complications are much less common in episcleritis and may occasionally include anterior uveitis; visual acuity is rarely affected. There is no rise in intraocular pressure in episcleritis [27, 28].

18.2.8 Anterior Segment Optical Coherence Tomography to Differentiate Episcleritis from Scleritis

Anterior segment OCT can differentiate episcleritis from scleritis and monitor the course of the disease. On SD-OCT, the conjunctival epithelium is seen as a low hyperreflective layer, with a highly reflective layer representing conjunctival stroma and episcleral complex under the conjunctival epithelium. This layer shows blood vessels that show a shadowing effect. The sclera is the thickest compact layer of moderate hyperreflectivity [50]. In episcleritis, the conjunctival-episcleral complex is thickened, there may also be some increase in the overall thickness of the sclera, but it is much less than seen in scleritis [50]. In episcleritis, there are no hyporeflective spaces in the scleral layers, but hyporeflective spaces may be seen in the episcleral tissue. While the overlying conjunctival epithelium does not show any alteration in thickness, there may be an associated hyporeflective space representing subconjunctival edema [51]. On the other hand, in scleritis, there is a significant increase in the thickness of the sclera with intrascleral hyporeflective spaces due to the accumulation of fluid and subconjunctival edema seen as increased hyporeflectivity [51]. The scleral fibres appear separated. Accumulation of inflammatory cells can be seen [32]. In necrotizing scleral nodules, the changes can be seen in the deeper sclera before these become visible on the surface of the sclera [32]. In necrotizing nodular scleritis, the nodule shows loss of lamellar pattern in the necrotic liquified centre and appears hyporeflective on OCT. This can be seen clearly on enface OCT scans as areas of hyporeflectivity [32]. Notably, OCT in nodular episcleritis may show thickening of the sclera, which is more than seen in diffuse scleritis [51].

18.2.9 Differentiating Infectious from Autoimmune Scleritis

It is important to recognize the infectious from autoimmune necrotizing scleritis since treatment for the two is diametrically opposite. Using corticosteroids or immunosuppressive therapy in infectious scleritis will lead to loss of the eye [49]. The presence of predisposing factors should alert to the possibility of infectious scleritis. These include a previous history of pterygium surgery, scleral buckle, vitreous surgery, cataract surgery, trauma, and contact lens wear [52]. Subtenon injections of corticosteroids may lead to opportunistic fungal scleritis [53]. There may be a concurrent or past history of herpes zoster Ophthalmicus or HSV keratitis and systemic tuberculosis. Bacterial infectious scleritis is often caused by Pseudomonas spp. or Staphylococcus spp. Infectious scleritis is characterized by mucopurulent discharge, hypopyon, and multiple pus points and may extend from purulent corneal ulcers. The infectious scleritis especially caused by pseudomonas may spread circumferentially around the globe leaving behind areas of scleral thinning. In a series of 21 patients reported from a tertiary referral centre in India, 38% were caused by a fungus alone or had mixed infection with a bacterial microbe. Nocardia was isolated in 24% of eyes. Eighty-six percent of eyes had a predisposing factor. There was associated endophthalmitis, serous retinal, or choroidal detachment. Infectious scleritis has a poor visual and anatomic outcome. Only 33% of eyes could salvage ≥20/200 visual acuity and nearly 20% were eviscerated [54]. Of 12 patients with infectious scleritis, three were caused by fungi. Six patients in this series had multifocal scleral abscesses caused by *Pseudomonas aeruginosa* (3), *Nocardia* (2), and *Klebsiella* spp. (1) [55]. The presenting visual acuity in these eyes is usually poor, and so is the outcome. Infectious scleritis often requires scrapping the scleral bed for microbiological testing. Scleritis caused by methicillin-resistant *Staphylococcus aureus* (MRSA) infection has been reported [56–58]. Fungal infection should be suspected in immune-mediated scleritis with exudative retinal detachment which is not responding to immunosuppressive therapy [59]. A scleral biopsy may be required to make a definitive diagnosis for a successful outcome in fungal scleritis [60]. For very aggressive infectious scleral abscesses, extensive debridement including full-thickness scleral dissection without scleral patch graft has led to favourable outcomes [61].

18.2.10 Pathogenesis of Scleritis

Why should the sclera, a predominantly avascular tissue, be a site of sight-threatening inflammation has defied explanation. The target antigen in scleritis may include collagen or proteoglycans. It mimics synovitis. It is generally believed that non-infectious scleritis is a polygenic autoimmune disease like rheumatoid arthritis [62]. Limited available pathological studies of necrotizing scleritis show evidence of polymorphonuclear cells, macrophages and CD20+ B cells and plasma cells, indicating an innate immune response. On the other hand, scleritis not associated with systemic inflammatory diseases shows a predominant T-cell response. There is evidence of immune complex deposition and vasculitis on pathology. Necrosis due to collagen lysis suggests a disbalance between the matrix metalloproteinase-8 and the tissue inhibitors of metalloproteinases [63]. Although type I collagen predominates in the sclera, there is also some component of type II collagen. A murine model of autoimmune arthritis-scleritis has been developed by twice immunizing the animals with type II collagen with complete Freund's adjuvant. Histopathology showed the presence of CD11b + and CD 138+ (myeloid lineage cells, macrophages, and plasma cells) more than CD4+ and CD8+ T lymphocytes, complement, IgG and IgM in the sclera in contact with the ciliary body. Blood and lymphatic vessels developed near the limbus [64, 65]. This model reinforces the clinical experience that therapies that target T cells are often ineffective in scleritis, but those which target the TNF and IL-6 are more effective in the treatment of anterior scleritis [64]. But for the systemic side effects, Tocilizumab, an IL-6 inhibitor, has been effective in refractory scleritis [66].

18.2.11 Pathology of Scleritis

An inadequate sample of the biopsied tissue limits histopathology studies of scleritis. The biopsy may be required for cases with an unusual presentation, suspected masquerade, or progression. In one of the largest studies, the pathology of scleritis associated with autoimmune diseases was characterized by necrosis surrounding granulomatous inflammation and vasculitis. None of them showed an attempt at healing by way of fibrosis. On the other hand, idiopathic scleritis showed predominantly a non-granulomatous inflammation around a small area of scleral necrosis and lymphoid follicles [20]. Based on histopathology, scleritis associated with RA could not be distinguished from that caused by other autoimmune disorders [67]. Infectious scleritis shows necrosis with signs of acute inflammation [68]. The fungal scleritis shows fungal hyphae, and the tubercular scleritis may show atypical mycobacteria [68].

18.2.12 Treatment of Episcleritis and Scleritis

Episcleritis is a benign self-limiting disease and should be treated with topical corticosteroids. Mild diffuse or nodular scleritis cases can be successfully treated with oral non-steroidal anti-inflammatory drugs (NSAIDs) supplemented with topical steroids [27, 28]. Using flurbiprofen for an average of 6 weeks led to the resolution of mild to moderate scleral inflammation, except in patients with associated systemic inflammatory diseases [69]. Failure to respond to this initial therapy prompted corticosteroids and immunosuppressive therapy [69]. Most patients with severe diffuse or nodular scleritis respond to corticosteroids with immunosuppressive therapy (Fig. 18.13) [27, 28]. Necrotising scleritis with lethal systemic inflammatory diseases requires biological agents. In a small, controlled trial, adalimumab combined with conventional therapy

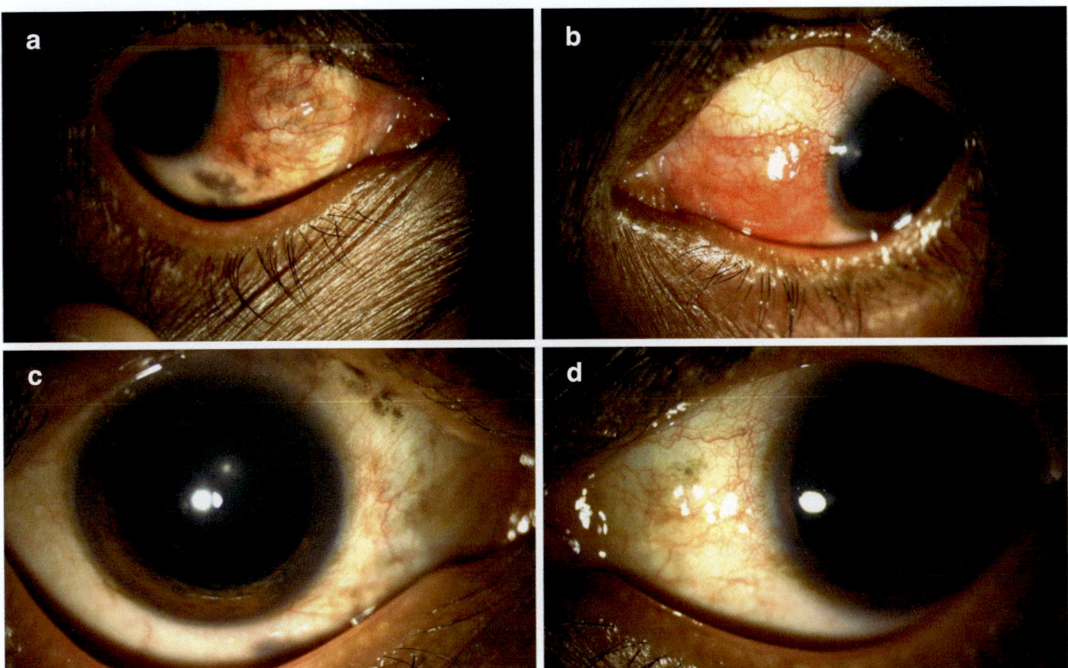

Fig. 18.13 A 36-year-old woman with bilateral anterior scleritis (**a**, **b**) complained of low backache and paraesthesias all over the body for 1 month. C-ANCA was positive. Rheumatological consultation revealed the diagnosis of pure motor axonal polyneuropathy. She received three doses of injection cyclophosphamide and oral corticosteroids. At three months, scleritis (**c**, **d**) was completely resolved

(Corticosteroids plus immunosuppressive therapy) led to a faster scleritis resolution than only conventional therapy alone. The use of adalimumab led to the early sparing of corticosteroids [70]. Rituximab is currently recommended for rheumatological disorders that are non-responsive to conventional therapies. In a review of 121 patients with scleritis, rituximab, administered as a third-line treatment, was well tolerated and led to an efficacious response. Most patients had an associated GPA (75 cases) or rheumatoid arthritis (15 cases). Infusion-related adverse reactions were noted in some patients [71].

Convenient twice-daily oral Tofacitinib, a JAK/STAT inhibitor drug, has successfully been used to treat recalcitrant scleritis [72]. However, it must be borne in mind that using biological agents has led to serious infections when used in rheumatoid arthritis [73]. JAK inhibitors double the rate of infections, especially the herpes zoster, compared to TNF-α inhibitors [74]. The incidence of HZ was 4.4 per 100 person-years in the RA-Tofacitinib program [75].

Compared to non-infectious uveitis, remission in anterior non-necrotizing scleritis takes much longer and requires slow taper even after achieving full remission, especially in bilateral cases and those associated with systemic inflammatory disease [76].

Using TNF-α inhibitors, NSAIDS, Hispanic race and association with SLE led to a faster corticosteroids-sparing remission of anterior scleritis [77]. In view of its well-known side effects, the use of cyclophosphamide is presently under question despite its efficacy in bringing about quick remission as effective alternative biological therapy is available. It should be reserved for only very severe cases that do not respond to the currently available immunosuppressive therapies, and rapid remission is desirable [78]. The initial treatment for patients with necrotizing scleritis with or without PUK should include intravenous cyclophosphamide bolus (0.7 gm/m^2) with intravenous methylprednisolone for 3 days or oral prednisolone at 1 mg/kg body weight [79]. By removing autoantibodies and immune complexes, plasmapheresis can lead to quick remission in remitting and relapsing scleritis [80]. Topical erythropoietin (3000 IU/mL) has been used four times daily to heal necrotizing scleritis of diverse etiologies [81]. Histopathological studies in a rabbit model of scleral necrosis demonstrated increased vascularization and reduced apoptosis following the application of topical erythropoietin, leading to faster healing of the scleral necrosis [82].

18.3 Cornea-Anatomical Considerations

The cornea is the anterior transparent continuation of the sclera and is the primary lens for transmitting light into the eye. It consists of five layers. The anterior-most is the 5–6 layered stratified epithelial layer followed by the Bowman's membrane-condensation of the anterior stromal fibres, corneal stroma, Descemet's membrane-the basement membrane, and the innermost is the single layer of post-mitotic endothelial cells. The stromal layer consists of densely packed parallel small collagen fibrils extending across the cornea. The small size and the lamellar arrangement provide for the transparency of the cornea. This layer also has extracellular matrix proteins, the proteoglycans, which provide structural stability and watch glass shape to the cornea. The cornea is avascular but has a rich nerve ending under the epithelial layer and intercellular junctions. Stroma also contains keratocytes that continuously constitute proteoglycans [1].

18.3.1 Epidemiology and Etiology of Peripheral Ulcerative Keratitis

The estimated incidence of PUK associated with systemic disorders was 3.01 per one million population in Yorkshire, UK. Of the 27 cases in the study period of 3 years, 21 were related to rheumatoid arthritis and five to Wegener's disease (presently renamed granulomatosis with polyangiitis). During the same time, the incidence of rheumatoid arthritis and Wegener's disease in this population was 12.5 and 8.5 per million. Peripheral corneal melt is a complication of long-standing rheumatoid arthritis; the average duration of RA was 20 years, and nearly 2/third of the patients had associated keratoconjunctivitis sicca. On the other hand, PUK was an early sign of Wegener's granulomatosis [83]. PUK is often seen in the inferior cornea or the interpalpebral aperture [84].

18.3.2 Systemic Associations of Peripheral Ulcerative Keratitis

PUK is frequently associated with serious systemic disorders, including rheumatoid arthritis (RA), granulomatosis with polyangiitis (GPA, Wegener's granulomatosis), and less commonly with relapsing polychondritis or SLE (Figs. 18.14, 18.15, and 18.16). Long-standing cases of RA are complicated by rheumatoid vasculitis, the life-threatening extraarticular complication which most frequently manifests in the skin (non-healing ulcers in legs and feet), gangrene of digits, mononeuritis complex in the peripheral nervous system, followed by ocular involvement in the form of episcleritis, scleritis, and PUK [85]. Extraarticular complications of RA in the eye are seen in up to 39% of patients with long-standing RA [86]. Besides the duration of RA, male sex and smoking are additional risk factors.

Besides rheumatoid arthritis and SLE, PUK is usually associated with small or medium-vessel vasculitis like GPA, ANCA-associated vasculitis, and Polyarteritis nodosa. Occasional cases of PUK have been reported in Giant cell arteritis [87]. Episcleritis and scleritis complicate most patients with relapsing polychondritis, an autoimmune disorder mainly involving type II

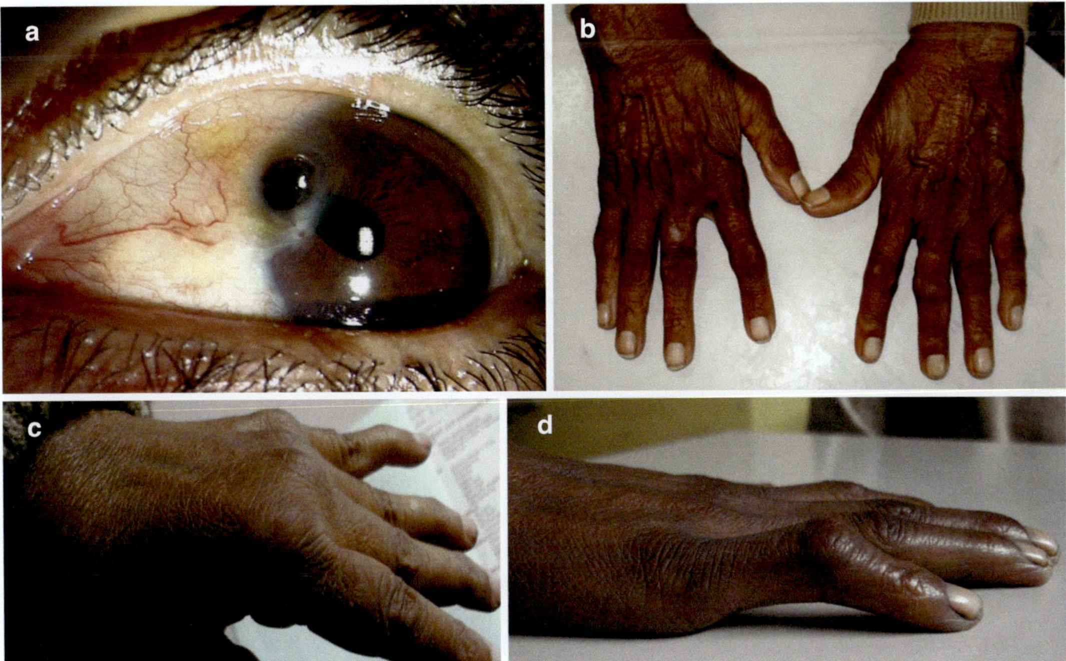

Fig. 18.14 Spontaneous gradual corneal melt with perforation in rheumatoid arthritis (**a**). A patient with early rheumatoid arthritis showing swelling of interphalangeal joints (**b**). Swan neck deformity of the little finger (**c**) and Boutonniere deformity in another patient with rheumatoid arthritis (**d**). Figures b, c and d reproduced with permission of the publishers from Bambery P, Sharm A, Gupta A and Gupta V (2009) Systemic examination and imaging in Gupta A, Gupta V, Herbort C, Khairallah M (eds) Uveitis: Text and Imaging 1st Edn. Jaypee Brothers Medical Publishers (P) Ltd., New Delhi. P. 288

collagen-containing cartilage of auricles, nose, trachea, and sclera. Necrotising scleritis and PUK may rarely be the first manifestation [88].

18.3.3 Peripheral Stromal Keratitis and Peripheral Ulcerative Keratitis

Nearly, one-third of the patients with scleritis and half of those with necrotizing scleritis have peripheral corneal inflammation. Sainz et al. [89] described three clinical phenotypes of peripheral corneal involvement seen within 2–3 mm of the limbus, (1) peripheral corneal thinning with intact corneal epithelium, (2) intact corneal epithelium but peripheral stromal keratitis due to inflammatory cells infiltration into the peripheral corneal stroma, and (3) peripheral ulcerative keratitis (PUK) which has an epithelial defect, with infiltration and ulceration of the stroma. PUK has well-defined borders on either side [89]. In a large retrospective study of episcleritis (85 patients) and sclerites (500 patients), PUK was seen in 7.4% of all scleritis cases, 35% of all necrotizing scleritis cases, and none in episcleritis. When PUK is associated with necrotizing scleritis, it is nearly always associated with inflammatory cells in the anterior chamber [27, 28].

Anterior segment optical coherence tomography (OCT) has been used to characterize the lesions of PUK. In the acute ulcerative stage, the epithelium is absent, with the underlying corneal stroma showing a scrambled heterogeneous appearance and the underlying unaffected stroma showing a normal homogeneous reflectivity. Upon healing, the corneal epithelium in PUK appears thickened and fills the area of the lost

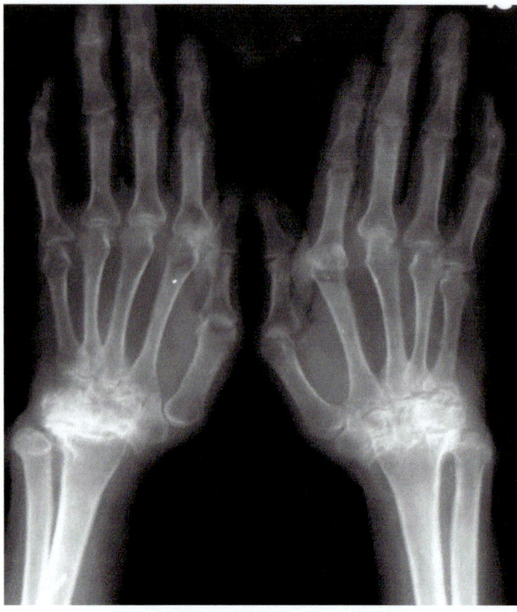

Fig. 18.15 X-ray hands in rheumatoid arthritis show extensive destruction of the wrist joint, with carpal bones almost being converted into a single mass. Images courtesy of Prof Pradeep Bambery, Ex-professor of Internal Medicine, Post Graduate Institute of Medical Education and Research, Chandigarh, India

stroma; the healed stroma appears smoother. A demarcation line separates the healed from the normal stroma [90].

Contrary to the reports from the Western world, a prospective report of 65 patients (76 eyes) with PUK from North India found more men than women (3:2); 83% were unilateral, 73% were from poor socioeconomic backgrounds, and the commonest cause was Mooren's ulcer (31.5%) followed by infections (19.7%) and collagen vascular disease (19.7%). Most of the infectious PUK was bacterial, and two were fungal and herpes [84]. In a series of 32 patients (48 eyes) from Western India, Mooren's ulcer was the most common PUK aetiology (34%) RA-associated PUK followed it at 19%, Herpes simplex keratitis, Meibomian gland disease (9% each), and GPA (6%). Half of the patients had bilateral PUK, and 58% of the eyes had severe disease [91].

Even syphilis may rarely present as bilateral PUK [92]. Bilateral HSV PUK is reported although rare [93, 94]. PUK may rarely be a primary manifestation of HIV infection [95]. AIDS

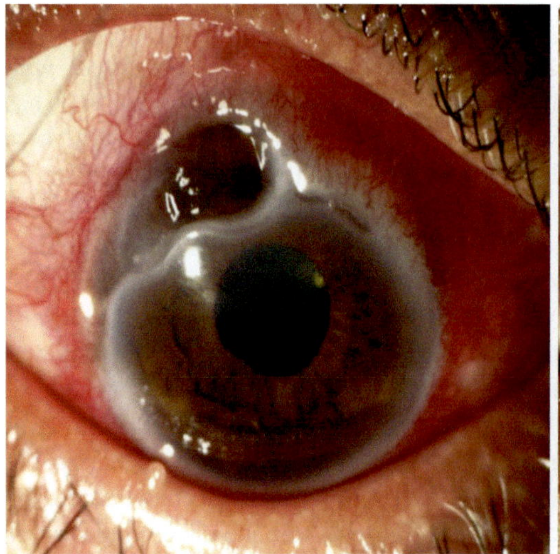

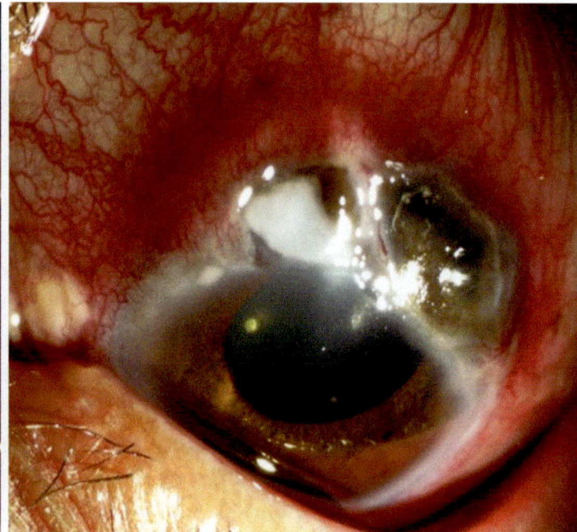

Fig. 18.16 Bilateral peripheral ulcerative keratitis in a patient with Rheumatoid arthritis. Images courtesy of Dr. Chintan Malhotra, Professor, Cornea, Lens and Refractive Surgery, Advanced Eye Centre, Post Graduate Institute of Medical Education and Research, Chandigarh, India

patients with varicella-zoster virus infection may have devastating corneal complications, including PUK [96]. Patients suffering from hepatitis B [97] or Hepatitis C infection may present with PUK [98].

Checkpoint inhibitors Ipilimumab and Nivolumab led to bilateral PUK with corneal perforation in a patient with metastatic melanoma [99].

18.3.4 Para Central Corneal Melt-Pathogenesis

RA-associated PUK must be differentiated from a paracentral corneal melt/perforation, a rare complication in RA unassociated with eye inflammation. The paracentral melts are almost always associated with aqueous deficiency DED or Sjogren syndrome (Fig. 18.17). The PUK and the paracentral melt, both sight-threatening complications of RA, may have different pathogenetic mechanisms [100]. In the corneal buttons removed during therapeutic corneal grafting, CD11c macrophages, CD3+ T-lymphocytes and only very few CD22 B cells were noted in the epithelium and the subepithelial stroma at the edges of the corneal melt. Anti-myeloperoxidase stain-positive cells (neutrophils) were seen in significant numbers. The immunopathology of the corneal buttons was highly suggestive of a cell-mediated T-cell response. The release of proteolytic enzymes from polymorphonuclear cells may also have been responsible for the corneal melts [100]. The consistent presence of T-cell infiltrates suggests that T-cell mediated response is primarily responsible for keratolysis [101]. One of the major complications of previously undiagnosed RA is corneal melt at the incision site following cataract surgery [102], especially in patients with sicca syndrome [103]. The sterile corneal ulceration may also follow using non-steroidal anti-inflammatory agents in cataract surgery in undiagnosed RA and dry eye cases. Even graft versus host disease may be complicated by PUK [104]. Although early diagnosis and the use of hydroxychloroquine, aspirin and biological agents in recent years have reduced the incidence of rheumatoid vasculitis, once it happens, it carries a mortality rate of nearly 60% within 5 years [105]. Thus, scleritis and PUK are the harbinger of life-threatening complications of RA [85] and necessitate a thorough systemic evaluation by a rheumatologist.

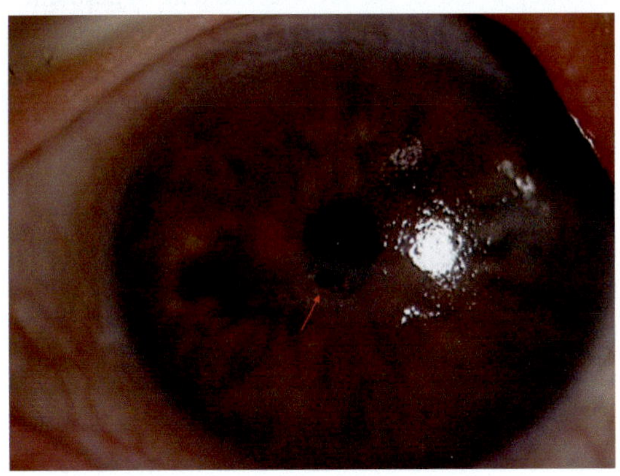

Fig. 18.17 Paracentral corneal thinning (red arrow) in a secondary Sjogren syndrome patient

18.3.5 Mooren's Ulcer

Mooren's ulcer is a painful, crescent-shaped peripheral ulcerative keratitis often seen in men who smoke, possibly unilateral or bilateral. The median age of the patients in India is 65 years [106]. Mooren's ulcer is seen in much younger in Africa [107]. It is not associated with any systemic inflammation or vasculitic disease. Unlike the Western world, Mooren's ulcer is the predominant cause of PUK in India and Africa. The edges overhang the ulcer, which tends to spread centrally and circumferentially. The base of the ulcer may show deep vessels. Significantly, there is no associated scleritis or scleral involvement in ulceration. In one of the largest series of Mooren's ulcers, 11% of the 242 eyes of 166 patients were already perforated at presentation. The major risk factors for Mooren's ulcer were corneal surgery and trauma in 22% and 17%, respectively [106]. Cataract surgery may be a risk factor [108]. However, successful cataract surgery can be carried out under adequate immunosuppression in Mooren's ulcer eyes [109]. The exact pathogenesis of Mooren's ulcer is not known. Pathology of the corneal buttons has shown infiltration by CD4+ and CD8+ T lymphocytes and CD19+/CD45+ B lymphocytes, and CD68+ macrophages, suggestive of both humoral and T-cell mediated adaptive immune response [110]. Similar cell infiltrates were found in the conjunctival submucosa adjacent to Mooren's ulcer [111]. Immunohistochemistry studies of corneal tissues of Mooren's ulcer detected GPR91, a succinate receptor, along with expression of IL-1β, VEGF, MMP-13, and p-p65, suggesting a role for GPR91-driven activation of NF-kB mediated inflammation in the causation of Mooren's ulcer [112].

18.3.6 Pathology of PUK

Histopathology studies of the excised conjunctiva and sclera from the PUK eyes revealed microangiopathy with immune complexes deposition in the vessel walls, fibrinoid necrosis of the vessel walls, and neutrophil monocytic infiltration. Immunoglobulins, including IgM, IgG, IgA, and complements, were seen in all cases of PUK. There was evidence of vasculitis and perivasculitis in nearly all the specimens [113]. These histopathological findings are characteristic of rheumatoid vasculitis seen in skin and other accessible sites for tissue biopsy [85].

18.3.7 Systemic Implications for PUK in Systemic Collagen Vascular Diseases

The development of PUK or necrotizing scleritis in collagen vascular diseases is a prognostic indicator for systemic outcomes. In a long-term study, nine of the 17 patients with RA who developed either PUK or necrotizing scleritis died within 10 years of conventional treatment. On the other hand, only one of the 17 patients who received long-term immunosuppressive therapy died in 10 years, and that too on immunosuppression withdrawal [114].

The major complication of the PUK is corneal perforation, which is often smaller than 1 mm or between 1 and 3 mm and rarely larger than 3 mm [115]. Perforation of peripheral ulcerative keratitis carries a poor visual outcome and a grave prognosis for life, especially if it is bilateral perforation (Fig. 18.16). Nearly, 25% of patients died within a year if it was unilateral, and 50% if it was a bilateral perforation [115].

18.3.8 Pathogenetic Mechanism for Peripheral Ulcerative Keratitis

Many autoimmune disorders such as rheumatoid arthritis (RA), primary Sjogren syndrome (pSS), granulomatosis with polyangiitis (GPA), SLE relapsing polychondritis or infections may lead to peripheral ulcerative keratitis (PUK). Keratoconjunctivitis sicca (KCS) is an inflammatory ocular surface disorder characterized by a deficiency of aqueous tears. While 10% of primary Sjogren syndrome patients get complicated by the development of KCS ([116], KCS due to secondary Sjogren syndrome (sSS) is seen in nearly 19.5% of patients with rheumatoid arthritis (RA) and 14% in patients with SLE. RA and SLE are 15 and 17 times more frequent in females [117]; hence, PUK is seen more often in women. However, it may have regional variations based on the etiological factors for PUK.

The pathogenesis of PUK is multifactorial. The key event in the KCS is the tear hyperosmolarity caused by an aqueous deficiency or evaporation of the aqueous layer due to an unstable tear film leading to activation of the conjunctival and corneal epithelial mitogen-activated protein kinase (MAPK) and NFkB pathways. These set the stage for releasing inflammatory cytokines, matrix metalloproteinases (MMPs) and the recruitment of inflammatory cells, primarily the polymorphonuclear cells that release proteolytic enzymes and chemokines that attract more inflammatory cells. The net result of these is the loss of both the epithelial and the goblet cells, compounding the insult and setting up a vicious cycle of chronic inflammation and dry eye [118] and lymphangiogenesis in the cornea.

The other factors include an immune complex-mediated vasculitis of the anterior ciliary arteries that supply the peripheral cornea. RA and SS are the commonest cause of PUK. Rheumatoid factor is an IgM antibody against the Fc region of IgG of several autoantigens and is found in 70–90% of patients with RA and pSS but is also present in low frequency in several other disorders and infections. It is mediated by a dysregulated B cell response leading to the formation of immune complexes and activation of complement pathway leading to infiltration of inflammatory cells, perivasculitis, vasculitis, and vascular occlusion [119].

Histopathological studies of PUK have shown occluded perilimbal vessels due to thrombosis by the deposition of immune complexes. This phenomenon has also been noted in fluorescein angiography studies of the anterior segment in patients with PUK which can demonstrate the configuration, patency and pattern of the peripheral limbal vessels [120].

Cornea is an avascular tissue and lacks lymphatic vessels and thus is an immune-privileged tissue. However, the blood vessels reach up to 0.5 mm of the peripheral cornea. The keratocytes lie inactivated in the normal corneal stroma but, when activated, may also serve as antigen-presenting cells and secrete matrix metalloproteinase-2, a collagenolytic enzyme. The keratocytes get activated by the inflammatory cytokines that are concentrated in the tears and superficial layer of the cornea. In the normal tissue of the cornea, tissue inhibitors of metalloproteinases-1 (TIMP-1) are expressed in abundance; however, these were found absent in RA-associated PUK areas, which stained strongly positive for activated macrophages and fibrocytes [121].

The corneal antigens are sequestrated from the immune system because of the absence of afferent lymphatic vessels in the cornea. However, when required, a rich network of the perilimbal conjunctival lymphoid tissue provides a ready source for the immune cells and cytokines.

In corneal infections, the polymorphonuclear cells invade the cornea and release cytokines and chemokines that attract more inflammatory cells and CD4+ cells. In response to the infection, blood vessels accompanied by lymphatic vessels grow into the cornea. Likely, the cytokines VEGF-C and VEGF-D induced by TNF-α, IL-6, and IL-1(innate immune system cytokines) promote corneal lymphangiogenesis [122, 123].

In RA patients, even without signs of sSS or overt inflammatory activity, significantly more Langerhans' cells (LC) were found, on vivo confocal microscopy, at the level of the basal epithelial layer in the peripheral and central cornea compared to the normal people. The LCs are highly active dendritic cells and were seen in various stages of activation, likely activated by the proinflammatory cytokines. The LC migrate into the peripheral and the central cornea from the perilimbal conjunctiva [124].

On the other hand, in dry eye disorders (DED), there is neo-lymphangiogenesis via the activation of Th17 cells. In DED, the blood vessels do not grow into the cornea. The availability of endothelial markers for the study of lymphatic endothelial cells has made it possible to demonstrate the development of lymphatic vessels in the cornea, creating an afferent path for the adaptive immune response [125].

In DED, the dendritic cells present corneal antigens to the regional lymph nodes. The naïve T cells are converted to corneal antigen-specific T effector cells, which reach the peripheral cornea via the limbal blood vessels (the efferent path).

Thus, there are multifactorial mechanisms involving the role of B and T cell-mediated immune response that cause the release of inflammatory cytokines and matrix metallic proteinases, leading to proteolysis, corneal thinning, and perforation.

18.3.9 Treatment of PUK

The main objective of treatment for PUK is to prompt quick healing and prevent perforation.

The secondary objectives are to prevent recurrences and restore the integrity of the globe and vision.

Several systemic or local infections/trauma disorders may lead to PUK and require a careful evaluation in consultation with a rheumatologist.

Corneal scraping for microscopy or culture may be required if bacterial infections are suspected. The conventional treatment has included topical antibiotics and tear substitutes. Using topical steroids alone should be avoided as these are often not helpful and may hasten corneal perforation in the event of HSV keratitis. Patients who develop PUK or paracentral corneal melts, especially following surgical procedures, respond best to topical 1–2% cyclosporin eye drops. If the PUK is associated with meibomitis or blepharitis, treating it with doxycycline is helpful as it reduces the MMPs and promotes healing.

However, most patients have associated collagen vascular diseases and require long-term immunosuppressive therapy, including oral corticosteroids. Patients presenting with RA-associated PUK should be given high-dose corticosteroids combined with IMT early in the course of the disease to prevent perforation of the cornea. Many of these already-known RA patients may be on maintenance therapy. The corticosteroids and IMT will need to be revised to their full dosage.

Early IMT prevents recurrences and complications and improves visual outcomes [126]. Mycophenolate 3 g daily or Methotrexate weekly is preferred. In RA, adalimumab can be given initially, and if there is no response, one can switch to infliximab or rituximab. If the patient fails to respond to rituximab, intravenous cyclophosphamide may be needed [127]. In PUK, due to GPA, the drug of choice is rituximab, and if there is no response, intravenous cyclophosphamide is required. All patients on biologic therapy maintain IMT with azathioprine [127].

PUK may remain refractory to treatment despite a good response in the systemic disease [128]. In patients with recalcitrant PUK, infliximab has been the most favoured primary biological therapy and has been FDA-approved to treat RA-associated scleritis for over 20 years. It binds soluble and transmembrane forms of TNF-α [129–131]. TNF-α inhibitor, infliximab, a chimeric monoclonal antibody, or adalimumab, a humanized IgG1 monoclonal antibody against TNF-α, prevent the proteolysis of the corneal stroma by downregulating the expression of MMPs and promote wound healing.

In a multicentric series of 34 patients, the patients received either anti-TNF-α agents (25), namely, adalimumab (16), infliximab (8), or etanercept (1) or other biological agents (9), namely, rituximab (7), tocilizumab (1), belimumab (1), or abatacept (1). Non-TNF-α agents were more effective than TNF-α inhibitors, as nearly half of those receiving the latter therapy had to be switched to other agents. None of the nine patients who received non-TNF-α agents required switching to a second agent [132].

Rituximab, an anti-CD20 agent, is currently preferred over cyclophosphamide for GPA and SLE. Rituximab effectively controlled corneal inflammation in seven patients with RA-associated PUK. Following its use, none of the patients developed any other vasculitic complication of RA [133].

Even in Mooren's ulcer, refractory to conventional treatment use of rituximab (two infusions of 1000 mg each at 2 weeks interval) led to complete resolution of the PUK. It has been recommended as a safe alternative to cyclophosphamide [134]. As mentioned above, the histopathology of the cornea in PUK closely resembles the B-cell-driven immune response seen in RA vasculitis, justifying the good outcome with rituximab. Using rituximab has, however, rarely led to PUK-like lesions [135, 136].

Tocilizumab, an IL-6 receptor-blocking antibody, has also been used in treating RA, as IL-6 is a key cytokine responsible for differentiating immune cells [137]. However, quiescent or partially active RA patients may develop PUK while receiving tocilizumab, suggesting either a paradoxical reaction to tocilizumab or insufficient control of disease activity [138, 139].

18.3.10 Adjunctive Local Treatment to Restore the Integrity of the Globe

Corneal perforation is an indicator of the severity of RA vasculitis. RA-associated corneal perforation often requires a corneal graft. In a UK ocular tissue transplantation database, only 42% of patients survived 5 years following a corneal graft for RA-associated corneal perforation. However, 85% of the deaths occurred within 2 years of the corneal graft. Only 48% of corneal grafts survived 5 years [140].

Many diverse adjunctive therapies prevent perforation or restore the globe's integrity. These include conjunctival resection at least 4 mm from the limbus and 2 mm circumferentially on either side of the PUK and are combined with an amniotic membrane graft. Cyanoacrylate or tissue glue with a bandage contact lens prevents or treats perforations <3 mm. Perforations larger than 3 mm require patch grafts [91]. Paracentral corneal melt associated with RA often responds best to topical cyclosporin. Still, if the perforation is large, it may require tissue adhesive with a bandage contact lens or penetrating corneal graft [100].

In corneal thinning, impending perforations and perforations, many options are available for tectonic support. However, no controlled trials are available to make strong recommendations. The current strategies are based on small case series or anecdotal cases. The subject was recently reviewed [141].

Lamellar tectonic grafts are preferred over penetrating grafts in corneal thinning as the latter often get rejected. Even the lamellar grafts may show opacification or melt in collagen vascular diseases [142]. Mushroom grafts may be preferred over full-thickness grafts [143]. Lamellar patch grafts have had a high success rate in tectonic support in patients with corneal thinning and perforations [144]. A multi-layered amniotic membrane grafting combined with conjunctival dissection has been used in PUK [145]. A suture-less and glueless multi-layered amniotic membrane graft under a bandage contact lens can prevent further thinning and perforation [146]. Multi-layered amniotic membrane accelerates healing and is a good option for corneal thinning and very small perforations to promote corneal healing and prevent further corneal melt. Still, it cannot provide tectonic support [141].

References

1. Riordan-Eva P. Chapter 1. Anatomy & embryology of the eye. In: Riordan-Eva P, Cunningham Jr ET, editors. Vaughan & Asbury's general ophthalmology, 18e. McGraw Hill; 2011. Accessed March 04, 2023. https://accessmedicine.mhmedical.com/content.aspx?bookid=387§ionid=40229318.
2. Atta G, Tempfer H, Kaser-Eichberger A, Traweger A, Heindl LM, Schroedl F. Is the human sclera a tendon-like tissue? A structural and functional comparison. Ann Anat. 2022;240:151858. https://doi.org/10.1016/j.aanat.2021.151858. Epub 2021 Nov 17. PMID: 34798297PMID: 24323074.
3. Schlereth SL, Kremers S, Schrödl F, Cursiefen C, Heindl LM. Characterization of antigen-presenting macrophages and dendritic cells in the healthy human sclera. Invest Ophthalmol Vis Sci. 2016;57(11):4878–85. https://doi.org/10.1167/iovs.15-18552. PMID: 27654414.
4. Schlereth SL, Karlstetter M, Hos D, Matthaei M, Cursiefen C, Heindl LM. Detection of pro- and anti-angiogenic factors in the human sclera. Curr Eye Res. 2019;44(2):172–84. https://doi.org/10.1080/02713683.2018.1540704. Epub 2018 Nov 9. PMID: 30358460.
5. Franz-Odendaal TA, Hall BK. Skeletal elements within teleost eyes and a discussion of their homology. J Morphol. 2006;267(11):1326–37. https://doi.org/10.1002/jmor.10479.
6. Chen K, Zhou Y, Sheng M, Li M. Culture and identification of multipotent stem cells in Guinea pig sclera. Int Ophthalmol. 2023;43(1):113–20. https://doi.org/10.1007/s10792-022-02393-4. Epub 2022 Jul 6.
7. Seko Y, Azuma N, Takahashi Y, Makino H, Morito T, Muneta T, Matsumoto K, Saito H, Sekiya I, Umezawa A. Human sclera maintains common characteristics with cartilage throughout evolution. PLoS One. 2008;3(11):e3709. https://doi.org/10.1371/journal.pone.0003709. Epub 2008 Nov 12. PMID: 19002264; PMCID: PMC2579486.
8. Xu TT, Reynolds MM, Hodge DO, Smith WM. Epidemiology and clinical characteristics of episcleritis and scleritis in Olmsted County, Minnesota. Am J Ophthalmol. 2020;217:317–24. https://doi.org/10.1016/j.ajo.2020.04.043. Epub 2020 May 11. PMID: 32437669; PMCID: PMC7492378.

9. Homayounfar G, Nardone N, Borkar DS, Tham VM, Porco TC, Enanoria WT, Parker JV, Vinoya AC, Uchida A, Acharya NR. Incidence of scleritis and episcleritis: results from the Pacific Ocular Inflammation Study. Am J Ophthalmol. 2013;156(4):752–8. https://doi.org/10.1016/j.ajo.2013.05.026. Epub 2013 Jul 24. PMID: 23891336; PMCID: PMC3852161.
10. Honik G, Wong IG, Gritz DC. Incidence and prevalence of episcleritis and scleritis in Northern California. Cornea. 2013;32(12):1562–6. https://doi.org/10.1097/ICO.0b013e3182a407c3.
11. Armbrust KR, Kopplin LJ. Characteristics and outcomes of patients with scleritis in the IRIS® registry (intelligent research in sight) database. Ophthalmol Sci. 2022;2(3):100178. https://doi.org/10.1016/j.xops.2022.100178. PMID: 36245751; PMCID: PMC9559886.
12. Berkenstock MK, Carey AR. Health system wide "big data" analysis of rheumatologic conditions and scleritis. BMC Ophthalmol. 2021;21(1):14. https://doi.org/10.1186/s12886-020-01769-3. PMID: 33407267; PMCID: PMC7788757.
13. Smith JR, Mackensen F, Rosenbaum JT. Therapy insight: scleritis and its relationship to systemic autoimmune disease. Nat Clin Pract Rheumatol. 2007;3(4):219–26. https://doi.org/10.1038/ncprheum0454. PMID: 17396107.
14. Sureja NP, Kalyan S, Patel MR. Recurrent scleritis as a presenting manifestation of asymptomatic occult Takayasu arteritis. Rheumatol Adv Pract. 2020;5(1):rkaa065. https://doi.org/10.1093/rap/rkaa065. PMID: 33615126; PMCID: PMC7882870.
15. Patel PR, Farrell MC, Peshtani A, Berkenstock MK. Bilateral anterior and posterior scleritis in a patient with acute myelogenous leukemia. Am J Ophthalmol Case Rep. 2022;26:101497. https://doi.org/10.1016/j.ajoc.2022.101497. PMID: 35372712; PMCID: PMC8971595.
16. Yan Y, Zhang Q. Bilateral posterior scleritis presenting as the first manifestation of immunoglobulin A nephropathy: case report and review of the literature. Ocul Immunol Inflamm. 2016;24(1):43–8. https://doi.org/10.3109/09273948.2014.964420. Epub 2014 Oct 7. PMID: 25290901.
17. Gonzalez-Gonzalez LA, Molina-Prat N, Doctor P, Tauber J, Sainz de la Maza MT, Foster CS. Clinical features and presentation of infectious scleritis from herpes viruses: a report of 35 cases. Ophthalmology. 2012;119(7):1460–4. https://doi.org/10.1016/j.ophtha.2012.01.033. Epub 2012 Mar 28.
18. Gungor IU, Ariturk N, Beden U, Darka O. Necrotizing scleritis due to varicella zoster infection: a case report. Ocul Immunol Inflamm. 2006;14(5):317–9. https://doi.org/10.1080/09273940600899890.
19. Hemady R, Sainz de la Maza M, Raizman MB, Foster CS. Six cases of scleritis associated with systemic infection. Am J Ophthalmol. 1992;114(1):55–62. https://doi.org/10.1016/s0002-9394(14)77413-6.
20. Rao NA, Marak GE, Hidayat AA. Necrotizing scleritis. A clinico-pathologic study of 41 cases. Ophthalmology. 1985;92(11):1542–9. PMID: 3878485.
21. Somkijrungroj T, Pimolrat W, Gonzales JA, Keenan JD, Margolis TP. Conjunctival sensation in scleritis. Ocul Immunol Inflamm. 2016;24(1):24–8. https://doi.org/10.3109/09273948.2015.1057598. Epub 2015 Dec 8. PMID: 26647348.
22. Patel SS, Saraiya NV, Tessler HH, Goldstein DA. Mycobacterial ocular inflammation: delay in diagnosis and other factors impacting morbidity. JAMA Ophthalmol. 2013;131(6):752–8. https://doi.org/10.1001/jamaophthalmol.2013.71.
23. Casey R, Flowers CW Jr, Jones DD, Scott L. Anterior nodular scleritis secondary to syphilis. Arch Ophthalmol. 1996;114(8):1015–6. https://doi.org/10.1001/archopht.1996.01100140223022.
24. Wilhelmus KR, Yokoyama CM. Syphilitic episcleritis and scleritis. Am J Ophthalmol. 1987;104(6):595–7. https://doi.org/10.1016/0002-9394(87)90170-x. PMID: 3688101.
25. Samalia P, Sims J, Niederer R. Necrotizing syphilitic scleritis: the resurgence of syphilis in New Zealand. Asia Pac J Ophthalmol (Phila). 2021;10(4):417. https://doi.org/10.1097/APO.0000000000000383. PMID: 34284458.
26. Fénolland JR, Bonnel S, Rambaud C, Froussart-Maille F, Rigal-Sastourné JC. Syphilitic scleritis. Ocul Immunol Inflamm. 2016;24(1):93–5. https://doi.org/10.3109/09273948.2014.916307. Epub 2014 May 15.
27. Sainz de la Maza M, Molina N, Gonzalez-Gonzalez LA, Doctor PP, Tauber J, Foster CS. Clinical characteristics of a large cohort of patients with scleritis and episcleritis. Ophthalmology. 2012a;119(1):43–50. https://doi.org/10.1016/j.ophtha.2011.07.013. Epub 2011 Oct 2. PMID: 21963265.
28. Sainz de la Maza M, Molina N, Gonzalez-Gonzalez LA, Doctor PP, Tauber J, Foster CS. Scleritis therapy. Ophthalmology. 2012b;119(1):51–8. https://doi.org/10.1016/j.ophtha.2011.07.043. Epub 2011 Oct 19. PMID: 22015381.
29. Magesan K, Surya J, Sridharan S, Nair V, Agarwal M, Agarwal AE, Biswas J, Dutta MP. Clinical profile of Scleritis presenting for the first time in the elderly. Ocul Immunol Inflamm. 2022;6:1–5. https://doi.org/10.1080/09273948.2022.2046792. Epub ahead of print.
30. Watson PG, Hayreh SS, Awdry PN. Episcleritis and scleritis. I. Br J Ophthalmol. 1968;52(3):278–9 contd. https://doi.org/10.1136/bjo.52.3.278. PMID: 5650814; PMCID: PMC506572.
31. Watson PG, Hayreh SS. Scleritis and episcleritis. Br J Ophthalmol. 1976;60(3):163–91. https://doi.org/10.1136/bjo.60.3.163. PMID: 1268179; PMCID: PMC1042706.
32. Watson P, Romano A. The impact of new methods of investigation and treatment on the understanding of the pathology of scleral inflammation. Eye

(Lond). 2014;28(8):915–30. https://doi.org/10.1038/eye.2014.110. Epub 2014 May 30. PMID: 24875228; PMCID: PMC4135249.

33. Cocho L, Gonzalez-Gonzalez LA, Molina-Prat N, Doctor P, Sainz-de-la-Maza M, Foster CS. Scleritis in patients with granulomatosis with polyangiitis (Wegener). Br J Ophthalmol. 2016;100(8):1062–5. https://doi.org/10.1136/bjophthalmol-2015-307460. Epub 2015 Nov 13.
34. Lavric A, Gonzalez-Lopez JJ, Majumder PD, Bansal N, Biswas J, Pavesio C, Agrawal R. Posterior scleritis: analysis of epidemiology, clinical factors, and risk of recurrence in a cohort of 114 patients. Ocul Immunol Inflamm. 2016;24(1):6–15. https://doi.org/10.3109/09273948.2015.1005240. Epub 2015 Jul 2.
35. Gupta A, Bansal RK, Bambery P. Posterior scleritis related fundal mass in a patient with rheumatoid arthritis. Scand J Rheumatol. 1992;21(5):254–6. https://doi.org/10.3109/03009749209099234.
36. Calthorpe CM, Watson PG, McCartney AC. Posterior scleritis: a clinical and histological survey. Eye (Lond). 1988;2(Pt 3):267–77. https://doi.org/10.1038/eye.1988.52.
37. Sin PY, Liu DT, Young AL. Nodular posterior scleritis mimicking choroidal tumor in a patient with systemic lupus erythematous: a case report and literature review. Asia Pac J Ophthalmol (Phila). 2016;5(5):324–9. https://doi.org/10.1097/APO.0000000000000165. PMID: 26692258.
38. Finger PT, Perry HD, Packer S, Erdey RA, Weisman GD, Sibony PA. Posterior scleritis as an intraocular tumour. Br J Ophthalmol. 1990;74(2):121–2. https://doi.org/10.1136/bjo.74.2.121. PMID: 2178679; PMCID: PMC1042007.
39. Sainz-de-la-Maza M, Molina N, Gonzalez-Gonzalez LA, Doctor PP, Tauber J, Foster CS. Scleritis associated with relapsing polychondritis. Br J Ophthalmol. 2016;100(9):1290–4. https://doi.org/10.1136/bjophthalmol-2015-306902. Epub 2016 Feb 17. PMID: 26888976.
40. Fukuda K, Mizobuchi T, Nakajima I, Kishimoto T, Miura Y, Taniguchi Y. Ocular involvement in relapsing polychondritis. J Clin Med. 2021;10(21):4970. https://doi.org/10.3390/jcm10214970. PMID: 34768492; PMCID: PMC8584789.
41. Majumder PD, Ali S, George A, Ganesh S, Biswas J. Clinical profile of scleritis in children. Ocul Immunol Inflamm. 2019;27(4):535–9. https://doi.org/10.1080/09273948.2017.1423333. Epub 2018 Jan 25.
42. Woon WH, Stanford MR, Graham EM. Severe idiopathic posterior scleritis in children. Eye (Lond). 1995;9(Pt 5):570–4. https://doi.org/10.1038/eye.1995.141. PMID: 8543074.
43. Levi M, Kodsi SR, Rubin SE, Lyons C, Golden R, Olitsky SE, Christiansen S, Alcorn DM. Ocular involvement as the initial manifestation of Wegener's granulomatosis in children. J AAPOS. 2008;12(1):94–6. https://doi.org/10.1016/j.jaapos.2007.09.006. Epub 2007 Dec 21.
44. Cheung CM, Chee SP. Posterior scleritis in children: clinical features and treatment. Ophthalmology. 2012;119(1):59–65. https://doi.org/10.1016/j.ophtha.2011.09.030. Epub 2011 Dec 3.
45. Wald KJ, Spaide R, Patalano VJ, Sugin S, Yannuzzi LA. Posterior scleritis in children. Am J Ophthalmol. 1992;113(3):281–6. https://doi.org/10.1016/s0002-9394(14)71579-x. PMID: 1543220.
46. Naseri A, Good WV, Cunningham ET. Herpes zoster virussclerokeratitis and anterior uveitis in a child following varicella vaccination. Am J Ophthalmol. 2003;135(3):415–7.
47. Tarsia M, Gaggiano C, Gessaroli E, Grosso S, Tosi GM, Frediani B, Cantarini L, Fabiani C. Pediatric scleritis: an update. Ocul Immunol Inflamm. 2023;31(1):175–84. https://doi.org/10.1080/09273948.2021.2023582. Epub 2022 Feb 28. PMID: 35226583.
48. McCluskey P, Wakefield D. Prediction of response to treatment in patients with scleritis using a standardised scoring system. Aust N Z J Ophthalmol. 1991;19(3):211–5. https://doi.org/10.1111/j.1442-9071.1991.tb00663.x.
49. Doshi RR, Harocopos GJ, Schwab IR, Cunningham ET Jr. The spectrum of postoperative scleral necrosis. Surv Ophthalmol. 2013;58(6):620–33. https://doi.org/10.1016/j.survophthal.2012.11.002. Epub 2013 Feb 12.
50. Preetam Peraka R, Murthy SI. Role of anterior segment optical coherence tomography in scleral diseases: a review. Semin Ophthalmol. 2023;38(3):238–47. https://doi.org/10.1080/08820538.2022.2112700. Epub 2022 Aug 22. PMID: 35996334.
51. Shoughy SS, Jaroudi MO, Kozak I, Tabbara KF. Optical coherence tomography in the diagnosis of scleritis and episcleritis. Am J Ophthalmol. 2015;159(6):1045–1049.e1. https://doi.org/10.1016/j.ajo.2015.03.004. Epub 2015 Mar 11. PMID: 25771347.
52. Murthy SI, Sabhapandit S, Balamurugan S, Subramaniam P, Sainz-de-la-Maza M, Agarwal M, Parvesio C. Scleritis: differentiating infectious from non-infectious entities. Indian J Ophthalmol. 2020;68(9):1818–28. https://doi.org/10.4103/ijo.IJO_2032_20. PMID: 32823398; PMCID: PMC7690484.
53. Todokoro D, Hoshino J, Yo A, Makimura K, Hirato J, Akiyama H. Scedosporium apiospermum infectious scleritis following posterior subtenon triamcinolone acetonide injection: a case report and literature review. BMC Ophthalmol. 2018;18(1):40. https://doi.org/10.1186/s12886-018-0707-4. PMID: 29433463; PMCID: PMC5809823.
54. Jain V, Garg P, Sharma S. Microbial scleritis-experience from a developing country. Eye (Lond). 2009;23(2):255–61. https://doi.org/10.1038/sj.eye.6703099. Epub 2008 Jan 25.
55. Pradhan ZS, Jacob P. Infectious scleritis: clinical spectrum and management outcomes in India. Indian

J Ophthalmol. 2013;61(10):590–3. https://doi.org/10.4103/0301-4738.121085. PMID: 24212312; PMCID: PMC3853459.
56. Feiz V, Redline DE. Infectious scleritis after pars plana vitrectomy because of methicillin-resistant Staphylococcus aureus resistant to fourth-generation fluoroquinolones. Cornea. 2007;26(2):238–40. https://doi.org/10.1097/01.ico.0000248383.09272.ee.
57. Goyal M, Murthy SI. Infectious scleritis due to methicillin-resistant Staphylococcus Aureus after dengue viral fever. Ocul Immunol Inflamm. 2022;30(6):1544–6. https://doi.org/10.1080/09273948.2021.1900877. Epub 2021 Apr 8.
58. Lee JE, Oum BS, Choi HY, Lee JS. Methicillin-resistant Staphylococcus aureus sclerokeratitis after pterygium excision. Cornea. 2007;26(6):744–6. https://doi.org/10.1097/ICO.0b013e31804e45ba.
59. Sawant SD, Biswas J. Fungal scleritis with exudative retinal detachment. Ocul Immunol Inflamm. 2010;18(6):457–8. https://doi.org/10.3109/09273948.2010.507129. Epub 2010 Sep 16. PMID: 20846054.
60. Bernauer W, Allan BD, Dart JK. Successful management of Aspergillus scleritis by medical and surgical treatment. Eye (Lond). 1998;12(Pt 2):311–6. https://doi.org/10.1038/eye.1998.71.
61. Karkhur S, Soni D, Sharma B. A novel technique of full-thickness scleral debridement in fulminant necrotising infectious scleritis and its outcomes-a consecutive case series. Int Ophthalmol. 2022;42(2):581–92.https://doi.org/10.1007/s10792--021-02030-6. Epub 2021 Oct 6.
62. Vergouwen DPC, Rothova A, Berge JCT, Verdijk RM, van Laar JAM, Vingerling JR, Schreurs MWJ. Current insights in the pathogenesis of scleritis. Exp Eye Res. 2020;197:108078. https://doi.org/10.1016/j.exer.2020.108078. Epub 2020 Jun 3. PMID: 32504648.
63. Wakefield D, Di Girolamo N, Thurau S, Wildner G, McCluskey P. Scleritis: immunopathogenesis and molecular basis for therapy. Prog Retin Eye Res. 2013;35:44–62. https://doi.org/10.1016/j.preteyeres.2013.02.004. Epub 2013 Feb 26. PMID: 23454614.
64. Nishio Y, Taniguchi H, Takeda A, Hori J. Immunopathological analysis of a mouse model of arthritis-associated scleritis and implications for molecular targeted therapy for severe scleritis. Int J Mol Sci. 2021;23(1):341. https://doi.org/10.3390/ijms23010341. PMID: 35008766; PMCID: PMC8745222.
65. Taniguchi H, Kitahara Y, Hori J. Long-term ocular analysis in murine model of anterior scleritis. Invest Ophthalmol Vis Sci. 2015;56:858.
66. Silpa-Archa S, Oray M, Preble JM, Foster CS. Outcome of tocilizumab treatment in refractory ocular inflammatory diseases. Acta Ophthalmol. 2016;94(6):e400–6. https://doi.org/10.1111/aos.13015. Epub 2016 Mar 24. PMID: 27010181.
67. Riono WP, Hidayat AA, Rao NA. Scleritis: a clinicopathologic study of 55 cases. Ophthalmology. 1999;106(7):1328–33. https://doi.org/10.1016/S0161-6420(99)00719-8. PMID: 10406616.
68. Hankins M, Margo CE. Histopathological evaluation of scleritis. J Clin Pathol. 2019;72(5):386–90. https://doi.org/10.1136/jclinpath-2018-205360. Epub 2019 Feb 5.
69. Agrawal R, Lee CS, Gonzalez-Lopez JJ, Khan S, Rodrigues V, Pavesio C. Flurbiprofen: a nonselective cyclooxygenase (COX) inhibitor for treatment of noninfectious, non-necrotizing anterior scleritis. Ocul Immunol Inflamm. 2016;24(1):35–42. https://doi.org/10.3109/09273948.2015.1032308. Epub 2015 Aug 26. PMID: 26308394; PMCID: PMC4813454.
70. Chen B, Yang S, Zhu L, Peng X, He D, Tao T, Su W. Adalimumab plus conventional therapy versus conventional therapy in refractory non-infectious scleritis. J Clin Med. 2022;11(22):6686. https://doi.org/10.3390/jcm11226686. PMID: 36431163; PMCID: PMC9697705.
71. Ng CC, Sy A, Cunningham ET Jr. Rituximab for non-infectious uveitis and Scleritis. J Ophthalmic Inflamm Infect. 2021;11(1):23. https://doi.org/10.1186/s12348-021-00252-4. PMID: 34396463; PMCID: PMC8364894.
72. Pyare R, Dutta Majumder P, Shah M, Kaushik V, Agarwal M, Biswas J. Tofacitinib in scleritis: a case series. Ocul Immunol Inflamm. 2022:1–7. https://doi.org/10.1080/09273948.2022.2113805. Epub ahead of print. PMID: 36126052.
73. Singh JA, Cameron C, Noorbaloochi S, Cullis T, Tucker M, Christensen R, Ghogomu ET, Coyle D, Clifford T, Tugwell P, Wells GA. Risk of serious infection in biological treatment of patients with rheumatoid arthritis: a systematic review and meta-analysis. Lancet. 2015;386(9990):258–65. https://doi.org/10.1016/S0140-6736(14)61704-9. Epub 2015 May 11. PMID: 25975452; PMCID: PMC4580232.
74. Favalli EG. Tofacitinib's infectious profile: concerns for clinical practice. Lancet Rheumatol. 2020;2(2):E65–7. https://doi.org/10.1016/S2665--9913(20)30001-1. Published Online January 13, 2020.
75. Winthrop KL, Yamanaka H, Valdez H, Mortensen E, Chew R, Krishnaswami S, Kawabata T, Riese R. Herpes zoster and tofacitinib therapy in patients with rheumatoid arthritis. Arthritis Rheumatol. 2014;66(10):2675–84. https://doi.org/10.1002/art.38745. PMID: 24943354; PMCID: PMC4285807.
76. Kempen JH, Pistilli M, Begum H, Fitzgerald TD, Liesegang TL, Payal A, Zebardast N, Bhatt NP, Foster CS, Jabs DA, Levy-Clarke GA, Nussenblatt RB, Rosenbaum JT, Sen HN, Suhler EB, Thorne JE, Systemic Immunosuppressive Therapy for Eye Diseases (SITE) Cohort Study Research Group. Remission of non-infectious anterior scleritis: inci-

dence and predictive factors. Am J Ophthalmol. 2021;223:377–95. https://doi.org/10.1016/j.ajo.2019.03.024. Epub 2019 Apr 3.

77. Abdel-Aty A, Kombo N. Factors affecting the resolution of acute non-infectious anterior scleritis. Br J Ophthalmol. 2022;106(12):1672–7. https://doi.org/10.1136/bjophthalmol-2021-318808. Epub 2021 Jul 1.
78. Wakefield D. Does cyclophosphamide still have a role in treating severe inflammatory eye disease? Ocul Immunol Inflamm. 2014;22(4):306–10. https://doi.org/10.3109/09273948.2013.854395. Epub 2013 Dec 11. PMID: 24329578.
79. Artifoni M, Rothschild PR, Brézin A, Guillevin L, Puéchal X. Ocular inflammatory diseases associated with rheumatoid arthritis. Nat Rev Rheumatol. 2014;10(2):108–16. https://doi.org/10.1038/nrrheum.2013.185. Epub 2013 Dec 10.
80. Preble JM, Lin X. Plasmapheresis as a viable treatment option for scleritis. Am J Ophthalmol Case Rep. 2022;27:101627. https://doi.org/10.1016/j.ajoc.2022.101627. PMID: 35782168; PMCID: PMC9243044.
81. Feizi S, Alemzadeh-Ansari M, Baradaran-Rafii A, Esfandiari H, Kheirkhah A. Topical erythropoietin for treatment of scleral necrosis. Ocul Immunol Inflamm. 2022;30(7-8):1701–6. https://doi.org/10.1080/09273948.2021.1934485. Epub 2021 Jun 14.
82. Feizi S, Kanavi MR, Safari S, Ebrahimi H, Javadi MA. Effects of topical erythropoietin on healing experimentally-induced avascular scleral damage in a rabbit model. Exp Eye Res. 2020;190:107898. https://doi.org/10.1016/j.exer.2019.107898. Epub 2019 Dec 19.
83. McKibbin M, Isaacs JD, Morrell AJ. Incidence of corneal melting in association with systemic disease in the Yorkshire Region, 1995-7. Br J Ophthalmol. 1999;83(8):941–3. https://doi.org/10.1136/bjo.83.8.941. PMID: 10413698; PMCID: PMC1723151.
84. Sharma N, Sinha G, Shekhar H, Titiyal JS, Agarwal T, Chawla B, Tandon R, Vajpayee RB. Demographic profile, clinical features and outcome of peripheral ulcerative keratitis: a prospective study. Br J Ophthalmol. 2015;99(11):1503–8. https://doi.org/10.1136/bjophthalmol-2014-306008. Epub 2015 May 2. PMID: 25935428.
85. Makol A, Matteson EL, Warrington KJ. Rheumatoid vasculitis: an update. Curr Opin Rheumatol. 2015;27(1):63–70. https://doi.org/10.1097/BOR.0000000000000126.
86. Wajnsztajn D, Nche E, Solomon A. Corneal complications of rheumatoid arthritis. Curr Opin Allergy Clin Immunol. 2022;22(5):304–13. https://doi.org/10.1097/ACI.0000000000000844. Epub 2022 Aug 16. PMID: 35980013.
87. Uchida S, Kaji Y, Ui M, Kawashima H, Usui T, Ohira Y. Peripheral ulcerative keratitis associated with large vessel vasculitis. Cureus. 2021;13(6):e15767. https://doi.org/10.7759/cureus.15767. PMID: 34290940; PMCID: PMC8290306.
88. Damian L, Pamfil C, Bucşa C, Nicula C, Mouthon L, Amoura Z, Cutolo M, Burmester GR, Fonseca JE, Grapini L, Arnaud L, Rednic S. Rare within rare. Necrotising scleritis and peripheral ulcerative keratitis: eye-threatening complications of relapsing polychondritis. Clin Exp Rheumatol 2022;40 Suppl 134(5):86–92. https://doi.org/10.55563/clinexprheumatol/27n7im. Epub 2022 Feb 24.
89. Sainz de la Maza M, Foster CS, Jabbur NS, Baltatzis S. Ocular characteristics and disease associations in scleritis-associated peripheral keratopathy. Arch Ophthalmol. 2002;120(1):15–9. https://doi.org/10.1001/archopht.120.1.15. PMID: 11786052.
90. Bonnet C, Debillon L, Al-Hashimi S, Hoogewoud F, Monnet D, Bourges JL, Brézin A. Anterior segment optical coherence tomography imaging in peripheral ulcerative keratitis, a corneal structural description. BMC Ophthalmol. 2020;20(1):205. https://doi.org/10.1186/s12886-020-01466-1. PMID: 32450833; PMCID: PMC7249626.
91. Kochhar S, Singh S, Desai B, Purohit D. Etiology, clinical profile, and treatment outcome of peripheral ulcerative keratitis. Saudi J Ophthalmol. 2022;36(1):90–4. https://doi.org/10.4103/sjopt.sjopt_38_20. PMID: 35971491; PMCID: PMC9375467.
92. Vignesh AP, Srinivasan R, Vijitha S. Ocular syphilis masquerading as bilateral peripheral ulcerative keratitis. Taiwan J Ophthalmol. 2016;6(4):204–5. https://doi.org/10.1016/j.tjo.2016.06.002. Epub 2016 Jul 16. PMID: 29018744; PMCID: PMC5525632.
93. Chranioti A, Malamas A, Metallidis S, Mataftsi A, Chalvatzis N, Ziakas N. Bilateral herpes simplex virus-related peripheral ulcerative keratitis leading to corneal perforation in a patient with primary herpes simplex virus infection. J Ophthalmic Vis Res. 2019;14(1):93–6. https://doi.org/10.4103/jovr.jovr_3_17. PMID: 30820293; PMCID: PMC638851.
94. Praidou A, Androudi S, Kanonidou E, Konidaris V, Alexandridis A, Brazitikos P. Bilateral herpes simplex keratitis presenting as peripheral ulcerative keratitis. Cornea. 2012;31(5):570–1. https://doi.org/10.1097/ICO.0b013e31822f3c18. PMID: 22378116.
95. Tavassoli S, Gunn D, Tole D, Darcy K. Peripheral ulcerative keratitis with corneal melt as the primary presentation in a case of human immunodeficiency virus. BMJ Case Rep. 2019;12(2):e226936. https://doi.org/10.1136/bcr-2018-226936. PMID: 30798272; PMCID: PMC6441276.
96. Neves RA, Rodriguez A, Power WJ, Muccioli C, Lane L, Belfort R Jr, Foster CS. Herpes zoster peripheral ulcerative keratitis in patients with the acquired immunodeficiency syndrome. Cornea. 1996;15(5):446–50.
97. Wei DW, Pagnoux C, Chan CC. Peripheral ulcerative keratitis secondary to chronic hepatitis B infection.

Cornea. 2017;36(4):515–7. https://doi.org/10.1097/ICO.0000000000001087. PMID: 27861312.

98. Pluznik D, Butrus SI. Hepatitis C-associated peripheral corneal ulceration: rapid response to intravenous steroids. Cornea. 2001;20(8):888–9. https://doi.org/10.1097/00003226-200111000-00023. PMID: 11685073.

99. Aschauer J, Donner R, Lammer J, Schmidinger G. Bilateral corneal perforation in Ipilimumab/Nivolumab - associated peripheral ulcerative keratitis. Am J Ophthalmol Case Rep. 2022;28:101686. https://doi.org/10.1016/j.ajoc.2022.101686. PMID: 36072439; PMCID: PMC9442328.

100. Kervick GN, Pflugfelder SC, Haimovici R, Brown H, Tozman E, Yee R. Paracentral rheumatoid corneal ulceration. Clinical features and cyclosporine therapy. Ophthalmology. 1992;99(1):80–8. https://doi.org/10.1016/s0161-6420(92)32006-8.

101. Kalsow CM, Ching SSST, Plotnik RD. Cellular infiltrate in rheumatoid arthritis-associated paracentral corneal ulceration. Ocul Immunol Inflamm. 2017;25(6):878–83. https://doi.org/10.1080/09273948.2016.1199707. Epub 2016 Aug 11. PMID: 27715362; PMCID: PMC6173203.

102. Akpek EK, Demetriades AM, Gottsch JD. Peripheral ulcerative keratitis after clear corneal cataract extraction(1). J Cataract Refract Surg. 2000;26(9):1424–7. https://doi.org/10.1016/s0886-3350(00)00359-x.

103. Perez VL, Azar DT, Foster CS. Sterile corneal melting and necrotizing scleritis after cataract surgery in patients with rheumatoid arthritis and collagen vascular disease. Semin Ophthalmol. 2002;17(3–4):124–30. https://doi.org/10.1076/soph.17.3.124.14786. PMID: 12759840.

104. Harada K, Mohamed YH, Uematsu M, Inoue D, Ueki R, Harada S, Imamura N, Miwako I, Kitaoka T. Three cases of acute sterile corneal melt after cataract surgery. Am J Ophthalmol Case Rep. 2018;13:62–5. https://doi.org/10.1016/j.ajoc.2018.12.004. PMID: 30582074; PMCID: PMC6297052.

105. Ntatsaki E, Mooney J, Scott DG, Watts RA. Systemic rheumatoid vasculitis in the era of modern immunosuppressive therapy. Rheumatology (Oxford). 2014;53(1):145–52. https://doi.org/10.1093/rheumatology/ket326. Epub 2013 Oct 8.

106. Srinivasan M, Zegans ME, Zelefsky JR, Kundu A, Lietman T, Whitcher JP, Cunningham ET Jr. Clinical characteristics of Moore's ulcer in South India. Br J Ophthalmol. 2007;91(5):570–5. https://doi.org/10.1136/bjo.2006.105452. Epub 2006 Oct 11. PMID: 17035269; PMCID: PMC1954782.

107. Fasina O, Ogundipe A, Ezichi E. Mooren'S ulcer in Ibadan, Southwest Nigeria. J West Afr Coll Surg. 2013;3(3):102–19. PMID: 25717466; PMCID: PMC4337214.

108. Acharya NR, Srinivasan M, Kundu A, Lietman TM, Whitcher JP, Cunningham ET Jr. Mooren's ulcer following extracapsular cataract extraction. Eur J Ophthalmol. 2008;18(3):351–5. https://doi.org/10.1177/112067210801800306.

109. Das S, Mohamed A, Sangwan VS. Clinical course and patient outcomes with Mooren ulcer who had cataract surgery. J Cataract Refract Surg. 2017;43(8):1044–9. https://doi.org/10.1016/j.jcrs.2017.05.034.

110. Lee HJ, Kim MK, Wee WR, Oh JY. Interplay of immune cells in Mooren ulcer. Cornea. 2015;34(9):1164–7. https://doi.org/10.1097/ICO.0000000000000471.

111. Shinomiya K, Ueta M, Sotozono C, Inatomi T, Yokoi N, Koizumi N, Kinoshita S. Immunohistochemical analysis of inflammatory limbal conjunctiva adjacent to Mooren's ulcer. Br J Ophthalmol. 2013;97(3):362–6. https://doi.org/10.1136/bjophthalmol-2012-302631. Epub 2013 Jan 3. PMID: 23292924.

112. Li L, Dong YL, Liu T, Luo D, Wei C, Shi WY. Increased succinate receptor GPR91 involved in the pathogenesis of Mooren's ulcer. Int J Ophthalmol. 2018;11(11):1733–40. https://doi.org/10.18240/ijo.2018.11.01. PMID: 30450301; PMCID: PMC6232339.

113. Messmer EM, Foster CS. Destructive corneal and scleral disease associated with rheumatoid arthritis. Medical and surgical management. Cornea. 1995;14(4):408–17. https://doi.org/10.1097/00003226-199507000-00010.

114. Foster CS, Forstot SL, Wilson LA. Mortality rate in rheumatoid arthritis patients developing necrotizing scleritis or peripheral ulcerative keratitis. Effects of systemic immunosuppression. Ophthalmology. 1984;91(10):1253–63. https://doi.org/10.1016/s0161-6420(84)34160-4.

115. Timlin HM, Hall HN, Foot B, Koay P. Corneal perforation from peripheral ulcerative keratopathy in patients with rheumatoid arthritis: epidemiological findings of the British Ophthalmological Surveillance Unit. Br J Ophthalmol. 2018;102(9):1298–302. https://doi.org/10.1136/bjophthalmol-2017-310671. Epub 2017 Dec 15. PMID: 29246891.

116. Akpek EK, Klimava A, Thorne JE, Martin D, Lekhanont K, Ostrovsky A. Evaluation of patients with dry eye for presence of underlying Sjögren syndrome. Cornea. 2009;28(5):493–7. https://doi.org/10.1097/ICO.0b013e31818d3846. PMID: 19421051; PMCID: PMC2693267.

117. Alani H, Henty JR, Thompson NL, Jury E, Ciurtin C. Systematic review and meta-analysis of the epidemiology of polyautoimmunity in Sjögren's syndrome (secondary Sjögren's syndrome) focusing on autoimmune rheumatic diseases. Scand J Rheumatol. 2018;47(2):141–54. https://doi.org/10.1080/03009742.2017.1324909. Epub 2017 Sep 20.

118. Bron AJ, de Paiva CS, Chauhan SK, Bonini S, Gabison EE, Jain S, Knop E, Markoulli M, Ogawa Y, Perez V, Uchino Y, Yokoi N, Zoukhri D, Sullivan DA. TFOS DEWS II pathophysiology report. Ocul Surf. 2017;15(3):438–510. https://doi.org/10.1016/j.jtos.2017.05.011. Epub 2017 Jul 20. Erratum in: Ocul Surf. 2019 Oct;17(4):842.

119. Gualtierotti R, Ciavarella T, Meroni L. Rheumatoid factors. In: Shoenfeld Y, Meroni PL, Gershwin ME, editors. Autoantibodies. 3rd ed. San Diego: Elsevier; 2014. p. 751–60. https://doi.org/10.1016/B978-0-444-56378-1.00089-7. https://www.sciencedirect.com/science/article/pii/B9780444563781000897.
120. Watson PG. Vascular changes in peripheral corneal destructive disease. Eye (Lond). 1990;4(Pt 1):65–73. https://doi.org/10.1038/eye.1990.7. PMID: 2323479.
121. Riley GP, Harrall RL, Watson PG, Cawston TE, Hazleman BL. Collagenase (MMP-1) and TIMP-1 in destructive corneal disease associated with rheumatoid arthritis. Eye (Lond). 1995;9(Pt 6):703–18. https://doi.org/10.1038/eye.1995.182. PMID: 8849537.
122. Tan KW, Chong SZ, Wong FH, Evrard M, Tan SM, Keeble J, Kemeny DM, Ng LG, Abastado JP, Angeli V. Neutrophils contribute to inflammatory lymphangiogenesis by increasing VEGF-A bioavailability and secreting VEGF-D. Blood. 2013;122(22):3666–77. https://doi.org/10.1182/blood-2012-11-466532. Epub 2013 Oct 10. PMID: 24113869.
123. Wang XL, Zhao J, Qin L, Qiao M. Promoting inflammatory lymphangiogenesis by vascular endothelial growth factor-C (VEGF-C) aggravated intestinal inflammation in mice with experimental acute colitis. Braz J Med Biol Res. 2016;49(5):e4738. https://doi.org/10.1590/1414-431X20154738. Epub 2016 Apr 8. PMID: 27074165; PMCID: PMC4830025.
124. Marsovszky L, Resch MD, Németh J, Toldi G, Medgyesi E, Kovács L, Balog A. In vivo confocal microscopic evaluation of corneal Langerhans cell density, and distribution and evaluation of dry eye in rheumatoid arthritis. Innate Immun. 2013;19(4):348–54. https://doi.org/10.1177/1753425912461677. Epub 2012 Nov 30.
125. Chauhan SK, Dohlman TH, Dana R. Corneal lymphatics: role in ocular inflammation as inducer and responder of adaptive immunity. J Clin Cell Immunol. 2014;5:1000256. https://doi.org/10.4172/2155-9899.1000256. PMID: 25580370; PMCID: PMC4287999.
126. Ruiz-Lozano RE, Ramos-Davila EM, Garza-Garza LA, Gutierrez-Juarez K, Hernandez-Camarena JC, Rodriguez-Garcia A. Rheumatoid arthritis-associated peripheral ulcerative keratitis outcomes after early immunosuppressive therapy. Br J Ophthalmol. 2023;107:1246. https://doi.org/10.1136/bjophthalmol-2022-321132. Epub ahead of print. PMID: 35418476.
127. Sura AA, McCallum RM. Peripheral ulcerative keratitis due to systemic diseases. Curr Opin Ophthalmol. 2022;33(6):543–50. https://doi.org/10.1097/ICU.0000000000000895. Epub 2022 Sep 19. PMID: 36165409.
128. Cordero-Coma M, Méndez RS, Blanco AC, Corral AL, Calleja-Antolín S, de Morales JM. Adalimumab for refractory peripheral ulcerative keratitis. J Ophthalmic Inflamm Infect. 2012;2(4):227–9. https://doi.org/10.1007/s12348-012-0080-z. Epub 2012 May 16. PMID: 22588776; PMCID: PMC3500990.
129. Huerva V, Ascaso FJ, Grzybowski A. Infliximab for peripheral ulcerative keratitis treatment. Medicine (Baltimore). 2014;93(26):e176. https://doi.org/10.1097/MD.0000000000000176. PMID: 25474432; PMCID: PMC4616390.
130. Odorcic S, Keystone EC, Ma JJ. Infliximab for the treatment of refractory progressive sterile peripheral ulcerative keratitis associated with late corneal perforation: 3-year follow-up. Cornea. 2009;28(1):89–92. https://doi.org/10.1097/ICO.0b013e318181a84f.
131. Thomas JW, Pflugfelder SC. Therapy of progressive rheumatoid arthritis-associated corneal ulceration with infliximab. Cornea. 2005;24(6):742–4. https://doi.org/10.1097/01.ico.0000154391.28254.1d. PMID: 16015096.
132. Dominguez-Casas LC, Sánchez-Bilbao L, Calvo-Río V, Maíz O, Blanco A, Beltrán E, Martínez-Costa L, Demetrío-Pablo R, Del Buergo MÁ, Rubio-Romero E, Díaz-Valle D, Lopez-Gonzalez R, García-Aparicio ÁM, Mas AJ, Vegas-Revenga N, Castañeda S, Hernández JL, González-Gay MA, Blanco R. Biologic therapy in severe and refractory peripheral ulcerative keratitis (PUK). Multicenter study of 34 patients. Semin Arthritis Rheum. 2020;50(4):608–15. https://doi.org/10.1016/j.semarthrit.2020.03.023. Epub 2020 May 15.s
133. Bonnet I, Rousseau A, Duraffour P, Pouchot J, Nguyen CD, Gabison E, Seror R, Marotte H, Mariette X, Nocturne G. Efficacy and safety of rituximab in peripheral ulcerative keratitis associated with rheumatoid arthritis. RMD Open. 2021;7(1):e001472. https://doi.org/10.1136/rmdopen-2020-001472. PMID: 33510042; PMCID: PMC7845725.
134. Guindolet D, Reynaud C, Clavel G, Belangé G, Benmahmed M, Doan S, Hayem G, Cochereau I, Gabison EE. Management of severe and refractory Mooren's ulcers with rituximab. Br J Ophthalmol. 2017;101(4):418–22. https://doi.org/10.1136/bjophthalmol-2016-308838. Epub 2016 Jul 22.
135. Goodisson LA, Bourne JT, Maharajan S. A case of bilateral peripheral ulcerative keratitis following treatment with rituximab. Rheumatology (Oxford). 2010;49(3):609–10. https://doi.org/10.1093/rheumatology/kep390. Epub 2009 Nov 27.
136. Mehta K, Gujjar AP, Babu K. Peripheral ulcerative keratitis in a young lady with systemic lupus erythematosus post rituximab infusion-a case report. Ocul Immunol Inflamm. 2022;30(6):1312–4. https://doi.org/10.1080/09273948.2022.2037654. Epub 2022 Feb 25.
137. Huang J, Chen Z, Zhao L, et al. Tocilizumab in rheumatoid arthritis-associated peripheral ulcerative keratitis: a 1-year follow-up case report. Rheumatol Autoimmun. 2022;2:45–50. https://doi.org/10.1002/rai2.12022.
138. Cohen F, Gabison EE, Stéphan S, Belkhir R, Nocturne G, Best AL, Haigh O, Barreau E, Labetoulle M,

Seror R, Rousseau A. Peripheral ulcerative keratitis in rheumatoid arthritis patients taking tocilizumab: paradoxical manifestation or insufficient efficacy? Rheumatology (Oxford). 2021;60(11):5413–8. https://doi.org/10.1093/rheumatology/keab093.

139. Wendling D, Dernis E, Prati C, Frisch E, Delbosc B. Onset of inflammatory eye disease under tocilizumab treatment for rheumatologic conditions: a paradoxical effect? J Rheumatol. 2011;38(10):2284. https://doi.org/10.3899/jrheum.110170. PMID: 21965707.
140. Stylianides A, Jones MN, Stewart RM, Murphy CC, Goodson NJ, Kaye SB. Rheumatoid arthritis-associated corneal ulceration: mortality and graft survival. Ophthalmology. 2013;120(4):682–6. https://doi.org/10.1016/j.ophtha.2012.09.050. Epub 2013 Jan 3. PMID: 23290983.
141. Sabhapandit S, Murthy SI, Sharma N, Sangwan VS. Surgical management of peripheral ulcerative keratitis: update on surgical techniques and their outcome. Clin Ophthalmol. 2022;16:3547–57. https://doi.org/10.2147/OPTH.S385782. PMID: 36274679; PMCID: PMC9579814.
142. Soong HK, Farjo AA, Katz D, Meyer RF, Sugar A. Lamellar corneal patch grafts in the management of corneal melting. Cornea. 2000;19(2):126–34. https://doi.org/10.1097/00003226-200003000-00002. PMID: 10746441.
143. Vanathi M, Sharma N, Titiyal JS, Tandon R, Vajpayee RB. Tectonic grafts for corneal thinning and perforations. Cornea. 2002;21(8):792–7. https://doi.org/10.1097/00003226-200211000-00013. PMID: 12410039.
144. Calli U, Genc S, Şalkacı O, Ömeroğlu A. Lamellar corneal patch grafts in the management of corneal thinning and perforations without using extra corneas. Semin Ophthalmol. 2022;37(1):3–6. https://doi.org/10.1080/08820538.2021.1896754. Epub 2021 Apr 6.
145. Eslami M, Benito-Pascual B, Goolam S, Trinh T, Moloney G. Case report: use of amniotic membrane for tectonic repair of peripheral ulcerative keratitis with corneal perforation. Front Med (Lausanne). 2022;27(9):836873. https://doi.org/10.3389/fmed.2022.836873. PMID: 35572993; PMCID: PMC9093648.
146. Lavaris A, Elanwar MFM, Al-Zyiadi M, Xanthopoulou PT, Kopsachilis N. Glueless and sutureless multi-layer amniotic membrane transplantation in a patient with pending corneal perforation. Cureus. 2021;13(7):e16678. https://doi.org/10.7759/cureus.16678. PMID: 34513346; PMCID: PMC8412217.

Lid Signs, Paralytic Squint, and Ocular Movement Disorders

19

19.1 Lids: Anatomical Considerations

The lids are tri-lamellar appendages which protect the eyeball from mechanical trauma and foreign bodies (Fig. 19.1). The anterior-most lamella consists of the skin, which continues with the skin of the face and the forehead. The skin of the lids is ~1 mm thick and is the thinnest in the body. Under the skin, a circumferentially oriented smooth muscle called orbicularis oculi lies that originates from the medial canthal ligament. It has two components, the palpebral (pretarsal and preseptal) and orbital. The pretarsal and preseptal components form the palpebral orbicularis oculi, which participate in spontaneous blinking. The orbital orbicularis oculi are used during voluntary blinking or forced eye closure [1]. The orbicularis oculi muscle fibres are inserted into the skin's connective tissue at the lateral canthus.

The middle lamella of the lid comprises the pretarsal fat, orbital septum, and the post-septal fat pad. The orbital septum is a barrier that divides the orbit into a pre-septal and a post-septal compartment. The orbital septum separates the orbital fat pad from a thin submuscular layer of fibro-adipose tissue that lies anterior to the orbital septum.

The tarsal plate, lid retractors, levator palpebrae superioris muscle (LPSM), and Muller's muscle form the inner lamella. The conjunctiva lines the inner lamella [2]. The tarsal plate is a thickened, tough fibrous membrane and is an extension of the orbital septum, which fuses with the orbital periosteum at the margin of the orbit. The tarsal plate is sickle-shaped in most and less commonly trapezoid or triangular [3]. The LPSM is the main retractor of the upper lid and contains fatigue-resistant muscle fibres [4]. It arises from the orbital surface of the lesser wing of the sphenoid bone lateral to the optic foramen and courses above the superior rectus, with which it also shares the fibrous sheath [5, 6]. It is 4 mm wide at the origin and progressively fans anteriorly; suddenly, the muscle fibres transition into aponeurosis (LA) 36 mm from its origin. The width of the aponeurosis is 18 mm at the transition site [5]. The anterior fascia of the LPSM is thickened and stretches from the trochlea to the lacrimal fascia and is called Whitnall's superior transverse ligament. It is present on the descending limb of LA after the culmination of the LPSM [7] and could not act as a pulley for the action of the LPSM. The LA splits into two layers; the anterior LA is reflected for a few mms and continues with the orbital septum. The posterior layer of the LA inserts into the anterior surface of the tarsal plate [2]. Throughout its extent, LA sends extensions through the orbicularis muscle into the overlying skin. These insertions of LA are responsible for forming the upper eyelid crease. Müller's tarsal

A. Gupta et al., *Ophthalmic Signs in Practice of Medicine*,
https://doi.org/10.1007/978-981-99-7923-3_19

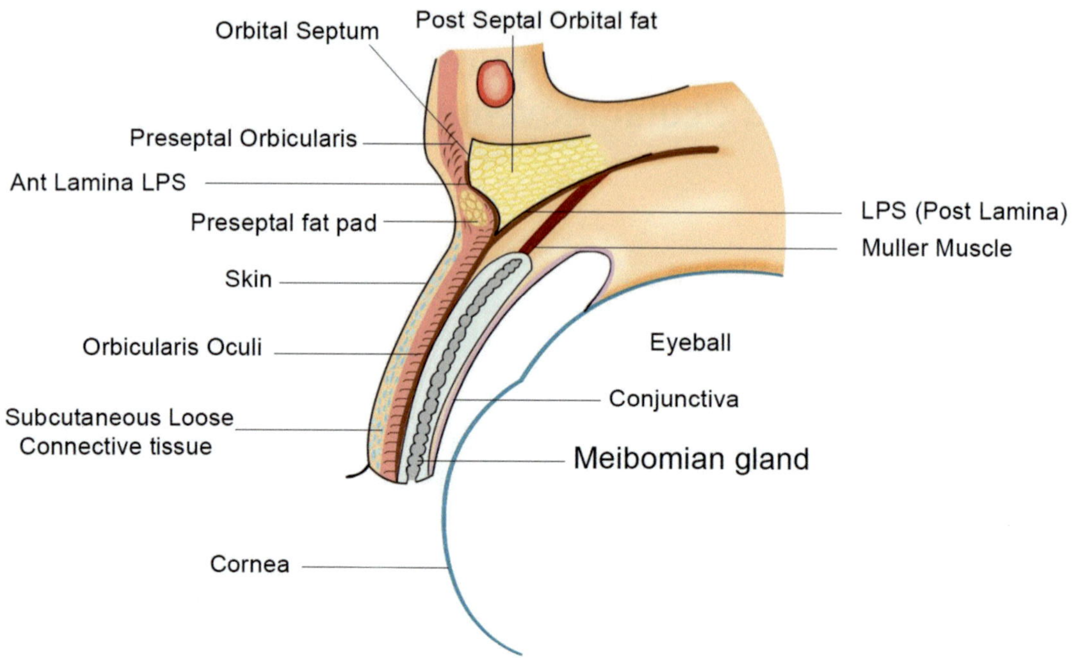

Fig. 19.1 Highly schematic representation of upper eyelid anatomy. Graphics by Kritika Thakur

muscle is smooth and innervated by sympathetic fibres. It arises from the LA undersurface as the LPSM transitions into LA and is inserted into the superior margin of the tarsal plate.

The tarsal plate in the lower lid is half the height of the upper tarsus. The lower retractors are rudimentary and include the capsulopalpebral fascia (counterpart of the LPSM) and the inferior tarsal muscle counterpart of Muller's muscle. The Muller's and inferior tarsal muscles are innervated by sympathetic fibres drawn from the superior cervical ganglion. The blood supply of the upper and lower lids is through the ophthalmic artery's medial and lateral palpebral arteries. The nerve supply of the LPSM is via the superior division of the oculomotor nerve. The orbicularis oculi are supplied by facial nerve branches (CN VII). During waking hours, the LPSM and the Muller muscle tone keep the eyes open and indicate alertness. The LPSM tone depends upon the vertical position of the eyes. In contrast, the tarsal muscles maintain their tone in all gaze directions [8]. There is a close relation between the level of alertness and the LPS tone. The LPS function is lost during sleep [1, 4]. Drooping of the eyelid (ptosis) results from decreased functioning of the LPSM rather than increased contraction of the orbicularis oculi muscle.

19.2 Anthropometry of Lids

The upper eyelid, by a windshield wiper movement, during each blink spreads the tear film over the cornea. The exposed gap between the open eyes' upper and lower lid margins, while looking in primary gaze, is called the palpebral fissure (Fig. 19.2). The normal height of the adult palpebral fissure is ~10 mm, and the width is ~30 mm (distance between the medial canthus and the lateral canthus). There are racial and gender differences in the height and width of the palpebral fissure. In a South Indian population, the average width was significantly longer in males (31.08 ± 1.79 mm males vs 29.90 ± 2.18 mm females). However, there was no difference in the height of the palpebral aperture that varied from 11.30 ± 1.66 mm in males and 11.58 ± 1.65 mm [9]. The lateral canthus is inclined slightly higher than the medial canthus and varies in various eth-

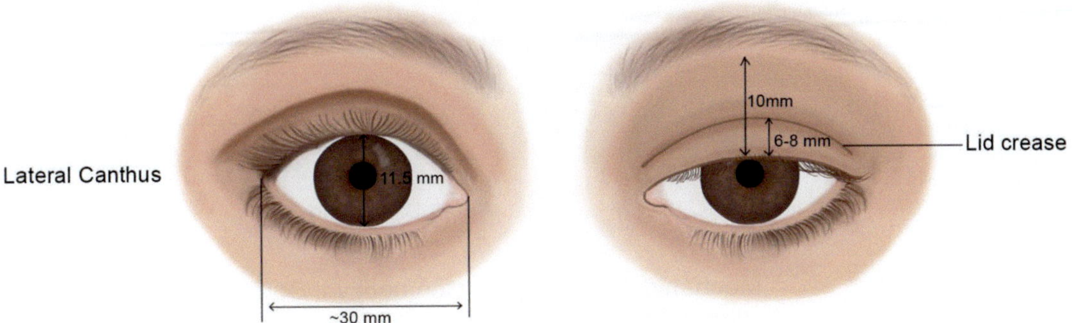

Fig. 19.2 Schematic representation of the anthropometry of the eyelids. Graphics by Kritika Thakur

nic populations. In the South Indian study, there was no significant difference in the degree of inclination (5.05 ± 2.47° in males and 6.1 ± 2.85° in females) [9]. The palpebral fissure inclination in North American whites (men 2.1° and women, 4.1°) [10] and in Koreans (men, 7.9° ± 2.4° and 8.8° ± 2.3° women,10.6°) [11].

The height of the upper eyelid is measured with the eyes open and looking in the primary gaze. It is the distance from the eyebrow's lower margin to the upper lid's margin. In the Indian population, it was 10.5 ± 0.8 mm for men and 9.3 ± 1.1 mm for women, showing an age-related increase [12]. The lid crease is the distance between the upper lid margin and a crease in its skin. It is formed by the extensions of the LPS aponeurosis to the skin through the orbicularis oculi. It is measured with the person looking down and measures 6–8 mm in men and 8–10 mm in women.

In the primary gaze, the upper lid covers the superior limbus by 0.5–1.00 mm while the lower lid is at the inferior limbus. All lid structures, except the conjunctiva, can be visualized on axial and sagittal MRI and CT scans. However, CT scans fail to show the tarsal muscles [13].

19.3 Lid Signs

Several lid signs provide a quick clue to the possible systemic severe disorders. The lid signs may occur in isolation or in association with ocular movement disorders.

19.3.1 Ptosis

Ptosis or blepharoptosis means drooping of either a unilateral or bilateral upper eyelid. Normal palpebral fissure is about 10 mm in height. The upper lid margin covers about 0.5–2 mm of the upper cornea, with a corneal reflex to upper lid margin (margin to reflex distance, or MRD) difference of ~4 mm. Two muscles, namely, the LPSM and Muller's muscle, elevate the lid and keep the eyes open.

When dealing with ptosis, it is most critical to determine whether ptosis was congenital or acquired. Thus, it is important to determine the age of onset of ptosis, whether it was present from birth or developed in old age. Abrupt onset ptosis often requires neuroimaging to rule out intracranial pathology, especially if it was painful at the onset. If the severity of ptosis varies with the time of the day is absent on waking up and worsens during the day, it is likely due to myasthenia gravis (MG).

19.3.1.1 Mechanical Ptosis

Mechanical lid drooping may result from many lid swellings and tumours that may vary from a benign chalazion to highly malignant lesions, which require complete evaluation for appropriate management. A chalazion is a common occurrence as a painless (unless infected) non-tender swelling, most often on the upper lid, chronic granulomatous inflammation of the meibomian gland due to obstruction to the outflow of the meibomian secretions in the tarsal plate. In old age, certain drugs like bortezomib, a proteasome

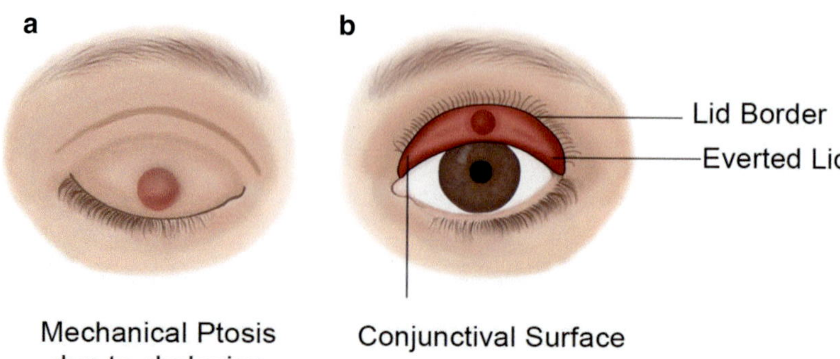

Fig. 19.3 Mechanical ptosis due to growth on the upper lid (**a**). The upper lid is everted and shows the bulge of the swelling on the conjunctival side (**b**). Graphics by Kritika Thakur

inhibitor used in patients with multiple myeloma, may lead to multiple chalazia in one or both eyes (Fig. 19.3) [14]. It appears as a smooth dome-shaped, painless swelling which, on eversion of the lid, reveals a swelling with a pale soft centre due to inspissated secretions which, on compression, may exude as a paste-like material from the opening of the Meibomian gland. The chalazia may grow in size, may get infected and become painful. These require incision and curettage from the conjunctival side, and if recurrent, the curetted material should be sent for pathological examination as meibomian gland carcinomas may mimic a chalazion. The other lid tumours include sebaceous gland carcinoma, Squamous cell carcinoma, Sturge-Weber syndrome, Neurofibromatosis, and dacryoadenitis.

19.3.1.2 Congenital Ptosis

The most common cause of ptosis is congenital; it may be unilateral or bilateral and is present from birth. The severity varies from mild to moderate to severe. If the drooping of the upper eyelid is ≤2 mm, it is classified as mild, between 3 and <4 mm is moderate, and ≥4 mm is severe (Fig. 19.4). In severe ptosis, the pupil is entirely covered with the ptotic lid. In congenital ptosis, the eyelid crease is absent, and when the patient is asked to look down, there is a lid lag. On the side of the ptosis, the eyebrow is raised as the frontalis muscle is activated to raise the upper lid. Moreover, the patients usually lift their chin to increase their field of vision. While measuring the MRD, the action of the frontalis muscle is carefully blocked by pressing it to give an accurate assessment of the MRD. Most often, the cause of congenital ptosis is myogenic, as the muscle fibres are replaced by fibrous tissue. Some important measurements include measuring the height of the palpebral aperture, MRD1 (distance from the upper lid margin to the centre of the pupil), and MRD2 (distance from the centre of the pupil to the lower lid margin). The lid margin to the upper lid skin crease distance (MCD) is also measured (Fig. 19.2). The LPS action is measured by asking the patient to look in an extreme downgaze, a transparent ruler is placed against the eye, frontalis muscle action is blocked, and the patient is asked to move the eye in an extreme upgaze. The movement of the lid margin against the ruler gives the action of LPS in mm. The LPS action is normal, if it is ≥15 mm; good, 12–14 mm; fair, 5–11 mm, and poor, ≤ 4 mm (Fig. 19.4). Other evaluations include a corrected visual acuity assessment of corneal sensations, and Schirmer's test, confirming the presence of Bell's phenomenon (on the forced closure of the lids, the eyeballs roll up and out). Jaw-winking phenomenon needs to be ruled out by asking the patient to mimic masticatory movements, which lift the ptotic eye due to synkinetic movements of the LPSM and the external pterygoid muscle [15].

There is no medical treatment for ptosis. Surgery is indicated for cosmetic reasons, abnormal head posture, amblyopia, and improvement of visual fields. In case squint is associated with ptosis, squint correction is done first. Mild ptosis can be left alone. Mild-to-moderate ptosis with good LPS action is usually subjected to a Fasanella-Servat procedure [16] involving resection of the tarsal plate (3 mm), Muller's muscle

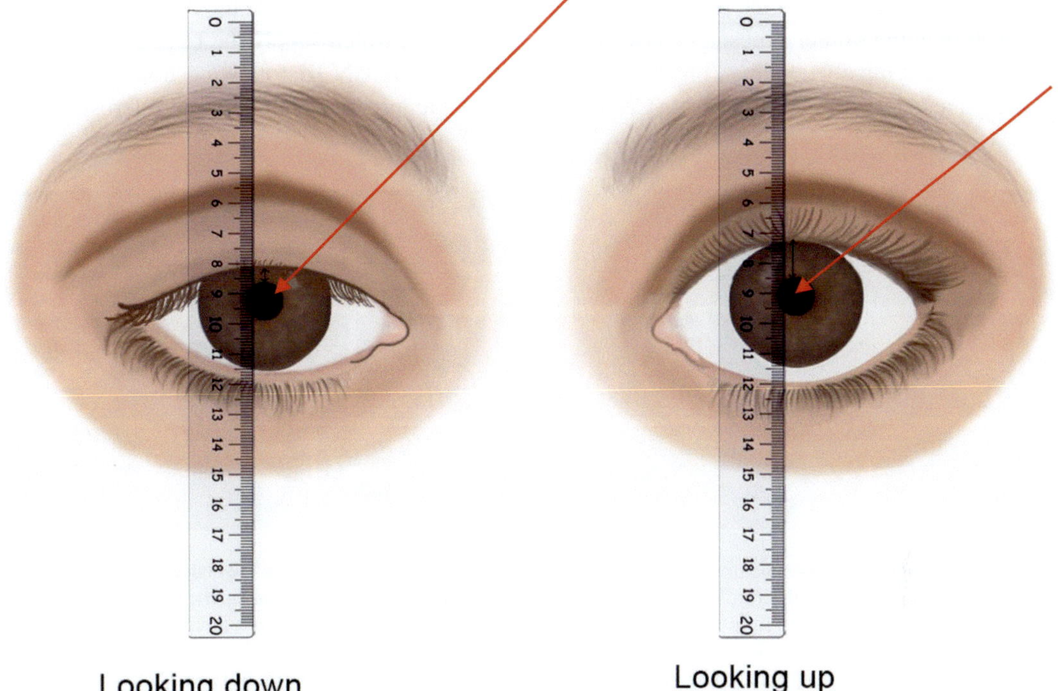

Fig. 19.4 Measuring the severity of the ptosis and LPS action with a transparent ruler: The patient is first asked to look in the primary gaze. The distance of the pupillary reflex to the upper lid margin is measured. For measuring the Levator Palpebrae Superioris (LPS) action, the patient is asked to look down. Distance from the central pupillary reflex to the margin of the upper lid is measured in down-gaze. The patient is then asked to look up after blocking the Frontalis muscle action by firmly pressing above the brow. A second reading of the distance between the pupillary reflex and the upper lid margin is noted. The difference between the two readings gives the action of the LPS muscle. Graphics by Kritika Thakur

and the conjunctiva and is done on an everted lid. Several variations and modifications have been made, and the exact way it functions is unknown, except that it shortens the tarsal plate and conjunctiva. Most excised tissue does not have LPS or Muller's muscle fibres. Patients with mild-to-moderate ptosis and fair LPS action are subjected to LPS resection and advancement from the skin side (Eversbusch approach) or the conjunctival approach (Blaskovics); the procedures are nearly 150 and 100 years old, respectively. A careful preoperative work-up and knowledge of anatomy are mandatory to achieve optimum results. The patients should not have dry eye or lagophthalmos and have intact Bell's phenomenon and normal ocular movements. The amount of LPS resection generally depends on the ptosis and the LPS action. It may vary from 8 to 30 mm (https://www.aao.org/education/oculoplastics-center/external-transcutaneous-levator-advancement-resect). Postoperatively, the eyes need frequent lubricants and ensuring no exposure of the cornea. If the LPS action is less <4 mm and the ptosis is severe, LPS resection is not done, and instead, a frontalis sling operation is advised, which carries lid lag as a major cosmetic blemish [17]. It is also the procedure of choice for Marcus Gunn (jaw winking with ptosis), traumatic ptosis or third nerve palsy. Children below the age of 3–4 years are not operated on for correction of ptosis unless there is a fear of amblyopia.

19.3.1.3 Neurogenic Ptosis

Neurogenic ptosis results from defects of innervation of the LPSM. The most common cause of neurogenic ptosis is CN III paresis/palsy

(Fig. 19.5). Horner's syndrome from sympathetic denervation of the Muller's muscles caused interruption of the sympathetic fibres (Fig. 19.6), Jaw-winking due to misdirected fibres from CN V (the mandibular division of the trigeminal nerve) (Fig. 19.7) which supply the LPSM, misdirected fibres of the CN III following trauma, ophthalmoplegic migraine, and multiple sclerosis [18].

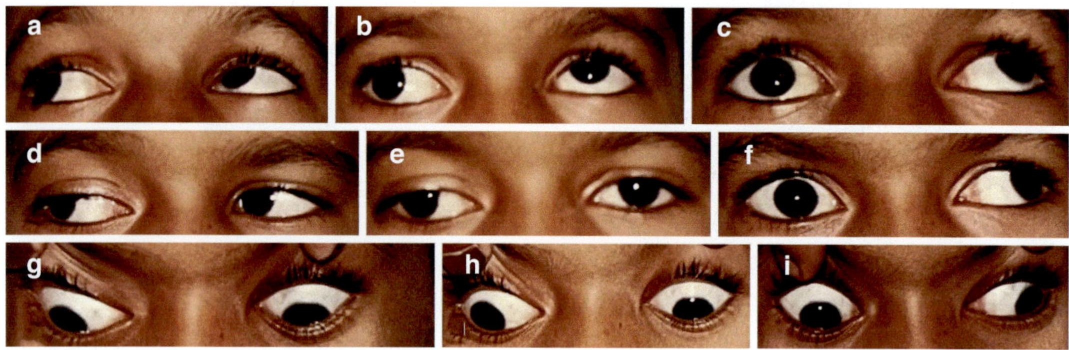

Fig. 19.5 The right eye shows neurogenic ptosis due to right congenital third nerve palsy (**e**). With left eye fixing, the right eye is divergent due to right medial rectus palsy (**e**) (primary deviation). When asked to look towards the left side, his right eye takes up fixation but fails to adduct (**f**). There is a significant increase in the divergent squint (**f**) (secondary deviation). In the right gaze, there is no squint (**d**). When asked to look up in different gazes, the right eye does not elevate in the abduction because of the superior rectus palsy (**a**, **b**) and in the left gaze also, it does not elevate because of the right inferior oblique palsy (**c**). The right eye shows limited downward movement due to right inferior rectus palsy (**g**, **h**, **i**). Images courtesy of Dr. Kanwar Mohan, Dr. Kanwar Mohan's Squint Centre, Chandigarh

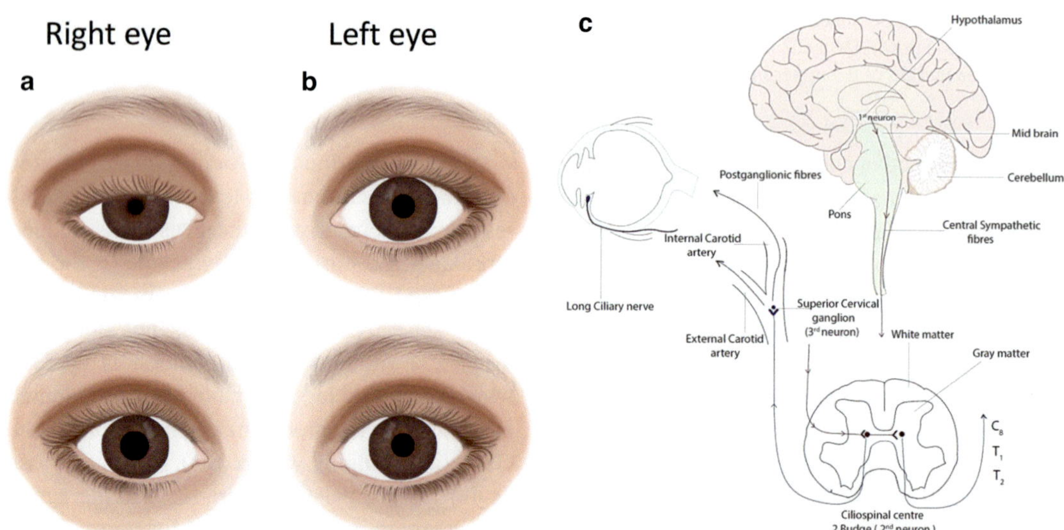

Fig. 19.6 Right eye Horner's syndrome**:** The right eye shows ptosis of both upper and lower lids. Note that in ptosis of the lower lid, the lower lid moves down. The pupil is miotic (right eye, **a**). The left eye is normal. The upper lid margin covers 0.5–1.5 mm of the upper limbus, while the lower lid just touches the limbus (left eye, **a**). Thirty minutes after the instillation of apraclonidine 0.5% eyedrops in both eyes, there is a remarkable improvement in ptosis of both lids in the right eye, and the pupil is dilated (right, **b**). This phenomenon is a sympathetic denervation hypersensitivity response seen in the right eye with Horner's syndrome. There is no change in the lids or the pupil in the left normal eye (left eye, **b**). The sympathetic pathway for ocular innervation is shown in Figure **c**. Graphics by Kritika Thakur

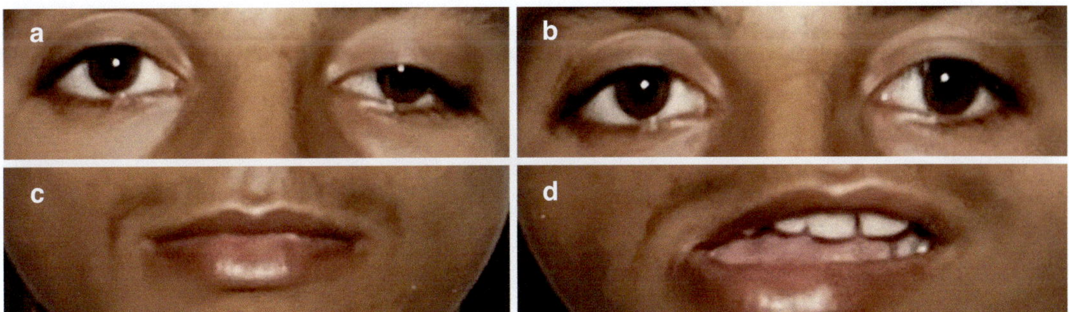

Fig. 19.7 Ptosis with Marcus-Gunn phenomenon: Left eye congenital ptosis (**a**) with mouth closed (**c**). Remarkable improvement in ptosis with the jaw movement (**b** and **d**). This is called the Marcus Gunn phenomenon. Images courtesy of Dr. Kanwar Mohan, Dr. Kanwar Mohan's Squint Centre, Chandigarh

19.3.1.4 Horner's Syndrome

The triad of Horner syndrome includes a small pupil, mild ptosis of the upper lid (<2 mm) and anhidrosis. Ptosis of the lower lid is caused by loss of the innervation of the retractors, and thus, the lower lid appears slightly elevated and is also called reverse ptosis. The apraclonidine (alpha 2-adrenergic agonist) test confirms the diagnosis of Horner's syndrome by demonstrating sympathetic denervation hypersensitivity. It may be negative in very early cases till degeneration of the nerves has set in. Within 30–40 min of the apraclonidine 0.5% eyedrop, there is dilatation of the affected pupil and elevation of the ptotic lid (Fig. 19.6).

Other ocular signs of Horner's syndrome include lower intraocular pressure in the ipsilateral eye. In the congenital Horner syndrome, the affected eyes have a lighter-coloured iris.

The central and preganglionic Horner syndrome produces significant anhidrosis of the face. The postganglionic Horner's syndrome does not cause anhidrosis as the sympathetic fibres meant for the sweat glands of the face leave the superior cervical ganglion along the branches of the external carotid artery https://eyewiki.aao.org/Horner_Syndrome.

The constellation of signs and the investigations to establish the cause depends on the level of injury and the cause of the Horner syndrome.

The most common cause of first neuron injury (central Horner's syndrome) is hemorrhagic stroke, demyelination, ischemia, syringomyelia (fluid-filled cysts in the spinal cord), arteriovenous malformations, meningitis, arachnoiditis, or cervical spinal injury.

The second neuronal Horner's syndrome results from interruption of preganglionic fibres due to lung cancer above the first rib (pancoast tumour, most of which are non-small cell adenocarcinomas and produce pain in the arm), cervical rib, supraclavicular nodes, aneurysm of the subclavian artery, injury to the brachial plexus or thoracic injury during surgical procedures.

The third neuronal postganglionic Horner's syndrome is caused by dissection of the internal carotid artery, skull-base fracture, herpes zoster, middle ear infections, migraine, cavernous sinus thrombosis, and temporal arteritis. Nearly, 1/3rd of the cases of Horner syndrome remain idiopathic.

The cause of Horner's syndrome may vary depending on where the patient first reports. Thus, most patients reporting first to Ophthalmology may be idiopathic, followed by surgical procedures and 3% due to undetected cancers [19]. A definitive cause was recognized in 61% of 159 apraclonidine-confirmed Horner syndrome cases. The most common cause was neck, chest, skull or paraspinal procedures, followed by cervical carotid dissection. In the pharmacologically unconfirmed cohort, tumours were next common to the procedures. In most cases, the cause of Horner's syndrome is known at presentation. If the cause is unknown prior to its diagnosis, a tumour or dissection of the aorta must be ruled out by appropriate imaging, CT angiography and CT chest [20].

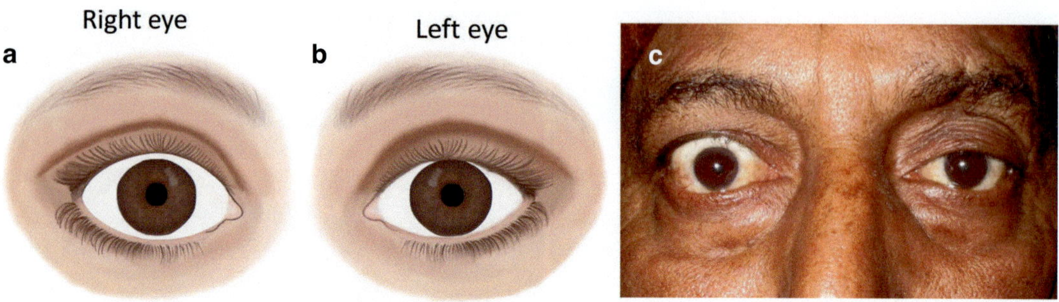

Fig. 19.8 *Lid retraction of the right upper lid*, Note the exposure of the sclera in the right eye due to lid retraction of both the upper and the lower eyelids (**a**). The left eye is normal (**b**). A euthyroid patient with unilateral thyroid eye disease shows lid retraction of the right upper lid. Image '**c**' courtesy of Dr. Manpreet Singh, Advanced Eye Centre, Post Graduate Institute of Medical Education and Research, Chandigarh. India. Graphics by Kritika Thakur

19.3.2 Lid Retraction of the Upper Eyelid

Retraction of the upper eyelid (UER) is the earliest sign of thyroid eye disease (TED), even when the patient has no symptoms (Fig. 19.8). In a review of community-based TED, nearly 90.8% of the 120 patients seen over 15 years had UER at diagnosis. In this cohort, 22% also had lower lid retraction (LER) [21]. The upper eyelid margin is retracted in the primary gaze, exposing the superior limbus giving a staring look [22]. Normally, the peak of the upper eyelid is slightly medial to the pupil, but in TED, the UER shows a temporal flare; the highest point of the upper lid margin peaks temporal to the pupil.

UER was believed to be a sign of sympathetic overactivity in Muller's tarsal muscle. Variable UER is likely due to increased adrenergic activity, especially in hyperthyroidism-associated TED. Usage of the topical adrenergic drug guanethidine led to the reversal of the UER [23]. Guanethidine is an antihypertensive drug available in several countries other than the USA.

In many cases, however, UER is seen only in one eye, defying explanation. In thyroid ophthalmopathy, the earliest inflammatory infiltration is seen in the inferior rectus muscle leading to a mechanical restriction of its action. Obeying Hering's law, UER may represent an overaction of the LPSM and the superior rectus (SR) [24].

UER possibly results from infiltration and expansion of the muscle volume in the LPSM/SR complex. In a 3D CT scan modelling of TED-associated UER without proptosis, an ipsilateral increase in the LPSM/SR volume was seen in 85% of the eyes. In the ULR eyes, without significant volume expansion in the LPSM/SR, a significant increase in the inferior rectus (IR) volume was seen in the contralateral eyes [25]. Persistent inflammation leads to increased fibrosis in these muscles, possibly leading to a permanent UER. Exophthalmos may itself lead to UER as the LA is put under stretch. However, not all patients show a reversal of UER following an orbital decompression of the proptosis [26].

In the natural course study of TED, without any intervention, 22.2% showed spontaneous resolution of the UER by 6 months, 37% by 1 year, and 49.4% by 2 years of follow-up. Improvement was seen in 70% in 1 year and 75% in 2 years [27].

In the lower lid, retraction (LER) leads to exposure of the lower sclera (scleral show) as the lid margin is pulled down. Some scleral show may be seen in normal, especially in older people and up to 2 mm of the scleral show may be taken as normal [28]. LER is a less frequent sign of TED and was seen only in 22% of the TED [21].

Both UER and LER may lead to lagophthalmos (inability to close the eyelids completely), conjunctival congestion, and irritation and carries a risk of exposure to keratitis.

UER may require full-thickness anterior blephratomy with mullerectomy in patients with lagophthalmos, exposure, dryness, congested eyes, or even aesthetic reasons [29]. Even a conjunctival approach may be followed for disinserting the attachment of the Muller muscles and the LA to the tarsal plate. The lateral canthal ligament is severed to control the lateral flare of the upper eyelid [30].

Non-surgical options include local injections of botulin toxin-A, hyaluronic acid, and triamcinolone acetonide into the supratarsal soft tissues [31].

19.3.2.1 Differential Diagnosis of Upper Lid Retraction

UER may occur due to neurogenic, myogenic, or mechanical causes. The commonest cause of neurogenic UER is seen in congenital or acquired unilateral or asymmetric bilateral ptosis, which causes pesudoretraction of the upper eyelid in the contralateral eye, respecting the Hering's law of equal innervation (Fig. 19.9). This phenomenon may be seen in 10–20% of the cases with ptosis [32]. If the ptotic eye happens to be the dominant eye, there is an urge to lift the eyelid, increasing motoneuronal inputs in the ptotic eye, which in the contralateral normal eye causes lid retraction. This retraction can be abolished by manually lifting the ptotic lid above the corneal limbus by the examiner, which should abolish the lid retraction [33, 34]. Covering the ptotic eye for 5 min can also abolish pesudoretraction [35]. Phenylephrine 2.5%, an adrenergic agonist in the ptotic eye, abolishes ptosis by acting on the Muller's muscle and is a widely used test. Simultaneously, it also abolishes the pseudo lid retraction.

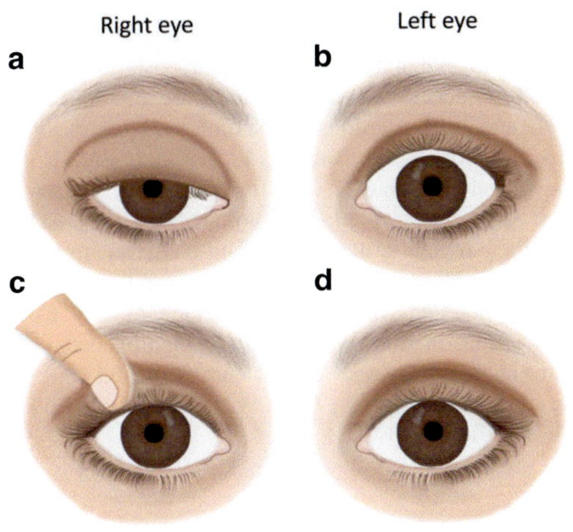

Fig. 19.9 Pesudoretraction of the left upper lid (**b**) due to ptosis of the right eye (**a**). Manually lifting the right upper eyelid (**c**) corrects the pseudo traction of the left upper lid (**d**). Graphics by Kritika Thakur

Other neurogenic causes of UER include ptosis in the contralateral eye due to Horner's syndrome, encephalitis, hydrocephalus, congenital ptosis with jaw winking (Marcus -Gunn), dehiscence of the LPS, facial nerve palsy, and aberrant regeneration in CNIII palsy [36]. Even ophthalmoplegic migraine may cause pesudoretraction of the contralateral eye [35].

Pathological lesions in the dorsal midbrain lead to symmetric bilateral UER, upward gaze palsy, convergence retraction nystagmus syndrome, and pseudo-Argyll-Robertson pupil [37–39]. The lid retraction worsens on up gaze and is minimized in downgaze. If there are associated neurological symptoms, like headache or ataxia, it calls for brain imaging to rule out a dorsal brain stem lesion.

Progressive supranuclear palsy (PSP), a rare degenerative disorder caused by midbrain atrophy, is characterized by vertical gaze palsy (downgaze first), upper lid retraction, blepharospasm and eye-opening and closing apraxia [40]. UER in these patients gives them a 'surprise' or 'staring' look and differentiates them from Parkinson's disease [8].

The most important cause of myogenic UER is TED, as discussed above. Uncommonly, MG may also cause UER, which is discussed later in the chapter.

A number of mechanical causes also may cause lid retraction, including orbital tumours, scleral buckling procedures, and inferior rectus recession [41]. For an exhaustive list of the differential diagnosis and classification of lid retraction, readers may refer to [36].

19.3.3 Lid Lag

Normally, the upper lid moves at the same velocity during upgaze as the eye movement because the vertical muscles and LPSM are linked in vertical movements. The premotor neuron for vertical movement is believed to be located in the rostral interstitial nucleus of the medial longitudinal fasciculus (riMLF) or just medial to it, the

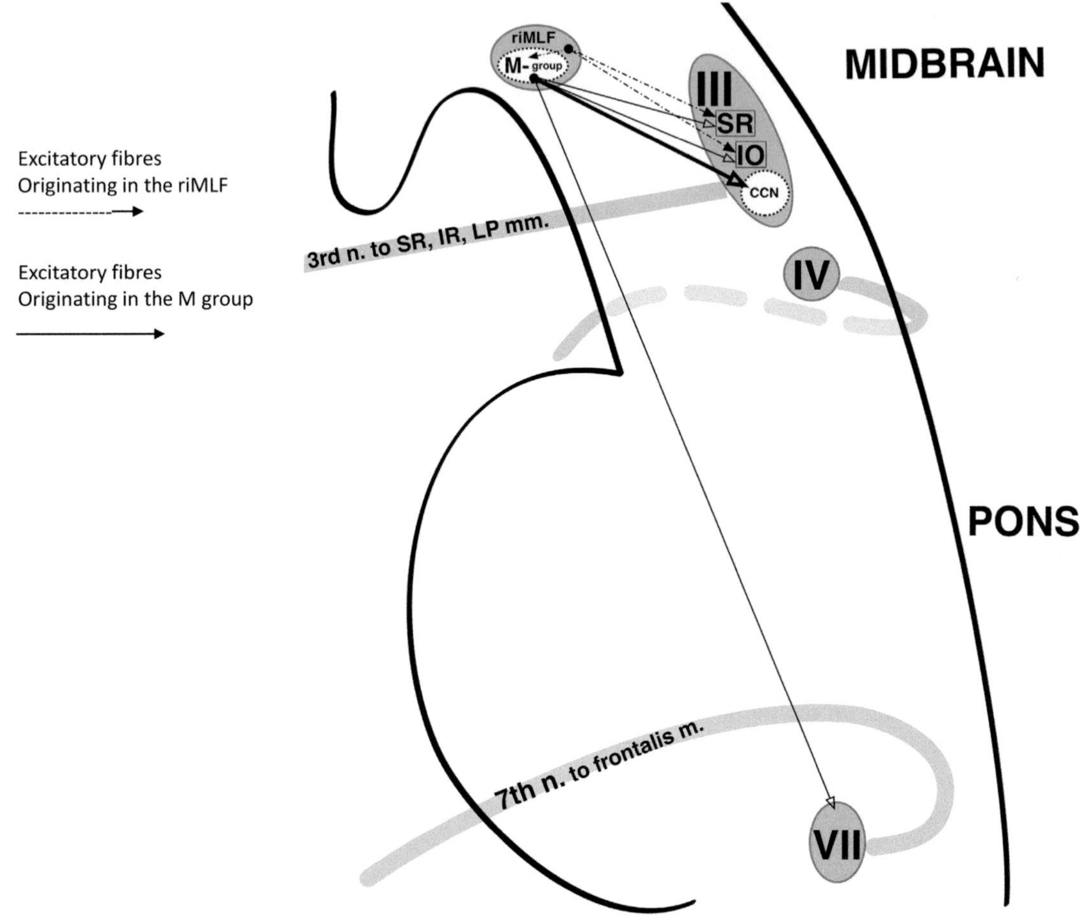

Fig. 19.10 *Supranuclear control of eyelid movement.* The midbrain's central caudal nucleus (CCN) contributes fibres to both oculomotor nerves and innervates both levator palpebrae superioris (LPS). During eye-opening, it maintains a tonic activity level that transiently increases with upward eye movements and decreases with downward eye movements. During a vertical saccade, the rostral interstitial nucleus of the medial longitudinal fasciculus (riMLF) is activated, and it provides excitatory input into the superior rectus (SR) and inferior oblique (IO) subnuclei of the oculomotor nerve to elevate the eyes. In addition, the riMLF activates the nearby M-group. The M-group provides a small amount of reinforcing excitation to the SR and IO subnuclei, but its primary excitatory output is to the CCN, increasing the firing rate, which produces eyelid elevation. The M-group also synapses on the facial nucleus, presumably to assist the frontalis in eyelid elevation when needed. The opposite occurs during a downgaze. Eyelid retraction in midbrain dysfunction occurs due to M-group overstimulation (in an attempt to overcome an upgaze palsy) or under inhibition (from injury to the nearby interstitial nucleus of Cajal and the nucleus of the posterior commissure. Reproduced with permission of the authors Drs Ali G. Hamedani (Department of Neurology, Hospital of the University of Pennsylvania, Philadelphia, PA, United States.) and Dr. Daniel R. Gold (Department of Neurology, Johns Hopkins Hospital, Baltimore, MD, United States) from their review article, Hamedani AG (Department of Neurology, Hospital of the University of Pennsylvania, Philadelphia, PA, United States.) and Dr. Gold DR. Eyelid Dysfunction in Neurodegenerative, Neurogenetic, and Neurometabolic Disease. Front Neurol. 2017 Jul 18;8:329. doi: 10.3389/fneur.2017.00329. PMID: 28769865; PMCID: PMC5513921

M group and interstitial nucleus of Cajal (inC), which excitatory sends signals to the motor neuron nucleus located in the central caudal nucleus which innervates the bilateral oculomotor nuclei. The M group also sends excitatory signals to the facial nerve nucleus, which supplies the frontalis muscle. Thus, the frontalis also provides a helping hand in elevating the upper lid during the elevation of the eyes [8] (Fig. 19.10). During the downward saccades, the inhibitory signals from

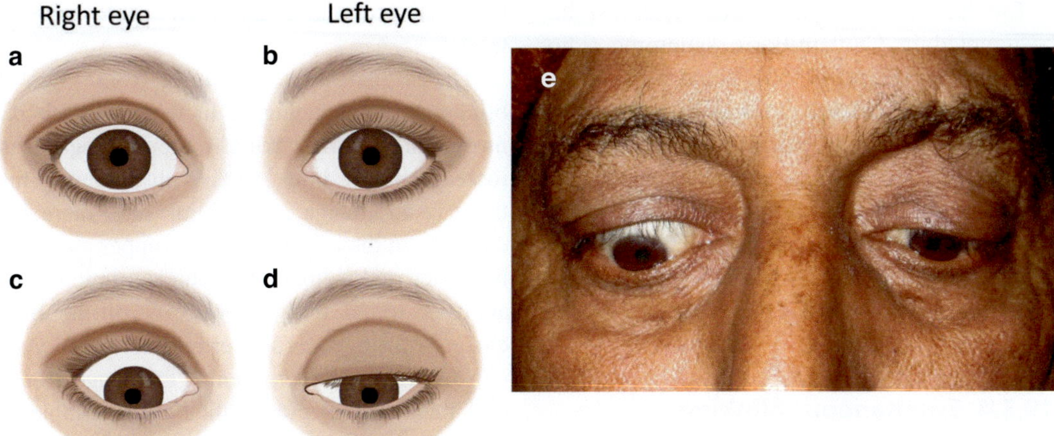

Fig. 19.11 *Lid lag*. In the Schematic representation, the right upper lid shows lid retraction in the primary gaze (**a**). The left eye is normal (**b**). On asking the patient to look down, the right upper lid does not follow the movement of the eyeball exposing the white sclera (**c**). The left upper lid moves down normally (**d**). A euthyroid patient with unilateral thyroid eye disease showing lid lag in the right eye. Note the normal downward movement of the left upper lid as the patient looks down (**e**). Image '**e**' courtesy of Dr. Manpreet Singh, Advanced Eye Centre, Post Graduate Institute of Medical Education and Research, Chandigarh. India. Graphics by Kritika Thakur

the premotor neurons (nuclei of the posterior commissure) lead to the relaxation of the LPSM and the superior rectus [42]. In UER, the LPS fails to keep pace with the downward movement of the eye, resulting in the upper lid margin maintaining a position higher than it should be. It results in the scleral show at the superior limbus. This phenomenon is termed lid lag (Fig. 19.11). Lid lag is an important sign of TED. Of the 105 patients with Graves' ophthalmopathy for which information was available, 35% had bilateral and 14% unilateral lid lag [21]. Notably, nearly 10% of normal people and, more commonly, those above 40 may have some degree of lid lag [43].

Lid lag needs to be differentiated from the von Graefe sign, which is also a sign of TED and is tested by asking the patient to look at a target brought down from the up gaze to the downgaze. A transient pause in the lid's downward movement is termed a positive von Graefe sign. von Graefe's sign is dynamic compared to the lid lag, which is a static, fixed position of the upper eyelid in downgaze. Lagophthalmos is an inability to close the eyes completely [44]. In a series of Graves' ophthalmopathy, lid lag was noted only in 8% of the patients, lagophthalmos in 16% and none in normal people. von Graefe's sign was more specific and noted in 36% of Graves' ophthalmopathy vs none in the normal [45].

19.3.3.1 Differential Diagnosis of Lid Lag

The association of acute onset ptosis, poor LPS action, and lid lag may be due to isolated LPS myositis. Such patients need orbital imaging to diagnose and respond well to oral corticosteroids [46].

In isolated bilateral lid retraction without signs and symptoms of TED, laboratory investigations are mandated to rule out TED. At the same time, dorsal midbrain lesions may cause these isolated UERs and call for brain imaging. The associated signs include vertical gaze limitation, slow pupil reactions, convergence retraction, nystagmus, and lid retraction [47]. Lid lag with lid retraction may occur in isolation without upgaze restriction in dorsal brain stem lesions [37, 38]. Pathology in the periaqueductal grey area suggests a premotor eyelid control centre in the nucleus of the posterior commissure [37, 38].

Isolated lid lag without lid retraction also calls for brain imaging. Lid retraction and lid lag dissociation may occur in pretectal pathology [48].

Lid lag accompanying facial weakness has been noted in Guillain-Barre syndrome (idiopathic polyneuritis) [49, 50]. Since the lid lag is seen on attempted lid closure, it may have a peripheral rather than central origin [50].

Isolated lid lag with spontaneous recovery in a few months has been reported in multiple sclerosis [51]. Isolated transient lid lag after forced looking in up gaze has been noted in ocular myasthenia gravis (OMG) [52].

19.3.4 Spontaneous Blinking

The LPSM is used for elevating the eyelids and the orbicularis oculi (OO) to close the lids. These two muscles act reciprocally. The normal motor tone in the LPSM keeps the eyes open. The LPSM tone is maintained by constant neural firing from the nucleus of the posterior commissure (nPC). During the blink, the firing from the nPC is interrupted, so the LPSM tone is lost. At the same time, there is firing from the nucleus of the facial nerve cells that subserve the palpebral oculi muscle contracting the palpebral part of the orbicularis and closing the eyelids. Within a very short span, firing in the OO stops, the nCP starts neural firing again, the LPSM regains its tone, and the eyes are opened. Simultaneously, the facial nucleus stops firing, and the eyes open again under the influence of the regained tone in the LPSM (Fig. 19.12).

The blink reflex is controlled by the superior colliculus, which is under the inhibitory control of the substantia nigra and is mediated through dopamine.

The decreased dopamine levels decrease the rates of spontaneous blinking, and increased levels increase the blinking rate [53].

The afferent inputs into the superior colliculus come from the trigeminal (cornea) and pretectal nuclei (visual). The corneal epithelium is the most densely innervated in the entire body and plays a major role in the blink rates. In dry eye disorder or irritant exposure, the blinking rate increases to maintain the normal tear film breakup time. With each upstroke of the upper lid, the meibomian secretions are spread over the tear film that prevents evaporation of the aqueous tears.

The normal blink rate varies from 15 to 20 blinks per minute, higher in women. With jaw movements, while talking, there is a significant increase in the blink rate. With ageing, while there is no change in the blink rate, there is a decrease in the excursion of the upper eyelids in both men and women. An optoelectronic motion analyser found that the velocity of the blink closure-opening was slower in older people, and closure was faster than opening for all age groups. Old men seldom closed their eyes completely [54].

In Parkinson's disease (PD), on the other hand, there is an increase in the activity of the substantia nigra, increasing the inhibitory control of the superior colliculus and leading to decreased blinking rate in these patients. If the spontaneous blink reflex decreases, the reflex blink increases [8]. In a systematic review and meta-analysis, nearly 61% of the patients with PD had lower blink rates, complained of dry eye symptoms, decreased aqueous secretion, showed a shorter tear film breakup time, and thinner cornea [55]. Tapping on the glabella (Glabellar reflex or reflex blinking) to elicit reflex blinking, although commonly used as a quick sign to diagnose PD, is an inconsistent test and cannot differentiate between PD and essential tremors [56]. The blink amplitude decreased when a high-speed blink reflex analysis system was used to test spontaneous blinking in PD. The pause between the closing and opening of eyelids increased in PD patients [57].

The blinking rate decreases in patients with PSP. When asked to blink as fast as possible, closing and opening were slower in patients with PSP than in normal persons. There was also a significant increase in the pause in spontaneous, voluntary, and reflex blinking than in normal persons indicating a widespread degeneration of the cortical, subcortical, and brain stem in PSP [58].

19.3.4.1 Apraxia of Eyelid Opening

First described in four patients by Goldstein and Cogan [59], apraxia of eyelid opening (AEO) is characterized by prolonged involun-

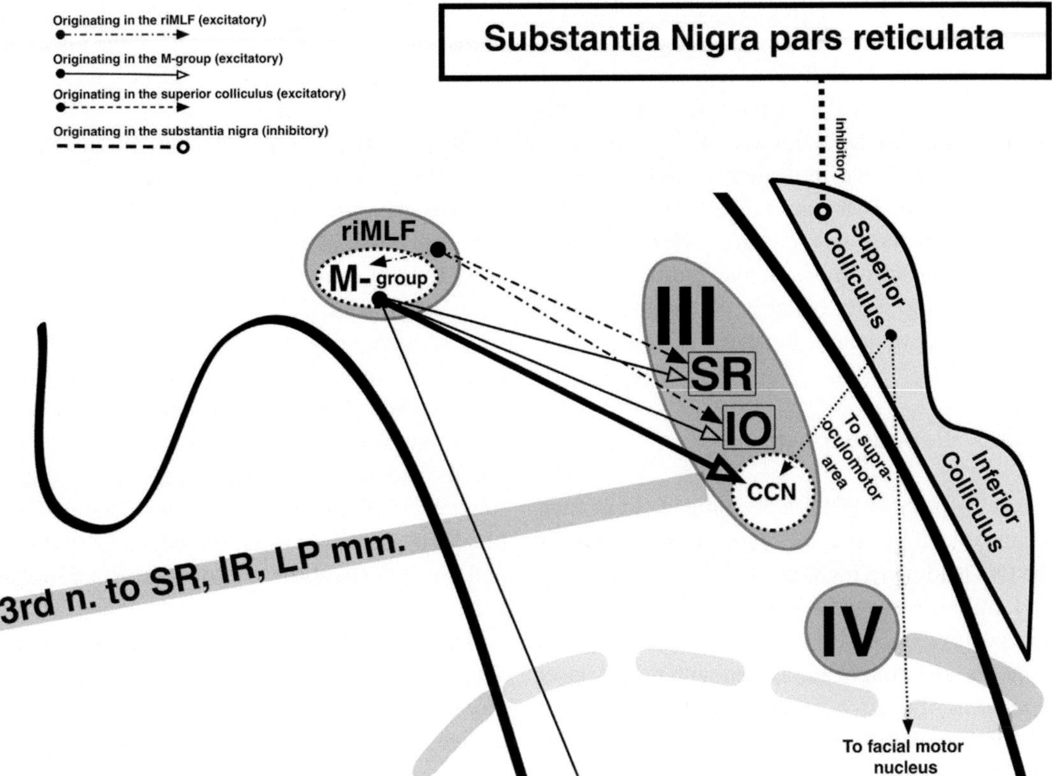

Fig. 19.12 During a blink, the LPSM stops firing and the orbicularis oculi (OO), innervated by the facial nerve, briefly contracts. This coordination of LPS and OO activity is thought to be mediated by the superior colliculus (SC). The SC projects to the supra oculomotor area directly overlying the CCN and to the facial nuclei and is inhibited by the pars reticulata of the substantia nigra (SNr). In Parkinsonism, increased SNr activity results in greater SC inhibition and reduced spontaneous blinking. Not shown are afferents from the trigeminal nucleus and pretectum to the SC, which mediate reflexive blinking to corneal stimulation and bright light, respectively. Reproduced with permission of the authors Drs Ali G. Hamedani (Department of Neurology, Hospital of the University of Pennsylvania, Philadelphia, PA, United States.) and Dr. Daniel R. Gold (Department of Neurology, Johns Hopkins Hospital, Baltimore, MD, United States) from their review article. Hamedani AG (Department of Neurology, Hospital of the University of Pennsylvania, Philadelphia, PA, United States.) and Dr. Gold DR. Eyelid Dysfunction in Neurodegenerative, Neurogenetic, and Neurometabolic Disease. Front Neurol. 2017 Jul 18;8:329. doi: 10.3389/fneur.2017.00329. PMID: 28769865; PMCID: PMC5513921

tary inhibition of the LPSM motor tone without concomitant contraction of the orbicularis oculi muscle. They first suggested that it was due to a supranuclear deficit and included one patient with Huntington's chorea and three suspected of PD.

On command to open eyes, the patient has difficulty initiating lid opening despite showing a strong frontalis muscle contraction. Once the eyes get opened, there is no ptosis. This is unlike in paralytic ptosis, where the patient cannot lift the upper eyelid. It can be differentiated from blepharospasm by lack of demonstrable orbicularis activity, even on electromyography. Any oculomotor or myogenic lesions are to be excluded [60]. AEO (Blepharocolysis, derived from Greek, blepharon meaning lid and analysis, meaning inhibition) can be isolated or seen in post-encephalitic PD, PD, or PSP [60].

In patients with stroke, AEO is seen exclusively in the right hemisphere infarction, suggesting that the right cerebral hemisphere controls the supranuclear eyelid movements. AEO indicates poor outcomes in such patients [61].

Functional MRI studies in healthy volunteers revealed activation of the (oculomotor fields), i.e., frontal eye field (FEF), supplementary eye field (SEF), and posterior parietal cortex (PPC) during winking (unilateral eye closure) and also during saccadic eye movements; however, only the FEF and SEF were activated during voluntary blinking (bilateral eye closure). FEF and SEF were significantly more active during winking than blinking [62]. Notably, winking did not cause any movement of the eyes.

19.3.5 Blepharospasm

Blepharospasm (BSP) is a dystonia in old women characterized by bilateral synchronous spasms of the OO leading to involuntary lid closure. It may be familial or sporadic dystonia. Family history was positive in 20% of the patients [63].

BSPs are strongly associated with recent onset symptoms of dry eye disorders, which may play a significant role in its pathogenesis [64]. Coffee drinking is protective in preventing the onset of BSP [65]. These risk factors were seen irrespective of the sporadic or familial cases, indicating that the two may share a common aetiology [65]. Increased exposure to sunlight may also be a risk factor [66].

In BSP, there is difficulty in opening the eyelids, and durations of the spasms may be very brief or longer. It is also associated with an increased blinking rate which may precede the onset of BSP. The BSP is often associated with a dry eye disorder, depression, or sleep disorder [67]. The BSP may be isolated in 50% of the patients associated with other focal dystonias involving facial and chewing muscles (Meige syndrome) in 31% [68, 69]. However, 50% of BSP patients showed the dystonia spread to neighbouring muscles, most commonly to the oromandibular muscles (masticatory muscles) and the neck muscles [70]. A positive family history of dystonia and head trauma are risk factors [70, 71]. BSP is believed to be a consequence of basal ganglia's malfunctioning neuronal circuit [67].

Patients use one or more sensory tricks to remission BSP, including pulling at the upper lid, walking, talking, and blowing cheeks, which may be seen in nearly 87% of the BSP [69]. Deep brain stimulation of the globus pallidus interna (one of the basal ganglia that control unwanted) movement) is emerging as a promising therapy in patients who do not respond to conventional therapy [71].

A subtype of BSP, pretarsal blepharospasm, may be seen, which responds best to pretarsal botulin toxin-A injections. Pretarsal blepharospasm results from the absence of reciprocal inhibition of LPSM and co-contraction of LPSM and the pretarsal OO. There is also an increased frequency of blinking in these patients. The blepharospasms are mild to moderate and do not pull down the eyebrows below the orbital margin [72].

There is a small chance of spontaneous remission of BSP within 5 years of the onset of the disease [73]. Using FL-41 rose-tinted glasses to reduce photophobia has significantly reduced the blinking rate and the BSP attacks. The pretarsal injections of botulin toxin-A in both lids may provide relief for 3–4 months [74]. More recently, topical application of glue to the eyelids, Frankincense from the Boswellia tree, led to the relief of BSP in two elderly patients with a significant reduction in the frequency of botulin toxin-A injections [75].

19.4 Extraocular Muscles-Anatomical Considerations

Six muscles extraocular muscles, including four recti and two obliques, move the eyeball. As the name suggests, the four recti are straight muscles from the origin to the insertion in the sclera. They arise from a collagenous ring, the annulus of Zinn, which encloses the optic foramen and the medial part of the superior orbital fissure. The recti are inserted at a variable distance from the limbus, and the imaginary line connecting the insertion is called the spiral of Tillaux. The respective median distances of the insertions from the corneal limbus are the medial rectus (MR) 5.5 mm, the inferior rectus (IR) 6.5 mm, the lateral rectus (LR) 6.9 mm, and the superior rectus (SR) 7.7 mm. The muscle belly of the MR is 37.6 + 4.6 mm, and the width at insertion is 10 ± 1.8 mm. The function of the MR muscle is to rotate the eye inwards or adduct around a vertical axis. The MR is supplied by the inferior branch of the CN III from its inner surface [76]. The nerve enters the muscle belly approximately 24 ± 2 mm from the insertion, divides into two branches, and then breaks into the plexus. The LR muscle abducts or rotates the eye outwards around a vertical axis. The CN VI (Abducens) innervates LR [77] (Fig. 19.13).

The superior and inferior recti are the elevator and depressor of the globe around a horizontal axis. The length of the SR is 41.8 mm, and the width is 10.6 mm at its insertion. The SR is aligned 23° from the visual axis. Therefore, when the globe is abducted, the main action of SR is the elevation of the eye (supraduction). In the primary gaze, besides elevation, it also adducts the globe (secondary action) and intorts (incycloduction around the Z axis) the globe (tertiary action). In the adducted position, it is a pure intortor. It gets its nerve supply from the superior division of the CN III, which also supplies the LPS muscle [78]. The IR muscle length is 40 mm, and its width at its insertion is 9.8 mm. The IR is aligned 23° from the visual axis. In the primary gaze, the primary action of IR is depression, in addition to adduction (secondary action) and extorter (excycloduction around a Z axis) of the globe (tertiary action). In the abducted position, its primary action is depression (infraduction) of the globe [79].

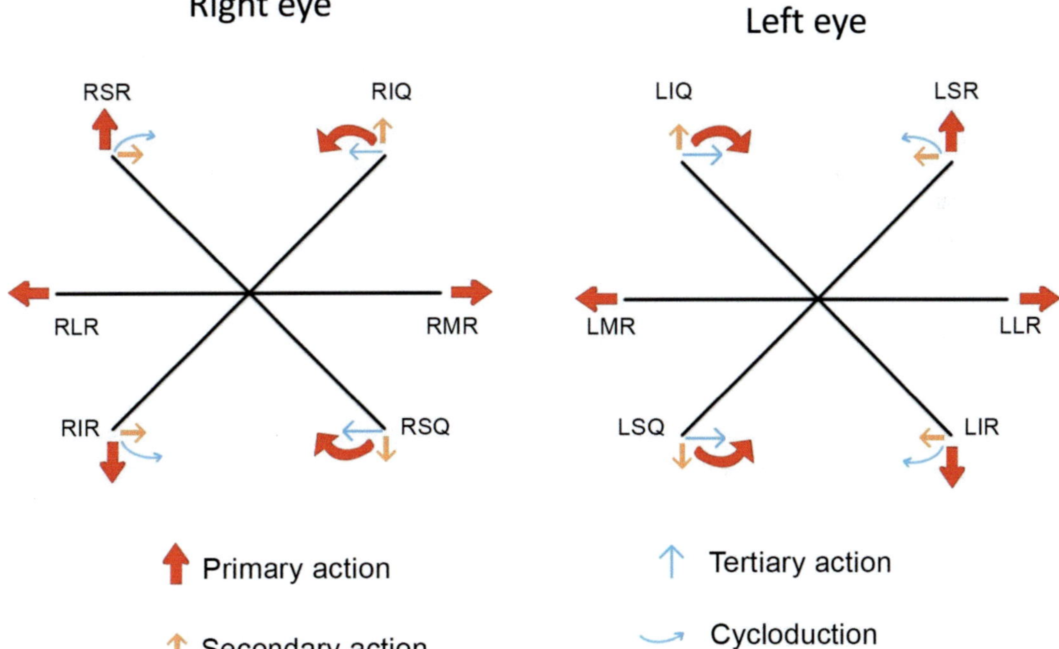

Fig. 19.13 A schematic to show the primary, secondary and tertiary actions. The thick red arrows show the primary action of extraocular muscles. Note the curved thick red arrows to show the primary action of the oblique muscles. The orange arrows show the secondary action of muscles, and the blue arrows show the tertiary action. *RSR* right superior rectus; *RLR* right lateral rectus; *RIR* right inferior rectus; *RIO* right inferior oblique; *RMR* right medial rectus; *RSQ* right superior oblique. Similar abbreviations are used for the left eye, *LSR* left superior rectus. Graphics by Kritika Thakur

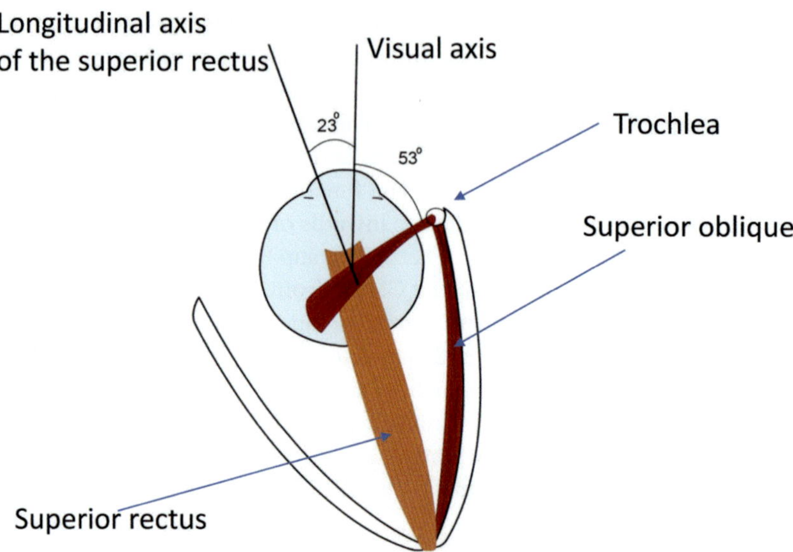

Fig. 19.14 Highly schematic diagram to show the angle formed by the superior rectus's longitudinal axis and the superior oblique's functional tendon with the visual axis. Graphics by Kritika Thakur

Compared to the other skeletal muscles of the body, the extraocular muscles have the richest nerve supply and is 1:3–1:5 per muscle fibre [80].

The superior oblique (SO) arises from the orbital surface of the lesser wing of the sphenoid medial to the optic foramen and courses forward along the medial wall of the orbit till the Trochlear pully located on the orbital plate of the frontal bone within the orbital rim. The SO becomes tendinous before the Trochlea and changes its course to move in the posterior and lateral directions. It crosses under the superior rectus and is inserted postero-lateral to the SR muscle insertion. It makes an angle of 53° with the visual axis. When the SO contracts, the Trochlea acts as the functional origin of the SO. The SO's tendon can slide easily through the Trochlea (Fig. 19.14). In the primary gaze, it is the intortor of the eye, depressor of the globe (secondary action), and abducts (tertiary action). When the eye is abducted, its main action is intorsion. In the adducted position, its main action is depression. This is the only muscle supplied by the CN IV, which emerges from the dorsal aspect of the midbrain.

The inferior oblique (IO) arises anteriorly from the orbital surface of the maxillary bone. It runs laterally and posteriorly, making an angle of 53° with the visual axis and courses below the inferior rectus to insert in the posterior lateral part of the globe. The inferior division of the CN III innervates it. In the primary position of the eye, IO is an extortor of the eye, besides elevation (secondary action) and abduction (tertiary action). When the eye is adducted, IO is an elevator of the eye. In the abducted position of the globe, its main action is extorsion.

19.5 Cranial Nerve Palsies

19.5.1 Oculomotor Nerve Paresis

The CN III emerges from the ventral aspect of the midbrain. As it courses forward in the interpeduncular fossa, it lies below the posterior cerebral artery and above the superior cerebellar artery. At this location, it is vulnerable to compression by a posterior communicating artery (PCA) aneurysm. As it proceeds to enter the cavernous sinus, it lies on the edge of the tentorium cerebelli. It becomes vulnerable to brain herniation in an acute rise in ICP due to subarachnoid haemorrhage. It pierces the dura mater to lie in the upper part of the lateral wall of the cavernous sinus, where it is vulnerable to compression by internal carotid artery aneurysms, the carotid-cavernous fistula and tumours.

The CN III divides into a superior and an inferior branch as it enters the orbit through the superior orbital fissure within the annulus of Zinn. All four recti, namely, the superior, lateral, inferior, and medial, originate from this tendinous ring at the orbital apex and span the orbital fissure. The superior branch innervates the superior rectus and LPSM and carries the sympathetic fibres destined for Muller's muscle. The inferior branch of the oculomotor nerve (CN III) innervates the inferior rectus, inferior oblique, and medial rectus through its inferior branches. Also, it carries preganglionic parasympathetic fibres to the ciliary ganglion, which innervates the sphincter pupillae and the ciliary muscles.

As it enters the orbit at its crowded apex, CN III branches are closely related to other important structures, such as the optic nerve, ophthalmic artery, and other cranial nerves (Figs. 19.15 and 19.16).

Thus, any pathology be the compression by aneurysms, tumours, metastatic lesions or inflammatory pathology along the entire route in the peduncular fossa, cavernous sinus or superior orbital fissure/anterior cavernous sinus, makes the CN III or its branches vulnerable. All these pathologies manifest as CN III paresis/palsy, which manifests as Ptosis accompanied by paresis of the muscles innervated by it. Sudden onset of painful diplopia, dilated, a non-reacting pupil with Ptosis needs urgent lesion localization, and brain imaging is mandated. However, in patients who present with painless ophthalmoplegia and Ptosis with pupil sparing, it is likely due to a compromized nutrient supply of the nerve. This is usually seen in patients who have cardiovascular risk factors such as diabetes, hypertension, atherosclerosis, and a history of smoking.

19.5.2 Recurrent Painful Ophthalmoplegic Neuropathy (Previously Labelled) Ophthalmoplegic Migraine)

Ophthalmoplegic migraine (OM) is a rare recurrent disorder seen in children. It is no longer classified as a migraine [81]. It is characterized by ipsilateral headache with ophthalmoplegia and usually presents with acute onset ptosis due to CN III paresis, the most common association of OM. The attack may last for a variable period lasting several hours, days, or weeks. Eventually, the muscle paresis improves spontaneously, but in rare cases, it may be permanent. Uncommonly, CN VI and rarely CN IV may also get involved. In patients with acute presentation, isolated contrast enhancement of the intracisternal segment of the CN III has been seen without any associated enhancement of the cavernous sinus or the adjacent structures. The enhancement was

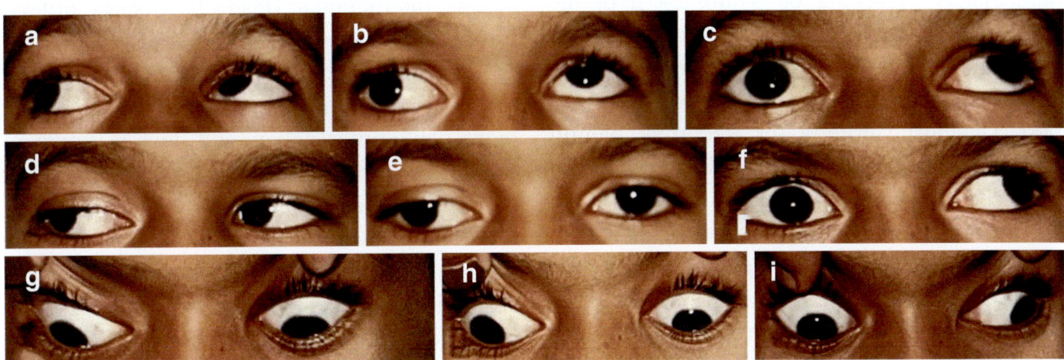

Fig. 19.15 *Right congenital third nerve palsy*. The right eye shows ptosis (**e**). With left eye fixing, the right eye is divergent due to right medial rectus palsy (**e**) (primary deviation). When asked to look towards the left side, his right eye takes up fixation but fails to adduct. There is a significant increase in the divergent squint (**f**) (secondary deviation). In the right gaze, there is no squint (**d**). When asked to look up in different gazes, the right eye does not elevate in the abduction because of the superior rectus palsy (**a**, **b**). The right eye does not elevate in the left gaze because of the right inferior oblique palsy (**c**). The right eye shows limited downward movement due to right inferior rectus palsy (**g**–**i**). Images courtesy of Dr. Kanwar Mohan, Dr. Kanwar Mohan's Squint Centre, Chandigarh

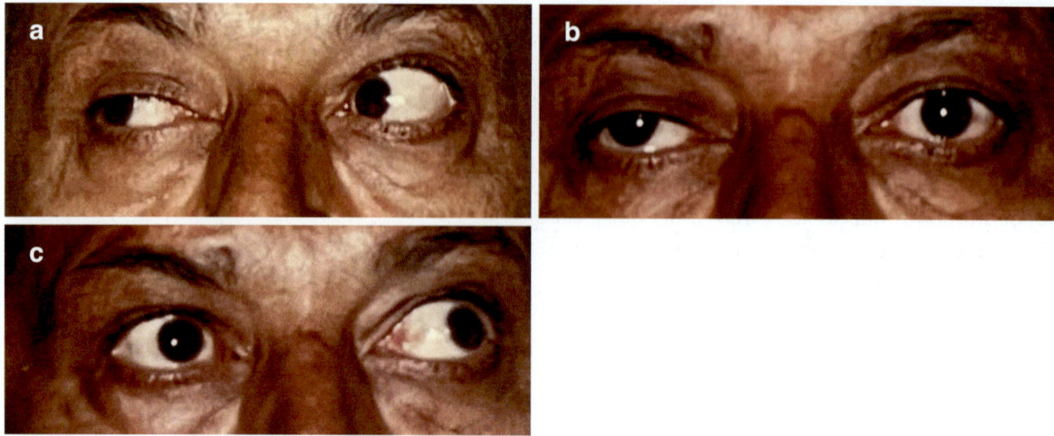

Fig. 19.16 Aberrant regeneration of third nerve following traumatic right third nerve palsy. Note ptosis and divergent squint in the primary position (**b**). In the right gaze, there is no squint, but the ptosis is still present (**a**). When the patient is asked to look to the left, the right upper lid is elevated due to aberrant regeneration (synkinesis) The right eye shows a recovery of adduction (**c**). Images courtesy of Dr. Kanwar Mohan, Dr. Kanwar Mohan's Squint Centre, Chandigarh

resolved in all patients within 7–9 weeks of the onset [82]. In recurrent OM, enhancement of the CN III may be seen only after several attacks [83].

In a study of 62 adult patients with OM observed over 10 years, more than 75% had a single attack of OM, and the others suffered two or more attacks. The most common CN involved was CN VI (56.5%), followed by CN III (33.9%), and the least common was CN IV (8.1%). Most patients had shown worsening migraine attacks immediately preceding or within 24 h of the onset of ophthalmoplegia. Interestingly none of these patients showed enhancement of the cranial nerves and responded well to corticosteroids [84]. Diagnostic criteria for Recurrent painful ophthalmoplegic Neuropathy by the International headache society include.

Unilateral headache (at least two attacks with an interval) accompanied by paresis of one, two or all of the oculomotor nerves, excluding any orbital or intracranial inflammation or mass lesion. Notably, headache may precede the onset of paresis by even 2 weeks. Gadolinium enhancement or nerve thickening can be demonstrated on MRI. Corticosteroid treatment leads to resolution [81].

19.5.3 Tolosa-Hunt Syndrome

The Tolosa-Hunt syndrome is a painful granulomatous inflammation of the soft tissues at the superior orbital fissure or the anterior cavernous sinus and may present as ptosis. It causes typical eyebrow or eye pain in the ipsilateral eye, which may precede the onset of paresis of either one or multiple oculomotor nerves. The granulomatous inflammation is demonstrable by either histopathology or MRI imaging (Fig. 19.17).

The International Headache Society criteria for the Tolosa-Hunt syndrome (THS) include (1) one or more episodes of orbital pain lasting for several weeks if untreated; (2) paresis of one or more oculomotor nerves and demonstration of orbital granulomatous pathology on MRI or biopsy; (3) paresis coincides with pain or follows it within 2 weeks; (4) pain and paresis are resolved within 3 days of starting adequate corticosteroid therapy; and (5) other pathologies have been excluded [81, 85]. The MRI may not always reveal the orbital/anterior cavernous sinus pathology in one-third of patients. Sympathetic involvement of the pupil may be occasionally seen. On the other hand, MRI may reveal other intracranial nerve pathologies, including systemic vasculitis,

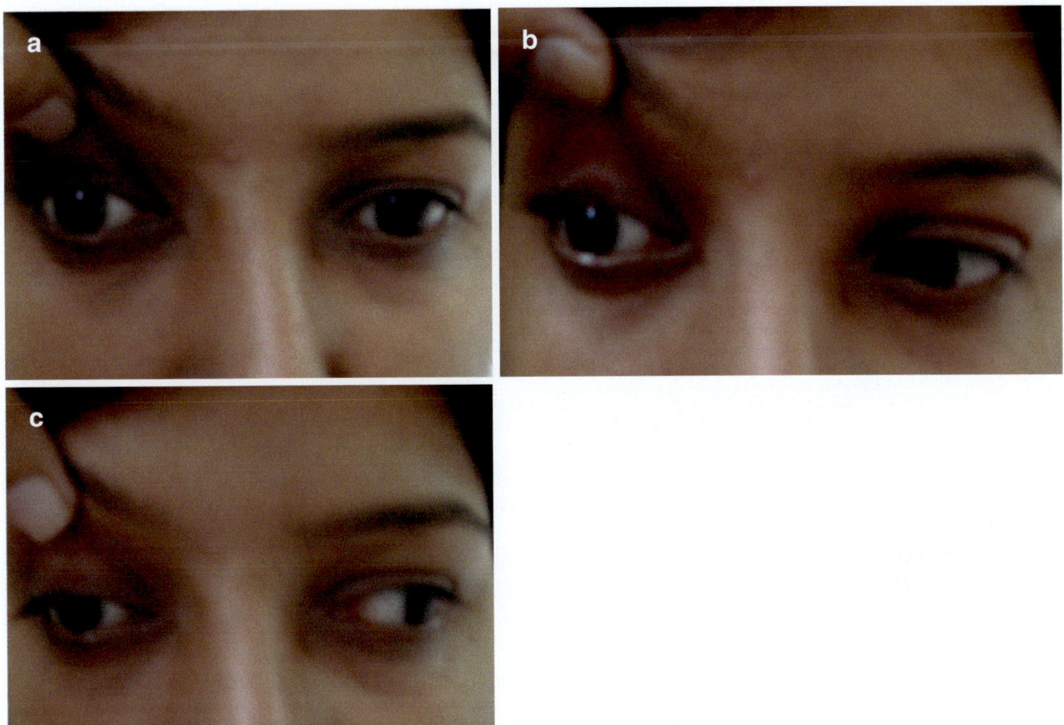

Fig. 19.17 *Tolosa-Hunt syndrome*: A 32-year-old woman presented with severe headache X 3–months; painful diplopia X 3 weeks, and complete ptosis right eye for 2 days. In the primary gaze, there is a right divergent squint (**b**), no squint in the right gaze (**a**, **b**) but no adduction of the right eye in the left gaze (**c**). The right upper lid was manually lifted to show the right eye's movement limitation. The right eye pupil was dilated and fixed. The right superior oblique was also paralysed. She responded to oral corticosteroids

sarcoidosis, basal meningitis, or tumours [81]. Clinically, the THS may be subdivided into benign, inflammatory, and symptomatic. Other cranial nerves, such as CN V, may be affected in 25–34% of cases, and 8–17% may have even optic nerve involvement [85]. Most patients recover on corticosteroid therapy but may show recurrence on stopping treatment.

19.5.4 Generalized Myasthenia Gravis

Generalized myasthenia gravis (gMG) is an autoimmune neuromuscular junction disorder characterized by the formation of autoantibodies to the Ach Receptor (AchR), which causes depletion of the AchR on the postsynaptic endplate of the muscle fibres. Patients present with symptoms suggestive of fatigue, which recover on resting. The three main affected organs include ocular, oropharyngeal, and generalized skeletal muscle. The ocular myasthenia gravis is class I in the Myasthenia Gravis Foundation of America classification [86]. However, ocular muscle weakness may also occur in all severity classes of gMG. The readers are encouraged to learn how to categorise various severity scores in patients with gMG [86] (Box 19.1).

Box 19.1 Myasthenia Gravis Foundation of America Clinical Classification

Class		Description
Class 1	Any ocular muscle weakness May have weakness of eye closure All other muscles strength is normal	
Class II	Mild weakness affecting other than ocular muscles May also have ocular muscle weakness of any severity	
	Class II a	Predominantly affecting limb, axial muscles, or both May also have lesser involvement of oropharyngeal muscles
	Class II b	Predominantly affecting oropharyngeal, respiratory muscles, or both May also have lesser or equal involvement of limb, axial muscles, or both
Class III	Moderate weakness affecting other than ocular muscles May also have ocular muscle weakness of any severity	
	Class III a	Predominantly affecting limb, axial muscles, or both May also have lesser involvement of oropharyngeal muscles
	Class III b	Predominantly affecting oropharyngeal, respiratory muscles, or both May also have lesser or equal involvement of limb, axial muscles, or both
Class IV	Severe weakness affecting other than ocular muscles May also have ocular muscle weakness of any severity	
	Class IV a	Predominantly affecting limb and/or axial muscles, May also have lesser involvement of oropharyngeal muscles
	Class IV b	Predominantly affecting oropharyngeal, respiratory muscles, or both May also have lesser or equal involvement of limb, axial muscles, or both
Class V	Defined by intubation, with or without mechanical ventilation, except when employed during routine postoperative management. The use of a feeding tube without intubation places the patient in class IV b	

Reproduced with permission of the publishers from Jaretzki A 3rd, Barohn RJ, Ernstoff RM, Kaminski HJ, Keesey JC, Penn AS, Sanders DB. Myasthenia gravis: recommendations for clinical research standards. Task Force of the Medical Scientific Advisory Board of the Myasthenia Gravis Foundation of America. Ann Thorac Surg. 2000 Jul;70(1):327-34. doi: 10.1016/s0003-4975(00)01595-2. PMID: 10921745.

However, 50% of patients with ocular myasthenia gravis (OMG) and 85% of the systemic MG show the presence of these antibodies to the AchR. The remaining 15% may show autoantibodies to membrane-bound muscle-specific tyrosine kinase (MuSK) or low-density lipoprotein receptor-related protein 4(LRRP-4) and agrin.

Acetylcholine (Ach) is in tiny vesicles in the motor neural endplate. The spontaneous release of a single packet containing Ach activates a voltage-gated calcium channel and a sudden release of Ach from the motor neural endplate at the neuromuscular junction. In a normal person, the Ach is received by the Ach receptor on the muscle fibres' motor endplate, and the excessive Ach is eliminated by acetylcholine esterase. A voltage-gated potassium channel activation repolarises the motor neuron endplate [87]. Reducing the number of available AchR on the postsynaptic membrane endplates means failure to generate a strong enough endplate potential leading to fatiguability of the skeletal muscles. Instead of anti-AchR antibodies, less than 10% of patients may show muscle-specific tyrosine kinase (MuSK) antibodies [87, 88]. MuSK is responsible for maintaining the AchR clusters.

Anticholinesterase inhibitor drugs prolong Ach's life at the neuromuscular junction for an adequate endplate potential in the muscle fibres. Short-acting acetylcholinesterase inhibitors (edrophonium) used in the past formed the basis of MG diagnosis. But this test has a low specificity and has been replaced by detecting specific antibodies and using a single fibre electromyography with high sensitivity and specificity for diagnosing OMG [89].

19.5.5 Ocular Myasthenia Gravis

OMG presents as ptosis, orbicularis weakness, and variable weakness of the extraocular muscles leading to variable diplopia (Fig. 19.18). Symptoms are maximum towards the evening. Sometimes, patients may present with unilateral ptosis, and the contralateral eye may show eyelid retraction. In the clinic, a simple test is to demonstrate Cogan's twitch. After looking down for 15 s, the patient is asked to look up and bring the eyes back to the primary gaze, when the upper lid may show retraction for a few seconds [90]. However, 75% of patients with OMG have a positive Cogan's lid twitch sign [90]. It is a highly specific test (99%). In another fatigue test, the patient is asked to stare at a distant light source without blinking for 1–2 min. If the lid droops, it strongly suggests OMG and calls for a tension test [91]. Ice-pack on the closed eye for 2 min can be done as cooling the neuromuscular junction improves muscle activity. It is a highly sensitive and specific test but is best for patients with unilateral or bilateral ptosis than extraocular involvement. In a small series, 80% of the patients with OMG showed positive ice-pack tests compared to nil non-OMG patients [92]. There was an improvement in the ptosis by 2.3 (± 1.5) mm by ice-pack, 1.3 (± 1.1) mm by rest, and 0.3 (± 1.4) mm by heat application [93].

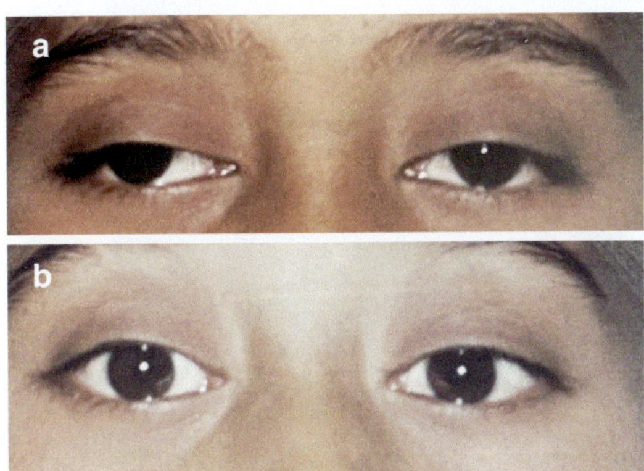

Fig. 19.18 *Ocular Myasthenia gravis*: A 13-year-old boy presented with ocular myasthenia gravis. Shows bilateral ptosis (**a**). Note that the right eye is divergent. His ptosis improved after intramuscular injection of neostigmine, and the eye became parallel (**b**). The neostigmine test involves an intramuscular injection of neostigmine 1 mg. The patient is given an intramuscular atropine injection to prevent complications of neostigmine. Neostigmine is an anticholinesterase and makes Ach available at the postsynaptic junction. Images courtesy of Dr. Kanwar Mohan, Dr. Kanwar Mohan's Squint Centre, Chandigarh

OMG is commonly associated with thyroid eye disease (TED). In a patient with OMG, if there is a lid retraction, it calls for investigations for thyroid eye disease. On the contrary, if a patient had been noted to have lid retraction due to TED, developing ptosis would indicate the onset of myasthenia. Apart from that, TED ptosis may be noted because of dermatochalasis or old age. Lid retraction is extremely uncommon in MG. In one study of 150 patients with OMG, only four had lid retraction. Lid retraction should be distinct from Cogan's lid twitch sign [94].

Elderly patients with OMG with severe symptoms, and positive for the AchR antibodies, show high tires, have thymomas or thymic hyperplasia run the risk of conversion to generalized MG. Nearly half the patients with OMG will progress to gMG, usually within the first year of diagnosis.

Most commonly, the patients are treated with corticosteroids, immunosuppressive therapy, plasma exchange, and rituximab. Thymectomy led to complete remission of OMG in 40% of patients below 40 [95, 96]. Newer treatment modalities for generalized MG have become available for AChR antibodies-positive patients. Soliris (eculizumab) blocks the cleavage of complement C5 and prevent the formation of membrane attack complex and was FDA approved in 2017 [97], and more recently, Vyvgart (**Efgartigimod alfa),** which blocks the neonatal Fc receptor of the antibodies to reduce a load of IgG [98] and Ultomiris (ravulizumab-cwvz) for control of gMG resistant to conventional therapies. For more detailed information, the readers are advised to review this article [99].

19.6 Paralytic Squint (Tropia)

All the extraocular muscles carry a motor tone which keeps the eyes in the primary position and are ensheathed in elastic and fibrous tissue, which keeps the eyes in position. Weakness of any muscle (decrease in the innervation) leads to loss of parallelism as the tone of the antagonist's muscle deviates the eye towards its field of action. Loss of parallelisms is called tropia or squint. It may be congenital or acquired. In congenital squint, also called concomitant or the combatants squint, the angle of deviation remains the same in all directions of gaze; images from the deviating eye are suppressed; hence, the patients do not have diplopia but lack binocular vision.

Double vision or diplopia is the most troublesome symptom of a paretic muscle because the image of the object of interest in the deviating eye is focused on the extrafoveal retina. The sharp and hazy images of the object are projected at a distance apart depending upon the direction of gaze and are seen as a double vision (diplopia). The separation of images is maximum in the field of action of the paretic muscle and absent in the opposite field.

The paresis of extraocular muscle/s leads to paretic or non-constant squint, and the angle of deviation is maximum in the field of action of the paretic muscle. If the RLR is paretic, it leads to inward deviation of the right eye by the unopposed action of the ipsilateral MR and is called right eye esotropia. The tropia is maximum in the direction of the action of the paretic muscle, i.e., in the right gaze in this example. There is no tropia when the eye is moved in the left gaze (opposite direction) (Fig. 19.19). Thus, the angle of deviation varies in different directions of gaze.

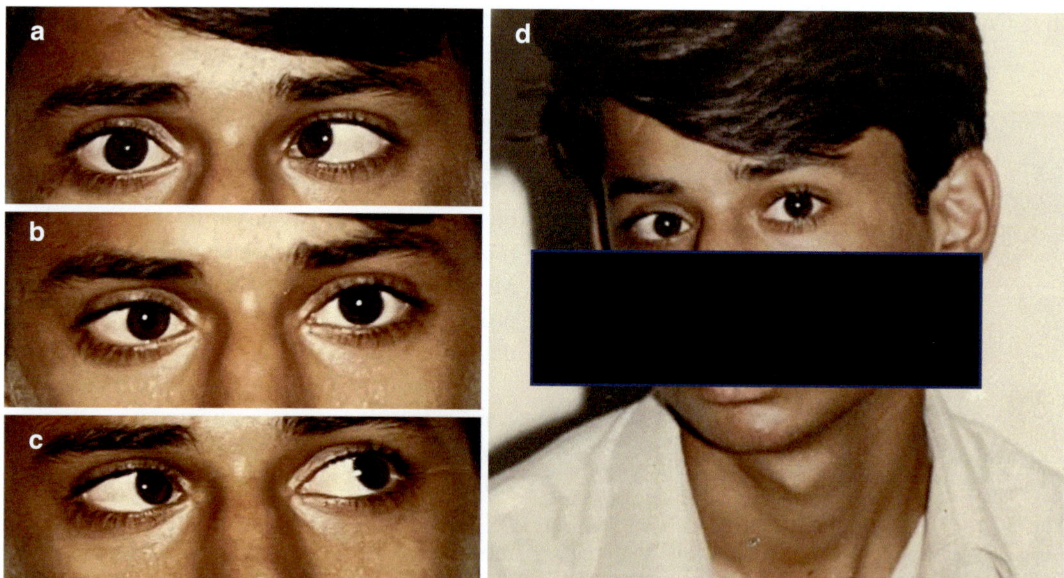

Fig. 19.19 *Traumatic right 6th nerve palsy*. In primary gaze, with left eye fixing, he shows right esotropia ~15° (primary deviation) (**b**). Looking to the right (**a**), he fails to abduct the right eye. The right eye is now fixing and there is a remarkable increase in left esotropia ~30 (secondary deviation) (**a**). Looking to the left, movements are normal, and no esotropia (**c**). The case illustrates secondary deviation more than the primary deviation in a paralytic squint. Note also the variable degree in a paralytic squint. To avoid diplopia, the patient has turned his head to the right (**d**). Images courtesy of Dr. Kanwar Mohan, Dr. Kanwar Mohan's Squint Centre, Chandigarh

Likewise, paresis of the MR leads to outward deviation by unopposed action of the ipsilateral lateral rectus and is called exotropia. Paresis of cyclovertical muscles produces more complex diplopia as the image from the paretic eye shows torsion.

19.6.1 Testing for the Paretic Muscle

While testing to identify the paretic muscle, the patient is asked to look at an object which is moved in all cardinal directions of the gaze. A cover test is performed to identify the paretic eye. As a first step, the patient is asked to fix a penlight in the primary gaze with one eye, and the other eye is covered with an occluder. On removing the occluder, the angle of deviation is assessed by the position of the corneal reflex of the penlight in the deviating eye. As a rough estimate, the corneal reflex in the deviating eye at the pupillary border is 15°, at the limbus is 45°, and in between is 30° (Hirschberg test). The deviation can be measured in prism dioptres by keeping prism in front of the good eye with the apex towards the direction of the squint (Krimsky test). The angle of deviation fixing with the good eye is called the primary deviation. In the second step, the good eye is covered, and the patient is asked to fix the light with the paretic eye; on removing the occluder, the angle of deviation of the good eye is measured. Measuring secondary deviation is easy if the paretic eye is dominant, as it tends to maintain fixation. If the paretic eye is non-dominant, it tends to lose fixation quickly, and one can note the degree of excursion. This is called secondary deviation. In paralytic squint, the secondary deviation is always greater than the primary deviation. This is following the Hering's law of equal innervation in the yoke muscles. When asked to fix an object with the paretic muscle in the primary position, the paretic muscle draws much more innervation to reach the primary gaze. The same amount is delivered to the non-paretic muscle, resulting in greater deviation.

19.6.2 Parks-Bielschowsky 3-Step Test-Diagnosing Paresis of a Cyclovertical Muscle

Paresis of a vertical muscle leads to vertical squint, elevation (hypertropia) in one eye and depression in the other. By convention, a notation indicates vertical squint; e.g., R/L indicates that the right eye is hypertropic and the left is hypotropic. Paresis of any of the four vertical muscles in each eye can produce either R/L or L/R hypertropia.

In the first step, hypertropia is assessed in the primary gaze. R/L hypertropia in the primary gaze indicates either a paresis of the right eye's depressors, i.e., RIR or RSO or the left eye's elevators, i.e., LSR or the LIO.

In the second step, the patient is asked to look to the right and then to the left and the hypertropia is assessed. If R/L increases in the left gaze, it rules out RIR and LIO. This is because, in the left gaze, the RIR (adducted position) and the LIO (abducted position) do not act, and their paresis cannot increase the hypertropia. This leaves the RSO or the LSR as the paretic muscle, depressor of the right and elevator of the left eye, respectively, in the left gaze.

In the third step, the patient is asked to tilt his head toward the shoulder on either side. In a normal person, on tilting the head to the right shoulder, the RSO/RSR intort the right eye, and the LIR/LIO extort the left eye to maintain the parallelism. In an RSO paresis, the R/L hypertropia increases on head tilt to the right due to the unopposed action of the RIO. In patients with bilateral SO paresis, the R/L hypertropia in the left and L/R hypertropia in the right gaze suggest bilateral involvement. Moreover, the Bielschowsky test is positive on titling the head to either side [100] (Fig. 19.20).

None of the unilateral SO palsy patients showed a positive Bielschowsky test on titling the head to either side [100]. The most common cause of unilateral SO palsy is congenital or trauma, while trauma is the main cause of bilateral SO palsy [100]. Since most patients with

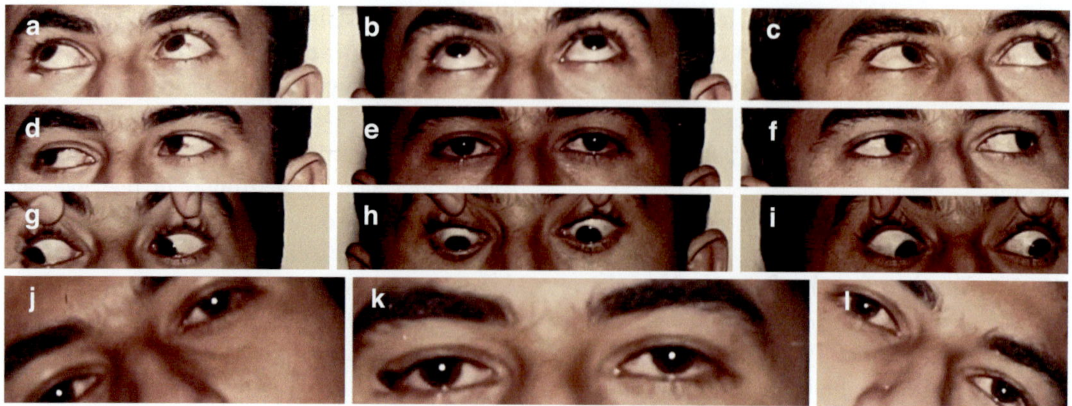

Fig. 19.20 *Superior oblique palsy of the left eye*. Note L/R hypertropia in the primary position (**e** and **k**), which increases in the right gaze due to unopposed action of the inferior oblique of the left eye (**d**). There is no restriction of upgaze (**a**, **b** and **c**). Note restriction of the left eye in down gaze (**h**). In the left down gaze, note the extorsion of the left eye as the light reflex has moved anti-clockwise (**i**) (cf from **h**). In the head tilt test, tilting the head to the right shoulder, there is no L/R hypertropia (**j**) but increases in the left head tilt (**l**).Images courtesy of Dr. Kanwar Mohan, Dr. Kanwar Mohan's Squint Centre, Chandigarh

acquired SO palsy and even 1/5th of the congenital SO palsy may complain of diplopia and tilted image, they may adopt a compensatory head posture, i.e., tilt the head towards the contralateral side to avoid diplopia [100].

When tested against gold standard atrophy of the SO muscle on MRI, the sensitivity of all three steps was sensitive only in 70% of the cases. Only two steps were positive in 28% of eyes [101]. Moreover, in a restrictive ophthalmopathy or Myasthenia gravis, the three steps test may be falsely positive [102].

19.6.3 Diplopia

Patients with acquired muscle paresis/palsy often complain of double vision (diplopia) when both eyes are open. Occasionally, monocular diplopia may be due to ocular causes, which can be excluded by asking the patient to cover each eye by turn and see if the diplopia persists. The patient may perceive one sharp and the other faded image of the same object; the latter belongs to the paretic eye. Next, the patient is asked whether the distance between the two images increases looking at a distant object (suggests paresis of the LR) or a near object (paresis of MR). The distance between the two images increases in the field of action of the paretic muscle. By asking the patient to wear Red-green goggles and showing a vertical slit light source in all cardinal gaze directions, crossed or non-crossed diplopia, increasing or decreasing the gap between the two images or even assessing a tilted image in cyclovertical muscle paresis can be assessed and charted. In horizontal diplopia, the esotropia causes an uncrossed diplopia, while the exotropia causes a crossed diplopia. Likewise, in hypertropia, the image from the paretic eye is below and above in a hypertrophic eye (https://eyewiki.aao.org/Basic_Approach_to_Diplopia). If the patient complains of vertical diplopia, the target slit light is kept horizontal. The patient is asked to draw using red-green markers on paper as he perceives the images in all the cardinal gaze directions.

19.6.4 Hess/Lees Screen/KM Digital Screen

It is based on the principle of foveal projection of the image when two different images are projected to the fovea (laparoscopy), one eye seeing one image and the other eye seeing the other image and the ability of the patient to fuse the two images. In non-constant squint, the chart can show the underacting or overacting muscle. Also, it can be used to note any improvement in paretic muscle or development of contractures in the overacting direct antagonistic muscle. The patient sits in front of the screen at a distance of 50 cm with his chin fixed on a chin rest to prevent head movement and wearing complimentary glasses (red-green), the right glass in front of the right eye. The room lights are dimmed. The two eyes can also be separated using a mirror, as in the Lees screen. A red dot is illuminated by the examiner on the screen, which can be seen by the patient only with the right eye. The dots are marked on the screen to form small squares that project 10^{Δ} at a 50 cm distance. The inner square isopter measures the muscle action in the 30^{Δ} and the outer square isopter measures 60^{Δ}. The patient is asked to use a green pointer light (seen only with the left eye) to coincide with the red dot. The examiner can switch on the red dots on the screen with a remote control and marks the patient's projections on a paper chart. Joining the dots gives the isopters of the activity of the extraocular muscles within 30^{Δ} of the fixation for which the head does need to move. The test is repeated with the red glass before the left eye [103]. It is a cumbersome test and has now been replaced by a digital KM screen developed by Konstantin Moutakis. It is done at a distance of 1 m and uses a digital screen 122 in in size. Like the Hess Screen, the patient sits in front of the screen wearing red-green goggles, red in front of the right eye. Two objects are presented on the screen, a dot and a circle. When the right eye is tested, the dot is red, and the ring is green. The patient is expected to drag and encircle the red dot using a laptop mouse. Once he has done it, he clicks the mouse. Twenty-five dots are plotted in the 15° and 30° square, ultimately getting a graph similar to the Hess chart that can be stored for future reference. To test the left eye, the dot's colour is changed to green, and the ring is red. Besides being less time-consuming, it can also test for torsions and several other parameters that are automatically calculated and provide comparable results with the Hess screen and the Lees screen [104].

19.7 Brief Physiological Considerations of Eye Movements

To bring an object of interest into focus at the fovea, the eyes, head, and body need to not only move fast but also well-regulated, controlled, and perfectly synchronized movement. When changing gaze from the primary position, the eyes must move fast to prevent the retina from losing focus on the object of interest. Moreover, the eyes should stop smoothly without oscillations at the end of the activity. The reticular formation in the brain stem performs these functions.

A densely packed collection of interconnected multipolar neurons, unmyelinated axons, dendrites and synapses control and coordinate the eye, head, body position, and movements. These cells form the brain stem's central core and continue down the spinal cord. These cells form a network lacking distinct boundaries and are called reticular formations. Well-designated nuclei with distinct boundaries lie in this mesh of cells. The function of the reticular formation is to receive signals from multiple sources, including the visual, auditory, vestibular and proprioceptive, as well as the oculomotor areas of the brain, namely the frontal eye field, supplementary eye field and posterior parietal cortex and pass them onto the premotor neurons. Medial longitudinal fasciculus (MLF) is a pair of highly myelinated fibres that lie ventral to the aqueduct in the dorsal brain stem and extends from its nucleus in the rostral interstitial nucleus of MLF (riMLF) in the subthalamic mesencephalon to the medulla oblongata. The riMLF has several ascending and descending pathways that transmit information from the frontal eye field to the PPRF, various nuclei of the oculomotor nerves and the vestibular nucleus. It carries pathways for all conjugate ocular movements, including saccades, pursuit, and vestibular-ocular reflex pathways (Fig. 19.21).

The reticular formation is the major centre for several vital functions such as cardiovascular, respiratory, consciousness, pain, sleep, and circadian rhythm, to name just a few. The reticular

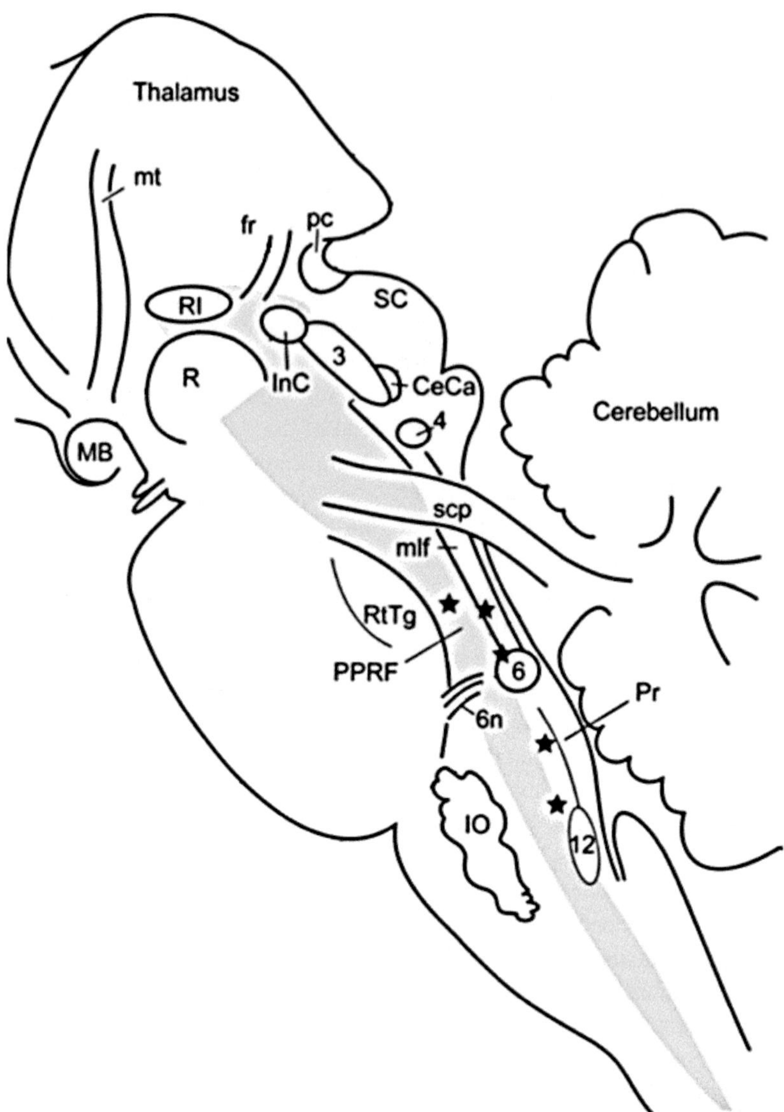

Fig. 19.21 A sagittal view of the human brainstem shows the reticular formation's location (shaded area) and several structures essential for controlling eye movements and gaze. The stars indicate the location of the cell groups of the paramedian tract. 3, oculomotor nucleus; 4, trochlear nucleus; 6, abducens nucleus; 6n, abducens nerve; 12, hypoglossal nucleus; *CeCa* central caudal nucleus; *fr* fasciculus retroflexus; *InC* interstitial nucleus of Cajal; *IO* inferior olive; *mlf* medial longitudinal fasciculus; *MB* mammillary body; *mt* mammillo-thalamic tract; *pc* posterior commissure; *PPRF* paramedian pontine reticular formation; *Pr* prepositus hypoglossal nucleus; *R* red nucleus; *RI* rostral interstitial nucleus of the medial longitudinal fasciculus; *RtTg* reticulotegmental nucleus of the pons; *SC* superior colliculus. Reproduced with permission from the authors Anja K E Horn and Christopher Adamcyzk (copyright holders). Chap. 9, Reticular formation, Eye movements, Gaze and Blinks. The Human Nervous System, Third Edition DOI: 10.1016/B978-0-12-374236-0.10009-4328. 2012. Elsevier Inc

formation also controls various motor movements and reflex actions.

The reticular formation lies in the tegmentum of the brain stem (the ventral aspect of the brain stem and medulla. Well-defined nuclei in this area include the red nuclei, substantia nigra, and oculomotor nuclei of CN III and IV at the midbrain level and the nuclei of CN V and VI at the level of Pons.

The reticular formation is divided into columns, and each column contains reticular cells assigned regulatory control of different vital functions. The reticular cells that control eye movements are located in the medial column ([105]). The reticular formation responsible for the vertical gaze is located in the midbrain. Those for the horizontal gaze are located in the paramedian pontine reticular formation (PPRF), while the gaze holding, and head movements are in the medullary pontine reticular formation [105].

The superior colliculus contains the premotor neurons for the various ocular movements. The descending tracts from the reticular formation to the spinal motor neurons control the body movements [106].

It is important to know the primary and secondary actions of the extraocular muscles to detect which muscle/s may be weak by asking the patient to move the eyes in different directions of gaze, called the cardinal positions. Looking straight ahead is the primary gaze, and looking left, right or up and down are the secondary positions.

The cardinal positions of gaze and the yoke muscles responsible for these positions include looking left (LLR, RMR), left and up (LSR, RIO), left and down (LIR, RSO); looking right (RLR, LMR), right and up (RSR, LIO); right and down (RIR, LSO) [107].

19.7.1 Movements of the Eye-Ductions

When tested in one eye at a time (the other eye is covered), eye movements are called ductions. The eye's movements are essentially rotations around imaginary axes (Fick's axes) passing through the geometric centre of the eye. When the eye rotates around a vertical 'Z' axis inward (towards the nose), it is called adduction. It is called abduction when the eye rotates outwards around the 'Z' axis. Abduction and adduction are horizontal eye movements by contraction of the lateral and medial rectus. The eye's upward rotation (elevation or supraduction) or downward rotation (depression or infraduction) occurs around a horizontal, 'X' axis. These are called vertical movements. In the primary gaze, the eye is elevated by the action of SR and IO. In the abducted eye position, SR is the only elevator of the eye, and the IO only extorts (excycloducts) the eyeball around a sagittal axis, the Y-axis. In the adducted position of the eye, the eye is elevated by the action of IO, and the SR intorts the eyeball. In the primary gaze, the IR and the SO are depressors of the eyeball. The IR is a depressor in the abducted eye position, and the SO intorts the eyeball. In the adducted position of the eye, the main depressor is the SO, and the IR extorts the eyeball. The SO is the key muscle while reading and going downstairs.

19.7.2 Conjugate Movements-Versions

Although the two eyes are situated a distance apart, the interpupillary distance between the two eyes varying from 53 to 75 mm (median 63 mm), the object of interest is focused on the fovea of each eye. It forms a somewhat disparate image in each eye, fused to be seen as a depth-resolved 3D image, called binocular vision. The striate cortex area V1 receives the images from the right and the left eye individually, but in the extrastriate area V2-LO, the images are fused and seen as the 'cyclopean' view [108].

If the object of interest moves, the eyes must move in the same direction without losing focus. Thus, on looking to the right, both eyes rotate around the vertical axis, the right eye abducting and the left eye adducting. This is called dextroversion. In this example, the two eyes rotate at almost the same degree using two different muscles, the right lateral rectus and the left medial rectus. This movement of the two eyes is called a conjugate movement, i.e., the two muscles are paired together for a specific movement and are also called yoke muscles. Conjugate movements of the eyes are called versions. When the eyes move to the left, the left eye's lateral rectus and the right eye's medial rectus act together, and the movement is called levoversion. For looking up and down, the movements are called supraver-

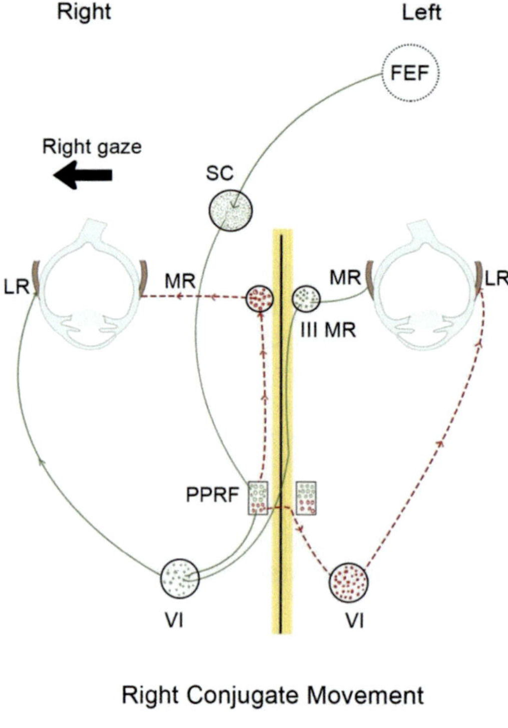

Fig. 19.22 Right eye conjugate movement is initiated from the left frontal eye field (FEF); the excitatory signals are sent to the right sixth nerve nucleus via the right superior colliculus (SC) and the right paramedian pontine reticular formation (PPRF). Signals also go to the contralateral, left medial rectus via the left third nerve subnucleus for the medial rectus. The right PPRF sends inhibitory signals to the left sixth nerve nucleus and the right third nerve subnucleus for the medial rectus to inhibit the right medial rectus and the left lateral rectus to allow the eyes to move in right gaze. Graphics by Kritika Thakur

sion and infraversion, respectively. When the eyes rotate around either a vertical or a horizontal axis, the position of the eyes is termed a secondary position (Fig. 19.22).

When the eyes move around both the vertical and the horizontal axis, the position of the eyes is called the tertiary position. For looking up and to the right (dextroelevation), the two muscles acting together are the right eye's SR and the left eye's IO. For looking up and to the left (levoelevation), the right eye's IO and the left eye's SR act in synergy. For looking down and to the right (dextrodepression), the right eye's IR and the left eye's SO will act together. Likewise, looking down and to the left (levodepression), the left eye's IR and the right eye's SO will act in synergy.

When one muscle contracts in response to increased motor innervation, its direct antagonist must relax similarly by inhibiting its innervation. This is Sherrington's reciprocal innervation law [109]. Looking to the right, the right LR contracts and the right MR relaxes by the same degree. In this conjugate movement, the RLR and RMR are antagonists. When converging, the MR of the two eyes contract to the same degree and synergise in this action. The net result is eye elevation when the SR and IO are stimulated. While elevating in the primary position, the adducting and intorting action of the SR is cancelled by the abducting and extorting action of the IO. Likewise, looking down, the IR and the SO synergise, and their respective secondary and tertiary actions cancel out. As SO and IO are antagonists, the rotational axis does not shift during horizontal eye movements [110]. One simple rule to remember is that superiors (SR and SO) are intortors while the inferiors (IR and IO) are extortors. The recti (SR and IR) are adductors, and the obliques (SO and IO) are abductors.

19.7.3 Vergence

Deconjugate movement of the eyes is called vergence. When both medial recti contract simultaneously, both eyes adduct, which is called convergence. Testing for the preservation of convergence is a helpful sign in gaze palsies since the subnucleus for the medial recti is located in the rostral midbrain, and the pathology affecting the MLF is located at the level of Pons. When both the lateral recti contract, they produce divergence of the eyes. Lesions located at the level of CN VI produce wall-eyed INO.

19.8 Supranuclear Control of Conjugate Ocular Movements (Gaze)

Many types of ocular movements keep the target focused on the fovea. Of these, the saccades are voluntary movements. Smooth pursuit movements track slow-moving objects moving at less than 40° per second, both in horizontal and vertical planes. The vestibular and optokinetic system keeps the target in focus when the head moves. The vergence is used to keep in focus the objects moving in anteroposterior axes [111]. The vestibulo-ocular reflex pathways which control the movements of the eyes when the head is turned or rotated are shown in Figs. 19.23 and 19.24.

19.8.1 Saccades

Saccades are rapid eye movements that bring into focus objects in the field of vision. These are the fastest movements and can move 500 per second [112].

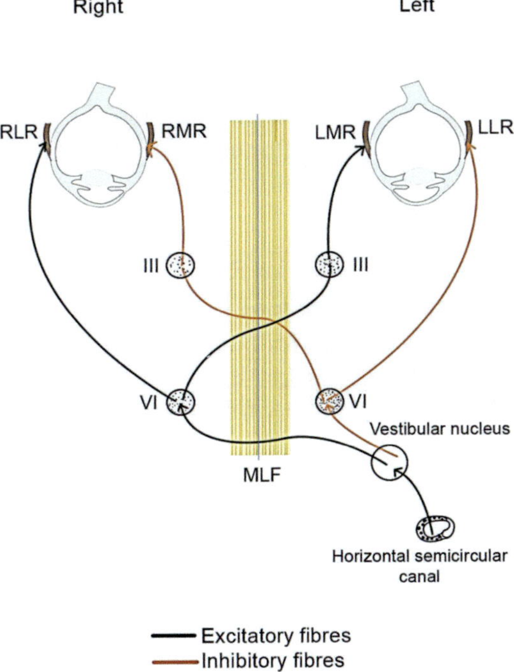

Fig. 19.23 Vestibulo-ocular reflex pathway. Head rotated to the left, and both eyes move in the right direction. Graphics by Kritika Thakur

Motor neurons for saccades are located in the nuclei of the extraocular muscles in the brain stem.

There are at least five types of neurons in the reticular formation for initiating and controlling eye saccades: the short-lead burst (excitatory and inhibitory burst) and long-lead burst neurons, omnipause neurons, burst tonic neurons, and tonic neurons. There are separate neurons for vertical and horizontal movements [105].

Omnidirectional pause neurons (OMN) are the most important neurons that regulate the excitatory signals from burst neurons. The OMNs bring about stability in the saccades. The neurotransmitter in most inhibitory neurons is γ-aminobutyric acid, except in omnidirectional pause neurons that transmit glycine [113]. The OPNs lie at the rostral end of the Abducens nucleus close to the midline [113] in the nucleus raphe interpositus.

For an ipsilateral horizontal saccade, the excitatory signal from the superior colliculus sends projections to the premotor excitatory burst neurons (EBN) in the PPRF, which excite the motor neurons in the ipsilateral CN VI nucleus and via the interneurons also excite the contralateral medial rectus neurons (subnucleus of CN III). Simultaneously, the EBN activate the inhibitory burst neurons in the contralateral CN VI to allow an ipsilateral horizontal conjugate movement of the eyes. A signal from the right FEF initiates a conjugate movement to the left.

For the vertical movements of the eyes, the premotor burst neurons (supra nuclear) are located in the rostral interstitial nucleus of the medial longitudinal fasciculus (riMLF) [114]. The riMLF also receives signals from the superior colliculus and the interstitial nucleus of Cajal (INC). It also receives inhibitory signals from the OMN located in the nucleus raphe interpositus in the pons, which help in the fixation of the eyes. For a down movement, the excitatory signals from the superior colliculus to the riMLF initiate signals to the INC and the motor neuron in the nuclei of CN IV and the inferior rectus. The contralateral INC also sends inhibitory signals to the

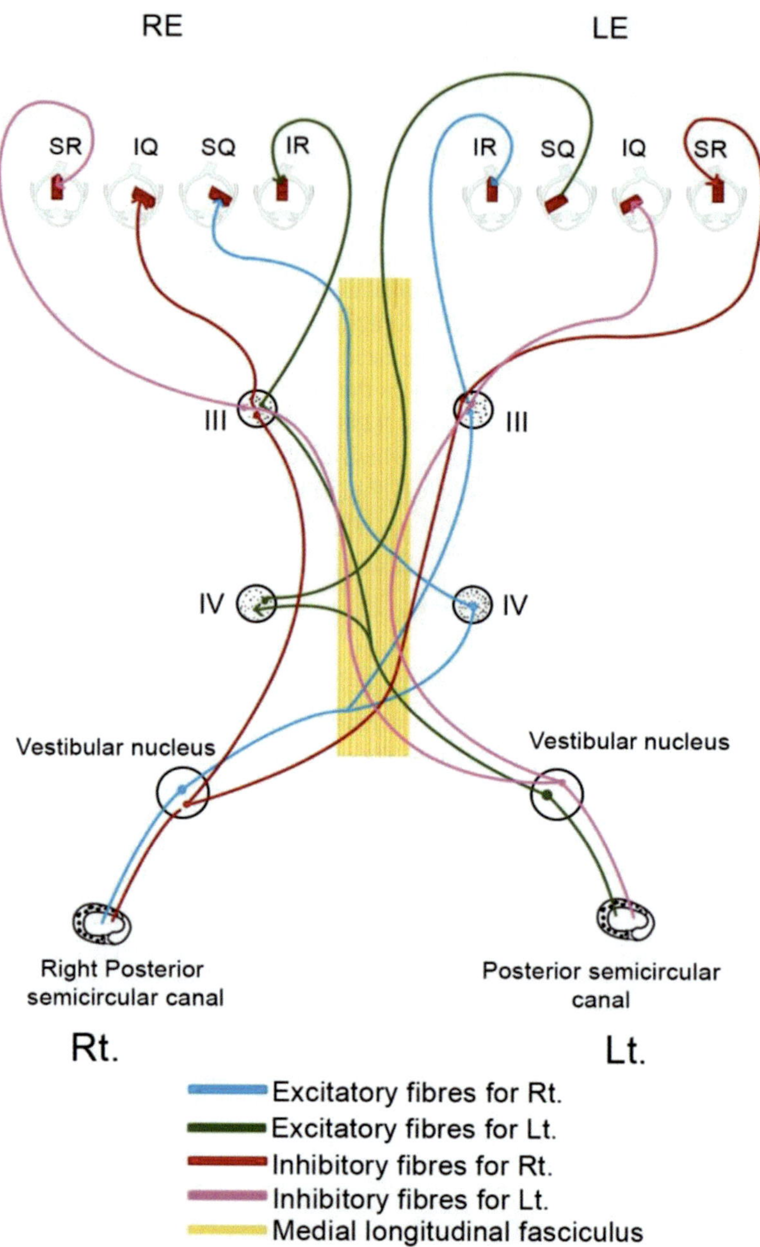

Fig. 19.24 Vestibulo-ocular reflex pathway. As the head is rotated up, the eyes move down by simultaneous activation of the bilateral posterior semicircular canals, which send signals to the vestibular nucleus. Excitatory signals go to the bilateral superior oblique and the inferior rectus muscles (Blue from the right and green from the left posterior semicircular canal. Simultaneously inhibitory signals are sent to both eyes' superior rectus and inferior oblique muscles (shown in red from the right and the pink fibres from the left posterior semicircular canal. Graphics by Kritika Thakur

motor neurons of the superior rectus and the inferior oblique nucleus [105].

In a monkey model, the destruction of unilateral PPRF formation led to the loss of ipsilateral rapid eye movement. Destruction of the bilateral rostral PPRF led to only the loss of rapid eye movement in horizontal gaze, and destruction of the bilateral caudal PPRF led to the loss of both horizontal and vertical rapid eye movements [115].

The neural integrators help to stabilise (hold) the image for clarity at the new position by providing feedback to the motor neurons on the velocity and the new position of the eye. The neural integrators for the horizontal saccades and smooth pursuit movements are located in the vestibular nucleus and the nucleus prepositus hypoglossi and those for the vertical movements in the interstitial nucleus of Cajal [116].

Horizontal and vertical saccades can be tested in the clinic by either verbal command or the patient can be asked to look at a target of his own volition. The patient can look at the nose of the examiner and the tip of a pencil held to the right, left, up, or down of the primary gaze of the patient. Any delay in the initiation of the saccade indicates oculomotor apraxia. Such patients tend to move their heads to look at the objects. This may also be associated with ataxia. This may be seen as congenital oculomotor apraxia [117] or acquired due to lesions in the cerebral cortex, frontal eye field or basal ganglia [118]. Smooth pursuit movements are also abnormal. The vestibulo-ocular reflex (VOR) movements are normal. The Doll's eye movement tests the VOR by quickly rotating the patient's head and noting the movement of the eyes in the opposite direction [112].

Besides the normal/abnormal initiation of the saccade, the examiner notes the speed and completion of the saccade, whether it is incomplete, i.e., conjugate movement fails to reach the target or overshoots the target. Incomplete saccades may be recorded in Parkinson's disease (PD), especially in self-paced testing in patients with advanced PD [119, 120]. The slow speed of the saccades with an associated upgaze palsy suggests progressive supranuclear palsy (PSP). Slow saccades are a hallmark of hereditary spinocerebellar ataxia [121]. Impaired signals from the contralateral superior colliculus or pathology directly involving the OPNs in the raphe interpositus may lead to impaired fixation and macrosaccadic oscillations due to loss of control on the premotor burst neurons in the PPRF [122]. Demyelinating lesions in the PPRF spreading to involve the OPN in the raphe interpositus may lead to impairment of vertical saccades, confirming the role of the inhibitory influence of OPN in controlling the vertical saccades [123].

19.8.2 Smooth Pursuit Movements

Once the saccadic movement has brought an object into focus at the fovea, smooth pursuit, with an initial delay of about 100 ms of the target movement, keeps it constantly focused if it is a moving object. Pursuit movements are slower than saccades. The latency is much reduced if the object moves in an anticipated trajectory [124]. Signals for the remembered objects moving to the right arise in the right FEF and moving to the left arise in the left FEF. The signals for the novel targets arise in the parietal cortex, the middle temporal visual area, which tracks the retinal image of the moving target, and the middle superior temporal area 1, which tracks the coordinates of the moving object in the extra personal space [124]. Besides the slipping image of the object on the fovea, the eye and head movements determine the gaze. Signals from the eye fields are projected to the superior colliculus and, from there, to the basal ganglia (caudate nucleus, putamen, globus pallidus, subthalamic nucleus, and substantia nigra).

The premotor neurons for ocular movements lie in the nucleus reticularis segments pontic (NRTP), a bridge between the basal ganglia and the cerebellum (flocculus-para flocculus complex and posterior vermis). The NRTP lies ventral to the most rostral end of the PPRF. The NRTP is heavily connected to the cerebellum. The pathways between these two control the movements [125]. Neurons in the rostral NRTP control the pursuit movements, while neurons in the caudal NRTP control the saccadic movements. Lesions in the frontal lobe, occipital cortex, thalamus, cerebellar, and brain stem lesions impair smooth pursuit movements [111]. The smooth pursuit movements are tested by slowly moving a pencil in the left or right gaze at a one-metre distance from the seated patient who follows the target without moving his head. Any loss of fixation and recovery saccades indicate impaired smooth movements. It can also be tested by using a pointer target fixed to the head and asking the patient to fix the target as the head moves. If there is no loss of fixation, it means the cancellation of the vestibulo-ocular reflex is intact. The pursuit movements and the cancellation of the VOR share the same pathways, and the impaired cancellation of VOR indicates defective pursuit movements [126].

19.8.3 Vestibulo-Ocular Reflexes

The vestibulo-ocular reflexes (VOR) are responsible for maintaining eye fixation on a fixed target during the rotational movements of the head. Rotation of the head stimulates the cupula, a cap-like membrane that senses the movement of the head and generates nerve impulses (movement of the endolymph in the semicircular canal is transmitted by the cupula to the hairy cells located in the ampulla, which stimulates the nerve). Movement of the cupula in the lateral (also called horizontal) semicircular canal sends signals to the CN VIII (vestibular nucleus) on the same side as the rotation of the head (Ipsilateral), which in turn activates the contralateral CN VI nucleus to initiate the saccade. At the same time, inhibitory impulses go to the contralateral vestibular nucleus. The CN VI nucleus also has interneurons which connect via the MLF with the ipsilateral subnucleus for the medial rectus (Fig. 19.23).

Defective or suppressed VOR leads to dizziness, nausea, imbalance, and vertigo, among other symptoms related to the inner ear. With the patient seated, he is asked to fix an object. Fixing the patient's head in both hands, the examiner quickly rotates the head in one direction by about 15–20°. Normally, the patient should not lose fixation on the object. However, if the fixation is lost and the patient has to move his eyes to regain fixation, he has an impaired VOR. The direction of the positive test suggests the side of the lesion. The important causes of impaired VOR include multiple sclerosis, ischemia, viral infections, and trauma.

Unilateral labyrinth pathologies affecting the lateral semicircular canal generate vestibular nystagmus when the head is rotated towards the side of the pathology, with the fast component away from the side of the pathology. Visual fixation suppresses peripheral vestibular nystagmus [126]. It can be tested by a modified head impulse test target fixed to the head at the end of a pointer and asking the patient to fix the target as the head is quickly moved. If there is no nystagmus, it means the cancellation of VOR and indicates impaired VOR. A healthy person needs to regain fixation and shows nystagmus. Since the peripheral vestibular nystagmus tends to disappear with time, such patients may be examined using Frenzel nystagmus goggles (+20D lenses with internal lighting to remove the visual fixation. Spontaneous nystagmus can be elicited [127]. Skull vibrations can exaggerate the peripheral vestibular nystagmus at the vertex of the skull or either of the mastoids using a muscle massager. The nystagmus has a slow phase towards the side of the lesion irrespective of the side of vibration [126]. The lesions of the vestibular nucleus also cause spontaneous contralesional nystagmus, whereas lesions of the nucleus propositus hypoglossal and the flocculus produce ipsilesional spontaneous nystagmus [126]. Central lesions produce gaze-changing nystagmus, right gaze right beating nystagmus, and left gaze produces left beating nystagmus. The presence of normal horizontal head impulse test, gaze changing nystagmus and skew deviation was highly sensitive and specific for a brain stem stroke [128].

During the downward rotation of the head, the anterior semicircular canal on each side stimulates the vestibular nucleus, sending signals to the contralateral subnucleus for the IO and the ipsilateral SR for initiating a saccade for the conjugate elevation of the eyes. During the upward rotation of the head, both posterior semicircular canals are stimulated, each sending signals to the ipsilateral vestibular nucleus, activating the contralateral subnucleus for the IR and the CN IV nucleus (SO for the downward movement of the eye) [129] (Fig. 19.24).

However, when walking, a person may need to move his eye and head in the same direction to see an approaching vehicle or look down to spot a pothole in the road ahead. Thus, he has to be able to suppress the VOR quickly. Old people or those with neurodegenerative disorders tend to fall because of the inability to suppress the VOR when the need arises [130].

19.8.4 Optokinetic Movement Reflex

The optokinetic reflex (OKR) movements combine a slow pursuit of a moving object in the periphery. As the object moves out of the fixation range, the eyes move back in a saccade to the original position. The OKR develops in infancy and stays throughout life. While the VOR is generated by brief but fast head movement, it is assisted by the OKN to maintain the image of the object on the fovea in the lighted environment. Unlike the small objects that generate smooth movements, the OKN is generated by the images cast on a large extrafoveal retinal area. The OKN can be tested by projecting images of moving vertical stripes in the field by asking a patient to count stripes on a rotating drum painted in stripes of different widths (Barany drum) in either direction. If the stripes are moving in the left direction, the eyes use smooth pursuit in the left gaze, but as soon as the stripe disappears, the eyes show a quick return using saccadic movement in the right direction. Left-moving stripes generate a right nystagmus (the direction of the fast component of the nystagmus gives the direction of the nystagmus). It can assess visual acuity by using drums with progressively smaller widths of stripes) in non-verbal children, the absence of OKN does not rule out cortical blindness. As a bedside tool, it has a limited role as the same information can be obtained by testing for pursuit movements. Demonstrating OKN can be used to discover if someone is faking blindness. Asymmetry of the OKN can detect unilateral cerebral lesions. It is absent on the side of the lesion. It can be used to demonstrate the upgaze palsy by moving the stripes to rotate in a downward direction [131]. Central lesions involving the pursuit, saccades, or vestibular pathways diminish or abolish the OKN [126].

19.9 Nystagmus

Nystagmus is a to-and-fro rhythmic oscillation of the eye, which may be acquired or congenital. Most often, nystagmus is bilaterally symmetric and conjugate. Most central nystagmus is horizontal but can be vertical or rarely torsional. Congenital (infantile) nystagmus is seen in children with defective fixation. It is pendular, which has equal to-and-fro movement of the eyes and has equal amplitude and velocity in either direction. The acquired nystagmus has a slow phase in one gaze direction and a quick recovery phase to bring the eye to the primary position. This is termed a 'jerk nystagmus'. The direction of the quick phase determines the direction of the jerk nystagmus; e.g., a quick phase in the right gaze is called right-beating nystagmus. The cause of the jerk nystagmus is mostly vestibular and neurological lesions. Most patients with acquired nystagmus complain of oscillopsia, the jumping images [132].

In a first-ever epidemiological study, the prevalence of congenital and acquired nystagmus was estimated to be 24 per ten thousand population [133]. The most common cause of nystagmus was neurological in 6.8, followed by bilateral congenital cataracts in 4.2 and achromatopsia in 3.4 per ten thousand population, respectively [133]. Nystagmus was significantly more common in the White ethnic population than the Asians.

Vestibular (VON), rotatory, and Optokinetic (OKN) are physiological nystagmus tests. The vestibular and the OKN have been discussed in the previous section. Caloric nystagmus is a type of VON, tested by circulating 50 mL of ice-cold water in the ear, which initiates jerk nystagmus with a slow phase toward the ear being tested. If tested negative, it is one of the several tests to declare a person brain dead [134]. A jerk nystagmus develops if a person is rotated, seated in a chair, and brought to a halt. The eyes show postrotatory jerk nystagmus beating in the opposite direction of rotation. The person perceives the surrounding objects revolving in the opposite direction of rotation.

See-saw nystagmus is a cyclical pendular nystagmus characterised by one eye showing elevation and intortion and the other showing depression and extorsion in one half of the cycle and showing a reversal in the second half. It may be caused by a large macroadenoma of the pituitary gland compressing the optic chiasma and accessory optic system and interrupting the signals to the interstitial nucleus of Cajal and the inferior olivary nucleus [135]. It is associated with bitemporal hemianopia. Pendular see-saw nystagmus associated with bitemporal hemianopia may follow head trauma [136]. Intrathecal methotrexate and irradiation for CNS lymphoma have resulted in see-saw nystagmus [137]. Arteriovenous malformations (Arnold-Chiari) in the sellar or parasellar region may also cause see-saw nystagmus [132]. Once a see-saw nystagmus is noted, it calls for a contrast-enhanced MRI [132].

Downbeat jerk nystagmus has a slow phase downwards and a fast up phase. It gets exaggerated in down, right, and left gazes. Patients may complain of vertigo and oscillopsia. Many lesions, including trauma, demyelinating disease, ischemia, paraneoplastic syndrome, and antibodies to glutamic acid decarboxylase 65, among others, may cause it [138].

A primary position upbeat nystagmus shows a slow downward drift followed by a quick up phase. It may be seen in the demyelinating lesion of the caudal pons [139] and may accompany internuclear ophthalmoplegia. For a more detailed discussion on nystagmus, the readers may refer to an extensive review on the subject [132, 140].

The congenital or infantile nystagmus is absent at birth but may develop over the next few months. The infantile nystagmus was previously called sensory nystagmus due to defective afferent visual pathway, as seen in foveal hypoplasia, albinism, optic disc aplasia, achromatopsia, Leber's congenital amaurosis [141]. Optical coherence tomography (OCT) is increasingly used to determine the ophthalmic cause of infantile nystagmus [142]. The infantile nystagmus is pendular and changes into a jerk type over the next 2–3 years. It is important to find the 'Null zone' where the amplitude of the nystagmus is minimal; it may be seen by moving the eyes in a specific or primary gaze. The children will adopt a head posture to minimise the movement of the eyes as the vision improves in the 'Null zone'. There are wide variations in the visual acuity of patients with nystagmus; most require low-vision aids to magnify the text.

Unlike vestibular nystagmus, which gets depressed by visual fixation, infantile nystagmus increases while fixing or pursuing objects [143]. Structural anomalies seen in nearly half the patients with infantile nystagmus do not allow the development of foveal pursuit movements, which allows the persistence of the subcortical accessory optic tract pathways, the nucleus of the optic tract-dorsal terminal nucleus (NOT-DTN). In normal children, the accessory optic tract pathway regresses once the foveal fixation movements develop [143].

19.10 Disorders of the Ocular Movements

19.10.1 Internuclear Ophthalmoplegia

Internuclear ophthalmoplegia (INO) is a horizontal gaze palsy due to a pathological lesion in the medial longitudinal fasciculus (MLF), which has interneurons (neurons that connect multiple neurons) for various oculomotor nuclei responsible for horizontal conjugate movements. The premotor neurons for the horizontal gaze are in the para-pontine reticular formation. They are activated by the frontal eye field signals that activate the CN VI nuclei to initiate the horizontal gaze. The MLF connects the CN VI nerve nucleus to the contralateral CN III subnucleus for the medial rectus located in the midbrain and initiates the horizontal saccade. A pathological lesion in the ipsilateral MLF leads to failure of adduction by the medial rectus. However, as the contralateral CN VI nucleus is not interrupted, the abduction of the contralateral eye remains intact (Fig. 19.25).

The INO may be isolated or associated with other neurological symptoms. In the elderly, the

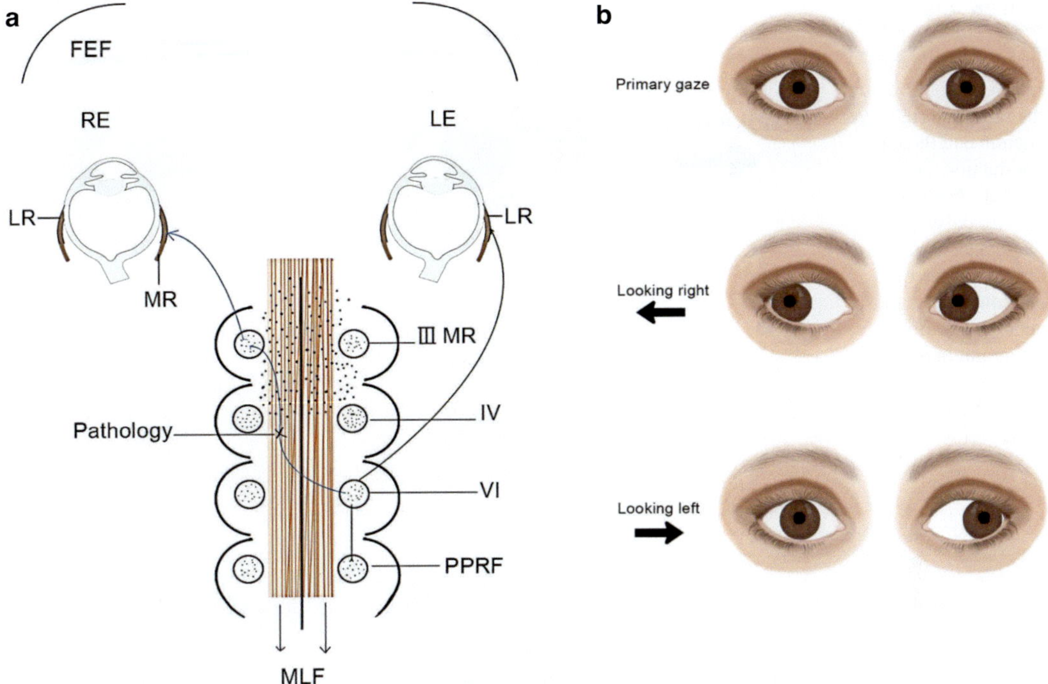

Fig. 19.25 *Right Internuclear ophthalmoplegia* resulting from a pathological lesion in the medial longitudinal fasciculus (MLF) which interrupts the excitatory signals to the right medial rectus (**a**). Clinically, the eyes are parallel in the primary gaze; there is no limitation of ocular movements looking in the right gaze, but in the left gaze, the right eye adduction is restricted, and the abducting left eye shows nystagmus (**b**). Graphics by Kritika Thakur

most common cause of INO is infarction in the dorsal pons (most often rostral than caudal) from atherosclerosis of the basilar artery, superior cerebellar artery, posterior cerebral artery or even the smaller penetrating branches [144]. The INO is most often unilateral and limits the adduction on the affected side and abduction nystagmus of the contralateral eye. The convergence of the eyes is maintained. Most unilateral INO cases are seen in men, while bilateral cases have no gender predilection. Most bilateral cases are due to multiple sclerosis and are seen in younger patients compared to unilateral cases [145]. Most patients have predisposing cardiovascular risk factors such as hypertension, diabetes mellitus, smoking, or stroke history [144]. Other causes of INO include multiple sclerosis, trauma, tumours, and infection [146, 147].

Patients with INO complain of sudden onset diplopia, worse when looking towards the contralateral side (opposite to the side with restricted adduction). The affected side may also have hyperopia with vertical diplopia/nystagmus, and pupils may be normal in 60% of the cases [145]. Systemic symptoms in some patients include headache, dysarthria and limb or gait ataxia [144].

Nearly, 72.5% of the INO lesions due to MS versus 90.5% in the INO due to stroke were seen in the MLF. Multiple lesions favour MS, while lesions at the level of mesencephalon favour stroke [148].

There is a spontaneous resolution of the isolated INO in about a month, but those associated with other neurological signs may last longer [144]. In a series of ischemic INO, 78.8% resolved within an average of 2.25 months, irrespective of the demonstrable ischemia on the MRI [149].

The other syndromes associated with INO are i) one-and-a-half syndrome, when there is a limitation of the ipsilateral adduction and inversive horizontal gaze palsy (Fig. 19.26). The lesion is

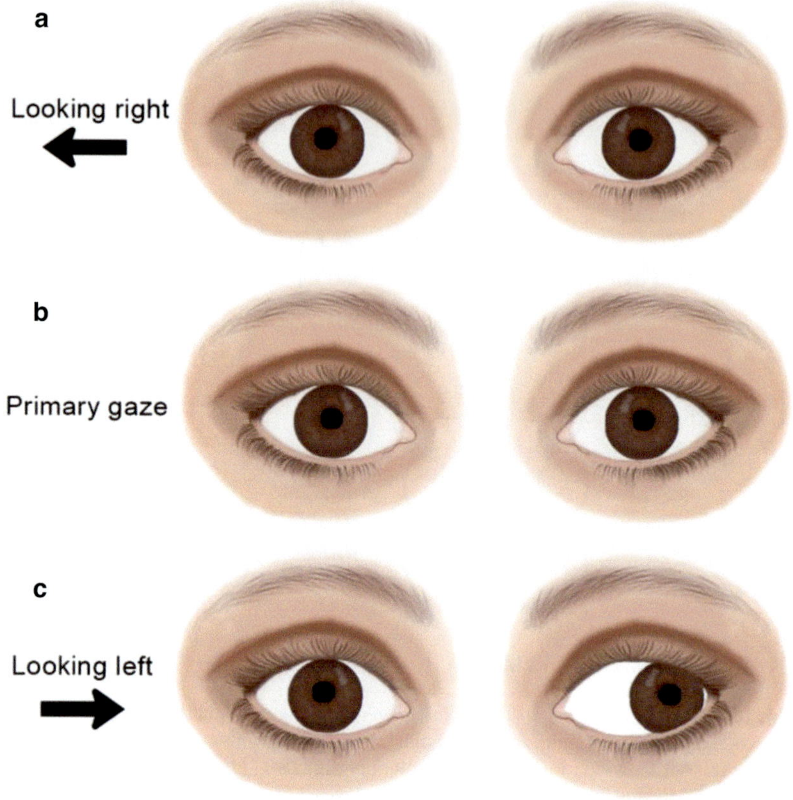

Fig. 19.26 *One-and-a-half syndrome*. In the primary gaze, the eyes are straight (**b**). Looking to the right, the right eye abduction and the left eye adduction are restricted, showing a right gaze palsy (**a**). In the left gaze, there is a restriction of the right adduction, but the left abduction is normal, showing internuclear ophthalmoplegia (**c**). Graphics by Kritika Thakur

more extensive and involves the MLF, CN VI nucleus and the PPRF [150].

If the lesion in the MLF is located between the CN III and CN IV nucleus, it results in hyperdeviation of the contralateral eye due to the non-activation of the SO. This is called INO with Trochlear syndrome [151]. A lesion involving bilateral MLF but sparing the CN nuclei leads to INO with the bilateral divergence of the eyes called the 'Wall-eyed' appearance INO [151].

References

1. Rucker JC. Normal and abnormal lid function. Handb Clin Neurol. 2011;102:403–23.
2. Kakizaki H, Malhotra R, Selva D. Upper eyelid anatomy: an update. Ann Plast Surg. 2009;63(3):336–43. https://doi.org/10.1097/SAP.0b013e31818b42f7. PMID: 19602949.
3. Coban I, Sirinturk S, Unat F, Pinar Y, Govsa F. Anatomical description of the upper tarsal plate for reconstruction. Surg Radiol Anat. 2018;40(10):1105–10. https://doi.org/10.1007/s00276-018-2064-7. Epub 2018 Jul 9. PMID: 29987378.
4. Porter JD, Burns LA, May PJ. Morphological substrate for eyelid movements: innervation and structure of primate levator palpebrae superioris and orbicularis oculi muscles. J Comp Neurol. 1989;287(1):64–81. https://doi.org/10.1002/cne.902870106. PMID: 2477400.
5. Lemke BN, Stasior OG, Rosenberg PN. The surgical relations of the levator palpebrae superioris muscle. Ophthalmic Plast Reconstr Surg. 1988;4(1):25–30. https://doi.org/10.1097/00002341-198801130-00004. PMID: 3154713.
6. Ng SK, Chan W, Marcet MM, Kakizaki H, Selva D. Levator palpebrae superioris: an anatomical update. Orbit. 2013;32(1):76–84. https://doi.org/10.3109/01676830.2012.736602. PMID: 23387464.
7. Ettl A, Zonneveld F, Daxer A, Koornneef L. Is Whitnall's ligament responsible for the curved course of the levator palpebrae superioris muscle? Ophthalmic Res. 1998;30(5):321–6. https://doi.org/10.1159/000055491. PMID: 9704336.
8. Hamedani AG, Gold DR. Eyelid dysfunction in neurodegenerative, neurogenetic, and neurometa-

bolic disease. Front Neurol. 2017;8:329. https://doi.org/10.3389/fneur.2017.00329. PMID: 28769865; PMCID: PMC5513921.

9. Vasanthakumar P, Kumar P, Rao M. Anthropometric analysis of palpebral fissure dimensions and its position in south Indian ethnic adults. Oman Med J. 2013;28(1):26–32. https://doi.org/10.5001/omj.2013.06. PMID: 23386941; PMCID: PMC3562989.
10. Farkas LG, Hreczko T, Katic M. Craniofacial norms in North American Caucasians from birth (one year) to young adulthood. In: Anthropometry of the head and face, vol. 2. New York: Raven Press; 1994. p. 241–312.
11. Park DH, Oh CH. Anthropometry of eyelids. In: Preedy V, editor. Handbook of anthropometry. New York, NY: Springer; 2012. https://doi.org/10.1007/978-1-4419-1788-1_35.
12. Patil SB, Kale SM, Math M, Khare N, Sumeet J. Anthropometry of the eyelid and palpebral fissure in an Indian population. Aesthet Surg J. 2011;31(3):290–4. https://doi.org/10.1177/1090820X11398475. PMID: 21385738.
13. Ferreira TA, Pinheiro CF, Saraiva P, Jaarsma-Coes MG, Van Duinen SG, Genders SW, Marinkovic M, Beenakker JM. MR and CT imaging of the normal eyelid and its application in eyelid tumors. Cancers (Basel). 2020;12(3):658. https://doi.org/10.3390/cancers12030658. PMID: 32178233; PMCID: PMC7139934.
14. Fraunfelder FW, Yang HK. Association between bortezomib therapy and eyelid chalazia. JAMA Ophthalmol. 2016;134(1):88–90. https://doi.org/10.1001/jamaophthalmol.2015.3963. PMID: 26469392.
15. Demirci H, Frueh BR, Nelson CC. Marcus Gunn jaw-winking synkinesis: clinical features and management. Ophthalmology. 2010;117(7):1447–52. https://doi.org/10.1016/j.ophtha.2009.11.014. Epub 2010 Feb 25. PMID: 20188419.
16. Fasanella RM, Servat J. Levator resection for minimal ptosis: another simplified operation. Arch Ophthalmol. 1961;65:493–6. https://doi.org/10.1001/archopht.1961.01840020495005. PMID: 13698293.
17. Vyas KS, Kim U, North WD, Stewart D. Frontalis sling for the treatment of congenital ptosis. Eplasty. 2016;16:ic12. PMID: 27110323; PMCID: PMC4828926.
18. Frueh BR. The mechanistic classification of ptosis. Ophthalmology. 1980;87(10):1019–21. https://doi.org/10.1016/s0161-6420(80)35135-x. PMID: 7017524.
19. Maloney WF, Younge BR, Moyer NJ. Evaluation of the causes and accuracy of pharmacologic localization in Horner's syndrome. Am J Ophthalmol. 1980;90(3):394–402. https://doi.org/10.1016/s0002-9394(14)74924-4. PMID: 7425056.
20. Sabbagh MA, De Lott LB, Trobe JD. Causes of Horner syndrome: a study of 318 patients. J Neuroophthalmol. 2020;40(3):362–9. https://doi.org/10.1097/WNO.0000000000000844. PMID: 31609831; PMCID: PMC7148177.
21. Bartley GB, Fatourechi V, Kadrmas EF, Jacobsen SJ, Ilstrup DM, Garrity JA, Gorman CA. Clinical features of Graves' ophthalmopathy in an incidence cohort. Am J Ophthalmol. 1996;121(3):284–90. https://doi.org/10.1016/s0002-9394(14)70276-4.
22. Bartley GB, Gorman CA. Diagnostic criteria for Graves' ophthalmopathy. Am J Ophthalmol. 1995;119(6):792–5. https://doi.org/10.1016/s0002-9394(14)72787-4.
23. Cant JS, Lewis DR, Harrison MT. Treatment of dysthyroid ophthalmopathy with local guanethidine. Br J Ophthalmol. 1969;53(4):233–8. https://doi.org/10.1136/bjo.53.4.233. PMID: 5818669; PMCID: PMC1207305.
24. Wesley RE, Bond JB. Upper eyelid retraction from inferior rectus restriction in dysthyroid orbit disease. Ann Ophthalmol. 1987;19(1):34–6, 40. PMID: 3827067.
25. Byun JS, Lee JK. Relationships between eyelid position and levator-superior rectus complex and inferior rectus muscle in patients with Graves' orbitopathy with unilateral upper eyelid retraction. Graefes Arch Clin Exp Ophthalmol. 2018;256(10):2001–8. https://doi.org/10.1007/s00417-018-4056-z. Epub 2018 Jun 29. PMID: 29959506.
26. Cruz AA, Ribeiro SF, Garcia DM, Akaishi PM, Pinto CT. Graves upper eyelid retraction. Surv Ophthalmol. 2013;58(1):63–76. https://doi.org/10.1016/j.survophthal.2012.02.007. PMID: 23217588.
27. Lee DC, Young SM, Kim YD, Woo KI. Course of upper eyelid retraction in thyroid eye disease. Br J Ophthalmol. 2020;104(2):254–9. https://doi.org/10.1136/bjophthalmol-2018-313578. Epub 2019 May 11. PMID: 31079052.
28. Ribeiro SF, Shekhovtsova M, Duarte AF, Velasco Cruz AA. Graves lower eyelid retraction. Ophthalmic Plast Reconstr Surg. 2016;32(3):161–9. https://doi.org/10.1097/IOP.0000000000000613. PMID: 26784547.
29. Guastella C, di Furia D, Torretta S, Ibba TM, Pignataro L, Accorona R. Upper eyelid retraction in Graves' ophthalmopathy: our surgical experience on 153 cases of full-thickness anterior blepharotomy with mullerectomy. Aesthet Plast Surg. 2022;46(4):1713–21. https://doi.org/10.1007/s00266-022-02770-5. Epub 2022 Feb 7. PMID: 35129648.
30. Perry JD, Hwang CJ. Invited discussion on: "upper eyelid retraction in Graves' ophthalmopathy: our surgical experience on 153 cases of full-thickness anterior blepharotomy with mullerectomy". Aesthet Plast Surg. 2022;46(4):1722–3. https://doi.org/10.1007/s00266-022-02875-x. Epub 2022 Apr 18. PMID: 35437666.
31. Osaki TH, Monteiro LG, Osaki MH. Management of eyelid retraction related to thyroid eye disease. Taiwan J Ophthalmol. 2022;12(1):12–21. https://

doi.org/10.4103/tjo.tjo_57_21. PMID: 35399960; PMCID: PMC8988987.

32. Zoumalan CI, Lisman RD. Evaluation and management of unilateral ptosis and avoiding contralateral ptosis. Aesthet Surg J. 2010;30(3):320–8. https://doi.org/10.1177/1090820X10374108. PMID: 20601555
33. Chen AD, Lai YW, Lai HT, Huang SH, Lee SS, Chang KP, Lai CS. The impact of Hering's law in blepharoptosis: literature review. Ann Plast Surg. 2016;76(Suppl 1):S96–100. https://doi.org/10.1097/SAP.0000000000000689. PMID: 26808763.
34. Gupta JS, Jain IS, Kumar K. Lid-retraction secondary to contralateral ptosis. Br J Ophthalmol. 1964;48(11):626–7. https://doi.org/10.1136/bjo.48.11.626. PMID: 14224935; PMCID: PMC506030.
35. Jain IS. Lid retraction in the non-paretic eye in acquired ophthalmoplegia. Br J Ophthalmol. 1963;47(12):757–9. https://doi.org/10.1136/bjo.47.12.757. PMID: 14186873; PMCID: PMC505887.
36. Bartley GB. The differential diagnosis and classification of eyelid retraction. Ophthalmology. 1996;103(1):168–76. https://doi.org/10.1016/s0161-6420(96)30744-6.
37. Galetta SL, Gray LG, Raps EC, Grossman RI, Schatz NJ. Unilateral ptosis and contralateral eyelid retraction from a thalamic-midbrain infarction. Magnetic resonance imaging correlation. J Clin Neuroophthalmol. 1993;13(4):221–4. PMID: 8113431.
38. Galetta SL, Gray LG, Raps EC, Schatz NJ. Pretectal eyelid retraction and lag. Ann Neurol. 1993;33(5):554–7. https://doi.org/10.1002/ana.410330522. PMID: 8498833.
39. Ortiz JF, Eissa-Garces A, Ruxmohan S, Cuenca V, Kaur M, Fabara SP, Khurana M, Parwani J, Paez M, Anwar F, Tamton H, Cueva W. Understanding Parinaud's syndrome. Brain Sci. 2021;11(11):1469. https://doi.org/10.3390/brainsci11111469. PMID: 34827468; PMCID: PMC8615667.
40. Friedman DI, Jankovic J, McCrary JA 3rd. Neuro-ophthalmic findings in progressive supranuclear palsy. J Clin Neuroophthalmol. 1992;12(2):104–9. PMID: 1629370.
41. Shome D, Toshniwal S, Jain V, Natarajan S, Vemuganti GK. Isolated upper eyelid retraction: a sign of idiopathic inflammatory orbital disease. Ophthalmic Plast Reconstr Surg. 2008;24(1):58–60. https://doi.org/10.1097/IOP.0b013e3181602213. PMID: 18209649.
42. Horn AK, Büttner-Ennever JA. Brainstem circuits controlling lid-eye coordination in monkey. Prog Brain Res. 2008;171:87–95. https://doi.org/10.1016/S0079-6123(08)00612-2. PMID: 18718286.
43. Jackson WP. Incidence of signs usually connected with thyrotoxicosis with special reference to lid lag. Br Med J. 1949;2(4632):847. https://doi.org/10.1136/bmj.2.4632.847. PMID: 18143463; PMCID: PMC2051467.
44. Harvey JT, Anderson RL. Lid lag and lagophthalmos: a clarification of terminology. Ophthalmic Surg. 1981;12(5):338–40. PMID: 7266976.
45. Gaddipati RV, Meyer DR. Eyelid retraction, lid lag, lagophthalmos, and von Graefe's sign quantifying the eyelid features of Graves' ophthalmopathy. Ophthalmology. 2008;115(6):1083–8. https://doi.org/10.1016/j.ophtha.2007.07.027. Epub 2007 Sep 27. PMID: 17900690.
46. Rice CD, Gray LD. Isolated levator myositis. Ophthalmic Plast Reconstr Surg. 1988;4(3):167–70. https://doi.org/10.1097/00002341-198804030-00009. PMID: 3154738.
47. Keane JR. The pretectal syndrome: 206 patients. Neurology. 1990;40(4):684–90. https://doi.org/10.1212/wnl.40.4.684. PMID: 2320246.
48. Galetta SL, Raps EC, Liu GT, Saito NG, Kline LB. Eyelid lag without eyelid retraction in pretectal disease. J Neuroophthalmol. 1996;16(2):96–8. PMID: 8797164.
49. Keane JR. Lid-lag in the Guillain-Barré syndrome. Arch Neurol. 1975;32(7):478–9. https://doi.org/10.1001/archneur.1975.00490490082009. PMID: 1137515.
50. Neetens A, Smet H. Lid lag in Guillain-Barré-Strohl syndrome. Arch Neurol. 1988;45(9):1046–7. https://doi.org/10.1001/archneur.1988.00520330142024. PMID: 3415523.
51. Kim N, Hwang JM. Isolated transient eyelid lag in multiple sclerosis. Neurol Sci. 2015;36(9):1711–2. https://doi.org/10.1007/s10072-015-2246-6. Epub 2015 May 16. PMID: 25981227.
52. Han SY, Kim US. Ocular myasthenia gravis presenting as transient eyelid lag. Graefes Arch Clin Exp Ophthalmol. 2013;251(9):2281–2. https://doi.org/10.1007/s00417-013-2279-6. Epub 2013 Feb 15. PMID: 23412394.
53. Taylor JR, Elsworth JD, Lawrence MS, Sladek JR, Roth RH, Redmond DE Jr. Spontaneous blink rates correlate with dopamine levels in the caudate nucleus of MPTP-treated monkeys. Exp Neurol. 1999;158(1):214–20. https://doi.org/10.1006/exnr.1999.7093. PMID: 10448434.
54. Sforza C, Rango M, Galante D, Bresolin N, Ferrario VF. Spontaneous blinking in healthy persons: an optoelectronic study of eyelid motion. Ophthalmic Physiol Opt. 2008;28(4):345–53. https://doi.org/10.1111/j.1475-1313.2008.00577.x. PMID: 18565090.
55. Nagino K, Sung J, Oyama G, Hayano M, Hattori N, Okumura Y, Fujio K, Akasaki Y, Huang T, Midorikawa-Inomata A, Fujimoto K, Eguchi A, Hurramhon S, Miura M, Ohno M, Hirosawa K, Morooka Y, Murakami A, Kobayashi H, Inomata

T. Prevalence and characteristics of dry eye disease in Parkinson's disease: a systematic review and meta-analysis. Sci Rep. 2022;12(1):18348. https://doi.org/10.1038/s41598-022-22037-y. PMID: 36319814; PMCID: PMC9626467.

56. Nuuttila S, Eklund M, Joutsa J, Jaakkola E, Mäkinen E, Honkanen EA, Lindholm K, Noponen T, Ihalainen T, Murtomäki K, Nojonen T, Levo R, Mertsalmi T, Scheperjans F, Kaasinen V. Diagnostic accuracy of glabellar tap sign for Parkinson's disease. J Neural Transm (Vienna). 2021;128(11):1655–61. https://doi.org/10.1007/s00702-021-02391-3. Epub 2021 Jul 30. PMID: 34328563; PMCID: PMC8536581.
57. Kimura N, Watanabe A, Suzuki K, Toyoda H, Hakamata N, Fukuoka H, Washimi Y, Arahata Y, Takeda A, Kondo M, Mizuno T, Kinoshita S. Measurement of spontaneous blinks in patients with Parkinson's disease using a new high-speed blink analysis system. J Neurol Sci. 2017;380:200–4. https://doi.org/10.1016/j.jns.2017.07.035. Epub 2017 Jul 29. PMID: 28870569.
58. Bologna M, Agostino R, Gregori B, Belvisi D, Ottaviani D, Colosimo C, Fabbrini G, Berardelli A. Voluntary, spontaneous and reflex blinking in patients with clinically probable progressive supranuclear palsy. Brain. 2009;132(Pt 2):502–10. https://doi.org/10.1093/brain/awn317. Epub 2008 Nov 29. PMID: 19043083.
59. Goldstein JE, Cogan DG. Apraxia of lid opening. Arch Ophthalmol. 1965;73:155–9. https://doi.org/10.1001/archopht.1965.00970030157003. PMID: 14237780.
60. Esteban A, Traba A, Prieto J. Eyelid movements in health and disease. The supranuclear impairment of the palpebral motility. Neurophysiol Clin. 2004;34(1):3–15. https://doi.org/10.1016/j.neucli.2004.01.002. PMID: 15030796.
61. Nersesjan V, Martens P, Truelsen T, Kondziella D. After stroke, apraxia of eyelid opening is associated with high mortality and right hemispheric infarction. J Neurol Sci. 2020;418:117145. https://doi.org/10.1016/j.jns.2020.117145. Epub 2020 Sep 19. PMID: 33007692.
62. van Koningsbruggen MG, Peelen MV, Davies E, Rafal RD. Neural control of voluntary eye closure: a case study and an fMRI investigation of blinking and winking. Behav Neurol. 2012;25(2):103–9. https://doi.org/10.3233/ben-2011-0355. PMID: 22530264; PMCID: PMC5294255.
63. Defazio G, Abbruzzese G, Aniello MS, Bloise M, Crisci C, Eleopra R, Fabbrini G, Girlanda P, Liguori R, Macerollo A, Marinelli L, Martino D, Morgante F, Santoro L, Tinazzi M, Berardelli A. Environmental risk factors and clinical phenotype in familial and sporadic primary blepharospasm. Neurology. 2011;77(7):631–7. https://doi.org/10.1212/WNL.0b013e3182299e13. Epub 2011 Jul 20. PMID: 21775731.
64. Martino D, Defazio G, Alessio G, Abbruzzese G, Girlanda P, Tinazzi M, Fabbrini G, Marinelli L, Majorana G, Buccafusca M, Vacca L, Livrea P, Berardelli A. Relationship between eye symptoms and blepharospasm: a multicenter case-control study. Mov Disord. 2005;20(12):1564–70. https://doi.org/10.1002/mds.20635. PMID: 16092106.
65. Defazio G, Martino D, Abbruzzese G, Girlanda P, Tinazzi M, Fabbrini G, Colosimo C, Aniello MS, Avanzino L, Buccafusca M, Majorana G, Trompetto C, Livrea P, Berardelli A. Influence of coffee drinking and cigarette smoking on the risk of primary late onset blepharospasm: evidence from a multicentre case control study. J Neurol Neurosurg Psychiatry. 2007;78(8):877–9. https://doi.org/10.1136/jnnp.2007.119891. Epub 2007 Jun 19. PMID: 17578856; PMCID: PMC2117757.
66. Molloy A, Williams L, Kimmich O, Butler JS, Beiser I, McGovern E, O'Riordan S, Reilly RB, Walsh C, Hutchinson M. Sun exposure is an environmental factor for the development of blepharospasm. J Neurol Neurosurg Psychiatry. 2016;87(4):420–4. https://doi.org/10.1136/jnnp-2014-310266. Epub 2015 Apr 22. PMID: 25904812.
67. Valls-Sole J, Defazio G. Blepharospasm: update on epidemiology, clinical aspects, and pathophysiology. Front Neurol. 2016;7:45. https://doi.org/10.3389/fneur.2016.00045. PMID: 27064462; PMCID: PMC4814756.
68. Ma H, Qu J, Ye L, Shu Y, Qu Q. Blepharospasm, oromandibular dystonia, and Meige syndrome: clinical and genetic update. Front Neurol. 2021;29(12):630221. https://doi.org/10.3389/fneur.2021.630221. PMID: 33854473; PMCID: PMC8039296.
69. Peckham EL, Lopez G, Shamim EA, Richardson SP, Sanku S, Malkani R, Stacy M, Mahant P, Crawley A, Singleton A, Hallett M. Clinical features of patients with blepharospasm: a report of 240 patients. Eur J Neurol. 2011;18(3):382–6. https://doi.org/10.1111/j.1468-1331.2010.03161.x. PMID: 20649903; PMCID: PMC3934127.
70. Berman BD, Groth CL, Sillau SH, Pirio Richardson S, Norris SA, Junker J, Brüggemann N, Agarwal P, Barbano RL, Espay AJ, Vizcarra JA, Klein C, Bäumer T, Loens S, Reich SG, Vidailhet M, Bonnet C, Roze E, Jinnah HA, Perlmutter JS. Risk of spread in adult-onset isolated focal dystonia: a prospective international cohort study. J Neurol Neurosurg Psychiatry. 2020;91(3):314–20. https://doi.org/10.1136/jnnp-2019-321794. Epub 2019 Dec 17. PMID: 31848221; PMCID: PMC7024047.
71. Pandey S, Sharma S. Meige's syndrome: history, epidemiology, clinical features, pathogenesis and treatment. J Neurol Sci. 2017;372:162–70. https://doi.org/10.1016/j.jns.2016.11.053. Epub 2016 Nov 23. PMID: 28017205.

72. Grandas F, Traba A, Perez-Sanchez JR, Esteban A. Pretarsal blepharospasm: clinical and electromyographic characteristics. Clin Neurophysiol. 2020;131(7):1678–85. https://doi.org/10.1016/j.clinph.2020.03.016. Epub 2020 Apr 2. PMID: 32280019.
73. Castelbuono A, Miller NR. Spontaneous remission in patients with essential blepharospasm and Meige syndrome. Am J Ophthalmol. 1998;126(3):432–5. https://doi.org/10.1016/s0002-9394(98)00099-3. PMID: 9744377.
74. Yen MT. Developments in the treatment of benign essential blepharospasm. Curr Opin Ophthalmol. 2018;29(5):440–4. https://doi.org/10.1097/ICU.0000000000000500. PMID: 29916840.
75. Baker MJ, Harrison AR, Lee MS. Possible role of frankincense in the treatment of benign essential blepharospasm. Am J Ophthalmol Case Rep. 2023;30:101848. https://doi.org/10.1016/j.ajoc.2023.101848.
76. Shin HJ, Lee SH, Ha TJ, Song WC, Koh KS. Intramuscular nerve distribution in the medial rectus muscle and its clinical implications. Curr Eye Res. 2019;44(5):522–6. https://doi.org/10.1080/02713683.2018.1562556. Epub 2019 Feb 27. PMID: 30624996.
77. Fernández Cabrera A, Suárez-Quintanilla J. Anatomy, head and neck: eye lateral rectus muscle. In: StatPearls [Internet]. Treasure Island (FL): StatPearls Publishing; 2022; 2023 Jan–. PMID: 30969543.
78. Shumway CL, Motlagh M, Wade M. Anatomy, head and neck: eye superior rectus muscle. In: StatPearls [Internet]. Treasure Island (FL): StatPearls Publishing; 2022; 2023 Jan–. PMID: 30252323.
79. Shumway CL, Motlagh M, Wade M. Anatomy, head and neck: eye inferior rectus muscle. In: StatPearls [Internet]. Treasure Island (FL): StatPearls Publishing; 2022; 2023 Jan–. PMID: 30085520.
80. Shumway CL, Motlagh M, Wade M. Anatomy, head and neck: eye medial rectus muscles. In: StatPearls [Internet]. Treasure Island (FL): StatPearls Publishing; 2022; 2023 Jan–. PMID: 30085568.
81. Headache Classification Committee of the International Headache Society (IHS). The international classification of headache disorders, 3rd edition (beta version). Cephalalgia. 2013;33(9):629–808. https://doi.org/10.1177/0333102413485658. PMID: 23771276.
82. Mark AS, Casselman J, Brown D, Sanchez J, Kolsky M, Larsen TC 3rd, Lavin P, Ferraraccio B. Ophthalmoplegic migraine: reversible enhancement and thickening of the cisternal segment of the oculomotor nerve on contrast-enhanced MR images. AJNR Am J Neuroradiol. 1998;19(10):1887–91. PMID: 9874541; PMCID: PMC8337745.
83. Bharucha DX, Campbell TB, Valencia I, Hardison HH, Kothare SV. MRI findings in pediatric ophthalmoplegic migraine: a case report and literature review. Pediatr Neurol. 2007;37(1):59–63. https://doi.org/10.1016/j.pediatrneurol.2007.03.008.
84. Lal V, Sahota P, Singh P, Gupta A, Prabhakar S. Ophthalmoplegia with migraine in adults: is it ophthalmoplegic migraine? Headache. 2009;49(6):838–50. https://doi.org/10.1111/j.1526--4610.2009.01405.x. Epub 2009 Apr 6. PMID: 19389140.
85. La Mantia L, Curone M, Rapoport AM, Bussone G, International Headache Society. Tolosa-Hunt syndrome: critical literature review based on IHS 2004 criteria. Cephalalgia. 2006;26(7):772–81. https://doi.org/10.1111/j.1468-2982.2006.01115.x. PMID: 16776691.
86. Jaretzki A 3rd, Barohn RJ, Ernstoff RM, Kaminski HJ, Keesey JC, Penn AS, Sanders DB. Myasthenia gravis: recommendations for clinical research standards. Task Force of the Medical Scientific Advisory Board of the Myasthenia Gravis Foundation of America. Ann Thorac Surg. 2000;70(1):327–34. https://doi.org/10.1016/s0003-4975(00)01595-2. PMID: 10921745.
87. Vincent A. Unravelling the pathogenesis of myasthenia gravis. Nat Rev Immunol. 2002;2(10):797–804. https://doi.org/10.1038/nri916. PMID: 12360217.
88. Phillips WD, Vincent A. Pathogenesis of myasthenia gravis: update on disease types, models, and mechanisms. F1000Res. 2016;5:F1000 Faculty Rev-1513. https://doi.org/10.12688/f1000research.8206.1. PMID: 27408701; PMCID: PMC4926737.
89. Giannoccaro MP, Di Stasi V, Zanesini C, Donadio V, Avoni P, Liguori R. Sensitivity and specificity of single-fibre EMG in the diagnosis of ocular myasthenia varies accordingly to clinical presentation. J Neurol. 2020;267(3):739–45. https://doi.org/10.1007/s00415-019-09631-3. Epub 2019 Nov 16. PMID: 31734908.
90. Singman EL, Matta NS, Silbert DI. Use of the Cogan lid twitch to identify myasthenia gravis. J Neuroophthalmol. 2011;31(3):239–40. https://doi.org/10.1097/WNO.0b013e3182224b92. PMID: 21654336.
91. Smith JL. Lids position in neuro-ophthalmological. J Clin Neuroophthalmol. 1987;7(3):149–50. https://collections.lib.utah.edu/ark:/87278/s6bp37xn/226458.
92. Golnik KC, Pena R, Lee AG, Eggenberger ER. An ice test for the diagnosis of myasthenia gravis. Ophthalmology. 1999;106(7):1282–6. https://doi.org/10.1016/S0161-6420(99)00709-5. PMID: 10406606.
93. Marinos E, Buzzard K, Fraser CL, Reddel S. Evaluating the temperature effects of ice and heat tests on ptosis due to Myasthenia Gravis. Eye (Lond). 2018;32(8):1387–91. https://doi.org/10.1038/s41433-018-0101-8. Epub 2018 May 10. PMID: 29743585; PMCID: PMC6085283.
94. Kansu T, Subutay N. Lid retraction in myasthenia gravis. J Clin Neuroophthalmol. 1987;7(3):145–50. PMID: 2958506.

95. Behbehani R. Ocular myasthenia gravis: a current overview. Eye Brain. 2023;15:1–13. https://doi.org/10.2147/EB.S389629. PMID: 36778719; PMCID: PMC9911903.
96. Liu X, Zhou W, Hu J, Hu M, Gao W, Zhang S, Zeng W. Prognostic predictors of remission in ocular myasthenia after thymectomy. J Thorac Dis. 2020;12(3):422–30. https://doi.org/10.21037/jtd.2020.01.17. PMID: 32274108; PMCID: PMC7139038.
97. Jiao L, Li H, Guo S. Eculizumab treatment for myasthenia gravis subgroups: 2021 update. J Neuroimmunol. 2022;362:577767. https://doi.org/10.1016/j.jneuroim.2021.577767. Epub 2021 Nov 18. PMID: 34823117.
98. Heo YA. Efgartigimod: first approval. Drugs. 2022;82(3):341–8. https://doi.org/10.1007/s40265-022-01678-3. Erratum in: Drugs. 2022 Apr;82(5):611. PMID: 35179720; PMCID: PMC8855644.
99. Narayanaswami P, Sanders DB, Wolfe G, Benatar M, Cea G, Evoli A, Gilhus NE, Illa I, Kuntz NL, Massey J, Melms A, Murai H, Nicolle M, Palace J, Richman D, Verschuuren J. International consensus guidance for management of myasthenia gravis: 2020 update. Neurology. 2021;96(3):114–22. https://doi.org/10.1212/WNL.0000000000011124. Epub 2020 Nov 3. PMID: 33144515; PMCID: PMC7884987.
100. von Noorden GK, Murray E, Wong SY. Superior oblique paralysis. A review of 270 cases. Arch Ophthalmol. 1986;104(12):1771–6. https://doi.org/10.1001/archopht.1986.01050240045037. PMID: 3789976.
101. Manchandia AM, Demer JL. Sensitivity of the three-step test in diagnosis of superior oblique palsy. J AAPOS. 2014;18(6):567–71. https://doi.org/10.1016/j.jaapos.2014.08.007. Epub 2014 Nov 12. PMID: 25459202; PMCID: PMC4268244.
102. Moster ML, Bosley TM, Slavin ML, Rubin SE. Thyroid ophthalmopathy presenting as superior oblique paresis. J Clin Neuroophthalmol. 1992;12(2):94–7. PMID: 1629377.
103. Roper-Hall G. The Hess screen test. Am Orthopt J. 2006;56:166–74. https://doi.org/10.3368/aoj.56.1.166. PMID: 21149145.
104. Thorisdottir RL, Sundgren J, Sheikh R, Blohmé J, Hammar B, Kjellström S, Malmsjö M. Comparison of a new digital KM screen test with conventional Hess and Lees screen tests in the mapping of ocular deviations. J AAPOS. 2018;22(4):277–280.e6. https://doi.org/10.1016/j.jaapos.2018.02.007. Epub 2018 May 28. PMID: 29852255.
105. Horn AK. The reticular formation. Prog Brain Res. 2006;151:127–55. https://doi.org/10.1016/S0079-6123(05)51005-7. PMID: 16221588.
106. Adamczyk C, Horn AKE. Reticular formation: eye movements, gaze and blinks. In: Mai JK, Paxinos G, editors. The human nervous system. 3rd ed) Chapter 9. Elsevier Inc.; 2012. p. 328–66.
107. Remington LA. Extraocular muscles. In: Clinical anatomy and physiology of the visual system. Elsevier; 2012. p. 182–201. https://doi.org/10.1016/b978-1-4377-1926-0.10010-4.
108. Barendregt M, Harvey BM, Rokers B, Dumoulin SO. Transformation from a retinal to a cyclopean representation in human visual cortex. Curr Biol. 2015;25(15):1982–7. https://doi.org/10.1016/j.cub.2015.06.003. Epub 2015 Jul 2.
109. Sherrington CS. Experimental note on two movements of the eye. J Physiol. 1894;17(1–2):27–9. https://doi.org/10.1113/jphysiol.1894.sp000517. PMID: 16992206; PMCID: PMC1514570.
110. Jampel RS. The fundamental principle of the action of the oblique ocular muscles. Am J Ophthalmol. 1970;69(4):623–38. https://doi.org/10.1016/0002-9394(70)91631-4. PMID: 4985568.
111. Vinny PW, Lal V. Gaze disorders: a clinical approach. Neurol India. 2016;64(1):121–8. https://doi.org/10.4103/0028-3886.173627. PMID: 26755003.
112. Termsarasab P, Thammongkolchai T, Rucker JC, Frucht SJ. The diagnostic value of saccades in movement disorder patients: a practical guide and review. J Clin Mov Disord. 2015;2:14. https://doi.org/10.1186/s40734-015-0025-4. PMID: 26788350; PMCID: PMC4710978.
113. Optican LM. The role of omnipause neurons: why glycine? Prog Brain Res. 2008;171:115–21. https://doi.org/10.1016/S0079-6123(08)00615-8. PMID: 18718289; PMCID: PMC2750832.
114. Büttner U, Büttner-Ennever JA, Henn V. Vertical eye movement related unit activity in the rostral mesencephalic reticular formation of the alert monkey. Brain Res. 1977;130(2):239–52. https://doi.org/10.1016/0006-8993(77)90273-6. PMID: 406969.
115. Henn V, Lang W, Hepp K, Reisine H. Experimental gaze palsies in monkeys and their relation to human pathology. Brain. 1984;107(Pt 2):619–36. https://doi.org/10.1093/brain/107.2.619. PMID: 6722520.
116. Sanchez K, Rowe FJ. Role of neural integrators in oculomotor systems: a systematic narrative literature review. Acta Ophthalmol. 2018;96(2):e111–8. https://doi.org/10.1111/aos.13307. Epub 2016 Nov 22. PMID: 27874249.
117. Cogan DG. A type of congenital ocular motor apraxia presenting jerky head movements. Am J Ophthalmol. 1953;36(4):433–41. https://doi.org/10.1016/0002-9394(53)90553-4. PMID: 13030653.
118. Chung PW, Moon HS, Song HS, Kim YB. Ocular motor apraxia after sequential bilateral striatal infarctions. J Clin Neurol. 2006;2(2):134–6. https://doi.org/10.3988/jcn.2006.2.2.134. Epub 2006 Jun 20. PMID: 20396497; PMCID: PMC2854953.
119. Briand KA, Strallow D, Hening W, Poizner H, Sereno AB. Control of voluntary and reflexive saccades in Parkinson's disease. Exp Brain Res. 1999;129(1):38–48. https://doi.org/10.1007/s002210050934. PMID: 10550501.

120. White OB, Saint-Cyr JA, Tomlinson RD, Sharpe JA. Ocular motor deficits in Parkinson's disease. II. Control of the saccadic and smooth pursuit systems. Brain. 1983;106(Pt 3):571–87. https://doi.org/10.1093/brain/106.3.571. PMID: 6640270.
121. Wadia NH, Swami RK. A new form of heredo-familial spinocerebellar degeneration with slow eye movements (nine families). Brain. 1971;94(2):359–74. https://doi.org/10.1093/brain/94.2.359. PMID: 5571047.
122. Averbuch-Heller L, Kori AA, Rottach KG, Dell'Osso LF, Remler BF, Leigh RJ. Dysfunction of pontine omnipause neurons causes impaired fixation: macrosaccadic oscillations with a unilateral pontine lesion. Neuroophthalmology. 1996;16(2):99–106. https://doi.org/10.3109/01658109609009668.
123. Rufa A, Cerase A, De Santi L, Mandalà M, Nuti D, Giorgio A, Annunziata P. Impairment of vertical saccades from an acute pontine lesion in multiple sclerosis. J Neuroophthalmol. 2008;28(4):305–7. https://doi.org/10.1097/WNO.0b013e318183bd26. PMID: 19145131.
124. Thier P, Ilg UJ. The neural basis of smooth-pursuit eye movements. Curr Opin Neurobiol. 2005;15(6):645–52. https://doi.org/10.1016/j.conb.2005.10.013. Epub 2005 Nov 3. PMID: 16271460.
125. Gibson AR, Horn KM, Pong M. Nucleus reticularis tegmenti pontis: a bridge between the basal ganglia and cerebellum for movement control. Exp Brain Res. 2023;241(5):1271–87. https://doi.org/10.1007/s00221-023-06574-0. Epub ahead of print. PMID: 37000205; PMCID: PMC10129968.
126. Chang T-P, Zee DS, Kheradmand A. Chapter 2. Technological Advances in testing the dizzy patient. In: Kesser BW, Tucker G, editors. Dizziness and vertigo across the lifespan. 1st ed. Elsevier; 2019. p. 9–30. https://doi.org/10.1016/b978-0-323-55136-6.00002-2.
127. Halmagyi GM, McGarvie LA, Strupp M. Nystagmus goggles: how to use them, what you find and what it means. Pract Neurol. 2020;20(6):446–50. https://doi.org/10.1136/practneurol-2020-002513. Epub 2020 Oct 28. PMID: 33115786.
128. Kattah JC, Talkad AV, Wang DZ, Hsieh YH, Newman-Toker DE. HINTS to diagnose stroke in the acute vestibular syndrome: three-step bedside oculomotor examination more sensitive than early MRI diffusion-weighted imaging. Stroke. 2009;40(11):3504–10. https://doi.org/10.1161/STROKEAHA.109.551234. Epub 2009 Sep 17. PMID: 19762709; PMCID: PMC4593511.
129. Frohman TC, Galetta S, Fox R, Solomon D, Straumann D, Filippi M, Zee D, Frohman EM. Pearls & Oy-sters: the medial longitudinal fasciculus in ocular motor physiology. Neurology. 2008;70(17):e57–67. https://doi.org/10.1212/01.wnl.0000310640.37810.b3. PMID: 18427066.
130. Srulijes K, Mack DJ, Klenk J, Schwickert L, Ihlen EA, Schwenk M, Lindemann U, Meyer M, Srijana KC, Hobert MA, Brockmann K, Wurster I, Pomper JK, Synofzik M, Schneider E, Ilg U, Berg D, Maetzler W, Becker C. Association between vestibulo-ocular reflex suppression, balance, gait, and fall risk in ageing and neurodegenerative disease: protocol of a one-year prospective follow-up study. BMC Neurol. 2015;15:192. https://doi.org/10.1186/s12883-015-0447-5. PMID: 26452640; PMCID: PMC4600299.
131. Furman JM. Optokinetic nystagmus. In: Aminoff MJ, Daroff RB, editors. Encyclopedia of the neurological sciences. 2nd ed. London: Elsevier/Academic Press; 2014. p. 687. https://doi.org/10.1016/b978-0-12-385157-4.00150-0.
132. Lee AG, Brazis PW. Localizing forms of nystagmus: symptoms, diagnosis, and treatment. Curr Neurol Neurosci Rep. 2006;6(5):414–20. https://doi.org/10.1007/s11910-996-0022-y. PMID: 16928352.
133. Sarvananthan N, Surendran M, Roberts EO, Jain S, Thomas S, Shah N, Proudlock FA, Thompson JR, McLean RJ, Degg C, Woodruff G, Gottlob I. The prevalence of nystagmus: the Leicestershire nystagmus survey. Invest Ophthalmol Vis Sci. 2009;50(11):5201–6. https://doi.org/10.1167/iovs.09-3486. Epub 2009 May 20. PMID: 19458336.
134. Goila AK, Pawar M. The diagnosis of brain death. Indian J Crit Care Med. 2009;13(1):7–11. https://doi.org/10.4103/0972-5229.53108. PMID: 19881172; PMCID: PMC2772257.
135. Yat-Ming Woo P, Takemura S, Ming-Yan Cheong A, Chi-Ho Chu A, Chan Y, Wong HT, Chan KY. Pendular seesaw nystagmus in a patient with a giant pituitary macroadenoma: pathophysiology and the role of the accessory optic system. J Neuroophthalmol. 2018;38(1):65–9. https://doi.org/10.1097/WNO.0000000000000575. PMID: 29135813.
136. Eggenberger ER. Delayed-onset seesaw nystagmus posttraumatic brain injury with bitemporal hemianopia. Ann N Y Acad Sci. 2002;956:588–91. https://doi.org/10.1111/j.1749-6632.2002.tb02890.x. PMID: 11960875.
137. Epstein JA, Moster ML, Spiritos M. Seesaw nystagmus following whole brain irradiation and intrathecal methotrexate. J Neuroophthalmol. 2001;21(4):264–5. https://doi.org/10.1097/00041327-200112000-00007. PMID: 11756856.
138. Chen Y, Morgan ML, Palau AE, Mudd JA, Lee AG, Barton JJ. Downbeat down south. Surv Ophthalmol. 2015;60(2):177–81. https://doi.org/10.1016/j.survophthal.2014.06.004. Epub 2014 Jul 2. PMID: 25109656.
139. Tilikete C, Milea D, Pierrot-Deseilligny C. Upbeat nystagmus from a demyelinating lesion in the caudal pons. J Neuroophthalmol. 2008;28(3):202–6. https://doi.org/10.1097/WNO.0b013e318183bd73. PMID: 18769284.
140. Konda S, Kamal S, Vickers A, Al Othman B, Kim JM. 2023. https://eyewiki.org/Nystagmus.
141. Penix K, Swanson MW, DeCarlo DK. Nystagmus in pediatric patients: interventions and patient-focused perspectives. Clin Ophthalmol. 2015;9:1527–36.

https://doi.org/10.2147/OPTH.S62786. PMID: 26345377; PMCID: PMC4551307.

142. Holmström G, Bondeson ML, Eriksson U, Åkerblom H, Larsson E. 'Congenital' nystagmus may hide various ophthalmic diagnoses. Acta Ophthalmol. 2014;92(5):412–6. https://doi.org/10.1111/aos.12250. Epub 2013 Jul 29. PMID: 23889849.
143. Brodsky MC, Dell'Osso LF. A unifying neurologic mechanism for infantile nystagmus. JAMA Ophthalmol. 2014;132(6):761–8. https://doi.org/10.1001/jamaophthalmol.2013.5833. PMID: 24525626.
144. Kim JS. Internuclear ophthalmoplegia as an isolated or predominant symptom of brainstem infarction. Neurology. 2004;62(9):1491–6. https://doi.org/10.1212/01.wnl.0000123093.37069.6d. PMID: 15136670.
145. Smith JW, Cogan DG. Internuclear ophthalmoplegia; a review of fifty-eight cases. AMA Arch Ophthalmol. 1959;61(5):687–94. PMID: 13636562.
146. Miley JT, Rodriguez GJ, Hernandez EM, Bundlie SR. Teaching NeuroImage: traumatic internuclear ophthalmoplegia. Neurology. 2008;70(1):e3–4. https://doi.org/10.1212/01.wnl.0000280462.85951.3c. PMID: 18166699.
147. Toral M, Haugsdal J, Wall M. Internuclear ophthalmoplegia. Eyerounds.org.posted June 8, 2017. Available from http://eyerounds.org/cases/252-internuclear ophthalmoplegia.htm.
148. Kleinsorge MT, Ebert A, Förster A, Weber CE, Roßmanith C, Platten M, Gass A, Eisele P. MRI topography of lesions related to internuclear ophthalmoplegia in patients with multiple sclerosis or ischemic stroke. J Neuroimaging. 2021;31(3):471–4. https://doi.org/10.1111/jon.12847. Epub 2021 Apr 1. PMID: 33793026.
149. Eggenberger E, Golnik K, Lee A, Santos R, Suntay A, Satana B, Vaphlades M, Stevens C, Kaufman D, Wall M, Kardon R. Prognosis of ischemic internuclear ophthalmoplegia. Ophthalmology. 2002;109(9):1676–8. https://doi.org/10.1016/s0161-6420(02)01118-1. PMID: 12208716.
150. Sharpe JA, Rosenberg MA, Hoyt WF, Daroff RB. Paralytic pontine exotropia. A sign of acute unilateral pontine gaze palsy and internuclear ophthalmoplegia. Neurology. 1974;24(11):1076–81. https://doi.org/10.1212/wnl.24.11.1076. PMID: 4472909.
151. Fiester P, Baig SA, Patel J, Rao D. An anatomic, imaging, and clinical review of the medial longitudinal fasciculus. J Clin Imaging Sci. 2020;10:83. https://doi.org/10.25259/JCIS_49_2020. PMID: 33408958; PMCID: PMC7771398.

20 Orbital Signs

20.1 Anatomical Considerations

The orbits, known as the eye sockets, are bony cavities located in the front of the skull and house the eyeballs and other associated structures. Orbits have proximity to paranasal sinuses and intracranial structures. The orbits are cone-shaped, wherein the medial walls are parallel while the lateral walls subtend an angle of 90°. The orbit volume is about 30 mL of which the eyeball contributes 6.5–7 mL. The mean anterior opening of the orbit is 35 mm high, 45 mm wide, and 45 mm deep [1].

The orbital rim protects the eyeball from injuries. The orbital rim is formed by the frontal bone superiorly, the zygomatic process of the frontal bone and the frontal process of the zygomatic bone laterally, the maxillary process of the frontal bone, and the frontal process of the maxillary bone medially. The inferior orbital rim is formed by the zygomatic and the maxillary bone.

The orbital cavity (Fig. 20.1) is formed by several skull bones, including the orbital plate of the frontal bone, which contributes to most of the orbital roof except posteriorly, where there is a small contribution by the lesser wind of the sphenoid, which harbours the optic canal. The orbit floor is formed by the maxillary bone, zygomatic and a small part of the orbital process of the palatine bone. It overlies the maxillary sinuses. The orbital plate of the maxillary bone is thin and vulnerable to fractures due to falls. From front to back, the medial wall of the orbit is formed by the frontal process of the maxillary bone, lacrimal bone, orbital plate of the ethmoid bone and the lesser wing of the sphenoid. The orbital plate of the ethmoid bone is called lamina papyracea. It is paper thin, is amenable to fractures and separates the paranasal sinuses from the intraorbital structures. The orbit's medial wall and the orbital plate of the maxilla are vulnerable to trauma. They may entrap the intraorbital contents, including the muscle sheaths. The medial rectus sheath in the medial wall fracture, the inferior oblique in the orbital floor fracture anteriorly, and the inferior rectus posteriorly (Fig. 20.1B). The lateral wall is thick and the strongest of all orbital walls and is formed by the zygomatic bone anteriorly and the greater wing of the sphenoid bone posteriorly. The main lacrimal gland is the most important structure in the lacrimal fossa near the roof of the orbit, located within the orbital rim, in the zygomatic process of the frontal bone. Orbital bones are covered with a loosely adherent tough connective tissue (periosteum) except at the orbital rim, fissures and the foramina where it is firmly adherent.

Many nerves, including the CN III, IV, and VI and branches of the CN V and blood vessels, including the ophthalmic artery, enter the orbit through Orbital Openings and Fissures. The most important nerve leaving the orbit is the optic nerve, which extends from the posterior surface of the sclera, courses through the intraorbital tis-

A. Gupta et al., *Ophthalmic Signs in Practice of Medicine*,
https://doi.org/10.1007/978-981-99-7923-3_20

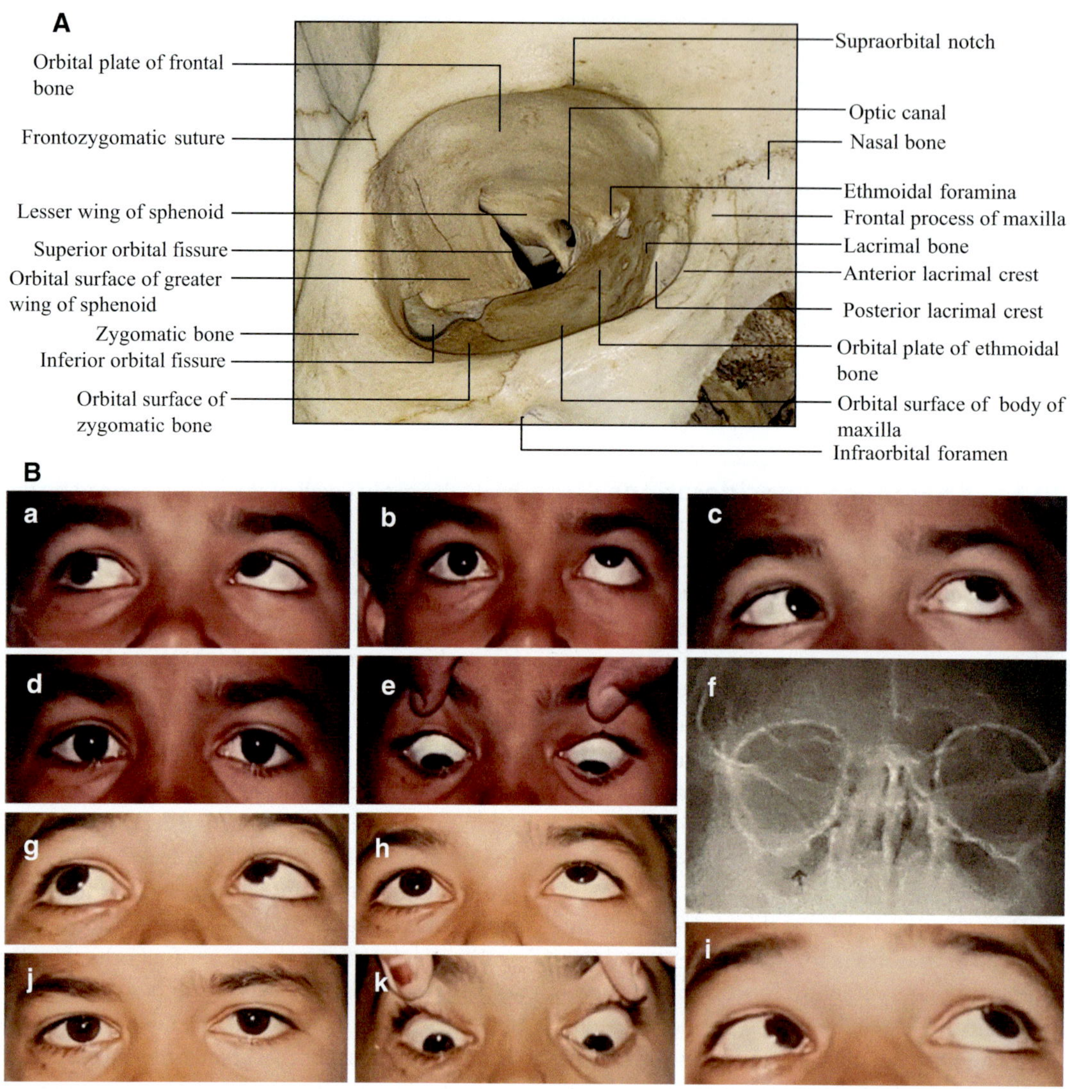

Fig. 20.1 (**A**) Anatomical aspects of the bones, fissures, and foramen. Image courtesy of Prof Daisy Sahney and Prof Anajli Agarwal, Department of Anatomy, Post Graduate Institute of Medical Education and Research, Chandigarh. (**B**) A child had a blowout fracture of the orbital floor of the right eye with entrapment of the inferior rectus. Right eye movements are restricted in the upgaze (**a**, **b**, and **c**). In the primary gaze, the eyes are parallel, and the downgaze is normal (**d** and **e**). An x-ray of the orbit shows a prolapse of the orbital contents into the right maxillary sinus (**f**). Following repair of the orbital floor, the movement of the right eye has improved in the upgaze (**g**, **h** and **i**). Postoperative primary position and downgaze are normal (**j** and **k**). Images courtesy of Dr. Kanwar Mohan, Dr. Kanwar Mohan's Squint Centre, Chandigarh

sues and exits the orbit through the optic foramen to pursue its intracranial course in the middle cranial fossa. The ophthalmic artery enters the orbit through the optic canal and lies below the optic nerve. In the optic canal, the optic nerve is in close proximity to the sphenoid and posterior ethmoidal air cells. The optic canal is a tight space, and the optic nerve is vulnerable to bone fracture and subdural hematoma formation due to indirect trauma sustained to the superior orbital rim.

20.1.1 Superior Orbital Fissure

The superior orbital fissure is located between the greater wing of the sphenoid laterally and its lesser wings medially and is the widest at its medial end. The optic canal is harboured by the lesser wing of the sphenoid. A tendinous ring of collagen, the annulus of Zinn, surrounds the optic canal and the middle part of the superior orbital fissure. Five extraocular muscles and the levator palpebrae superioris arise from the annulus. The inferior oblique muscle is an exception and arises in the anterior orbit from the orbital plate of the maxillary bone. The most important structures that course through the annulus are the optic nerve, the ophthalmic artery, and the sympathetic fibres. The superior and inferior divisions of CN III, nasociliary nerve, CN VI and the superior ophthalmic vein pass through the middle part of the superior orbital fissure. The parasympathetic fibres enter the orbit along with the inferior division of CN III. Other important nerves that pass through the lateral half of the superior orbital fissure include the lacrimal and frontal branches of the CN V, CN IV (trochlear nerve), and the superior ophthalmic vein [1]. The inferior ophthalmic vein exits the orbit from the medial end of the superior orbital fissure.

20.1.2 Inferior Orbital Fissure

The inferior orbital fissure is located between the maxilla and the greater wing of the sphenoid bone; it allows for the passage of nerves and blood vessels that includes the inferior ophthalmic vein that joins the pterygoid venous plexus, infraorbital nerve, infraorbital artery and vein, and the zygomatic branch of the maxillary division of CN V. Orbital cavity communicates with the infratemporal fossa and the pterygoid fossa through the inferior orbital fissure [2]. The infraorbital nerve and vessels course through the infraorbital groove and exit the orbit through the infraorbital foramen located just below the orbital rim.

20.1.3 Contents of the Orbit

Major contents of the orbit include the eyeball, the extraocular muscles, nerves, vessels, connective tissue and fat. An orbit is a confined space, and any increase in the volume of its contents—by inflammation, hemorrhage, infiltrations, tumours or vascular malformations pushes (protrudes) the eyeball forward. It is called proptosis if there is an abnormal or pathological protrusion. The term exophthalmos is used specifically in the context of thyroid eye disease.

20.1.4 Spaces of the Orbit

There are three major orbital spaces. These are the (1) intraconal space, the space behind the eyeball and enclosed by the extraocular muscles and their intermuscular connective tissue septa; (2) the extraconal (peripheral orbital) space lies outside the muscle cone and extends up to the orbital bones' periosteum, bound anteriorly by the orbital septum; and (3) the subperiosteal space lies between the orbital bones and the periorbita. In addition to these spaces in the orbital cavity, the subarachnoid space surrounds the optic nerve and the subtenon space between the eyeball and the tenon's capsule.

20.1.5 Spaces of the Orbit and Orbital Pathologies

As stated above, the orbit is a confined space, and any lesion in orbit tends to push the eyeball forward and, in the direction, opposite the pathology's site. How the eyeball is proptosed or protrudes from the orbit depends on the location of the pathological lesion in the orbital spaces. Different lesions affect different spaces and help the physician narrow the differential diagnosis. Most of the vascular malformations, cavernous hemangiomas or tumours arising from the optic nerve (glioma) or its meningeal sheaths (optic nerve sheath meningioma) are located in the intraconal space, pushing the eyeball forward and causing an axial proptosis. Thyroid-associated orbitopathy expands the orbital spaces and the extraocular muscles and causes axial proptosis. Infiltrative lymphomas, pseudotumors, rhabdomyosarcoma (affects the extraocular muscle), and lacrimal gland lesions are present in the extraconal space. Such lesions cause asymmetric proptosis depending upon the site of the lesion. Lesions arising from the bones or extending from the sinuses lie in the subperiosteal space, where the periosteum forms a tough barrier to prevent the spread of malignancy or infection into the peripheral orbital space.

20.2 Measurement of the Proptosis

The protrusion of the eyeball is measured from the deepest point in the lateral orbital rim to the apex of the Cornea using Hertel's exophthalmometer. The normal values vary in different ethnic populations. Usually, up to 21 mm is taken as the upper limit of normal [3]. A difference of >2 mm between the two eyes is considered abnormal protrusion [3]. The mean normal values were 16.5 mm for adult white men and 18.5 mm for adult black men. Women had ~1 mm less than men [4]. They considered the normal range as 11.3–21.7 mm for white men and 12.3–24.7 mm for black men. Corresponding values for women were 10.7 to 20.1 mm (white) and 12.6–23 mm (black) [4]. Pseudoexophthalmosis may occur due to high myopia, buphthalmos, and total ophthalmoplegia [4]. Several factors, including age, gender, race, height, weight, interpupillary distance, and body mass index, may affect the normal exophthalmometry values [5]. The exophthalmometer values can be calculated using CT scans of the orbit with high accuracy, reproducibility, and concordant with the manual methods [6–8].

20.3 Orbital Signs

Many diseases produce distinct orbital signs that provide clues to the possible underlying severe systemic disorders, including thyroid eye disease, orbital inflammations, hemorrhage, benign or malignant tumors, infiltrative disorders, and vascular malformations. Orbital fractures are commonly associated with violent assault, non-violent facial trauma, and motor vehicle accidents [9, 10] and are not discussed in this chapter.

Nearly, 2/3rd of orbital lesions are benign, and 1/3rd are malignant [11]. Some common lesions in orbit are vasculogenic (cavernous hemangiomas, lymphangioma, orbital varix, and carotid-cavernous fistula), infiltrative lymphomas and leukaemia, inflammatory, thyroid-associated orbitopathy (TAO) and secondary orbital involvement from the neighbouring structures [11]. In a large series (excluding TAO) of orbital pathologies requiring biopsy over 20 years, inflammatory lesions simulating tumours were at 13%, lacrimal fossa lesions at 13% and leukaemia and lymphoma at 10% and vasculogenic lesions at 6%, half of which were due to cavernous hemangioma [12].

20.4 Thyroid Eye Disease

Graves' ophthalmopathy, thyroid associated orbitopathy, or thyroid eye disease affects nearly 25–50% of the patients with Graves' disease [13]. It is an autoimmune disorder of the thyroid gland characterized by the formation of antibodies against thyroid-stimulating hormone (thyrotropin) receptors (TSHR) and the insulin-like growth factors-1 receptor (IGF-1R). The antibodies against TSHR are either stimulating, blocking (these compete with the TSH to bind with the TSHR) or neutral [14]. In hyperthyroidism, stimulating antibodies are formed. Patients with hyperthyroidism present with tremors, heat sensitivity, loss of weight, loose motions, arrhythmias, anxiety, and visible goitre, among others. TED is the most prominent feature of Graves' disease.

20.4.1 Pathogenesis of Thyroid-Associated Orbitopathy

Thyrotropin (thyroid stimulating hormone, TSH) is secreted by the anterior pituitary gland, which binds with its receptors on the thyroid and regulates thyroid hormone production. TSHR are present in a variety of cells in extra thyroid tissues, including the orbital fibroblasts, adipocytes, osteoblasts, cardiomyocytes, and embryonic stem cells and likely regulate the growth of various organs [14]. Thyrotropin receptor-stimulating antibodies act as TSH agonists and stimulate thyroid hormone formation, resulting in hyperthyroidism. In orbit, these TSHR-Ab (TSH agonists) act on the orbital fibroblasts, converting them into adipocytes and producing hyaluronic acid (non-sulphated glycosaminoglycan, GAG) [15]. Fibroblasts are phenotypically a heterogeneous population of cells with different properties. When appropriately stimulated, the orbital fibroblasts that show CD 90+ surface marker (a stem cell marker), Thy-1(+), can differentiate into myofibroblasts. The Thy-1(−) fibroblasts differentiate into adipocytes [16]. Subsequently, connective tissue and adipose tissue specimens from patients with Graves' orbitopathy were found positive for the Thy-1 surface marker [17]. Hyaluronic acid is a hydrophilic compound that absorbs water and increases the volume of the extraocular muscles and the orbital adipose tissue [13]. The orbital fibroblasts also express insulin-like growth factor-1 receptors (IGF-1R) receptors. It is believed that genetic and epigenetic polymorphisms may account for nearly 30% of the risk of Graves' disease and orbitopathy [18].

Immunohistochemical studies in TAO have shown a perivascular collection of plasma cells and lymphocytes, diffuse fibrosis in massively swollen extraocular muscles with collection GAGs of fibroblastic origin [19].

The orbital fibroblasts are unique, showing an exaggerated response to TSH analogues and expressing inflammatory cytokines [20]. CD40-CD154 overexpression has been shown in the orbital fibroblasts of patients with TAO. CD 154 is a ligand for CD40 (expressed on the surface of antigen-presenting cells.) It is a protein belonging to the TNF-α superfamily and binds to CD 40 receptors. This pathway is involved not only in B-cell activation but also the T-cells activation. CD40-CD154 pathway leads to hyperexpression of IL6, IL8, and monocyte chemoattractant protein-1 (MCP-1) from the orbital fibroblasts [9, 10]. Cytokine IL-1β produces significantly more Il-6 and IL-8 from orbital fibroblasts in patients with TAO [9, 10].

The primary event in TAO is the activation of CD34+ fibroblasts. CD34+ fibroblasts are constitutively present in tissues in various organs, express MHC-class II antigens, and serve as antigen-presenting cells. In the normal orbital tissues, CD34+ fibroblasts are absent, and in patients with TAO, these likely get infiltrated from the circulation. The orbital fibroblasts express TSHR and the Insulin-like growth factor-1 receptor (IGF-1R). The orbital fibroblasts are activated by IGF-1R antibodies and the TSHR antibodies and differentiate into myofibroblasts and adipocytes. These cells also produce GAGs. The TSHR-stimulating antibodies bind the TSHR leading to the expression of thyrotropin, thyroglobulin, and thyroperoxidase (all thyroid antigens) by the activated orbital fibroblasts. The activated fibroblasts produce IL-6, IL-8, and MCP-1 and set up a chain of inflammatory reactions involving both the stimulation of B lymphocytes by T cells to produce antibodies by the plasma cells but also infiltration of T-cells mediated inflammation [11].

The levels of TSHR on thyrocytes (thyroid follicular cells) are 11 times higher than on the orbital fibroblasts taken from patients with thyroid-associated orbitopathy (TAO). At the same time, the levels of IGF-1R are three times higher in the orbital fibroblasts compared to control fibroblasts. On confocal microscopy, TSHR and IGF-1Rβ colocalize on the fibroblasts' surface perinuclear cytoplasm, suggesting that IGF-1R may play a major role in the TAO [21]. It has been shown that in TAO, IGF-1 enhances the expression of TSHR on the orbital fibroblasts [22].

Current understanding of the role of IGF-1R in the pathogenesis of TAO has led to the development of antibodies against IGF-1R, teprotumumab (Tepezza). It was approved in January 2020 for treating TAO of less than 9 months [11]. In the pivotal trial, 83% who received the drug showed proptosis reduction of ≥2 mm versus 10% in the placebo group. Minor adverse events were seen in most patients whether or not receiving the drug. Serious adverse events, including infusion reactions, diarrhoea or Hashimoto's encephalopathy, were seen in 4% [11].

20.4.2 Ophthalmic Signs of Thyroid Eye Disease

20.4.2.1 Lid Retraction of the Upper Eyelid

Retraction of the upper eyelid (UER) is the earliest sign of thyroid eye disease (TED), even when the patient has no symptoms. In a review of community-based TED, nearly 90.8% of the 120 patients seen over 15 years had UER at diagnosis. In this cohort, 22% also had lower lid retraction (LER) [23]. The upper eyelid margin is retracted in the primary gaze, exposing the superior limbus giving a staring look (Fig. 20.2a) [24]. Normally, the peak of the upper eyelid is slightly medial to the pupil, but in TED, the UER shows a temporal flare; the highest point of the upper lid margin peaks temporal to the pupil.

UER was believed to be a sign of sympathetic overactivity in Muller's tarsal muscle. Variable UER is likely due to increased adrenergic activity, especially in hyperthyroidism-associated TED. Using the topical adrenergic drug guanethidine led to the reversal of the UER [25]. Guanethidine is an antihypertensive drug available in several countries other than the USA.

In many cases, however, UER is seen only in one eye, defying explanation (Fig. 20.2a). In thyroid ophthalmopathy, the earliest inflammatory infiltration is seen in the inferior rectus muscle leading to a mechanical restriction of its action. Obeying Hering's law, UER may represent an overaction of the LPSM and the superior rectus (SR) [26].

UER possibly results from infiltration and expansion of the muscle volume in the LPSM/SR complex. In a 3-D CT scan modelling of TED-associated UER without proptosis, an ipsilateral increase in the LPSM/SR volume was seen in 85% of the eyes. In the ULR eyes, without significant volume expansion in the LPSM/SR, a significant increase in the inferior rectus (IR) volume was seen in the contralateral eyes [27]. Persistent inflammation leads to increased fibrosis in these muscles, possibly leading to a permanent UER. Exophthalmos may itself lead to UER as the LA is put under stretch. However, not all patients show a reversal of UER following an orbital decompression of the proptosis [28].

In the natural course study of TED, without any intervention, 22.2% showed spontaneous resolution of the UER by 6 months, 37% by 1 year, and 49.4% by 2 years of follow-up. Improvement was seen in 70% in 1 year and 75% in 2 years [29].

In the lower lid, retraction (LER) leads to exposure of the lower sclera (scleral show) as the lid margin is pulled down. Some scleral show may be seen in normal, especially in older people and up to 2 mm of the scleral show may be taken as normal [30]. LER is a less frequent sign of TED and was seen only in 22% of the TED [23].

Both UER and LER may lead to lagophthalmos (inability to close the eyelids completely), conjunctival congestion, and irritation and carries a risk of exposure to keratitis.

UER may require full-thickness anterior blepharotomy with mullerectomy in patients with lagophthalmos, exposure, dryness, congested eyes, or even aesthetic reasons [31]. Even a conjunctival approach may be followed for disinserting the attachment of the Muller muscles and the LA to the tarsal plate. The lateral canthal ligament is severed to control the lateral flare of the upper eyelid [32].

Non-surgical options include local injections of botulin toxin-A, hyaluronic acid, and triamcinolone acetonide into the supratarsal soft tissues [33].

20.4.2.2 Lid Lag

Normally, the upper lid moves at the same velocity during upgaze as the eye movement because the vertical muscles and LPSM are linked in vertical movements. The premotor neuron for vertical movement is believed to be located in the rostral interstitial nucleus of the medial longitudinal fasciculus (riMLF) or just medial to it, the M group and interstitial nucleus of Cajal (inC), which excitatory sends signals to the motor neuron nucleus located in the central caudal nucleus

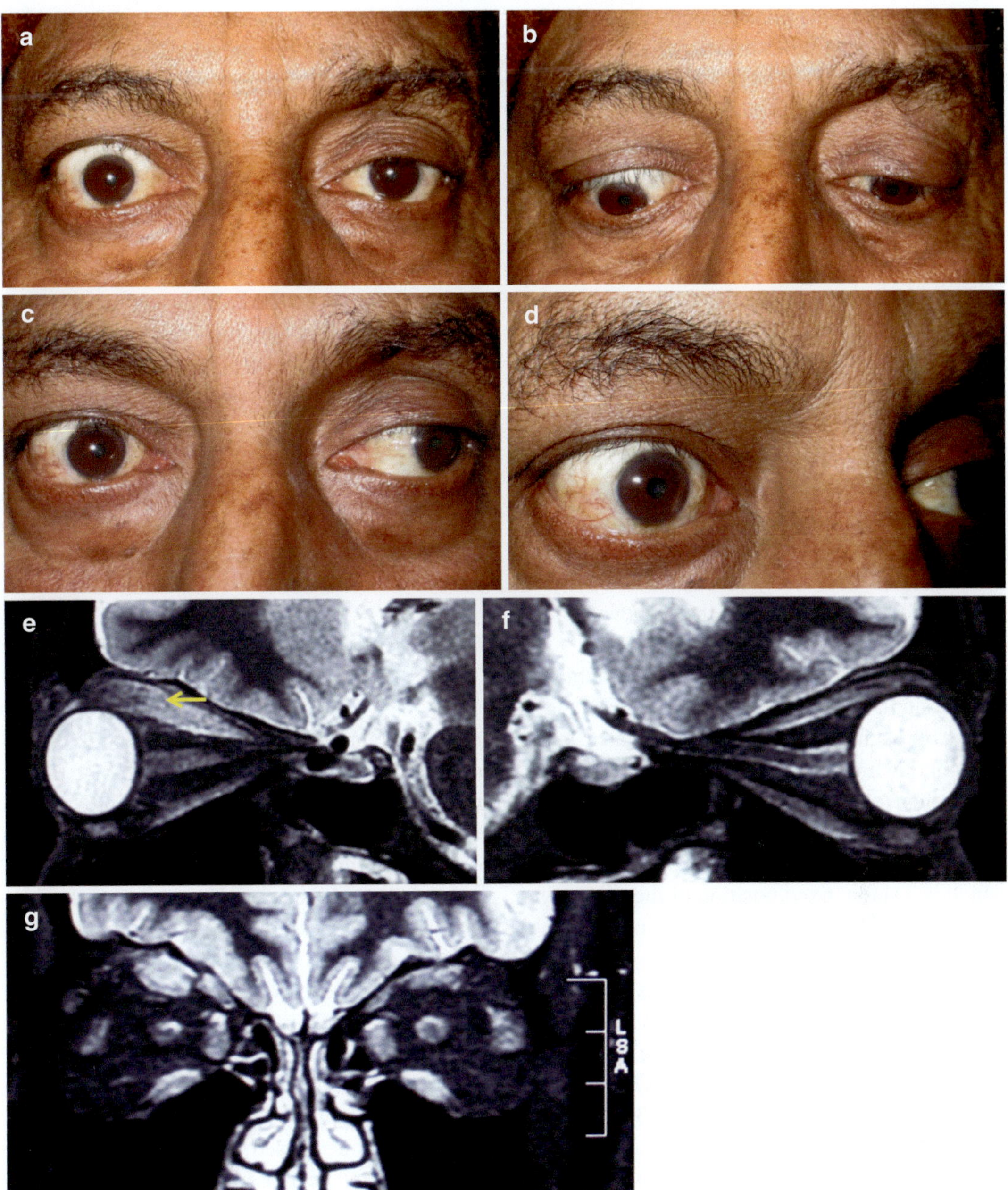

Fig. 20.2 (**a–d**) Thyroid-associated Ophthalmopathy (**a–d**): A 58-year-old euthyroid smoker presented with unilateral proptosis, eyelid retraction and eyelid lag. He demonstrates the classical signs of TAO, Dalrymple's sign (**a**), Eyelid lag (**b**), Ballet's sign- the medial rectus restriction (**c**), Goldzeiher's sign-congestion over lateral rectus insertion (**d**). MR imaging (**e–g**): Sagittal section of the right orbit shows the thickening of the right superior rectus/LPS complex (yellow arrow in **e**). It is hyperintense due to inflammation compared to the left orbit (**f**). Coronal section shows hyperintensity in the right superior rectus/LPS complex, and medial and inferior rectus muscles in the right orbit. In the left orbit, hyperintensity is noted in the medial and inferior rectus (**f**). Images courtesy of Dr. Manpreet Singh, Advanced Eye Centre, Post Graduate Institute of Medical Education and Research, Chandigarh, India

which innervates the bilateral oculomotor nuclei. The M group also sends excitatory signals to the facial nerve nucleus, which supplies the frontalis muscle. Thus, the frontalis also provides a helping hand in elevating the upper lid during the elevation of the eyes [34]. During downward saccades, the inhibitory signals from the premotor neurons (nuclei of the posterior commissure) lead to the relaxation of the LPSM and the superior rectus [35]. In UER, the LPS fails to keep pace with the downward movement of the eye, resulting in the upper lid margin maintaining a position higher than it should be. It results in the scleral show at the superior limbus (Fig. 20.2b). This phenomenon is termed lid lag. Lid lag is an important sign of TED. Of the 105 patients with Graves' ophthalmopathy for which information was available, 35% had bilateral and 14% unilateral lid lag [23]. Notably, nearly 10% of normal people and, more commonly, those above 40 may have some degree of lid lag [36].

Lid lag needs to be differentiated from the von Graefe sign, which is also a sign of TED and is tested by asking the patient to look at a target brought down from the up gaze to the downgaze. A transient pause in the lid's downward movement is termed a positive von Graefe sign. Von Graefe's sign is dynamic compared to the lid lag, which is a static, fixed position of the upper eyelid in downgaze. Lagophthalmos is an inability to close the eyes completely [37]. In a series of Graves' ophthalmopathy, lid lag was noted only in 8% of the patients, lagophthalmos in 16% and none in normal people. von Graefe's sign was more specific and noted in 36% of Graves' ophthalmopathy vs none in the normal [38].

20.4.2.3 Orbital Signs of Thyroid-Associated Orbitopathy (Ophthalmopathy)

As discussed above, lid retraction is the earliest sign of thyroid-associated ophthalmopathy (TAO). TAO can be diagnozed if lid retraction presents with abnormal thyroid functions, restriction of extraocular movements (Fig. 20.2c) or evidence of compressive optic neuropathy or exophthalmos. In the absence of lid retraction, a diagnosis can be made if other signs listed above are present. If other signs of TAO are present, a ptosis or normal lid should raise the suspicion of associated ocular myasthenia gravis (discussed above in the lid retraction section) [24]. Besides the lid signs, TAO is characterized by proptosis, periorbital edema, conjunctival congestion and chemosis, and restriction of eye movements resulting in diplopia and pain (Figs. 20.2, 20.3, and 20.4). TAO may lead to lagophthalmos (inability to close the eyes) and exposure keratitis in severely affected patients. The vision may be threatened due to compressive optic neuropathy. Any vision impairment, abnormal pupillary reactions, impaired colour vision or visual field defects and corneal ulceration call for urgent interventions to prevent imminent blindness.

20.4.3 Evaluation of the Patient with Thyroid Orbitopathy

It is important to seek the history of smoking and other autoimmune diseases in patients or family members. Patients are assessed clinically on disease activity by (1) pain behind the globe, (2) pain in the movement of the eyes, (3) redness of eyelids, (4) eyelid edema, (5) redness of the conjunctiva, (6) redness of the caruncle, and (7) conjunctival chemosis. Each item is given a score of 1. If the score exceeds ≥3/7, it is considered a clinically active disease [39].

A 10-point scoring system involves objectively evaluating exophthalmos, including increased proptosis by 2 mm on Hertel's exophthalmometry, decreased visual acuity by two or more lines, and decreased eye movements in any direction by 8°. These three additional items require a previous examination. Any change in the last 1–3 months is noted for the above-listed items [39, 40]. In addition to the above signs and symptoms, a note is made of photophobia, watering, and grittiness; the palpebral aperture's height and intercanthal distance; lid signs, squint, restriction of movement >8°; RAPD, colour vision, and visual field defects [41].

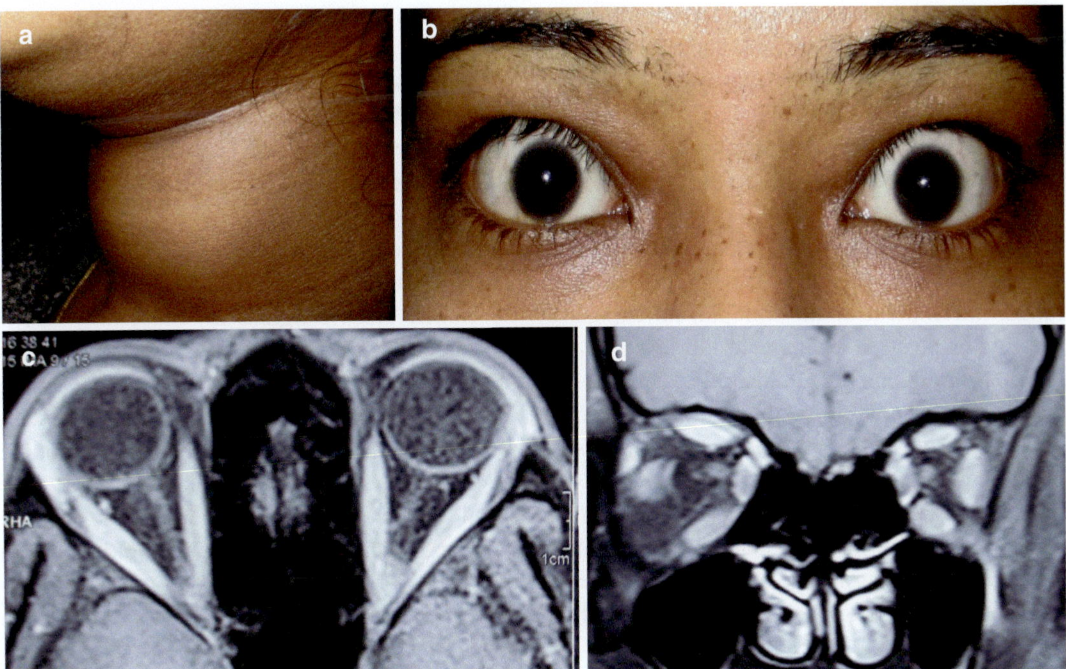

Fig. 20.3 Bilateral thyroid-associated orbitopathy (TAO) in a 16-year-old girl with thyrotoxic goiter (**a**) with clinical features of TAO-bilateral proptosis, eyelid retraction (**b**). MRI orbits show hyperintense fusiform enlarged muscles with sparing of tendons (**c**). Coronal sections show enlarged recti and superior obliques (**d**). Images courtesy of Dr. Manpreet Singh, Advanced Eye Centre, Post Graduate Institute of Medical Education and Research, Chandigarh, India

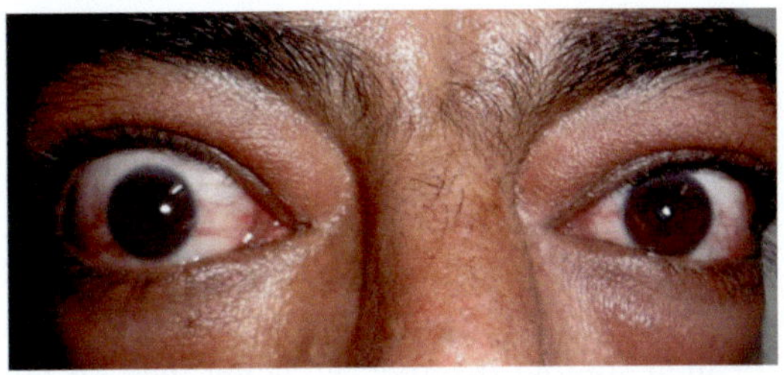

Fig. 20.4 A young patient of TAO with proptosis, prominent lid retraction and periocular swelling right > left eye. Images courtesy of Prof. Usha Singh, Advanced Eye Centre, Post Graduate Institute of Medical Education and Research, Chandigarh

20.4.3.1 NOSPECS Classification

An ad hoc committee of the American thyroid association gave one of the earliest classifications of TAO. A simple, easy-to-remember classification indicated a stepwise increase in the TAO's severity [42]. Grade 0-N (no signs or symptoms), Grade 1-O (only lid signs, lid retraction, lid lag and staring gaze), Grade 2-S (symptoms and signs of soft tissue inflammation), Grade 3-P (proptosis), Grade 4-E (restriction of extraocular movements), Grade 5-C (Corneal involvement), and Grade 6-S (sight-threatening due to optic neuropathy). Each class included the signs and symptoms of the previous class. Some years later, this classification was revized to be more elaborate in classes 2–6. Class 2 was graded as 0 (absent), mild, moderate, and severe. Class 3 (Proptosis) was further graded o (absent), a (3–4 mm), b (4–7 mm), and c (8 mm or more). Class 4 (extraocular movements) was o (absent), a (restrictions in extreme gaze), b (evident restrictions, and c (no movements, frozen globe). Class 5 (Corneal involvement) 0 (absent), a (stippling), b (corneal ulceration), and c (cloudy cornea, perforation). Class 6 0 (absent), a (visual acuity 20/20 to 20/60 with optic disc pallor, edema or visual field defect), b (Visual acuity 20/70 to 20/200), c (Visual acuity less than 20/200, No light perception) [43]. The NOSPECS classification has been criticized for being too simplified in its approach to a highly variable and complex disease [44].

20.4.3.2 Classification of the Severity of Thyroid-Associated Orbitopathy

TAO is classified as mild if the lid retraction is <2 mm, proptosis <3 mm of the expected normal range, intermittent or no diplopia, no exposure keratitis or positive response to lubricants. TAO has no or minimal effect on daily life activities.

TAO is moderate to severe if lid retraction is ≥2 mm, proptosis is ≥3 mm, signs of soft tissue inflammation are present, and diplopia. The TAO impacts daily life but is not sight-threatening.

The severity of the TAO can be more reliably classified by measuring the metabolic target volume and total lesion glycolysis on ^{18}F-FDG-PET/MRI scan [45].

TAO is very severe if TAO is sight-threatening because of corneal ulceration or optic neuropathy [39, 46]. Men above 50, unstable thyroid functions, those who have received radioactive iodine, smokers, diabetics, and those with progressive diplopia and soft tissue inflammation signs, orbital pain, the restricted elevation of the eyes and lagophthalmos are at a higher risk of developing a severe TAO [39].

Patients of GD who develop any sudden deterioration of vision, loss of colour vision, corneal ulceration or globe luxation require an emergency referral [41].

20.4.4 Laboratory Evaluation of Thyroid-Associated Orbitopathy

Includes testing for T3, T4, TSH, Thyrotropin receptor antibodies (TRAb), and TPO. Higher titers of TRAb determined by serial dilutions of serum can differentiate patients with only Graves' disease (GD) and TAO (Graves' orbitopathy, Fig. 20.3) as the titers remain positive at much higher dilution in TAO (75% + at 1:243 in TAO vs none >1:9 dilution in GD) [47]. Compared to the TR inhibitory immunoglobulins, TR stimulation antibodies were significantly associated with TAO [48].

20.4.5 Prevention of Thyroid-Associated Orbitopathy

In a large cohort of patients with Graves' disease, 8.8% of patients with Graves' Disease ($n = 8404$) developed TAO. Surgical thyroidectomy had a 74% decreased hazard of developing TAO compared to those who received radioactive iodine [49]. Care should be taken in patients with Graves' disease who receive radioactive iodine so that patients do not become hypothyroid. They should receive preventive corticosteroids. Those who smoke should refrain from smoking. There is some evidence that statins and no other lipid-lowering agents may have a protective role in the development of TAO in patients with Graves' disease [50]. A 40% hazard reduction was seen in patients who received statins for at least ≥60 days vs less than 60 days of non-use in the past year [49]. Selenium 100 μg twice a day may be considered for six months in patients with mild TAO [51].

20.4.6 Treatment of Thyroid-Associated Orbitopathy

20.4.6.1 Mild TAO

Patients with TAO should preferably be managed in specialized clinics. Patients should be treated for their thyroid disorder, knowing they do not become hypothyroid. Patients must refrain from smoking. Topical lubricating drops and gels should suffice at this stage [46]. Selenium 100 μg may be used twice a day for 6 months.

20.4.6.2 Moderate to Severe Thyroid Associated Orbitopathy

The standard of care for active TAO is intravenous methylprednisolone pulse therapy at 0.5 g/weekly for 6 weeks, followed by 0.25 g/weekly for another 6 weeks. The cumulative dose should not exceed 4.5 g for most cases [46]. (Fig. 20.5) A cumulative dose of 8.0 g should not be

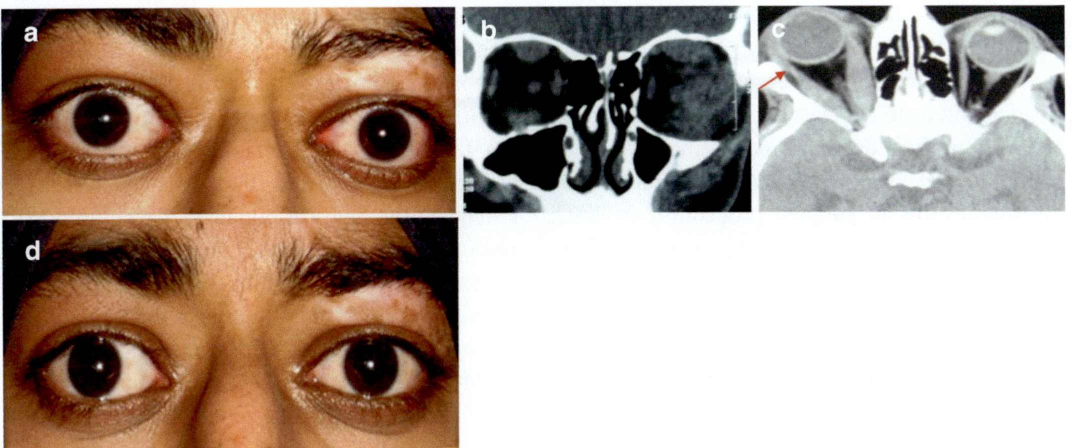

Fig. 20.5 Thyroid-associated Ophthalmopathy: A Young male with acute onset proptosis, lid retraction and conjunctival injection (**a**). The coronal view of the CT scan shows enlarged superior and inferior recti (**b**). The axial section shows right-sided proptosis more than the left and bulky extraocular muscles sparing the tendon characteristic of thyroid eye disease (**c**, red arrow). After treatment with three doses of intravenous methylprednisolone, the same patient showed decreased proptosis, resolution of lid retraction and conjunctival injection (**d**). Images courtesy of Prof. Usha Singh, Advanced Eye Centre, Post Graduate Institute of Medical Education and Research, Chandigarh

exceeded [39]. A recent meta-analysis found that the IVMP therapy vs placebo showed clinically insignificant improvement in proptosis and modest response in diplopia. Proptosis and diplopia respond significantly to teprotumumab compared to IVMP [52].

Of the various immunomodulatory therapies, the drug of choice is mycophenolate mofetil alone or in combination with corticosteroids. Cyclosporine or azathioprine can be considered second-line immunomodulatory therapy and oral corticosteroids. Rituximab or tocilizumab can be a good second-line drug in patients who do not have optic neuropathy due to TAO [46]. It should be administered by experienced physicians. Tepezza (teprotumumab), a humanized monoclonal IGF-1R blocking antibody, has been FDA-approved for treating TAO of a short duration of fewer than 9 months. It carries nearly an 80% response rate. However, patients must be warned of potential side effects like hearing loss and tinnitus. The treating physician must discuss the risk-benefit and cost-efficacy of each therapy with the patients. Radiotherapy is usually reserved for patients who show progressive diplopia. Radiation therapy should be used cautiously in diabetic patients and those younger than 35 to prevent the development/progression of diabetic retinopathy and secondary tumours, respectively [39].

20.4.6.3 Sight Threatening Thyroid-Associated Orbitopathy

Sight-threatening TAO due to optic neuropathy requires urgent care with 0.5–1.0 g methylprednisolone daily for 3 days. If the patient does not show improvement by 2 weeks, orbital decompression should be considered. It is recommended that deep decompression of the medial wall and the orbital floor should be considered for reducing compression at the orbital apex in patients with compressive optic neuropathy [39]. Other indications for surgical decompression include imminent corneal perforation, globe luxation and steroid-unresponsive optic neuropathy. Patients with inactive TAO often require surgery to reduce exophthalmos, fat prolapse, squint or lid repair. The surgical technique includes most commonly only the lateral wall, or in severe cases, two walls (lateral plus medial wall) or two-and-a-half walls (lateral, medial and medial half of the orbital floor). The reduction in proptosis is maximum (median 7.6 mm) with the two-and-a-half wall decompression, 4.2 mm with lateral wall decompression, and least with a medial one-and-a-half wall (2.9 mm) [53]. Significant post-surgical complications included numbness (25%), new diplopia (19%), squint surgery (34%), lid surgery (25%) and vary with different procedures [53]. Readers interested in learning the steps of various surgical orbital decompression may refer to Jefferis et al. [53]. For more comprehensive information on all surgical procedures in TAO, we suggest that readers refer to this review [54].

20.5 Infiltrative Lesions of Extraocular Muscles

Orbital metastasis from hematogenous malignancies is rare and forms about 9% of all orbital metastasis [55].

Bilateral leukemic infiltrates in all the extraocular muscles may produce bilateral proptosis with conjunctival chemosis and must be differentiated from TAO. Unlike TAO, the patients with leukemic infiltrates of extraocular muscles do not show restriction of ocular movements, lid retraction or lid lag [56]. Although rare, bilateral enlargement of all the extraocular muscles due to haematological malignancies and lymphomas must be kept in the differential diagnosis of proptosis [57]. An inguinal rhabdomyosarcoma may metastasise to all the extraocular muscles and cause their enlargement [58]. Rhabdomyosarcoma may metastasise to a single extraocular muscle [59].

20.6 Causes of Extraocular Muscles Enlargement

20.6.1 Orbital Myositis

Most cases of inflammatory orbital myositis involve more often one or uncommonly more than one extraocular muscle, unilateral (more common) or bilateral and cause acute onset of painful diplopia. Proptosis may or,may not be present. However, 62.5% of such cases were due to acute non-specific inflammation, and 32.5% were due to low-grade progressive myositis[55]. Generally, female preponderance is observed in non-specific myositis [60].

Restriction of movement is more commonly seen in the direction of action of the affected muscle and less commonly in the opposite direction [61].

Expansion of extraocular muscles is observed in ultrasonography and other imaging modalities. On T1-weighted MR imaging, the affected muscle is isointense, but the affected muscle is enhanced on contrast-enhanced T-weighted MRI with fat suppression [62]. Unlike in TAO, the extraocular muscle tendons thicken in nearly half of the patients with orbital myositis. The tendons were thickened in 6% of patients with TAO [63].

Multiple muscle involvement and bilaterality are risk factors for recurrences [55]. Rarely sarcoidosis and SLE may also present as orbital myositis. Rarely, IgG4-related inflammatory disease may manifest as enlargement of extraocular muscles (Fig. 20.6) and thickening of the infraorbital nerve [64]. Extraocular muscle enlargement may also be seen in growth hormone-secreting pituitary adenomas [65]. In recent years, Graves' orbitopathy has been associated with raised serum levels of IgG4 in nearly 17.5% of patients especially young patients with higher clinical activity scores. These patients may show eosinophilia in the peripheral blood. They respond well to antithyroid therapies but run the risk of developing hypothyroidism [66].

Inflammatory Orbital myositis responds rapidly to the use of corticosteroids. All non-responder patients must undergo muscle biopsy to rule out metastatic and malignant infiltrative pathologies [56, 67, 68]. In recurrent cases, tacrolimus has been used successfully [69].

20.6.1.1 Measuring the Diameter of the Extraocular Muscles

The muscle diameters for the lateral and medial rectus muscles are measured in an axial CT scan at the maximum thickness diagonal to the long axis of the muscle. The inferior rectus and superior rectus/levator palpebrae superioris (superior muscle group) are measured in coronal sections [70, 71].

20.6.2 IgG4-Related Ophthalmic Disease (IgG4-ROD)

IgG4-related inflammatory disorders are autoimmune diseases characterized by multiorgan

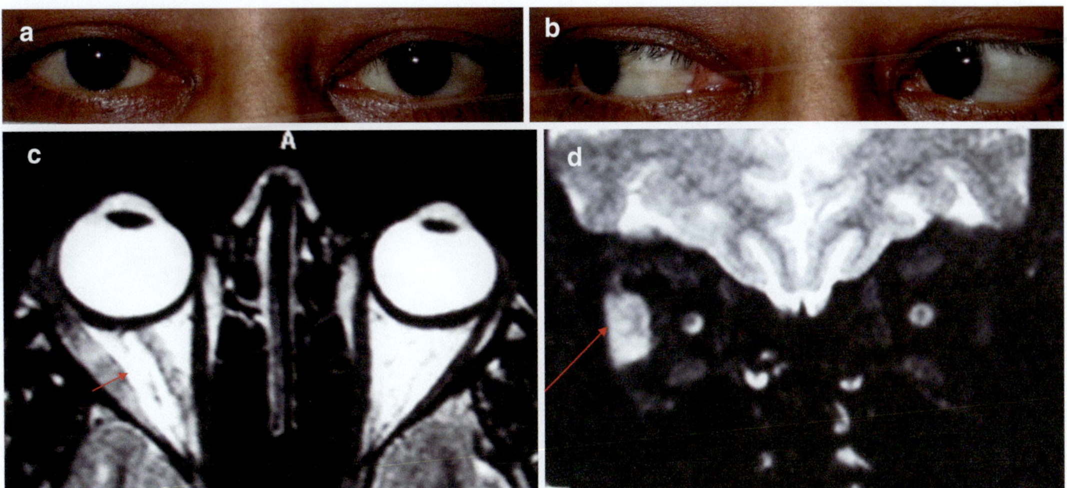

Fig. 20.6 Myositis: A 45-year-old woman presented with pain and diplopia in the right gaze. Right abduction was normal (**a**, **b**). Contrast-enhanced MRI orbits show right lateral rectus thickening and irregular hyperintensity with contrast enhancement and tendon involvement (red arrow, **c**). Fat-suppressed images show similar features in the coronal section (red arrow, **d**). She did not have any other organ involvement. Her serology was positive for IgG4 at 1130 mg/dL (normal <135 mg/dL) and was considered a possible IgG4-related Myositis. She was treated with oral corticosteroids with a good response. Images courtesy of Dr. Manpreet Singh, Advanced Eye Centre, Post Graduate Institute of Medical Education and Research, Chandigarh, India

involvement, infiltration of tissues with lymphatic and IgG4+ plasma cells, and fibrotic occlusions of veins. The IgG4 levels are elevated. They account for many idiopathic orbital inflammations and lymphoid hyperplasia [72, 73]. Ophthalmic involvement may occur in up to 1/4th of all IgG4-related diseases [74]. Commonly involved extraocular tissues include the lacrimal gland, orbital soft tissues, conjunctiva, and myositis [75] (Fig. 20.6).

The consensus criteria for the IgG4-ROD includes a demonstration of histopathology of orbital tissues at least two of (1) dense lymphoplasmacytic cells infiltration, (2) storiform (cartwheel type) fibrosis, (3) obliterative phlebitis. For the lacrimal gland, any of these suffices to diagnose IgG-4-related dacryoadenitis. IgG4+ plasma cells to IgG+ cells ratio > 40% highly suggest the IgG4-ROD [76]. Comprehensive criteria also include IgG4 levels ≥135 mg/dL. Clinically suspected cases of orbital inflammation with elevated IgG4 levels are possible IgG4-ROD, while in the presence of clinical, pathological, and serological criteria, a definitive diagnosis of IgG4-ROD can be made [77].

IgG4 levels are markers for the corticosteroid response and recurrence of the disease. Higher levels are associated with systemic involvement [78]. In steroid-resistant patients, rituximab is a good alternative [74]. The differential diagnosis includes granulomatosis with polyangiitis, Sjogren syndrome, lymphoma, and sarcoidosis.

20.7 Orbital Lymphoma

Orbital lymphomas are the most common cancers of the orbit with several histopathological subtypes that may show regional variations (Figs. 20.7, 20.8, and 20.9). Of all the non-Hodgkin lymphomas, more than 90% are B-cell lymphomas, and most are diffuse large B-cell lymphomas. [79]. In the Asian-Chinese population, the most common variant was extranodal mucosa-associated lymphoid tissue lymphoma (MALT-lymphoma) followed by diffuse large B-cell lymphoma (DLBCL), follicular cell lymphoma, and small lymphocytic lymphoma [80]. In a study from the United States, MALT-lymphoma was seen in nearly 50% of the patients

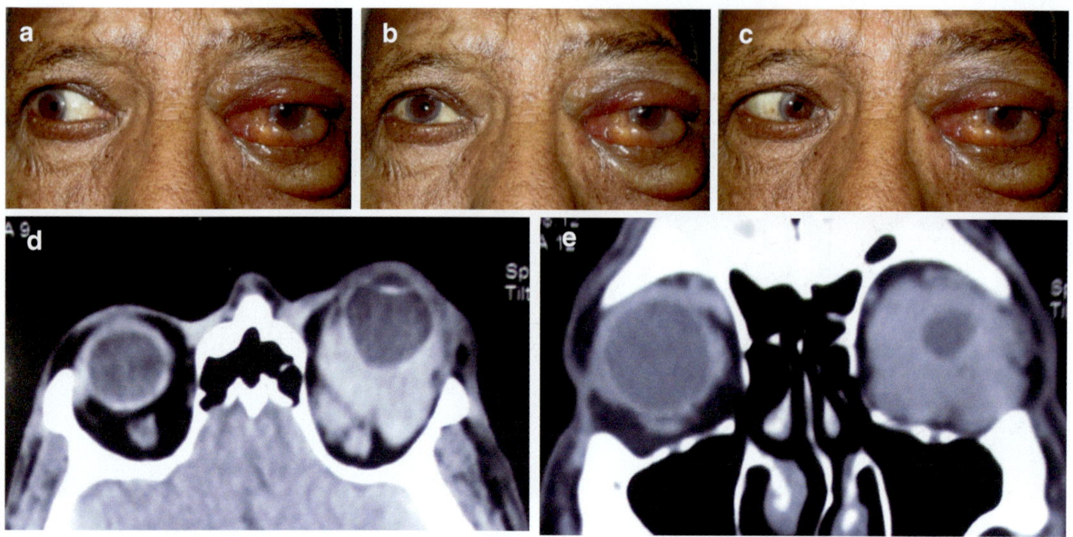

Fig. 20.7 Orbital lymphoma: A 69-year-old man with left proptosis, orbital sulcus fullness, cutaneous erythema and subconjunctival mass (**a**). Left eye movements were restricted in all gazes (**b**, **c**). CT scan orbits show enhancing mass moulding around the left globe (**d**). The coronal section shows non-discernable recti from the ill-defined homogenous mass (**e**). Images courtesy of Dr. Manpreet Singh, Advanced Eye Centre, Post Graduate Institute of Medical Education and Research, Chandigarh, India

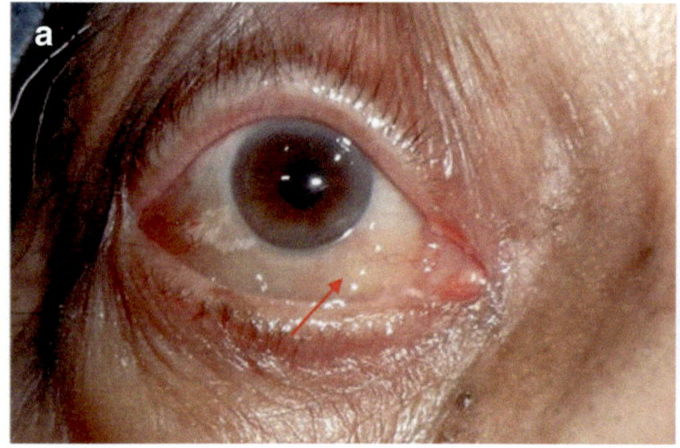

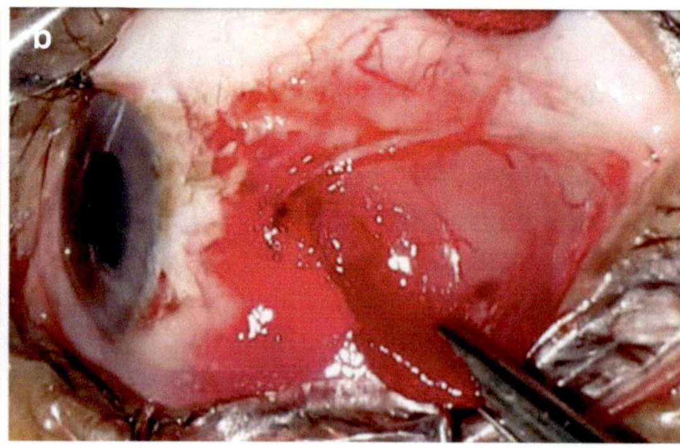

Fig. 20.8 Orbital lymphoma presenting as a subconjunctival mass lesion. An 85-year-old patient presented with a pale pink subconjunctival mass in the inferior quadrant salmon-pink 'fleshy' patch (red arrow, **a**). A clinical sign of orbital lymphoma. An incisional biopsy was taken for histopathological and Immunohistochemistry (**b**). Images courtesy of Prof. Usha Singh, Advanced Eye Centre, Post Graduate Institute of Medical Education and Research, Chandigarh, India

and over 90% of them survived 10 years. DLBCL was seen in nearly 20% and carried the worse outcome and only about 2/3rd survived 10 years. Older age, male sex and DLBCL subtype carried a higher risk of worse outcomes [81]. Of the 2211 orbital lymphoma cases reported over 24 years, 97% were B-cell type, 59% were extranodal marginal zone lymphoma, DLBCL (23%), follicular (9%) and mantle cell lymphoma (5%) [82].

The most common site is the orbit followed by conjunctiva and lacrimal glands and the least common in the eyelids [80]. Orbital lymphomas are most often unilateral and present most often as proptosis, diplopia, pain, ptosis, limitation of

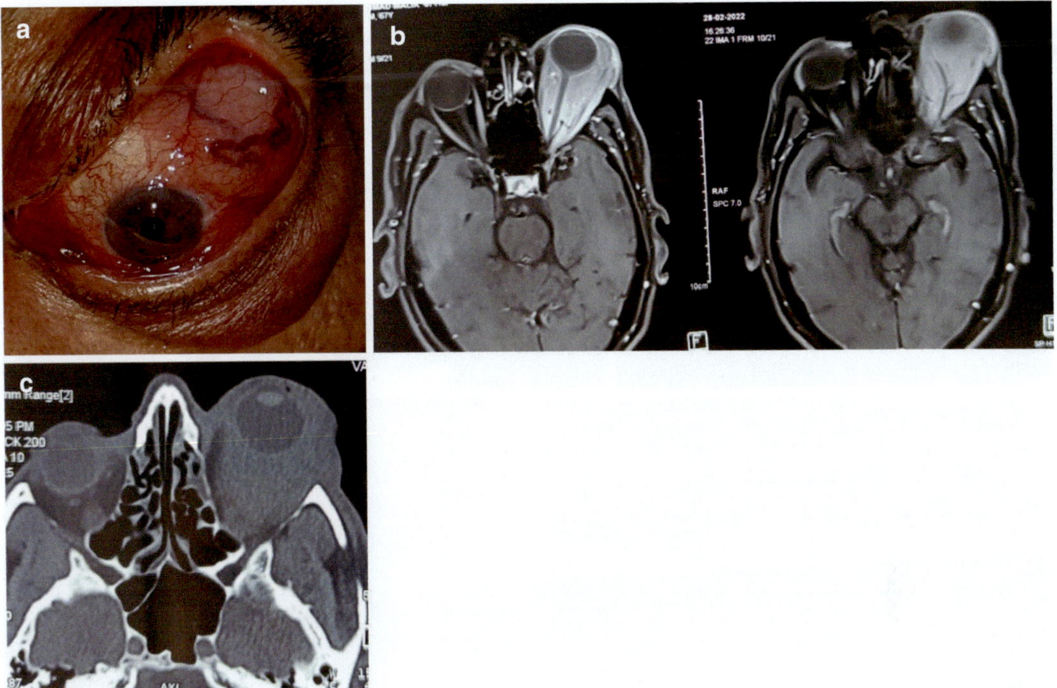

Fig. 20.9 Orbital lymphoma presenting as a subconjunctival mass lesion. A 65-year-old man presented with gradually progressive forward protrusion and redness of the left eye for 7–8 months. The left eye showed a salmon-pink subconjunctival mass in the superotemporal part of the bulbar conjunctiva (**a**). The MRI (**b**) and CT scans (**c**) of orbits showed a diffuse ill-defined intra and extraconal orbital mass without any orbital bony changes or indentation of the left eyeball. A biopsy of the mass was confirmatory of low-grade B cell non-Hodgkin lymphoma. Images courtesy of Dr. Pankaj Gupta, Advanced Eye Centre, Post Graduate Institute of Medical Education and Research, Chandigarh

movements, and conjunctival chemosis (Figs. 20.7, 20.8, and 20.9). These are most often seen in the extraconal orbital space (72%) and lacrimal gland (51%) less commonly in the intraconal space. These may infiltrate the conjunctiva and the eyelids. Most patients require a CT scan, MR Imaging, whole-body FDG-PET/CT and bone marrow biopsy. These are well-circumscribed, homogeneous lesions on CT/MRI of the orbit and tend to wrap around normal anatomical structures [83].

Histopathological examination of the biopsy requires immunohistochemical staining, in addition to the haematoxylin and eosin, for subtyping of the lymphomas. Most of these require radiation therapy alone for Stage 1E (confined to the orbital adnexa) or combined with chemotherapy and surgery [82, 84]. Chemotherapy is often used in high-grade or disseminated lymphomas. Rituximab has substantially improved the outcome of B-cell lymphomas [82].

20.8 Orbital Metastasis

Orbits get involved in cancer metastasis, most often as a part of disseminated disease. The most common cancers metastasising to the orbit include breast, prostate, lung, and skin melanomas [85]. Neuroblastoma is a childhood cancer, with 90% of cases occurring before the age of 10 years. The presentation to the ophthalmologists can be variable from asymptomatic to vision-threatening proptosis and ecchymosis [86] (Fig. 20.10). In a recent review of the literature, the most frequent primary site was (36.3%), mel-

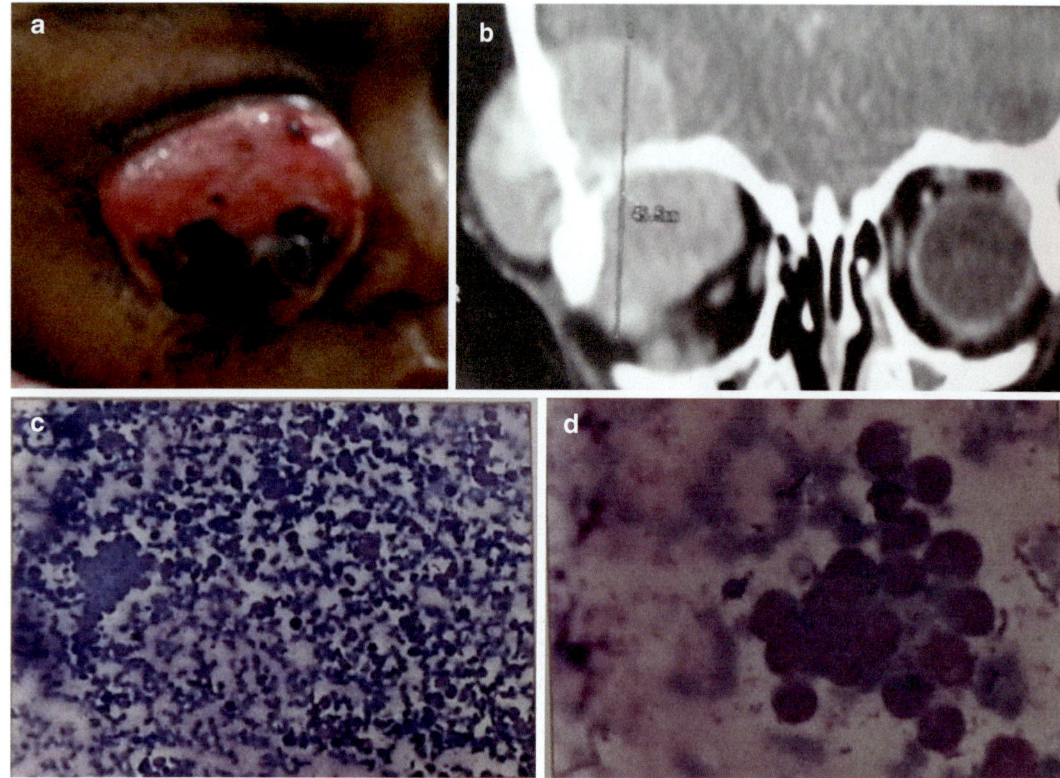

Fig. 20.10 Biopsy-proven Neuroblastoma: A 3-year-old male with rapidly progressive painless axial proptosis, decreased vision, and swelling in the temporal region over 2 months (**a**) CT scan coronal section shows an enhancing well-defined mass around the right greater wing of the sphenoid and frontal bone involving the roof of orbit with bony erosions and spiculations, extensions in the extradural, intra-orbital region and scalp with compression of brain parenchyma (**b**). Low (**c**) and high-power smear (**d**) reveal discrete, and clusters of round to oval hyperchromatic and pleomorphic cells with scanty cytoplasm forming pseudo-rosettes compatible with poorly differentiated neuroblastoma. Images courtesy of Dr. Shweta Chaurasia, Advanced Eye Centre, Post Graduate Institute of Medical Education and Research, Chandigarh

anoma (10.1%) and prostate (8.3%). Proptosis (52.3%) was the most frequent presentation followed by a relative afferent pupillary defect (38.7%). The soft tissues often infiltrate with metastatic cancer cells [87].

A thorough search for the primary cancer is needed. In nearly 20–30%, orbital metastasis may be the first cancer presentation; in 10%, the primary site may never be found [85, 87]. 7–12% of all lung adenocarcinomas may metastasize to the orbits [88].

These lesions may present as orbital apex syndrome [89]. FDG-PET/ CT is useful in locating the primary site [90, 91]. Besides, the FDG-PET/CT helps determine the total disease burden [90, 91].

20.9 Lacrimal Gland Granulomas and Tumours

The lacrimal gland may be involved in several inflammatory, infiltrative, epithelial and malignant tumours. The inflammatory and infiltrative pathologies tend to be bilateral and remain confined to the lacrimal gland without affecting the adjacent bone (Figs. 20.11 and 20.12). The benign epithelial tumours may cause expansion of the lacrimal fossa while the malignant tumours cause bony erosion. Benign and malignant tumours are unilateral. Malignant lesions progress fast and are painful [92].

The lacrimal glands may be involved in autoimmune disorders including granulomatosis with

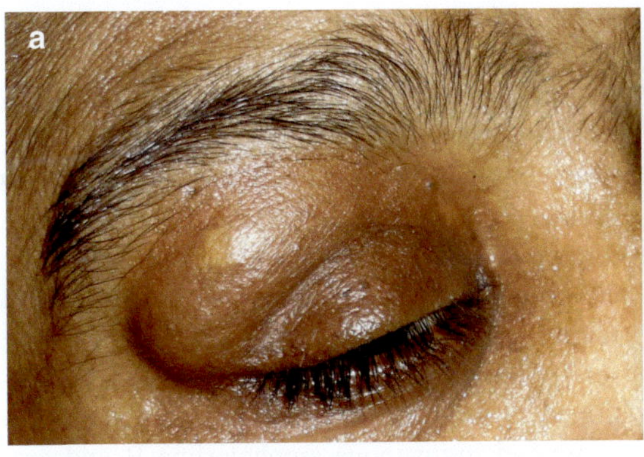

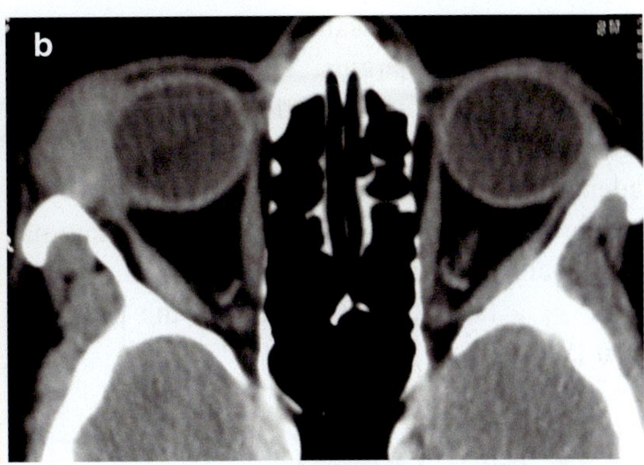

Fig. 20.11 Lacrimal gland tumour: The right eye of a 56-year-old female showed swelling in the lacrimal gland region (**a**). CT axial section shows an enhancing soft tissue lesion in the superolateral quadrant of the right eye in the lacrimal fossa in the extra-coronal location with an infero-medial displacement of the globe with a maintained fat plane. The lacrimal gland is not seen separately without fat stranding and the normal adjacent bone (**b**). It is likely to be a pleomorphic adenoma of the lacrimal gland neoplasm. Images courtesy of Dr. Shweta Chaurasia, Advanced Eye Centre, Post Graduate Institute of Medical Education and Research, Chandigarh

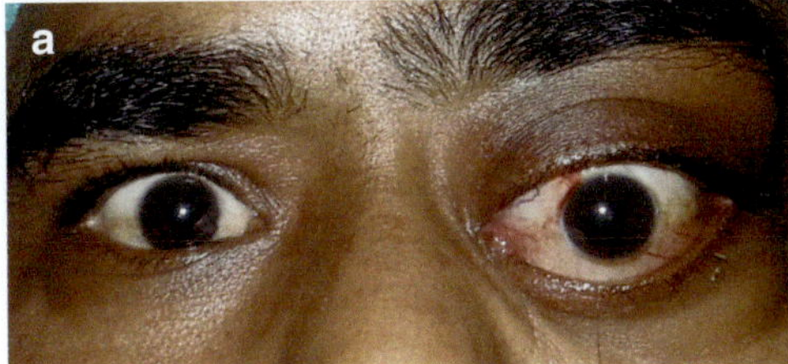

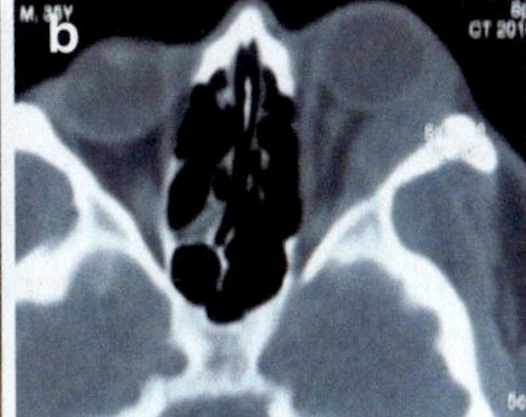

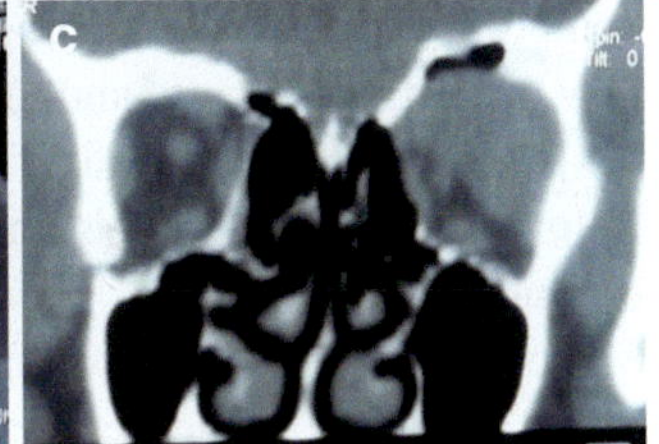

Fig. 20.12 Lacrimal gland tumour: A 40-year male with gradually progressive, painless axial proptosis over 2 years developed progressively decreasing vision over 2 months (**a**). Proptosis resisted retropulsion and had no increase in Valsalva manoeuvre or straining. CT scan axial (**b**) and coronal (**c**) show a solid mass in the lacrimal gland with bone re-modelling suggestive of lacrimal gland neoplasm. Images courtesy of Dr. Shweta Chaurasia, Advanced Eye Centre, Post Graduate Institute of Medical Education and Research, Chandigarh

polyangiitis, sarcoidosis, IgG4 disease or Sjogren syndrome. A pleiomorphic adenoma is the most common benign tumour involving the lacrimal gland; it is more often unilateral and present as a slowly progressive, painless mass lesion in the lacrimal fossa and displaces the globe down and nasally with restriction of the ocular movements. The symptoms are usually present for more than a year. The development of facial anaesthesia and pain indicates a malignant change in the tumour. These tumours should not be biopsied but excized [93]. However, there is not much evidence of malignant transformation of the biopsied pleomorphic adenomas and this prohibition against biopsy may not be valid [94]. Fine needle aspiration biopsy (25G) for cytopathological diagnosis is almost 99% sensitive in accurately diagnosing orbital pathologies and should be preferred over the open incisional biopsy that violates the capsule of the pleomorphic adenoma [95]. Recurrences following complete excision of the pleomorphic adenoma even with an attenuated thin capsule even in long-term follow up are exceptional, and these patients may not need to be kept under follow-up [96]. Most pleomorphic adenomas arise from the orbital part of the lacrimal glands. Adenomas arising from the palpebral part of the lacrimal gland are very rare [97]. Saving the palpebral part of the gland can prevent the development of dry eye following surgery.

The malignant epithelial tumours of the lacrimal gland or the transformation of the benign into malignant form have a shorter duration of symptoms. On CT scan the malignant lesions have ill-defined margins. These are unlikely to have calcification compared to the pleomorphic adenomas or the recurrence of the pleomorphic adenomas. The bony erosions are more likely in malignant and recurrent pleomorphic adenoma. Malignant lesions will likely show a 'wedge sign' or a tail-like extension into the posterior obit [98].

20.10 Orbital Granulomas

The fungal granulomas in orbit are mostly caused by Aspergillus and Mucormycosis that invade the orbit from paranasal sinuses and are labelled sino-orbital fungal infections. The major risk factors for fungal granuloma are diabetes, immunocompromized host, haematological malignancies, HIV, organ transplant, and marijuana smoking [99]. In immunocompromized patients and those following organ transplants, invasive fungal sino-orbital infections are more likely to be Mucormycosis and are often fatal [100].

On CT imaging these appear as heterogenous enhancing soft tissue lesions and appear hypointense on MRI [99]. Invasive fungal sinusitis has been reported in immunocompetent patients presenting solely with proptosis, the fullness of the eyelids, and chronic pain (Fig. 20.13) [101]. These infections may present as orbital apex syndrome [102]. The use of corticosteroids can be disastrous [103]. These patients need aggressive treatment including surgical debridement and intravenous and oral antifungal agents [104]. The role of surgery in these patients has been questioned in the past in view of good response to combined intravenous amphotericin B and oral itraconazole or voriconazole [105].

A high index of clinical suspicion, orbital imaging and confirmation with microbiology and histopathology is critical in the management. The recent coronavirus epidemic led to a spate of Rhino-orbital cerebral Mucormycosis (ROCM) worldwide, especially In India. In a series of 243 patients with ROCM, the median time to the onset was 20 days from the diagnosis of COVID-19, 94.5% had diabetes, and 54% had received corticosteroids or other immunomodulatory agents [106]. Mucormycosis is an angioinvasive fungus; more than 90% are caused by Rhizopus spp. A number of risk factors including

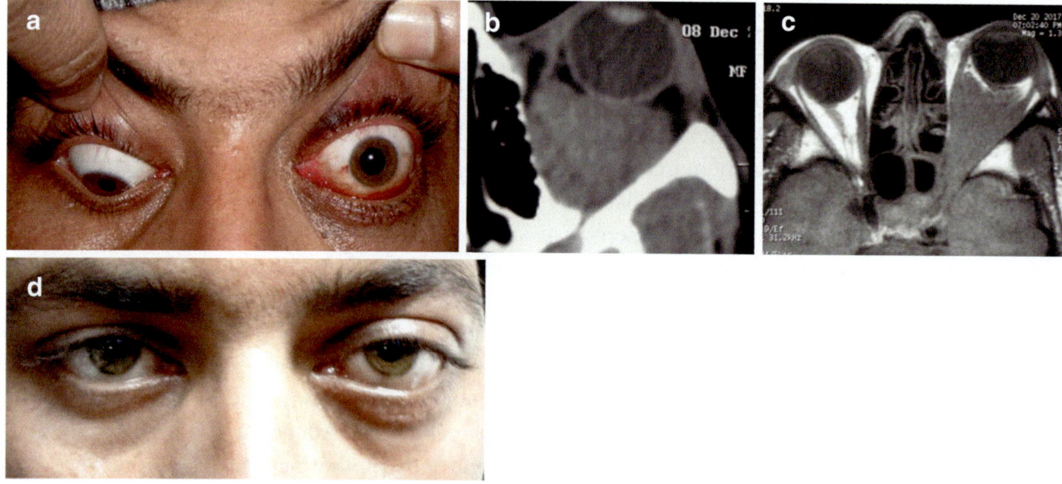

Fig. 20.13 Fungal granuloma: A 22-year-old immunocompetent male presented with subacute proptosis of 1-month duration associated with diminution of vision in the left eye, conjunctival congestion and restriction of extraocular motility (**a**). A CT scan of orbits shows left eye proptosis with a retrobulbar mass lesion in the intraconal space (**b**). The medial orbital wall is breached, with the mass being continuous in the ethmoid sinus (**b**). MRI shows its extension till the orbital apex and infiltration into the orbital fat (**c**). The same patient 4 months later, after orbital-sinus mass debulking and oral antifungal therapy with itraconazole (**d**). Histopathology confirmed aspergillus fungal infection. Images courtesy of Prof. Usha Singh, Advanced Eye Centre, Post Graduate Institute of Medical Education and Research, Chandigarh

diabetic ketoacidosis, increased free iron levels, and non-functional leucocytes may be responsible [106]. The presenting features include facial pain, stuffiness of the nose, lid edema, diplopia, restriction of eye movements, proptosis, and loss of vision. Black eschar due to gangrene of the nose, face or palate is a tell-tale signature of the disease. ROCM has been staged depending on the involvement of various tissues. In stage 1, the disease is confined to the nose; in stage 2, the paranasal sinuses are involved; in stage 3, the orbit gets invaded; in stage 4, when it invades the CNS [107]. For a detailed staging description and management strategies, the readers may refer to Honavar [107].

The key to saving the life and disfigurement of these patients is early diagnosis, endoscopic evaluation biopsy, debridement, and aggressive antifungal therapy. Immediate treatment with intravenous liposomal amphotericin B. Extensive debridement of the nose, sinuses and even exenteration of the orbit if extensively involved [107].

20.11 Tuberculosis of the Orbit

Tuberculosis of the orbit is a rare disease which may affect the periosteum or the orbital bones and may or may not have concurrent pulmonary tuberculosis [108] (Fig. 20.14). It should be con-

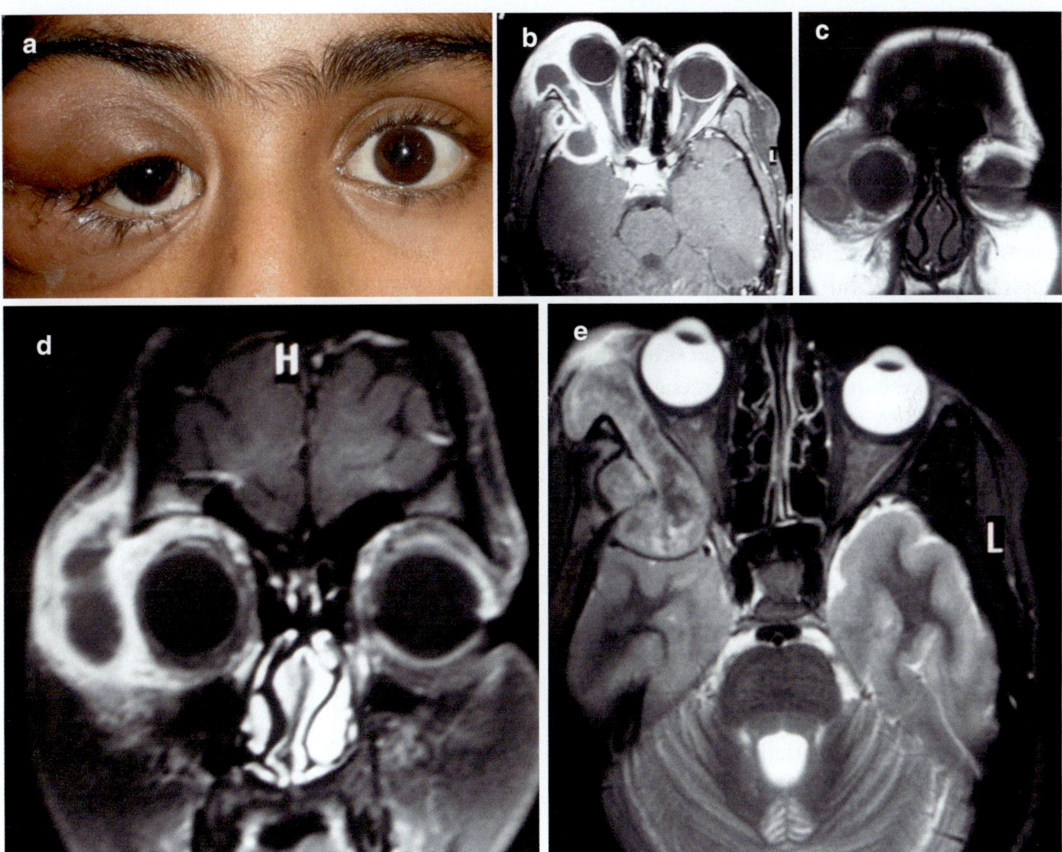

Fig. 20.14 Orbital tuberculosis: (**a**) A12-year female with proptosis with redness and boggy swelling on the temporal side (**a**). Pre-contrast T1 MRI scan axial (**b**) and coronal (**c**) scan. Post-contrast T1 MRI coronal scan (**d**) and the T2 MRI axial scan (**e**) show a peripheral enhancing soft tissue mass lesion in retro-orbital extra-conal space extending into right lateral peri-orbital space causing extrinsic compression of the underlying brain parenchyma involving the right greater wing of sphenoid (CT correlation revealed destruction of the right greater wing of sphenoid with sclerosis, periosteal reaction and surrounding hypodense soft tissue not shown) compatible with orbital tuberculosis. Images courtesy of Dr. Shweta Chaurasia, Advanced Eye Centre, Post Graduate Institute of Medical Education and Research, Chandigarh

sidered in the differential diagnosis of inflammatory lesions of the orbit especially in TB-endemic regions of the world. The diagnosis of orbital TB is difficult. In a review of the literature, most of the reported cases were isolated cases or short case series; it presented as periostitis, orbital cold abscess, TB granuloma with or without bony involvement and dacryoadenitis [109]. The nasolacrimal duct with overlying skin may be involved. It may present as orbital osteomyelitis and periorbital cellulitis [110] or have an intracranial extension [111]. On a CT scan, bony destruction is noted. Contrast-enhanced CT may show an enhancing preseptal tissue edema which continues into the extraconal orbital space. Serial imaging can monitor treatment efficacy [112]. The diagnosis is made on histopathology [109].

20.12 Orbital Granulomatosis with Polyangiitis

Orbital soft tissues are a common site of granulomatosis with polyangiitis (GPA) apart from the respiratory tracts and the kidneys. In the eye, GPA may cause scleritis and peripheral ulcerative keratitis. GPA may affect the orbit and the nasolacrimal system [113]. Early recognition and treatment of GPA are crucial. GPA may extend into the orbit from the neighbouring paranasal sinuses or nasopharynx. The patients present with orbital pain, redness and epiphora. Proptosis may or may not be painful. Movement of the eyes may be restricted. GPA may present with dacryoadenitis [114]. Another feature is socket contracture characterized by enophthalmos following proptosis due to increased fibrosis in the orbital tissues [115]. A biopsy is mandated to make the diagnosis. However, the triad of vasculitis, granulomatous inflammation and necrosis may not be seen in 50% of the cases [116]. While a number of autoimmune markers are ordered for orbital inflammations including angiotensin-converting enzyme, antinuclear antibodies, anti-neutrophilic cytoplasmic antibodies, anti-double stranded DNA antibodies, extractable nuclear antigens, anti-cyclic citrullinated peptide, only 1/3rd may be positive for a specific inflammation. Most of the orbital inflammations remain non-specific and require a biopsy with immunohistochemical studies [117].

20.13 Vascular Malformations of the Orbit

20.13.1 Carotid-Cavernous Fistula

A carotid-cavernous fistula (CCF) is an abnormal communication between the internal carotid artery (ICA) and the cavernous sinus or between the dural branches of the ICA, the external carotid artery or both and accordingly has been classified in type A to D [118]. Type A CCF is a high-flow communication following a tear of the ICA wall into the cavernous sinus and usually follows head trauma or spontaneous rupture of an ICA aneurysm into the cavernous sinus. It results in a sudden onset of pulsatile proptosis and significant engorgement of the conjunctival and episcleral vessels (Figs. 20.15, 20.16, and 20.17). Patients usually complain of the sudden occurrence of a buzzing sound in their head occurring with the onset of proptosis. Type B, C, and D CCFs occur spontaneously and are low-flow and may result in conjunctival congestion or episcleral injection and may be mistaken for conjunctivitis or episcleritis. These dural fistulas have an insidious onset and are seen almost always in old hypertensive women [118]. Type A fistulas do not close spontaneously and require em-bolization of the fistula. Types B, C and D dural CCF may resolve spontaneously.

20.13.2 Other Orbital Malformations: (Figs. 20.18, 20.19, and 20.20)

20.13.2.1 Orbital Varices

Orbital varices are congenital dilated thin-walled venous channel malformations in the

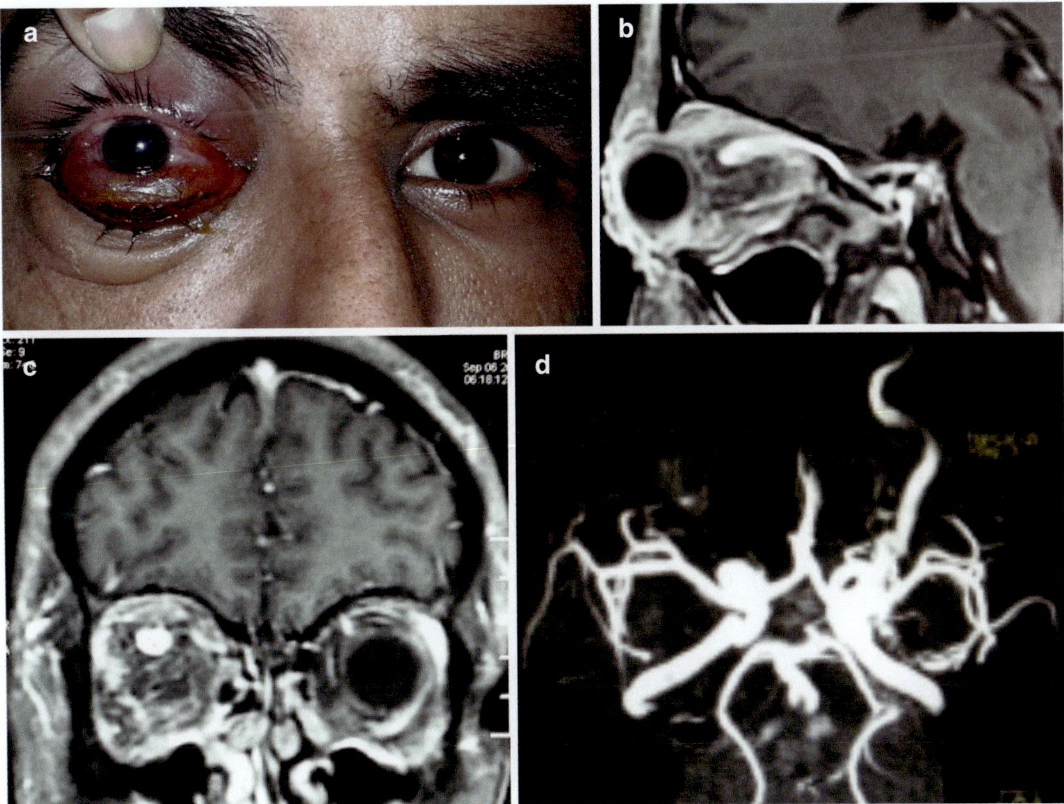

Fig. 20.15 Carotid-cavernous fistula: A 34-year-old patient with a history of head trauma presented with sudden onset of right eye redness, pain, decreased sensation over the right side of the face, progressive proptosis and vision loss. Examination revealed pulsatile exophthalmos, chemosis, dilated episcleral vessels, and ophthalmoplegia involving the pupil with a bruit on auscultation (**a**). On T1-MRI, sagittal (**b**) and coronal sections (**c**) reveal markedly dilated superior ophthalmic vein (SOV). MRA confirmed the diagnosis of Carotid-cavernous fistula (**d**). Images courtesy of Dr. Shweta Chaurasia, Advanced Eye Centre, Post Graduate Institute of Medical Education and Research, Chandigarh

orbit which do not anastomose with the arteriolar system and cause a non-pulsatile intermittent proptosis (Fig. 20.18). The proptosis increases on bending over, coughing or during the Valsalva manoeuvre [119]. The varices may cause orbital bone defects [120]. The varices may show the formation of phleboliths (Fig. 20.18). The orbital varices may be rarely associated (4.5%) with midline encephalocele, medial orbital wall defects or defects in the greater wing of the sphenoid [121]. This calls for caution when operating on the orbital varices. Inflammation of the orbital varices may lead to recurrent meningitis [121].

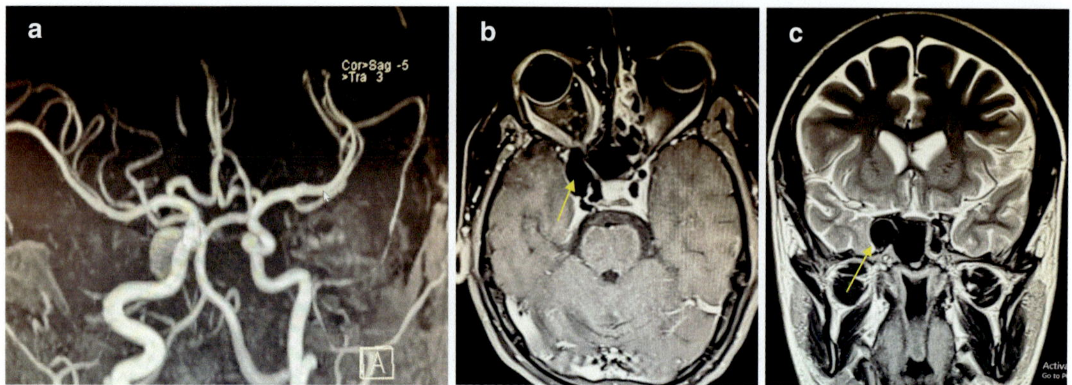

Fig. 20.16 Carotid-cavernous fistula: A 32-year-old man with a history of blunt trauma to the head and orbits presented with right eye mild proptosis with congestion and pain. MR angiography orbits and brain coronal section show communication between the cavernous part of the ICA and the right cavernous sinus (**a**). MRI orbits T1 axial scan (**b**) and T2 Coronal scan (**c**): The right cavernous sinus is expanded (yellow arrows in b and c). There is an enlargement of extraocular muscles and congestion in the retrobulbar fat. Features suggest a CCF with communication between the right ICA and the cavernous sinus. Images courtesy of Dr. Kasturi Bhattacharjee Sri Sankaradeva Nethralaya, Guwahati, India

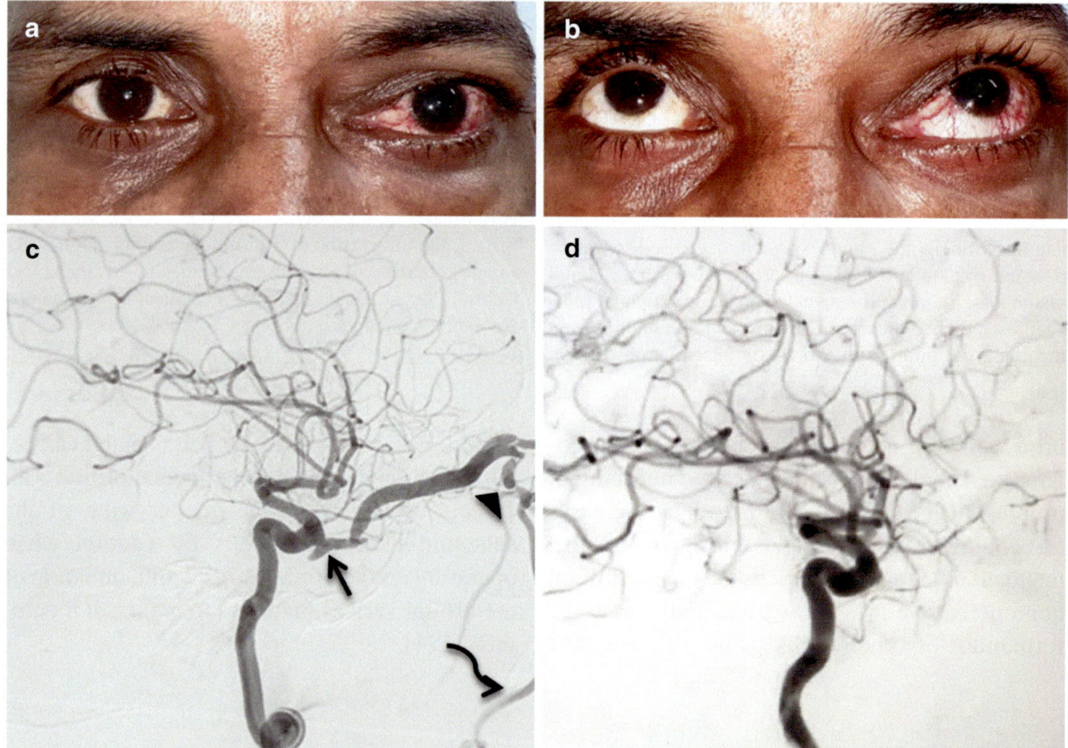

Fig. 20.17 Carotid-cavernous fistula: A 52-year-old male presented 8 months after trauma to the left forehead region. Left eye examination shows a scar above the brow, proptosis, exotropia, dilated pupil, dilated tortuous conjunctival vessels (**a**, **b**). He had raised intraocular pressure in the left eye. Digital subtraction angiogram revealed a Carotico-cavernous fistula It shows a fistulous communication between the cavernous segment of the left internal carotid artery and the superior ophthalmic vein draining into the angular and left facial veins (**c**). Following embolization, the fistula closed with restoration of normal circulation (**d**), the Images courtesy of Prof. Usha Singh, Advanced Eye Centre, Post Graduate Institute of Medical Education and Research, Chandigarh

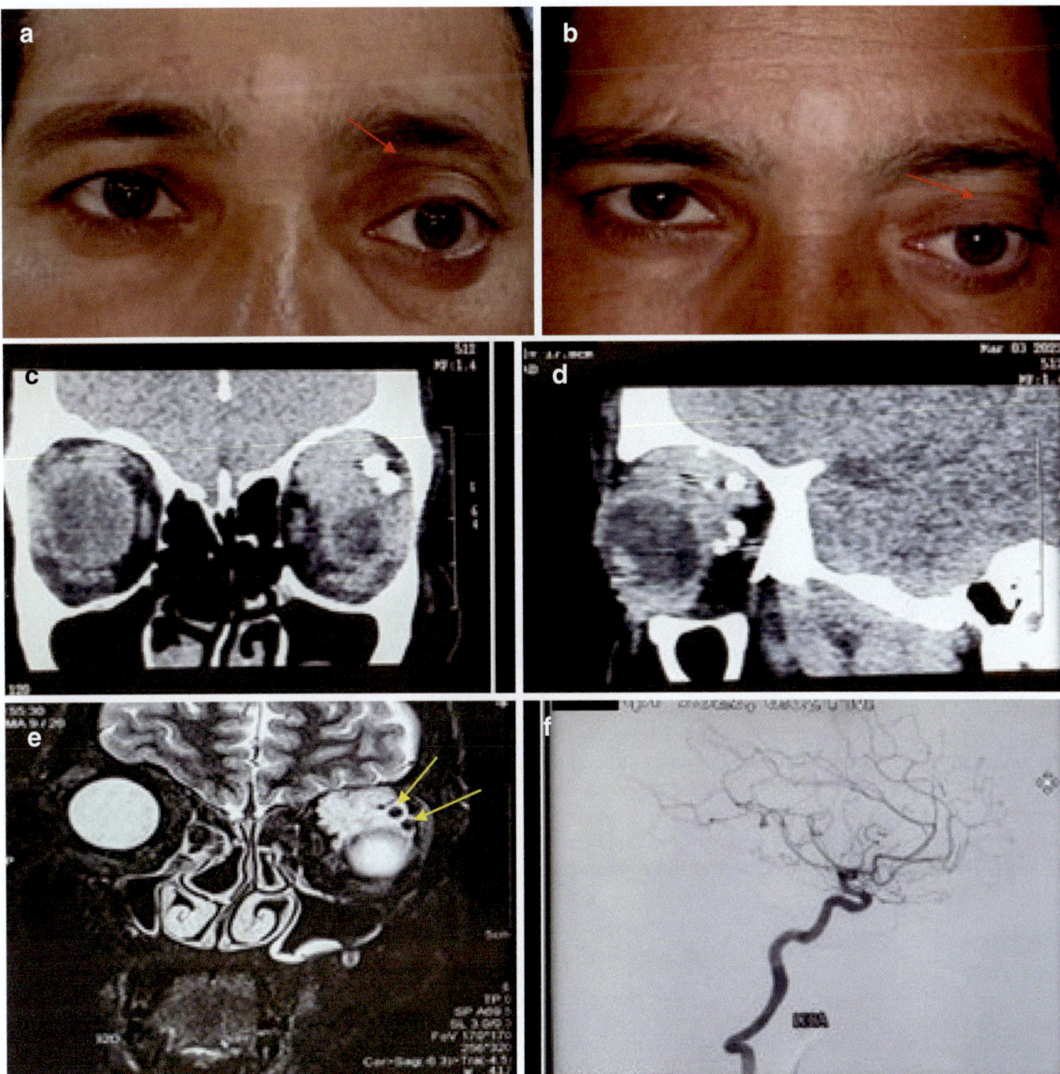

Fig. 20.18 Orbital varix: A 45-year-old female presented with outward protrusion of the left eye for 1 year (**a**). Increased fullness of the superior sulcus and inferior dystopia was noticed on the Valsalva manoeuvre (**b**, arrow, cf. **a**). Contrast-enhanced CT scan of the orbit in coronal view shows a solid mass in the superior and lateral aspect of the left eye with dense calcifications within it, s/o phleboliths (**c**). On the sagittal view, the mass extends intracranially (**d**). On T2 weighted MRI, the extent of the lobulated hyperintense mass is better defined, along with the presence of phleboliths appearing as rounded signal voids (yellow arrows, (**e**). The Left Internal Carotid Artery digital subtraction angiogram in lateral view showed no dilated arterial feeders (**f**). Images courtesy of Prof. Usha Singh, Advanced Eye Centre, Post Graduate Institute of Medical Education and Research, Chandigarh

20.13.2.2 Arteriovenous Malformations

Arteriovenous malformations (AVM) are high-flow congenital malformations that tend to grow with time (Figs. 20.19 and 20.20). These may be intraorbital or extra-orbital. In the AVM, the arterial blood flows directly into the venous system causing a pulsatile proptosis. There may be hemorrhage into the AVM. On CT angiography, there is uniform enhancement. MRI may show flow voids. Doppler scans will show the pulsatile nature of the lesion [122]. Because of the risk of intraoperative bleeding, the adnexal AVM are first embolized and then excized surgically [123, 124].

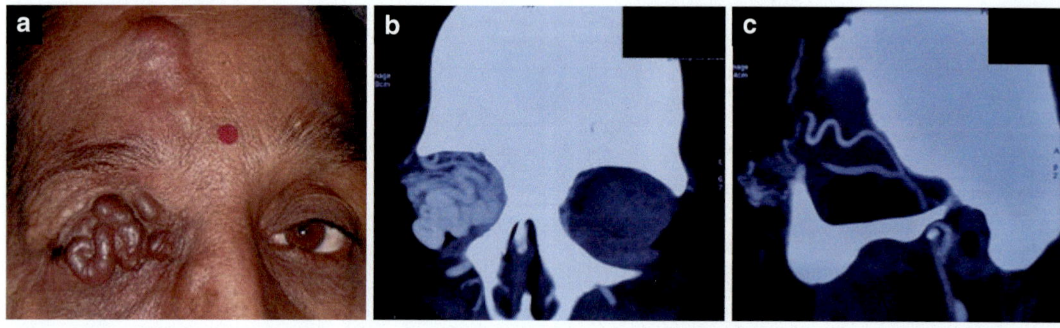

Fig. 20.19 AV malformation: A 53-year-old woman presented with swelling over her forehead for 20 years with the involvement of the right upper lid with serpentine swelling for 7 years (**a**) Palpation revealed a soft cystic compressible swelling with a bag of worms feel, audible bruit and pulsations. On CT angiography, intensely enhancing tangle of vessels are seen over the right upper lid leading into a nidus with predominant arterial feeders from branches of the right superficial temporal artery and ophthalmic artery with venous drainage into angular and superficial temporal veins (**b**, **c**). Images courtesy of Prof. Usha Singh, Advanced Eye Centre, Post Graduate Institute of Medical Education and Research, Chandigarh

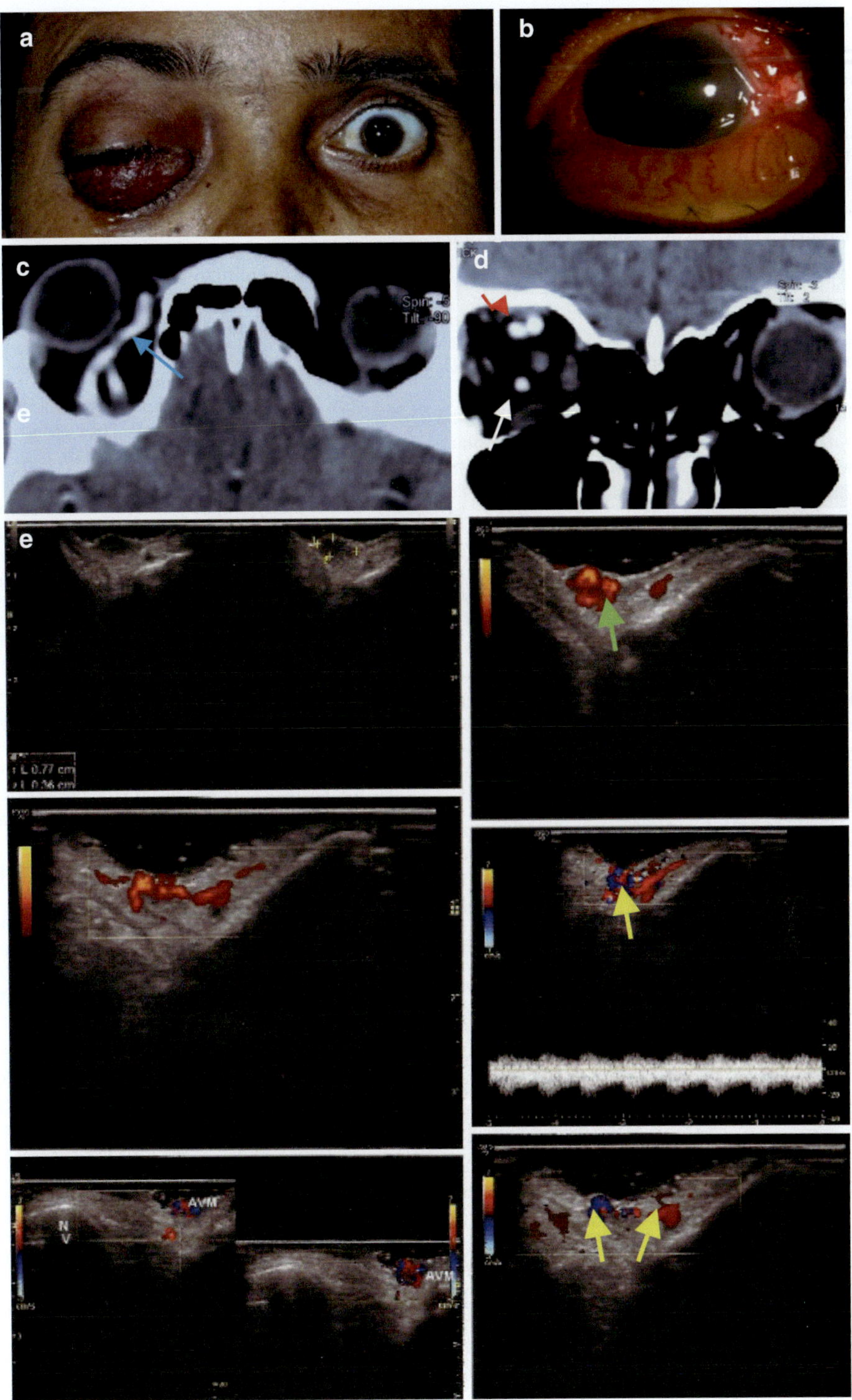

Fig. 20.20 AV malformation: A 40-year-old woman with right eye pulsatile proptosis and severe chemosis (**a**) Slit-lamp photograph shows dilated cork-screw-like episcleral vessels with chemosis (**b**). CT axial scan shows right proptosis with the dilated superior ophthalmic vein (**c**), blue arrow), and coronal scan (**d**) shows both dilated superior (red arrow) and inferior ophthalmic veins (white arrow). The colour Doppler study shows increased flow within the mass (green arrow). Pulse Doppler study shows bi-directional flow (yellow arrows) suggestive of arterio-venous malformation (**e**). Images courtesy of Dr. Kasturi Bhattacharjee, Sri Sankaradeva Nethralaya, Guwahati, Assam, India

References

1. Shumway CL, Motlagh M, Wade M. Anatomy, head and neck, orbit bones. In: StatPearls [Internet]. Treasure Island (FL): StatPearls Publishing; 2022; 2023 Jan–. PMID: 30285385.
2. Rootman J, Rootman DB, Stewart B, Diniz SB, Roelofs KA, Cohen LM, Claire CS, Eran A, Kaplan B, Marom A. Orbital fissures: inferior orbital fissure. In: Simon GB, Greenberg G, Prat DL, editors. Atlas of orbital imaging. Cham: Springer; 2022. p. 69–74. https://doi.org/10.1007/978-3-030-62426-2_91.
3. Wright JE. Proptosis. Ann R Coll Surg Engl. 1970;47(6):323–34. PMID: 5536948; PMCID: PMC2387903.
4. Migliori ME, Gladstone GJ. Determination of the normal range of exophthalmometric values for black and white adults. Am J Ophthalmol. 1984;98(4):438–42. https://doi.org/10.1016/0002-9394(84)90127-2. PMID: 6486215
5. Revankar S, Mehta A. Determination of exophthalmometry values in the North Indian population. Indian J Ophthalmol. 2022;70(8):3083–7. https://doi.org/10.4103/ijo.IJO_489_22. PMID: 35918977; PMCID: PMC9672748.
6. Huh J, Park SJ, Lee JK. Measurement of proptosis using computed tomography based three-dimensional reconstruction software in patients with Graves' orbitopathy. Sci Rep. 2020;10(1):14554. https://doi.org/10.1038/s41598-020-71098-4. PMID: 32883985; PMCID: PMC7471301.
7. Park NR, Moon JH, Lee JK. Hertel exophthalmometer versus computed tomography scan in proptosis estimation in thyroid-associated orbitopathy. Clin Ophthalmol. 2019;13:1461–7. https://doi.org/10.2147/OPTH.S216838. PMID: 35008259; PMCID: PMC8750198.
8. Zhang Y, Rao J, Wu X, Zhou Y, Liu G, Zhang H. Automatic measurement of exophthalmos based orbital CT images using deep learning. Front Cell Dev Biol. 2023;11:1135959. https://doi.org/10.3389/fcell.2023.1135959. PMID: 36910161; PMCID: PMC9998665.
9. Hwang CJ, Afifiyan N, Sand D, Naik V, Said J, Pollock SJ, Chen B, Phipps RP, Goldberg RA, Smith TJ, Douglas RS. Orbital fibroblasts from patients with thyroid-associated ophthalmopathy overexpress CD40: CD154 hyper induces IL-6, IL-8, and MCP-1. Invest Ophthalmol Vis Sci. 2009a;50(5):2262–8. https://doi.org/10.1167/iovs.08-2328. Epub 2008 Dec 30. PMID: 19117935; PMCID: PMC2752347.
10. Hwang K, You SH, Sohn IA. Analysis of orbital bone fractures: a 12-year study of 391 patients. J Craniofac Surg. 2009b;20(4):1218–23. https://doi.org/10.1097/SCS.0b013e3181acde01. PMID: 19553835.
11. Shields JA, Shields CL, Scartozzi R. Survey of 1264 patients with orbital tumors and simulating lesions: the 2002 Montgomery Lecture, part 1. Ophthalmology. 2004;111(5):997–1008. https://doi.org/10.1016/j.ophtha.2003.01.002. PMID: 15121380.
12. Shields JA, Bakewell B, Augsburger JJ, Flanagan JC. Classification and incidence of space-occupying lesions of the orbit. A survey of 645 biopsies. Arch Ophthalmol. 1984;102(11):1606–11. https://doi.org/10.1001/archopht.1984.01040031296011. PMID: 6497741.
13. Bahn RS, Heufelder AE. Pathogenesis of Graves' ophthalmopathy. N Engl J Med. 1993;329(20):1468–75. https://doi.org/10.1056/NEJM199311113292007.
14. Michalek K, Morshed SA, Latif R, Davies TF. TSH receptor autoantibodies. Autoimmun Rev. 2009;9(2):113–6. https://doi.org/10.1016/j.autrev.2009.03.012. Epub 2009 Mar 27. PMID: 19332151; PMCID: PMC3753030.
15. Garrity JA, Bahn RS. Pathogenesis of graves ophthalmopathy: implications for prediction, prevention, and treatment. Am J Ophthalmol. 2006;142(1):147–53. https://doi.org/10.1016/j.ajo.2006.02.047. PMID: 16815265; PMCID: PMC3960010.
16. Koumas L, Smith TJ, Feldon S, Blumberg N, Phipps RP. Thy-1 expression in human fibroblast subsets defines myofibroblastic or lipofibroblastic phenotypes. Am J Pathol. 2003;163(4):1291–300. https://doi.org/10.1016/S0002-9440(10)63488-8. PMID: 14507638; PMCID: PMC1868289.
17. Khoo TK, Coenen MJ, Schiefer AR, Kumar S, Bahn RS. Evidence for enhanced Thy-1 (CD90) expression in orbital fibroblasts of patients with Graves' ophthalmopathy. Thyroid. 2008;18(12):1291–6. https://doi.org/10.1089/thy.2008.0255. PMID: 18976167; PMCID: PMC2857447.
18. Neag EJ, Smith TJ. 2021 update on thyroid-associated ophthalmopathy. J Endocrinol Invest. 2022;45(2):235–59.https://doi.org/10.1007/s40618--021-01663-9. Epub 2021 Aug 20. PMID: 34417736; PMCID: PMC9455782.
19. Hufnagel TJ, Hickey WF, Cobbs WH, Jakobiec FA, Iwamoto T, Eagle RC. Immunohistochemical and ultrastructural studies on the exenterated orbital tissues of a patient with Graves' disease. Ophthalmology. 1984;91(11):1411–9. https://doi.org/10.1016/s0161-6420(84)34152-5. PMID: 6240008.
20. Dik WA, Virakul S, van Steensel L. Current perspectives on the role of orbital fibroblasts in the pathogenesis of Graves' ophthalmopathy. Exp Eye Res. 2016;142:83–91. https://doi.org/10.1016/j.exer.2015.02.007.
21. Tsui S, Naik V, Hoa N, Hwang CJ, Afifiyan NF, Sinha Hikim A, Gianoukakis AG, Douglas RS, Smith TJ. Evidence for an association between thyroid-stimulating hormone and insulin-like growth factor 1 receptors: a tale of two antigens implicated in Graves' disease. J Immunol. 2008;181(6):4397–405. https://doi.org/10.4049/jimmunol.181.6.4397. PMID: 18768899; PMCID: PMC2775538.

22. Paik JS, Kim SE, Kim JH, Lee JY, Yang SW, Lee SB. Insulin-like growth factor-1 enhances the expression of functional TSH receptor in orbital fibroblasts from thyroid-associated ophthalmopathy. Immunobiology. 2020;225(2):151902. https://doi.org/10.1016/j.imbio.2019.151902. Epub 2019 Dec 25. PMID: 31899052.
23. Bartley GB. The differential diagnosis and classification of eyelid retraction. Ophthalmology. 1996;103(1):168–76. https://doi.org/10.1016/s0161-6420(96)30744-6.
24. Bartley GB, Gorman CA. Diagnostic criteria for Graves' ophthalmopathy. Am J Ophthalmol. 1995;119(6):792–5. https://doi.org/10.1016/s0002-9394(14)72787-4.
25. Cant JS, Lewis DR, Harrison MT. Treatment of dysthyroid ophthalmopathy with local guanethidine. Br J Ophthalmol. 1969;53(4):233–8. https://doi.org/10.1136/bjo.53.4.233. PMID: 5818669; PMCID: PMC1207305.
26. Wesley RE, Bond JB. Upper eyelid retraction from inferior rectus restriction in dysthyroid orbit disease. Ann Ophthalmol. 1987;19(1):34–6, 40. PMID: 3827067.
27. Byun JS, Lee JK. Relationships between eyelid position and levator-superior rectus complex and inferior rectus muscle in patients with Graves' orbitopathy with unilateral upper eyelid retraction. Graefes Arch Clin Exp Ophthalmol. 2018;256(10):2001–8. https://doi.org/10.1007/s00417-018-4056-z. Epub 2018 Jun 29.
28. Cruz AA, Ribeiro SF, Garcia DM, Akaishi PM, Pinto CT. Graves upper eyelid retraction. Surv Ophthalmol. 2013;58(1):63–76. https://doi.org/10.1016/j.survophthal.2012.02.007.
29. Lee DC, Young SM, Kim YD, Woo KI. Course of upper eyelid retraction in thyroid eye disease. Br J Ophthalmol. 2020;104(2):254–9. https://doi.org/10.1136/bjophthalmol-2018-313578. Epub 2019 May 11. PMID: 31079052.
30. Ribeiro SF, Shekhovtsova M, Duarte AF, Velasco Cruz AA. Graves lower eyelid retraction. Ophthalmic Plast Reconstr Surg. 2016;32(3):161–9. https://doi.org/10.1097/IOP.0000000000000613. PMID: 26784547.
31. Guastella C, di Furia D, Torretta S, Ibba TM, Pignataro L, Accorona R. Upper eyelid retraction in Graves' ophthalmopathy: our surgical experience on 153 cases of full-thickness anterior blepharotomy with mullerectomy. Aesthet Plast Surg. 2022;46(4):1713–21. https://doi.org/10.1007/s00266-022-02770-5. Epub 2022 Feb 7. PMID: 35129648.
32. Perry JD, Hwang CJ. Invited discussion on: "upper eyelid retraction in Graves' ophthalmopathy: our surgical experience on 153 cases of full-thickness anterior blepharotomy with mullerectomy". Aesthet Plast Surg. 2022;46(4):1722–3. https://doi.org/10.1007/s00266-022-02875-x. Epub 2022 Apr 18. PMID: 35437666.
33. Osaki TH, Monteiro LG, Osaki MH. Management of eyelid retraction related to thyroid eye disease. Taiwan J Ophthalmol. 2022;12(1):12–21. https://doi.org/10.4103/tjo.tjo_57_21. PMID: 35399960; PMCID: PMC8988987.
34. Hamedani AG, Gold DR. Eyelid dysfunction in neurodegenerative, neurogenetic, and neurometabolic disease. Front Neurol. 2017;8:329. https://doi.org/10.3389/fneur.2017.00329. PMID: 28769865; PMCID: PMC5513921.
35. Horn AK, Büttner-Ennever JA. Brainstem circuits controlling lid-eye coordination in monkey. Prog Brain Res. 2008;171:87–95. https://doi.org/10.1016/S0079-6123(08)00612-2. PMID: 18718286.
36. Jackson WP. Incidence of signs usually connected with thyrotoxicosis with special reference to lid lag. Br Med J. 1949;2(4632):847. https://doi.org/10.1136/bmj.2.4632.847. PMID: 18143463; PMCID: PMC2051467.
37. Harvey JT, Anderson RL. Lid lag and lagophthalmos: a clarification of terminology. Ophthalmic Surg. 1981;12(5):338–40. PMID: 7266976.
38. Gaddipati RV, Meyer DR. Eyelid retraction, lid lag, lagophthalmos, and von Graefe's sign quantifying the eyelid features of Graves' ophthalmopathy. Ophthalmology. 2008;115(6):1083–8. https://doi.org/10.1016/j.ophtha.2007.07.027. Epub 2007 Sep 27. PMID: 17900690.
39. Burch HB, Perros P, Bednarczuk T, Cooper DS, Dolman PJ, Leung AM, Mombaerts I, Salvi M, Stan MN. Management of thyroid eye disease: a consensus statement by the American Thyroid Association and the European Thyroid Association. Thyroid. 2022;32(12):1439–70. https://doi.org/10.1089/thy.2022.0251. Epub 2022 Dec 8. PMID: 36480280; PMCID: PMC9807259.
40. Mourits MP, Koornneef L, Wiersinga WM, Prummel MF, Berghout A, van der Gaag R. Clinical criteria for the assessment of disease activity in Graves' ophthalmopathy: a novel approach. Br J Ophthalmol. 1989;73(8):639–44. https://doi.org/10.1136/bjo.73.8.639. PMID: 2765444; PMCID: PMC1041835.
41. European Group on Graves' Orbitopathy (EUGOGO), Wiersinga WM, Perros P, Kahaly GJ, Mourits MP, Baldeschi L, Boboridis K, Boschi A, Dickinson AJ, Kendall-Taylor P, Krassas GE, Lane CM, Lazarus JH, Marcocci C, Marino M, Nardi M, Neoh C, Orgiazzi J, Pinchera A, Pitz S, Prummel MF, Sartini MS, Stahl M, von Arx G. Clinical assessment of patients with Graves' orbitopathy: the European Group on Graves' orbitopathy recommendations to generalists, specialists and clinical researchers. Eur J Endocrinol. 2006;155(3):387–9. https://doi.org/10.1530/eje.1.02230.
42. Werner SC. Classification of the eye changes of Grave's disease. J Clin Endocrinol Metab. 1969;29(7):982–4. https://doi.org/10.1210/jcem-29-7-982. PMID: 5819411.

43. Werner SC. Modification of the classification of the eye changes of Graves' disease: recommendations of the Ad Hoc Committee of the American Thyroid Association. J Clin Endocrinol Metab. 1977;44(1):203–4. https://doi.org/10.1210/jcem-44-1-203. PMID: 576230.
44. Frueh BR. Why the NOSPECS classification of Graves' eye disease should be abandoned, with suggestions for the characterization of this disease. Thyroid. 1992;2(1):85–8. https://doi.org/10.1089/thy.1992.2.85.
45. Weber M, Deuschl C, Bechrakis N, Umutlu L, Antoch G, Eckstein A, Binse I, Oeverhaus M. 18 F-FDG-PET/MRI in patients with Graves' orbitopathy. Graefes Arch Clin Exp Ophthalmol. 2021;259(10):3107–17. https://doi.org/10.1007/s00417-021-05339-1. Epub 2021 Aug 18. PMID: 34406498; PMCID: PMC8478760.
46. Bartalena L, Kahaly GJ, Baldeschi L, Dayan CM, Eckstein A, Marcocci C, Marinò M, Vaidya B, Wiersinga WM, EUGOGO †. The 2021 European Group on Graves' orbitopathy (EUGOGO) clinical practice guidelines for the medical management of Graves' orbitopathy. Eur J Endocrinol. 2021;185(4):G43–67. https://doi.org/10.1530/EJE-21-0479.
47. Kahaly GJ, Wüster C, Olivo PD, Diana T. High titers of thyrotropin receptor antibodies are associated with orbitopathy in patients with graves disease. J Clin Endocrinol Metab. 2019;104(7):2561–8. https://doi.org/10.1210/jc.2018-02705. PMID: 30753531.
48. Sarić Matutinović M, Kahaly GJ, Žarković M, Ćirić J, Ignjatović S, Nedeljković BB. The phenotype of Graves' orbitopathy is associated with thyrotropin receptor antibody levels. J Endocrinol Investig. 2023;46:2309. https://doi.org/10.1007/s40618-023-02085-5. Epub ahead of print. PMID: 37020104.
49. Stein JD, Childers D, Gupta S, Talwar N, Nan B, Lee BJ, Smith TJ, Douglas R. Risk factors for developing thyroid-associated ophthalmopathy among individuals with graves disease. JAMA Ophthalmol. 2015;133(3):290–6. https://doi.org/10.1001/jamaophthalmol.2014.5103. PMID: 25502604; PMCID: PMC4495733.
50. Nilsson A, Tsoumani K, Planck T. Statins decrease the risk of orbitopathy in newly diagnosed patients with Graves Disease. J Clin Endocrinol Metab. 2021;106(5):1325–32. https://doi.org/10.1210/clinem/dgab070. PMID: 33560351.
51. Bartalena L, Baldeschi L, Boboridis K, Eckstein A, Kahaly GJ, Marcocci C, Perros P, Salvi M, Wiersinga WM, European Group on Graves' Orbitopathy (EUGOGO). The 2016 European Thyroid Association/European Group on Graves' Orbitopathy guidelines for the management of graves' orbitopathy. Eur Thyroid J. 2016;5(1):9–26. https://doi.org/10.1159/000443828. Epub 2016 Mar 2. PMID: 27099835; PMCID: PMC4836120.
52. Douglas RS, Dailey R, Subramanian PS, Barbesino G, Ugradar S, Batten R, Qadeer RA, Cameron C. Proptosis and diplopia response with teprotumumab and placebo vs the recommended treatment regimen with intravenous methylprednisolone in moderate to severe thyroid eye disease: a meta-analysis and matching-adjusted indirect comparison. JAMA Ophthalmol. 2022;140(4):328–35. https://doi.org/10.1001/jamaophthalmol.2021.6284. PMID: 35175308; PMCID: PMC8855315.
53. Jefferis JM, Jones RK, Currie ZI, Tan JH, Salvi SM. Orbital decompression for thyroid eye disease: methods, outcomes, and complications. Eye (Lond). 2018;32(3):626–36. https://doi.org/10.1038/eye.2017.260. Epub 2017 Dec 15. PMID: 29243735; PMCID: PMC5848288.
54. Baeg J, Choi HS, Kim C, Kim H, Jang SY. Update on the surgical management of Graves' orbitopathy. Front Endocrinol (Lausanne). 2023;13:1080204. https://doi.org/10.3389/fendo.2022.1080204. PMID: 36824601; PMCID: PMC9941741.
55. Lacey B, Chang W, Rootman J. Nonthyroid causes of extraocular muscle disease. Surv Ophthalmol. 1999;44(3):187–213.https://doi.org/10.1016/s0039--6257(99)00101-0. PMID: 10588439.
56. Leung V, Maietta A, Kalin-Hajdu E. Bilateral enlargement of all extraocular muscles. JAMA Ophthalmol. 2021;139(3):359–60. https://doi.org/10.1001/jamaophthalmol.2020.4679. PMID: 33443567.
57. McCoskey M, Reshef ER, Wolkow N, Yoon MK. Bilateral enlargement of all extraocular muscles: a presenting ophthalmic sign of hematologic malignancy. Orbit. 2022;22:1–4. https://doi.org/10.1080/01676830.2022.2090014. Epub ahead of print. PMID: 35734822.
58. Gupta P, Singh U, Singh SK, Kapoor R, Gupta V, Das A. Bilateral symmetrical metastasis to all extraocular muscles from distant rhabdomyosarcoma. Orbit. 2010;29(3):146–8. https://doi.org/10.3109/01676830903294917. PMID: 20497080.
59. McCarty ML, Wilson MW, Ibrahim F, Fuller CE, Kun LE, Haik BG. Primary perineal alveolar rhabdomyosarcoma metastatic to an extraocular muscle. Ophthalmic Plast Reconstr Surg. 2003;19(4):333–5. https://doi.org/10.1097/01.IOP.0000075798.91711.68. PMID: 12878888.
60. Scott IU, Siatkowski RM. Idiopathic orbital myositis. Curr Opin Rheumatol. 1997;9(6):504–12. https://doi.org/10.1097/00002281-199711000-00005. PMID: 9375279.
61. Kang MS, Yang HK, Kim N, Hwang JM. Clinical features of ocular motility in idiopathic orbital myositis. J Clin Med. 2020;9(4):1165. https://doi.org/10.3390/jcm9041165. PMID: 32325733; PMCID: PMC7231042.
62. Rana K, Juniat V, Patel S, Selva D. Extraocular muscle enlargement. Graefes Arch Clin Exp Ophthalmol. 2022;260(11):3419–35. https://doi.org/10.1007/s00417-022-05727-1. Epub 2022 Jun 17. PMID: 35713708; PMCID: PMC9581877.

63. Ben Simon GJ, Syed HM, Douglas R, McCann JD, Goldberg RA. Extraocular muscle enlargement with tendon involvement in thyroid-associated orbitopathy. Am J Ophthalmol. 2004;137(6):1145–7. https://doi.org/10.1016/j.ajo.2004.01.033.
64. Wu N, Sun FY. Clinical observation of orbital IgG4-related diseases. Exp Ther Med. 2019;17(1):883–7. https://doi.org/10.3892/etm.2018.7002. Epub 2018 Nov 21. PMID: 30651876; PMCID: PMC6307391.
65. Coutu B, Alvarez DA, Ciurej A, Moneymaker K, White M, Zhang C, Drincic A. Extraocular muscle enlargement in growth hormone-secreting pituitary adenomas. AJNR Am J Neuroradiol. 2022;43(4):597–602. https://doi.org/10.3174/ajnr.A7453. Epub 2022 Mar 17. PMID: 35301224; PMCID: PMC8993204.
66. Olejarz M, Szczepanek-Parulska E, Dadej D, Sawicka-Gutaj N, Domin R, Ruchała M. IgG4 as a biomarker in Graves' orbitopathy. Mediat Inflamm. 2021;2021:5590471. https://doi.org/10.1155/2021/5590471. PMID: 34220335; PMCID: PMC8213474.
67. Abouelatta MM, Shalaby OE, Awara AM, Kikkawa DO, Liu CY, Eldesouky MA. Role of muscle biopsy in diagnosis of extraocular muscles enlargement. Int Ophthalmol. 2023;43(3):717–23. https://doi.org/10.1007/s10792-022-02470-8. Epub 2022 Aug 30.
68. Lucarelli KM, Chen KG, Akella SS. An unusual case of severe bilateral extraocular muscle enlargement. JAMA Ophthalmol. 2022;140(7):738–9. https://doi.org/10.1001/jamaophthalmol.2022.0265. PMID: 35511150.
69. Zheng Y, Zhang YX, Ding MP. Treatment of idiopathic orbital myositis with frequent relapses: first case with tacrolimus and review of literature. J Neuroimmunol. 2020;346:577316. https://doi.org/10.1016/j.jneuroim.2020.577316. Epub ahead of print. PMID: 32668345.
70. Dagi LR, Zoumalan CI, Konrad H, Trokel SL, Kazim M. Correlation between extraocular muscle size and motility restriction in thyroid eye disease. Ophthalmic Plast Reconstr Surg. 2011;27(2):102–10. https://doi.org/10.1097/IOP.0b013e3181e9a063.
71. Ozgen A, Ariyurek M. Normative measurements of orbital structures using CT. AJR Am J Roentgenol. 1998;170(4):1093–6. https://doi.org/10.2214/ajr.170.4.9530066. PMID: 9530066.
72. Andrew NH, Sladden N, Kearney DJ, Selva D. An analysis of IgG4-related disease (IgG4-RD) among idiopathic orbital inflammations and benign lymphoid hyperplasias using two consensus-based diagnostic criteria for IgG4-RD. Br J Ophthalmol. 2015;99(3):376–81. https://doi.org/10.1136/bjophthalmol-2014-305545. Epub 2014 Sep 2.
73. Wu A, Andrew NH, McNab AA, Selva D. IgG4-related ophthalmic disease: pooling of published cases and literature review. Curr Allergy Asthma Rep.2015;15(6):27.https://doi.org/10.1007/s11882--015-0530-4. PMID: 26141575.
74. Wallace ZS, Deshpande V, Stone JH. Ophthalmic manifestations of IgG4-related disease: single-center experience and literature review. Semin Arthritis Rheum. 2014;43(6):806–17. https://doi.org/10.1016/j.semarthrit.2013.11.008. Epub 2013 Nov 15. PMID: 24513111.
75. Park J, Lee MJ, Kim N, Kim JE, Park SW, Choung HK, Khwarg SI. Risk factors for extraophthalmic involvement and treatment outcomes in patients with IgG4-related ophthalmic disease. Br J Ophthalmol. 2018;102(6):736–41. https://doi.org/10.1136/bjophthalmol-2017-310584. Epub 2017 Sep 28. PMID: 28972022.
76. Deshpande V, Zen Y, Chan JK, Yi EE, Sato Y, Yoshino T, Klöppel G, Heathcote JG, Khosroshahi A, Ferry JA, Aalberse RC, Bloch DB, Brugge WR, Bateman AC, Carruthers MN, Chari ST, Cheuk W, Cornell LD, Fernandez-Del Castillo C, Forcione DG, Hamilos DL, Kamisawa T, Kasashima S, Kawa S, Kawano M, Lauwers GY, Masaki Y, Nakanuma Y, Notohara K, Okazaki K, Ryu JK, Saeki T, Sahani DV, Smyrk TC, Stone JR, Takahira M, Webster GJ, Yamamoto M, Zamboni G, Umehara H, Stone JH. Consensus statement on the pathology of IgG4-related disease. Mod Pathol. 2012;25(9):1181–92. https://doi.org/10.1038/modpathol.2012.72. Epub 2012 May 18.
77. Umehara H, Okazaki K, Masaki Y, Kawano M, Yamamoto M, Saeki T, Matsui S, Yoshino T, Nakamura S, Kawa S, Hamano H, Kamisawa T, Shimosegawa T, Shimatsu A, Nakamura S, Ito T, Notohara K, Sumida T, Tanaka Y, Mimori T, Chiba T, Mishima M, Hibi T, Tsubouchi H, Inui K, Ohara H. Comprehensive diagnostic criteria for IgG4-related disease (IgG4-RD), 2011. Mod Rheumatol. 2012;22(1):21–30. https://doi.org/10.1007/s10165--011-0571-z. Epub 2012 Jan 5. PMID: 22218969.
78. Woo YJ, Kim JW, Yoon JS. Clinical implications of serum IgG_4 levels in patients with IgG_4-related ophthalmic disease. Br J Ophthalmol. 2017;101(3):256–60. https://doi.org/10.1136/bjophthalmol-2016-308592. Epub 2016 May 23. PMID: 27215743.
79. Ko BS, Chen LJ, Huang HH, Wen YC, Liao CY, Chen HM, Hsiao FY. Subtype-specific epidemiology of lymphoid malignancies in Taiwan compared to Japan and the United States, 2002–2012. Cancer Med. 2018;7(11):5820–31. https://doi.org/10.1002/cam4.1762. Epub 2018 Oct 9. PMID: 30460792; PMCID: PMC6246924.
80. Hsu CR, Chen YY, Yao M, Wei YH, Hsieh YT, Liao SL. Orbital and ocular adnexal lymphoma: a review of epidemiology and prognostic factors in Taiwan. Eye (Lond). 2021;35(7):1946–53. https://doi.org/10.1038/s41433-020-01198-y. Epub 2020 Sep 29. PMID: 32994547; PMCID: PMC8225637.
81. Ahmed OM, Ma AK, Ahmed TM, Pointdujour-Lim R. Epidemiology, outcomes, and prognostic factors of orbital lymphoma in the United States. Orbit.

2020;39(6):397–402. https://doi.org/10.1080/01676830.2019.1704032. Epub 2020 Jan 2.
82. Olsen TG, Heegaard S. Orbital lymphoma. Surv Ophthalmol. 2019;64(1):45–66. https://doi.org/10.1016/j.survophthal.2018.08.002. Epub 2018 Aug 23. PMID: 30144455.
83. Vogele D, Sollmann N, Beck A, Haggenmüller B, Schmidt SA, Schmitz B, Kapapa T, Ozpeynirci Y, Beer M, Kloth C. Orbital tumors-clinical, radiologic and histopathologic correlation. Diagnostics (Basel). 2022;12(10):2376. https://doi.org/10.3390/diagnostics12102376. PMID: 36292065; PMCID: PMC9600631.
84. Olsen TG, Holm F, Mikkelsen LH, Rasmussen PK, Coupland SE, Esmaeli B, Finger PT, Graue GF, Grossniklaus HE, Honavar SG, Khong JJ, McKelvie PA, Mulay K, Sjö LD, Vemuganti GK, Thuro BA, Heegaard S. Orbital lymphoma-an international multicenter retrospective study. Am J Ophthalmol. 2019;199:44–57. https://doi.org/10.1016/j.ajo.2018.11.002. Epub 2018 Nov 10. PMID: 30419193.
85. Shields JA, Shields CL, Brotman HK, Carvalho C, Perez N, Eagle RC Jr. Cancer metastatic to the orbit: the 2000 Robert M. Curts Lecture. Ophthalmic Plast Reconstr Surg. 2001;17(5):346–54. https://doi.org/10.1097/00002341-200109000-00009. PMID: 11642491.
86. Ahmed S, Goel S, Khandwala M, Agrawal A, Chang B, Simmons IG. Neuroblastoma with orbital metastasis: ophthalmic presentation and role of ophthalmologists. Eye (Lond). 2006;20(4):466–70. https://doi.org/10.1038/sj.eye.6701912.
87. Palmisciano P, Ferini G, Ogasawara C, Wahood W, Bin Alamer O, Gupta AD, Scalia G, Larsen AMG, Yu K, Umana GE, Cohen-Gadol AA, El Ahmadieh TY, Haider AS. Orbital metastases: a systematic review of clinical characteristics, management strategies, and treatment outcomes. Cancers (Basel). 2021;14(1):94. https://doi.org/10.3390/cancers14010094. PMID: 35008259; PMCID: PMC8750198.
88. Soeroso NN, Tarigan SP, Saragih W, Sari ND, Lubis N, Lubis H. Lung adenocarcinoma presenting with an orbital metastasis. Respir Med Case Rep. 2018;25:116–8. https://doi.org/10.1016/j.rmcr.2018.08.005. PMID: 30112271; PMCID: PMC6091225.
89. Ookuma T, Kikuchi R, Takoi H, Toriyama K, Abe S. Orbital apex syndrome associated with intraorbital metastasis of lung cancer. Respirol Case Rep. 2022;10(4):e0922. https://doi.org/10.1002/rcr2.922. PMID: 35251665; PMCID: PMC8886096.
90. Manohar K, Mittal BR, Bhattacharya A, Gupta A. Orbital metastases as presenting sign of lung carcinoma: detection of primary malignancy and disease burden by F-18 FDG PET/CT. Nucl Med Mol Imaging. 2012a;46(1):73–5. https://doi.org/10.1007/s13139-011-0123-7. Epub 2012 Jan 4. PMID: 24900036; PMCID: PMC4042977.
91. Manohar K, Mittal BR, Kulkarni P, Singh N, Bhattacharya A, Gupta A. Usefulness of F-18 FDG PET/CT as one-stop-shop imaging modality for diagnosis of occult primary and estimation of disease burden in patients with intraocular masses. Clin Nucl Med. 2012b;37(2):200–3. https://doi.org/10.1097/RLU.0b013e31823e9d69. PMID: 22228354.
92. Kim JS, Liss J. Masses of the lacrimal gland: evaluation and treatment. J Neurol Surg B Skull Base. 2021;82(1):100–6. https://doi.org/10.1055/s-0040-1722700. Epub 2021 Feb 18. PMID: 33777623; PMCID: PMC7987400.
93. Rose GE, Wright JE. Pleomorphic adenoma of the lacrimal gland. Br J Ophthalmol. 1992;76(7):395–400. https://doi.org/10.1136/bjo.76.7.395. PMID: 1320923; PMCID: PMC504299.
94. Lai T, Prabhakaran VC, Malhotra R, Selva D. Pleomorphic adenoma of the lacrimal gland: is there a role for biopsy? Eye (Lond). 2009;23(1):2–6. https://doi.org/10.1038/eye.2008.16. Epub 2008 Mar 7. PMID: 18327162.
95. Kopp ED, Sahlin S, Tani E, Skoog L, Seregard S. Fine-needle aspiration biopsy in lacrimal gland pleomorphic adenoma. Eye (Lond). 2010;24(2):386. https://doi.org/10.1038/eye.2009.97. Epub 2009 May 1. PMID: 19407844.
96. Currie ZI, Rose GE. Long-term risk of recurrence after intact excision of pleomorphic adenomas of the lacrimal gland. Arch Ophthalmol. 2007;125(12):1643–6. https://doi.org/10.1001/archopht.125.12.1643.
97. Vangveeravong S, Katz SE, Rootman J, White V. Tumors arising in the palpebral lobe of the lacrimal gland. Ophthalmology. 1996;103(10):1606–12. https://doi.org/10.1016/s0161-6420(96)30456-9. PMID: 8874433.
98. Young SM, Kim YD, Shin HJ, Imagawa Y, Lang SS, Woo KI. Lacrimal gland pleomorphic adenoma and malignant epithelial tumours: clinical and imaging differences. Br J Ophthalmol. 2019;103(2):264–8. https://doi.org/10.1136/bjophthalmol-2017-311538. Epub 2018 Apr 21. PMID: 29680804.
99. Johnson TE, Casiano RR, Kronish JW, Tse DT, Meldrum M, Chang W. Sino-orbital aspergillosis in acquired immunodeficiency syndrome. Arch Ophthalmol. 1999;117(1):57–64. https://doi.org/10.1001/archopht.117.1.57. PMID: 9930161.
100. Trief D, Gray ST, Jakobiec FA, Durand ML, Fay A, Freitag SK, Lee NG, Lefebvre DR, Holbrook E, Bleier B, Sadow P, Rashid A, Chhabra N, Yoon MK. Invasive fungal disease of the sinus and orbit: a comparison between mucormycosis and Aspergillus. Br J Ophthalmol. 2016;100(2):184–8. https://doi.org/10.1136/bjophthalmol-2015-306945. Epub 2015 Jun 25. PMID: 26112869.

101. Alsulaiman HM, Elkhamary SM, Alrajeh M, Al-Alsheikh O, Al-Ghadeer H. Invasive sino-orbital aspergillosis with brain invasion in an immunocompetent pregnant patient. Am J Ophthalmol Case Rep. 2021;24:101210. https://doi.org/10.1016/j.ajoc.2021.101210. PMID: 34611568; PMCID: PMC8476652.
102. Chang YM, Chang YH, Chien KH, Liang CM, Tai MC, Nieh S, Chen YJ. Orbital apex syndrome secondary to aspergilloma masquerading as a paranasal sinus tumor: a case report and literature review. Medicine (Baltimore). 2018;97(30):e11650. https://doi.org/10.1097/MD.0000000000011650. PMID: 30045315; PMCID: PMC6078660.
103. Mukherjee B, Raichura ND, Alam MS. Fungal infections of the orbit. Indian J Ophthalmol. 2016;64(5):337–45. https://doi.org/10.4103/0301-4738.185588. PMID: 27380972; PMCID: PMC4966370.
104. Adulkar NG, Radhakrishnan S, Vidhya N, Kim U. Invasive sino-orbital fungal infections in immunocompetent patients: a clinico-pathological study. Eye (Lond). 2019;33(6):988–94. https://doi.org/10.1038/s41433-019-0358-6. Epub 2019 Feb 14. PMID: 30765886; PMCID: PMC6707179.
105. Pushker N, Meel R, Kashyap S, Bajaj MS, Sen S. Invasive aspergillosis of orbit in immunocompetent patients: treatment and outcome. Ophthalmology. 2011;118(9):1886–91. https://doi.org/10.1016/j.ophtha.2011.01.059. Epub 2011 Jun 12. PMID: 21665281.
106. Vadivel S, Gowrishankar M, Vetrivel K, Sujatha B, Navaneethan P. Rhino orbital cerebral mucormycosis in Covid-19 crisis. Indian J Otolaryngol Head Neck Surg. 2023;75(Suppl 1):1014–20. https://doi.org/10.1007/s12070-023-03474-1. Epub 2023 Feb 23. PMID: 36855632; PMCID: PMC9948777.
107. Honavar SG. Code mucor: guidelines for the diagnosis, staging and management of rhino-orbito-cerebral mucormycosis in the setting of COVID-19. Indian J Ophthalmol. 2021;69(6):1361–5. https://doi.org/10.4103/ijo.IJO_1165_21. PMID: 34011699; PMCID: PMC8302268.
108. Khalil M, Lindley S, Matouk E. Tuberculosis of the orbit. Ophthalmology. 1985;92(11):1624–7. https://doi.org/10.1016/s0161-6420(85)33818-6. PMID: 4080333.
109. Madge SN, Prabhakaran VC, Shome D, Kim U, Honavar S, Selva D. Orbital tuberculosis: a review of the literature. Orbit. 2008;27(4):267–77. https://doi.org/10.1080/01676830802225152. PMID: 18716964.
110. Bhattacharya S, Raina UK, Gupta SK, Mishra M, Saini V, Kumar B. Tubercular osteomyelitis of the orbit presenting as periorbital cellulitis. J Ophthalmic Vis Res. 2022;17(1):146–9. https://doi.org/10.18502/jovr.v17i1.10181. PMID: 35194506; PMCID: PMC8850846.
111. Diyora B, Giri SA, Bhende B, Giri D, Kukreja S, Sharma A. Orbital tuberculosis with intracranial extension. J Neurosci Rural Pract. 2018;9(4):636–8. https://doi.org/10.4103/jnrp.jnrp_70_18. PMID: 30271066; PMCID: PMC6126309.
112. Sohail M, Maniar A, Winn BJ, Patel S, Famuyide A, Dagi Glass LR. Orbital tuberculosis: a case report and update on the role of imaging in treatment. Orbit. 2022:1–6. https://doi.org/10.1080/01676830.2022.2126499. Epub ahead of print. PMID: 36154445.
113. Pakrou N, Selva D, Leibovitch I. Wegener's granulomatosis: ophthalmic manifestations and management. Semin Arthritis Rheum. 2006;35(5):284–92. https://doi.org/10.1016/j.semarthrit.2005.12.003. PMID: 16616151.
114. Hibino M, Kondo T. Dacryoadenitis with ptosis and diplopia as the initial presentation of granulomatosis with polyangiitis. Intern Med. 2017;56(19):2649–53. https://doi.org/10.2169/internalmedicine.8761-16. Epub 2017 Sep 6. PMID: 28883246; PMCID: PMC5658534.
115. Talar-Williams C, Sneller MC, Langford CA, Smith JA, Cox TA, Robinson MR. Orbital socket contracture: a complication of inflammatory orbital disease in patients with Wegener's granulomatosis. Br J Ophthalmol. 2005;89(4):493–7. https://doi.org/10.1136/bjo.2004.050039. PMID: 15774931; PMCID: PMC1772590.
116. Kalina PH, Lie JT, Campbell RJ, Garrity JA. Diagnostic value and limitations of orbital biopsy in Wegener's granulomatosis. Ophthalmology. 1992;99(1):120–4. https://doi.org/10.1016/s0161--6420(92)32028-7. PMID: 1741123.
117. Ang T, Juniat V, Selva D. Autoimmune markers in screening for orbital inflammatory disease. Eye (Lond). 2023;37(6):1088–93. https://doi.org/10.1038/s41433-022-02068-5. Epub 2022 Apr 19. PMID: 35440697; PMCID: PMC10102185.
118. Barrow DL, Spector RH, Braun IF, Landman JA, Tindall SC, Tindall GT. Classification and treatment of spontaneous carotid-cavernous sinus fistulas. J Neurosurg. 1985;62(2):248–56. https://doi.org/10.3171/jns.1985.62.2.0248.
119. Howells MS, Sharma R. Orbital varices. BMJ Case Rep. 2019;12(12):e232887. https://doi.org/10.1136/bcr-2019-232887. PMID: 31818898; PMCID: PMC6904158.
120. Islam N, Mireskandari K, Rose GE. Orbital varices and orbital wall defects. Br J Ophthalmol. 2004a;88(6):833–4. https://doi.org/10.1136/bjo.2003.024547. PMID: 15148222; PMCID: PMC1772180.
121. Islam N, Mireskandari K, Burton BJ, Rose GE. Orbital varices, cranial defects, and encephaloceles: an unrecognized association. Ophthalmology. 2004b;111(6):1244–7. https://doi.org/10.1016/j.ophtha.2003.10.022. PMID: 15177979.

122. Rootman J. Vascular malformations of the orbit: hemodynamic concepts. Orbit. 2003;22(2):103–20. https://doi.org/10.1076/orbi.22.2.103.14311. PMID: 12789590.
123. Mukherjee B, Vijay V, Halbe S. Combined approach to management of periocular arteriovenous malformation by interventional radiology and surgical excision. Indian J Ophthalmol. 2018;66(1):151–4. https://doi.org/10.4103/ijo.IJO_663_17. PMID: 29283148; PMCID: PMC5778556.
124. Capasso R, Russo C, Iuliano A, Cocozza S, Pontillo G, Tortora F, Strianese D, Elefante A, Briganti F. Upper eyelid isolated arterio-venous malformation treated with embolization in a patient with Keloid-Prone skin. Ophthalmic Plast Recofnstr Surg. 2020;36(5):e116–9. https://doi.org/10.1097/IOP.0000000000001620. PMID: 32205780.

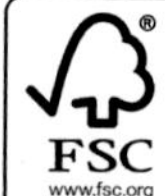

MIX
Papier aus verantwortungsvollen Quellen
Paper from responsible sources
FSC® C105338

If you have any concerns about our products,
you can contact us on
ProductSafety@springernature.com

In case Publisher is established outside the EU,
the EU authorized representative is:
Springer Nature Customer Service Center GmbH
Europaplatz 3, 69115 Heidelberg, Germany

Printed by Libri Plureos GmbH
in Hamburg, Germany